Mosby's Manual of Diagnostic and Laboratory Tests

Kathleen Deska Pagana, PhD, RN

Associate Professor
Department of Nursing
Lycoming College
Williamsport, Pennsylvania

Timothy James Pagana, MD, FACS

Surgical Oncologist
Williamsport, Pennsylvania

Illustrated

Mosby
A Harcourt Health Sciences Company
St. Louis London Philadelphia Sydney Toronto

Mosby
A Harcourt Health Sciences Company

Publisher: Nancy L. Coon
Editor: Loren Wilson
Developmental Editor: Brian Dennison
Project Manager: John Rogers
Designer: Liz Rudder
Design Manager: Yael Kats
Manufacturing Manager: Don Carlisle
Illustrator: Mark Swindle
Photographer: Pat Wilson
Cover Photo: Pete Saloutos/The Stock Market
Credits for all borrowed figures and tables appear before the index.

Printed in the United States of America

Mosby, Inc.
11830 Westline Industrial Drive
St. Louis, Missouri 63146

Library of Congress Cataloging-in-Publication Data

Pagana, Kathleen Deska
Mosby's manual of diagnostic and laboratory tests
Kathleen Deska Pagana, Timothy James Pagana.
p. cm.
Includes bibliographical references.
ISBN 0-8151-5586-7
1. Diagnosis, Laboratory–Handbooks, manuals, etc. 2. Diagnosis, Radioscopic–Handbooks, manuals, etc. 3. Reference values (Medicine)–Handbooks, manuals, etc. I. Pagana, Timothy James, 1949- . II. Title.
[DNLM: 1. Diagnosis, Laboratory–Methods–handbooks. QY 39 P128m 1998]
RB38.2.P34 1998
616.07'56–dc21
DNLM/DLC 97-40589

00 01 02/9 8 7 6 5 4 3 2 1

This book is dedicated to all healthcare workers who continually seek knowledge to improve their care of the sick.

Preface

This book provides the user with an up-to-date, extensive manual that allows rapid access to clinically relevant laboratory and diagnostic tests. A unique feature of this manual is its consistent format, which provides a comprehensive approach to laboratory and diagnostic tests. Tests are categorized according to either the method of testing (e.g., x-ray, ultrasound, nuclear scan) or the type of specimen (e.g., blood, urine, stool) used for testing. Each chapter of this book is based on this categorization. Each chapter begins with an alphabetical listing of all tests in the chapter to aid the user in locating discussions quickly. An overview follows the list and contains general information concerning test methods and related patient care.

Chapter One includes a discussion of guidelines for proper test preparation and performance. Universal precautions and other clinically important information for the healthcare provider are included to ensure accurate diagnostic and laboratory testing. This information is essential for healthcare economics so that tests are performed in a timely fashion and do not need to be repeated because of problems in patient preparation, test procedure, and/or specimen handling. Communication and collaboration with other healthcare providers are emphasized.

Throughout the book, information is explained in a comprehensive manner to enhance full understanding of each particular test. Every feature of test discussion is geared to provide complete information in a sequence that best simulates priorities in clinical practice. The following information is provided, whenever possible, for a thorough understanding of each diagnostic test:

- **Name of test**. Tests are listed by their complete name. A complete list of abbreviations and alternate test names follows each main entry.
- **Normal findings**. Normal values are listed, when applicable, for the infant, child, adult, and elderly person. Also, where appropriate, values are separated into male and female categories. We realize that normal ranges of laboratory tests vary significantly, depending on the method of testing and the particular laboratory. For this reason, we strongly encourage the user to check the normal values at the institution where the test is performed. This should be relatively easy because most laboratory reports indicate normal values.
- **Critical values**. These values give an indication of results that are well outside the usual range of normal. These results generally require immediate intervention.

- **Indications**. This section describes the main uses for each test. Emphasis is placed on the type of patient signs and symptoms that lead to the indications for each test.
- **Test explanation**. This section provides a comprehensive description of each test. The explanation includes fundamental information about basic pathophysiology related to the test methods, what diseases the test results may indicate, and the location where the test is generally performed. Also, in this section, patient sensation, test duration, and the type of healthcare professional involved in the testing are described.
- **Contraindications**. This information alerts the user to patients who should not have the test performed. As in other segments of the book, each contraindication is fully explained with an in-depth rationale. Patients frequently highlighted in this section include those who are pregnant, who are allergic to iodinated or contrast dye, or who have bleeding disorders.
- **Potential complications**. This section alerts the user to potential problems that will necessitate astute post-testing assessments and interventions. Not only is each complication fully explained in detail, but patient symptoms and appropriate interventions are described. For example, a potential complication of an IVP is renal failure, especially in the elderly patient. An appropriate intervention may be to hydrate the patient before the test and force fluids afterwards.
- **Interfering factors**. This section includes a thorough discussion of factors that can invalidate or alter the test results. An important feature of this section is the inclusion of drugs that can interfere with test results. Drugs that increase or decrease test values are indicated by a drug icon (✱) for quick access.
- **Procedure and patient care**. This section emphasizes the role of nurses and other healthcare providers in diagnostic and laboratory testing by addressing psychosocial and physiologic interventions. Patient education and rationales are thoroughly discussed. For quick location of essential information concerning the testing procedure, this section is divided into *before*, *during*, and *after* time sequences.

  Before. This section addresses the need to explain the procedure and to allay patient concerns or anxieties. Dietary restrictions, bowel preparations, baseline pretest assessment, and the need for informed consent are discussed.

  During. This section provides a complete and thorough description of the testing procedure, alternate procedures, and methods of testing. In most instances, a step-by-step description of testing procedures is provided. This information is important because all healthcare providers involved in the particular test should have a good understanding of what the procedure entails in order to assist more completely in the testing process.

  After. This section includes vital information that the nurse or other healthcare provider should know concerning post-procedure care of the patient. This includes specific post-test assessment, medication administration, recognition of post-test complications (with suggestions for nursing interventions), home care, and follow-up information.
- **Test results and clinical significance**. As the name implies, this section describes the significance of the test findings. A unique feature of this manual, in comparison to

other books on diagnostic and laboratory tests, is an extensive discussion of the pathophysiology of the disease process and how it relates to the test result. This provides enhanced understanding of the diagnostic test and better understanding of many disease processes.

- **Related tests**. This section, another unique feature of the text, includes a list of tests that are related to the main test under discussion. This includes tests that provide similar information, tests that provide confirmatory information, or other tests used to evaluate the same organ, disease process, or symptom complex. A short description and page numbers for all related tests are included for ease in cross-referencing. This provides the reader with a broader understanding of diagnostic testing and indicates where the reader may go to obtain more information on the topic of interest.

This logical format emphasizes clinically relevant information. The clarity of the format will facilitate a full understanding of content essential to both students and healthcare providers and its uniformity will allow the user to quickly recognize where information of interest may be found.

Multiple colors have been used to help locate tests, highlight critical information, and generally improve the readability of the text. Also, another key feature is the use of color photographs and illustrations throughout the book. Many tables are also included to simplify or summarize complex material regarding clinical care, test categories, or disease processes.

Feature boxes are used throughout the book in order to highlight and summarize important clinical data. They allow the reader to assimilate important information at a glance. There are three types of feature boxes: clinical priorities, age-related concerns, and home care responsibilities. *Clinical Priorities* emphasize pertinent information specific to understanding and performing a particular test. For example, coagulation studies need to be assessed prior to invasive studies (e.g., liver biopsy) that may cause bleeding. Chest x-rays should be performed after procedures (e.g., pleural biopsy) that may cause a pneumothorax. *Age-Related Concerns* primarily address pediatric and geriatric priorities. For example, the risk of dye-induced renal failure is emphasized in the dehydrated elderly patient scheduled for an IVP. The bowel preparation for children of different ages is described in the barium enema study. *Home Care Responsibilities* focus on factors that need to be addressed after a test is performed. With an increasing number of procedures being performed on an out-patient basis, the patient has the responsibility for detecting problems and knowing what to do when they occur. Often, the patient returns home with instructions or guidelines for recognizing problems (such as infection, bleeding, urinary retention).

Appendix A *Alphabetical Listing of Tests*, helps the user locate specific tests at a glance. **Appendix B** *List of Tests by Body System*, familiarizes the user with other related studies the patient or client may need or the user may want to review. This information should be especially useful for students and healthcare providers working in specialized areas. For example, all tests related to infertility are listed in the reproductive system section. **Appendix C** contains a list of *Abbreviations for Diagnostic and Laboratory Tests*. Finally, a comprehensive index includes the names of all tests and their synonyms and other relevant terms found within the tests. *Typical Abbreviations and Units of Measurement* are located on the inside cover.

We sincerely thank our editors for their enthusiasm and continual support. We invite comments from users of this book so that we may improve our goal of providing useful and relevant diagnostic and laboratory test information to users of future editions.

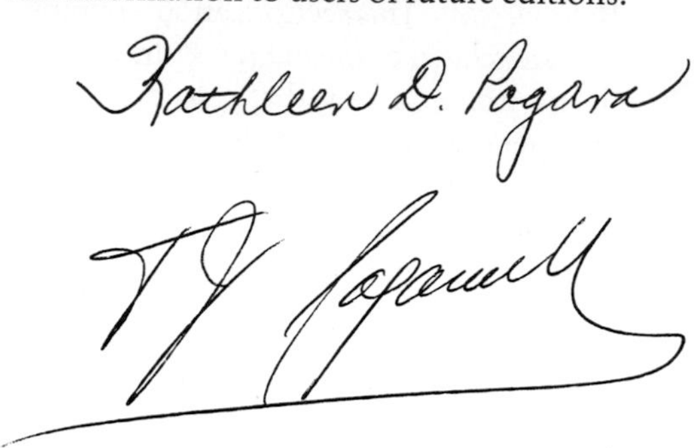

Contents

Mosby's Manual of Diagnostic and Laboratory Tests

1 Guidelines for Proper Test Preparation and Performance

A complete evaluation of patients with signs or symptoms of disease usually requires a thorough history and physical examination as well as efficient diagnostic testing. The correct use of diagnostic testing can confirm or eliminate the presence of disease and improve the cost efficiency of screening tests in a community of people without signs or symptoms of disease. Finally, appropriate and thoughtfully timed use of diagnostic testing allows monitoring of disease and treatment.

Furthermore, health care economics demands that laboratory and diagnostic testing be performed accurately and in a timely fashion. Tests should not have to be repeated because of improper patient preparation, test procedures, and/or specimen collection technique. The following guidelines will describe the responsibilities of health care providers to ensure safety and accuracy in diagnostic testing.

Patient education is the single most important factor in ensuring accuracy and success of test results. All phases (before, during, and after) of the testing process must be thoroughly explained to the patient. A complete understanding of these factors is essential to the development of nursing processes and standards of care for diagnostic testing.

The interpretation of diagnostic testing is no longer left to the physician alone. In today's complex environment of high-tech testing and economic restrictions, individuals representing many health care professions must be able to interpret diagnostic tests to develop a timely and effective treatment plan.

Universal precautions

The spread of hepatitis B virus (HBV) and human immunodeficiency virus (HIV) has made all health care organizations aware of the need to protect health care providers. This threat prompted the Centers for Disease Control (CDC) to release its guidelines for universal precautions in 1987 (Box 1-1). This policy recommends that blood and body fluid precautions be used for all patients regardless of their infection status. All patients should be considered potentially infectious. The universal precautions apply to all blood and tissues. Serous fluids such as pleural, peritoneal, amniotic, cerebrospinal, and synovial fluids are included. Semen and vaginal secretions should also be considered hazardous. Other clinical specimens (e.g., sputum, stool, urine) are of less concern, and the universal precautions apply only if these specimens contain visible amounts of blood.

These precautions require the use of protective barriers (gloves, gowns, masks, protective eyewear) to avoid skin and mucous membrane exposure to blood and body fluids. A fundamental principle of universal precautions is frequent handwashing between patients and when gloves are changed. All specimens should be collected and transported in containers that prevent leakage. Blood-tinged stains or spills must be decontaminated immediately. All needles and other sharp items must be handled carefully and discarded in puncture-resistant containers. Needles should not be recapped, broken, bent, or removed from a syringe to avoid the risk of puncturing the finger or hand. Special reusable needles are placed in metal containers for transport to a special area for sterilization or disinfection.

Vaccination against HBV is another safety precaution recommended by the CDC.

Proper sequencing and scheduling of tests

Because of the cost and complexity of laboratory and diagnostic testing, it is important that tests be scheduled in the most efficient sequential manner. Since one type of test can interfere with another, certain guidelines apply when multiple tests must be performed in

Box 1-1 Universal Precautions *

These precautions have been mandated by the Occupation Safety and Health Administration (OSHA). Their purpose is to protect health care workers from contracting illnesses from the specimens they handle, the patients they care for, and the environment in which they work. They can be summarized as follows:

- Wear gowns, gloves, protective eyewear, face masks, and protective clothing (including laboratory coat) whenever exposed to blood or other body fluids.
- If the health care worker's skin is opened, gloves should be worn whenever direct patient care is performed.
- Mouth-to-mouth emergency resuscitation equipment should be available in strategic locations. The mouthpieces should be individualized for each health care worker. Ambu bags are preferable. Saliva is considered an infectious fluid.
- Dispose all sharp items in puncture-resistant containers.
- Do not "recap," bend, break, or remove needles from syringes.
- Immediately remove gloves that have a hole or tear in them.
- All disposed patient-related wastes must be labeled as a "biohazard."
- All specimens must be transported in leakproof containers.
- Eating, drinking, applying cosmetics, or handling contact lenses is prohibited in patient care areas.
- Presume all patients have HBV and HIV.
- If a health care worker has experienced an exposure incident to blood or other body fluids (e.g., needlestick), testing of the health care worker and the patient for HBV and HIV is necessary.

*Centers for Disease Control, 1987

a limited amount of time. X-ray examinations that do not require contrast material should precede examinations that do require contrast media. X-ray studies using barium should be scheduled after ultrasonography studies. For example, x-ray studies using barium should follow x-rays using iodine contrast dye (such as intravenous pyelography [IVP]), which should follow x-ray studies using no contrast because contrast agents can obscure visualization of other body areas on subsequent x-ray tests. Also, stool specimens should be collected before x-ray studies using barium.

Test sequencing affects the ability to efficiently perform tests in a limited time period. An essential component of this process is communication and collaboration with other health care workers in numerous departments.

Before the test

Patient preparation is vital to the success of any diagnostic test. Patient education is essential and will be discussed later in this chapter. Development of and adherence to patient care guidelines in regard to patient preparation for the test require an understanding of the procedure. A thorough history to identify *contraindications* to the specific test is vital. Recognition of patients at risk for *potential complications* and counseling the patient about those complications is important. The fears and concerns of the patient should be elicited and addressed prior to testing. Documentation and a thorough understanding of ongoing factors (e.g., medications, previous test, other variables as discussed later in this chapter) that could *interfere* with the test results are essential to avoid misinterpretation of diagnostic testing.

Pretest preparation procedures must be followed closely. Dietary restriction is often an important factor in preparing the patient for tests. Studies requiring fasting should be performed as early in the morning as possible to diminish patient discomfort. Adherence to dietary restriction is important for test accuracy in some cases. Many blood tests and procedures require fasting. Studies such as a barium enema, colonoscopy, upper GI series, and IVP are more accurate if the patient has been on NPO status for several hours prior to the test. Sometimes dietary restrictions are important for safety, especially if a sedative is to be administered during testing. For example, upper GI endoscopy requires that the patient remain NPO for 8 to 12 hours before the test to prevent gagging, vomiting, and aspiration. Bowel preparation is necessary for many procedures designed to evaluate the mucosa of the GI tract.

Equally important to total patient care is the coordination of ongoing therapy (e.g., physical therapy, administration of medications, other diagnostic testing). Finally, correct timing of testing is key to accurate interpretation of results. For example, blood samples for cortisol, parathormone, and fasting glucose levels (among others) must be obtained in the early morning hours.

Patient identification

Proper identification of the patient is a critical safety factor. The conscious patient should be asked to state his or her full name. The name should be verified by checking the identification band and requisition slip. The identity of an unconscious patient should be verified by family or friends. No specimens should be collected or procedure performed without properly identifying the patient. Costly tests on the wrong patient are useless and may instigate legal action. Confusion can occur when patients with the same name are on the same nursing unit. Most units have some type of warning or "name alert" to address this concern.

Patient education

Once the patient is properly identified and the proper test or procedure is scheduled, patient education begins. Patients want to know what tests they are having and why they are needed. An informed patient is less apprehensive and more cooperative. Patient education helps ensure that the test will not need to be repeated because of improper preparation. Fasting requirements and bowel preparations must be clearly explained to the patient. Written instructions are essential. Sometimes medications may need to be discontinued for a period of time before certain tests. This information should be determined in consultation with the physician. Medications that are not discontinued are often listed on the requisition to aid in interpretation of test results.

Variables affecting test results

Many laboratory tests are affected by individual variables that must be considered in test result interpretation. Several of these key variables are discussed below.

Age. Pediatric reference values differ from adult values. For some tests, values vary according to the week of life of the infant. For example, in the first week of life, newborns have elevated levels of serum bilirubin, growth hormone, blood urea nitrogen (BUN), and fetal hemoglobin. They have decreased levels of cholesterol and haptoglobin. Healthy newborns also have increases in total white blood cells and decreases in IgM and IgA immunoglobulins. For some tests, children have different reference values based on their developmental stage. For example, alkaline phosphatase levels in children are much higher than adult values because of rapid bone growth.

Age-related changes are also apparent in the middle adult and older adult years. For example, albumin and total protein levels begin to decline in the mid-adult years. Reference values for cholesterol and triglyceride levels begin to increase in the mid-adult years. Creatinine clearance levels decrease with age relative to changes in glomerular filtration rate.

Gender. Sex is another variable that affects values in men and women. Differences are usually related to increased muscle mass in men and differences in hormonal secretion. For example, men usually have higher reference values for hemoglobin, blood urea nitrogen, serum creatinine, and uric acid. Males also have higher serum levels of cholesterol and triglycerides as compared with premenopausal women. Sex-specific hormones will also differ, with men having higher testosterone levels and women having higher levels of estrogens, follicle-stimulating hormone, and luteinizing hormones.

Race. Generally race has little effect on laboratory values. It has a greater effect on genetic diseases, such as sickle cell anemia in blacks and thalassemia in those with origins near the Mediterranean Sea.

Pregnancy. Many endocrine, hematologic, and biochemical changes occur during pregnancy. Pregnant women have increased levels of cholesterol, triglycerides, lactic dehydrogenase, alkaline phosphatase, and aspartate aminotransferase. They may have lower values of hemoglobin, hematocrit, serum creatinine, urea, glucose, albumin, and total protein.

Food ingestion. Several serum values are markedly affected by food. For example, levels of glucose and triglycerides rise after a meal. To avoid the effects of diet on laboratory tests, many tests are obtained when the patient is in the fasting state.

Posture. Changes in body position affect the concentration of several components in the peripheral blood. Therefore it is often important to note whether the patient was in the supine, sitting, or standing position when blood was drawn. Examples of laboratory values affected by posture include norepinephrine, epinephrine, renin, aldosterone, protein, and potassium.

During testing

Often many different health care professionals are necessary to successfully perform a diagnostic procedure. The health care provider's knowledge of the procedure will be a major determinant of the success of the procedure. Furthermore, the presence of a knowledgeable and supportive health care provider during any procedure is invaluable to the patient and to the accuracy of the test.

Specimen collection

Protocols and guidelines are available for each type of specimen collection. These are essential for appropriate preparation and collection. For example, the selection of the color-coded tube varies with the type of blood test needed. Guidelines for the collection of a 24-hour urine collection must be followed to obtain a representative urine sample. These and other examples are described in detail in the following chapter overviews.

Transport and processing of the specimen

Preparing the patient and collecting the specimen are essential. Getting the specimen to the laboratory in an acceptable state for examination is just as important. In general, the specimen should be transported to the laboratory as soon as possible after collection. Delays may result in rejection of the specimen.

A note about SI units

The International System of Units (SI units) is a system of reporting laboratory values in terms of standardized international measures. This system is currently used in many countries, and it is expected to be adopted worldwide. Throughout this book results are given in conventional units and SI units when possible.

After the test

Posttest care is an important aspect of total patient care. Attention should be directed to the patient's concerns about possible results or the difficulties of the procedure. Appropriate treatment subsequent to testing must be provided. For example, after a barium test, a cathartic is indicated. However, if a bowel obstruction has been identified, catharsis is contraindicated.

Recognition and rapid institution of treatment of complications (e.g., bleeding, shock, bowel perforation) is often vital in caring for the patient who has just had a diagnostic procedure. Procedures often require heavy sedation or a surgical procedure. In these situations, aftercare is similar to postoperative care.

Reporting test results

Although proper patient preparation and skill and accuracy in performing test procedures are vital, timeliness in reporting test results is no less essential. To be clinically useful, results must be reported promptly. Delays in reporting test results can make the data useless. The data must be included in the appropriate medical record and presented in a manner that is clear and easily interpreted. As in all phases of testing, communication among health professionals is important. Health care providers need to understand the significance of test results. For example, often nurses on the evening shift may be the first to see the results of a culture and sensitivity report on a patient with a urinary tract infection. If the results indicate that the infecting organism is not sensitive to the prescribed antibiotic, the doctor should be informed and an appropriate antibiotic order obtained.

The impact of an abnormal test result on the patient must always be appreciated and support for concerns provided. Ethical standards for disclosure of test results must be strictly adhered to. The physician usually communicates the test results to the patient and family, but occasionally the nurse must provide that information. Knowledge of the implications of various test results and an understanding of the disease process are as important as the communicative skills required to inform the patient and the family.

Succinct documentation of test results may be required before the "official" result is included in the patient's chart. Here again, a thorough understanding of the test is essential. Adequate follow-up is as important as all previously mentioned factors for successful diagnostic testing. The patient must be educated regarding home care, the next doctor's visit, and treatment options.

• • •

Knowledgeable interpretation of diagnostic tests is key for effective collaboration among health care providers if the most efficient patient care is to be provided. The safety and success of diagnostic testing often depend on the nurse and other health care professionals. The safety of the patient and health care professionals depends on the creation of practice guidelines and standards of care. These can only be effectively developed with a thorough understanding of laboratory and diagnostic testing.

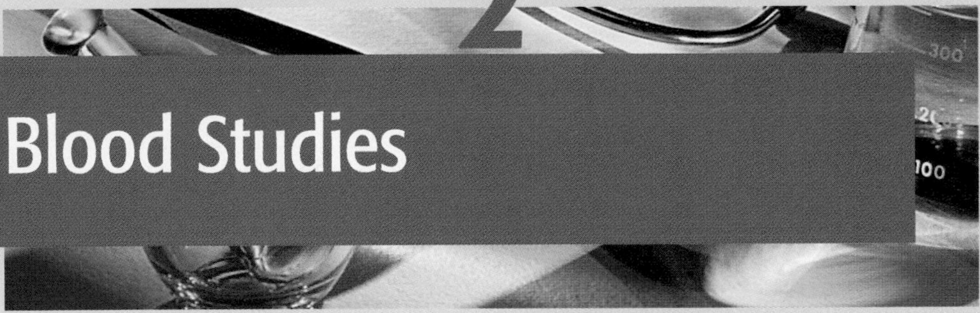

2 Blood Studies

TESTS

Overview

Reasons for Obtaining Blood Tests

Blood is the body fluid most frequently used for analytic purposes. Blood studies are used to assess a multitude of body processes and disorders. Common studies assess the quantity of red and white blood cells, as well as the levels of enzymes, lipids, clotting factors, hormones, and breakdown products (such as urea nitrogen). Most blood studies are performed for one of the following reasons:

1. To establish a diagnosis (e.g., high blood urea nitrogen and creatinine levels are indicative of renal failure).
2. To rule out a clinical problem (e.g., hypokalemia is ruled out with a normal potassium level).
3. To monitor therapy (e.g., glucose levels are used to monitor treatment of diabetic patients, and partial thromboplastin time values are used to regulate heparin therapy).
4. To establish a prognosis (e.g., declining CD4 counts reflect a poor clinical prognosis for the AIDS patient).
5. To screen for disease (e.g., prostate-specific antigen levels are used to detect prostate cancer).
6. To determine effective drug dosage and to prevent toxicity. (Peak and trough levels are drawn at designated time periods, see p. 195.)

Methods of Blood Collection

There are three general methods for obtaining blood: venous, arterial, and skin puncture. Blood collected from these sites differs in several important aspects. For example, arterial blood is oxygenated by the lungs and pumped from the heart to body organs and tissues. It is essentially uniform in its composition throughout the body. Venous blood composition varies depending on the metabolic activity of the organ or tissue being perfused. Venous blood is oxygen deficient in comparison to arterial blood. Variations between arterial and venous blood are often seen in measurements of pH, CO_2 concentration, and glucose, lactic acid, and ammonia levels. On the other hand, blood obtained by skin puncture is a mixture of arterial and venous blood. Skin puncture blood also includes intracellular and interstitial fluid. By far the most common access for blood withdrawal is venous puncture.

Venous Puncture

Background information The ease of obtaining venous blood makes this the primary source of blood collection. It is relatively free of any complications. Venipuncture is usually obtained by drawing a specimen of blood from a superficial vein (Figure 2-1). The site most often used is the antecubital fossa of the arm, because there are

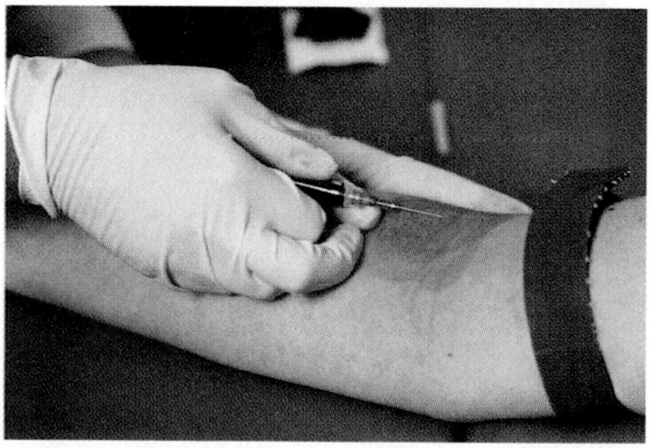

Figure 2-1 Performing venipuncture.

several large superficial veins at that location. The basilic, cephalic, and median cubital veins are the most commonly used sites. Veins of the wrist, hands, or ankles can also be used. When venous puncture cannot be performed on the upper extremities, the femoral vein is the most easily accessible for puncture.

Collection tubes Venipuncture is usually accomplished using needles attached to glass tubes under specified vacuum. A needle and a syringe can also be used to collect the blood sample and then to inject it into the appropriate tube. Tubes come in various sizes (2, 3, 5, 7, 10, and 15 ml). The rubber stoppers are color-coded to distinguish whether the tube is a plain tube (e.g., no preservatives or anticoagulants added), whether the tube contains a specific anticoagulant (such as heparin, oxalate, citrate, or ethylenediaminetetraacetic acid salts), or whether the tube is chemically clean (e.g., iron determination). Depending on the tests needed, the analysis is performed on whole blood, serum, or plasma. A centrifuge is used to separate the blood components and to obtain either serum or plasma. Whole blood collected without an anticoagulant yields *serum,* whereas whole blood collected with an anticoagulant yields *plasma.* Plasma contains fibrinogen, which is missing from serum.

The selection of the color-coded tube is based on the requirements of the test. Charts are available from the laboratory that indicate the type of tube needed for a particular blood test. Colors may vary according to the laboratory. A representative chart is shown in Table 2-1.

The recommended order of draw must be followed when collecting multiple tubes of blood. Specimens should be drawn into nonadditive tubes (e.g., red top) before tubes are drawn that contain additives. The tubes should be filled in the following order:

1. Blood culture tubes first (to maintain sterility)
2. Nonadditive tubes (e.g., red top)
3. Coagulation tubes (e.g., blue top)
4. Heparin tubes (e.g., green top)

Table 2-1 Common blood collection tubes

Color	Additive	Purpose	Examples
Red top	None	To allow blood sample to clot. This permits separation of serum when the serum needs to be tested	Chemistry Bilirubin Blood urea nitrogen Calcium
Purple or lavender top	Ethylenediamine tetraacetic acid (EDTA)	To prevent blood from clotting	Hematology Complet blood count Platelet count
Gray top	Sodium fluoride oxalate	To prevent glycolysis	Chemistry Glucose Lactose tolerance
Green top	Heparin	To prevent blood from clotting when plasma needs to be tested	Chemistry Ammonia Carboxyhemoglobin
Blue top	Sodium citrate	To prevent blood from clotting when plasma needs to be tested	Hematology Prothrombin time Partial thromboplastin time

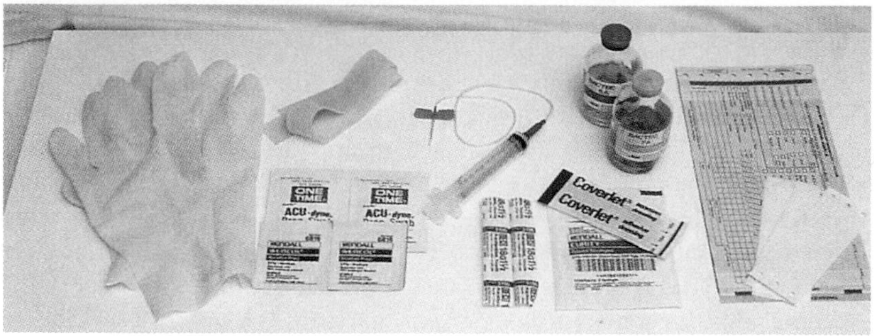

Figure 2-2 Equipment for blood collection.

5. EDTA-K3 tubes (e.g., lavender top)
6. Oxalate-fluoride tubes (e.g., gray top)

Technique

Before

- Identify the patient. Assemble all equipment and supplies and put on gloves (Figure 2-2).
- Explain the procedure to the patient. Explain that mild, brief discomfort may result from the needlestick.
- If fasting is required, verify that this requirement has been followed.

During

- Position the patient properly for easy access to the antecubital fossa.
- Ask the patient to make a fist to distend the veins.
- Select a vein for venipuncture.
- Apply a tourniquet several inches above the puncture site.
- Cleanse the venipuncture site (usually with 70% isopropanol alcohol). Allow the area to dry.
- Perform the venipuncture by entering the skin with the needle bevel up and the needle at approximately a 15° angle to the skin.
- If using a *Vacutainer,* ease the tube forward in the holder as soon as the needle is in the vein. When the tube is filled, remove it. Another tube can then be inserted into the holder. If using a *syringe,* pull back on the barrel with slow, even tension as blood fills the syringe. Transfer the blood to the appropriate color tubes.
- Release the tourniquet when the blood begins to flow.

After

- After the blood is drawn, place a cotton ball over the site. Withdraw the needle and apply pressure to the site. A Band-Aid applied over the cotton ball usually stops the bleeding.
- Mix tubes with the additives by gently rolling the tubes. Do not vigorously shake the tubes. Specimens collected in the syringe should be transferred to appropriate test tube containers.
- Properly dispose of contaminated materials, such as needles, syringes, and cotton balls (Figure 2-3).

- Initial the label and record the date and time of blood collection. Attach a label to each vial of blood.
- Arrange for prompt delivery of the blood specimen to the laboratory.
- If the patient fasted before the test, remove diet restrictions.

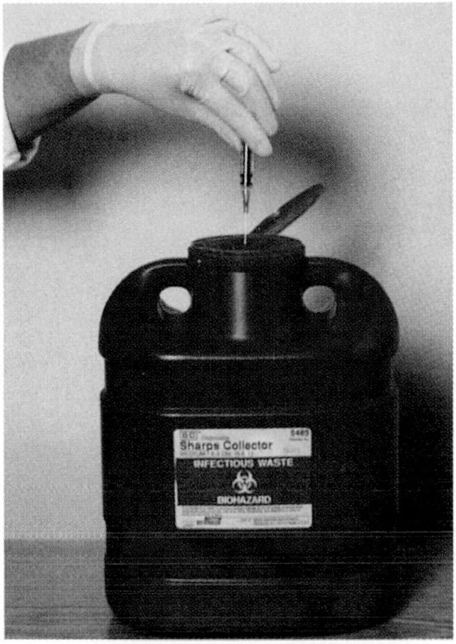

Figure 2-3 Proper disposal of needles.

Potential complications

- *Bleeding:*
  After the specimen is drawn, apply pressure or a pressure dressing to the venipuncture site. Assess the venipuncture site for bleeding.
- *Hematoma:*
  Hematomas can form under the skin when the vein continues to leak blood. This results in a large, bruised area. This can usually be prevented by applying pressure to the venipuncture site until clotting occurs. If a hematoma does occur, reabsorption of the blood can be enhanced by the application of warm compresses.
- *Infection:*
  Instruct the patient to assess the venipuncture site for redness, pain, swelling, or tenderness. This is more common in immunocompromised patients or patients who have had lymph node dissection above the venipuncture site.
- *Dizziness and fainting:*
  If this occurs, prevent injury by helping the patient to a sitting or reclining position. Lowering the head between the knees or using smelling salts can also help.

Preventing interfering factors

- Hemolysis may result from vigorous shaking of a blood specimen. This may invalidate test results.
- Collect the blood specimen from the arm without an IV device if possible. IV infusion can influence test results. If it is necessary to draw blood from the arm with an IV device, never draw blood above the IV needle site. Satisfactory samples may be obtained by drawing the blood below the IV needle after turning the IV infusion off for 2 minutes before the venipuncture. Select a vein other than the one with the IV device and draw 5 ml of blood. Discard this sample before drawing blood for analysis.
- Do not use the arm with the dialysis arteriovenous fistula for a venipuncture unless the physician specifically authorizes it.
- Because of the risk of cellulitis, specimens should not be taken from the side on which an axillary lymph node dissection has been performed.
- To obtain valid results, do not fasten the tourniquet for longer than 1 minute. Prolonged tourniquet application can cause stasis, localized acidemia, and hemoconcentration.

Drawing blood from an indwelling venous catheter Follow the unit guidelines for drawing blood from an indwelling venous catheter, such as a central venous catheter or a peripherally inserted central catheter. Guidelines will specify the amount of blood to be drawn from the catheter and discarded before blood is collected for laboratory studies. The guidelines also indicate the amount and type of solution needed to flush the catheter to prevent it from being clogged by blood.

Drawing a panel of blood studies Blood tests are often part of a panel or group of specified tests. This is because patterns of abnormalities may be more useful than single test changes. Common panels of blood tests include the following:

Blood chemistry screen

Sodium
Potassium
Chloride
CO_2
Blood urea nitrogen (BUN)
Creatinine

Complete blood count (CBC) and differential

Red blood cell (RBC) count
Hemoglobin
Hematocrit
RBC indices
White blood cell (WBC) count and differential
Blood smear
Platelet count

Coagulation tests

Prothrombin time (PT)
Partial thromboplastin time (PTT)
Bleeding time
Platelet count

Lipid profile

Cholesterol
High-density lipoproteins (HDL)
Low-density lipoproteins (LDL)
Very-low-density lipoproteins (VLDL)

Lipid profile, cont'd

Apolipoproteins
Triglycerides

Liver function tests

Bilirubin
Aspartate aminotransferase (AST) (formerly serum glutamic-oxaloacetic transaminase [SGOT])
Alanine aminotransferase (ALT) (formerly serum glutamic-pyruvic transaminase [SGPT])
Gamma-glutamyl transpeptidase (GGT)
5′-Nucleotidase
Leucine aminopeptidase (LAP)
Alkaline phosphatase (ALP)

Renal function tests

BUN
Creatinine
Creatinine clearance

Thyroid panel

Radioactive iodine uptake (RAIU)
Thyroxine (T_4)
Free thyroxine index
Triiodothyronine (T_3)
T_3 uptake test
Thyroid-stimulating hormone (TSH)
Thyrotropin-releasing hormone (TRH)

Arterial Puncture

Background information Arterial blood is used to measure oxygen, CO_2, and pH. These are often referred to as arterial blood gases (ABGs) and are described on p. 97. If a patient will require frequent sampling, an indwelling arterial catheter is usually placed. Arterial puncture is used for single or infrequent sampling.

Arterial punctures are more difficult to perform than venipuncture. They also cause a significant amount of patient discomfort. The brachial and radial arteries are the arteries most often used for arterial puncture. The femoral artery is usually avoided because bleeding occurs more often after the procedure and may not be noted because it is hidden by bed covers. Large amounts of blood could be lost before blood loss is detected.

Technique

Before

- Explain the procedure to the patient. Inform the patient why this blood test is necessary. Tell the patient that the test causes more discomfort than a venipuncture.
- Notify the laboratory before drawing arterial blood samples so the necessary equipment can be calibrated before the blood sample arrives.
- Perform the *Allen test* to assess collateral circulation before performing the arterial puncture on the radial artery. To perform the Allen test, make the patient's hand blanch by obliterating both the radial and ulnar pulses. Then release the pressure over the ulnar artery only. If flow through the ulnar artery is good, flushing will be observed immediately. The Allen test is then positive and the radial artery can be used for venipuncture. If the Allen test is negative (no flushing), repeat it on the other arm. If the results are negative in both arms, choose another artery for puncture. The Allen test is important because it ensures collateral circulation to the hand if thrombosis of the radial artery occurs after the puncture.

During

- Cleanse the arterial site with 70% isopropyl alcohol. Allow the site to dry.
- Attach a 20-gauge needle to a syringe containing approximately 0.2 ml of heparin. Insert the needle at a 45° to 60° angle into the skin over the palpable artery (Figure 2-4).
- After drawing approximately 3 to 5 ml of blood, remove the needle and apply pressure to the arterial site for 3 to 5 minutes. Expel any air bubbles in the syringe.
- Cap the syringe and gently rotate to mix the blood and the heparin.

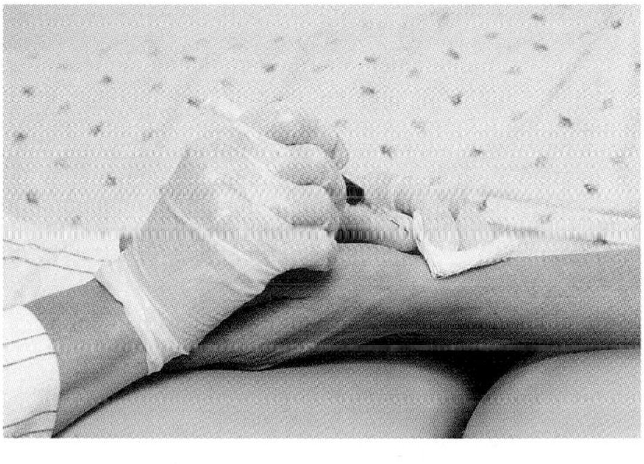

Figure 2-4 Drawing arterial blood. Note that the needle is at a 45° angle.

After

- Indicate on the laboratory slip if the patient is receiving any oxygen therapy or is attached to a ventilator.
- Place the arterial blood on ice and immediately take it to the chemistry laboratory for analysis.
- If the patient has an abnormal clotting time or is taking anticoagulants, apply pressure for approximately 15 minutes.

Potential complications

- *Arterial thrombosis*
  Thrombosis can result and impair arterial circulation. This can result in ischemia or necrosis of tissue on the extremity.
- *Hematoma formation*
  Pressure must be applied to the arterial puncture site for at least 3 to 5 minutes to prevent hematoma formation (longer if the patient is anticoagulated). If a hematoma results, warm compresses will enhance absorption of the blood.
- *Bleeding*
  The site must be carefully assessed for bleeding. An arterial puncture can cause rapid bleeding. This is especially important if the patient has an abnormal clotting time or is taking anticoagulants.

Skin Puncture

Background information Skin puncture (sometimes called capillary puncture) is the method of choice for obtaining blood from pediatric patients, especially infants, because large amounts of blood required for repeated venipuncture could result in anemia. However, skin punctures are also used in adult patients.

Common puncture sites include the fingertips, earlobes, and heel surfaces. The fingertips are often used in adults and small children. The heel is the most commonly used site for infants. The earlobe can be used to obtain blood in adults and older pediatric patients. The earlobe can also be used to obtain arterialized capillary blood as a possible substitute for arterial blood in determining the pH, PCO_2 and PO_2.

With changes in the health care economics and delivery, the use of skin punctures will probably increase. Blood monitoring will be increasingly performed in outpatient settings. Clinical laboratory tests will be performed more frequently at the bedside using a skin puncture.

Technique

Before

- Identify the patient. Explain the procedure to the patient and/or family. Assemble all supplies. Put on gloves.
- Select an appropriate puncture site. For *infants,* the lateral or medial heel surface is commonly used. For *older* infants, children, or adults, the lateral aspect of the second, third, or fourth fingertip may be used to avoid the central tip of the fingers where the nerve supply is more dense.

During

- Warm the puncture site with a warm, moist towel to increase blood flow.
- Cleanse the puncture site with 70% isopropyl alcohol. Allow the site to dry.
- Make the puncture with a sterile lancet.
- Discard the first drop of blood by wiping it away with a sterile pad.
- Do not milk the site, as this may hemolyze the specimen and introduce excess tissue fluid. Also avoid using excess pressure on the fingers during blood collection. This may cause hemolysis of the sample.
- Collect the specimen in capillary tubes or on special filter papers.
- If using capillary tubes, seal the capillary tubes by inserting clay into the end of the micropipette.

After

- Initial the blood label and record the time and date of blood collection. Indicate that the blood was collected by skin puncture.
- Arrange for prompt transportation of the blood specimen to the laboratory.

Potential complications

- *Infection:*
  Assess the skin puncture site for redness, swelling, pain, or tenderness. Although this is a serious complication, the incidence is very low.
- *Hematoma and bruising:*
  Check the skin puncture site for discoloration, bruising, or swelling. Look for bleeding onto the skin. Avoid frequent skin punctures or excessive squeezing of the tissue during blood collection to prevent this problem.

Timing of Blood Collection

Although many blood specimens can be obtained randomly, some must be drawn at specific times. For example, lipoproteins (see p. 289) should be drawn after a 12- to 14-hour fast (except for water), because food can alter lipoprotein values. Because glucose levels are related to food intake, fasting blood glucose specimens require an 8-hour fast. Glucose tolerance tests (see p. 233) require a fasting blood glucose level and a glucose level drawn at 30 minutes, 1 hour, 2 hours, 3 hours, and sometimes 4 hours after glucose administration.

Specimens for therapeutic drug monitoring (see p. 194) must be obtained at specific times determined by the method of drug delivery (e.g., intravenous or oral), dosage interval, absorption characteristics of the drug, and half-life of the drug. Drug monitoring is especially important in patients taking medications (such as antiarrhythmics, bronchodilators, antibiotics, anticonvulsants, and cardiotonics), because the margin of safety between therapeutic and toxic levels may be narrow. Blood levels can be taken at the drug's *peak level* (highest therapeutic concentration) or at the drug's *trough level* (lowest therapeutic concentration). Peak levels are useful when testing for toxicity, and trough levels are useful for demonstrating a satisfactory therapeutic level.

Transport and Processing of Blood Specimens

Once blood specimens are obtained, they should be promptly transported to the laboratory. Because the blood cells continue to live in the collection tubes, they will metabolize some of the components in the blood. This can result in alterations in the concentration of some blood components prior to analysis in the laboratory. Therefore blood specimens should be delivered to the laboratory for processing within 1 hour, depending

Box 2-1 Criteria for rejection of blood sample

- Improper sample identification
- Wrong collection tube used
- Insufficient blood quantity
- Hemolyzed blood sample
- Improper transport of sample
- Insufficient filling of anticoagulated tube

on the test. Stat specimens should be delivered immediately after being drawn. Laboratories have written criteria for rejecting a specimen as unsuitable for testing. Box 2-1 lists common reasons for rejecting a blood specimen.

In general, specimens should be tested within 1 hour of collection. If this is not possible, the sample may need to be refrigerated or frozen depending on the compound for testing. Some blood specimens must be sent by mail or special courier from physicians' offices or small hospitals to large reference laboratories. As a result, delays of 24 hours may occur prior to specimen analysis.

After testing, the remainder of the blood sample should be saved by the laboratory along with the original sample for 24 hours to be retested if needed to verify discrepant results. These samples can also be used for additional tests ordered by the physician. If the "add-on" request can be performed, the patient is spared additional venipunctures. With retesting or "add-on" requests, the stability of the requested serum constituent becomes an important consideration.

Multiphasic screening machines can perform many blood tests quickly and simultaneously using a very small blood sample. An example of this is the sequential multiple analyzer (SMA), which is the name of one instrument used for automatically testing a specific group of tests. An SMA-12 performs 12 tests, whereas an SMA-6 performs six tests. The advantage of these machines is that results are available quickly and the cost is cheaper per individual test in comparison with the panel of tests included in the SMA group.

Reporting of Results

Although accuracy and processing are the prerequisites of good laboratory practice, timeliness in reporting results is essential. To be clinically useful, a test result must be reported promptly. Delays in reporting a result can make the data useless. The report must also be entered in the appropriate medical record and must be presented in a manner that is clear and easily interpreted.

The results should include the test results, reporting units, and reference ranges. It is important to note that normal ranges for laboratory tests vary from institution to institution. Often serial listing of results is useful for tests in which trends and values make interpretation easier. Comments may be added to help interpret test results. For example, the technologist would indicate if the sample was hemolyzed.

Because acronyms are used to shorten test names, these code names must be understood for proper interpretation. For example, the acronym LAP could stand for leucine amino peptidase or for leukocyte alkaline phosphatase.

Proper reporting of a "critical" or "panic" value is essential. These values are results well outside the usual range of normal and generally require immediate intervention. A good example of this is high or low potassium levels. If these results were phoned to a physician or nurse, verification of this notification must be properly documented.

Acetylcholine Receptor Antibody
(AChR Ab, Anti–Acetylcholine Receptor Antibody)

Normal Findings

≤0.03 nmol/L or negative

Indications

Antibodies to AChR are used to diagnose acquired myasthenia gravis (MG) and also to monitor patient response to immunosuppressive therapy.

Test Explanation

Antibodies to AChR occur in over 85% to 90% of patients with acquired MG, and 63% of patients with only ocular MG have elevated levels. The presence of this antibody is virtually diagnostic of MG. The measured titer does not correspond well with the severity of MG. In an individual patient with MG, however, antibody levels are particularly useful in monitoring response to immunosuppressive therapy. As the patient improves, antibody titer decreases. This test is also used in patients who are suspected of having a thymoma, because 59% of these patients have MG. Because congenital MG is not an autoimmune disease, this antibody test is not helpful in the diagnosis of congenital MG.

This antibody blocks neuromuscular transmission by interfering with the binding of AChR sites on the muscle membrane and preventing muscle contraction. It is this phenomenon that characterizes MG. There are three different AChR antibodies that test for MG. The AChR-binding antibody is most commonly used. If this test is negative and the diagnosis of MG is highly suspected, the AChR-modulating antibody is used and may be more sensitive. Furthermore, a positive modulating antibody test may indicate subclinical MG, contraindicating the use of curare-like drugs during surgery. The AChR-blocking antibody is the least sensitive test (positive in only 61% of patients with MG), but it can be quantified more accurately. The blocking and modulating antibodies are not often positive for about 1 year after onset of MG symptoms. The most commonly used method for the detection of these AChR antibodies is radioimmunoassay.

Interfering Factors

- False-positive results may occur in patients with amyotrophic lateral sclerosis who have been treated with cobra venom.
- ✗ The use of muscle relaxant drugs (metacurine and succinylcholine) or penicillamine may also cause false-positive results.
- ✗ Immunosuppressive drugs may suppress the formation of these antibodies in patients with subclinical MG.

Procedure and Patient Care

Before

- Explain the procedure to the patient.
- Tell the patient that no fasting is required.

- Inform the patient that the blood sample is usually sent to a reference laboratory. It will take several days before the results are available.

During

- Collect a venous blood sample in a red-top tube.
- List on the laboratory slip all medications that the patient has taken in the last few days.

After

- Apply pressure or a pressure dressing to the venipuncture site.
- Assess the venipuncture site for bleeding.

Test Results and Clinical Significance

Increased levels

MG
Ocular MG
Thymoma *59% of patients with thymoma have MG and 10% of MG patients have a thymoma.*

Related Tests

- Antistriated muscle antibody (antistriational antibody): This is a serum antibody titer that has been reported to be positive in 95% of patients with MG and thymoma and in 30% of patients with thymoma without MG.
- Cholinesterase (p. 147): Patients with an acquired or congenital deficiency of this enzyme will experience acute MG-like muscle paralysis when a depolarizing agent, such as succinylcholine, is used for anesthesia induction.

Acid Phosphatase (Prostatic Acid Phosphatase [PAP], Tartrate-Resistant Acid Phosphatase [TRAP])

Normal Findings

Adult/elderly: 0.11-0.60 U/L (Roy, Brower, Hayden, 37° C) or 0.11-0.60 U/L (SI units)
Child: 8.6-12.6 U/ml (30° C)
Newborn: 10.4-16.4 U/ml (30° C)

Indications

Total acid phosphatase and specifically the PAP isoenzyme is primarily used to diagnose and stage prostatic carcinoma and to monitor the efficacy of treatment.

Test Explanation

Usually (but not always) elevated levels are seen in patients with prostatic cancer that has metastasized beyond the capsule to other parts of the body, especially bone. The degree of elevation indicates the extent of disease. Since PAP is not elevated in early-stage prostate disease, this test is not recommended for screening. If the prostate tumor is successfully treated by surgery, radiation, or hormone manipulation, PAP levels decrease in several days. Rising levels of PAP may indicate a recurrent tumor.

Because acid phosphatase is also found at high concentrations in seminal fluid, this test can be performed on vaginal secretions to investigate alleged rape. High levels of acid phosphatase also exist in white blood cells (mostly monocytes and lymphocytes). They are helpful in determining the clinical course of patients with lymphoproliferative diseases and hairy cell leukemia. Acid phosphatase is a lysosomal enzyme. Therefore lysosomal storage diseases (such as Gaucher's disease and Niemann-Pick disease) are associated with elevated levels.

In males, one half of the total acid phosphatase (nearly all of the PAP) is found in the prostate gland. Lesser amounts are found in the liver, spleen, blood cells, and bone marrow. In females, total acid phosphatase is from the liver, red blood cells, and platelets (PAP is negligible). The isoenzymes of acid phosphatase are determined by electrophoresis. As mentioned above, the most clinically significant isoenzyme is PAP. It is more accurate than total acid phosphatase in patients with prostatic cancer but less accurate than the prostate-specific antigen (PSA) (p. 356).

Acid phosphatase can be identified by cellular hydrolysis of naphthol phosphoric acid. The optimal pH for this reaction is on the acid side. When tartaric acid is added to the solution, hydrolysis of the substance by acid phosphatase is inhibited in prostate cells but not in the cells of hairy cell leukemia. The identification of tartrate-resistant acid phosphatase (TRAP) is therefore helpful in the diagnosis of hairy cell leukemia (and occasionally other lymphoproliferative diseases). It is important to note, however, that the specimens of 5% of patients with hairy cell leukemia are not tartrate resistant. In the past decade, radioimmunoassay and enzyme-linked immunosorbent assay kits have been used to determine acid phosphatase levels (specifically PAP). These methods are more accurate than the biochemical methods previously described.

Interfering Factors

- Falsely high levels of acid phosphatase (and specifically PAP) may occur in males after a digital rectal examination or after instrumentation of the prostate (e.g., cystoscopy) because of prostatic stimulation. Elevated levels of 25% to 50% may occur for up to 48 hours after prostate manipulation. The test should be repeated if elevated levels occur after a rectal or prostate examination.
- Alkaline and acid phosphatase are very similar enzymes that function at different pH levels. Any condition associated with very high levels of alkaline phosphatase may falsely indicate high acid phosphatase levels.
- Drugs that may cause *elevated* levels of acid phosphatase include androgens (in females), clofibrate (Atromid-S), and alglucerase.
- Drugs that may cause *decreased* levels include fluorides, phosphates, oxalates, heparin, and alcohol.

Procedure and Patient Care

Before

- Explain the procedure to the patient.
- Tell the patient that no food or drink restrictions are necessary.
- Remember that some laboratories request notification before the blood sample is drawn so that immediate attention (1 hour) can be given to the sample.

During

- Collect approximately 5 to 10 ml of blood in a red-top tube.
- Avoid hemolysis. Red blood cells contain acid phosphatase.
- Note on the laboratory slip if the patient has had a prostatic or rectal examination or instrumentation of the prostate within the past 24 to 48 hours.

After

- Apply pressure or a pressure dressing to the venipuncture site.
- Assess the venipuncture site for bleeding.
- Promptly deliver the specimen to the lab.
- Do not leave the specimen at room temperature for 1 hour or longer, because the enzyme is heat and pH sensitive and acid phosphatase activity will decrease. Once the specimen is received by the laboratory, the use of a preservative and prompt refrigeration are important.

Test Results and Clinical Significance

Increased levels

Prostatic carcinoma
Benign prostatic hypertrophy
Prostatitis
Acid phosphatase and specifically PAP exist in the lysosomes of prostate cells. Diseases affecting prostate tissue will destroy those cells and the lysosomal contents will spill into the bloodstream where they will be detected.

Multiple myeloma
Paget's disease
Hyperparathyroidism
Metastasis to the bone
Because acid phosphatase exists in the lysosomes of the bone marrow, diseases affecting the bone will be associated with elevated blood levels.

Multiple myeloma
Sickle cell crisis
Thrombocytosis
Because acid phosphatase exists in the lysosomes of blood cells, diseases affecting blood cells will be associated with elevated blood levels.

Lysosomal disorders (e.g., Gaucher's disease) *Because acid phosphatase exists in the lysosomes of many tissues affected by these diseases, elevated blood levels can be expected.*

Renal diseases
Liver diseases, such as cirrhosis
Because acid phosphatase is present in these organs, diseases affecting these organs will be associated with elevated blood levels.

Related Tests

- Prostate-specific antigen (PSA) (p. 356): This is a more specific test for prostatic cancer.
- Alkaline phosphatase (p. 42): This is a similar enzyme that is more easily identified in an alkaline environment. It is useful in the evaluation of diseases of the liver and bone.

Adrenocorticotropic Hormone
(ACTH, Corticotropin)

Normal Findings

AM: 15-100 pg/ml or 10-80 ng/L (SI units)
PM: <50 pg/ml or <50 ng/L (SI units)

Indications

The serum ACTH study is a test of anterior pituitary gland function that affords the greatest insight into the causes of either Cushing's syndrome (overproduction of cortisol) or Addison's disease (underproduction of cortisol).

Test Explanation

An elaborate feedback mechanism for cortisol coordinates the function of the hypothalamus, pituitary gland, and adrenal glands. ACTH is an important aspect of this mechanism. Corticotropin-releasing hormone (CRH) is made in the hypothalamus. This stimulates ACTH production in the anterior pituitary gland, which in turn stimulates the adrenal cortex to produce cortisol. The rising levels of cortisol act as a negative feedback and curtail further production of CRH and ACTH

In the patient with Cushing's syndrome an elevated ACTH level can be caused by a pituitary ACTH-producing tumor or a nonpituitary (ectopic) ACTH-producing tumor, usually in the lung, pancreas, thymus, or ovary. ACTH levels over 200 pg/ml usually indicate ectopic ACTH production. If the ACTH level is below normal in a patient with Cushing's syndrome, an adrenal adenoma or carcinoma is probably the cause of the hyperfunction (Table 2-2).

In patients with Addison's disease an elevated ACTH level indicates primary adrenal gland failure, as in adrenal gland destruction caused by infarction, hemorrhage, or autoimmunity; surgical removal of the adrenal gland; congenital enzyme deficiency; or adrenal suppression after prolonged ingestion of exogenous steroids. If the ACTH level

Table 2-2 Cortisol/ACTH levels in diagnosis of adrenal dysfunction

Disease	Cortisol level	ACTH level
Cushing's syndrome Adrenal micronodular hyperplasia Adrenal tumor (adenoma, cancer)	High	Low
Cushing's syndrome Cushing's disease (ACTH-producing pituitary tumor) Ectopic ACTH-producing tumor (e.g., lung cancer)	High	High
Addison's disease Adrenal gland failure (e.g., infarction, hemorrhage, or congenital adrenal hyperplasia)	Low	High
Hypopituitarism	Low	Low

is below normal in a patient with adrenal insufficiency, hypopituitarism is most probably the cause of the hypofunction (Table 2-2).

ACTH can be directly measured by immunoassay in many large reference laboratories, but smaller laboratories usually are not equipped for this test. Thus it requires several days to obtain results. ACTH levels exhibit diurnal variations that correspond to cortisol levels. Levels in evening (8 to 10 PM) samples are usually one half to two thirds of morning (4 to 8 AM) specimens. This diurnal variation is lost when disease (especially neoplasm) affects the pituitary or adrenal glands. Likewise, stress can blunt or eliminate this normal diurnal variation.

ACTH is measured in amniotic fluid when anencephaly is suspected. Decreased levels are noted in anencephalic fetuses. (See discussion of amniocentesis on p. 560.)

Interfering Factors

- Stress (trauma, pyrogen, hypoglycemia), menses, and pregnancy cause increased levels of cortisol. This is accomplished through elevation of ACTH.
- Recently administered radioisotope scans can affect levels measured by radioimmunoassay or immunoradiometry.
- Drugs that may cause *increased* levels include estrogens, ethanol, vasopressin, aminoglutethimide, amphetamines, insulin, metyrapone, levodopa, and spironolactone.
- Exogenously administered corticosteroids *decrease* ACTH levels.

✓ CLINICAL PRIORITIES

- Evaluate the patient for stress factors that could invalidate test results.
- Remember there is a diurnal variation in ACTH levels that corresponds to cortisol levels. With a normal sleep pattern, levels are highest in the morning and lowest in the evening.

Procedure and Patient Care

Before

- Explain the procedure to the patient. Allow plenty of time to answer questions so that the patient's stress is diminished as much as possible.
- Keep the patient on NPO status after midnight the day of the test.
- Evaluate the patient for stress factors that would invalidate the test results.
- Evaluate the patient for sleep pattern abnormalities. With a normal sleep pattern, the ACTH level is highest between 4 AM and 8 AM and lowest around 9 PM.
- Assess the patient for self-administration of drugs that could affect test results.

During

- Collect approximately 20 ml of heparinized venous blood in a green-top tube or as required by your reference laboratory.
- Chill the blood tube to prevent enzymatic degradation of ACTH.

After

- Place the specimen in ice water and send it to the chemistry laboratory immediately. ACTH is a very unstable peptide in plasma and should be stored at minus 20° C to prevent artificially low values.
- Apply pressure or a pressure dressing to the venipuncture site.
- Assess the venipuncture site for bleeding.

Test Results and Clinical Significance

Increased levels

Addison's disease (primary adrenal insufficiency)
Adrenogenital syndrome (congenital adrenal hyperplasia)
The adrenal glands are not making enough cortisol for the body's needs. The reduced serum cortisol level is a strong stimulus to pituitary production of ACTH.

Cushing's disease (pituitary-dependent adrenal hyperplasia)
Ectopic ACTH syndrome
Stress
ACTH is overproduced as a result of neoplastic overproduction of ACTH in the pituitary or elsewhere in the body by an ACTH-producing cancer. Stress is a potent stimulus to ACTH production.

Decreased levels

Secondary adrenal insufficiency (pituitary insufficiency)
Hypopituitarism
The pituitary gland is incapable of producing adequate ACTH.

Adrenal adenoma or carcinoma
Cushing's syndrome
Exogenous steroid administration
Overproduction or availability of cortisol is a strong inhibitor to pituitary production of ACTH.

Related Tests

- Cortisol, blood and urine (p. 167 and 827): Cortisol is a hormone produced by the adrenal gland and is the main determinant of Cushing's syndrome (overproduction) or Addison's disease (underproduction).
- Adrenocorticotropic hormone (ACTH) stimulation (p. 26): This test is used to determine the cause of adrenal insufficiency.
- Dexamethasone suppression (p. 187): This test is used to determine the cause of Cushing's syndrome.
- Metyrapone (p. 306): This test is used to determine the cause of Cushing's syndrome.

Adrenocorticotropic Hormone Stimulation
(ACTH Stimulation, Cortisol Stimulation, Cosyntropin)

Normal Findings

Rapid test: cortisol levels increase >7 mg/dl above baseline
24-hour test: cortisol levels >40 μg/dl
3-day test: cortisol levels >40 μg/dl

Indications

This test evaluates the ability of the adrenal gland to respond to ACTH administration. It is useful in evaluating the cause of adrenal insufficiency and also in evaluating patients with cushingoid symptoms.

Test Explanation

This test is performed on patients found to have adrenal insufficiency. An increase in plasma cortisol levels after the infusion of an "ACTH-like" drug indicates that the adrenal gland is normal and capable of functioning if stimulated. In that case the cause of adrenal insufficiency would lie within the pituitary gland (hypopituitarism, which is called secondary adrenal insufficiency). If little or no rise in cortisol levels occurs after the administration of the ACTH-like drug, the adrenal gland is the source of the problem and cannot secrete cortisol. This is called primary adrenal insufficiency (Addison's disease), which may be caused by adrenal hemorrhage, infarction, autoimmunity, metastatic tumor, surgical removal of the adrenal glands, or congenital adrenal enzyme deficiency.

This test can also be used to evaluate patients with Cushing's syndrome. Patients with Cushing's syndrome caused by bilateral adrenal hyperplasia have an exaggerated cortisol elevation in response to the administration of the ACTH-like drug. Those experiencing Cushing's syndrome as a result of hyperfunctioning adrenal tumors (which are usually autonomous and relatively insensitive to ACTH) have little or no increase in cortisol levels over baseline values.

Cosyntropin (Cortrosyn) is a synthetic subunit of ACTH that has the same corticosteroid-stimulating effect as endogenous ACTH in healthy persons. During this test, cosyntropin is administered to the patient, and the ability of the adrenal gland to respond is measured by plasma cortisol levels.

The *rapid stimulation test* is only a screening test. A normal response excludes adrenal insufficiency. An abnormal response, however, requires a 1- to 3-day prolonged ACTH stimulation test to differentiate primary insufficiency from secondary insufficiency. It should be noted that the adrenal gland can also be stimulated by insulin-induced hypoglycemia as a stressing agent. When insulin is the stimulant, cortisol and glucose levels are measured.

Interfering Factors

- Drugs that may cause artificially *increased* cortisol levels include prolonged corticosteroid administration, estrogens, and spironolactone.

Procedure and Patient Care

Before

- Have the patient remain on NPO status after midnight the day of the test.

During

Rapid Test

- Obtain a baseline plasma cortisol level less than 30 minutes prior to cosyntropin administration.
- Administer an IV injection of cosyntropin (250 μg) over a 2-minute period. An IM injection may also be used.
- Measure plasma cortisol levels 30 and 60 minutes after drug administration. Serum or heparinized blood is acceptable.

24-hour Test

- Obtain a baseline plasma cortisol level.
- Start an IV infusion of synthetic cosyntropin in 1 L of saline solution administered at a rate of 2 U/hr for 24 hours.
- After 24 hours, obtain another plasma cortisol level.

3-day Test

- Obtain a baseline plasma cortisol level.
- Administer 25 U of cosyntropin IV over an 8-hour period on 2 to 3 consecutive days.
- Plasma cortisol is then measured at 12, 24, 36, 48, 60, and 72 hours after the start of the test.

After

- Apply pressure or a pressure dressing to the venipuncture site.
- Check the venipuncture site for bleeding.

Test Results and Clinical Significance

Exaggerated response

Cushing's syndrome
Bilateral adrenal hyperplasia
Adrenal insufficiency
Secondary adrenal insufficiency caused by hypopituitarism, exogenous steroid ingestion, or endogenous steroid production from nonendocrine tumor

Normal or below normal response

Cushing's syndrome
Adrenal adenoma, adrenal carcinoma, ACTH-producing tumor, chronic steroid ingestion
Adrenal insufficiency
Primary adrenal insufficiency (Addison's disease) caused by adrenal infarction, hemorrhage, infection, or metastatic tumor to adrenal gland
Congenital enzyme adrenal insufficiency, surgical removal of adrenal gland, and ingestion of drugs, such as mitotane, metyrapone, or aminoglutethimide

Related Tests

- Cortisol (p. 167): Cortisol is a hormone produced by the adrenal gland and is the main determinant of Cushing's syndrome (overproduction) or Addison's disease (underproduction).
- Adrenocorticotropic hormone (ACTH) (p. 23): This test is used to determine the cause of Cushing's syndrome or Addison's disease.
- Dexamethasone suppression (p. 187): This test is used to determine the cause of Cushing's syndrome.
- Metyrapone (p. 306): This test is used to determine the cause of Cushing's syndrome.

Agglutinin, Febrile/Cold

Normal Findings

Febrile (warm) agglutinins: no agglutination in titers ≤1:80
Cold agglutinins: no agglutination in titers ≤1:16

Indications

Febrile agglutinin serologic studies are used to diagnose infectious diseases such as salmonellosis, rickettsial diseases, brucellosis, and tularemia. Neoplastic diseases, such as leukemias and lymphomas, are also associated with febrile agglutinins. Appropriate antibiotic treatment of the infectious agent is associated with a drop in the titer activity of febrile agglutinins. *Cold* agglutinins occur in patients who are infected by other agents, most notably *Mycoplasma pneumoniae.* Other diseases include influenza, mononucleosis, rheumatoid arthritis, lymphomas, and hemolytic anemia.

Test Explanation

The febrile and cold agglutinins are antibodies that cause RBCs to aggregate at high or low temperatures, respectively. They are believed to be due to infection by organisms with antigenic groups similar to some of those found on the RBCs. Agglutination may occur normally in concentrated serum (less than 1:32 dilution). Agglutination occurring at titers greater than 1:16 for cold agglutinins and 1:80 for febrile agglutinins is considered abnormal and diagnostic of the infectious agent or disease with which the agglutinins are associated. Agglutinins in high titers can attack RBCs and cause hemolytic anemias. Cold agglutinins are often obtained during the suspected acute phase of the disease and are repeated during the convalescence phase (7 to 10 days later). A fourfold or higher increase in antibody titer is considered diagnostic for the associated infectious diseases. Titer elevation is directly related to severity of infection. High titers of either cold or warm agglutinins can interfere with blood typing, crossmatching, and transfusion. In the elderly, agglutinins can persist for years following an associated illness.

Temperature regulation is critical when performing these tests. For cold agglutinins, the red-top tube is previously warmed to over 37° C; for febrile agglutinins, the red-top tube is cooled. The specimen is taken to the laboratory immediately so that no hemolysis will occur. Under no circumstances should the cold agglutinin specimen be refrigerated or the febrile agglutinin be heated. At the laboratory the cold agglutinin specimen is chilled and evaluated for agglutination of RBCs. The febrile agglutinin specimen is heated and also inspected for agglutination of RBCs. Serial dilutions are performed to detect the dilution at which agglutination occurs.

Interfering Factors

- Some antibiotics (penicillin and cephalosporins) can interfere with the development of cold agglutinins.

Procedure and Patient Care

Before

- Explain the procedure to the patient.
- Tell the patient that no fasting is required.

During

- Collect approximately 7 ml of venous blood in a red-top tube (warmed or cooled; see previous discussion).

After

- Apply pressure or a pressure dressing to the venipuncture site.
- Observe the venipuncture site for bleeding.
- Immediately transport the specimen to the laboratory.

Test Results and Clinical Significance

Increased cold agglutinins

Viral illness–rapid rise (7 days) peaking at 14 days and falling at 25 days
Mycoplasma pneumoniae
Infectious mononucleosis
Influenza
Nonbacterial infection
Collagen vascular diseases (e.g., scleroderma, rheumatoid arthritis)
Cirrhosis
Leukemia, lymphoma, multiple myeloma
These diseases are associated with very high titers of cold agglutinins.

Increased febrile agglutinins

Salmonella, rickettsia, brucellosis, tularemia

AIDS Serology (Acquired Immunodeficiency Serology, AIDS Screen, Human Immunodeficiency Virus (HIV) Antibody, Western Blot for HIV and Antibody, Enzyme-Linked Immunosorbent Assay [ELISA] for HIV and Antibody)

Normal Findings No evidence of HIV antigen or antibodies

Indications

These tests are used to diagnose HIV virus infection. They are also used to screen blood and organ donors for the presence of HIV virus.

Test Explanation

Tests used to detect the antibody to HIV, which is the virus that causes AIDS, were first licensed by the Food and Drug Administration in 1985 for the screening of blood and plasma donors. The HIV virus is also known as human T-lymphotrophic virus, type III (HTLV-III), or the lymphadenopathy-associated virus (LAV). There are two types of HIV viruses (types 1 and 2). Type 1 is most prevalent in the United States and western Europe. Type 2 is mostly limited to western African nations.

Since 1985 millions of HIV antibody tests have been performed in laboratories of blood and plasma collection centers, in counseling centers, and in clinical screening facilities. Those at high risk for AIDS include sexually active male homosexuals and bisexual men and women with multiple partners, IV drug abusers, persons receiving blood products containing HIV, and infants exposed to the virus during gestation and delivery. Accurate test results depend on the intrinsic quality of the tests and the technical expertise of those performing the tests.

Because of the medical and social significance of a positive test for HIV antibody, test results must be accurate and their interpretation correct. Therefore the U.S. Public Health

Service has emphasized that an individual can be said to have serologic evidence of HIV infection only after an enzyme immunoassay (EIA) screening test is repeatedly reactive and another test, such as the Western blot or immunofluorescence assay, validates the results. However, a positive EIA that is not confirmed by the Western blot test or immunofluorescence should not be considered negative. Repeat testing is required in 3 to 6 months. A person with positive HIV test results does not have AIDS until the clinical criteria are fulfilled.

ELISA, which tests for antibodies to HIV in serum or plasma, is the most widely used serologic test for AIDS. It is important to reiterate that ELISA detects antibodies to HIV. Because it does not detect viral antigens, it cannot detect infection in its earliest stage (before antibodies are formed). ELISA is used for clinical diagnosis, screening blood and blood products, and testing individuals who believe they may be infected with HIV.

The sensitivity (i.e., probability that the test results will be reactive if the specimen is a true positive) of the ELISA test is approximately 99% for blood from persons infected with HIV for 12 weeks or more. The probability of a false-negative test is remote except during the first few weeks after infection before detectable antibodies appear.

The specificity (probability that test results will be nonreactive if the specimen is a true negative) of the ELISA test is approximately 99% for repeatedly reactive tests. To increase the specificity of serologic tests further, a supplemental test (most often the Western blot test) is performed to validate repeatedly reactive ELISA results. The sensitivity of the blot test is comparable to or greater than a repeatedly reactive ELISA. A repeatedly reactive ELISA and a positive Western blot test are highly predictive of HIV infection. Negative tests tend to eliminate HIV infection in high-risk individuals.

The diagnostic test described above detects HIV infection based on demonstration of antibodies to HIV. Recently it has become possible to diagnose HIV infection by the direct detection of HIV or one of its components. New tests are now available in the research laboratory and are of considerable help when the Western blot test results are indeterminate. The simplest of these tests is the *p24 antigen* capture assay. This is an ELISA type assay that detects the viral protein p24 in the peripheral blood of HIV-infected individuals, where it exists either as a free antigen or complexed to anti-p24 antibodies.

The p24 antigen may be detectable as early as 2 to 6 weeks after infection. An equilibrium exists between p24 antigen and anti-p24 antibodies throughout the course of HIV infection. During the first few weeks of infection before the development of an immune response, there is a sharp increase in p24 antigen levels. These levels decline after the development of anti-p24 antibodies. Later in HIV disease, p24 antigen levels again become detectable.

The p24 antigen test is currently being used to assess the antiviral activity of experimental HIV therapies. The p24 antigen test can also be used to diagnose neonatal HIV infection, detect HIV before seroconversion, and determine the progression of AIDS.

Home kits are now available that provide anonymous registration and pretest counseling via a toll-free call. Sample collection in the privacy of one's home, laboratory processing, and posttest counseling are components of this home-testing process.

Interfering Factors

- False-positive results can occur in patients who have autoimmune disease, lymphoproliferative disease, leukemia, lymphoma, or syphilis or those who are alcoholics.

- False-negative results can occur in the early incubation stage or the end-stage of AIDS. Tests for HIV antigen should be performed at this stage.

Procedure and Patient Care

Before

- Explain the procedure to the patient.
- Obtain an informed consent as required by law.
- Tell the patient that no fasting or preparation is required.
- Maintain a nonjudgmental attitude toward the patient's sexual practices and allow the patient ample time to express his or her concerns regarding the results.

During

- Observe universal blood and body precautions. Wear gloves when handling blood products from all patients.
- Collect 7 ml of peripheral venous blood in a red-top tube. The blood is usually sent to an outside laboratory for testing, although testing kits are becoming increasingly available for hospital laboratories and even in homes.
- If the patient wishes to remain anonymous, use a number with the patient's name and record it accurately.
- Note that if the ELISA is repeatedly reactive (i.e., test is positive twice consecutively), the Western blot test is performed on the same blood sample.
- If the Western blot test is equivocal, collect a second serum specimen 2 to 4 months later for testing.

After

- Apply pressure or a pressure dressing to the venipuncture site.
- Assess the site for bleeding.
- Inform the patient to observe the venipuncture site for infection. Patients with AIDS are immunocompromised and susceptible to infection.
- Follow the institution's policy regarding test result reporting.
- Do not give results over the telephone. Remember that positive results may have devastating consequences.
- Explain to the patient that a positive Western blot test merely implies exposure to and presence of the AIDS virus within the body. It does not mean that the patient has clinical AIDS. Not all patients with positive antibodies will acquire the disease.

✓ CLINICAL PRIORITIES

- Do not give the test results over the telephone. Positive results may have devastating consequences, including loss of job, insurance, relationships, and housing.
- Encourage patients testing positive to inform their sexual partners so they can be tested.
- Inform patients testing positive that subsequent sexual contact will put partners at high risk for contracting AIDS.

- Encourage patients testing positive to identify their sexual contacts so that they can be informed and tested.
- Inform the patient that subsequent sexual contact will put new partners at high risk for contracting AIDS.
- Provide patient education regarding safe sexual practices.

Test Results and Clinical Significance

Increased levels

AIDS
AIDS-related complex

Related Tests

- Lymphocyte immunotyping (AIDS-T lymphocyte markers) (p. 301): This test quantifies the number of CD4 and CD8 lymphocytes in an HIV-positive patient. These tests are predictive of the disease course and prognosis.

Alanine Aminotransferase (ALT, Formerly Serum Glutamic-Pyruvic Transaminase [SGPT])

Normal Findings

Elderly: may be slightly higher than adult
Adult/child: 5-35 IU/L or 8-20 U/L (SI units)
Values may be higher in men and in African-Americans.
Infant: may be twice as high as adult

Indications

This test is used to identify hepatocellular diseases of the liver. It is also an accurate monitor of improvement or worsening of these diseases. In jaundiced patients an abnormal ALT will incriminate the liver rather than RBC hemolysis as a source of the jaundice.

Test Explanation

ALT is found predominantly in the liver; lesser quantities are found in the kidneys, heart, and skeletal muscle. Injury or disease affecting the liver parenchyma will cause a release of this hepatocellular enzyme into the bloodstream, thus elevating serum ALT levels. Most ALT elevations generally are caused by liver dysfunction. Therefore this enzyme is not only sensitive but also quite specific for hepatocellular disease. In hepatocellular disease other than viral hepatitis the ALT/AST ratio (DeRitis ratio) is less than 1. In viral hepatitis the ratio is greater than 1. This is helpful in the diagnosis of viral hepatitis.

Interfering Factors

- Previous IM injections may cause elevated levels.
- Drugs that may cause *increased* ALT levels include acetaminophen, allopurinol, aminosalicylic acid, ampicillin, azathioprine, carbamazepine, cephalosporins, chlordiazepoxide, chlorpropamide, clofibrate, cloxacillin, codeine, dicumarol, indomethacin, isoniazid (INH), methotrexate, methyldopa, nafcillin, nalidixic acid, nitrofurantoin, oral contraceptives, oxacillin, phenothiazines, phenylbutazone, phenytoin, procainamide, propoxyphene, propranolol, quinidine, salicylates, tetracyclines, and verapamil.

Procedure and Patient Care

Before

- Explain the procedure to the patient.
- Tell the patient that no fasting is required.

During

- Collect approximately 7 to 10 ml of blood in a red-top tube and send it to the laboratory for analysis.
- Indicate on the laboratory slip any medications that might affect the test results.

After

- Apply pressure or a pressure dressing to the venipuncture site.
- Assess the venipuncture site for bleeding. Patients with liver dysfunction often have prolonged clotting times.

Test Results and Clinical Significance

Significantly increased levels

Hepatitis
Hepatic necrosis
Hepatic ischemia

Moderately increased levels

Cirrhosis
Cholestasis
Hepatic tumor
Hepatotoxic drugs
Obstructive jaundice
Severe burns
Trauma to striated muscle

Mildly increased levels

Myositis
Pancreatitis
Myocardial infarction
Infectious mononucleosis
Shock

Injury or disease affecting the liver, heart, or skeletal muscles will cause a release of this enzyme into the bloodstream, thus elevating serum ALT levels.

Related Tests

- Aspartate aminotransferase (AST) (p. 105): This is another enzyme predominantly existing in the liver.

- Gamma-glutamyl transpeptidase (GGTP) (p. 219): This is another enzyme predominantly existing in the liver.
- Alkaline phosphatase (p. 42): This is another enzyme predominantly existing in the liver.
- 5′-Nucleotidase (p. 312): This is another enzyme predominantly existing in the liver.
- Creatine phosphokinase (CPK) (p. 173): This enzyme is used similarly to AST and exists predominantly in heart and skeletal muscle.
- Lactic dehydrogenase (LDH) (p. 278): This is an intracellular enzyme used to support the diagnosis of injury or disease involving the heart, liver, RBCs, kidneys, skeletal muscle, brain, and lungs.
- Leucine aminopeptidase (p. 286): This enzyme is specific to the hepatobiliary system. Diseases affecting that system will cause elevation of this enzyme.

Aldolase

Normal Findings

Adult: 3.0-8.2 Sibley-Lehninger U/dl or 22-59 mU at 37° C (SI units)
Child: approximately two times adult
Newborn: approximately four times adult

Indications

This test is used to aid in the diagnosis and surveillance of skeletal muscle diseases.

Test Explanation

Serum aldolase is very similar to the enzymes aspartate aminotransferase (AST) (see p. 105) and creatine phosphokinase (CPK) (see p. 173). Aldolase is an enzyme used in the glycolytic breakdown of glucose. As with AST and CPK, aldolase is present in most tissues of the body. This test is most useful for identifying muscular or hepatic cellular injury or destruction. The serum aldolase level is very high in patients with muscular dystrophies, dermatomyositis, and polymyositis. Levels also are increased in patients with gangrenous processes, muscular trauma, and muscular infectious diseases (e.g., trichinosis). Elevated levels are also noted in chronic hepatitis, obstructive jaundice, and cirrhosis.

Neurologic diseases causing weakness can be differentiated from muscular causes of weakness with this test. Normal values are seen in patients with such neurologic diseases as poliomyelitis, myasthenia gravis, and multiple sclerosis. Elevated aldolase levels are seen in patients with primary muscular disorders.

Interfering Factors

- Previous IM injections may cause elevated levels.
- Drugs that may cause *increased* aldolase levels include hepatotoxic agents.
- Drugs that may cause *decreased* levels include phenothiazine.

Procedure and Patient Care

Before

- Explain the procedure to the patient.
- Note that a short period of fasting usually will provide more accurate results.

During

- Collect 7 to 10 ml of blood in a red-top tube.
- Indicate on the laboratory slip any drugs that may affect test results.

After

- Apply pressure or pressure dressing to the venipuncture site.
- Observe the venipuncture site for bleeding.

Test Results and Clinical Significance

Increased levels

MUSCULAR DISEASES

Muscular dystrophy (highest aldolase levels associated with Duchenne's muscular dystrophy)
Dermatomyositis
Polymyositis

MUSCLE INJURY

Muscular trauma (examples include severe crush injuries, muscular infections [such as trichinosis], delirium tremens, severe burns)
Gangrenous/ischemic processes (such as prolonged shock)
Diseases or injury to muscle causes lysis of the muscle cells. Intracellular enzymes such as aldolase spill out into the bloodstream and are detected at elevated levels.

HEPATOCELLULAR DISEASES

Hepatitis
Cirrhosis
Diseases of the liver cause lysis of the liver cells. Intracellular enzymes such as aldolase spill out into the bloodstream and are detected at elevated levels.

MYOCARDIAL INFARCTION

Infarction of heart muscle causes lysis of the muscle cells. Intracellular enzymes such as aldolase spill out into the bloodstream and are detected at elevated levels.

Decreased levels

Muscle wasting diseases
Late muscular dystrophy
As muscle mass decreases, aldolase values decrease.

Hereditary fructose intolerance *Without an adequate source of glycogen (i.e., fructose), normal levels of aldolase are not needed.*

Related Tests

- Creatine phosphokinase (CPK) (p. 173): CPK is another muscular enzyme and is more frequently used for identifying cardiac and skeletal injury.

Aldosterone

Normal Findings

Blood

Supine: 3-10 ng/dl or 0.08-0.30 nmol/L (SI units)
Upright (sitting for at least 2 hours)
  Female: 5-30 ng/dl or 0.14-0.80 nmol/L (SI units)
  Male: 6-22 ng/dl or 0.17-0.61 nmol/L (SI units)
  Child/adolescent
    1 week-1 year: 1-160 ng/dl
    1-3 years: 5-60 ng/dl
    3-5 years: 5-80 ng/dl
    5-7 years: 5-50 ng/dl
    7-11 years: 5-70 ng/dl
    11-15 years: 5-50 ng/dl
  Newborn: 5-60 ng/dl

Urine

2-80 mg/24 hr or 5.5-72.0 nmol/24 hr (SI units)

Indications

This test is used to diagnose hyperaldosteronism. To differentiate primary aldosteronism (adrenal pathology) from secondary aldosteronism (extra-adrenal pathology), plasma renin must be performed simultaneously.

Test Explanation

Aldosterone, a hormone produced by the adrenal cortex, is a potent mineralocorticoid. Production of aldosterone is regulated primarily by the renin-angiotensin system. This system works as follows: a decreased effective renal blood flow triggers pressure-sensitive renal glomeruli elements to release renin. The renin then stimulates the liver to secrete angiotensin I, which is converted to angiotensin II in the lung and kidney. Angiotensin II is a potent stimulator of aldosterone (see Figure 2-15, p. 381).

Secondarily, aldosterone is stimulated by adrenocorticotropic hormone (ACTH), low serum sodium levels, and high serum potassium levels. Aldosterone in turn stimulates the renal tubules to absorb sodium (water follows) and to secrete potassium in the urine. In this way, aldosterone regulates serum sodium and potassium levels. Because water follows sodium transport, aldosterone also partially regulates water absorption (and plasma volume).

Increased aldosterone levels are associated with primary aldosteronism in which a tumor (usually an adenoma) of the adrenal cortex (Conn's syndrome) or bilateral adrenal nodular hyperplasia causes increased production of aldosterone. The typical pattern for primary aldosteronism is an increased aldosterone level and a decreased renin level. The renin level is low because the increased aldosterone level "turns off" the renin-angiotensin system. Patients with primary aldosteronism characteristically have hypertension, weakness, polyuria, and hypokalemia.

Increased aldosterone levels also occur with secondary aldosteronism caused by non-adrenal conditions. These include the following:

Renal vascular stenosis or occlusion
Hyponatremia (from diuretic or laxative abuse) or low salt intake
Hypovolemia
Pregnancy or use of estrogens
Malignant hypertension
Potassium loading
Generalized fluid overload (edema) (e.g., congestive heart failure, cirrhosis, nephrotic syndrome)

In secondary aldosteronism, aldosterone levels and renin levels are high.

The aldosterone assay can be performed on a 24-hour urine specimen or a plasma blood sample. The advantage of the 24-hour urine sample is that short-term fluctuations are eliminated. Plasma values are more convenient to sample, but they are affected by short-term fluctuations. Factors that can rapidly cause fluctuation in aldosterone levels include the following:

Diurnal variation: Peak aldosterone levels occur in early morning. In late afternoon the levels are cut in half.

Body position: In the upright position, plasma aldosterone levels are greatly increased.

Diet: Levels of both urine and plasma aldosterone are increased by low-sodium diets and are decreased by high-sodium diets. (Diets high and low in potassium have the opposite affect.)

A 24-hour urine collection is therefore much more reliable because the effect of these interfering factors is dampened.

Primary aldosteronism can be diagnosed by demonstrating little or no increase in renin levels after aldosterone stimulation (using salt restriction as the stimulant). This is because aldosterone is already maximally secreted by the pathologic adrenal gland. Also, patients with primary aldosteronism fail to suppress aldosterone after saline infusion (1.5 to 2.0 L of normal saline solution infused between 8 and 10 AM). Aldosterone can be measured in blood obtained from adrenal venous sampling (see pp. 887-890). In this situation, high levels from the right and left adrenal veins are diagnostic of bilateral adrenal hyperplasia. Unilateral high aldosterone levels are found in patients with aldosterone-producing tumors of the adrenal gland or renal artery stenosis. Renin levels are usually obtained at the same time. High unilateral renin levels with unilateral high aldosterone levels indicate renal artery stenosis. Aldosterone-producing tumors of the adrenal gland are characterized by unilateral high adrenal vein aldosterone and low renin levels.

Interfering Factors

- Strenuous exercise and stress can stimulate adrenocortical secretions and increase aldosterone levels.
- Excessive licorice ingestion can cause decreased levels, because it produces an aldosterone-like effect.
- Values are influenced by posture, diet, pregnancy, and diurnal variations.
- Position can significantly affect aldosterone levels.
- Because the test is usually performed by radioimmunoassay, recently administered radioactive medications will affect test results.
- Drugs that may cause *increased* levels include diazoxide (Hyperstat), hydralazine (Apresoline), nitroprusside (Nipride), diuretics, laxatives, potassium, and spironolactone.
- Drugs that may cause *decreased* levels include fludrocortisone (Florinef), propranolol (Inderal), and angiotensin-converting inhibitor (e.g., captopril) as well as licorice.

✓ CLINICAL PRIORITIES

- Aldosterone levels exhibit a diurnal variation, with peak levels occurring early in the morning and lower levels in the late afternoon.
- Body position affects aldosterone levels. Levels are greatly increased in the upright position. Usually patients should be sitting up for at least 2 hours before blood is drawn.
- Levels of both urine and plasma aldosterone are increased by low-sodium diets and are decreased by high-sodium diets. Patients should maintain a normal sodium diet (approximately 3 g/day) for at least 2 weeks prior to blood or urine collection.

Procedure and Patient Care

Before

- Explain the procedure for blood collection to the patient. Usually the patient is asked to be in the upright position (at least sitting) for at least 2 hours before blood is drawn. Occasionally blood will be drawn again before the patient gets out of bed. Inform nonhospitalized patients when to arrive at the laboratory and to maintain the upright position for at least 2 hours.
- Tell the patient that no fasting is necessary.
- Explain the procedure for collecting a 24-hour urine sample.
- Give the patient verbal and written instructions regarding dietary and medication restrictions.
- Instruct the patient to maintain a normal sodium diet (approximately 3 g/day) for at least 2 weeks before blood or urine collection.
- Have the patient ask the physician whether drugs that alter sodium, potassium, and fluid balance (e.g., diuretics, antihypertensives, steroids, oral contraceptives) should be withheld. Test results will be more accurate if these are suspended at least 2 weeks before either the blood or urine test.

- Inform the patient that renin inhibitors (e.g., propranolol) should not be taken 1 week before the test if confirmed by the physician.
- Tell the patient to avoid licorice for at least 2 weeks before the test because of its aldosterone-like effect.

During (blood collection)

- Collect approximately 5 to 10 ml of venous blood in a gold-top (serum separator) tube. For hospitalized patients, the sample is occasionally drawn first with the patient in the supine position. A second specimen (upright sample) is collected 4 hours later after the patient has been up and moving.
- Obtain the specimen in the morning.
- Indicate on the laboratory slip if the patient was supine or standing during the venipuncture.
- Handle the blood specimen gently. Rough handling may cause hemolysis and alter the test results.
- Transport the specimen on ice to the laboratory.
- List on the laboratory slip any medications that can affect test results.
- Indicate the source of the specimen (i.e., peripheral or adrenal vein).

During (urine collection)

- Instruct the patient to begin the 24-hour urine collection after discarding the first morning specimen. This is the start time of the 24-hour collection.
- Collect all urine passed over the next 24 hours into a container containing a boric acid preservative.
- Instruct the patient to void before defecating so that the urine is not contaminated by feces.
- Remind the patient not to put toilet paper in the collection container.
- Keep the urine specimen on ice or keep it refrigerated during the 24 hours.
- Collect the last specimen as close as possible to the end of the 24 hours.

After (blood collection)

- Apply pressure or a pressure dressing to the venipuncture site.
- Assess the venipuncture site for bleeding.

After (urine collection)

- Transport the urine specimen promptly to the laboratory.

Test Results and Clinical Significance

Increased levels

PRIMARY ALDOSTERONISM

Aldosterone-producing adrenal adenoma (Conn's disease)
Adrenal cortical nodular hyperplasia
Bartter's syndrome (renal wasting of potassium associated with poor sodium tubule absorption)
Aldosterone is produced in abnormally high quantities by the pathologic adrenal gland. This is reflected in serum and urine levels.

SECONDARY ALDOSTERONISM

Hyponatremia
Hyperkalemia
Diuretic ingestion resulting in hypovolemia and hyponatremia
Laxative abuse
These are all direct stimulants of aldosterone.

Stress
Malignant hypertension
Generalized edema (from congestive heart failure, nephrotic syndrome, cirrhosis)
Renal arterial stenosis
Pregnancy and oral contraceptives
Hypovolemia or hemorrhage
The renin-angiotensin system is stimulated in these conditions. Renin levels are high, and aldosterone secretion is stimulated.

Cushing's disease *Abnormally high ACTH levels secreted by a pituitary adenoma act as a direct stimulant to aldosterone.*

Decreased levels

Aldosterone deficiency
Renin deficiency *This is very rare and results in aldosterone deficiency.*
Steroid therapy *ACTH is suppressed and therefore aldosterone is suppressed.*
Addison's disease *The adrenal cortex is not functional and therefore aldosterone cannot be secreted.*

Patients on a high-sodium diet
Hypernatremia
Hypokalemia
Addison's disease
The above act as potent inhibitors to aldosterone secretion.

Toxemia of pregnancy
Antihypertensive therapy *Some antihypertensive medications inhibit aldosterone secretion.*

Related Tests

- Sodium, serum (p. 396) , urine (p. 851), and potassium, serum (p. 342), urine (p. 847): These are direct measurements of these electrolytes.
- Adrenocorticotropic hormone (ACTH) (p. 23): This is a test of anterior pituitary gland function.
- Renin assay (p. 380): This test is helpful in the differential diagnosis of primary vs. secondary aldosteronism.

Alkaline Phosphatase (ALP)

Normal Findings

Elderly: slightly higher than adult
Adult: 30-85 ImU/ml or 42-128 U/L (SI units)
Child/adolescent
  <2 years: 85-235 ImU/ml
  2-8 years: 65-210 ImU/ml
  9-15 years: 60-300 ImU/ml
  16-21 years: 30-200 ImU/ml

Indications

ALP is used to detect and monitor diseases of the liver or bone.

Test Explanation

Although ALP is found in many tissues, the highest concentrations are found in the liver, biliary tract epithelium, and bone. The intestinal mucosa and placenta also contain ALP. This phosphatase enzyme is called alkaline because its function is increased in an alkaline (pH of 9 to 10) environment. This enzyme test is important for detecting liver and bone disorders. Within the liver, ALP is present in Kupffer's cells. These cells line the biliary collecting system. This enzyme is excreted into the bile. Enzyme levels of ALP are greatly increased in both extrahepatic and intrahepatic obstructive biliary disease and cirrhosis. Other liver abnormalities, such as hepatic tumors, hepatoxic drugs, and hepatitis, cause smaller elevations in ALP levels. Reports have indicated that the most sensitive test to indicate tumor metastasis to the liver is the ALP.

Bone is the most frequent extrahepatic source of ALP; new bone growth is associated with elevated ALP levels. Pathologic new bone growth occurs with osteoblastic metastatic (e.g., breast, prostate) tumors. Paget's disease, healing fractures, rheumatoid arthritis, hyperparathyroidism, and normal-growing bones are sources of elevated ALP levels as well.

Isoenzymes of ALP are also used to distinguish between liver and bone diseases. These isoenzymes are most easily differentiated by the heat stability test and electrophoresis. The isoenzyme of liver origin (ALP1) is heat stable; the isoenzyme of bone origin (ALP2) is inactivated by heat. The detection of isoenzymes can help differentiate the source of the pathologic condition associated with the elevated total ALP. ALP1 would be expected to be high when liver disease is the source of the elevated total ALP. ALP2 would be expected to be high when bone disease is the source of the elevated total ALP. Another way to separate the source of elevated ALP is to simultaneously test for 5′-nucleotidase. This later enzyme is made predominantly in the liver. If total ALP and 5′-nucleotidase are concomitantly elevated, the disease is in the liver. If 5′-nucleotidase is normal, the bone is the most probable source.

In pregnancy the placenta produces ALP. In certain persons with type B and O blood, the ALP is elevated. Fibroblasts in granulation tissue within a healing wound can produce ALP.

Age-related concerns

- *Young children* have increased ALP levels because their bones are growing. This increase is magnified during the "growth spurt," which occurs at different ages in males and females.

Interfering Factors

- Recent ingestion of a meal can increase this ALP level.
- Age: Young children with rapid bone growth have increased ALP levels. This is most magnified during the growth spurt. Females and males differ in age of growth spurt.
- Drugs that may cause *elevated* ALP levels include albumin made from placental tissue, allopurinol, antibiotics, azathioprine, colchicine, fluorides, indomethacin, isoniazid (INH), methotrexate, methyldopa, nicotinic acid, phenothiazine, probenecid, tetracycline, and verapamil.
- Drugs that may cause *decreased* levels include arsenicals, cyanides, fluorides, nitrofurantoin, oxalates, and zinc salts.

Procedure and Patient Care

Before

- Explain the procedure to the patient.
- Tell the patient that fasting is preferred but not required. Overnight fasting may be required for isoenzymes. The ALP level is generally higher after eating.

During

- Collect approximately 7 to 10 ml of blood in a red-top tube.
- List on the laboratory slip any medications that can affect test results.

After

- Apply pressure or a pressure dressing to the venipuncture site.
- Assess the venipuncture site for bleeding. Patients with liver dysfunction often have prolonged clotting times.

Test Results and Clinical Significance

Increased levels

Primary cirrhosis
Intrahepatic or extrahepatic biliary obstruction
Primary or metastatic liver tumor
ALP is found in the liver and biliary epithelium. It is normally excreted into the bile. Obstruction, no matter how mild, will cause elevations in ALP.

Normal pregnancy (third trimester, early postpartum period) *The ALP comes from the placenta and from the new bone growth that occurs during this time.*

Normal bones of growing children
Metastatic tumor to the bone
Healing fracture
Hyperparathyroidism
Paget's disease
Rheumatoid arthritis
The ALP comes from the bone in the above-noted diseases.

Intestinal ischemia or infarction
Myocardial infarction
Sarcoidosis

Decreased levels

Hypophosphatemia *There is insufficient phosphate to make ALP.*
Malnutrition
Milk-alkali syndrome
Pernicious anemia
Scurvy (vitamin C deficiency)

Related Tests

- Alanine aminotransferase (ALT) (p. 33): This liver enzyme can aid in the differential diagnosis of causes of ALP elevation. If the ALT is elevated along with the ALP, hepatocellular disease is suspected.
- Aspartate aminotransferase (AST) (p. 105): This liver enzyme can aid in the differential diagnosis of causes of ALP elevation. If the AST is elevated along with the ALP, hepatocellular disease is suspected.
- Gamma-glutamyl transferase (GGT) (p. 219): This liver enzyme can aid in the differential diagnosis of causes of ALP elevation. If the GGT is elevated along with the ALP, diseases affecting the biliary tree are suspected.
- 5′-Nucleotidase (p. 312): This liver enzyme can aid in the differential diagnosis of causes of ALP elevation. If the 5′-nucleotidase is elevated along with the ALP, diseases affecting the biliary tree are suspected.
- Acid phosphatase (p. 20): This bone enzyme can aid in the differential diagnosis of causes of ALP elevation. If the acid phosphatase is elevated along with the ALP, bone disease is suspected.
- Creatine phosphokinase (CPK) (p. 173): This enzyme exists predominantly in heart and skeletal muscle.
- Lactic dehydrogenase (LDH) (p. 278): This intracellular enzyme is used to support the diagnosis of injury or disease involving the heart, liver, red blood cells, kidneys, skeletal muscle, brain, and lungs.
- Leucine aminopeptidase (p. 286): This enzyme is specific to the hepatobiliary system. Diseases affecting that system will cause elevation of this enzyme.

Alpha$_1$-Antitrypsin (AAT, A1AT)

Normal Findings

>250 mg/dl or 0.8-2.1 g/L (SI units)

Indications

Serum AAT determinations are obtained in patients with a family history of emphysema, because there is a familial tendency for a deficiency of this antienzyme. Deficient or absent serum levels of this enzyme can cause the early onset of disabling emphysema. A similar deficiency in AAT is seen in children with cirrhosis and other liver diseases.

AAT is also an acute-phase reactant protein that is elevated in the presence of inflammation, infection, or malignancy. It is not specific as to the source of the inflammatory process.

Test Explanation

AAT inactivates endoproteases (protein catabolic enzymes that are released in the body by degenerating and dying cells), such as trypsin and neutrophil elastase, that can break down elastic fibers and collagen, especially in the lung. Deficiencies of AAT can be genetic or acquired. Genetic typing has shown that most persons have two AAT "M" genes (designated as MM,) and AAT levels over 250 mg/dl. "Z" and "S" genes are typically associated with alterations in serum levels of AAT. Individuals who are ZZ or SS homozygous always have serum levels below 50 mg/dl and often near zero.

Acquired deficiencies in AAT can occur in patients with protein-deficiency syndromes (e.g., malnutrition, liver disease, nephrotic syndrome, neonatal respiratory distress syndrome). People with AAT deficiency develop severe panacinar (although usually more severe in the lower third of the lungs) emphysema in the third or fourth decade of life. Their major clinical symptoms usually include progressive dyspnea with minimal coughing. Chronic bronchitis is prominent in those patients with deficient AAT levels who smoke. Bronchiectasis can also occur in these patients.

Individuals who are MZ or MS heterozygous have serum levels of AAT between 50 and 250 mg/dl. Approximately 5% to 14% of the adult population have this heterozygous state, which is considered to be a risk factor for emphysema. AAT is now qualitatively measured using immunochemical methods. Quantification is possible but rarely useful with phenotyping. Routine serum protein electrophoresis is a good screening test for AAT deficiency, because AAT accounts for about 90% of the protein in the alpha$_1$-globulin region on electrophoresis.

Interfering Factors

- Serum levels of AAT can double during pregnancy.
- Drugs that may cause *increased* levels include oral contraceptives.

Procedure and Patient Care

Before

- Explain the procedure to the patient.
- Note that no fasting is usually required. Verify this with the laboratory performing the study.

During

- Collect approximately 5 to 10 ml of blood in a red-top tube.

After

- Apply pressure or a pressure dressing to the venipuncture site.
- Observe the venipuncture site for bleeding.
- If the results show the patient is at risk for emphysema, begin patient teaching. Include such factors as avoidance of smoking, infection, and inhaled irritants; proper nutrition; adequate hydration; and education about the disease process of emphysema.
- If the test is positive, genetic counseling is indicated. Other family members should be tested to determine their and their children's risks.

Test Results and Clinical Significance

Increased levels

Acute and chronic inflammatory disorders
Stress
Infection
Thyroid infections
Because AAT is an acute-phase reactant protein, elevated levels can be expected when the body is subjected to any inflammatory reaction or stress.

Decreased levels

Early onset of emphysema (adults)
Neonatal respiratory distress syndrome
Cirrhosis (children)
These diseases are a result of endoproteases working uninhibited (no AAT available) within the body. Collagen is broken down, setting up the destruction of lung and liver structures.

Low serum proteins *Diseases such as malnutrition, end-stage cancer, nephrotic syndrome, protein-losing enteropathy, and hepatic failure are associated with lack of protein synthesis. AAT is a protein and therefore will not be produced in adequate quantities in these diseases.*

Related Tests

- C-reactive protein (p. 172): This also is an acute-phase reactant protein.
- Erythrocyte sedimentation rate (p. 199): This also is an acute-phase reactant protein.

Alpha-Fetoprotein (AFP, Alpha$_1$-fetoprotein)

Normal Findings

Adult: <40 ng/ml or <40 mg/L (SI units)
Child less than 1 year: <30 ng/ml
Ranges are stratified by weeks of gestation and vary according to different laboratories.

Indications

This test can be used as a tumor marker to identify cancers, such as hepatomas. It is also used in the diagnosis of fetal body wall defects, such as neural tube defects.

Test Explanation

AFP is an oncofetal protein normally produced by the fetal liver and yolk sac. It is the dominant fetal serum protein in the first trimester of life and diminishes to very low levels by the age of 1 year. Normally it is found in very low levels in the adult. Increased serum levels of AFP are found in as many as 90% of patients with hepatomas. The higher the AFP level, the greater the tumor burden. A decrease in AFP is seen if the patient is responding to antineoplastic therapy. AFP is not specific for hepatomas, although extremely high levels (above 500 ng/ml) are diagnostic for hepatoma. Other neoplastic conditions, such as nonseminomatous germ cell tumors and teratomas of the testes, yolk sac and germ cell tumors of the ovaries, and to a lesser extent Hodgkin's disease, lymphoma, and renal cell carcinoma, are also associated with elevated AFP levels. With improved methods of detection (such as radioimmunoassay and enzyme immunoassay), AFP can also be detected in the serum of patients with cancer of the stomach, colon, breast, and lung. Noncancerous causes of elevated AFP levels occur in patients with cirrhosis or chronic active hepatitis.

AFP is also helpful in the diagnosis of fetal body wall defects. The most notable of these is neural tube defects, which can vary from a small myelomeningocele to anencephaly. Although not widely used in the United States, AFP levels can be used for widespread screening for neural tube defects. If a fetus has an open body wall defect, fetal serum AFP leaks out into the amniotic fluid and is picked up by the maternal serum. Normally AFP from fetal sources can be detected in the amniotic fluid or the mother's blood after 10 weeks of gestation. Peak levels occur between 16 and 18 weeks. With neural tube defects, AFP leaks out of the fetal serum through the neural tube defect and into the amniotic fluid. Maternal serum reflects that change in amniotic AFP levels. When elevated maternal serum AFP levels are identified, further evaluation with repeat serum AFP levels, amniotic fluid AFP levels, and ultrasound is warranted. Other examples of fetal body wall defects would include omphalocele and gastroschisis. Elevated serum AFP levels in pregnancy may also indicate multiple pregnancy, fetal distress, fetal congenital abnormalities, or intrauterine death. Low AFP levels after correction for age of gestation, maternal weight, race, and presence of diabetes are found in mothers carrying a fetus with trisomy 21 (Down syndrome).

Interfering Factors

- Fetal blood contamination, which may occur during amniocentesis, can cause increased AFP levels.
- Multiple pregnancies can cause increased levels.
- Recent administration of radioisotopes can affect values because results are determined by radioimmunoassay.

Procedure and Patient Care

If an AFP test is to be performed on amniotic fluid, follow "Procedure and Patient Care" for amniocentesis, p. 564.

Before

- Explain the procedure to the patient.
- Tell the patient that no food or fluid restriction is required.

During

- Collect approximately 7 to 10 ml of blood in a red-top tube.

After

- Apply pressure or a pressure dressing to the venipuncture site.
- Assess the venipuncture site for bleeding.
- Include the gestational age on the laboratory slip.

Test Results and Clinical Significance

Increased maternal serum levels

Neural tube defects (e.g., anencephaly, encephalocele, spina bifida, myelomeningocele)
Abdominal wall defects (e.g., gastroschisis, omphalocele)
If a fetus has an open body wall defect, fetal serum AFP leaks out into the amniotic fluid and is picked up by the maternal serum.

Multiple pregnancy *Large quantities are made by the multiple fetuses.*
Threatened abortion
Fetal distress or congenital anomalies
Fetal death

Increased nonmaternal levels

Primary hepatocellular cancer (hepatoma)
Germ cell or yolk sac cancer of the ovary
Embryonal cell or germ cell tumor of the testes
Other cancers (e.g., stomach, colon, lung, breast, lymphoma)
Liver cell necrosis (e.g., cirrhosis, hepatitis)
Cancers contain undifferentiated cells that may carry the surface markers of their fetal predecessors.

Decreased maternal levels

Trisomy 21 (Down syndrome)
Fetal wastage

Related Tests

- Tumor markers: carcinoembryonic antigen (CEA) (p. 137), CA-125 (p. 125), CA15-3 (p. 123), prostate specific antigen (PSA) (p. 356), CA 19-9 (p. 121): These are other tumor markers used for detection and surveillance of various cancers.
- Amniocentesis (p. 560): This is a procedure to obtain amniotic fluid for evaluation of fetal health.

Ammonia

Normal Findings

Adult: 15-110 mg/dl or 47-65 mmol/L (SI units)
Child: 40-80 mg/dl
Newborn: 90-150 mg/dl

Indications

Ammonia is used to support the diagnosis of severe liver diseases (fulminant hepatitis or cirrhosis), and for surveillance of these diseases. Ammonia levels are also used in the diagnosis and follow-up of hepatic encephalopathy.

Test Explanation

Ammonia is a by-product of protein catabolism. Most of it is made by bacteria acting on proteins present in the gut. By way of the portal vein, it goes to the liver where it is normally converted into urea and then secreted by the kidneys. Ammonia cannot be catabolized in the presence of severe hepatocellular dysfunction. Furthermore, when portal blood flow to the liver is altered (e.g., in portal hypertension), ammonia cannot reach the liver to be catabolized. Ammonia blood levels rise. Congenital enzymatic defects in the urea cycle also can cause a rise in ammonia levels. Finally, impaired renal function diminishes excretion of ammonia, and the blood levels rise. High levels of ammonia result in encephalopathy and coma. Arterial ammonia levels are more reliable than venous levels but more difficult to obtain and are therefore not routinely used.

Interfering Factors

- Hemolysis increases ammonia levels because the RBCs have about three times the ammonia level content of plasma.
- Muscular exertion can increase ammonia.
- Cigarette smoking can produce significant increases in ammonia levels within 1 hour of inhalation.
- Ammonia levels may be factitiously increased if the tourniquet is too tight for too long.

- Drugs that may cause *increased* ammonia levels include acetazolamide, alcohol, ammonium chloride, barbiturates, narcotics, parenteral nutrition, and diuretics (loop, thiazide).
- Drugs that may cause *decreased* levels include broad-spectrum antibiotics (e.g., neomycin), lactulose, levodopa, lactobacillus, and potassium salts.

Procedure and Patient Care

Before

- Explain the procedure to the patient.
- Note that no fasting is usually required.

During

- Collect approximately 5 to 7 ml of blood in a green-top tube. Note that some institutions require the specimen be sent to the laboratory in an iced container.
- List on the laboratory slip any drugs that can affect test results.
- Avoid hemolysis and send the specimen promptly to the laboratory.

After

- Apply pressure or a pressure dressing to the venipuncture site.
- Assess the venipuncture site for bleeding. Many patients with liver disease have prolonged clotting times.

Test Results and Clinical Significance

Increased levels

Primary hepatocellular disease
Reye's syndrome
Asparagine intoxication
There are not enough functioning liver cells to metabolize the ammonia.

Portal hypertension
Severe heart failure with congestive hepatomegaly
The portal blood flow from the gut to the liver is altered. The ammonia cannot get to the liver to be metabolized for excretion. Furthermore, the ammonia from the gut is rapidly shunted around the liver (by way of gastroesophageal varices) and into the systemic circulation.

Hemolytic disease of newborn (erythroblastosis fetalis) *RBCs contain high amounts of ammonia. The newborn liver is not mature enough to metabolize all the ammonia presented to it by the hemolysis that occurs in this disease.*

GI bleeding with mild liver disease
GI obstruction with mild liver disease
Ammonia production is increased because the bacteria have more protein (blood) to catabolize. An impaired liver may not be able to keep up with the increased load of ammonia presented to it.

Hepatic encephalopathy and hepatic coma *These neurologic states are a result of ammonia acting as false neurotransmitters. The brain cannot function properly.*

Genetic metabolic disorder of urea cycle *Ammonia is catabolized by the urea cycle. Disruption of that cycle will inhibit excretion of ammonia and levels can be expected to rise.*

Decreased levels

Essential or malignant hypertension
Hyperornithinemia

Amylase

Normal Findings

Adult: 56-190 IU/L, 80-150 Somogyi units/dl, or 25-125 U/L (SI units)
Newborn: 6-65 U/L
Values may be slightly increased during normal pregnancy and in the elderly.

Critical Values

More than three times the upper limit of normal (depending on the method)

Indications

This test is used to detect and monitor the clinical course of pancreatitis. It is frequently ordered when a patient presents with acute abdominal pain.

Test Explanation

The serum amylase test, which is easy and rapidly performed, is most specific for pancreatitis. Amylase is normally secreted from pancreatic acinar cells into the pancreatic duct and then into the duodenum. Once in the intestine it aids in the catabolism of carbohydrates (starch) to their component simple sugars. Damage to pancreatic acinar cells (as in pancreatitis) or obstruction of the pancreatic duct flow (as in pancreatic carcinoma or common bile duct gallstones) causes an outpouring of this enzyme into the intrapancreatic lymph system and the free peritoneum. Blood vessels draining the free peritoneum and absorbing the lymph pick up the excess amylase. An abnormal rise in the serum level of amylase occurs within 12 hours of the onset of disease. Because amylase is rapidly cleared (2 hours) by the kidney, serum levels return to normal 48 to 72 hours after the initial insult. Persistent pancreatitis, duct obstruction, or pancreatic duct leak (e.g., pseudocysts) will cause persistent elevated serum amylase levels.

Although serum amylase is a sensitive test for pancreatic disorders, it is not specific. Other nonpancreatic diseases can cause elevated amylase levels in the serum. For example, during bowel perforation, intraluminal amylase leaks into the free peritoneum and is picked up by the peritoneal blood vessels. This results in an elevated serum amylase level. A penetrating peptic ulcer into the pancreas will also cause elevated amylase levels. Duodenal obstruction can be associated with less significant elevations in amylase. Because salivary glands contain amylase, elevations can be expected in patients with parotiditis (mumps). Amylase is also found in low levels in the ovaries and skeletal muscles. Ectopic pregnancy and severe diabetic ketoacidosis are also associated with hyperamylasemia.

Patients with chronic pancreatic disorders (e.g., chronic pancreatitis) that have resulted in pancreatic cell destruction or patients with massive hemorrhagic pancreatic necrosis often do not have high amylase levels, because there may be so few pancreatic cells left to make amylase.

Interfering Factors

- IV dextrose solutions can lower amylase levels and cause a false-negative result.
- Serum lipemia factitiously decreases amylase with the current laboratory methods.
- Drugs that may cause *increased* serum amylase levels include aminosalicylic acid, aspirin, azathioprine, corticosteroids, dexamethasone, ethyl alcohol, glucocorticoids, iodine-containing contrast media, loop diuretics (e.g., furosemide), methyldopa, narcotic analgesics, oral contraceptives, and prednisone.
- Drugs that may cause *decreased* levels include citrates, glucose, and oxalates.

Procedure and Patient Care

Before

- Explain the procedure to the patient.
- Tell the patient that no fasting is required.

During

- Collect 5 to 7 ml of venous blood in a red-top tube.
- Indicate on the laboratory slip any medications that may affect test results.

After

- Apply pressure or a pressure dressing to the venipuncture site.
- Check the venipuncture site for bleeding.

Test Results and Clinical Significance

Increased levels

Acute pancreatitis
Chronic relapsing pancreatitis
Damage to pancreatic acinar cells, as in pancreatitis, causes an outpouring of amylase into the intrapancreatic lymph system and the free peritoneum. Blood vessels draining the free peritoneum and absorbing the lymph pick up the excess amylase.

Penetrating peptic ulcer into the pancreas
GI disease
In patients with perforated peptic ulcer, necrotic bowel, perforated bowel, or duodenal obstruction, amylase leaks out of the gut and into the free peritoneal cavity. The amylase is picked up by the blood and lymphatics of the peritoneum, where levels are demonstrated in excess.

Acute cholecystitis
Parotiditis (mumps)
Ruptured ectopic pregnancy
Amylase is also present in the salivary glands, gallbladder, and fallopian tubes. Diseases affecting these organs will be associated with elevated levels of amylase.

Renal failure *Amylase is cleared by the kidney. Renal diseases will reduce excretion of amylase.*
Diabetic ketoacidosis
Pulmonary infarction
After endoscopic retrograde pancreatography

Related Tests

- Urine amylase (p. 818): Amylase can be detected in the urine long after serum amylase has cleared. If serum amylase levels are normal and pancreatitis is suspected, the period of peak amylase levels may have passed. Elevated amylase levels may still be found in the urine.
- Lipase (p. 287): Lipase is similar to amylase except that it is more specific for the pancreas.

Androstenedione

Normal Findings

<250 ng/dl

Critical Values

>1000 ng/dl

Indications

This test is used for evaluating virilizing syndromes.

Test Explanation

Androstenedione is a precursor of cortisol, aldosterone, testosterone, and estrogen. This hormone is important for the diagnosis of virilizing syndromes, especially in the female. In the adrenal glands of females, androstenedione is converted to the above-noted hormones. In the female peripheral tissues and ovaries, androstenedione is converted into testosterone and estrogen. In females, 50% to 60% of testosterone is made in the peripheral tissues, 30% is produced in the adrenal gland, and 20% is produced in the ovary.

Tumors of the adrenal glands (cancers, adenomas) or ovaries (stroma tumors) can secrete large amounts of androstenedione, which is then converted into large amounts of testosterone relative to normal. In the adult female this can cause virilizing symptoms such as hirsutism, change in voice, and sterility. Children with congenital adrenal hyperplasia have enzyme defects that affect conversion of androstenedione to cortisol. Excess androstenedione is built up. As adrenocorticotropic (ACTH) levels increase, androstenedione production is stimulated and levels increase still further. Again, this hormone is converted into a relatively high level of testosterone by the peripheral tissues. Pseudohermaphroditism results in female children. In male children with similar congenital defects, precocious puberty will become obvious. Adult female patients with Cushing's syndrome experience virilization through the same pathophysiologic process.

Patients with polycystic ovary syndrome (Stein-Leventhal syndrome) may also have elevated levels of testosterone precursors, including androstenedione.

Interfering Factors

- A radioactive scan performed 1 week before the test may invalidate the test results, because this assay is usually performed by radioimmunoassay.
- Drugs that may *increase* levels of androstenedione are corticotropin, clomiphene, and metyrapone.
- Steroids may *decrease* levels of androstenedione.

Procedure and Patient Care

Before

- Explain the procedure to the patient.
- Tell the patient that the specimen should be collected 1 week before or after the menstrual period.
- Note that fasting is preferable.
- Since peak production of androstenedione is around 7 AM, blood should be drawn around that time.

During

- Collect one red-top tube of venous blood.
- Indicate the date of the last menstrual period on the laboratory form.

After

- Apply pressure or a pressure dressing to the venipuncture site.
- Assess the venipuncture site for bleeding.

Test Results and Clinical Significance

Increased levels

Adrenal tumor *The tumor makes large amounts of androstenedione, which is then converted by ovaries and fatty tissue to testosterone and estrogen. The relatively high level of testosterone causes the virilizing signs.*

Congenital adrenal hyperplasia *This disease is characterized by enzyme defects that prevent conversion of androstenedione to cortisol. Androstenedione levels are increased.*

Ectopic ACTH-producing tumors
Cushing's disease
ACTH stimulates the adrenal to make large amounts of hormones, including androstenedione.

Cushing's syndrome *Large amounts of hormones, including androstenedione, are made in the adrenal gland.*
Stein-Leventhal syndrome
Ovarian sex cord tumor

Decreased levels

Primary or secondary adrenal insufficiency
Ovarian failure
Oophorectomy
There is a decreased production and conversion of androstenedione.

Related Tests

- Testosterone (p. 405): This is a direct measurement of testosterone.
- Estradiol (p. 202): This is a direct measurement of one of the conjugated estrogens.
- Cortisol, blood (p. 167): This is a direct measurement of cortisol, the major adrenal glucocorticosteroid.

Angiotensin-Converting Enzyme
(ACE, Serum Angiotensin-Converting Enzyme [SACE], Peptidyldipeptide Hydrolase)

Normal Findings 23-57 U/ml (over 20 years of age)

Indications

ACE is used to detect and monitor the clinical course of sarcoidosis (a granulomatous disease that affects many organs, especially the lungs). Furthermore, it is used to differentiate between sarcoidosis and other granulomatous diseases. It is also used to differentiate active and dormant sarcoid disease.

Test Explanation

ACE is found in pulmonary epithelial cells and converts angiotensin I to angiotensin II (a potent vasoconstrictor). Angiotensin II is a significant stimulator of aldosterone. ACE is vital in the renin/aldosterone mechanism and therefore important in controlling blood pressure. Despite this, ACE is not very helpful in the evaluation of hypertension. Its value is in the detection of sarcoidosis.

Elevated ACE levels are found in a high percentage of patients with sarcoidosis. This test is primarily used in patients with sarcoidosis to evaluate the severity of disease and the response to therapy. Levels are especially high with active pulmonary sarcoidosis and can be normal with inactive (dormant) sarcoidosis. Elevated ACE levels also occur in conditions other than sarcoidosis, including Gaucher's disease (a rare familial lysosomal disorder of fat metabolism), leprosy, alcoholic cirrhosis, active histoplasmosis, tuberculosis, Hodgkin's disease, myeloma, scleroderma, pulmonary embolism, and idiopathic pulmonary fibrosis. An ACE assay can be performed using spectrophotometry or radioimmunoassay.

Interfering Factors

- Patients under 20 years of age normally have very high ACE levels.
- Hemolysis or hyperlipidemia may factitiously decrease ACE levels.
- Drugs that may cause *decreased* ACE levels include ACE inhibitor antihypertensives and steroids.

Procedure and Patient Care

Before

- Explain the procedure to the patient.
- Tell the patient that no fasting is required.

During

- Collect approximately 5 ml of blood in a red-top tube.
- Note on the laboratory slip if the patient is taking steroids.

After

- Apply pressure or a pressure dressing to the venipuncture site.
- Assess the venipuncture site for bleeding.

Test Results and Clinical Significance

Increased levels

Sarcoidosis *This is the disease for which this test is primarily performed. The more severe the sarcoidosis, the greater the likelihood that ACE will be increased.*

Other rare diseases that have been found to be associated with ACE elevations include Gaucher's disease, tuberculosis, leprosy, alcoholic cirrhosis, active histoplasmosis, Hodgkin's disease, myeloma, idiopathic pulmonary fibrosis, diabetes mellitus, primary biliary cirrhosis, amyloidosis, hyperthyroidism, scleroderma, and pulmonary embolism.

Related Tests

- Kveim test: This is a skin test for sarcoidosis that is rarely performed today.

Anion Gap (AG, R Factor)

Normal Findings

8-16 mEq/L (if potassium is used in the calculation)
8-12 mEq/L (if potassium is not used in the calculation)

Indications

Calculation of the AG assists in the evaluation of patients with acid-base disorders. It is used to attempt to identify the potential cause of the disorder. It can also be used to monitor therapy for acid-base abnormalities.

Test Explanation

The AG is the difference between the cations and the anions in the extracellular space.

$$\text{Anion gap} = (\text{Sodium} + \text{Potassium}) - (\text{Chloride} + \text{Bicarbonate})$$

In some laboratories the potassium is not factored in. The normal value is adjusted downward if potassium is eliminated from the equation. Normally the AG is created by the small amounts of anions in the blood, such as lactate, phosphates, sulfates, and proteins.

This calculation can help identify the cause of metabolic acidosis. As acids such as lactic acid or ketoacids accumulate in the bloodstream, bicarbonate levels diminish to regulate the pH within the blood. The bicarbonate mixes with the hydrogen in the blood to form water and CO_2. The acid anion combines with sodium to form a new salt, which is excreted in the urine. Mathematically, when bicarbonate decreases, the AG increases. If bicarbonate is lost from the extracellular space through diarrhea or increased excretion by a diseased kidney, the AG will increase.

Diseases that increase bicarbonate in the bloodstream will decrease the AG. Metabolic alkalosis results from excessive loss of acid from the GI tract, or excessive reabsorption of bicarbonate by the kidneys will increase bicarbonate and decrease AG.

Interfering Factors

- Drugs that *increase* AG include carbonic anhydrase inhibitors (e.g., acetazolamide), salicylate, spironolactone, triamterene, and methanol.
- Drugs that *decrease* AG include carbenicillin, penicillin phosphate, diuretics, antacids, licorice, and carbenoxolone.

Procedure and Patient Care

Before

- Explain the procedure to the patient.
- Tell the patient that foods or fluids are not restricted.

During

- Collect 5 to 10 ml of venous blood in a red- or green-top tube.
- If the patient is receiving an IV infusion, obtain the blood from the opposite arm.
- List on the laboratory slip any drugs that may affect test results.

After

- The sodium, potassium, chloride and bicarbonate levels are determined by an automated multichannel analyzer. The AG is then calculated as indicated above.
- Apply pressure or a pressure dressing to the venipuncture site.
- Assess the venipuncture site for bleeding.

Test Results and Clinical Significance

Increased levels

Lactic acidosis
Diabetic ketoacidosis
Alcoholic ketoacidosis
Starvation
Acids within the blood are accumulated. The hydrogen combines with the bicarbonate to maintain a homeostatic pH. Bicarbonate levels diminish and AG rises.

Renal failure *Phosphate, sulfates, and other acids accumulate in the blood as a result of poor excretion of these acids. The hydrogen combines with the bicarbonate to maintain a homeostatic pH. Bicarbonate levels diminish and AG rises.*
Renal tubular acidosis *Bicarbonate is lost through the kidney. Bicarbonate levels diminish and AG rises.*
Increased GI losses of bicarbonate (e.g., diarrhea, fistulas) *Bicarbonate is lost through the GI tract. Bicarbonate levels diminish and AG rises.*
Hypoaldosteronism *Aldosterone stimulates acid secretion in the distal renal tubule in exchange for sodium. With deficient quantities of aldosterone, acid builds up and is combined with bicarbonate. Bicarbonate levels diminish and AG rises.*

Decreased levels

Excess alkali ingestion *With the excessive use of antacids or bicarbonates, the AG decreases.*
Multiple myeloma *The M-chain component of the proteins produced by the neoplastic plasma cells are cationic, causing a retention of chloride to maintain electrical neutrality. As the chloride increases, the AG decreases.*
Chronic vomiting or gastric suction *Gastric acids are lost, causing an increased bicarbonate level and a decreased AG.*
Hyperaldosteronism *Aldosterone stimulates acid excretion in the distal renal tubule, causing an increased bicarbonate level and a decreased AG.*

Related Tests

- Electrolytes (sodium [p. 396], potassium [p. 342], chloride [p. 141], bicarbonate [p. 133]): Measurement of these electrolytes is necessary to calculate the AG.
- Arterial blood gases (ABG) (p. 97): This is the method by which acid-base balance is identified and evaluated.

Anticardiolipin Antibody (ACA, aCL Antibodies)

Normal Findings

<23 g/L for IgG anticardiolipin antibodies
<11 mg/L for IgM anticardiolipin antibodies

Indications

This test is positive in some patients with systemic lupus erythematosus (SLE). The presence of this antibody places the patient at higher risk for "antiphospholipid syndrome" (i.e., venous or arterial thrombosis, thrombocytopenia, recurrent spontaneous abortions). This test is performed on patients with SLE to determine if the patient is at risk for developing the above-noted complications.

Test Explanation

Antiphospholipid antibodies include anticardiolipin antibodies and the "lupus anticoagulant." The lupus anticoagulant derived its name from its association with SLE and can act as an anticoagulant to prolong the phospholipid-dependent coagulation test (such as partial thromboplastin time). It is present in half of the patients with SLE. Despite its name, it is not associated with bleeding tendencies. Anticardiolipin antibodies (IgG, IgM) are found in approximately 40% of patients with SLE. SLE patients who are positive for anticardiolipin antibodies and the lupus anticoagulant are at higher risk for antiphospholipid antibody syndrome. The clinical features include venous and arterial thrombosis, neuropsychiatric disorders, recurrent spontaneous abortion, and thrombocytopenia. Strokes in young adults have been associated with elevated levels of these antibodies. Both antibodies may be found in patients with drug-induced lupus and nonautoimmune diseases (e.g., syphilis, acute infection) and in the normal elderly person.

Interfering Factors

- Patients who have or had syphilis infections can have a cross reaction to the radiolabeled antibody used for radioimmune assay or the antibody used for enzyme-linked immunosorbent assay. These patients therefore will have a false-positive result.
- The transient presence of these antibodies can occur in patients with infections, AIDS, inflammation, autoimmune diseases, or cancer.
- False-positive results have been seen in patients who take medications such as chlorpromazine, procainamide, phenytoin (Dilantin), penicillin, hydralazine, and quinidine.

Procedure and Patient Care

Before

- Explain the procedure to the patient.
- Tell the patient that no fasting is required.

During

- Collect a venous blood sample according to the laboratory protocol.

After

- Apply pressure or a pressure dressing to the venipuncture site.
- Assess the venipuncture site for bleeding.

Test Results and Clinical Significance

Increased levels

SLE lupus

A patient is considered positive and therefore at risk for the antiphospholipid syndrome if either anticardiolipin antibodies or the lupus anticoagulant is present.

Antiphospholipid syndrome

Related Tests

- Anti-DNA antibody (p. 68): This test is used to diagnose SLE.
- Antinuclear antibody (p. 76): This test is used to diagnose SLE.

Anticentromere Antibody
(Centromere Antibody)

Normal Findings

Negative (If positive, serum will be titrated.)
Weak positive: positive screening titer (1:40 for HEp-2 cells, 1:20 for kidney cells)
Moderately positive: one dilution above screening titer
Strong positive: two dilutions above screening titer

Indications

This test is used to support the diagnosis of CREST syndrome.

Test Explanation

A centromere is the region of the chromosome referred to as the primary constriction that divides the chromosome into arms. During cell division the centromere exists in the pole of the mitotic spindle.

Anticentromere antibodies are a form of antinuclear antibodies. They are found in a very high percentage of patients with CREST syndrome, a variant of scleroderma. CREST is characterized by calcinosis, Raynaud's phenomenon, esophageal dysfunction, sclerodactyly, and telangiectasia. Anticentromere antibodies, on the contrary, are present in only a small minority of patients with scleroderma, a disease that is difficult to differentiate from CREST. No correlation exists between antibody titer and severity of CREST disease.

Procedure and Patient Care

Before

- Explain the procedure to the patient.
- Tell the patient that no fasting is usually required.

During

- Collect one red-top tube of venous blood.

After

- Apply pressure or a pressure dressing to the venipuncture site.
- Assess the venipuncture site for bleeding.

Test Results and Clinical Significance

Positive

CREST syndrome

Related Tests

- Antinuclear antibody (p. 76): This test is used to diagnose autoimmune-related diseases.

Antideoxyribonuclease-B Titer

(Anti DNase-B [ADB], ADNase-B)

Normal Findings

Adult: 85 U
Child:
Preschool: 60 U
School age: 170 U

Indications

This test is performed to indicate previous infection of group A beta-hemolytic *Streptococcus*. This is important in patients suspected of having acute rheumatic fever (ARF) or acute glomerulonephritis.

Test Explanation

Like the antistreptolysin O titer (ASO) test, this immunologic test also detects antigens produced by group A streptococci and is elevated in most patients with ARF or post-streptococcal glomerulonephritis. This test is often run concurrently with the ASO; subsequent testing is usually performed to detect differences in the acute and convalescent blood samples. A rise in the titer of two or more dilution increments between acute and convalescent sera is significant and indicates that a streptococcal infection has occurred. The American Heart Association does not recommend performing only this test in the evaluation of patients with ARF. It may be more sensitive than ASO, but its results are too variable. ASO is the recommended test, but when done together, the combination testing kit (Streptozyme) is better than either the ASO or ADB alone.

Interfering Factors

- Drugs that may *decrease* test results include some antibiotics.

Procedure and Patient Care

Before

- Explain the procedure to the patient.
- Inform the patient that no fasting is required.

During

- Collect one red-top tube of venous blood.

After

- Apply pressure to the venipuncture site after the blood is drawn.
- Assess the site for bleeding.

Test Results and Clinical Significance

Increased levels

Acute rheumatic fever
Poststreptococcal glomerulonephritis

Related Tests

- Antistreptolysin O titer (ASO) (p. 85): This is another, yet less variable, test to detect previous streptococcal infection.

Antidiuretic Hormone
(ADH, Vasopressin, Arginine Vasopressin [AVP])

Normal Findings

1-5 pg/ml or 1.5 ng/L (SI units)

Indications

ADH levels are tested in patients suspected of having diabetes insipidus or the syndrome of inappropriate ADH (SIADH). It is often performed in patients who complain of polyuria or polydipsia and are found to have marked variations in blood and urine osmolarity or sodium levels.

Test Explanation

ADH, also known as vasopressin, is formed by the hypothalamus and stored in the posterior pituitary gland. It controls the amount of water reabsorbed by the kidney. ADH release is stimulated by an increase in serum osmolality or a decrease in intravascular blood volume. Physical stress, surgery, and even high levels of anxiety may also stimulate ADH release. On release of ADH more water is reabsorbed from the glomerular filtrate at the level of the distal convoluted renal tubule and collecting ducts. This increases the amount of free water within the bloodstream and causes highly concentrated urine.

With low ADH levels, water is excreted, thereby producing hemoconcentration and a more dilute urine. Diabetes insipidus (DI) occurs when ADH secretion is inadequate or when the kidney is unresponsive to ADH stimulation. Inadequate ADH secretion is usually associated with central neurologic abnormalities (neurogenic DI), such as trauma, tumor, or inflammation of the brain (hypothalamus). Surgical ablation of the pituitary gland will also result in the neurogenic form of DI; such patients excrete large volumes of free water in the dilute urine. Their blood is hemoconcentrated, producing a strong thirst.

Primary renal diseases may make the renal collecting system less sensitive to ADH stimulation (nephrogenic DI). Again, in this instance, dilute urine may be produced by excretion of high volumes of free water. To differentiate ADH deficiency (neurogenic DI) from renal resistance to ADH (nephrogenic DI), a water deprivation ADH stimulation (p. 453) test is performed. Water intake is restricted during this test. Urine osmolality is measured. Vasopressin is administered. In neurogenic DI there is no rise in urine osmolality after water restriction, but there is a rise after vasopressin is given. In nephrogenic DI there is no rise in urine osmolality after water deprivation or vasopressin administration. The diagnosis indicated by this test can be corroborated by a serum ADH level. ADH levels are low in neurogenic DI. ADH levels are high in nephrogenic DI.

High serum ADH levels are also associated with SIADH. In response to this inappropriately high level of ADH secretion, water is reabsorbed by the kidneys greatly in excess of normal amounts. Thus the patient becomes very hemodiluted and the urine concentrated. Blood levels of important serum ions diminish, causing severe neurologic, cardiac, and metabolic alterations. The most frequent cause of SIADH is the paraneoplastic syndrome of ectopic ADH production. The most common tumors associated with SIADH include carcinoma of the lung and thymus, lymphomas, leukemia, and carcinomas of the pancreas, urologic tract, and intestine. SIADH is also associated with pulmonary diseases (e.g., tuberculosis, bacterial pneumonia), severe stress (e.g., surgery, trauma), CNS tumor, infection, or trauma. Patients with myxedema or Addison's disease also can experience SIADH.

Interfering Factors

- Patients with dehydration, hypovolemia, or stress may have increased ADH levels.
- Patients with overhydration, decreased serum osmolality, and hypervolemia may have decreased ADH levels.
- Use of a glass syringe or collection tube causes degradation of ADH.
- Drugs that *increase* ADH levels include acetaminophen, barbiturates, cholinergic agents, estrogen, nicotine, oral hypoglycemic agents, some diuretics (e.g., thiazides), cyclophosphamide, narcotics, and tricyclic antidepressants.
- Drugs that *decrease* ADH levels include alcohol, beta-adrenergic agents, morphine antagonists, and phenytoin (Dilantin).

Procedure and Patient Care

Before

- Explain the procedure to the patient.
- Ensure that the patient is adequately hydrated. Tell the patient to fast for 12 hours.
- Evaluate the patient for high levels of physical or emotional stress.

During

- Collect approximately 7 ml of venous blood in a prechilled plastic anticoagulant tube while the patient is in the sitting or recumbent position.
- Record on the laboratory slip any drugs that may alter test results.

After

- Apply pressure or a pressure dressing to the venipuncture site.
- Assess the venipuncture site for bleeding.
- The specimen is centrifuged at low temperatures in the laboratory. The serum is frozen and sent to a reference laboratory on dry ice for testing.

Test Results and Clinical Significance

Increased levels

SIADH
CNS tumors or infection
Pneumonia or pulmonary tuberculosis
Ectopic ADH secretion (usually from lung cancer)
Endocrinopathies, such as myxedema or Addison's disease
The above-noted diseases have been implicated to be associated with inappropriate high levels of ADH. Patients experience dilutional hyponatremia, hypo-osmolality, and concentrated urine.

Nephrogenic DI caused by primary renal diseases *Because of primary renal disease, the kidneys cannot respond to ADH. The patient becomes hemoconcentrated and hyperosmolar. As a result, ADH is maximally stimulated, yet the kidneys cannot respond.*

Postoperative days 1 to 3
Severe physical stress (e.g., trauma, pain, prolonged mechanical ventilation)
Stress in a potent stimulator (through the autonomic nervous system) of ADH.

Hypovolemia
Dehydration
Decreased blood volume is a potent direct stimulator of ADH.

Acute porphyria

Decreased levels

Neurogenic (or central) DI caused by CNS trauma, tumor, or infection
Surgical ablation of pituitary gland
The hypothalamus or pituitary ADH–secreting cells are destroyed by the above-noted disease processes.

Hypervolemia *Increased blood volume is an inhibitor of ADH secretion.*
Decreased serum osmolality caused by overhydration nephrotic syndrome, psychogenic polydipsia, IV overinfusion of non-salt-containing fluid *Decreased serum osmolality is an inhibitor of ADH secretion.*

Related Tests

- Water deprivation (p. 453): This test is helpful in differentiation of the causes of polyuria (neurogenic DI, nephrogenic DI, psychogenic polydipsia).
- Serum osmolality (p. 313): This test is a measurement of solute load in the serum.
- Urine osmolality (p. 842): This test is a measurement of solute load in the urine.
- Serum sodium (p. 396): This is a direct measurement of sodium level in the blood.
- Urine sodium (p. 851): This is a direct measurement of sodium level in the urine.
- Antidiuretic hormone suppression (p. 65): This test is used to differentiate SIADH from other causes of hyponatremia or edematous states.

Antidiuretic Hormone Suppression
(ADH Suppression, Water Load)

Normal Findings

65% of water load excreted in 4 hours
80% of water load excreted in 5 hours
Urine osmolality (in second hour): ≤100 mmol/kg
Urine to serum (U/S) osmolality ratio: >100
Urine specific gravity: <1.003

Indications

This test is used to differentiate the syndrome of inappropriate ADH (SIADH) from other causes of hyponatremia or edematous states listed in Box 2-2.

Test Explanation

This test is used to evaluate the possibility of SIADH in patients with electrolyte abnormalities (such as hyponatremia) or edematous states. Usually this test is performed concomitantly with measurements of urine and serum osmolality. Patients with SIADH will excrete none or very little of the water load. Furthermore, their urine osmolality will never be less than 100, and the U/S ratio is greater than 100. Patients with hyponatremia, other edematous states, or chronic renal diseases will excrete up to 80% of the water load and will develop midrange osmolality results.

Box 2-2 Causes of hyponatremia or edema

HYPONATREMIA
SIADH
Primary (or psychogenic) polydipsia
Adrenal insufficiency
Excessive sodium loss (vomiting, diarrhea, diuretics, excessive sweating)
Pseudohyponatremia associated with excessive nonionic solute load (e.g., hyperglycemia, hyperlipidemia, hyperproteinemia)
Sick cell syndrome associated with chronic debilitating diseases

EDEMATOUS STATES
Congestive heart failure
Cirrhosis
Nephrosis
Myxedema

Contraindications

- Patients with severe pain, nausea, stress, hypovolemia, or hypotension, because ADH is already near maximally stimulated

Potential Complications

- Water intoxication in patients with SIADH, because they are not able to excrete the water load. Symptoms would include anorexia, nausea, vomiting, abdominal cramps, confusion, irritability, convulsions, and coma.

Interfering Factors

- Patients with dehydration, hypovolemia, hypotension, or stress may have increased ADH levels.
- Drugs that *increase* ADH levels include acetaminophen, barbiturates, cholinergic agents, estrogen, nicotine, oral hypoglycemic agents, some diuretics (e.g., thiazides), cyclophosphamide, narcotics, and tricyclic antidepressants.

Procedure and Patient Care

Before

- Explain the procedure to the patient.
- Ask the patient to fast after midnight prior to the test.
- The test is begun early in the morning.
- Inform the patient of the early signs of water intoxication and instruct the patient to inform you if any occur.

- Place the patient in the recumbent position. The response to water loading in the upright position is reduced since this position is associated with increased ADH.
- One hour before the test administer 300 ml of water to replace fluids lost overnight. This is not part of the water load.
- Obtain a baseline serum sodium or a serum sodium level 24 hours before the test. If the sodium concentration is above a safe level (125 mmol/L), the test can proceed. If not, the test should be canceled until the sodium is brought to a safe level by water restriction or saline infusion. This precaution will minimize the risk of water intoxication.

During

- Administer water (20 ml/kg body weight up to 1500 ml) in 10 to 20 minutes.
- Collect urine every hour for 6 hours and send it for specific gravity and osmolality measurements. (Discard the first morning specimen.)
- Obtain blood for osmolality hourly or at specified times in serum (red top) or heparinized (green top) tube.

After

- Observe for signs of water intoxication.
- If water load clearance does not occur, be sure to instruct the patient to restrict water ingestion. Some patients must be admitted for observation.

Test Results and Clinical Significance

SIADH

Water excretion: none or very little of the water load
Urine osmolality: >100
Urine specific gravity: >1.020
U/S ratio: >90

Other hyponatremic or edematous states (see Box 2-2)

Water excretion: up to 80% of water load
Urine osmolality: <300
Urine specific gravity: >1.020
U/S ratio: 90

Related Tests

- Antidiuretic hormone (p. 62): This is a serum assay for direct measurement of ADH. This test is used in the differential diagnosis of neurogenic diabetes insipidus, nephrogenic diabetes insipidus, or psychogenic polydipsia.
- Serum osmolality (p. 313): This test is a measurement of solute load in the serum.
- Urine osmolality (p. 842): This test is a measurement of solute load in the urine.
- Serum sodium (p. 396): This is a direct measurement of sodium level in the blood.
- Urine sodium (p. 851): This is a direct measurement of sodium level in the urine.
- ADH stimulation (water deprivation) (p. 65): This is a test to assist in the differential diagnosis of diabetes insipidus.

Anti-DNA Antibody (Antideoxyribonucleic Acid Antibodies, Antibody to Double-Stranded DNA, Anti-Double-Stranded DNA [Anti-ds-DNA], DNA Antibody, Native Double-Stranded DNA)

Normal Findings

Negative: <70 U
Borderline: 70-200 U
Positive: >200 U

Indications

The anti-DNA antibody test is useful for the diagnosis and follow-up of systemic lupus erythematosus (SLE).

Test Explanation

This antibody is found in approximately 65% to 80% of patients with active SLE and rarely in patients with other diseases. High titers are characteristic of SLE. Low to intermediate levels of this antibody may be found in patients with other rheumatic diseases and in those with chronic hepatitis, infectious mononucleosis, and biliary cirrhosis. The anti-DNA titer decreases with successful therapy and increases with exacerbation of SLE and especially with the onset of lupus glomerulonephritis. Near-negative values are seen in patients with dormant SLE.

The anti-DNA antibody is a subtype of the *antinuclear antibodies* (ANA) (p. 76). There are two types of anti-DNA antibodies. The first and most popular is the antibody against double-stranded DNA (anti-ds-DNA). The second type is the antibody against single-stranded DNA (anti-ss-DNA). This is less sensitive and specific for SLE but is positive in other autoimmune diseases. These antibody-antigen complexes that occur with autoimmune disease are not only diagnostic but are major contributors to the disease process. These complexes induce the complement system, which then may cause local or systemic tissue injury.

There are currently several radioimmunoassay methods for measuring anti-DNA antibodies. The Farr method is the oldest and is more sensitive than the lupus erythematosus prep. It detects anti-ds-DNA and anti-ss-DNA antibodies. As a result, its specificity is not great.

Interfering Factors

- A radioactive scan performed within 1 week before the test may alter the test results.
- Drugs that may cause *increased* levels include hydralazine and procainamide.

Procedure and Patient Care

Before

- Explain the procedure to the patient.
- Tell the patient that no fasting is required.

During

- Collect one red-top tube of venous blood.

After

- Apply pressure or a pressure dressing to the venipuncture site.
- Assess the venipuncture site for bleeding.

Test Results and Clinical Significance

Increased levels

SLE
Other autoimmune diseases, such as rheumatic fever
Chronic hepatitis
Infectious mononucleosis
Biliary cirrhosis

Related Tests

- Antinuclear antibody (p. 76): This is another antibody associated with SLE.

Antiextractable Nuclear Antigen

(Anti-ENA, Antibodies to Extractable Nuclear Antigens, Antiribonucleoprotein [Anti-RNP], Anti-Smith [Anti-SM])

Normal Findings

Negative

Indications

The anti-ENAs are used to assist in the diagnosis of systemic lupus erythematosus (SLE) and mixed connective tissue disease (MCTD) and to eliminate other rheumatoid diseases.

Test Explanation

Anti-ENAs are a type of antinuclear antibodies to certain nuclear antigens that consist of RNA and protein. The antigen is extracted from the thymus using phosphate-buffered saline solutions and therefore is sometimes referred to as saline-extracted antigen. The most common ENAs are Smith (SM) and ribonucleoprotein (RNP) types.

The anti-SM antibody is present in about 30% of patients with SLE and in about 8% of patients with MCTD diseases. However, it is not present in patients with most other rheumatoid-collagen diseases.

The anti-RNP antibody is reported in nearly 100% of patients with MCTD disease and in about 25% of patients with SLE, discoid lupus, and progressive systemic sclerosis (scleroderma). In high titers, anti-RNP is suggestive of MCTD.

Two other antibodies to ENAs are anti-SS-A and anti-SS-B (see p. 84) and are used mainly in the diagnostic evaluation of Sjögren's syndrome.

Procedure and Patient Care

Before

- Explain the procedure to the patient.
- Tell the patient that no fasting is required.

During

- Collect a venous blood sample in a red-top tube.

After

- Apply pressure or a pressure dressing to the venipuncture site.
- Assess the venipuncture site for bleeding.
- Check the venipuncture site for infection. Patients with autoimmune disease are immunocompromised.

Test Results and Clinical Significance

Increased anti-SM antibodies

SLE

Increased anti-RNP antibodies

MCTD
SLE
Discoid lupus scleroderma
The absence of anti-SM antibodies and the presence of anti-RNP antibodies help to delineate mixed connective tissue disease serologically from SLE and other autoimmune diseases.

Related Tests

- Antinuclear antibody (p. 76): This is another antibody associated with SLE.
- Anti-DNA antibody (p. 68): This is another test used to diagnose SLE.

Antiglomerular Basement Membrane Antibody (Anti-GBM Antibody, AGBM, Glomerular Basement Antibody, Goodpasture's Antibody)

Normal Findings

Tissue

Negative: No immunofluorescence is noted on the renal or lung tissue basement membrane.

Blood

Negative: <20 U
Borderline: 20-100 U
Positive: >100 U

Indications

This test is used to detect the presence of circulating glomerular basement membrane antibodies commonly present in autoimmune-induced nephritis (Goodpasture's syndrome).

Test Explanation

Goodpasture's syndrome is an autoimmune disease characterized by the presence of circulating antibodies against an antigen in the renal glomerular basement membrane and the pulmonary alveolar basement membrane. These immune complexes activate the complement system and thereby cause tissue injury. Patients with this problem usually display a triad of glomerulonephritis (hematuria), pulmonary hemorrhage (hemoptysis), and antibodies to basement membrane antigens. This is a rare form of glomerular nephritis. About 60% to 75% of patients with immune-induced glomerular nephritis have pulmonary complications.

With the use of immunohistochemistry and now with radioimmunoassay, antibodies also can be demonstrated in the glomeruli, renal tubular basement membrane, and the pulmonary capillary basement membranes. Lung or renal biopsies are required to demonstrate these antibodies in tissue. Serum assays are a faster and more reliable method for diagnosing Goodpasture's syndrome, especially in patients in whom renal or lung biopsy may be difficult or contraindicated. Furthermore, serum levels can be used in monitoring response to therapy (plasmapheresis or immunosuppression).

Procedure and Patient Care

Before

- Explain the procedure to the patient.
- Tell the patient to fast for 8 hours before the test. Water is permitted.
- If a lung biopsy or kidney biopsy will be used to collect the specimen, explain these procedures to the patient.

During

- Collect one red-top tube of venous blood.

After

- Apply pressure or a pressure dressing to the venipuncture site.
- Assess the venipuncture site for bleeding.

Test Results and Clinical Significance

Positive

Goodpasture's syndrome
Autoimmune glomerulonephritis
Lupus nephritis

Related Tests

- Lung biopsy (p. 662): This is a test in which lung tissue is obtained for microscopic evaluation.
- Kidney biopsy (p. 674): This is a test in which renal tissue is obtained for microscopic evaluation.

Antimitochondrial Antibody (AMA)

Normal Findings
No AMAs at titers >1:5

Indications

The AMA test is used primarily to aid in the diagnosis of primary biliary cirrhosis.

Test Explanation

AMA is an anticytoplasmic antibody directed against a lipoprotein in the mitochrondrial membrane. Normally the serum does not contain AMA at a titer greater than 1:5. AMAs are found in 94% of patients with primary biliary cirrhosis. This disease may be an autoimmune disease that occurs predominantly in young or middle-aged women. It has a slow progressive course marked by elevated liver enzymes, especially alkaline phosphatase and gamma-glutamyl transpeptidase, and a positive AMA test. Liver biopsy (see p. 662) is usually required to confirm the diagnosis because the AMA test can be positive in patients with chronic active hepatitis, drug-induced cholestasis, autoimmune hepatitis (e.g., scleroderma, systemic lupus erythematosus), extrahepatic obstruction, or acute infectious hepatitis. There are subgroups of AMA. The M-2 subgroup is suspected to be highly specific for primary biliary cirrhosis. For the AMA test, immunofluorescent assay or enzyme-linked immunosorbent assay techniques are used.

Procedure and Patient Care

Before

- Explain the procedure to the patient.
- Tell the patient that no fasting or special preparation is required.

During

- Collect 7 to 10 ml of venous blood in a red-top tube.

After

- Apply pressure or a pressure dressing to the venipuncture site.
- Check the venipuncture site for bleeding. Patients with jaundice often have bleeding disorders associated with vitamin K deficiency.

Test Results and Clinical Significance

Increased levels

Primary biliary cirrhosis *AMA test is positive in 90% to 100% of patients.*
Chronic active hepatitis *AMA test is positive in 30% of patients.*

Systemic lupus erythematosus
Syphilis
Drug-induced cholestasis
Autoimmune hepatitis (e.g., scleroderma, systemic lupus erythematosus)
Extrahepatic obstruction
Acute infectious hepatitis
AMA test is positive in 2% to 5% of patients.

Related Tests

- Anti-smooth muscle antibody (p. 81): This is another anticytoplasmic antibody that usually is present in patients with chronic active hepatitis and in 30% of patients with primary biliary cirrhosis.
- Alkaline phosphatase (p. 42): Although alkaline phosphatase (ALP) is found in many tissues, the highest concentrations are found in the liver, biliary tract epithelium, and bone.
- Gamma-glutamyl transpeptidase (p. 219): This enzyme is found in the liver and is used to detect liver cell dysfunction and cholestasis.

Antimyocardial Antibody (AMA)

Normal Findings Negative (If positive, serum will be titrated.)

Indications

This test is used to detect an autoimmune source of myocardial injury and disease. AMAs may be detected in rheumatic heart disease, cardiomyopathy, postthoracotomy syndrome, and after myocardial infarction. This test is not only used in the detection of an autoimmune cause for these conditions but also for monitoring response to treatment.

Test Explanation

A positive AMA test is associated with several forms of heart disease. AMAs may be detected prior to the development of clinical symptoms of heart disease. An immunologic basis has been suspected in rheumatic heart disease for a long time. Research has now documented the presence of serum antibodies against myocardial components and deposition of immunoglobulin and complement in lesional areas. Antibodies against heart muscle are also found in 20% to 40% of patients after cardiac surgery and in a smaller number of patients after myocardial infarction. These antibodies are usually associated with pericarditis that follows the myocardial injury associated with cardiac surgery or myocardial infarction (Dressler's syndrome). AMAs have also been detected in patients with cardiomyopathy. Their role in this latter disease is unknown.

This test is performed by indirect immunofluorescent technique. The patient's serum is added to a rat heart muscle extract. Antigen-antibody immune complexes are identified by immunofluorescent antihuman antibodies. Positive results (increased immunofluorescence) are reported in titers.

Procedure and Patient Care

Before

- Explain the procedure to the patient.
- Tell the patient that no fasting or special preparation is necessary.

During

- Collect a venous blood sample in a red-top tube of blood.

After

- Apply pressure or a pressure dressing to the venipuncture site.
- Check the venipuncture site for bleeding.

Test Results and Clinical Significance

Increased levels

Rheumatic heart disease

Streptococcal infection *The myocardial antigen may be associated with* Streptococcus *because the antibody may occur in patients with other streptococcal diseases.*

Postthoracotomy (cardiac surgery) syndrome

After myocardial infarction (Dressler's syndrome) *Myocardial injury occurs and the antibody develops. The antibody-antigen complex may incite the pericarditis that follows the myocardial injury.*

Cardiomyopathy *The association of cardiomyopathy and AMA is unknown. Whether the antibodies cause or contribute to the development of cardiomyopathy is being studied.*

Antineutrophil Cytoplasmic Antibody
(ANCA)

Normal Findings
Negative

Indications

This blood test is used to assist in the diagnosis of Wegener's granulomatosis (WG). It also is used to follow the course of the disease, to monitor the response to therapy, and to provide early detection of relapse.

Test Explanation

WG is a regional systemic vasculitis in which the small arteries of the kidneys, lungs, and upper respiratory tract (nasopharynx) are damaged by a granulomatous inflammation. Diagnosis can be made by biopsy of clinically affected tissue. Serologic testing has begun to play a key role in the diagnosis of WG and other systemic vasculitis syndromes. Most patients with WG have circulating autoantibodies against neutrophil cytoplasm, which are useful in the diagnosis.

ANCAs are antibodies directed against cytoplasmic components of neutrophils. They are detected by the fluorescent antibody method. There are two types of antineutrophil cytoplasmic antibodies. The C-ANCA pattern is highly specific (95% to 99%) for WG and is seen as diffuse granular staining of the cytoplasm. When the disease is limited to the respiratory tract, the C-ANCA is positive in only about 65% of patients. Nearly all patients with WG limited to the kidney do not have a positive C-ANCA result. When WG is inactive, the percentage of positive tests drops to about 30%.

The second type of ANCA is P-ANCA, which produces a perinuclear pattern of staining in the neutrophil cytoplasm. The P-ANCA pattern is found in 50% of patients with WG localized in the kidney. It also occurs in patients with non-WG glomerulonephritis. As many as 75% of patients with ulcerative colitis or sclerosing cholangitis will have a positive P-ANCA test. In 50% of patients with autoimmune hepatitis or Churg-Strauss vasculitis, the P-ANCA test will be positive.

Procedure and Patient Care

Before

- Explain the procedure to the patient.
- Tell the patient that no fasting is required.

During

- Collect venous blood in the tube specified by the laboratory performing the test.

After

- Apply pressure or a pressure dressing to the venipuncture site.
- Observe the venipuncture site for bleeding.

Test Results and Clinical Significance

Increased levels

WG
Microscopic polyarteritis
Idiopathic crescentic glomerulonephritis
Ulcerative colitis
Primary sclerosing cholangitis
Autoimmune hepatitis
Churg-Strauss vasculitis
Active viral hepatitis
Crohn's disease
The mechanism by which these antibodies are associated with these diseases is unknown.

Antinuclear Antibody (ANA)

Normal Findings Negative (titer <1:20)

Indications

ANAs are used to diagnose systemic lupus erythematosus (SLE) and other autoimmune diseases. These antibodies are primarily used to screen for SLE. Because almost all patients with SLE develop autoantibodies, a negative ANA test excludes the diagnosis. If the ANA test is positive, other antibody studies must be done to corroborate the diagnosis.

Test Explanation

Autoantibodies are directed to nuclear material (ANAs) or to cytoplasm material (anticytoplasmic antibodies) (Tables 2-3 and 2-4). Many abnormal antibodies are present in patients with autoimmune (rheumatic) diseases. ANA is a group of protein antibodies that react against cellular nuclear material. ANA is quite sensitive for detecting SLE. Positive results occur in approximately 95% of patients with this disease; however, many other rheumatic diseases are also associated with ANA (Table 2-5). ANA, therefore, is not a specific test for SLE (Table 2-6).

Several different patterns of fluorescence are seen under the ultraviolet microscope. When combined with the specific subtype of ANA, the pattern can increase specificity of the ANA subtypes for the various autoimmune diseases (Figure 2-5). In general, the higher the titer of a certain ANA antibody known to be associated with a certain autoimmune disease, the more likely that disease exists and the more active the disease is. As the diseases becomes less active after therapy, the ANA titers can be expected to fall. As one can see from Table 2-5,

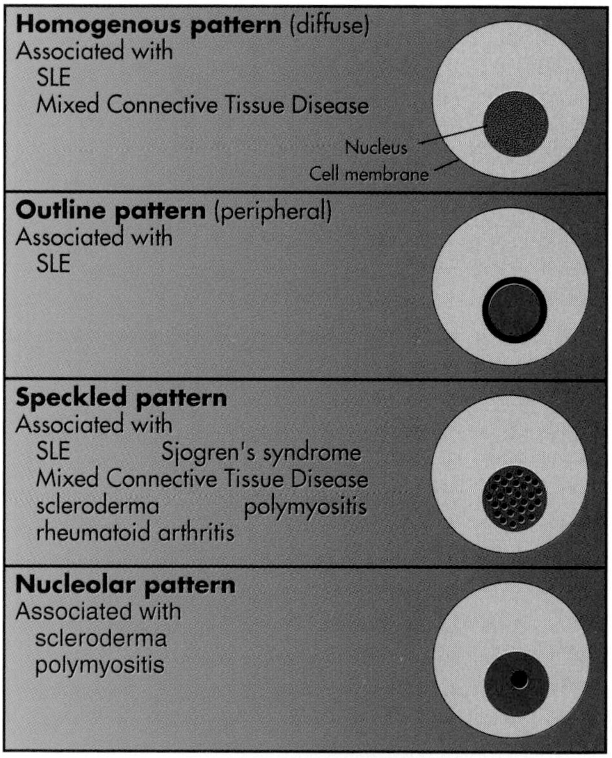

Figure 2-5 Patterns of immunofluorescent staining for antinuclear antibodies (ANAs).

Table 2-3 Common antinuclear antibodies and diseases they cause

Common antinuclear antibodies	Disease
Anti-sNP	SLE
Anti-ENA	SLE, MCTD
Anti-Smith	SLE
Anti-RNP	MCTD, SLE, PSS
Antinucleolar	PSS, SLE
Anticentromere	CREST syndrome
Anti-ss-A (Ro) and Anti-ss-B (La)	Sjögren's syndrome, SLE
Rheumatoid arthritis precipitin	RA, Sjögren's syndrome
Anti-scleroderma-70	PSS
Anti-Jo-1	Polymyositis, dermatomyositis

SLE = systemic lupus erythematosus; MCTD = mixed connective tissue disease; PSS = progressive systemic sclerosis (scleroderma); CREST = calcinosis, Raynaud's, esophageal dysfunction, sclerodactyly, telangiectasia; RA = rheumatoid arthritis.

Table 2-4 Common anticytoplasmic antibodies and diseases they cause

Common Anticytoplasmic Antibody	Disease
Antimitochrondial	Primary biliary cirrhosis
Antineutrophil cytoplasmic	Wegener's granulomatosis
Antimicrosomal	Chronic active hepatitis
Antiribosomal	SLE

Table 2-5 Autoimmune disease and positive antibodies

Autoimmune disease	Positive antibodies
SLE	ANA, SLE prep, dsDNA, ssDNA, anti-DNP, SS-A
Drug Induced SLE	ANA
Sjögren's syndrome	RF, ANA, SS-A, SS-B
Scleroderma	ANA, Scl-70, RNA, dsDNA
Raynaud's disease	ACA, Scl-70
Mixed connective tissue disease	ANA, RNP, RF, ssDNA
Rheumatoid arthritis	RF, ANA, RANA, RAP
Primary biliary cirrhosis	AMA
Thyroiditis	Antimicrosomal, antithyroglobulin
Chronic active hepatitis	ASMA

Table 2-6 Disease and percent of patients with ANAs

Disease	ANA positive (%)
SLE	95
Progressive systemic sclerosis (scleroderma)	70
Rheumatoid arthritis	30
Sjögren's syndrome	60
Dermatomyositis	30
Polyarteritis	10

none of the ANA subtypes are exclusive for any one autoimmune disease.

Often the ANA test is used to screen patients with suspected SLE. If the ANA test is negative, the patient probably does not have SLE. If positive, other corroborative serologic tests are performed (Table 2-5). About 5% of patients with SLE have a negative ANA test.

ANA is a gamma globulin and usually belongs to more than one class of immunoglobulins. The test can be performed by fluorescent testing, enzyme-linked immunosorbent assay, and enzyme immunoassay. Usually the patient's serum is combined with nuclear material derived from an animal liver or other such tissue. For fluorescent testing, fluorescein-labeled antihuman serum is mixed with the patient's serum and the animal nuclear material. If positive, the radiolabeled antihuman antibody should attach to the patient's ANA. This fluorescein will then be seen under the ultraviolet microscope. The pattern is noted. The patient's serum is serially diluted, and the ANA test is carried out with each dilution. The most dilute serum in which ANA is detected is called the titer. The test is considered positive if ANA is found in a titer with a dilution of greater than 1:32.

Interfering Factors

- Drugs that may cause a *false-positive* ANA test include acetazolamide, aminosalicylic acid, chlorprothixene, chlorothiazides, griseofulvin, hydralazine, penicillin, phenylbutazone, phenytoin, procainamide, streptomycin, sulfonamides, and tetracyclines.
- Drugs that may cause a *false-negative* test include steroids.

Procedure and Patient Care

Before

- Explain the procedure to the patient.
- Tell the patient that no fasting or preparation is required.

During

- Collect 7 to 10 ml of venous blood in a red-top tube.
- Indicate on the laboratory slip any drugs that may affect the test results.

After

- Apply pressure or a pressure dressing to the venipuncture site.
- Assess the venipuncture site for bleeding.
- Because they are usually immunocompromised, instruct patients with an autoimmune disease to check for signs of infection at the venipuncture site. These patients often take steroids that further compromise their immune system.

Test Results and Clinical Significance

Increased levels

SLE *The signs and symptoms of this disease are vague and nonspecific. This disease is associated with a significant production of various autoimmune antibodies. Any organ in the patient's body can be the target of these autoantibodies. The immune complexes incite the complement system and thereby create tissue damage.*

Rheumatoid arthritis *The autoimmune response is targeted to the synovial tissues.*
Periarteritis (polyarteritis) nodosa *The autoimmune response is targeted to the small vessels of various organs.*
Dermatomyositis
Polymyositis *The autoimmune response is targeted to the skeletal muscle.*
Scleroderma *The autoimmune response is targeted to the endothelium of blood vessels. Fibrosis occurs. This combined with deposit of collagen-related tissue creates the organ changes seen in the skin, GI tract, and other internal organs.*
Sjögren's syndrome *The autoimmune response is targeted to the exocrine glands (lacrimal and salivary).*
Raynaud's phenomenon *This phenomenon is characterized by episodic digital ischemia as manifested by blanching and then cyanosis of the fingers in cold temperatures followed by rubor on rewarming. It is associated with many autoimmune diseases. The term "Raynaud's disease" refers to this phenomenon without an associated autoimmune disease.*
Other immune diseases
Leukemia
Infectious mononucleosis
Myasthenia gravis
Cirrhosis
Chronic hepatitis

Related Tests

- Anticentromere antibody (p. 60): This test is used to diagnose CREST syndrome.
- Anti-DNA antibody (p. 68): This test is used to diagnose SLE.
- Antiextractable nuclear antigen (ENA) (p. 69): This test is used to diagnose SLE and mixed connective tissue disease.
- Antiscleroderma-70 (p. 79): This test is used to diagnose scleroderma.

Antiscleroderma Antibody
(Scl-70 Antibody, Scleroderma Antibody)

Normal Findings

Negative

Indications

This antibody is diagnostic for scleroderma (progressive systemic sclerosis [PSS]) and is present in 45% of patients with that disease.

Test Explanation

Scl-70 antibody is an antinuclear antibody. On the fluorescent antinuclear antibody test, using the ultraviolet microscope, the pattern created is specific for the Scl-70 antibody. The pattern is a speckled group of dots throughout the nucleus. The test can be performed by fluorescent testing, enzyme-linked immunosorbent assay, and enzyme immunoassay. Progressive serial dilutions are carried out.

PSS is a multisystem disorder characterized by inflammation with subsequent fibrosis of the small blood vessels in skin and visceral organs, including the heart, lungs, kidneys, and GI tract. A collagen-like substance is also deposited into the tissue of these organs. In general, the higher the titer of Scl-70 antibody, the more likely that PSS exists and the more active the disease is. As the disease becomes less active because of therapy, the Scl-70 antibody titers can be expected to fall.

The absence of this antibody does not exclude the diagnosis of scleroderma. The antibody is rather specific for PSS but is occasionally seen in other autoimmune diseases, such as systemic lupus erythematosus, mixed connective tissue disease (MCTD), Sjögren's syndrome, polymyositis, and rheumatoid arthritis.

Interfering Factors

- Drugs that may cause *increased* levels include aminosalicylic acid, isoniazid, methyldopa, penicillin, propylthiouracil, streptomycin, and tetracycline.

Procedure and Patient Care

Before

- Explain the procedure to the patient.
- Tell the patient that no fasting is required.

During

- Collect a venous sample of blood in a red-top tube.

After

- Apply pressure or a pressure dressing to the venipuncture site.
- Assess the venipuncture site for bleeding.

Test Results and Clinical Significance

Positive

Scleroderma (PSS)

CREST syndrome *CREST is a variant of scleroderma. In both of these diseases the autoimmune response is targeted to the endothelium of blood vessels. Fibrosis occurs. This, combined with deposit of collagen-related tissue, creates the organ changes seen in the skin, GI tract, and other internal organs.*

Related Tests

- Antinuclear antibody (p. 76): This group of antibodies is used to diagnose systemic lupus erythematosus and other autoimmune diseases such as PSS.

Anti-Smooth Muscle Antibody (ASMA)

Normal Findings

No ASMAs at titers >1:20

Indications

The ASMA is used primarily to aid in the diagnosis of autoimmune chronic active hepatitis (CAH), which has also been referred to as "lupoid" CAH.

Test Explanation

ASMA is an anticytoplasmic antibody directed against actin, a cytoskeletal protein. Normally the serum does not contain ASMA at a titer greater than 1:20. ASMA is the most commonly recognized autoantibody in the setting of CAH. It appears in 70% to 80% of patients with CAH. Patients with some types of CAH do not test positive for ASMA antibodies. This disease may be an autoimmune disease that occurs predominantly in adult women. The clinical presentation of CAH is similar to that of viral hepatitis. That clinical picture, along with serologic and pathologic criteria, must exist for over 6 months to be classified as CAH.

ASMA is not specific for CAH and can be positive in patients with viral infections, malignancy, multiple sclerosis, primary biliary cirrhosis, and *Mycoplasma* infections. Usually the titer of ASMA is low in these diseases. With CAH, the titer is usually higher than 1:160. The titers are not helpful in predicting prognosis, nor do they indicate response to therapy. For the ASMA test, immunofluorescent assay or enzyme-linked immunosorbent assay techniques are used.

Procedure and Patient Care

Before

- Explain the procedure to the patient.
- Tell the patient that no fasting or special preparation is required.

During

- Collect 7 to 10 ml of venous blood in a red-top tube.

After

- Apply pressure or a pressure dressing to the venipuncture site.
- Check the venipuncture site for bleeding. Patients with jaundice often have bleeding disorders associated with vitamin K deficiency.

Test Results and Clinical Significance

Increased levels

CAH

Mononucleosis hepatitis

ASMA is positive in 70% to 80% of patients.

Primary biliary cirrhosis
Viral hepatitis
Multiple sclerosis
Malignancy
Intrinsic asthma
ASMA is positive in about 30% of patients.

Related Tests

- Liver enzymes, such as alkaline phosphatase (ALT) (p. 42) and aspartate aminotransferase (AST) (p. 105): These enzymes exist within the hepatocytes and are elevated in patients with hepatitis.
- Antimitochrondrial antibody (p. 72): This is an antibody that is most frequently associated with primary biliary cirrhosis. Positive titers of AMA are found in 30% of the patients with CAH.

Antispermatozoal Antibody (Sperm Agglutination and Inhibition, Sperm Antibodies, Antisperm Antibodies, Infertility Screen)

Normal Findings

Negative

Indications

The antispermatozoal antibody test is an infertility screening test used to detect the presence of sperm antibodies. Antibodies directed toward sperm antigens can result in diminished fertility.

Test Explanation

This test is commonly used in the evaluation of an infertile couple. Antisperm antibodies may be found in the blood of men with blocked efferent ducts of the testes (a common cause of low sperm counts or poor sperm mobility) and in 30% to 70% of men who have had a vasectomy. Reabsorption of sperm from the blocked ducts results in the formation of autoantibodies to sperm as a result of sperm antigens interacting with the immune system. These antibodies can be agglutinins or cytotoxic. The IgA antisperm antibodies to the sperm tail are associated with poor motility and poor penetration of cervical mucus. IgG antisperm antibodies are associated with blockage of sperm-ovum fusion. High titers of IgG autoantibodies are often associated with postvasectomy degeneration of the testes, which explains why 50% of males remain infertile after successful repair of vasectomy.

In men, high serum titers of antispermatozoal antibody are considered strong evidence of infertility. Low titers are of unknown significance, because this is not an uncommon finding in normal fertile males. Serum antispermatozoal antibodies are found in nearly 20% of women. However, many of these women become pregnant. The significance of this antibody in women, therefore, is uncertain.

Antispermatozoal antibodies can also be detected in the sperm of infertile males and in the cervical mucus of infertile females. It is often necessary to identify these antibodies in the serum and other body fluids in the thorough evaluation of infertility.

Procedure and Patient Care

Before

- Explain the procedure to the patient.

For a sperm specimen:

- Inform the man that a semen specimen should be collected after avoiding ejaculation for at least 3 days.
- Give the male patient the proper container for the sperm collection.
- If the specimen is to be collected at home, be certain the patient is told that it must be taken to the laboratory for testing within 2 hours of collection.

During

- Collect a venous blood sample of approximately 7 to 10 ml from both the male and the female patient in red-top tubes.
- For a sperm specimen, collect the ejaculate in a plastic container.
- For a vaginal mucus specimen, collect 1 ml of cervical mucus and place it in a plastic vial.

After

- Apply pressure or a pressure dressing to the venipuncture sites.
- Check the venipuncture sites for bleeding.
- For a sperm, blood, or cervical specimen, the specimen is placed in a plastic vial, frozen, and sent to a reference laboratory on dry ice.
- Instruct the couple when and how to obtain the test results.

Test Results and Clinical Significance

Infertility *Antispermatozoal antibodies may be present in the male or the female and may inhibit the number or motility of sperm or the ability of the sperm to penetrate the ovum.*

Blocked efferent ducts in the testes *This is considered to be a common cause of male infertility. Reabsorption of sperm from the blocked ducts results in the formation of autoantibodies to sperm as a result of sperm antigens interacting with the immune system.*

Vasectomy *Reabsorption of sperm from the occluded vas deferens results in the formation of autoantibodies to sperm as a result of sperm antigens interacting with the immune system.*

Related Tests

- Sims-Huhner test (p. 602): This test consists of a postcoital examination of the cervical mucus to measure the ability of the sperm to penetrate the mucus and maintain motility. It is used in the diagnostic workup of infertility. This analysis is also helpful in documenting cases of suspected rape by testing the vaginal and cervical secretions for sperm.
- Luteinizing hormone assay and follicle-stimulating hormone (p. 296): These hormones are useful for determining the pituitary effect on gonadal function and spermatogenesis.
- Semen analysis (p. 599): This test is used to evaluate the quality of sperm. Semen analysis is used to evaluate an infertile couple and to document the adequacy of operative vasectomy.

Anti–SS-A (Ro), Anti–SS-B (La), and Anti–SS-C Antibody
(Anti-Ro, Anti-La, Sjögren's Antibodies)

Normal Findings
Negative

Indications

These three antinuclear antibodies are used to diagnose Sjögren's syndrome.

Test Explanation

Ro, La, and SS-C antibodies are a subtype of antinuclear antibodies (ANA) (see Table 2-3, p. 77) and react to nuclear antigens extracted from human B lymphocytes. Ro and La produce a speckled immunofluorescent pattern when seen under the ultraviolet microscope. They are strongly associated with Sjögren's syndrome. This disease is an immunologic abnormality characterized by progressive destruction of the lacrimal and salivary exocrine glands leading to mucosal and conjunctival dryness. This disease can occur by itself (primary) or in association with other autoimmune diseases, such as systemic lupus erythematosus (SLE), rheumatoid arthritis (RA), and scleroderma. In the latter case it is referred to as secondary Sjögren's syndrome.

Anti–SS-A antibodies may be found in approximately 60% to 70% of patients with primary Sjögren's syndrome. Anti–SS-B antibodies may be found in approximately 50% to 60% of patients with primary Sjögren's syndrome. When anti–SS-A and SS-B antibodies are positive, Sjögren's syndrome can be diagnosed accurately. These antibodies are more rarely found when secondary Sjögren's syndrome is associated with RA. In fact, SS-B is only found in primary Sjögren's syndrome. However, anti–SS-C is positive in about 75% of patients with RA or patients with secondary Sjögren's syndrome associated with RA. Yet anti–SS-A and anti–SS-B are almost never found in patients with Sjögren's syndrome associated with RA. Therefore these antibodies are also useful in differentiating primary from secondary Sjögren's syndrome.

SS-A can also be found in 25% of patients with SLE. This is particularly useful in "ANA-negative" patients with SLE, because these antibodies are present in the majority of such patients. Anti–SS-B is never found in patients with SLE. In general, the higher the titer of anti–SS antibodies, the more likely that Sjögren's syndrome exists and the more active the disease is. As Sjögren's syndrome becomes less active with therapy, the anti-SS antibodies titers can be expected to fall.

Procedure and Patient Care

Before

- Explain the procedure to the patient.
- Tell the patient that no fasting is required.

During

- Collect a venous blood sample in a red-top tube.

After

- Apply pressure or a pressure dressing to the venipuncture site.
- Assess the venipuncture site for bleeding.
- Check the venipuncture site for infection. Patients with autoimmune disease have a compromised immune system.

Test Results and Clinical Significance

Positive

Sjögren's syndrome *When high titers of anti–SS-A or anti–SS-B are present, Sjögren's syndrome can be diagnosed with confidence.*
RA *When high titers of anti–SS-C are present, RA with or without Sjögren's syndrome can be diagnosed with confidence.*
ANA-negative SLE *Anti–SS-A will be positive in most of these patients.*
Neonatal lupus *Anti–SS-A will be positive in 95% of these patients.*

Related Tests

- Antinuclear antibody (ANA) (p. 76): This test is used to diagnose SLE and other autoimmune diseases.
- Anticentromere antibody (p. 60): This test is used to diagnose CREST syndrome.
- Anti-DNA antibody (p. 68): This test is used to diagnose SLE.
- Antiextractable nuclear antigen (ENA) (p. 69): This test is used to diagnose SLE and mixed connective tissue disease.
- Antiscleroderma (p. 79): This test is used to diagnose scleroderma.

Antistreptolysin O Titer (ASO Titer)

Normal Findings

Adult/elderly: 160 Todd units/ml
Child
6 months to 2 years: 50 Todd units/ml
2-4 years: 160 Todd units/ml
5-12 years: 170-330 Todd units/ml
Newborn: similar to mother's value

Indications

This test is used primarily to determine whether a previous *Streptococcus* infection has caused a poststreptococcal disease, such as glomerulonephritis, rheumatic fever, bacterial endocarditis, and scarlet fever. Levels are highest in glomerulonephritis and rheumatic fever.

Test Explanation

The ASO titer is a serologic procedure demonstrating the reaction of the body to infection caused by group A beta-hemolytic streptococci. The *Streptococcus* organism produces an enzyme called streptolysin O, which has the ability to destroy (lyse) red blood corpuscles. Because streptolysin O is antigenic, the body reacts by producing ASO, a neutralizing antibody. ASO appears in the serum 1 week to 1 month after the onset of a streptococcal infection; a high titer is not specific for a certain type of poststreptococcal disease (i.e., rheumatic fever vs. glomerulonephritis) but merely indicates that a streptococcal infection is or has been present. When ASO elevation is seen in a patient with glomerulonephritis or endocarditis, one can safely assume that the disease was caused by streptococcal infection. ASO is of no value for diagnosing acute streptococcal infection. Cultures for streptococci are required for that. However, cultures are useless during the latent period of the poststreptococcal disease (about 2 to 3 weeks after initial infection). ASO is very helpful at this point. Serial ASO testing may be performed to detect the difference between the acute and convalescent blood sample. Serial rising titers of ASO over several weeks, followed by a slow fall in titers, is much more significant in the diagnosis of a previous streptococcal infection than is a single titer. The highest incidence of positive results is during the third week after the onset of acute symptoms of the streptococcal disease. By 6 months, only about 30% of patients have abnormal titers.

Another immunologic test, antideoxyribonuclease-B (anti-DNase-B) (p. 61), also detects antigens produced by group A streptococci. The anti-DNase-B level is elevated in most patients with acute rheumatic fever and poststreptococcal glomerulonephritis. When ASO and anti-DNase-B are performed concurrently, 95% of previous streptococcal infections are detected. If both are repeatedly negative, there is no reason to suspect the symptoms are caused by a poststreptococcal disease. The Streptozyme test is often used as a screening test to detect any one of multiple streptococcal-induced antibodies.

Interfering Factors

- Increased beta-lipoprotein levels can neutralize streptolysin O and can cause a false-positive ASO titer.
- Drugs that may cause *decreased* ASO levels include antibiotics and adrenocorticosteroids. Antibiotics reduce the number of streptococci and thereby suppress ASO production. Steroids are immunosuppressive and thereby suppress ASO production.

Procedure and Patient Care

Before

- Explain the procedure to the patient.
- Tell the patient that no fasting is required.

During

- Collect approximately 5 to 10 ml of blood in a red-top tube.
- Avoid hemolysis of the blood specimen.
- Note on the laboratory slip any medications that may affect the test results.

After

- Apply pressure or a pressure dressing to the venipuncture site.
- Observe the venipuncture site for bleeding.
- Note that repeat ASO testing may be done to determine the highest level of increase.

Test Results and Clinical Significance

Increased levels

Acute streptococcal infection *ASO titers will not have developed during the early days of the infection. It is only after the second week of an untreated infection that the ASO will rise.*

Acute rheumatic fever
Bacterial endocarditis
ASO titers are highest in these diseases.

Acute glomerulonephritis *As many as 50% to 75% of these patients will not have high ASO titers.*

Scarlet fever
Streptococcal pyoderma
ASO is often not elevated in these diseases.

Related Tests

- Antideoxyribonuclease-B titer (p. 61): Like the ASO test, this immunologic test also detects antigens produced by group A streptococci and is positive in most patients with acute rheumatic fever or poststreptococcal glomerulonephritis.

Antithrombin III

(AT-III, Functional Antithrombin III Assay, Heparin Cofactor, Immunologic Antithrombin III, Serine Protease Inhibitor)

Normal Findings

Plasma: 50% of control value
Serum: 15%-34% lower than plasma value
Immunologic: 17-30 mg/dl
Functional: 80%-120%
Values vary according to laboratory methods.

Indications

This test is used to evaluate patients suspected of having hypercoagulable states. It is also used to help identify the cause of heparin resistance in patients receiving heparin therapy.

Test Explanation

AT-III is an $alpha_2$-globulin produced in the liver. It inhibits the serine proteases involved in coagulation (II, X, IX, XI, XII). In normal homeostasis the coagulation system results from a balance between AT-III and thrombin. A deficiency of AT-III increases coagulation or the tendency toward thrombosis. A hereditary deficiency of AT-III is characterized by a predisposition toward thrombus formation. This is passed on as an autosomal dominant abnormality. Individuals with hereditary AT-III deficiency typically develop thromboembolic events in their early twenties. These thrombotic events are usually venous. Acquired AT-III deficiency may be seen in patients with cirrhosis, liver failure, advanced carcinoma, nephrotic syndrome, disseminated intravascular coagulation (DIC), and acute thrombosis. AT-III is also decreased as much as 30% in pregnant women and those who take estrogens.

AT-III provides most of the anticoagulant effect of heparin. Heparin requires AT-III to express its effect. Patients who are deficient in AT-III may be heparin resistant and require unusually high doses for an anticoagulation effect. In general, patients respond to heparin if more than 60% of normal AT-III levels exists.

There are two methods of testing for AT-III. The first is a "functional" assay and measures AT-III activity. The second is an "immunologic" assay and actually quantifies the AT-III level. There are two types of inherited AT-III syndromes identified by using both of these methods. In type I the immunologic assay is reduced (decreased amount of AT-III), but the functional assay is normal (AT-III activity is normal). In type II the immunologic assay is normal (normal levels of AT-III), but the functional assay is low (AT-III activity is reduced).

Asymptomatic individuals with an antithrombin deficiency should receive prophylactic anticoagulation to increase their antithrombin levels before any medical/surgical interventions in which inactivity increases the risk of thrombosis. Increased levels of AT-III may occur in patients with acute hepatitis, obstructive jaundice, vitamin K deficiency, and kidney transplantation.

Interfering Factors

- Drugs that may cause *increased* levels include anabolic steroids, androgens, oral contraceptives (containing progesterone), and sodium warfarin.
- Drugs that may cause *decreased* levels include fibrinolytics, heparin, L-asparaginase, and oral contraceptives (containing estrogen).

Procedure and Patient Care

Before

- Explain the procedure to the patient.
- Tell the patient that no fasting is required.

During

- Collect a venous blood sample in a blue- or red-top tube.

After

- Apply pressure or a pressure dressing to the venipuncture site.
- Assess the venipuncture site for bleeding. Patients receiving heparin therapy may develop a hematoma at the venipuncture site.
- Send the specimen to the laboratory immediately after collection.

Test Results and Clinical Significance

Increased levels

Kidney transplant
Acute hepatitis
Obstructive jaundice
Vitamin K deficiency
The exact mechanisms for increased levels in these states is not known.

Decreased levels

DIC
Hypercoagulation states (e.g., deep vein thrombosis)
In these diseases the AT-III is consumed by the thrombotic process.

Hepatic disorders (especially cirrhosis) *AT-III is a protein whose synthesis is reduced by liver dysfunction*
Nephrotic syndrome
Protein-wasting diseases (malignancy)
Proteins are either lost or otherwise used up and the amino acid pool is depleted. Therefore AT-III cannot be made.

Hereditary familial deficiency of AT-III *Inadequate amounts of AT-III or adequate amounts of inactive AT-III are made. Anticoagulation is inhibited and thrombotic events occur.*

Antithyroglobulin Antibody
(Thyroid Autoantibody, Thyroid Antithyroglobulin Antibody, Thyroglobulin Antibody)

Normal Findings

Titer <1:100

Indications

This test is primarily used in the differential diagnosis of thyroid diseases, such as Hashimoto's thyroiditis and chronic lymphocytic thyroiditis (in children).

Test Explanation

There are several antibodies to various thyroid gland components. The two most common include antithyroglobulin antibody and antithyroid microsomal antibody. Antithyroglobulin antibody occurs when thyroglobulin, which normally exists in the blood (as a

Table 2-7 Thyroid diseases and the incidence of antithyroid antibodies

Disease	Antithyroglobulin antibody (%)	Antimicrosomal antibody (%)
Hashimoto's thyroiditis	70	95
Graves' disease	55	75
Myxedema	55	75
Nontoxic goiter	5-50	27
Thyroid cancer	20	20
Normal male	2	3
Normal female	10	15

thyroid hormone carrier) and in the thyroid, acts as an immune-stimulating antigen. Autoantibodies are developed and react against the thyroglobulin in the thyroid cells. This leads to thyroid inflammation and destruction.

Although many different thyroid diseases are associated with elevated antithyroglobulin antibody levels, the most frequent is chronic thyroiditis (Hashimoto's thyroiditis in the adult and lymphocytic thyroiditis in children and young adults) (Table 2-7). The level must be extremely high to confirm the diagnosis of Hashimoto's thyroiditis. This antibody is present in only about 50% of patients with Hashimoto's thyroiditis. Both Hashimoto's and lymphocytic thyroiditis have been associated with other autoimmune (collagen vascular) diseases. The antithyroglobulin antibody test is usually performed in conjunction with the antithyroid microsomal antibody test. When this is done, the specificity and sensitivity are greatly increased.

A small percentage of the normal population have antithyroglobulin antibodies. Normally women tend to have higher levels than men. Blood levels can be determined by latex agglutination, immunofluorescence, or radioimmunoassay.

Interfering Factors

- Normal individuals, especially elderly women, may have antithyroglobulin antibodies.

Procedure and Patient Care

Before

- Explain the procedure to the patient.
- Tell the patient that no fasting is required.

During

- Collect approximately 3 to 5 ml of blood in a red-top tube.

After

- Apply pressure or a pressure dressing to the venipuncture site.
- Assess the venipuncture site for bleeding.

Test Results and Clinical Significance

Increased levels

Chronic thyroiditis (Hashimoto's thyroiditis) *Antithyroglobulin antibodies attack the globulin in the thyroid cells. The immune complex creates an inflammatory and destructive process in the gland, which is mediated through the complement system.*
Rheumatoid arthritis
Rheumatoid-collagen disease
The association with other autoimmune diseases is well known; however the mechanism of this association has not been elucidated.

Pernicious anemia *Antiparietal cell antibodies have been associated with the presence of antithyroglobulin antibodies.*
Thyrotoxicosis
Hypothyroidism
Thyroid carcinoma
Thyroglobulin, which leaks out of the thyroid as a result of these destructive diseases, stimulates the immune system to produce antithyroglobulin antibodies.

Myxedema *The antithyroid microsomal antibodies destroy the thyroid cell, resulting in hypofunction of the gland.*

Related Tests

- Antithyroid microsomal antibody (p. 92): This antibody is used in conjunction with antithyroglobulin antibody to support the diagnosis of thyroid diseases.
- Long-acting thyroid stimulator (LATS) (p. 294): This and other thyroid-stimulating immunoglobulins are used to support the diagnosis of Graves' disease, especially when the diagnosis is complex.
- Thyrotropin-releasing hormone (p. 415): This test assists in the evaluation of patients with hyper- and hypothyroidism. It is especially helpful in the differential diagnosis of hypothyroidism.
- Thyroid-stimulating hormone (p. 410): This test is used to diagnose primary hypothyroidism and to differentiate it from secondary (pituitary) and tertiary (hypothalamus) hypothyroidism.
- Thyroid-stimulating hormone stimulation (p. 413): This test is also used to differentiate primary from secondary (and tertiary) hypothyroidism.
- Thyroxine-binding globulin (p. 421): This major thyroid hormone protein carrier is measured for evaluation of patients who have abnormal total thyroxine (T_4) and triiodothyronine (T_3) levels. When it is performed concurrently with a T_4/T_3 test, T_4 and T_3 levels can be more easily interpreted.
- Thyroxine (p. 417): This is one of the first tests done to assess thyroid function. It is used to diagnose thyroid function and to monitor replacement and suppressive therapy.
- Triiodothyronine (p. 435): A T_3 test is used to evaluate thyroid function, primarily to diagnose hyperthyroidism. It is also used to monitor thyroid replacement and suppressive medical therapy.

- Thyroxine index, free (p. 426): This test is used to evaluate thyroid function. It corrects for changes in thyroid hormone–binding serum proteins that can affect total T_4 levels. It is used to diagnose hyper- and hypothyroidism.
- Thyroxine, free (p. 423): This test is used to evaluate thyroid function in patients who may have protein abnormalities that could affect total T_4 levels. It is used to diagnose thyroid function and to monitor replacement and suppressive therapy.
- Triiodothyronine uptake (p. 438): This test is an indirect measurement of total T_4.

Antithyroid Microsomal Antibody
(Antimicrosomal Antibody, Microsomal Antibody, Thyroid Autoantibody, Thyroid Antimicrosomal Antibody)

Normal Findings
Titer <1:100

Indications

This test is primarily used in the differential diagnosis of thyroid diseases, such as Hashimoto's thyroiditis and chronic lymphocytic thyroiditis (in children).

Test Explanation

Thyroid microsomal antibodies are commonly found in patients with various thyroid diseases. They are present in 70% to 90% of patients with Hashimoto's thyroiditis. Microsomal antibodies are produced in response to microsomes escaping from the thyroid epithelial cells surrounding the thyroid follicle. These escaped microsomes then act as antigens and stimulate the production of antibodies. These immune complexes initiate inflammatory and cytotoxic effects on the thyroid follicle. This test is often performed in conjunction with the antithyroglobulin antibody test, which greatly increases the specificity and sensitivity.

Although many different thyroid diseases are associated with elevated antimicrosomal antibody levels, the most frequent is chronic thyroiditis (Hashimoto's thyroiditis in the adult and lymphocytic thyroiditis in children and young adults) (Table 2-7, p. 90). Both of these chronic inflammatory diseases have been associated with other autoimmune (collagen vascular) diseases. Twelve percent of normal females and 1% of normal males have positive antimicrosomal antibodies.

Procedure and Patient Care

Before

- Explain the procedure to the patient.
- Tell the patient that no fasting is required.

During

- Collect approximately 3 to 5 ml of venous blood in a red-top tube.

After

- Apply pressure or a pressure dressing to the venipuncture site.
- Assess the venipuncture site for bleeding.

Test Results and Clinical Significance

Increased levels

Chronic thyroiditis (Hashimoto's thyroiditis) *Antimicrosomal antibodies attack the microsome in the thyroid cells. The immune complex creates an inflammatory and destructive process in the gland, which is mediated through the complement system.*

Rheumatoid arthritis
Rheumatoid-collagen disease
The association with other autoimmune diseases is well known. The mechanism of this association, however, is not well known.

Pernicious anemia *Antiparietal cell antibodies have been associated with the presence of antimicrosomal antibodies.*

Thyrotoxicosis
Hypothyroidism
Thyroid carcinoma
Microsomes that leak out of the thyroid as a result of the presence of these destructive diseases stimulate the immune system to produce antimicrosomal antibodies.

Myxedema
Antithyroid microsomal antibodies destroy the thyroid cell, resulting in hypofunction of the gland.

Related Tests

- Antithyroglobulin antibody (p. 89): This test is primarily used in the differential diagnosis of thyroid diseases such as Hashimoto's thyroiditis.

Apolipoprotein (Apolipoprotein A-I [Apo A-I], Apolipoprotein B [Apo B], Lipoprotein [a] [Lp(a)])

Normal Findings

Apo A-I

Adult/elderly
- Male: 75-160 mg/dl
- Female: 80-175 mg/dl

Child/adolescent
- 6 months-4 years
  - Male: 67-167 mg/dl
  - Female: 60-148 mg/dl
- 5 to 17 years: 83-151 mg/dl
- Newborn
  - Male: 41-93 mg/dl
  - Female: 38-106 mg/dl

Apo B

Adult/elderly
- Male: 50-125 mg/dl
- Female: 45-120 mg/dl

Child/adolescent
- 6 months-3 years: 23-75 mg/dl
- 5-17 years
  - Male: 47-139 mg/dl
  - Female: 41-132 mg/dl

Newborn: 11-31 mg/dl

Apo A-I/apo B ratio

Male: 0.85-2.24
Female: 0.76-3.23

Lipoprotein (a)

Caucasian (5th-95th percentile)
Male: 2.2-49.4 mg/dl
Female: 2.1-57.3 mg/dl
African-American (5th-95th percentile)
Male: 4.6-71.8 mg/dl
Female: 4.4-75.0 mg/dl

Indications

This test is used to evaluate the risk of atherogenic heart and peripheral vascular diseases. These levels may be better indicators of atherogenic risks than high-density lipoprotein [HDL], low-density lipoprotein [LDL], and very-low-density lipoprotein [VLDL].

Test Explanation

The protein component of lipoproteins, which plays an important role in lipid transport, is composed of several specific polypeptides called apolipoproteins. Apolipoproteins are also involved in binding lipoproteins to lipoprotein receptors at the cell surface, thus facilitating lipid uptake by cells.

Apolipoprotein A (apo A) is the major polypeptide component of HDL. Apo A has two major forms: apo A-I, which constitutes about 75% of the apo A in HDL, and apo A-II, which constitutes about 20% of the total HDL protein. In general, as HDL levels increase, apo A-I values increase. Since apo A-I reflects the HDL content of the serum and HDL levels are greater in females, apo A-I values are also higher in women than in men. Some believe apo A-I is a better index of atherogenic risk than HDL.

Apo B is the major polypeptide component of LDL and makes up about 80% of that protein. Forty percent of the protein portion of VLDL is composed of apo B. Apo B has been shown to exist in two forms: apo B-100 and apo B-48. Apo B-100 is synthesized in the liver and found in lipoproteins of endogenous origin (VLDL and LDL). Apo B-100 is the principal transport mechanism for endogenous cholesterol. Apo B-100 has an affinity for the LDL receptor located on cell surfaces in peripheral tissues and is involved with cellular deposition of cholesterol. Because of this, some believe that apo B-100 may be a better indicator of atherosclerotic heart disease than LDL. The second apo B component is apo B-48, which is of intestinal origin and found mainly in chylomicrons. Apo B-48 serves to transport ingested lipids through the intestines and into the bloodstream.

Lp(a) (referred to as "lipoprotein little a") is another lipoprotein. The two polypeptide components of Lp(a) are apo(a) and an LDL-like protein containing apo B-100. Recent research has suggested that increased levels of Lp(a) may be an independent risk factor for atherosclerosis. It has been shown that apo(a) is a deformed relative of plasminogen, the precursor of the proteolytic enzyme plasmin, which is responsible for dissolving fibrin clots. This strong resemblance between apolipoprotein and plasminogen may provide a link between lipids, the clotting mechanism, and atherogenesis. Microthrombi containing fibrin on the vessel wall become incorporated into the atherosclerotic plaque. It is suggested that Lp(a) may insinuate itself into the arterial wall following endothelial damage, inhibiting the cleavage of fibrin in microthrombi by competing with plasminogen for access to fibrin. Atherosclerotic damage of the arterial wall soon follows, leading to occlusive disease or aneurysm.

Quantification of apolipoproteins is beginning to be performed as a routine clinical procedure. However, unsolved methodologic problems within apolipoprotein immunoassays produce significant variability. Several studies have indicated that apo A-I and apo B are better determinants of atherosclerotic disease than are lipid or lipoprotein determinants. Decreased levels of apo A-I and increased levels of apo B-100 are associated with increased risk of coronary heart disease. Reports also indicate that a low ratio of apo A-I to apo B may be a good predictor of coronary heart disease. Individuals with increased concentrations of Lp(a) appear to have a significantly higher risk for coronary heart disease.

These and other apolipoproteins are associated with the identification of other maladies. For example, the apo E4 gene has been proposed as a risk factor for Alzheimer's disease. Familial hypercholesterolemia, some forms of renal failure, nephrotic syndrome, and estrogen depletion in women over the age of 50 years may be associated with increased levels of Lp(a).

Interfering Factors

Apo A-I

- Physical exercise may increase apo A-I levels.
- Smoking may decrease levels.
- Diets high in carbohydrates or polyunsaturated fats may decrease apo A-I levels.
- Drugs that may *increase* apo A-I levels include carbamazepine, estrogens, ethanol, lovastatin, niacin, oral contraceptives, phenobarbital, pravastatin, and simvastatin.
- Drugs that may *decrease* apo A-I levels include androgens, beta blockers, diuretics, and progestins.

Apo B

- Diets high in saturated fats and cholesterol may increase apo B levels.
- Drugs that may *increase* apo B levels include androgens, beta blockers, diuretics, ethanol, and progestins.
- Drugs that may *decrease* apo B levels include cholestyramine, estrogen (postmenopausal women), lovastatin, simvastatin, neomycin, niacin, and thyroxine.

Lipoprotein (a)

- Drugs that may *decrease* Lp(a) include estrogens, niacin, neomycin, and stanozolol.

CLINICAL PRIORITIES

- Apolipoproteins may be better indicators of atherogenic risks than HDL, LDL, and VLDL.
- Decreased levels of apo A-1 and increased levels of apo B-100 are associated with an increased risk of coronary artery disease.
- Research has suggested that increased levels of Lp(a) are associated with a high risk of coronary artery disease.
- Test preparation requires a 12- to 14-hour fast before testing. Only water is permitted.

Procedure and Patient Care

Before

- Explain the procedure to the patient.
- Instruct the patient to fast for 12 to 14 hours before testing. Only water is permitted.
- Inform the patient that smoking is prohibited.

During

- Collect venous blood in a red-top tube.
- Indicate on the laboratory slip any drugs that may affect test results.

After

- Apply pressure or a pressure dressing to the venipuncture site.
- Observe the venipuncture site for bleeding.

Test Results and Clinical Significance *

Increased apo A-I
Familial hyperalphalipoproteinemia
Pregnancy
Weight reduction

Decreased apo A-I
Coronary artery disease
Ischemic coronary disease
Myocardial infarction
Familial hypoalphalipoproteinemia
Fish eye disease
Uncontrolled diabetes mellitus
Tangier disease
Nephrotic syndrome
Chronic renal failure
Cholestasis
Hemodialysis

Increased apo B
Hyperlipoproteinemia (types IIa, IIb, IV, V)
Nephrotic syndrome
Pregnancy
Hemodialysis
Biliary obstruction
Coronary artery disease
Diabetes
Hypothyroidism
Anorexia nervosa

Decreased apo B
Tangier disease
Hyperthyroidism
Malnutrition
Inflammatory joint disease
Chronic pulmonary disease
Weight reduction
Chronic anemia
Reye's syndrome

Increased Lp(a)
Premature coronary artery disease
Stenosis of cerebral arteries
Uncontrolled diabetes mellitus
Severe hypothyroidism
Familial hypercholesterolemia
Chronic renal failure
Estrogen depletion

Decreased Lp(a)
Alcoholism
Malnutrition
Chronic liver hepatocellular disease

*The pathophysiology of these observations has not been well defined.

Related Tests

- Lipoprotein (p. 289): This is a test also used to assess the risk of atherogenic vascular disease.

Arterial Blood Gases (Blood Gases, ABG)

Normal Findings

pH (arterial)

Adult/child: 7.35-7.45
Newborn: 7.32-7.49
2 months-2 years: 7.34-7.46

pH (venous) 7.31-7.41

Pco_2 (arterial)

Adult/child: 35-45 mm Hg (torr)
Child <2 years: 26-41 mm Hg (torr)

Pco_2 (venous) 40-50 mm Hg (torr)

HCO_3^-

Adult/child: 21-28 mEq/L
Newborn/infant: 16-24 mEq/L

Po_2 (arterial)

Adult/child: 80-100 mm Hg (torr)
Newborn: 60-70 mm Hg (torr)

Po_2 (venous) 40-50 mm Hg (torr)

O_2 saturation

Elderly: 95%
Adult/child: 95% to 100%
Newborn: 40% to 90%

O_2 content (arterial) 15-22 vol%

O_2 content (venous) 11-16 vol%

Critical Values

pH: <7.25, >7.55
Pco_2: <20, >60
HCO_3^-: <15, >40
Po_2 (arterial): <40
O_2 saturation: 75% or lower
Base/Excess ± 3mEq/L

Indications

Measurement of ABGs provides valuable information in assessing and managing a patient's respiratory (ventilation) and metabolic (renal) acid-base and electrolyte homeostasis. It is also used to assess the adequacy of oxygenation.

Test Explanation

ABGs are used to monitor patients on ventilators, monitor critically ill nonventilator patients, establish preoperative baseline parameters, and regulate electrolyte therapy. Although O_2 saturation monitors can accurately indicate O_2, ABGs are still used to monitor O_2 flow rates in the hospital and at home. ABGs are often performed in conjunction with pulmonary function studies.

pH

The pH is the negative logarithm of the hydrogen ion concentration in the blood. It is inversely proportional to the actual hydrogen ion concentration. Therefore, as the hydrogen ion concentration decreases, the pH increases, and vice versa. The acids normally found in the blood include carbonic acid (H_2CO_3), dietary acids, lactic acid, and ketoacids. The pH is a measure of alkalinity (pH >7.4) and acidity pH <7.35). In respiratory or metabolic alkalosis the pH is elevated; in respiratory or metabolic acidosis the pH is decreased. The pH is usually calculated by a machine that directly measures pH.

PCO_2

The PCO_2 is a measure of the partial pressure of CO_2 in the blood. CO_2 is carried in the blood as follows: 10% in the plasma and 90% in the RBCs. PCO_2 is a measurement of ventilation. The faster and more deeply the patient breathes, the more CO_2 is blown off, and PCO_2 levels drop. PCO_2 is therefore referred to as the *respiratory* component in acid-base determination, because this value is primarily controlled by the lungs. As the CO_2 level increases, the pH decreases. The CO_2 level and the pH are inversely proportional. The PCO_2 in the blood and the cerebrospinal fluid is a major stimulant to the breathing center in the brain. As PCO_2 levels rise, breathing is stimulated. If PCO_2 levels rise too high, breathing cannot keep up with the demand to blow off or ventilate. As PCO_2 levels rise further, the brain is depressed and ventilation decreases further, causing coma.

The PCO_2 level is elevated in primary respiratory acidosis and decreased in primary respiratory alkalosis (Table 2-8). Because the lungs compensate for primary metabolic acid-base derangements, PCO_2 levels are affected by metabolic disturbances as well. In meta-

Table 2-8 Normal values for ABGs and abnormal values in uncompensated acid-base disturbances

Acid-base disturbance	pH	PCO_2 (mm Hg)	HCO_3^- (mEq/L)	Common cause
None (normal values)	7.35-7.45	35-45	22-26	
Respiratory acidosis	↓	↑	Normal	Respiratory depression (drugs, CNS trauma) Pulmonary disease (pneumonia, chronic obstructive pulmonary disease, respiratory underventilation)
Respiratory alkalosis	↑	↓	Normal	Hyperventilation (emotions, pain, respiratory overventilation)
Metabolic acidosis	↓	Normal	↓	Diabetes, shock, renal failure, intestinal fistula
Metabolic alkalosis	↑	Normal	↑	Sodium bicarbonate overdose, prolonged vomiting, nasogastric drainage

Table 2-9 Acid-base disturbances and compensatory mechanisms

Acid-base disturbance	Mode of compensation
Respiratory acidosis	Kidneys will retain increased amounts of HCO_3^- to increase pH.
Respiratory alkalosis	Kidneys will excrete increased amounts of HCO_3^- to lower pH.
Metabolic acidosis	Lungs "blow off" CO_2 to raise pH.
Metabolic alkalosis	Lungs retain CO_2 to lower pH.

bolic acidosis the lungs attempt to compensate by blowing off CO_2 to raise pH. In metabolic alkalosis the lungs attempt to compensate by retaining CO_2 to lower pH (Table 2-9).

HCO_3^- or CO_2 content

Most of the CO_2 content in the blood is HCO_3^-. The bicarbonate ion (HCO_3^-) is a measure of the *metabolic (renal)* component of the acid-base equilibrium. It is regulated by the kidney. This ion can be measured directly by the bicarbonate value or indirectly by the CO_2 content (see p. 133). It is important not to confuse CO_2 content with PCO_2. CO_2 content is an indirect measurement of HCO_3^-. PCO_2 is a direct measurement of the tension of CO_2 in the blood and is regulated by the lungs.

As the HCO_3 level increases, the pH also increases; therefore the relationship of bicarbonate to pH is directly proportional. HCO_3^- is elevated in metabolic alkalosis and decreased in metabolic acidosis (Table 2-8). The kidneys also are used to compensate for primary respiratory acid-base derangements. For example, in respiratory acidosis the kidneys attempt to compensate by reabsorbing increased amounts of HCO_3^-. In respiratory alkalosis the kidneys excrete HCO_3^- in increased amounts in an attempt to lower pH through compensation (Table 2-9). In diabetic ketoacidosis, HCO_3^- ion does decrease, because it is used directly to neutralize the plasma diabetic acids.

PO_2

This is an indirect measure of the O_2 content of the arterial blood. PO_2 is a measure of the tension (pressure) of O_2 dissolved in the plasma. This pressure determines the force of O_2 to diffuse across the pulmonary alveoli membrane. The PO_2 level is decreased in:

1. Patients who are unable to oxygenate the arterial blood because of O_2 diffusion difficulties (e.g., pneumonia, shock lung, congestive failure)
2. Patients in whom venous blood mixes prematurely with arterial blood (e.g., congenital heart disease)
3. Patients who have underventilated and overperfused pulmonary alveoli (pickwickian syndrome; i.e., obese patients who cannot breathe properly when in the supine position or in patients with significant atelectasis)

PO_2 is one of the measures used to determine the effectiveness of O_2 therapy.

O_2 saturation

O_2 saturation is an indication of the percentage of hemoglobin saturated with O_2. When 92% to 100% of the hemoglobin carries O_2, the tissues are adequately provided with O_2, assuming normal O_2 dissociation. As the PO_2 level decreases, the percentage of hemoglobin saturation also decreases. This decrease (see an oxyhemoglobin-dissociation curve) is linear to a certain value. However, when the PO_2 level drops below 60 mm Hg, small decreases in the PO_2 level will cause large decreases in the percentage of hemoglobin saturated with O_2. At O_2 saturation levels of 70% or lower the tissues are unable to extract enough O_2 to carry out their vital functions.

O_2 saturation is calculated by the blood gas machine using the following formula:

$$\text{Percentage of } O_2 \text{ saturation} = 100 \times \frac{\text{Volume of } O_2 \text{ content Hgb}}{\text{Volume of } O_2 \text{ Hgb capacity}}$$

Pulse oximetry is a noninvasive method of determining O_2 saturation. This can be done easily and continuously. This machine measures O_2 saturation. It actually measures all forms of O_2-saturated hemoglobin, including carboxyhemoglobin (which rises during smoke inhalation or after using some inhalants). Therefore, in cases of carbon monoxide poisoning when carboxyhemoglobin is high, oximetry will indicate an inaccurately high O_2 saturation. During oximetry monitoring a small cliplike sensor is applied to the tip of the finger or earlobe. The oximeter transmits light from one side and records the amount of light on the other side, thus determining O_2 saturation.

O_2 content

This is a calculated number that represents the amount of O_2 in the blood. The formula for calculation is

$$O_2 \text{ content} = O_2 \text{ saturation} \times \text{Hgb} \times 1.34 + PO_2 \times 0.003$$

Nearly all O_2 in the blood is bound to hemoglobin. O_2 content decreases with the same diseases that diminish PO_2.

Base excess/deficit

This number is calculated by the blood gas machine using the pH, PCO_2, and the hematocrit. It represents the amount of buffering anions in the blood. HCO_3^- is the largest of these. Others include hemoglobin, proteins, phosphates, etc. Base excess is a way to take all of these anions into account when determining acid/base treatment based on the *metabolic* component. A negative-base excess (deficit) indicates metabolic acidosis (e.g., lactic acidosis). A positive-base excess indicates metabolic alkalosis or compensation to prolonged respiratory acidosis.

Alveolar (A) to arterial (a) O_2 difference (A-a gradient)

This is a calculated number that indicates the difference between alveolar O_2 and arterial O_2. The normal value is less than 10 mm Hg (torr). If the A-a gradient is abnormally high, there is either a problem in diffusing O_2 across the alveolar membrane (thickened edematous alveoli) or unoxygenated blood is mixing with the oxygenated blood. Thickened alveolar membranes can occur in patients with pulmonary edema, pulmonary fibrosis, and acute respiratory distress syndrome (ARDS). Mixing of unoxygenated blood occurs in patients with congenital cardiac septal defects, arterial-venous shunts, or underventilated alveoli that are still being perfused (atelectasis, mucus plug, etc).

Interpretation of ABG levels can seem difficult but is really quite easy when one follows a system of evaluation (see Table 2-8). One such system is as follows:

1. Evaluate the pH.
   If the pH is <7.4, acidosis is present.
   If the pH is >7.4, alkalosis is present.
2. Next look at the Pco_2.
   A. If the Pco_2 is high in a patient who has been said to have acidosis (by step 1), the patient has respiratory acidosis (RA).
   B. If the Pco_2 is low in a patient who has been said to have acidosis (by step 1), the patient has metabolic acidosis (MA) and is compensating for that situation by blowing off CO_2.
   C. If the Pco_2 is low in a patient who has been said to have alkalosis (by step 1), the patient has respiratory alkalosis (RAl).
   D. If the Pco_2 is high in a patient who has been said to have alkalosis (by step 1), the patient has metabolic alkalosis (MAl) and is compensating for that situation by retaining CO_2.
3. Next look at the bicarbonate ion (HCO_3^-).
   In patient A, HCO_3^- can be expected to be high in an attempt to compensate for the RA.
   In patient B, HCO_3^- can be expected to be low as a reflection of the MA.
   In patient C, HCO_3^- can be expected to be low to compensate for the RAl.
   In patient D, HCO_3^- can be expected to be high as a reflection of the MAl.

Contraindications

Arterial access should *not* be performed if:

- There is no palpable pulse.
- Cellulitis or open infection is present in the area considered for access.
- The Allen test is negative, indicating that there is no ulnar artery. If the radial artery is used for access, thrombosis may occur and jeopardize the viability of the hand.
- There is an arteriovenous (AV) fistula proximal to the site of proposed access.
- The patient has a severe coagulopathy.

Potential Complications

- Occlusion of the artery used for access (It is preferable to avoid use of end arteries such as the brachial or femoral artery.)
- Penetration of other important structures anatomically juxtaposed to the artery (eg., nerve)

Interfering Factors

- O_2 saturation can be falsely increased by the inhalation of carbon monoxide, which increases the carboxyhemoglobin level.
- In patients with chronic obstructive pulmonary disease (COPD), the stimulus to breathe is not triggered by CO_2 levels (as normal) but by O_2 levels. If a large amount of O_2 is provided to these patients, they will no longer be driven to breathe and will hypoventilate.
- Respiration can be inhibited by the use of sedative-hypnotics or narcotics. Overdosage of these drugs can cause hypoventilation in patients with normal lungs.

CLINICAL PRIORITIES

- Perform the Allen test to assess collateral circulation before performing the arterial puncture on the radial artery. A positive Allen test ensures collateral circulation to the hand if thrombosis of the radial artery should follow the puncture.
- Arterial puncture should not be performed on an arm with an AV fistula or shunt.
- After the arterial blood is obtained, apply pressure to the puncture site for 3 to 5 minutes to avoid hematoma formation. If the patient has an abnormal clotting time or is taking anticoagulants, apply pressure for approximately 15 minutes.

Procedure and Patient Care

Before

- Explain the procedure to the patient.
- Notify the laboratory before drawing ABGs so that the necessary equipment can be calibrated before the blood sample arrives.
- Perform the Allen test to assess collateral circulation before performing the arterial puncture on the radial artery (Figure 2-6). To perform the Allen test, make the patient's hand blanch by obliterating both the radial and the ulnar pulses and then release the pressure over the ulnar artery only. If flow through the ulnar artery is good, flushing can be seen immediately. The Allen test is then positive, and the radial artery can be used for puncture. If the Allen test is negative (no flushing), repeat it on the other arm. If both arms give a negative result, choose another artery (femoral) for puncture.
- Note that the Allen test ensures collateral circulation to the hand if thrombosis of the radial artery should follow the puncture.

During

- Note that arterial blood can be obtained from any area of the body where strong pulses are palpable, usually from the radial, brachial, or femoral artery. The artery chosen for access should have adequate collateral vessels, be easily accessible, and be surrounded by few other vital structures.
- Cleanse the arterial site carefully with an antiseptic such as alcohol or povidone-iodine.
- Consider injecting 0.5 ml of lidocaine in the skin overlying the access site.
- Attach a 20-gauge needle to a syringe containing approximately 0.2 ml of heparin.
- After drawing 3 to 5 ml of blood, remove the needle and apply pressure to the arterial site for 3 to 5 minutes.
- Expel any air bubbles in the syringe.

After

- Place the arterial blood on ice and immediately take it to the chemistry or pulmonary laboratory for analysis.

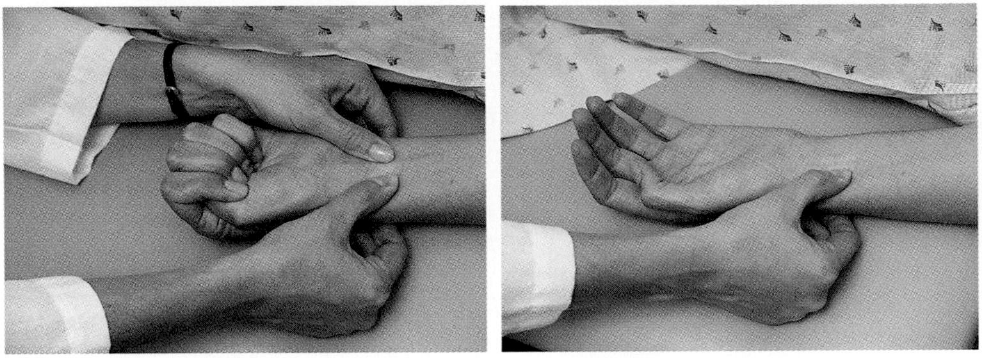

A B

Figure 2-6 The Allen test for evaluating collateral circulation of the radial artery. **A,** *Step 1,* While the patient's fist is closed tightly, obliterate both the radial and ulnar arteries simultaneously. Instruct the patient to relax the hand, and watch for blanching of the palm and fingers. **B,** *Step 2,* Release the obstructing pressure from only the ulnar artery. Wait 15 seconds, observing the hand for flushing caused by capillary refilling. This indicates a positive Allen test, verifying that the ulnar artery alone is capable of supplying the entire hand. If flushing does not occur within 15 seconds, the Allen test is negative and the radial artery cannot be used.

- Hold pressure or apply pressure or a pressure dressing to the arterial puncture site for 3 to 5 minutes to avoid hematoma formation.
- Assess the puncture site for bleeding. Remember that an artery rather than a vein has been accessed.
- If the patient has an abnormal clotting time or is taking anticoagulants, apply pressure for a longer period (approximately 15 minutes).

Test Results and Clinical Significance (see Table 2-8)

Increased A-a O_2 gradient

Mucus plug, bronchospasm, atelectasis, pneumothorax, pulmonary edema, ARDS
Nonventilated lung tissue is still perfused. The perfused blood does not get oxygenated, however, because there is no ventilation in that area of the lung to bring O_2 to the blood. The perfused, yet unoxygenated blood mixes with the oxygenated blood in the pulmonary veins. By dilution, the O_2 content of the mixed blood returning to the heart is lowered. The arterial blood is therefore lowered.

Atrial or ventricular cardiac septal defects, emboli *The unoxygenated blood gains access to the oxygenated blood by direct shunting. By dilution, the O_2 content of the mixed blood returning to the heart is lowered. The arterial blood is therefore lowered.*

Increased P_{CO_2}

COPD (bronchitis, emphysema)

Oversedation, head trauma, overoxygenation in a patient with COPD or pickwickian syndrome

Reduced ventilation causes increased levels of P_{CO_2}.

Decreased PCO_2

Hypoxemia, pulmonary emboli *Hypoxemia drives the respiratory center to increase ventilation. With increased ventilation, PCO_2 levels decrease.*

Anxiety, pain, pregnancy *These situations are associated with rapid ventilation. With increased ventilation, PCO_2 levels decrease.*

Increased PO_2 and O_2 content

Polycthemia *The amount of hemoglobin is significantly increased. O_2 content, which saturates that hemoglobin, is also increased.*

Increased inspired O_2, hyperventilation *With increased alveolar O_2 caused by breathing more rapidly or increasing the O_2 in the inspired air, the PO_2 and O_2 content can be expected to increase.*

Decreased PO_2 and O_2 content

Anemias *The amount of hemoglobin is significantly reduced. O_2 content, which saturates that hemoglobin, is also reduced.*

Mucus plug, bronchospasm, atelectasis, pneumothorax, pulmonary edema, ARDS, restrictive lung disease

Atrial or ventricular cardiac septal defects, emboli

See above rationale under increased A-a O_2 gradient

Inadequate O_2 in inspired air (suffocation)

Severe hypoventilation states, such as oversedation or neurologic somnolence

Without air exchange, PO_2 levels fall.

Increased HCO_3^-

Chronic vomiting or chronic high-volume gastric suction

Aldosteronism

Use of mercurial diuretics

Important acid hydrogen ions are lost. HCO_3^- ions are relatively high. This causes metabolic alkalosis.

COPD *HCO_3^- ions are increased to compensate for chronic hypoventilation (high PCO_2). Compensation occurs for respiratory acidosis.*

Decreased HCO_3^-

Chronic and severe diarrhea

Chronic use of loop diuretics

Persistent loss of base ions, including HCO_3^-, occurs. Most of the CO_2 content is HCO_3^-.

Starvation

Diabetic ketoacidosis

Acute renal failure

Ketoacids are built up. HCO_3^- neutralizes these acids. HCO_3^- levels therefore drop.

Increased pH (alkalosis)

METABOLIC ALKALOSIS

Hypokalemia, hypochloremia, chronic and high-volume gastric suction, chronic vomiting

Aldosteronism
Use of mercurial diuretics
Important acid hydrogen ions are lost. HCO_3^- *ions are relatively high.*

RESPIRATORY ALKALOSIS

Hypoxemic states, such as chronic heart failure, cystic fibrosis, carbon monoxide poisoning, pulmonary emboli, shock, acute severe pulmonary diseases *With hypoxemia, breathing is accelerated.* CO_2 *is blown off.*
Anxiety neuroses, pain, pregnancy *These situations are associated with hyperventilation. With hyperventilation,* CO_2 *is blown off.*

Decreased pH (acidosis)

METABOLIC ACIDOSIS

Ketoacidosis
Lactic acidosis
Acid anions build up. Acidosis occurs.

Severe diarrhea
Renal failure
Important base ions are lost. Acid ions are relatively increased and acidosis occurs.

RESPIRATORY ACIDOSIS

Respiratory failure Pco_2 *builds up, causing acidosis.*

Related Tests

- Pulmonary function tests (p. 1016): This is measurement of lung volume, which aids in the diagnosis and treatment of obstructive and restrictive lung diseases.
- pH, fetal scalp (p. 324): Measurement of fetal scalp blood pH provides valuable information on fetal acid-base status. This screening test is useful clinically for diagnosing fetal distress.

Aspartate Aminotransferase (AST, Formerly Serum Glutamic-Oxaloacetic Transaminase [SGOT])

Normal Findings

Age	Normal Value (U/L)
0-5 days	35-140
<3 yr	15-60
3-6 yr	15-50
6-12 yr	10-50
12-18 yr	10-40
Adult	5-40 IU/L
Adult	8-20 U/L (SI units)
Females	Slightly higher than males
Elderly	Slightly higher than adults

Indications

This test is used in the evaluation of patients with suspected coronary occlusive heart disease or suspected hepatocellular diseases.

Test Explanation

This enzyme is found in very high concentrations within highly metabolic tissue, such as the heart muscle, liver cells, skeletal muscle cells, and to a lesser degree in the kidneys, pancreas, and red blood cells. When disease or injury affects the cells of these tissues, the cells lyse. The AST is released, picked up by the blood, and the serum level rises. The amount of AST elevation is directly related to the number of cells affected by the disease or injury. Furthermore, the elevation depends on the length of time that the blood is drawn after the injury. AST is cleared from the blood in a few days. Serum AST levels become elevated 8 hours after cell injury, peak at 24 to 36 hours, and return to normal in 3 to 7 days. If the cellular injury is chronic, levels will be persistently elevated.

AST is one of the enzymes tested in the cardiac enzyme series. Although not specific for myocardial injury, when observed with the enzymes creatine phosphokinase (CPK) and lactic dehydrogenase, it is useful in the diagnosis of a myocardial infarction (MI). It aids in determining the timing of a recent MI and in determining the extent of the MI. In the case of an acute MI, the AST level rises within 6 to 10 hours after an MI, peaks at 12 to 48 hours, and returns to normal in 3 to 4 days assuming further cardiac injury does not occur. A second rise is AST would indicate extension or progression of myocardial injury despite therapy. Myocardial injuries such as angina, pericarditis, or rheumatic carditis do not increase the AST level.

As with CPK, serial determinations of AST are necessary in determining the timing, initiation, and resolution of an MI. Unlike the isoenzyme CPK-MB, however, AST is much less specific for infarction of myocardial muscle cells.

Because AST also exists within the liver cells, diseases that affect the hepatocyte will cause elevated levels of this enzyme. In acute hepatitis, AST levels can rise 20 times the normal value. In acute extrahepatic obstruction (e.g., gallstone), AST levels quickly rise to 10 times the normal and swiftly fall. In cirrhotic patients the level of AST depends on the amount of active inflammation.

Serum AST levels are often compared with alanine aminotransferase (ALT) levels. The AST/ALT ratio is usually greater than 1 in patients with alcoholic cirrhosis, liver congestion, and metastatic tumor of the liver. Ratios less than 1 may be seen in patients with acute hepatitis, viral hepatitis, or infectious mononucleosis. The ratio is less accurate if AST levels exceed 10 times normal.

Patients with acute pancreatitis, acute renal diseases, musculoskeletal diseases, or trauma may have a transient rise in serum AST. Patients with red blood cell abnormalities such as acute hemolytic anemia and severe burns also can have elevations of this enzyme. AST levels may be decreased in patients with beriberi or diabetic ketoacidosis and in patients who are pregnant.

Interfering Factors

- Pregnancy may cause decreased AST levels.
- Exercise may cause increased levels.

- Drugs that may cause *increased* levels include antihypertensives, cholinergic agents, coumarin-type anticoagulants, digitalis preparations, erythromycin, isoniazid, methyldopa, oral contraceptives, opiates, salicylates, hepatotoxic medications, and verapamil.
- Levels are falsely *decreased* in patients with pyridoxine deficiency (beriberi, pregnancy), severe long-standing liver disease, uremia, or diabetic ketoacidosis.

Procedure and Patient Care

Before

- Explain the procedure to the patient.
- Discuss with the patient the need and reason for frequent venipunctures in diagnosing MI.
- Avoid giving the patient any IM injection.
- If possible, hold drugs that could interfere with test results for 12 hours before the test.

During

- Collect a venous sample of blood in a red-top tube. This is usually done daily for 3 days and then again in 1 week.
- Rotate the venipuncture site.
- Avoid hemolysis.
- Indicate on the laboratory slip any drugs that may cause false-positive results.
- Record the time and date of any IM injection given.
- Record the exact time and date when the blood test is performed. This aids in the interpretation of the temporal pattern of enzyme elevations.

After

- Apply pressure or a pressure dressing to the venipuncture site.
- Observe the venipuncture site for bleeding.

Test Results and Clinical Significance

Increased levels

HEART DISEASES

Myocardial infarction
Cardiac operations
Cardiac catheterization and angioplasty
These diseases cause heart cell injury. The cells die and lysis of the cell occurs. The contents of the cell (including AST) are spewed out and are collected into the blood. Elevated AST levels thereby occur.

LIVER DISEASES

Hepatitis
Hepatic cirrhosis
Drug-induced liver injury
Hepatic metastasis
Hepatic necrosis (initial stages only)

Hepatic surgery
Infectious mononucleosis with hepatitis
Hepatic infiltrative process (e.g., tumor)
These diseases cause liver cell injury. The cells die and lysis of the cell occurs. The contents of the cell (including AST) are spewed out and are collected into the blood. Elevated AST levels thereby occur.

SKELETAL MUSCLE DISEASES

Skeletal muscle trauma
Recent noncardiac surgery
Multiple traumas
Severe, deep burns
Progressive muscular dystrophy
Recent convulsions
Heat stroke
Primary muscle diseases (e.g., myopathy, myositis)
These diseases cause muscle cell injury. The cells die and lysis of the cell occurs. The contents of the cell (including AST) are spewed out and are collected into the blood. Elevated AST levels thereby occur.

OTHER DISEASES

Acute hemolytic anemia
Acute pancreatitis
These diseases cause cell injury in these tissues. The cells die and lysis of the cell occurs. The contents of the cell (including AST) are spewed out and are collected into the blood. Elevated AST levels thereby occur.

Decreased levels

Acute renal disease
Beriberi
Diabetic ketoacidosis
Pregnancy
Chronic renal dialysis

Related Tests

- Creatine phosphokinase (CPK) (see p. 173): This enzyme is used similarly to AST and exists predominantly in heart and skeletal muscle.
- Alanine aminotransferase (ALT) (see p. 33): This enzyme is used similarly to AST and exists predominantly in the liver.
- Lactic dehydrogenase (LDH) (p. 278): This is an intracellular enzyme used to support the diagnosis of injury or disease involving the heart, liver, red blood cells, kidneys, skeletal muscle, brain, and lungs.
- Leucine aminopeptidase (LAP) (see p. 286): This enzyme is specific to the hepatobiliary system. Diseases affecting that system will cause elevation of this enzyme.
- Gamma-glutamyl transpeptidase (GGTP) (p. 219): This is another enzyme predominantly existing in the liver.
- Alkaline phosphatase (p. 42): This is another enzyme predominantly existing in the liver.
- 5′-Nucleotidase- (p. 312): This is another enzyme predominantly existing in the liver.

Bilirubin

Normal Findings

Blood

Adult/elderly/child
Total bilirubin: 0.3-1.0 mg/dl or 5.1-17.0 μmol/L (SI units)
Indirect bilirubin: 0.2-0.8 mg/dl or 3.4-12.0 μmol/L (SI units)
Direct bilirubin: 0.1-0.3 mg/dl or 1.7-5.1 μmol/L (SI units)
Newborn total bilirubin: 1.0-12 mg/dl or 17.1-205 μmol/L (SI units)

Urine 0-0.02 mg/dl

Critical Values

Adult: >12 mg/dl
Newborn: >15 mg/dl (immediate treatment required to avoid kernicterus)

Indications

This test is used to evaluate liver function. It is a part of the evaluation of adult patients with hemolytic anemias and newborns with jaundice.

Test Explanation

Bile, which is formed in the liver, has many constituents, including bile salts, phospholipids, cholesterol, bicarbonate, water, and bilirubin. Bilirubin metabolism begins with the breakdown of RBCs in the reticuloendothelial system (mostly the spleen) (Figure 2-7). Hemoglobin is released from RBCs and broken down to heme and globin molecules. Heme is then catabolized to form biliverdin, which is transformed to bilirubin. This form of bilirubin is called unconjugated (indirect) bilirubin. In the liver, indirect bilirubin is conjugated with a glucuronide molecule, resulting in conjugated (direct) bilirubin. The conjugated bilirubin is then excreted from the liver cells and into the intrahepatic canaliculi, which eventually lead to the hepatic ducts, the common bile duct, and the bowel.

Jaundice is the discoloration of body tissues caused by abnormally high blood levels of bilirubin. This yellow discoloration is recognized when the total serum bilirubin exceeds 2.5 mg/dl. Jaundice results from a defect in the normal metabolism or excretion of bilirubin. This defect can occur at any stage of heme catabolism.

Physiologic jaundice of the newborn occurs if the newborn's liver is immature and does not have enough conjugating enzymes. This results in a high circulating blood level of unconjugated bilirubin, which can pass through the blood-brain barrier and deposit in the brain cells of the newborn, causing encephalopathy (kernicterus). In newborns, if bilirubin levels are greater than 15 mg/dl, immediate treatment is required to avoid mental retardation. This may include exchange transfusions. High levels of bilirubin in the newborn are often treated with light therapy.

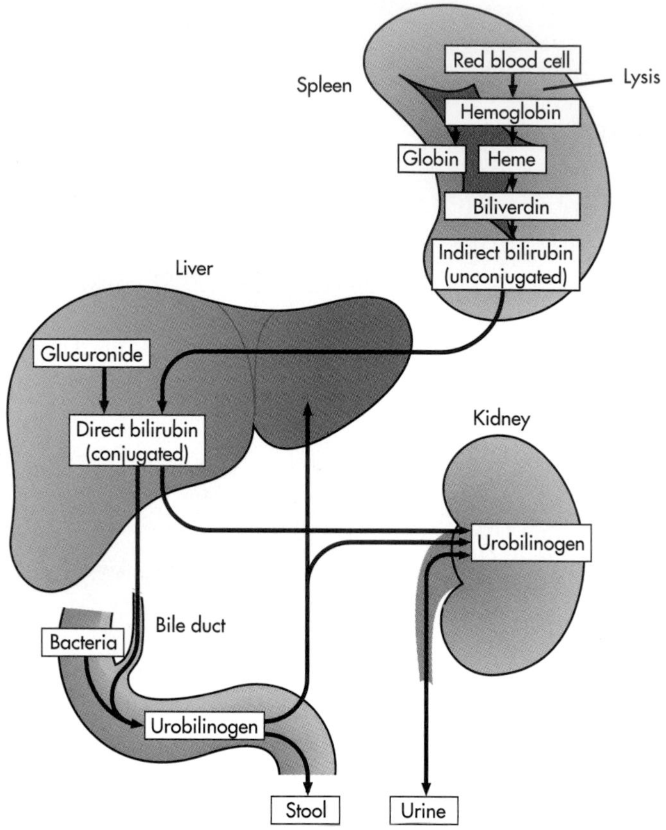

Figure 2-7 Bilirubin metabolism and excretion.

If the defect in bilirubin metabolism occurs after addition of glucuronide, conjugated (direct) hyperbilirubinemia will result. Obstruction of the bile duct by a gallstone is the classic example of obstructed bilirubin excretion causing a direct hyperbilirubinemia.

Once the jaundice is recognized either clinically or chemically, it is important (for therapy) to differentiate whether it is predominantly caused by indirect (unconjugated) or direct (conjugated) bilirubin. This in turn will help differentiate the etiology of the defect. In general, jaundice caused by hepatocellular dysfunction (e.g., hepatitis) results in elevated levels of indirect bilirubin. This dysfunction usually cannot be repaired surgically. On the other hand, jaundice resulting from extrahepatic dysfunction (e.g., gallstones, tumor blocking the bile ducts) results in elevated levels of direct bilirubin; this type of jaundice usually can be resolved by open surgery or endoscopic surgery.

The total serum bilirubin level is the sum of the conjugated (direct) and unconjugated (indirect) bilirubin. These are separated out when "fractionation or differentiation" of the total bilirubin to its direct and indirect parts is requested from the laboratory (Figure 2-8). Normally the indirect (unconjugated) bilirubin makes up 70% to 85% of the total bilirubin. In patients with jaundice, when more than 50% of the bilirubin is direct (con-

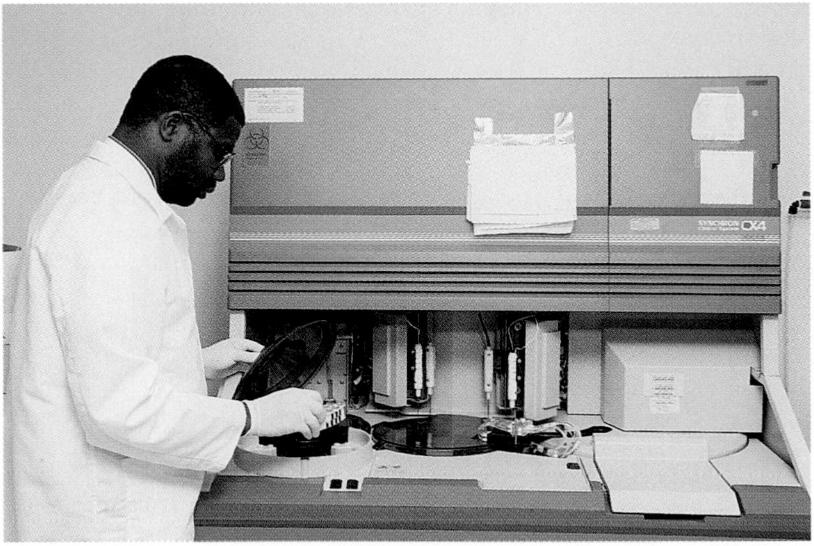

Figure 2-8 Medical technologist performing a test to measure serum bilirubin levels.

jugated), it is considered a direct hyperbilirubinemia from gallstones, tumor, inflammation, scarring, or obstruction of the extrahepatic ducts. Indirect hyperbilirubinemia is diagnosed when less than 15% to 20% of the total bilirubin is direct bilirubin. Diseases that typically cause this form of jaundice include accelerated erythrocyte (RBC) hemolysis, hepatitis, or drugs.

Delta bilirubin is a form of bilirubin that is covalently bound to albumin. It has a longer half-life than the other bilirubins; therefore it remains elevated during the convalescent phases of hepatic disorders when the conjugated bilirubin has typically returned to normal. It can be derived by the following calculation:

Total bilirubin − Direct (conjugated) bilirubin + Indirect (unconjugated) bilirubin

When the defect in bilirubin metabolism occurs after conjugation, elevated levels of direct (conjugated) bilirubin occur. Unlike the unconjugated form, direct bilirubin is water soluble and can be excreted into the urine. Therefore bilirubin in urine suggests disease affecting bilirubin metabolism after conjugation or defects in excretion (e.g., gallstones). There may be a small amount of bilirubin in the urine. Testing for bilirubin in the urine is a part of routine urine analysis.

Interfering Factors

- Blood hemolysis and lipemia can produce erroneous results.
- Drugs that may cause *increased blood* levels of total bilirubin include allopurinol, anabolic steroids, antibiotics, antimalarials, ascorbic acid, azathioprine, chlorpropamide (Diabinese), cholinergics, codeine, dextran, diuretics, epinephrine, meperidine,

methotrexate, methyldopa, monoamine oxidase inhibitors, morphine, nicotinic acid (large doses), oral contraceptives, phenothiazines, quinidine, rifampin, salicylates, steroids, sulfonamides, theophylline, and vitamin A.

- Drugs that may cause *increased urine* bilirubin levels include allopurinol, antibiotics, barbiturates, chlorpromazine, diuretics, oral contraceptives, phenazopyridine (Pyridium), steroids, and sulfonamides.
- Drugs that may cause *decreased blood* levels of total bilirubin include barbiturates, caffeine, penicillin, and salicylates (high dose).
- Drugs that can cause *false-negative* results in urine levels include indomethacin (Indocin) and ascorbic acid (vitamin C).
- Drugs that can cause *false-positive* results in the urine level include "pyridium-like" drugs and urochromes. These drugs can color the urine yellow or orange and foil the color analysis tests. Bilirubin is not stable in urine, especially when exposed to light.

Procedure and Patient Care

Before

- Explain the procedure to the patient.
- Note that fasting requirements vary among different laboratories. Some require keeping the patient on NPO status after midnight the day of the test except for water.

During

For Blood

- Collect 5 to 7 ml of venous blood in a red-top tube.
- Use a heel puncture for blood collection in infants.
- Prevent hemolysis of blood during phlebotomy.
- Do not shake the tube, because inaccurate test results may occur.
- Protect the blood sample from bright light. Prolonged exposure (over 1 hour) to sunlight or artificial light can reduce bilirubin content.
- List on the laboratory slip any drugs that may affect test results.

For Urine

- Note that this is a spot urine test.
- Collect at least 10 ml of urine for quick, simple testing.
- Use reagent strips (e.g., Multistix) or tablets (e.g., Icotest) for quick, simple testing.

For Urine Testing With Multistix Reagent Strips

- Note that this is a firm, plastic strip with seven separate areas for testing pH, protein, glucose, ketones, bilirubin, blood, and urobilinogen.
- For testing bilirubin, obtain a fresh urine specimen and examine it as soon as possible.
- Immerse the dipstick in the well-mixed urine and then remove immediately to avoid dissolving other reagents.
- Tap the dipstick against the rim of the urine container to remove excess urine.
- Hold the strip horizontally and compare it with the color chart on the label of the bottle after 20 to 30 seconds, according to directions. Results are given in the range of 0 to 3.

For Urine Testing With Icotest Tablets

- Place 5 drops of urine on the special test mat.
- Add 2 drops of water. The bilirubin test is positive if the mat turns blue or purple within 30 seconds.
- Note that this test is considered more sensitive than reagent strips for detecting bilirubin.

After

For Blood

- Apply pressure or a pressure dressing to the venipuncture site.
- Assess the venipuncture site for bleeding. Patients who are jaundiced may have prolonged clotting times.

For Urine

- Do not reuse reagent strips or Icotest tablets.
- Whether using strips or tablets or if sending the urine to the laboratory, list any medications that may affect test results.

Test Results and Clinical Significance

Increased blood levels of conjugated (direct) bilirubin

Gallstones
Extrahepatic duct obstruction (tumor, inflammation, gallstone, scarring, surgical trauma)
These diseases cause a blockage of the bile ducts. Bile, containing bilirubin, cannot be excreted. Blood levels rise.

Extensive liver metastasis *The intrahepatic ducts or hepatic ducts become obstructed because of tumor. Bile, containing bilirubin, cannot be excreted. Blood levels rise.*

Cholestasis from drugs *Some drugs inhibit the excretion of bile from the hepatocyte into the bile canaliculi. Bile, containing bilirubin, cannot be excreted. Blood levels rise.*

Dubin-Johnson syndrome
Rotor's syndrome
Congenital defects in enzyme quantity inhibit metabolism and excretion of bilirubin. Blood levels rise.

Increased blood levels of unconjugated (indirect) bilirubin

Erythroblastosis fetalis
Transfusion reaction
Sickle cell anemia
Hemolytic jaundice
Hemolytic anemia
Pernicious anemia
Large-volume blood transfusion
Resolution of large hematoma
RBC destruction occurs. Large amounts of heme are available for catabolism into bilirubin. This quantity exceeds the liver's capability to conjugate bilirubin. Indirect (unconjugated) bilirubin levels rise.

Hepatitis
Cirrhosis
Sepsis
Neonatal hyperbilirubinemia
The diseased, injured, or immature liver cannot conjugate the bilirubin presented to it. Indirect (unconjugated) bilirubin levels rise.

Crigler-Najjar syndrome
Gilbert syndrome
Congenital enzyme deficiencies interrupt conjugation of bilirubin. Indirect (unconjugated) bilirubin levels rise.

Increased urine levels of bilirubin

Gallstones
Extrahepatic duct obstruction (tumor, inflammation, gallstone, scarring, surgical trauma)
Extensive liver metastasis
Cholestasis from drugs
Dubin-Johnson syndrome
Rotor's syndrome
Defects in bilirubin metabolism and excretion, as discussed earlier, inhibit intestinal excretion of bilirubin. The above-noted diseases are associated with direct (conjugated) hyperbilirubinemia. The conjugated bilirubin is water soluble and is excreted, in a small part, in the urine.

Related Tests

- Liver enzymes such as alkaline phosphatase (ALP) (p. 42), lactic dehydrogenase (LDH) (p. 278), aspartate aminotransferase (AST) (p. 105), alanine aminotransferase (ALT) (p. 33), and 5′-nucleotidase (p. 312) are very helpful in the evaluation of the liver.
- Complete blood count (p. 162), haptoglobin (p. 247), and other blood tests are helpful in the evaluation of hemolytic anemias.

Bleeding Time (Ivy Bleeding Time)

Normal Findings 1-9 minutes (Ivy method)

Critical Values >15 minutes on repeated evaluation

Indications

The bleeding time test is used to evaluate the vascular and platelet factors associated with hemostasis. It is frequently performed on preoperative patients to ensure adequate hemostasis.

Test Explanation

When vascular injury occurs, the first hemostatic response is a spastic contraction of the lacerated microvessels. Next, platelets adhere to the wall of the vessel at the area of laceration in an attempt to plug the hole. Failure of either process results in a prolonged bleeding time. If platelets are present in inadequate quantities (usually less than 50,000), the bleeding time will be prolonged. If the platelet function is inadequate (as in patients with uremia or after recent ingestion of aspirin), the bleeding time will be prolonged. If vessel constriction is inadequate (such as in the elderly or in patients with increased capillary fragility), the bleeding time will be prolonged.

For this study, a small, standard superficial incision is made in the forearm, and the time required for the bleeding to stop is recorded. This is called the bleeding time. Normal values vary according to the method used; the Ivy bleeding time test is most often used today. Because vessel constriction and platelet adherence are not affected by coagulation (intrinsic and extrinsic system), defects in this part of hemostasis will not affect the bleeding time. Therefore this test only evaluates platelet function and quantity and vascular constriction capability. This is not an accurate test of platelet number. This can better be quantified by a direct platelet count.

A single prolonged bleeding time does not prove with certainty that an abnormality exists. A larger vessel could potentially be lacerated during the test and bleeding time prolonged not because of a defect in hemostasis, but rather because the caliber of the vessel is too large to stop bleeding without pressure. Therefore abnormal bleeding times should be repeated to ensure accuracy. Test performance may also vary among technicians, thereby altering results. Prolonged values occur in the following:

1. Patients with decreased platelet counts or function
2. Patients with disseminated intravascular coagulation (DIC) resulting from consumption of platelets
3. Patients with uremia, because the platelets are reduced in number and function
4. Patients with warfarin (Coumadin) overdosage
5. Patients with increased capillary fragility secondary to collagen vascular disease, Cushing's disease, or Henoch-Schönlein syndrome (purpura)
6. Patients ingesting antiinflammatory drugs (e.g., aspirin, indomethacin)

Contraindications

- Patients with known low platelet counts
- Patients who are unable to cooperate
- Patients who cannot have a blood pressure cuff placed on the arm (e.g., those with cellulitis)
- Patients with a history of keloid formation (They must be told of the potential for scar.)
- Patients with senile skin changes (Their capillaries are fragile and vessel constriction is inadequate.)
- Patients who have had an axillary lymph node dissection (eg., breast cancer patients) (Avoid the arm on that side.)

Potential Complications

- Skin infection
- Excessive bleeding from test site

Interfering Factors

- Aggressively wiping the site of laceration can prolong the test results.
- Extremes in body temperatures can alter results. High temperatures can prolong results; low body temperatures can factitiously shorten results.
- Drugs that may cause *increased* bleeding times include alcohol, anticoagulants, dextran, indomethacin, salicylates, streptokinase, allopurinol, some antibiotics, halothane, nonsteroidal antiinflammatory drugs, urokinase, and warfarin.

Procedure and Patient Care

Before

- Explain the procedure to the patient.
- Obtain a consent form if required by the institution.
- Tell the patient that no fasting is required.
- Obtain a drug history to detect if the patient has recently had aspirin, anticoagulants, alcohol, or any other medications that may affect test results.
- Inform the patient that minor discomfort may occur with this test because of the skin laceration.

During

- Note the following procedural steps:
  1. The skin of the inner part of the forearm is cleansed with alcohol or povidone-iodine (Betadine).
  2. A blood pressure cuff is applied on the arm above the elbow, inflated to 40 mm Hg, and maintained at this pressure during the study.
  3. A small laceration is then made 1-mm deep into the skin, and the time is recorded.
  4. Bleeding ensues, and the blood is wiped clean at 30-second intervals.

5. When no new bleeding occurs, the time is again noted.
6. The interval from the beginning to the end of bleeding is calculated. This is the bleeding time.
7. The blood pressure cuff is then removed, and an adhesive dressing is applied to the patient's arm.
8. If bleeding persists for more than 10 minutes, the test is stopped and a pressure dressing is applied.

- Indicate on the laboratory slip any medications that may affect test results.
- Note that this test is usually performed by a laboratory technician in less than 10 minutes.

After

- Apply pressure or a pressure dressing to the puncture site.
- Assess the puncture site for bleeding.
- Abnormal results should be rechecked.

Test Results and Clinical Significance

Prolonged times or increased values

Bone marrow failure
Primary or metastatic tumor infiltration of bone marrow
Thrombocytopenia
Leukemia
Production of platelets is diminished and quantity decreases.

Hypersplenism *Platelets are consumed (extracted from the bloodstream) by the enlarged spleen.*

von Willebrand's disease
Glanzmann's thrombasthenia
Uremia
Bernard-Soulier syndrome
Platelet function (adherence to the vessel wall to form a plug) is reduced.

DIC *Platelets are consumed and quantities decrease.*
Cushing's disease
Collagen vascular disease
Henoch-Schönlein syndrome
Severe liver disease
Capillary fragility abnormalities and purpuras
Connective tissue disorder
Hereditary telangiectasia
The microvessels are too fragile and are incapable of constricting adequately to allow hemostasis.

Related Tests

- Platelet count (p. 337): This is a direct measurement of platelet number.
- Platelet volume, mean (p. 340): This is a direct measurement of platelet volume.
- Platelet aggregation (p. 333): This is a direct measurement of platelet function.

- Platelet antibody (p. 335): This test identifies antiplatelet antibodies that destroy the platelet.
- Tourniquet test (p. 428): This test evaluates capillary fragility.
- Thrombin time (p. 408): This is a test of the fibrinogen-to-fibrin reaction.
- Prothrombin time (p. 366): This test is used to evaluate the adequacy of the extrinsic system and common pathway in the clotting mechanism.
- Coagulating factor concentration (p. 154): This is a quantitative measurement of specific coagulation factors.
- Partial thromboplastin time (p. 319): This test is used to evaluate the intrinsic system and the common pathway of clot formation. It is most commonly used to monitor heparin therapy.

Blood Typing

Normal Findings Compatibility

Indications

This test is used to determine the blood type of the patient prior to donating or receiving blood and to determine the blood type of expectant mothers to assess the risks of Rh incompatibility between mother and newborn.

Test Explanation

With blood typing, ABO and Rh antigens can be detected in the blood of prospective blood donors and potential blood recipients. This test is also used to determine the blood type of expectant mothers and newborns. The ABO system, Rh factors, and blood cross-matching are reviewed below.

ABO system

Human blood is grouped according to the presence or absence of these antigens. The two major antigens, A and B, form the basis of the ABO system. The surface membranes of group A RBCs contain A antigens; group B RBCs contain B antigens on their surface; group AB RBCs have both A and B antigens; and group O RBCs have neither A nor B antigens (Table 2-10). In general, a person will not have antibodies to match the surface antigen on their RBCs. That is, persons with group A antigen (type A) blood will not have anti-A antibodies. However, they may have anti-antibodies. The opposite is true for persons with group B antigens. Group O blood may have both anti-A and anti-B antibodies. Blood transfusions are actually transplantations of tissue (blood) from one person to another. It is important that the recipient not have antibodies to the donor's RBCs. If this were to occur, there could be a hypersensitivity reaction, which can vary from mild fever

Table 2-10 Blood types

Blood type (ABO, Rh)	Antigens present	Antibodies possibly present	Percent of general population
O, +	Rh	A, B	35
O, − *	None	A, B, Rh	7
A, +	A, Rh	B	35
A, −	A	B, Rh	7
B, +	B, Rh	A	8
B, −	B	A, Rh	2
AB, +†	A, B, Rh	None	4
AB, −	A, B	Rh	2

*Universal donor.
†Universal recipient.

to anaphylaxis with severe intravascular hemolysis. If donor ABO antibodies are present against the recipient antigens, usually only minimal reactions occur unless the recipient is immunocompromised.

Persons with group O blood are considered universal donors, because they do not have antigens on their RBCs. Persons with group AB blood are considered universal recipients because they have no antibodies to react to the transfused blood. Group O blood is often transfused in emergent situations where rapid life-threatening blood loss occurs and immediate transfusion is required. There is no time for crossmatching (about 20 minutes). The chance of a transfusion reaction is least with type O.

Rh factors

The presence or absence of Rh antigens on the surface of RBCs determines the classification of Rh positive or Rh negative. Rh factor is the next most important antigen associated with a blood transfusion after ABO compatibility. The major Rh factor is Rh_oD. There are several minor Rh factors. If Rh_oD is absent, the minor Rh antigens are tested. If negative, the patient is considered Rh negative (Rh−). The incidence of each blood type is noted in Table 2-10

Rh− persons may develop antibodies to Rh antigens if exposed to Rh positive (Rh+) blood by prior transfusions or fetal-maternal blood mixing. All women who are pregnant should have a blood typing and Rh factor determination. If the mother's blood is Rh−, the father's blood should also be typed. If his blood is Rh+, the woman's blood should be examined for the presence of Rh antibodies (by the indirect Coombs' test). If the initial screening is negative (no antibodies to Rh found), the test is repeated at 28 to 30 weeks and 36 weeks of pregnancy. If these tests are also negative, the fetus is not at risk. However, if the test is positive, the fetus is at risk for hemolytic disease of the newborn (erythroblastosis fetalis). In this disease the mother is Rh− and the fetus is Rh+. Any fetal bleeding that occurs can sensitize the mother to form anti-Rh antibodies. These antibodies cross the placenta and hemolyze the fetal RBCs. Problems ranging from mild fetal anemia to in utero fetal death could occur. The severity of the hemolytic anemia can be evaluated by determining the quantity of bilirubin in the amniotic fluid (amniocentesis).

Hemolytic disease of the newborn can be prevented by Rh typing during pregnancy. If the mother is Rh−, she should be advised that she is a candidate for RhoGAM (Rh immunoglobulin that "neutralizes" the Rh antigen) after the delivery. RhoGAM can reduce the chance of fetal hemolytic problems during subsequent pregnancies.

Blood crossmatching

Although typing for the major ABO and Rh antigens is no guarantee that a reaction will not occur, it does greatly reduce the possibility of such a reaction. Many potential minor antigens are not routinely detected during blood typing. If allowed to go unrecognized, these minor antigens also can initiate a blood transfusion reaction. Therefore blood is not only typed but also crossmatched to identify a mismatch of blood caused by minor antigens. Crossmatching consists of the mixing of the recipient's serum with the donor's RBCs in saline solution followed by the addition of Coombs' serum (indirect Coombs' test). Only blood products containing RBCs need to be crossmatched. Plasma products do not need to be crossmatched but should be ABO compatible because other cells (WBCs and platelets) have ABO antigens.

Homologous (donor and recipient are different people) and directed (recipient chooses the donor) blood donation must be rigorously tested prior to transfusion (Box 2-3). Autologous (recipient and donor is the same person) blood transfusions, however, are not subject to that same testing. It is important to note, however, that autologous blood transfusion is not 100% safe. As a result of the additives used for banking purposes, blood and hypersensitivity reactions can still occur.

Finally, one must be aware of graft-versus-host disease in which donor lymphocytes included in the blood transfusion may engraft and multiply in the recipient. These lymphocytes can react against the recipient's tissues. This is most common among immunocompromised patients. Pretransfusion radiation will avoid this problem.

Interfering Factors

- Non-ABO or non-Rh (D) minor antibodies can interfere with obtaining an adequate crossmatch.

Box 2-3 Blood tests required on donated blood

ABO typing
Rh typing
Rh antibody screen
Hepatitis B surface antigen
Hepatitis B core antigen
Hepatitis C antibody
Syphilis
HIV testing antibody 1 and 2
HIV antigen
HTLV 1 testing
Liver hepatocellular enzyme (ALT)

Procedure and Patient Care

Before

- Explain the procedure to the patient.
- Tell the patient that no fasting is required.

During

- Collect approximately 7 to 14 ml of venous blood in a red-top tube. (This may vary among laboratories.)
- Avoid hemolysis.
- Label the blood tube appropriately before sending it to the laboratory.

After

- Apply pressure or a pressure dressing to the venipuncture site.
- Assess the venipuncture site for bleeding.

Test Results and Clinical Significance

ABO type
Rh type
Crossmatch compatibility

Related Tests

- Coombs' test, indirect (p. 165): This test detects circulating antibodies against RBCs.
- Amniocentesis (p. 560): This is a test of amniotic fluid, which may demonstrate some evidence of hemolytic disease of the newborn.

CA 19-9 Tumor Marker (Cancer Antigen 19-9)

Normal Findings <37 U/ml

Indications

CA 19-9 antigen is a tumor marker used for the diagnosis of patients with pancreatic or hepatobiliary cancer, evaluation of response to treatment, and surveillance.

Test Explanation

CA 19-9 is a carbohydrate cell-surface antigen. It exists on the surface of cancer cells. Although initially thought to be specific for colorectal cancer, it is now used primarily in the evaluation of patients with pancreatic or hepatobiliary cancers. In the diagnosis of pancreatic carcinoma, for example, the presence of a pancreatic mass or biliary obstruction and greatly elevated CA 19-9 levels would support the diagnosis of pancreatic cancer over benign pancreatitis. Likewise, patients whose presenting symptoms are ascites, jaundice, and elevated CA 19-9 levels would be suspected of having hepatobiliary cancer. CA 19-9 levels, however, may not be elevated in all patients with pancreatic carcinoma. Approximately 70% of patients with pancreatic carcinoma and 65% of patients with hepatobiliary cancer have elevated levels.

CA 19-9 levels are used in the posttreatment surveillance of those who have had pancreatic or hepatobiliary cancers. In the few patients with pancreatic or biliary cancer who have a good response to surgery, chemotherapy, or radiation therapy, a decline in serum levels of CA 19-9 will confirm this response. A rapid rise in CA 19-9 levels may be associated with recurrent or progressive tumor growth. Mildly elevated levels may exist in patients with gastric cancer, colorectal cancer, hepatoma, and even in 6% to 7% of patients with non-GI malignancies. Patients who have pancreatitis, gallstones, cirrhosis, inflammatory bowel disease, or cystic fibrosis also can have minimally elevated levels of CA 19-9.

Because of its lack of sensitivity and specificity, CA 19-9 is not effective in screening for pancreatobiliary tumors in the general population.

CLINICAL PRIORITIES

- CA 19-9 is *not* used as a screening test for pancreatic or hepatobiliary tumors because of its lack of sensitivity and specificity.
- CA 19-9 is used to support the diagnosis of pancreatic or hepatobiliary tumors and to monitor patients' response to treatment.

Procedure and Patient Care

Before

- Explain the procedure to the patient.
- Tell the patient that no fasting is required.

During

- Collect 7 to 10 ml of blood in a red-top tube.
- Have the blood sent to a central diagnostic laboratory for CA 19-9 determinations. The results are available to the local hospital in 7 to 10 days.

After

- Apply pressure or a pressure dressing to the venipuncture site.
- Observe the venipuncture site for bleeding.

Test Results and Clinical Significance

Increased levels

Pancreatic carcinoma
Hepatobiliary carcinoma
Pancreatitis

Cholecystitis
Cirrhosis
Gastric cancer
Colorectal cancer
Gallstones
Lung cancer
CA 19-9 antigen is released from the surface of the cancer cell and leaks into the bloodstream where it can be detected.

Related Test

- Carcinoembryonic antigen (CEA) (p. 137): This is another tumor marker that is elevated in patients with pancreatobiliary cancer.

CA 27.29 and CA 15-3 Tumor Marker
(Cancer Antigen 15-3)

Normal Findings

CA 27.29: <38 U/ml
CA 15-3: <22 U/ml

Indications

The CA 15-3 and CA 27.29 antigens are tumor-associated serum markers available for staging breast cancer and monitoring its treatment.

Test Explanation

Carcinoembryonic antigen, the most widely used tumor marker, is limited by poor sensitivity and specificity for patients with breast cancer. Most recently monoclonal antibody technology has permitted the development of CA 15-3 and CA 27.29 antigens. These antigens are not as sensitive for the diagnosis of primary breast cancer as other tumor markers are for their respective tumors. That is, CA 15-3 and CA 27.29 levels are high in only 50% of patients who have a localized breast cancer or a small tumor burden. Eighty percent of patients with metastatic breast cancer, however, do have elevated CA 15-3 levels and 65% have elevated CA 27.29 levels; therefore the usefulness of these antigen tests as a screening technique in early breast cancers (the most common cancer of women) is quite limited.

Benign breast disease and nonbreast malignancies (e.g., lung, pancreas, ovary, prostate) also can cause elevation of these antigen levels. These antigens are useful in monitoring the patient's response to therapy of metastatic breast cancer. A partial or complete response to treatment will be confirmed by declining levels. Likewise, a persistent rise in these antigen levels despite therapy strongly suggests progressive disease.

CA 15-3 or CA 27.29 levels cannot be used in the surveillance of patients who have had a complete response to breast cancer surgery, radiation therapy, or chemotherapy. The high sensitivity and low specificity noted with these markers often inaccurately suggest recurrent disease when none is present. Other benign diseases may be found instead. The use of these antigens should be limited to monitoring the treatment of advanced disease. CA 15-3 was the first breast tumor marker available. It is not FDA approved. It is usually performed by a reference laboratory using competitive inhibition radioimmune assay. The CA 27.29 marker has recently received FDA approval. The test is done by immunoradiometric assay.

CLINICAL PRIORITIES

- CA 27.29 and CA 15-3 tumor markers are *not* used for screening of *early* breast cancers.
- These tumor antigens are used for monitoring the patient's response to therapy for metastatic breast cancer. Declining levels suggest a good response to therapy; rising levels suggest disease progression.

Interfering Factors

- Some of the other benign and malignant diseases associated with elevations of these antigens include cancer of the lung, ovary, pancreas, prostate, and colon; fibrocytic disease of the breast; cirrhosis; and hepatitis.

Procedure and Patient Care

Before

- Explain the procedure to the patient.
- Tell the patient that no fasting is required.

During

- Collect 7 to 10 ml of venous blood in a red-top tube.
- Have the blood sample sent to a central diagnostic laboratory for CA 15-3 determinations. The results are available to the local hospital in 7 to 10 days.

After

- Apply pressure or a pressure dressing to the venipuncture site.
- Observe the venipuncture site for bleeding.

Test Results and Clinical Significance

Increased levels

Metastatic breast cancer *Breast cancer antigens on the surface of the breast cancer cell leak into the bloodstream where they can be detected.*

Related Tests

- Carcinoembryonic antigen (CEA) (p. 137): This is another tumor marker used in the monitoring of breast cancer.

CA-125 Tumor Marker (Cancer Antigen-125)

Normal Findings 0-35 U/ml

Indications

CA-125 is used in the detection of ovarian cancer. It is also used to determine the extent of disease and to monitor the response to treatment.

Test Explanation

This tumor marker has a high degree of sensitivity and specificity for ovarian cancer. Just as alpha-fetoprotein (AFP) and human chorionic gonadotropin (HCG) are accurate tumor markers for germ cell tumors of the ovary, CA-125 is an extremely accurate marker for nonmucinous epithelial tumors of the ovary. It is elevated in over 80% of women with ovarian cancer.

The CA-125 marker can be used in many ways. By and of itself, it cannot be used to diagnose ovarian cancer, but it helps support the diagnosis of ovarian cancer. For example, a greatly elevated CA-125 level in women who have abdominal distention, ascites, and a palpable pelvic mass is strong confirmation that the underlying etiology is an epithelial ovarian malignancy.

The CA-125 serum tumor marker is also used to determine a patient's response to therapy. Comparative serial testing will show a progressive decline in CA-125 levels for patients responding to treatment. Also, CA-125 tumor markers can predict whether or not a second-look (repeat) diagnostic laparotomy will be positive. A second-look laparotomy will detect a residual tumor in 97% of patients whose CA-125 level is greater than 35 U/ml, whereas only 56% of patients with ovarian cancer whose CA-125 level is less than 35 U/ml will have a positive second-look laparotomy. A precipitous fall in CA-125 after two courses of chemotherapy is an accurate predictor of a complete response to chemotherapy and is used as a good prognostic sign.

Finally, CA-125 determinations can be used in posttreatment surveillance of patients with ovarian cancer. In a patient who has had a complete response to radiation therapy, chemotherapy, or surgery, a delayed rise in the CA-125 level is an early predictor of a recurrent tumor in 93% of patients. Abnormal levels can antedate the appearance of obvious recurrent ovarian cancer by 2 to 7 months.

CA-125 is not an effective screening test for the asymptomatic general public because of its lack of specificity. It is used in "high-risk" women who have a strong family history of ovarian cancer. Elevated levels in the general population indicate that either benign or malignant disease is present in 95% of patients.

Other tumors and benign processes can cause elevated CA-125 levels as well. Diseases that affect the peritoneum, such as cirrhosis, pancreatitis, peritonitis, endometriosis, and pelvic inflammatory disease, can cause elevated levels of CA-125. Other malignancies occurring in the female genital tract, pancreas, colon, lung, and breast can also be associated with elevated levels of this protein. A total of 1% to 2% of the normal population have CA-125 levels in excess of 35 U/mL.

CLINICAL PRIORITIES

- CA-125 is used in detecting ovarian cancer and in determining its extent and response to treatment.
- CA-125 is *not* an effective screening test for asymptomatic women because of its lack of specificity. It is used in "high-risk" women with a strong history of ovarian cancer.
- CA-125 levels can be used to determine the need for a second-look (repeat) diagnostic laparotomy in women being followed after ovarian cancer therapy.

Interfering Factors

- The first trimester of pregnancy and normal menstruation may be associated with mild elevations of CA-125 levels.
- Patients with benign peritoneal diseases (e.g., cirrhosis, endometriosis) will have mildly increased levels.

Procedure and Patient Care

Before

- Explain the procedure to the patient.
- Tell the patient that no fasting or sedation is required.

During

- Collect 7 to 10 ml of blood in a red-top tube.
- Have the blood sent to a central diagnostic laboratory for determination of CA-125 level.
- The results are available to the local hospital in 3 to 7 days.

After

- Apply pressure or a pressure dressing to the venipuncture site.
- Observe the venipuncture site for bleeding.
- Provide emotional support to the patient. Cancer testing is very stressful.

Test Results and Clinical Significance

Increased levels

MALIGNANT DISORDERS

Cancer of the ovary

Cancer of the pancreas
Cancer of the colon
Cancer of the lung
Peritoneal carcinomatosis
Cancer of the nonovarian female genital tract
Cancer of the breast
Lymphoma
The CA-125 antigen from the surface ovarian cancer cells leaks into the blood where it can be detected.

BENIGN DISORDERS

Cirrhosis
Peritonitis
Pregnancy
Endometriosis
Pancreatitis
Pelvic inflammatory disease
The mechanism of elevated CA-125 in these diseases is not known.

Related Tests

- Carcinoembryonic antigen (CEA) (p. 137): This tumor marker can be elevated in ovarian epithelial tumors.
- Alpha-fetoprotein (p. 47): This tumor is elevated in nonepithelial ovarian tumors.
- Human chorionic gonadotropin (p. 348): This tumor is elevated in nonepithelial ovarian tumors.

Calcitonin (Human Calcitonin [HCT], Thyrocalcitonin)

Normal Findings

Basal

Males: ≤19 pg/ml or 19 ng/L (SI units)
Females: ≤14 pg/ml or 14 ng/L (SI units)

Calcium infusion (2.4 mg/kg)

Males: ≤190 pg/ml or 190 ng/L
Females: ≤130 pg/ml or 130 ng/L

Pentagastrin injection (0.5 mg/kg)

Males: ≤110 pg/ml or 110 ng/L
Females: ≤30 pg/ml or 30 ng/L

Indications

This test is usually indicated to evaluate persons with suspected medullary carcinoma of the thyroid. Calcitonin is useful in monitoring response to therapy and predicting recurrences of medullary thyroid cancer. It is also useful as a screening test for those with a family history of medullary cancer.

Test Explanation

Calcitonin is a hormone secreted by the parafollicular or C cells. Secretion is stimulated by elevated serum calcium levels. Calcitonin contributes to calcium homeostasis. It decreases serum calcium levels by inhibiting bone resorption and increasing calcium excretion by the kidneys.

This test is usually used in the evaluation of patients with or suspected to have medullary carcinoma of the thyroid. Seventy-five percent of these patients have hypersecretion of calcitonin despite normal serum calcium levels. Calcitonin is useful in monitoring response to therapy and predicting recurrences of medullary thyroid cancer. It is also useful as a screening test for those with a family history of medullary cancer and therefore at high risk (20%) for medullary cancer. This is a cancer of the thyroid with a familiar tendency and if found late has a poor prognosis. Routine screening for elevated calcitonin levels can detect medullary cancer early and improve chances for cure. Calcitonin can be used as a tumor marker in monitoring patients with medullary cancer of the thyroid. Increases in calcitonin levels herald progression of the cancer. Declining levels indicate tumor regression. C-cell hyperplasia, a benign calcitonin-producing disease that also has a familial tendency, is also associated with elevated calcitonin levels.

Equivocal elevations in calcitonin levels should be followed with further provocative testing using pentagastrin or calcium to stimulate calcitonin secretion. Pentagastrin stimulation involves an IV infusion over 5 to 10 seconds with blood samples drawn before the injection and at 90 seconds, 2 minutes, and 5 minutes following the infusion. The calcium infusion test can be performed in a variety of ways but is most commonly administered over a 1-minute interval with baseline and 5- and 10-minute postinfusion blood levels. With medullary cancer of the thyroid, the provocative tests can cause the calcitonin to rise significantly (often greater than 1000 mg/L).

Elevated levels of calcitonin also may be seen in people with cancer of the lung, breast, and pancreas. This is probably a form of paraneoplastic syndrome in which there is an ectopic production of calcitonin by the nonthyroid cancer cells.

Interfering Factors

- Levels are often elevated in normal pregnant females and in newborns.
- Drugs that may cause *increased* levels include calcium, cholecystokinin, epinephrine, glucagon, pentagastrin, and oral contraceptives.

Procedure and Patient Care

Before

- Explain the procedure to the patient.

- Tell the patient that an overnight fast is required. Water is permitted.

During

- Collect a venous sample of blood in a heparinized green-top or a chilled red-top tube according to the laboratory's protocol.
- The specimen should be placed on ice immediately. The blood is frozen and sent to a reference laboratory.

After

- Apply pressure or a pressure dressing to the venipuncture site.
- Assess the venipuncture site for bleeding.
- Tell the patient that results may not be available for several days since this test is often sent to a reference laboratory for analysis.

Test Results and Clinical Significance

Increased levels

Medullary carcinoma of thyroid
G-cell hyperplasia
Calcitonin is secreted by the thyroid in these diseases despite high calcium blood levels. These abnormalities are not responsive to the normal regulatory feedback mechanisms.

Oat cell carcinoma of lung
Breast carcinoma
Pancreatic cancer
These cancers can act as an autonomous ectopic site of calcitonin production.

Primary hyperparathyroidism
Secondary hyperparathyroidism as a result of chronic renal failure
These states are associated with high serum calcium levels. High calcitonin levels may be compensatory.

Pernicious anemia
Zollinger-Ellison syndrome
Several endocrine familial and nonfamilial multiple endocrinopathies (APUDomas) may be associated with high calcitonin levels.

Alcoholic cirrhosis *The mechanism is not well defined. Perhaps the liver cannot metabolize hormones well and high levels of calcitonin result.*
Thyroiditis

Related Tests

- Calcium, blood (p. 130): This is a direct measurement of the serum calcium level.

Calcium, Blood (Total/Ionized Calcium, Ca^{++})

Normal Findings

Age	mg/dl	mmol/L
	TOTAL CALCIUM	
< 10 days	7.6-10.4	1.9-2.60
Umbilical	9.0-11.5	2.25-2.88
10 days-2 years	9.0-10.6	2.3-2.65
Child	8.8-10.8	2.2-2.7
Adult*	9.0-10.5	2.25-2.75
	IONIZED CALCIUM	
Newborn	4.20-5.58	1.05-1.37
2 months-18 years	4.80-5.52	1.20-1.38
Adult	4.5-5.6	1.05-1.30

*Values tend to decrease in the elderly.

Critical Values

Total calcium: <6.0 or >13 mg/dl or <1.5 or >3.25 mmol/L (SI units)
Ionized calcium: <2.2 or >7.0 mg/dl or <0.78 or >1.58 mmol/L (SI units)

Indications

The serum calcium test is used to evaluate parathyroid function and calcium metabolism by directly measuring the total amount of calcium in the blood. Serum calcium levels are used to monitor patients with renal failure, renal transplantation, hyperparathyroidism, and various malignancies. They are also used to monitor calcium levels during and after large-volume blood transfusions.

Test Explanation

Serum calcium is necessary in many metabolic enzymatic pathways. It is vital for muscle contractility, cardiac function, neural transmission, and blood clotting. The serum calcium test is used to evaluate parathyroid function and calcium metabolism by directly measuring the total amount of calcium in the blood. The bone and the teeth act as a reservoir for calcium. When blood levels decrease, parathyroid hormone (PTH) release is stimulated. This hormone acts on the reservoirs to release calcium into the blood. About one half of the total calcium exists in the blood in its free (ionized) form, and about one half exists in its protein-bound form (mostly with albumin). The serum calcium level is a measure of both. As a result, when the serum albumin level is low (as in malnourished patients), the serum calcium level will also be low, and vice versa. As a rule of thumb, the total serum calcium level decreases by approximately 0.8 mg for every 1-g decrease in the serum albumin level. Serum albumin should be measured with serum calcium.

The ionized form of calcium also can be measured by ion-selective electrode techniques or can be calculated from several available formulas. An advantage of measuring the ionized form is that it is unaffected by changes in serum albumin levels. Some physicians consider measurement of ionized calcium more sensitive and reliable than that of total calcium in the detection of primary hyperparathyroidism. Other physicians, however, do not agree. Many laboratories do not have the equipment to perform the ionized calcium assay. Certainly, when albumin levels are variable, measurement of ionized calcium can allow more accurate calcium replacement therapy if needed. This is especially true during open heart surgery, major organ transplantation, and renal dialysis.

When the serum calcium level is elevated on at least three separate determinations, the patient is said to have hypercalcemia. Symptoms of hypercalcemia may include anorexia, nausea, vomiting, somnolence, and coma. The most common cause of hypercalcemia is hyperparathyroidism. Parathormone causes elevated calcium levels by increasing GI absorption, decreasing urinary excretion, and increasing bone resorption. Malignancy, the second most common cause of hypercalcemia, can cause elevated calcium levels in two main ways. First, tumor metastasis (myeloma, lung, breast, renal cell) to the bone can destroy the bone, causing resorption and pushing calcium into the blood. Second, the cancer (lung, breast, renal cell) can produce a PTH-like substance that drives the serum calcium up (ectopic PTH). Excess vitamin D ingestion can increase serum calcium by increasing renal and GI absorption. Granulomatous infections such as sarcoidosis and tuberculosis are associated with hypercalcemia.

In some instances a normal serum calcium does not preclude hypercalcemia. For example, if the serum calcium is normal in a patient with reduced serum albumin (the calcium should be reduced in these patients), hypercalcemia should be suspected. A similar situation exists in patients with chronic renal failure. These patients have high phosphate levels and other anions that tend to chronically lower serum calcium. As a result, PTH is persistently stimulated to increase calcium levels. The calcium levels return to normal in time, but that "normal" level actually represents a "high" level when one considers that it should be low in these individuals. This is the classic case of secondary hyperparathyroidism.

Hypocalcemia occurs in patients with hypoalbuminemia. The most common causes of hypoalbuminemia are malnutrition (especially in alcoholics) and large-volume IV infusions. Because one-half of the calcium is bound to albumin, when albumin is low, calcium should be expected to be low. Large blood transfusions are associated with low serum calcium levels, because the citrate additives used in banked blood for anticoagulation bind the free calcium in the recipient's bloodstream. Intestinal malabsorption, renal failure, rhabdomyolysis, alkalosis, and acute pancreatitis (due to saponification of fat) are also known to be associated with low serum calcium levels. Hypomagnesemia can be associated with refractory hypocalcemia. Symptoms of hypocalcemia include nervousness, excitability, and tetany.

Interfering Factors

- Vitamin D intoxication may cause increased serum calcium levels.
- Excessive ingestion of milk may cause increased levels.
- Serum pH can affect calcium values. A decrease in pH causes increased calcium levels.

- Prolonged tourniquet time will lower pH and factitiously increase calcium levels.
- There is normally a small diurnal variation in calcium, with peak levels occurring around 9 PM.
- Hypoalbuminemia is associated with decreased levels of total calcium.
- Drugs that may cause *increased* levels include calcium salts, hydralazine, lithium, thiazide diuretics, PTH, thyroid hormone, alkaline antacids, calcium salts, ergocalciferol, androgens, and vitamin D.
- Drugs that may cause *decreased* levels include acetazolamide, anticonvulsants, asparaginase, aspirin, calcitonin, cisplatin, corticosteroids, heparin, laxatives, loop diuretics, magnesium salts, thiazide diuretic, estrogens, albuterol, and oral contraceptives.

Procedure and Patient Care

Before

- Explain the procedure to the patient.
- Tell the patient that no fasting is required; however, the serum calcium may be part of a multichemical analysis in which fasting is required for the other studies.

During

- Collect approximately 7 ml of venous blood in a red-top tube.
- Avoid prolonged tourniquet use.
- List on the laboratory slip any medications that may affect test results.

After

- Apply pressure or a pressure dressing to the venipuncture site.
- Assess the venipuncture site for bleeding.

Test Results and Clinical Significance

Increased levels (hypercalcemia)

Hyperparathyroidism
Nonparathyroid PTH-producing tumor (e.g., lung or renal carcinoma)
Parathormone or a similar hormone mobilizes calcium stores from the bone to the blood.

Metastatic tumor to bone
Paget's disease of bone
Prolonged immobilization
Bone destruction or thinning pushes calcium from the bone and into the blood.

Milk-alkali syndrome *With increased ingestion of milk products or antacids (which contain calcium), the serum calcium level can be elevated.*

Vitamin D intoxication *Vitamin D works synergistically with PTH to increase serum calcium.*

Lymphoma
Granulomatous infections such as sarcoidosis and tuberculosis.
These diseases are associated with enhanced levels of vitamin D, which works synergistically with PTH to increase serum calcium.

Addison's disease *Glucocorticosteroids inhibit vitamin D activity. When steroid activity is decreased, vitamin D action is enhanced. Vitamin D works synergistically with PTH to increase serum calcium.*
Acromegaly
Hyperthyroidism

Decreased levels (hypocalcemia)

Hypoparathyroidism *PTH acts to increase serum calcium. If PTH levels are reduced, serum calcium declines.*

Renal failure
Hyperphosphatemia secondary to renal failure
Excess anions, present in patients with renal failure, bind serum calcium.

Rickets
Vitamin D deficiency
Vitamin D acts synergistically with PTH. PTH acts to increase serum calcium. Without that synergism, calcium levels decline.

Osteomalacia
Malabsorption
Less calcium is available to the blood.

Pancreatitis
Fat embolism
Pancreatitis is associated with saponification (binding of calcium to fats) of the peripancreatic tissue. This reduces the calcium from the blood.

Alkalosis *High pH in the blood drives the calcium to intracellular spaces. Blood levels decline.*

Related Tests

- Parathyroid hormone (p. 316): This is a measurement of PTH, which increases serum calcium levels.
- Albumin (p. 358): This is a direct measurement of serum albumin. Albumin has a major effect on serum calcium metabolism.

Carbon Dioxide Content (CO_2 Content, CO_2-Combining Power, Bicarbonate [HCO_3^-])

Normal Findings

Adult/elderly: 23-30 mEq/L or 23-30 mmol/L (SI units)
Child: 20-28 mEq/L
Infant: 20-28 mEq/L
Newborn: 13-22 mEq/L

Critical Values $<$6 mEq/L

Indications

The CO_2 content is a measure of CO_2 in the blood. In the peripheral venous blood this is used to assist in evaluating the pH status of the patient and to assist in evaluation of electrolytes.

Test Explanation

The serum CO_2 test is usually included with other electrolyte assessments. It is usually performed using a multiphasic testing machine that also measures sodium, potassium, chloride, BUN, and creatinine. It is important not to confuse this test with Pco_2. This CO_2 content measures H_2CO_3, dissolved CO_2 and the bicarbonate ion (HCO_3^-) that exists in the serum. Because the amounts of H_2CO_3 and dissolved CO_2 in the blood are so small, CO_2 content is an indirect measure of HCO_3^- anion. HCO_3^- anion is second in importance to the chloride ion in electrical neutrality (negative charge) of extracellular and intracellular fluid; it plays a major role in acid-base balance.

Levels of HCO_3^- are regulated by the kidneys. Increases occur with alkalosis, and decreases occur with acidosis. This test as it is performed on arterial blood is discussed further on p. 97. When CO_2 content is measured in the laboratory with other serum electrolytes, air affects the specimen and the CO_2 partial pressure can be altered. Therefore venous blood specimens are not highly accurate for measuring true CO_2 content or HCO_3^-. It is primarily used as a rough guide as to acid-base balance.

Interfering Factors

- Underfilling the tube with blood allows CO_2 to escape from the serum specimen and may significantly reduce HCO_3^- values.
- Drugs that may cause *increased* serum CO_2 and HCO_3^- levels include aldosterone, barbiturates, bicarbonates, ethacrynic acid, hydrocortisone, loop diuretics, mercurial diuretics, and steroids.
- Drugs that may cause *decreased* levels include methicillin, nitrofurantoin (Furadantin), paraldehyde, phenformin, tetracycline, thiazide diuretics, and triamterene.

Procedure and Patient Care

Before

- Explain the procedure to the patient.
- Tell the patient that no fasting is required.

During

- Collect approximately 7 to 10 ml of venous blood in a red- or green-top tube.

After

- Apply pressure or a pressure dressing to the venipuncture site.
- Assess the venipuncture site for bleeding.

Test Results and Clinical Significance

Increased levels

Severe vomiting
High-volume gastric suction
Aldosteronism
Use of mercurial diuretics
Important acid hydrogen ions are lost. HCO_3^- ions are relatively high.

Chronic obstructive pulmonary disease *HCO_3^- ions are increased to compensate for chronic hypoventilation (high Pco_2). This is compensation for respiratory acidosis.*
Metabolic alkalosis *Metabolic alkalosis is defined by an increased amount of HCO_3^- anions in the blood.*

Decreased levels

Chronic diarrhea
Chronic use of loop diuretics
Persistent loss of base ions, including HCO_3^-. Most of the CO_2 content is HCO_3^-.

Renal failure
Diabetic ketoacidosis
Starvation
Ketoacids and other anions are built up. HCO_3^- neutralizes these acids. HCO_3^- levels therefore drop.

Metabolic acidosis *Metabolic acidosis is defined by a decreased amount of HCO_3^- anions in the blood.*
Shock *Lactic acid builds up and is buffered by the HCO_3^-, therefore HCO_3^- levels diminish.*

Related Tests

- Arterial blood gases (p. 97): This is a battery of arterial blood tests that are used to evaluate acid-base homeostasis. CO_2 content and HCO_3^- are components of that test.

Carboxyhemoglobin
(COHb, Carbon Monoxide [CO])

Normal Findings

Nonsmoker: <3% of total hemoglobin
Light smoker: 2%-5%
Heavy smoker: 5%-10%
Newborn: ≥12%

Critical Values >20%

Indications This test is used to detect CO poisoning.

Test Explanation

This test measures the amount of serum COHb, which is formed by the combination of CO and hemoglobin (Hgb). CO combines with Hgb 200 times more readily than O_2 can combine with Hgb (oxyhemoglobin). This results in fewer Hgb bonds available to combine with O_2. Furthermore, when CO occupies the O_2-binding sites, the hemoglobin molecule is changed so as to bind the remaining O_2 more tightly. This greater affinity of CO for Hgb and change in O_2-binding strength does not allow the O_2 to readily pass from the RBCs to the tissue. Less O_2 is therefore available for tissue cell respiration. This results in hypoxemia. CO poisoning is documented by Hgb analysis for COHb. A specimen should be drawn as soon as possible after exposure, because CO is rapidly cleared from the Hgb by breathing normal air. O_2 saturation studies and oximetry are inaccurate in CO-exposed patients, because they measure all forms of O_2-saturated hemoglobin, including COHb. In these circumstances the results will be normal, even though the patient is hypoxemic.

This test can also be used to evaluate patients with complaints of headache, irritability, nausea, vomiting, and vertigo, who may have been, unknowingly, exposed to CO. Its greatest use, however, is in patients exposed to smoke inhalation, exhaust fumes, and fires. Other sources of CO include tobacco smoke, petroleum and natural gas fuel fumes, automobile exhaust, unvented natural-gas heaters, and defective gas stoves. Symptoms of CO poisoning correlated with blood levels are shown in Table 2-11. CO toxicity is treated by administering high concentrations of O_2 to displace the COHb.

✓ CLINICAL PRIORITIES

- CO combines with Hgb 200 times more readily than O_2 can combine with Hgb. This results in hypoxemia.
- CO poisoning is documented by the COHb test. Specimens should be drawn as soon as possible after exposure, because CO is rapidly cleared from the Hgb by breathing normal air.
- CO toxicity is treated by administration of high concentrations of O_2 to displace the COHb.

Table 2-11 Symptoms of CO poisoning by level of Hgb saturation

CO-saturated Hgb (%)	Symptoms
10	Slight dyspnea
20	Headache
30	Irritability, disturbed judgment, memory loss
40	Confusion, weakness, dimness of vision
50	Fainting, ataxia, collapse
60	Coma
>60	Death

Procedure and Patient Care

Before

- Explain the procedure to the patient or the family.
- Obtain the patient history relative to any possible source of CO inhalation.
- Assess the patient for signs and symptoms of mild CO toxicity (e.g., headache, weakness, dizziness, malaise, dyspnea) and moderate to severe CO toxicity (e.g., severe headache, bright-red mucous membranes, cherry-red blood). Maintain patient safety precautions if confusion is present.

During

- Collect approximately 5 to 10 ml of venous blood in a lavender- or green-top tube.

After

- Apply pressure or a pressure dressing to the venipuncture site.
- Assess the venipuncture site for bleeding.
- Treat the patient as indicated by the physician. Usually the patient receives high concentrations of O_2.
- Encourage respirations to allow the patient to clear CO from the Hgb.

Test Results and Clinical Significance

Increased levels

CO poisoning

Related Tests

- Oximetry (p. 1013): This test is used to easily and continuously monitor O_2 saturation of Hgb.
- Oxygen saturation (p. 97): This test measures the amount of Hgb saturated by O_2.

Carcinoembryonic Antigen (CEA)

Normal Findings

<5 ng/ml or 0.0-2.5 mg/L (SI units)

Indications

This tumor marker is used for determining the extent of disease and prognosis in patients with cancer (especially GI or breast). It is also used in monitoring the disease and its treatment.

Test Explanation

CEA is a protein that normally occurs in fetal gut tissue. By birth, detectable serum levels disappear. In the early 1960s CEA was found to exist in the bloodstream of adults who had colorectal tumors. It was originally thought to be a specific indicator of the presence of colorectal cancer. Subsequently, however, this tumor marker has been found in patients who have a variety of carcinomas (e.g., breast, pancreatic, gastric, hepatobiliary), sarcomas, and even many benign diseases (e.g., ulcerative colitis, diverticulitis, cirrhosis). Chronic smokers also have elevated CEA levels.

Because the CEA level can be elevated in both benign and malignant diseases, it is not a specific test for colorectal cancer. Furthermore, not all colorectal cancers produce CEA. Therefore CEA is not a reliable screening test for the detection of colorectal cancer in the general population. Its use is limited to determining the prognosis and monitoring the response of tumor to antineoplastic therapy in a patient with cancer. This is especially helpful in patients with breast and GI cancers. The initial pretreatment CEA level is an indicator of tumor burden and therefore prognosis. Patients with smaller and early-stage tumors are likely to have low CEA levels, if not normal CEA levels. Patients with more advanced or metastatic tumors are likely to have high CEA levels. A drastic reduction of the preoperative CEA to normal levels indicates complete eradication of the tumor. Therefore this test is used to determine the efficacy of treatment.

This test also is used in the surveillance of patients with cancer. A steadily rising CEA level is occasionally the first sign of tumor recurrence. This makes CEA testing very valuable in the follow-up of patients who have already had potentially curative therapy. It is important to reiterate that many (about 20%) patients with advanced breast or GI tumors may not have elevated CEA levels.

CEA can also be detected in body fluids other than blood. Its presence in those body fluids indicates metastasis. This test is commonly performed on peritoneal fluid or chest effusions. Elevated CEA levels in these fluids indicate metastasis to the peritoneum or pleural, respectively. Likewise, elevated CEA levels in the CSF indicate CNS metastasis.

Interfering Factors

- Smokers tend to have higher CEA levels than nonsmokers.
- Benign diseases (e.g., cholecystitis, colitis, diverticulitis) and especially liver diseases (e.g., hepatitis, cirrhosis) are also associated with elevated CEA levels.

Procedure and Patient Care

Before

- Explain the procedure to the patient.
- Tell the patient that no fasting is required.

During

- Collect a peripheral blood specimen. The collecting tube varies according to the commercial laboratory. (The two most frequently used laboratories for this test are Abbott Laboratories and Roche Laboratories.) Diagnostic kits are now available so that CEA can be tested at most local hospitals.
- Indicate on the laboratory slip if the patient smokes or has diseases that can affect test results.

After

- Apply pressure or a pressure dressing to the venipuncture site.
- Observe the venipuncture site for bleeding.

Test Results and Clinical Significance

Increased levels

Cancer (GI, breast, lung, pancreatic, hepatobiliary) *The cancer cells produce CEA on their cell surface. By a yet unrecognized mechanism, the CEA leaks into the bloodstream. Elevated levels result.*
Inflammation (colitis, cholecystitis, pancreatitis, diverticulitis)
Cirrhosis
Peptic ulcer
The mechanism by which benign diseases produce CEA is unknown.

Related Tests

- CA 27.29 and CA 15-3 (p. 123): These antigens are tumor-associated serum markers available for staging breast cancer and monitoring the treatment of the disease.
- CA 19-9 (p. 121): This tumor marker is elevated in pancreatobiliary tumors and colorectal tumors.

Ceruloplasmin (Cp)

Normal Findings

Adults: 23-43 mg/dl
Neonates: 2-13 mg/dl

Indications

This test is an acute-phase reactant protein and can indicate an acute illness. However, its primary use is in the diagnosis of preclinical states of Wilson's disease.

Test Explanation

Cp is an alpha$_2$-globulin that binds copper for transport within the bloodstream after it is absorbed from the GI tract. Levels are decreased in most instances of Wilson's disease, which is an inherited disorder. Patients who are homozygous for this disease make very little Cp. High unbound copper blood levels result and are toxic to tissues. The copper is deposited in the eye, brain, liver, and kidney. Wilson's disease is fatal unless early treatment is instituted. If this disease is identified before significant copper deposits affect major organs, the ravages of the disease can be avoided. Cp levels are obtained in children at high risk for the disease. Teenagers and young adults with hepatitis, cirrhosis, or recurrent neuromuscular incoordination (signs compatible with Wilson's disease) should also have this test. Early detection is important, because therapy is effective in most cases.

Cp is also an acute-phase reactant protein that becomes elevated during stress, infection, and pregnancy. However, it rises more slowly than other acute-phase reactants, such as C-reactive protein, and erythrocyte sedimentation rate.

Interfering Factors

- Values are increased during pregnancy.
- Drugs that may cause *increased* levels include estrogen, birth control pills, tamoxifen, methadone, and phenytoin.

Procedure and Patient Care

Before

- Explain the procedure to the patient.
- Tell the patient that no fasting is required.

During

- Collect venous blood in a red-top tube.
- Keep the specimen on ice.

After

- Apply pressure or a pressure dressing to the venipuncture site.
- Assess the venipuncture site for bleeding.
- Medical follow-up and genetic counseling are indicated when Wilson's disease is confirmed.

Test Results and Clinical Significance

Increased levels

Pregnancy
Thyrotoxicosis
Cancer
Acute inflammatory reaction (e.g., infection, rheumatoid arthritis)
Biliary cirrhosis
These diseases induce the synthesis of Cp as an acute-phase reactant.

Copper intoxication *Copper elevation will stimulate Cp in normal people.*

Decreased levels

Wilson's disease *Patients with this disease have homozygous or heterozygous genes and are unable to make Cp. Homozygous patients have lower Cp levels than heterozygous patients.*

Normal infants (6 months) *Young infants normally are unable to make adequate amounts of acute-phase reactant proteins (alpha$_2$-globulins) until they are 6 months of age.*

Nephrotic syndrome

Sprue
These are protein-losing diseases. Cp is a protein that is lost in these diseases and therefore blood levels fall.

Kwashiorkor
Starvation
Nutritional deficiencies are associated with low serum proteins, including Cp.

Menkes' (kinky-hair) syndrome *This is an inherited disorder associated with defects in the production of alpha$_2$-globulins such as Cp.*

Related Tests

- C-reactive protein (p. 172): This is a test for an acute-phase reactant protein.
- Erythrocyte sedimentation rate (p. 199): This is a test for an acute-phase reactant protein.

Chloride, Blood (Cl)

Normal Findings

Adult/elderly: 90-110 mEq/L or 98-106 mmol/L (SI units)
Child: 90-110 mEq/L
Newborn: 96-106 mEq/L
Premature infant: 95-110 mEq/L

Critical Values <80 or >115 mEq/L

Indications

This test is performed as a part of multiphasic testing for what is usually called "electrolytes." By itself, not much information is obtained. However, with interpretation of the other electrolytes, chloride can give an indication of acid-base balance and hydrational status.

Test Explanation

Chloride is the major extracellular anion. Its primary purpose is to maintain electrical neutrality, mostly as a salt with sodium. It follows sodium (cation) losses and accompanies sodium excesses in an attempt to maintain electrical neutrality. For example, when aldosterone encourages sodium reabsorption, chloride follows to maintain electrical neutrality. Because water moves with sodium and chloride, chloride also affects water balance. Finally, chloride also serves as a buffer to assist in acid-base balance. As carbon dioxide (and H cation) increases, bicarbonate must move from the intracellular space to the extracellular space. To maintain electrical neutrality, chloride will shift back into the cell.

Hypochloremia and hyperchloremia rarely occur alone and usually are part of parallel shifts in sodium or bicarbonate levels. Signs and symptoms of hypochloremia include hyperexcitability of the nervous system and muscles, shallow breathing, hypotension, and tetany. Signs and symptoms of hyperchloremia include lethargy, weakness, and deep breathing.

Interfering Factors

- Excessive infusions of saline solution can result in increased chloride levels.
- Drugs that may cause *increased* serum chloride levels include acetazolamide, ammonium chloride, androgens, chlorothiazide, cortisone preparations, estrogens, guanethidine, hydrochlorothiazide, methyldopa, and nonsteroidal antiinflammatory drugs.
- Drugs that may cause *decreased* levels include aldosterone, bicarbonates, corticosteroids, cortisone, hydrocortisone, loop diuretics, thiazide diuretics, and triamterene.

Procedure and Patient Care

Before

- Explain the procedure to the patient.
- Tell the patient that no fasting is required.

During

- Collect 5 to 10 ml of venous blood in a red- or green-top tube.

After

- Apply pressure or a pressure dressing to the venipuncture site.
- Assess the venipuncture site for bleeding.

Test Results and Clinical Significance

Increased levels (hyperchloremia)

Dehydration *Chloride ions are more concentrated in the blood.*
Excessive infusion of normal saline solution *Intake of chloride exceeds output, and blood levels rise.*

Metabolic acidosis
Renal tubular acidosis
Cushing's syndrome
Kidney dysfunction
Hyperparathyroidism
Eclampsia
Chloride urinary excretion is decreased.

Respiratory alkalosis *Chloride is driven out of the cell in place of* HCO_3^-.

Decreased levels (hypochloremia)

Overhydration
Syndrome of inappropriate secretion of antidiuretic hormone (SIADH)
Chloride is diluted.

Congestive heart failure *Chloride is retained with sodium retention but is diluted by excess total body water.*

Vomiting or prolonged gastric suction
Chronic diarrhea or high-output GI fistula
Chloride cation is high in the stomach and GI tract because of HCl acid produced in the stomach.

Chronic respiratory acidosis
Metabolic alkalosis
Chloride is driven into the cell to compensate for the HCO_3^- that leaves the cell to maintain pH neutrality.

Salt-losing nephritis
Addison's disease
Diuretic therapy
Hypokalemia
Aldosteronism
Chloride excretion is increased.

Burns *Sodium and chloride losses from the massive burn can be great.*

Related Tests

- Sodium, potassium, bicarbonate (pp. 396, 342, 133): These are other electrolytes commonly measured with chloride.
- Chloride, urine (p. 827): This is a measurement of chloride in the urine.

Cholesterol

Normal Findings

Adult/elderly: <200 mg/dl or 5.20 mmol/L (SI units)
Child: 120-200 mg/dl
Infant: 70-175 mg/dl
Newborn: 53-135 mg/dl

Indications

Cholesterol testing is used to determine the risk for coronary heart disease (CHD). It is also used for evaluation of hyperlipidemias.

Test Explanation

Cholesterol is the main lipid associated with arteriosclerotic vascular disease. Cholesterol, however, is required for the production of steroids, sex hormones, bile acids, and cellular membranes. Most of the cholesterol we eat comes from foods of animal origin. The liver metabolizes the cholesterol to its free form, and cholesterol is transported in the bloodstream by lipoproteins. Nearly 75% of the cholesterol is bound to low-density lipoproteins (LDL), and 25% is bound to high-density lipoproteins (HDLs). Cholesterol, therefore, is the main component of LDL and only a minimal component of HDL and very-low-density lipoprotein (VLDL). It is the LDL that is most directly associated with increased risk of CHD.

The purpose of cholesterol testing is to identify patients at risk for arteriosclerotic heart disease. Cholesterol testing is usually done as a part of lipid profile testing, which also evaluates lipoproteins and triglycerides, because, by itself, cholesterol is not a totally accurate predictor of heart disease. There is considerable overlap in what are considered "normal" and "high-risk" levels. "Normal" levels have been derived from a group of patients who have no obvious evidence of CHD. However, this may not be accurate since these patients may have preclinical CHD and may not truly reflect a "no-risk" population.

There is considerable variation in cholesterol levels. Day-to-day cholesterol values in the same individual can vary by 15%. An 8% difference can even be identified within the same day. Positional changes can affect these levels. Levels can decrease by as much as 15% in the recumbent position. As a result, hospitalized patients can be expected to have lower levels than outpatients. Because of these significant variabilities, elevated results should be corroborated by repeating the study. The two results should be averaged to obtain an accurate cholesterol level for risk assessment.

Because the liver is required to metabolize ingested cholesterol products, subnormal cholesterol levels are indicative of severe liver diseases. Furthermore, because our main

Table 2-12 ***Total cholesterol as an indicator of CHD in mg/100 ml (SI units: mmol/L)****

Age (yr)	Low risk	Moderate risk	High risk
2-19	<170 (4.4)	171-185	>185 (4.8)
20-29	<200 (5.5)	201-220	>220 (5.7)
30-39	<220 (5.7)	221-240	>240 (6.2)
>40	<240 (6.2)	241-260	>260 (6.8)

*When cholesterol testing is combined with lipoproteins, risk of CHD can be more accurately calculated.

Table 2-13 ***Cholesterol-to-HDL ratio as an indicator of risk of CHD****

	Ratio	
Risk	Male	Female
One-half average	3.4	3.3
Average	5.0	4.4
2 × average	10.0	7.0
3 × average	24.0	11.0

*When cholesterol testing is combined with lipoproteins, risk of CHD can be more accurately calculated.

source of cholesterol is our diet, malnutrition is also associated with low cholesterol levels. Certain illnesses can affect cholesterol levels. For example, patients with an acute myocardial infarction may have as much as a 50% reduction in cholesterol level for as long as 6 to 8 weeks.

In 1984 the National Institutes of Health developed a consensus statement in regard to total cholesterol levels and risk of CHD (Table 2-12). The cholesterol-to-HDL ratio has been used to assess the risk of CHD (Table 2-13).

Familial hyperlipidemias and hyperlipoproteinemias are often associated with high cholesterol.

Interfering Factors

- Pregnancy is usually associated with elevated cholesterol levels.
- Oophorectomy and postmenopausal status are associated with increased levels.
- Recumbent position is associated with decreased levels.
- Drugs that may cause *increased* levels include adrenocorticotropic hormone, anabolic steroids, beta-adrenergic blocking agents, corticosteroids, epinephrine, oral contraceptives, phenytoin (Dilantin), sulfonamides, thiazide diuretics, cyclosporine, and vitamin D.
- Drugs that may cause *decreased* levels include allopurinol, androgens, bile salt–binding agents, captopril, chlorpropamide, clofibrate, colchicine, colestipol, erythromycin, isoniazid, liothyronine (Cytomel), lovastatin (Mevacor), monoamine oxidase inhibitors, neomycin (oral), niacin, and nitrates.

CLINICAL PRIORITIES

- Cholesterol testing is usually done as part of lipid profile testing, which also evaluates lipoproteins and triglycerides.
- Because of considerable variations in cholesterol values, elevated results should be verified by repeating the test.
- Test preparation usually requires a 12- to 14-hour fast after eating a low-fat meal. Only water is permitted.

Procedure and Patient Care

Before

- Instruct the patient to fast 12 to 14 hours after eating a low-fat meal before testing. Only water is permitted. Actually, cholesterol levels increase only minimally after a meal. However, early-morning fasting cholesterol levels are more easily compared when performed serially. Furthermore, lipoproteins, which are often ordered simultaneously, are affected by a previous meal. Therefore fasting is usually requested.
- Indicate to the patient that dietary intake for 2 weeks before testing will affect results. It is suggested that the patient eat a normal diet for at least 1 week before testing.
- Tell the patient that no alcohol should be consumed 24 hours before the test.

During

- Collect 5 to 10 ml of blood in a red-top tube.
- Indicate on the laboratory slip any drugs that may affect cholesterol levels.
- The fingerstick method is also often used for mass screening. There is less than a 5% difference in cholesterol measurements with these two methods.

After

- Apply pressure or a pressure dressing to the venipuncture site.
- Assess the venipuncture site for bleeding.
- Instruct patients with high levels regarding the following:
  Low-cholesterol diet
    Avoid animal fats.
    Replace saturated fats with polyunsaturated fats.
    Increase ingestion of fruits and vegetables.
  Exercise
  Appropriate body weight

Test Results and Clinical Significance

Increased levels

Familial hypercholesterolemia
Familial hyperlipidemia
Enzymatic deficiencies in lipid metabolism are associated with elevated cholesterol.

Increased cholesterol levels are associated with hypothyroidism, uncontrolled diabetes mellitus, nephrotic syndrome, pregnancy, high-cholesterol diet, xanthomatosis, hypertension, myocardial infarction, atherosclerosis, biliary cirrhosis, and extrahepatic biliary, stress, and nephrotic syndrome.
The pathophysiology of the association of cholesterol with these diseases is not well known. The association has been made by observation.

Decreased levels

Malabsorption
Malnutrition
Advanced cancer
Most of the cholesterol is synthesized from fat eaten in the diet. When dietary intake is decreased, fat levels and subsequently cholesterol levels fall.

Decreased levels of cholesterol are also associated with hyperthyroidism, cholesterol-lowering medication, pernicious anemia, hemolytic anemia, sepsis/stress, liver disease, and acute myocardial infarction.
The pathophysiology of the association of cholesterol with these diseases is not well known. The association has been made by observation.

Related Tests

- Apolipoprotein (p. 93): These polypeptides are associated with lipoproteins and have been used as accurate indicators of risk for CHD.

- Lipoprotein (p. 289): HDL and LDL play an important role in the transport of lipids in the bloodstream. They, too, have been used in the assessment of risk for CHD.
- Triglyceride (p. 432): This test is a measure of total triglycerides in the blood. It is a part of the lipid profile.

Cholinesterase
(CHS, Pseudocholinesterase, Cholinesterase RBC, Red Cell Cholinesterase, Acetylcholinesterase)

Normal Findings

0.5-1.5 mg/dl or 5-15 mg/L (SI units)
7-19 U/ml or 7-19 kU/L (SI units)

Values vary with laboratory test methods.

Indications

This test is done to identify patients with pseudocholinesterase deficiency prior to anesthesia or to identify patients who may have phosphate poisoning.

Test Explanation

Cholinesterases hydrolyze acetylcholine and also other choline esters and thereby regulate nerve impulse transmission at the nerve synapse and neuromuscular junction. There are two types of cholinesterases: acetylcholinesterase, also known as "true cholinesterase," and pseudocholinesterase. True cholinesterase exists primarily in the RBCs and nerve tissue. It is not in the serum. Pseudocholinesterase, on the other hand, exists in the serum. Deficiencies in either of these enzymes can be acquired or congenital.

Because succinylcholine (a muscle relaxant commonly used during anesthesia induction) is inactivated by pseudocholinesterase, people with an inherited pseudocholinesterase enzyme deficiency exhibit increased sensitivity to the effects of succinylcholine. Prolonged muscle paralysis and apnea occur after anesthesia. This situation can be avoided by measuring pseudocholinesterase directly on all patients with a family history of prolonged apnea after surgery.

A common form of acquired cholinesterase deficiency, either true or pseudocholinesterase, is overexposure to pesticides or organophosphates. Measurement of true cholinesterase is more valuable in cases of suspected prolonged overexposure because RBC levels take longer to decrease than serum pseudocholinesterase and take longer to return to normal after exposure. Persons with jobs associated with chronic exposure to these chemicals are often monitored by frequent testing of cholinesterase levels. Other potential causes include chronic liver diseases, malnutrition, and hypoalbuminemia. If an abnormally low level of cholinesterase is found, inhibition using dibucaine can indicate whether the cause is acquired (reduced inhibition) or congenital (no inhibition).

Interfering Factors

- Pregnancy decreases test values.
- Drugs that may cause *decreased* values include atropine, caffeine, codeine, estrogens, morphine sulfate, neostigmine, oral contraceptives, phenothiazines, theophylline, quinidine, steroids, and vitamin K. It is important to recognize that pseudocholinesterase levels cannot be measured in postoperative patients in the recovery room if the patient is not regaining muscular function, because often one or more of the above drugs may be given during the surgery and could invalidate the results.

Procedure and Patient Care

Before

- Explain the procedure to the patient.
- Tell the patient that no fasting is required.
- If the test is done to identify the presurgical patient who may be at risk for cholinesterase deficiency, be sure the test is done several days prior to the planned surgery.
- It may be recommended to withhold medications that could alter test results for 12 to 24 hours before the test.

During

- Collect a venous blood sample in a red-top tube.
- Include a listing of all medications taken by the person with the laboratory requisition slip.

After

- Apply pressure or a pressure dressing to the venipuncture site.
- Assess the venipuncture site for bleeding.

Test Results and Clinical Significance

Increased Levels

Reticulocytosis *Increased RBC precursors are associated with higher levels of true cholinesterase.*

Hyperlipidemia
Nephrosis
Diabetes
Increased levels are observed without any known pathophysiology.

Decreased levels

Poisoning from organic phosphate insecticides *These chemicals inhibit the activity of cholinesterases.*
Hepatocellular disease
Persons with congenital enzyme deficiency *Cholinesterases are not synthesized.*
Malnutrition and other forms of hypoalbuminemia *Albumin is important in the transport and function of cholinesterases.*

Related Tests

- Acetylcholine receptor antibody (p. 19): This is a measurement of an antibody that blocks the activity of cholinesterases. It is commonly found in patients with myasthenia gravis.

Chromosome Karyotype
(Blood Chromosome Analysis, Chromosome Studies, Cytogenetics, Karyotype)

Normal Findings

Female: 44 autosomes, 2 X chromosomes; karyotype: 46,XX
Male: 44 autosomes, 1 X, 1 Y chromosome; karyotype: 46,XY

Indications

This test is used to study an individual's chromosome makeup to determine chromosomal defects associated with disease or the risk of developing disease.

Test Explanation

The term "karyotyping" refers to the arrangement of cell chromosomes from the largest to the smallest to analyze their number and structure. Variations in either can produce numerous developmental abnormalities and diseases. A normal karyotype of chromosomes consists of a pattern of 22 pairs of autosomal chromosomes and a pair of sex chromosomes: XY for the male and XX for the female. Chromosomal karyotype abnormalities can be congenital or acquired. These karyotype abnormalities can occur because of duplication, deletion, translocation, reciprocation, or genetic rearrangement.

Chromosome karyotyping is useful in evaluating congenital anomalies, mental retardation, growth retardation, delayed puberty, infertility, hypogonadism, primary amenorrhea, ambiguous genitalia, chronic myelogenous leukemia, neoplasm, recurrent miscarriage, prenatal diagnosis of serious congenital diseases (especially when advanced maternal age is a factor), Turner's syndrome, Klinefelter's syndrome, Down syndrome, and other suspected genetic disorders. The products of conception also can be studied to determine the cause of stillbirth or miscarriage.

The most common form of karyotyping is performed by banding techniques. This technique provides a method of pairing similar chromosomes based on their size, location of the centromere (constriction that divides the chromosome into long and short arms) and other constrictions, ratio of long to short arms, satellite DNA, and banding patterns. With this method, a characteristic karyotype is determined. An extensive nomenclature system for the types has been developed.

Special chromosome studies can be performed on cells grown in special medium to identify certain chromosome abnormalities. DNA testing has recently become possible through the use of DNA probes and DNA linkage studies. Recurrent amino acid patterns are identified with this type of testing. They may be associated with or be near a particular gene. With these techniques, certain genes, pathologic and otherwise, can be recognized. The exact relationship of a genetic defect to a particular disease is still unknown. Not only is the pathophysiology unknown, but the frequency of clinically significant disease for any genetic defect is unknown. For example, it is not known how many women with the BRCA 1 (breast cancer) gene on the 17q chromosome will, indeed, develop breast cancer. Only long-term studies will answer these difficult questions even after the genetic and chromosome codes have been worked out.

Procedure and Patient Care

Before

- Explain the procedure to the patient.
- Determine how the specimen will be collected.
- Obtain preparation guidelines from the laboratory if indicated.
- Many patients are fearful of the test results and require considerable emotional support.
- In some states, informed consent is required.

During

- Specimens for chromosome analysis can be obtained from numerous sources. Leukocytes from a peripheral venipuncture site are the most easily obtained and most often used for this study.
- Bone marrow biopsies and surgical specimens also can sometimes be used as sources for analysis.
- During pregnancy, specimens can be collected by amniocentesis (see p. 560) and chorionic villus sampling (see p. 1006).
- Fetal tissue or products of conception can be studied as well to determine the reason for the loss of the fetus.
- Smears and stains of buccal mucosal cells are less costly but not as accurate as other tissue for karyotyping.

After

- Aftercare depends on how the specimen was collected.
- Inform the patient that test results are generally not available for weeks to several months.
- If an abnormality is identified, often the entire family line must be tested. This can be exhaustive and expensive.
- If the test results show an abnormality, encourage the patient to verbalize his or her feelings. Provide emotional support.

Test Results and Clinical Significance

Abnormal findings

Chromosome abnormalities can be a cause of congenital anomalies, mental retardation, growth retardation, delayed puberty, infertility, hypogonadism, primary amenorrhea, ambiguous genitalia, chronic myelogenous leukemia, neoplasm, recurrent miscarriage, pre-

Table 2-14 Common chromosome abnormalities

Chromosome abnormality	Clinical manifestation or syndrome
Trisomy 21	Down
Single X	Turner's
Extra X in male (XXY)	Klinefelter's
5p deletion	Cat-cry
15q deletion	Prader-Willi
3q trisomy	Cornelia de Lange's
Fragile X	Mental retardation
X centromere dislocation	Roberts'
Philadelphia	Chronic myelogenous leukemia, acute myelogenous leukemia

natal diagnosis (e.g., Down syndrome, Tay-Sachs disease, sickle cell anemia) in situations of advanced maternal age, Turner's syndrome, Klinefelter's syndrome, and Down syndrome. (See Table 2-14 for some of the commonly known abnormalities.)

Related Tests

- Barr body analysis (p. 638): This is an inexpensive test for detecting chromatin material (X chromatin).

Clot Retraction
(Whole-Blood Clot Retraction Test)

Normal Findings

50%-100% clot retraction in 1-2 hours
Complete retraction within 24 hours

Indications

This is a qualitative assessment of platelet number and function.

Test Explanation

The clot retraction test is used to evaluate bleeding disorders. Clot retraction is prolonged in thrombocytopenia (i.e., decreased platelet count) and Glanzmann's thrombasthenia (abnormal platelet function). Blood is collected in a tube free of anticoagulants. The time required to form a clot and for the edges of the clot to retract from the sides of the glass tube is the clot retraction time. The clot should be separate from the clear serum. It should maintain its shape (a mold of the glass tube) after being removed from the tube. If the platelet count is reduced or the function of the platelets is inadequate, the clot may

Table 2-15 **Minimum concentration of coagulation factors required for adequate fibrin production**

Factor	Minimal hemostatic level (mg/dl)	Blood components*
I	60-100	C, FFP, FWB
II	10-15	P, WB, FFP, FWB
V	5-10	FFP, FWB
VII	5-20	P, WB, FFP, FWB
VIII	30	C, FFP, VIII CONC
IX	30	FFP, FWB
X	8-10	P, WB, FFP, FWB
XI	25	P, WB, FFP, FWB

*Blood components capable of providing specific factor: C = cryoprecipitate; FFP = fresh frozen plasma; FWB = fresh whole blood (<24 hours old); P = unfrozen banked plasma; WB = banked whole blood; VIII CONC = factor VIII concentrate.

only be weakly formed and may have very little if any retraction from the tube side walls. On removal, the clot will be shapeless and dissipate. Clot retraction is rarely used today because of the availability of accurate platelet counts and more accurate methods of determining platelet dysfunction.

If fibrinolysins are present, no clot retraction will occur. This test is only reliable if the hematocrit and fibrinogen (factor I) concentration (Table 2-15) are within normal limits. If the hematocrit is high (polycythemia or hemoconcentration), clot retraction is reduced. If fibrinogen is reduced, clot retraction will be shortened. Poor whole-blood clot retraction also occurs in patients with thrombasthenia (abnormal platelets) and Waldenström's macroglobulinemia.

Contraindications

- Patients with low platelet counts
- Patients with hypofibrinogenemia
- Patients taking aspirin

In patients with the above-noted conditions, the clot retraction can be expected to be prolonged.

Interfering Factors

- With uremia, the platelet function is reduced and clot retraction can be expected to be prolonged.
- When the hematocrit is high, serum volume is reduced and clot retraction will decrease.
- If fibrinolysis is present (e.g., disseminated intravascular coagulation), clot retraction may not be noticed as lysis takes place simultaneously.
- Drugs that may *prolong* test results include aspirin and nonsteroidal antiinflammatory agents.

Procedure and Patient Care

Before

- Explain the procedure to the patient.
- Tell the patient that no fasting is required.

During

- Avoid excessive probing during venipuncture if a coagulation disorder is suspected.
- Collect approximately 5 to 7 ml of venous blood in a red-top tube.
- Avoid hemolysis.
- Indicate on the laboratory slip if the patient is taking aspirin or a nonsteroidal antiinflammatory agent.

After

- Transport the specimen to the laboratory within 1 hour of collection.
- Apply pressure or a pressure dressing to the venipuncture site.
- Assess the venipuncture site for bleeding and bruising.

Test Results and Clinical Significance

Increased clot retraction

Severe anemia *The red cellular component of blood is decreased, allowing for a smaller clot that is more easily formed.*

Hypofibrinogenemia *Fibrin degradation is an important stimulant to the plasminogen fibrinolytic system. Without fibrinogen, fibrinolysis is reduced and clot retraction is increased.*

Decreased or poor clot retraction

Thrombocytopenia
von Willebrand's disease
Thrombasthenia (abnormal platelets)
Waldenström's macroglobulinemia
Reduced platelet number or function is associated with poor clot retraction.

Related Tests

- Platelet count (p. 337): This is a direct measurement of platelet number.
- Euglobulin lysis time (p. 207): This is a measurement of the fibrinolytic system.
- Platelet aggregation (p. 333): This is a measurement of platelet function.
- Platelet antibody (p. 335): This test provides identification of antibodies directed against platelets.
- Bleeding time (p. 115): This test of coagulation is affected by platelet number and function.
- Platelet volume, mean (p. 340): This is a measurement of the size of the platelets. It is helpful in the evaluation of thrombocytopenia.

Coagulating Factor Concentration
(Factor Assay, Coagulating Factors, Blood-Clotting Factors)

Normal Findings

Factor	Normal value (% of "normal")
II	80-120
V	50-150
VII	65-140
VIII	55-145
IX	60-140
X	45-155
XI	65-135
XII	50-150

Indications

The coagulating factor concentration test measures the concentration of specific coagulating factors in the blood.

Test Explanation

These tests measure the quantity of each specific factor suspected to be responsible for suspected defects in hemostasis. Testing is available to measure the quantity of the factors listed in Table 2-16. When these factors exist in concentrations below their "minimal he-

Table 2-16 ***Coagulation factors***

Factor	Name	Quantitation available	Abnormal coagulation tests associated with deficiency
I	Fibrinogen	Yes	
II	Prothrombin	Yes	Prothrombin time
III	Tissue factor or thromboplastin	No	Prothrombin time
IV	Calcium	Yes	
V	Proaccelerin	Yes	Prothrombin time, activated partial thromboplastin time
VII	Stable factor	Yes	Prothrombin time
VIII	Antihemophilic factor	Yes	Activated partial thromboplastin time
IX	Christmas factor	Yes	Activated partial thromboplastin time
X	Stuart factor	Yes	Prothrombin time, activated partial thromboplastin time
XI	Plasma thromboplastin antecedent	Yes	Activated partial thromboplastin time
XII	Hageman factor	Yes	Activated partial thromboplastin time, whole-blood clotting
XIII	Fibrin-stabilizing factor	No	

mostatic level," clotting will be impaired. These minimal hemostatic levels vary according to the factor involved (see Table 2-15). Their replacement blood components are also listed in Table 2-15 (see p. 152).

Deficiencies of these factors may be a result of inherited genetic defects, acquired diseases, or drug therapy. Common medical conditions associated with decreased factor concentrations are listed in Table 2-17. It is important to identify the exact factor or factors involved in the coagulating defect so that appropriate blood component replacement can be administered (Figure 2-9).

Table 2-17 ***Conditions that may result in coagulation factor deficiency***

Condition	Diminished factors
Liver disease	I, II, V, VII, IX, X, XI
Disseminated intravascular coagulation	I, V, VIII
Fibrinolysis	I, V, VIII
Congenital deficiency	I, II, V, VII, VIII, IX, X, XI, XII
Heparin administration	II
Warfarin ingestion	II, VII, IX, X, XI
Autoimmune disease	VIII
Vitamin K deficiency or maldigestion	II, VII, IX, X, XI

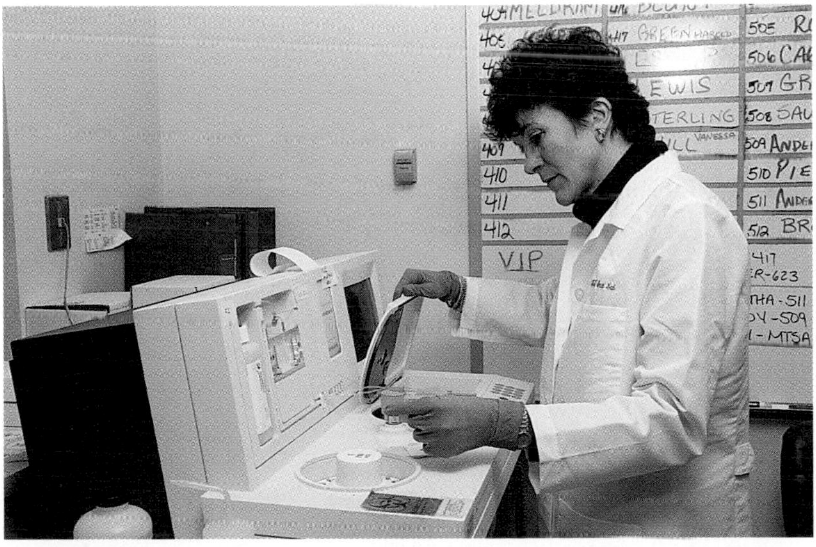

Figure 2-9 Laboratory analysis of coagulating factor concentration.

The hemostasis and coagulation system is a homeostatic balance between factors encouraging clotting and factors encouraging clot dissolution. The first reaction of the body to active bleeding is blood vessel constriction. In small-vessel injury this may be enough to stop bleeding. In large-vessel injury, hemostasis is required to form a clot that will durably plug the hole until healing can occur. The primary phase of the hemostatic mechanism involves platelet aggregation to the blood vessel (Figure 2-10). Secondary hemostasis then occurs. The first phase of reactions is called the intrinsic system. Factor XII and other proteins form a complex on the subendothelial collagen in the injured blood vessel. Through a series of reactions, activated factor XI (XIa) is formed and activates factor IX (IXa). In a complex formed by factors VIII, IX, and X, activated X (Xa) is formed.

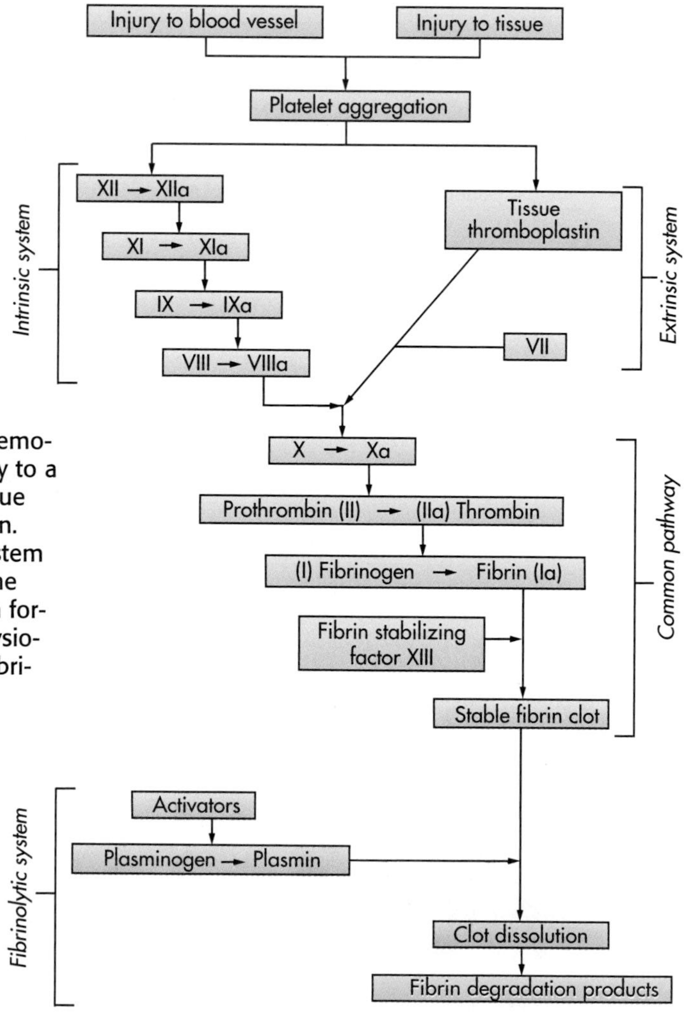

Figure 2-10 Process of hemostasis and fibrinolysis. Injury to a blood vessel surface or tissue initiates platelet aggregation. The intrinsic or extrinsic system is activated and activates the common pathway for fibrin formation. Finally, fibrin is physiologically dissolved by the fibrinolytic system.

At the same time the extrinsic system is activated and a complex is formed between tissue thromboplastin (factor III) and factor VII (which is exposed after cellular injury). Activated factor VII (VIIa) results. Factor VIIa can directly activate factor X. Alternatively, VIIa can activate factors IX and X together.

The final step is a common pathway whereby prothrombin is converted to thrombin on the surface of the aggregated platelets. The main purpose of thrombin is to convert fibrinogen to fibrin, which is polymerized into a stable gel. Factor XIII crosslinks the fibrin polymers to a stable clot.

Almost immediately, three major activators of the fibrinolytic system act on plasminogen, which had previously been absorbed into the clot, to form plasmin. Plasmin degenerates the fibrin polymer into fragments, which are cleared by macrophages.

Roman numerals have been assigned by the order in which the factor had been identified, not by their order in the above-noted hemostatic mechanism. (See Table 2-16 for a list of factor names and for routine coagulation test abnormalities associated with factor deficiency.)

Fibrinogen, like many other of the coagulation proteins, is considered an acute-phase reactant protein and is elevated in many severe illnesses. It is also considered a risk factor for coronary heart disease and stroke. Prothrombin is a vitamin K–dependent vitamin. Its production in the liver requires vitamin K. This vitamin is fat soluble and is dependent on bile for absorption. Bile duct obstruction or malabsorption will cause a vitamin K deficiency and result in a reduced quantity of prothrombin and other vitamin K–dependent factors (VII, IX, X). It usually takes about 3 weeks before body stores of vitamin K are exhausted.

Factor VIII is actually a complex molecule with two components. The first component is related to hemophilia A and is involved in the hemostatic mechanism as described above. The second component is the von Willebrand's factor and is related to von Willebrand's disease. This second component is involved in platelet adhesion and aggregation. Patients with factor XII deficiency have been observed to have an increased risk of myocardial infarction and venous thrombosis.

Interfering Factors

- Many of these proteins are heat sensitive, and their levels will be decreased the longer the specimen is kept at room temperatures.
- Pregnancy or the use of contraceptive medication can increase levels of several of these factors, especially VIII and IX. A mild deficiency could be masked.
- Many of these protein coagulation factors are acute-phase reactant proteins. Acute illness, stress, exercise, or inflammation could raise levels.

Procedure and Patient Care

Before

- Explain the procedure to the patient.
- Tell the patient that no fasting is required.

During

- Collect approximately 7 to 10 ml of venous blood in a blue-top tube.

After

- Apply pressure or a pressure dressing to the venipuncture site.
- Assess the venipuncture site for bleeding, especially if the patient has had other episodes of clotting deficiency.
- Deliver the blood specimen to the laboratory as soon as possible.
- Freeze the specimen if testing is not going to be done immediately since these proteins are very labile.

Test Results and Clinical Significance

Fibrinogen

Increased levels

Acute inflammatory reactions
Trauma
Fibrinogen is an acute-phase reactant protein.

Coronary heart disease
Cigarette smoking
Elevated fibrinogen levels are merely an observation with no known pathophysiology.

Decreased levels

Liver disease (hepatitis or cirrhosis) *Fibrinogen is not made in adequate volume.*

Consumptive coagulopathy (disseminated intravascular coagulation)
Action of fibrinolysins
Fibrinolysins act to destroy fibrinogen in the serum.

Prothrombin

Decreased levels

Vitamin K deficiency
Liver disease
Synthesis is diminished.

Proaccelerin

Decreased levels

Liver disease *Synthesis is diminished.*

Proconvertin stable factor

Decreased levels

Inherited deficiency
Vitamin K deficiency
Liver disease
Coumadin therapy
Synthesis is diminished.

Antihemophilic factor

Increased levels

Acute inflammatory reactions
Trauma/stress

Pregnancy
Factor VIII is an acute-phase reactant protein.

Decreased levels

Inherited deficiency (hemophilia A) *Hemophilia A is controlled by a sex-linked gene on the X chromosome. Females are rarely affected, because the other X chromosome has a normal gene.*
Consumptive coagulation *This factor is used up and synthesis cannot match the demand.*

von Willebrand's factor

Decreased levels (von Willebrand's disease)

Inherited deficiency
Autoimmune disease
Von Willebrand's factor is reduced in quantity.

Christmas factor

Decreased levels

Inherited deficiency (hemophilia B)
Liver disease
Nephrotic syndrome
Coumadin therapy
Synthesis is diminished.

Consumptive coagulation *This factor is used up and synthesis cannot match the demand.*

Stuart factor

Decreased levels

This is an inherited deficiency.

Hageman factor

Decreased levels

Inherited deficiency
Vitamin K deficiency
Liver disease
Coumadin therapy
Synthesis is diminished.

Consumptive coagulation *This factor is used up and synthesis cannot match the demand.*

Related Tests

- Bleeding time (p. 115): This test is used to evaluate the vascular and platelet factors associated with hemostasis.
- Thrombin time (p. 408): This test is used to evaluate the fibrinogen portion of the hemostatic mechanism.
- Partial thromboplastin time, activated (p. 319): This test is used to evaluate the intrinsic system and the common pathway of clot formation.
- Prothrombin time (p. 366): This test is used to evaluate the adequacy of the extrinsic system and common pathway in the clotting mechanism.
- Fibrinogen (p. 215): This is a separate discussion on this coagulating factor.

Complement Assay

Normal Findings

Total complement: 75-160 U/ml or 75-160 U/L (SI units)
C3: 55-120 mg/dl or 0.55-1.20 g/L (SI units)
C4: 20-50 mg/dl or 0.20-0.50 g/L (SI units)

Indications

Measurements of complement are used primarily to diagnose angioedema and to monitor the activity of disease in patients with systemic lupus erythematosus (SLE), nephritis, membranoproliferative nephritis, or poststreptococcal nephritis.

Test Explanation

Serum complement is a group of globulin proteins that act as enzymes. These enzymes facilitate the immunologic and inflammatory response. The complement system is important for destroying foreign cells and isolating "foreign" antigens. The total complement, sometimes labeled CH_{50}, is made up of nine major components, C1 through C9. Besides these major components, there are some subcomponents and "inhibitor" components involved in the system. Classic complement activation starts when an IgM or IgG antibody binds with the C1q subcomponent of C1. C1 activates C4, which activates C2 and so on to C9. There are also alternative pathways for the activation of this system.

Once activated, complement acts to increase vascular permeability, allowing antibodies and WBCs to be delivered to the area of the immune/antigen complex. Complement also acts to increase chemotaxis (attracting WBCs to the area), phagocytosis, and immune adherence of the antibody to antigen. These processes are vitally important in the normal inflammatory response.

Total complement can be measured by hemolytic tests. For this test, the patient's blood is mixed with antibody-coated RBCs of sheep. The end point is when 50% of the RBCs are lysed. The patient's blood is serially diluted and results are reported in complement units per milliliter. Usually specimens for complement assays must be sent out to reference laboratories. These tests assess the overall function of the entire complement system. The C3 and C4 components can be quantitated by direct immunologic measurement. These subcomponent are measured when total complement has been found to be reduced. C3 makes up the majority of the component of complement. It is made in the liver and to a lesser degree in the spleen, skin, and other lymphoid nodules. C4 is made in the bone and lung.

Reduced complement levels can be congenital, as in hereditary angioedema. Hereditary angioedema is a congenital lack of a C1 "inhibitor" (often called C1 esterase). The complement system is overly activated and the complement components are "consumed" or used up. Serum levels fall.

Acquired complement deficiency occurs with diseases that are associated with increased antibody/antigen complexes. Here again, these complexes serve to act as complement activators. If the presence of these complexes is chronic, the complement system is overly activated and the complement components are consumed or used up. Serum levels fall. Diseases associated with immune complexes such as described include serum sickness, lupus erythematosus, infectious endocarditis, renal transplant rejection, vasculitis, and some forms of glomerulonephritis. When these diseases are successfully treated, complement levels can be expected to return to normal.

Complement components are increased following the onset of various acute or chronic inflammatory diseases or acute tissue damage. This is very similar to an acute-phase reactant protein.

Interfering Factors

- C3 is very unstable at room temperatures. If the specimen is left standing for more than 1 hour, complement levels could be falsely low. The serum should be separated out and frozen immediately when the specimen is received.

Procedure and Patient Care

Before

- Explain the procedure to the patient.
- Tell the patient that no fasting or special preparations are required.

During

- Collect 7 to 10 ml of venous blood in a red-top tube.

After

- Apply pressure or a pressure dressing to the venipuncture site.
- Observe the venipuncture site for bleeding.

Test Results and Clinical Significance

Increased levels

Rheumatic fever (acute)
Myocardial infarction (acute)
Ulcerative colitis
Inflammatory illnesses, stress, and trauma
Complement can develop very similarly to an acute-phase reactant protein. With these illnesses, complement is increased.

Cancer *The pathophysiology of this observation is unknown.*

Decreased levels

Hereditary angioedema *Hereditary angioedema is a congenital lack of a C1 "inhibitor" (often called C1 esterase). The complement system is overly activated and the complement components are consumed or used up. Serum levels fall.*

Severe liver diseases such as hepatitis or cirrhosis *The liver is the site of synthesis of many of the complement components. Synthesis is decreased in the presence of liver disease. Serum levels fall.*

Autoimmune disease (SLE, glomerulonephritis, lupus nephritis, rheumatoid arthritis [severe and active], Sjögren's syndrome)
Serum sickness (immune complex disease)
Renal transplant rejection (acute)
These diseases are associated with the increased presence of antibody/antigen complexes, which serve to act as complement activators. The complement system is overly activated and complement components are consumed. Serum levels fall.

Protein malnutrition
Anemia
Malnutrition
These diseases are associated with protein depletion. Complement is a protein and its synthesis can be expected to be reduced in these illnesses.

Infection such as gram-negative sepsis or bacterial endocarditis
Glomerulonephritis, specifically poststreptococcal and membranoproliferative
Alternate pathways of complement activation occur. The complement system is overly activated and complement components are consumed. Serum levels fall.

Complete Blood Count and Differential Count (CBC and Diff)

The CBC and differential count are a series of tests of the peripheral blood that provide a tremendous amount of information about the hematologic system and many other organ systems. They are inexpensively, easily, and rapidly performed as a screening test. The CBC and differential count include automated multimeasurement of the following studies (Figure 2-11), which are discussed separately:

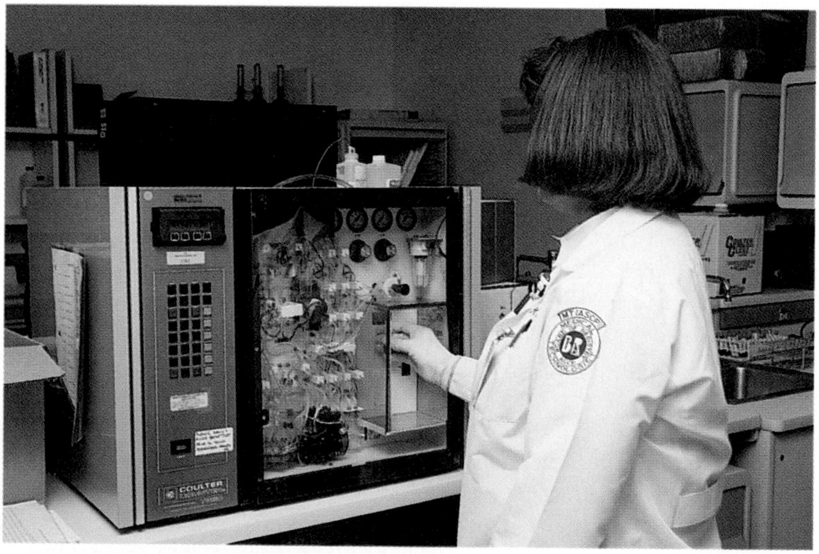

Figure 2-11 Medical technologist performing a CBC.

Red blood cell count (see p. 372)
Hemoglobin (see p. 254)
Hematocrit (see p. 251)
Red blood cell indices (see p. 375)
Mean corpuscular volume (MCV)
Mean corpuscular hemoglobin (MCH)
Mean corpuscular hemoglobin concentration (MCHC)
White blood cell count and differential count (see p. 455)
Neutrophils (polynucleated cells or "polys," segmented cells or "segs," band cells, stab cells)
Lymphocytes
Monocytes
Eosinophils
Basophils
Blood smear (see p. 641)
Platelet count (see p. 337)

Coombs' Test, Direct (Direct Antiglobulin Test)

Normal Findings Negative; no agglutination

Indications

This test is performed to identify hemolysis (lysis of RBCs) or to investigate hemolytic transfusion reactions.

Test Explanation

Most of the antibodies to RBCs are directed against the ABO/Rh blood grouping antigens, such as that observed in hemolytic anemia of the newborn (erythroblastosis fetalis) or blood transfusion of incompatible blood. When a transfusion reaction occurs, Coombs' test can detect the patient's antibodies coating the transfused RBCs. Coombs' test is therefore useful in evaluating suspected transfusion reactions.

Non-blood grouping antigens can develop on the RBC membrane and stimulate formation of antibodies. Drugs such as levodopa or methyldopa can do this. Also, in some diseases, antibodies not originally directed against the patient's RBCs can attach to the RBCs and cause hemolysis, which can be detected by the direct Coombs' test. Examples of the latter would include:

Antibodies developed in reaction to drugs such as penicillin
Autoantibodies formed in various autoimmune diseases
Antibodies developed in some patients with advanced cancer (e.g., lymphoma)

Frequently the production of these autoantibodies against RBCs is not associated with any identifiable disease, and the resulting hemolytic anemia is therefore called idiopathic.

The direct Coombs' test must be performed on a clotted blood specimen to obtain the patient's RBCs for testing. The test can be done in either a test tube or on a slide. Serum for Coombs' testing is prepared by injecting human antibodies (IgG/IgM) into a rabbit. The rabbit produces antibodies to human globulin (antibodies). This rabbit serum is called Coombs' serum. The direct Coombs' test demonstrates that RBCs have been attacked by antibodies in the patient's bloodstream. The RBCs of patients suspected of having antibodies against RBCs are washed to eliminate any excess free gamma globulins. Coombs' serum is added to the RBCs. If the RBCs have antibodies on them, Coombs' serum will cause agglutination. The greater the quantity of antibodies against RBCs, the more clumping occurs. This test is read as *positive* with clumping on a scale of trace to 4. If the RBCs are not coated with autoantibodies against RBCs (immunoglobulins), agglutination will not occur; this is a *negative* test.

Interfering Factors

- Drugs that may cause *false-positive* results include ampicillin, captopril, cephalosporins, chlorpromazine (Thorazine), chlorpropamide, hydralazine, indomethacin (Indocin), insulin, isoniazid (INH), levodopa, methyldopa (Aldomet), penicillin, phenytoin (Dilantin), procainamide, quinidine, quinine, rifampin, streptomycin, sulfonamides, and tetracyclines.

Procedure and Patient Care

Before

- Explain the procedure to the patient.
- Tell the patient that no fasting is required.

During

- Collect approximately 5 to 7 ml of venous blood in a red- or lavender-top tube.
- Use venous blood from the umbilical cord to detect the presence of antibodies in the newborn.
- List on the laboratory slip all medications that the patient has taken in the last few days.

After

- Apply pressure or a pressure dressing to the venipuncture site.
- Assess the venipuncture site for bleeding.

Test Results and Clinical Significance

Erythroblastosis fetalis
Incompatible blood transfusion reaction
Antibodies to the patient's RBCs have been created by mixing of incompatible blood grouping antigens.

Lymphoma
Autoimmune hemolytic anemia (rheumatoid/collagen diseases, e.g., systemic lupus erythematosus, rheumatoid arthritis)
Autoantibodies formed in these illnesses attach to RBCs.

Mycoplasmal infection
Infectious mononucleosis
In these illnesses, antibodies develop and for unknown reasons attach to the RBCs.

Hemolytic anemia after heart bypass *Autoantibodies formed during the use of the heart/lung bypass machine attach to RBCs.*

Adult hemolytic anemia (idiopathic) *Autoantibodies not otherwise associated with any other disease attach to RBCs.*

Related Tests

- Coombs' test, indirect (below): This test is used to detect antibodies against RBCs in the serum. It is most commonly used for screening potential blood recipients.

Coombs' Test, Indirect
(Indirect Antiglobulin Test, Blood Antibody Screening)

Normal Findings Negative; no agglutination

Indications

This test is used to detect antibodies against RBCs in the serum. This laboratory method is used most commonly for screening potential blood recipients.

Test Explanation

The indirect Coombs' test detects circulating antibodies against RBCs. The major purpose of this test is to determine if the patient has minor serum antibodies (other than the major ABO/Rh system) to RBCs before receiving a blood transfusion. Therefore this test is the "screening" portion of the "type and screen" routinely performed for blood compatibility testing (crossmatching in the blood bank). This test is also used to detect other agglutinins, such as cold agglutinins that are associated with mycoplasmal infections.

Coombs' serum for Coombs' testing is prepared by injecting human antibodies (IgG/IgM) into a rabbit. The rabbit produces antibodies to human globulin (antibodies). This rabbit serum is called Coombs' serum. Unlike the direct Coombs' test performed on the patient's RBCs, this test is performed on the patient's serum. In this test a small amount of the recipient's serum is added to RBCs containing known antibodies on their surface. This is the first stage. In the second stage of the test, Coombs' serum is added after the test RBCs have been washed of any free globulins. If antibodies exist in the patient's serum, agglutination occurs. In blood transfusion screening, visible agglutination indicates that the recipient has antibodies to the donor's RBCs. If the recipient has no antibodies against the donor's RBCs, agglutination will not occur; transfusion should then proceed safely without any transfusion reaction. Circulating antibodies against RBCs also may occur in an Rh-negative pregnant woman who is carrying an Rh-positive fetus.

Interfering Factors

- Drugs that may cause false-positive results include antiarrhythmics, antituberculins, cephalosporins, chlorpromazine (Thorazine), insulin, levodopa, methyldopa (Aldomet), penicillins, phenytoin (Dilantin), quinidine, sulfonamides, and tetracyclines.

✓ CLINICAL PRIORITIES

- This test is the "screening" portion of the "type and screen" routinely performed for blood compatability testing.
- If the recipient of the blood transfusion has antibodies to the donor's RBCs, agglutination occurs. The blood cannot be used for that recipient.
- If the recipient has no antibodies to the donor's RBCs, agglutination will not occur. Transfusion should then proceed safely without any transfusion reaction.

Procedure and Patient Care

Before

- Explain the procedure to the patient.
- Tell the patient that no fasting is required.

During

- Collect approximately 7 ml of venous blood in a red-top tube.
- List on the laboratory slip all medications that the patient has taken in the last few days.

After

- Apply pressure or a pressure dressing to the venipuncture site.
- Assess the venipuncture site for bleeding.
- Remember that if this antibody screening test is positive, antibody identification is then done.

Test Results and Clinical Significance

Incompatible crossmatched blood *Anti-ABO/Rh antigens in the donor blood cross-react with the patient's serum.*

Maternal anti-Rh antibodies
Erythroblastosis fetalis
Anti-ABO/Rh antibodies result from previous exposure to RBCs of noncompatible blood.

Acquired hemolytic anemia
Presence of specific cold agglutinin antibody *Drugs and other illnesses are associated with the development of antibodies detected in the patient's serum.*

Related Tests

- Coombs' test, direct (p. 163): This test is performed to identify hemolysis (lysis of RBCs) or to investigate hemolytic transfusion reactions.

Cortisol, Blood (Hydrocortisone, Serum Cortisol)

Normal Findings

Adult/elderly
  8 AM: 6-28 mg/dl or 170-625 nmol/L (SI units)
  4 PM: 2-12 mg/dl or 80-413 nmol/L (SI units)
Child 1-16 years
  8 AM: 3-21 mg/dl
  4 PM: 3-10 mg/dl
Newborn: 1-24 mg/dl

Indications

This test is a measure of serum cortisol. It is performed on patients who are suspected to have hyper- or hypofunctioning adrenal glands.

Test Explanation

An elaborate feedback mechanism for cortisol coordinates the function of the hypothalamus, pituitary gland, and adrenal glands. Corticotropin-releasing hormone (CRH) is made in the hypothalamus. This stimulates adrenocorticotropic hormone (ACTH) production in the anterior pituitary gland. ACTH stimulates the adrenal cortex to produce cortisol. The rising levels of cortisol act as a negative feedback to curtail further production of CRH and ACTH. Cortisol is a potent glucocorticoid released from the adrenal cortex. This hormone affects the metabolism of carbohydrates, proteins, and fats. It has a profound effect on glucose serum levels. Cortisol tends to increase glucose by stimulating gluconeogenesis from glucose stores. It also inhibits the effect of insulin and thereby inhibits glucose transport into the cells.

The best method of evaluating adrenal activity is by directly measuring plasma cortisol levels. Normally cortisol levels rise and fall during the day; this is called the diurnal variation. Cortisol levels are highest around 6 to 8 AM and gradually fall during the day, reaching their lowest point around midnight. Sometimes the earliest sign of adrenal hyperfunction is only the loss of this diurnal variation, even though the cortisol levels are not yet elevated. For example, individuals with Cushing's syndrome often have upper normal plasma cortisol levels in the morning and do not exhibit a decline as the day proceeds. High levels of cortisol indicate Cushing's syndrome, and low levels of plasma cortisol are suggestive of Addison's disease.

For this test, blood is usually collected at 8 AM and again at around 4 PM. The 4 PM value is anticipated to be one third to two thirds of the 8 AM value. Normal values may be transposed in individuals who have worked during the night and slept during the day for long periods of time.

Interfering Factors

- Pregnancy is associated with increased levels.
- Physical and emotional stress can elevate cortisol levels. Stress stimulates the pituitary-cortical mechanism and thereby stimulates cortisol production.
- Drugs that may cause *increased* levels include estrogen, oral contraceptives, amphetamines, cortisone, and spironolactone (Aldactone).
- Drugs that may cause *decreased* levels include androgens, aminoglutethimide, betamethasone and other exogenous steroid medications, danazol, lithium, levodopa, metyrapone, and phenytoin (Dilantin).

CLINICAL PRIORITIES

- Cortisol levels are affected by a diurnal variation, with peak levels occurring around 6 to 8 AM and the lowest levels around midnight.
- Blood levels are usually drawn at 8 AM and again around 4 PM. The 4 PM level is usually one third to two thirds of the morning level.
- Physical and emotional stress can elevate cortisol levels.

Procedure and Patient Care

Before

- Explain the procedure to the patient to minimize anxiety.
- Assess the patient for signs of physical stress (e.g., infection, acute illness) or emotional stress and report these to the physician.

During

- Collect approximately 7 to 10 ml of venous blood in a red- or green-top tube in the morning after the patient has had a good night's sleep.
- Collect another blood sample at about 4 PM.
- Indicate on the laboratory slip the time of the venipuncture and any drugs that may affect test results.

After

- Apply pressure or a pressure dressing to the venipuncture site.
- Observe the venipuncture site for bleeding.

Test Results and Clinical Significance

Increased levels

Cushing's disease
Ectopic ACTH-producing tumors
Stress
ACTH is overproduced as a result of neoplastic overproduction of ACTH in the pituitary or elsewhere in the body by an ACTH-producing cancer. Stress is a potent stimulus to ACTH production. Cortisol rises as a result.

Cushing's syndrome (adrenal adenoma or carcinoma) *The neoplasm produces cortisol without regard to the normal feedback mechanism.*
Hyperthyroidism *The metabolic rate is increased and cortisol levels rise accordingly to maintain the elevated glucose needs.*
Obesity *All sterols are increased in the obese, perhaps because fatty tissue may act as a depository or site of synthesis.*

Decreased levels

Adrenal hyperplasia *The congenital absence of important enzymes in the synthesis of cortisol prevents adequate serum levels.*
Addison's disease *As a result of hypofunctioning of the adrenal gland, cortisol levels drop.*
Hypopituitarism *ACTH is not produced by the pituitary gland, which is destroyed by disease, neoplasm, or ischemia. The adrenal gland is not stimulated to produce cortisol.*
Hypothyroidism *Normal cortisol levels are not required to maintain the reduced metabolic rate of hypothyroid patients.*

Related Tests

- Adrenocorticotropic hormone (ACTH) stimulation (p. 26): This test is used for the differential diagnosis of Cushing's syndrome or Addison's disease.
- Adrenocorticotropic (ACTH) hormone (p. 23): The serum ACTH study is a test of anterior pituitary gland function that affords the greatest insight into the causes of either Cushing's syndrome (overproduction of cortisol) or Addison's disease (underproduction of cortisol).
- Dexamethasone suppression tests (p. 187): This test is important for diagnosing Cushing's syndrome and distinguishing its cause.
- Urinary cortisol (p. 827): This test is a measure of urinary cortisol. It is performed on patients who are suspected to have hyper- or hypofunctioning adrenal glands.

C-Peptide (Connecting Peptide Insulin, Insulin C-Peptide, Proinsulin C-Peptide)

Normal Findings

Fasting: 0.78-1.89 ng/ml or 0.26-0.62 nmol/L (SI units)
1 hour after glucose load: 5-12 ng/ml

Indications

This test is used to evaluate diabetic patients and to identify patients who secretly self-administer insulin. C-peptide is also helpful in monitoring patients with insulinomas.

Test Explanation

C-peptide (connecting peptide) is a protein that connects the beta and alpha chains of proinsulin. In the beta cells of the islet of Langerhans of the pancreas, the chains of proinsulin are separated during the conversion of proinsulin to insulin and C-peptide. C-peptide is released into the portal vein in nearly equal amounts. Because it has a longer half-life than insulin, more C-peptide exists in the peripheral circulation. In general, C-peptide levels correlate with insulin levels in the blood, except possibly in islet cell tumors and in obese patients. The capacity of the pancreatic beta cells to secrete insulin can be evaluated by directly measuring either insulin or C-peptide. In most cases, direct measurement of insulin is more accurate. However, in some instances, direct measurement of insulin does not accurately assess the patient's insulin generating capability. C-peptide levels more accurately reflect islet cell function in the following situations:

1. Patients with diabetes who are treated with insulin and who have antiinsulin antibodies. This most often occurs in patients treated with old bovine or pork insulin. These antibodies falsely increase insulin levels.
2. Patients who secretly administer insulin to themselves (factitious hypoglycemia). Insulin levels will be elevated. Direct insulin measurement in these patients tends to be high, because the insulin measured is self-administered exogenous insulin. But C-peptide levels in that same specimen will be low, because exogenously administered insulin suppresses endogenous insulin (and C-peptide) production.
3. Diabetic patients who are taking insulin. The exogenously administered insulin suppresses endogenous insulin production. Insulin levels only measure the exogenously administered insulin and do not accurately reflect true islet cell function. C-peptide would be a more accurate test of islet cell function. This is performed to see if the diabetes is in remission and the patient may not need exogenous insulin.

The C-peptide test is indicated for the clinical situations described above. Further, C-peptide is used in evaluating patients who are suspected to have an insulinoma. It can differentiate patients with insulinoma from patients with factitious hypoglycemia. In the latter patients, C-peptide levels are suppressed by exogenous insulin challenge. In patients with an autonomous secreting insulinoma, C-peptide levels are not suppressed. Furthermore, C-peptide can be used to monitor treated patients with insulinoma. A rise in C-peptide levels indicates a recurrence or progression of the insulinoma. Likewise, some clinicians use C-peptide testing as an indicator of the adequacy of therapeutic surgical pancreatectomy in patients with pancreatic tumors. C-peptide can also be used to diagnose "insulin resistance" syndrome.

Interfering Factors

- Because the majority of C-peptide is degraded in the kidney, renal failure can cause increased levels of C-peptide.

- Drugs that may cause *increased* levels of C-peptide include oral hypoglycemic agents (e.g., sulfonylureas).

Procedure and Patient Care

Before

- Explain the procedure to the patient.
- Instruct the patient to fast for 8 to 10 hours before the test. Only water is permitted.

During

- Collect venous blood in one red-top tube.

After

- Apply pressure or a pressure dressing to the venipuncture site.
- Assess the venipuncture site for bleeding.

Test Results and Clinical Significance

Increased levels

Insulinoma *Insulin and C-peptide are made concomitantly by the neoplastic cells.*
Pancreas transplant *Excess C-peptide is produced by the transplanted islet cells.*
Renal failure *C-peptide is removed from the blood by the kidneys. Diminished kidney function will lead to elevated levels.*
Administration of oral hypoglycemic agents *Oral hypoglycemic agents stimulate insulin and C-peptide synthesis.*

Decreased levels

Factitious hypoglycemia
Diabetes mellitus
The self-administered insulin suppresses endogenous insulin and C-peptide production.

Total pancreatectomy *All islet cells have been surgically removed. C-peptide production ceases.*

Related Tests

- Glucose, blood (p. 225): This is a measurement of serum glucose.
- Glucagon (p. 223): This is a direct measurement of glucagon, an islet cell hormone that acts to increase serum glucose levels.
- Glycosylated hemoglobin (p. 238): This is a test to measure the amount of glycosylated hemoglobin, which is an indirect measure of the chronic state of glucose levels.
- Insulin assay (p. 272): This is a direct measurement of insulin, an islet cell hormone that acts to decrease serum glucose levels.

C-Reactive Protein (CRP)

Normal Findings <0.8 mg/dl

Indications

C-reactive protein is an acute-phase reactant protein used to indicate an inflammatory illness

Test Explanation

CRP is a nonspecific, acute-phase reactant protein used to diagnose bacterial infectious disease and inflammatory disorders, such as acute rheumatic fever and rheumatoid arthritis. It is also elevated when there is tissue necrosis. CRP levels do not consistently rise with viral infections. CRP is an abnormal protein produced primarily by the liver during an acute inflammatory process. A positive test result indicates the presence, but not the cause, of an acute inflammatory reaction. The synthesis of CRP is initiated by antigen-immune complexes, bacteria, fungi, and trauma. CRP is functionally analogous to immunoglobulin G, except that it is not antigen specific. CRP interacts with the complement system.

The CRP test is a more sensitive and rapidly responding indicator than the erythrocyte sedimentation rate (ESR). In an acute inflammatory change, CRP shows an earlier and more intense increase than ESR; with recovery, the disappearance of CRP precedes the return of ESR to normal. The CRP also disappears when the inflammatory process is suppressed by antiinflammatory agents, salicylates, or steroids.

This test is also useful in evaluating patients with an acute myocardial infarction. The level of CRP correlates with peak levels of the MB isoenzyme of creatine kinase (see p. 173), but CRP peaks occur 18 to 72 hours later. Failure of CRP to normalize may indicate ongoing damage to the heart tissue. Levels are not elevated in patients with angina.

This test also may be used postoperatively to detect wound infections. CRP levels increase within 4 to 6 hours after surgery and generally begin to decrease after the third postoperative day. Failure of the levels to fall is an indicator of complications, such as infection or pulmonary infarction.

Interfering Factors

- An intrauterine device may cause positive test results because of tissue inflammation.
- Drugs that may cause *increased* levels include oral contraceptives.
- Drugs that may cause *decreased* levels include nonsteroidal antiinflammatory agents, salicylates, and steroids.

Procedure and Patient Care

Before

- Explain the procedure to the patient.

- Tell the patient that fasting usually is not required; however, some laboratories require a 4- to 12-hour fast. Water is permitted.

During

- Collect one red-top tube of venous blood.

After

- Apply pressure or a pressure dressing to the venipuncture site.
- Assess the venipuncture site for bleeding.

Test Results and Clinical Significance

Increased levels

Acute, noninfectious inflammatory reaction (e.g., arthritis, acute rheumatic fever, Reiter's syndrome, Crohn's disease)
Collagen vascular diseases (e.g., vasculitis syndrome, lupus erythematosus)
Tissue infarction or damage (e.g., acute myocardial infarction, pulmonary infarction, kidney or bone marrow transplant rejection, soft tissue trauma)
Bacterial infections such as postoperative wound infection, urinary tract infection, or tuberculosis
Malignant disease
Bacterial infection (e.g., tuberculosis)

Related Tests

- Erythrocyte sedimentation rate (p. 199): This is also an acute-phase reactant protein. It is a nonspecific test used to detect inflammatory, infectious, and necrotic processes.
- Complement assay (p. 160): Not only are some of the complement components acute-phase reactants proteins, but C-reactive protein interacts with this complex immune system
- Fibrinogen (p. 215): This is an important part of the hemostatic mechanism. It is also an acute-phase reactant protein.

Creatine Phosphokinase
(CPK, CP, Creatine Kinase [CK])

Normal Findings

Total CPK

Adult/elderly
Male: 12-70 U/ml or 55-170 U/L (SI units)
Female: 10-55 U/ml or 30-135 U/L (SI units)
Values are higher after exercise.

Newborn: 68-580 U/L (SI units)

Isoenzymes

CPK-MM: 100%
CPK-MB: 0%
CPK-BB: 0%

Indications

This test is used to support the diagnosis of myocardial infarction. It can also indicate neurologic or skeletal muscle diseases.

Test Explanation

CPK is found predominantly in the heart muscle, skeletal muscle, and brain. Serum CPK levels are elevated when these muscle or nerve cells are injured. CPK levels can rise within 6 hours after damage. If damage is not persistent, the levels peak at 18 hours after injury and return to normal in 2 to 3 days.

To test specifically for myocardial muscle injury, electrophoresis is performed to detect the three CPK isoenzymes: CPK-BB (CPK1), CPK-MB (CPK2), and CPK-MM (CPK3). The CPK-MB isoenzyme portion appears to be specific for myocardial cells. CPK-MB levels rise 3 to 6 hours after infarction occurs. If there is no further myocardial damage, the level peaks at 12 to 24 hours and returns to normal 12 to 48 hours after infarction. CPK-MB levels do not usually rise with transient chest pain caused by angina, pulmonary embolism, or congestive heart failure. One can expect to see a rise in CPK-MB in patients with unstable angina, shock, malignant hyperthermia, myopathies, or myocarditis. Very small amounts of CPK-MB also exist in skeletal muscle. Severe injury to skeletal muscle can be significant enough to raise the CPK-MB isoenzyme above normal. To avoid the misdiagnosis of myocardial injury, a *relative index* is calculated to determine whether myocardial injury has occurred. This relative index is a mathematic calculation of the ratio of CPK-MB to total CPK. A relative index of greater than 2.5 is highly suggestive of myocardial injury.

The CPK-MB isoenzyme level is helpful in both quantifying the degree of myocardial infarction and timing the onset of infarction. With the more frequent use of thrombolytic therapy for myocardial infarction, the CPK-MB isoenzyme is often used to determine appropriateness of thrombolytic therapy. High CPK-MB levels would suggest that significant infarction has already occurred, thereby precluding the benefit of thrombolytic therapy.

Because the CPK-BB isoenzyme is predominantly found in the brain and lung, injury to either of these organs (e.g., cerebrovascular accident, pulmonary infarction) will be associated with elevated levels of this isoenzyme.

The CPK-MM isoenzyme normally comprises almost all of the circulatory total CPK enzymes in healthy people. When the total CPK level is elevated as a result of increases in CPK-MM, injury to or disease of the skeletal muscle is present. Examples of this include myopathies, vigorous exercise, multiple IM injections, electroconvulsive therapy, cardioversion, chronic alcoholism, or surgery. Because CPK is made only in the skeletal muscle, the normal value of total CPK (and therefore CPK-MM) varies according to a person's muscle mass. Large muscular people may normally have a CPK level in the high range of normal.

Table 2-18 ***Timing of appearance and disappearance of commonly used cardiac enzymes***

	Hours		Days
Enzyme	Starts to rise	Peaks	Returns to normal
Total CPK	4-6	24	3-4
CK-MB	4	18	2
AST	8	24-48	4
LDH	24	72	8-9
Troponin T	4-6	10-24	10
Troponin I	4-6	10-24	4

Each isoenzyme has been found to have isoforms. The CPK-MM isoforms MM1 and MM3 are most useful for cardiac disease. An MM3/MM1 ratio of greater than 1 suggests acute myocardial injury. A CPK-MB ratio of MB2/MB1 greater than 1 also indicates acute myocardial injury.

CPK is the main cardiac enzyme studied in patients with heart disease. Because its blood clearance and metabolism are well known, its frequent determination (on admission and at 12 hours and 24 hours) can accurately reflect timing, quantity, and resolution of a myocardial infarction. Lactic dehydrogenase (LDH) and aspartate aminotransferase (AST) are also important enzymes used to confirm a myocardial infarction. The clearance characteristics of each enzyme are noted in Table 2-18.

New blood assays for cardiac markers have promised to rapidly and accurately detect acute myocardial infarction in the emergency room. One of these new assays is troponin. *Troponin* is a protein complex consisting of three isotypes (T, I, and C). Troponin T and troponin I have the potential to become better diagnostic markers for acute myocardial infarction than existing enzymes (such as CPK-MB), because these new cardiac isotypes are distinctly different from skeletal isotypes. Monoclonal antibodies to cardiac troponin have been developed that do not cross-react with skeletal muscle forms. At the present time, troponins are mainly used in emergency departments with a cardiac center where the patient can be monitored for several hours while awaiting test results. Then a decision can be made regarding admission to the cardiac care unit or discharge to home.

Interfering Factors

- IM injections can cause elevated CPK levels.
- Strenuous exercise and recent surgery may cause increased levels.
- Early pregnancy may produce decreased levels.
- Muscle mass is directly related to a patient's normal CPK level.
- Drugs that may cause *increased* levels include amphotericin B, ampicillin, some anesthetics, anticoagulants, aspirin, clofibrate, dexamethasone (Decadron), furosemide (Lasix), captopril, colchicine, alcohol, lovastatin, lithium, lidocaine, propranolol, succinylcholine, and morphine.

Procedure and Patient Care

Before

- Explain the procedure to the patient.
- Discuss with the patient the need and reason for frequent venipuncture in diagnosing myocardial infarction.
- Avoid IM injections in patients with cardiac disease. These injections may falsely elevate the total CPK level.
- Tell the patient that no food or fluid restrictions are necessary.

During

- Collect a venous blood sample in a red-top tube. This is usually done initially and 12 hours later, followed by daily testing for 3 days and then at 1 week.
- Rotate the venipuncture sites.
- Avoid hemolysis.
- Record the time and date of any IM injection.
- Record the exact time and date of venipuncture on each laboratory slip. This aids in the interpretation of the temporal pattern of enzyme elevations.

After

- Apply pressure or a pressure dressing to the venipuncture site.
- Observe the venipuncture site for bleeding.

CLINICAL PRIORITIES

- Avoid IM injections in patients with cardiac disease. IM injections can cause elevated CPK levels.
- The CPK-MB isoenzyme is helpful in both quantifying the degree of myocardial infarction and timing the onset of the infarction.
- The CPK-MB isoenzyme is often used to determine the appropriateness of thrombolytic therapy. High levels may indicate that significant infarction has already occurred, thus precluding a benefit from thrombolytic therapy.

Test Results and Clinical Significance

Increased levels of total CPK

Diseases or injury affecting the heart muscle, skeletal muscle, and brain.

Increased levels of CPK-BB isoenzyme

Diseases that affect the CNS (e.g., brain injury, brain cancer, cerebrovascular accident [stroke], subarachnoid hemorrhage, seizures, shock, Reye's syndrome) and electroconvulsive therapy

Adenocarcinoma (especially breast and lung) *The pathophysiology of this observation is not known.*

Pulmonary infarction *The lung tissue has small amounts of CPK-BB. With cellular injury of this organ, the contents of the cell, including CPK, spill out into the bloodstream, causing elevated CPK-BB isoenzyme levels.*

Increased levels of CPK-MB isoenzyme

Acute myocardial infarction
Cardiac aneurysm surgery
Cardiac defibrillation
Myocarditis
Ventricular arrhythmias
Cardiac ischemia
Any disease or injury to the myocardium causes CPK-MB to spill out of the damaged cells and into the bloodstream, producing elevated CPK-MB isoenzyme levels.

Increased levels of CPK-MM isoenzyme

Rhabdomyolysis
Muscular dystrophy
Myositis
Diseases affecting skeletal muscle cause CPK-MM to spill out of the damaged cells and into the bloodstream, producing elevated CPK-MM isoenzyme levels.

Recent surgery
Electromyography
IM injections
Crush injuries
Injury affecting skeletal muscle causes CPK-MM to spill out of the damaged cells and into the bloodstream, producing elevated CPK-MM isoenzyme levels.

Delirium tremens
Malignant hyperthermia
Recent convulsions
Electroconvulsive therapy
Shock
Anoxic injury from lack of blood supply or repetitive muscular motion can cause injury to skeletal muscle. This causes CPK-MM to spill out of the damaged cells and into the bloodstream, producing elevated CPK-MM isoenzyme levels.

Hypokalemia
Hypothyroidism
These diseases have a metabolic effect on skeletal muscle. Muscle injury results. This causes CPK-MM to spill out of the damaged cells and into the bloodstream, producing elevated CPK-MM isoenzyme levels.

Related Tests

- Aspartate aminotransferase (AST) (p. 105): Elevated levels of this enzyme indicate cardiac injury. It is not specific to the heart, however.
- Lactic dehydrogenase (LDH) (p. 278): This intracellular enzyme is used to support the diagnosis of injury or disease involving the heart, liver, red blood cells, kidneys, skeletal muscle, brain, and lungs.

- Alanine aminotransferase (ALT) (see p. 33): This enzyme is used similarly to AST and exists predominantly in the liver.
- Leucine aminopeptidase (LAP) (see page 286): This enzyme is specific to the hepatobiliary system. Diseases affecting that system will cause elevation of this enzyme.
- Gamma-glutamyl transpeptidase (GGTP) (p. 219): This is another enzyme predominantly existing in the liver.
- Alkaline phosphatase (p. 42): This is another enzyme predominantly existing in the liver.
- 5′-Nucleotidase (p. 312): This is another enzyme predominantly existing in the liver.

Creatinine, Blood (Serum Creatinine)

Normal Findings

Elderly: Decrease in muscle mass may cause decreased values.
Adult
  Female: 0.5-1.1 mg/dl or 44-97 μmol/L (SI units)
  Male: 0.6-1.2 mg/dl or 53–106 μmol/L (SI units)
Adolescent: 0.5-1.0 mg/dl
Child: 0.3-0.7 mg/dl
Infant: 0.2-0.4 mg/dl
Newborn: 0.3-1.2 mg/dl

Critical Values

>4 mg/dl (indicates serious impairment in renal function)

Indications

Creatinine is used to diagnose impaired renal function.

Test Explanation

This test measures the amount of creatinine in the blood. Creatinine is a catabolic product of creatine phosphate, which is used in skeletal muscle contraction. The daily production of creatine, and subsequently creatinine, depends on muscle mass, which fluctuates very little. Creatinine, as BUN, is excreted entirely by the kidneys and therefore is directly proportional to renal excretory function. Thus, with normal renal excretory function, the serum creatinine level should remain constant and normal. Only renal disorders, such as glomerulonephritis, pyelonephritis, acute tubular necrosis, and urinary obstruction, will cause an abnormal elevation in creatinine. There are slight increases in creatinine levels after meals, especially after ingestion of large quantities of meat. Furthermore, there may be some diurnal variation in creatinine (nadir at 7 AM and peak at 7 PM).

The serum creatinine test, as with the BUN, is used to diagnose impaired renal function. Unlike the BUN, however, the creatinine level is affected minimally by hepatic function. The serum creatinine level has much the same significance as the BUN level but tends to rise later. Therefore elevations in creatinine suggest chronicity of the disease process. In general, a doubling of creatinine suggests a 50% reduction in the glomerular

Age-related concerns

- The elderly and young children normally have lower creatinine levels as a result of reduced muscle mass. This may potentially mask renal disease in patients of these age groups.

filtration rate. The creatinine level is interpreted in conjunction with the BUN. These tests are referred to as *renal function studies.*

Interfering Factors

- A diet high in meat content can cause transient elevations of serum creatinine.
- Drugs that may *increase* creatinine values include aminoglycosides (e.g., gentamicin), cimetidine, heavy-metal chemotherapeutic agents (e.g., cisplatin), and other nephrotoxic drugs such as cephalosporins (e.g., cefoxitin).

Procedure and Patient Care

Before

- Explain the procedure to the patient.
- Tell the patient that no fasting is required.

During

- Collect approximately 5 ml of blood in a red-top tube.
- For pediatric patients, blood is usually drawn from a heel stick.

After

- Apply pressure or a pressure dressing to the venipuncture site.
- Observe the venipuncture site for bleeding.

Test Results and Clinical Significance

Increased levels

Diseases affecting renal function, such as glomerulonephritis, pyelonephritis, acute tubular necrosis, urinary tract obstruction, reduced renal blood flow (e.g., shock, dehydration, congestive heart failure, atherosclerosis), diabetic nephropathy, nephritis *With these illnesses, renal function is impaired and creatinine levels rise.*

Rhabdomyolysis *Injury of the skeletal muscle causes myoglobin to be released in the bloodstream. Large amounts are nephrotoxic. Creatinine levels rise.*

Acromegaly
Gigantism
These diseases are associated with increased muscle mass, which causes the "normal" creatinine level to be high.

Decreased levels

Debilitation
Decreased muscle mass (e.g., muscular dystrophy, myasthenia gravis)
These diseases are associated with decreased muscle mass, which causes the "normal" creatinine level to be low.

Related Tests

- Blood urea nitrogen (BUN) (p. 443): This is a test of renal function. Unlike creatinine, there are many nonrenal factors that can alter this test result.
- Creatinine clearance (p. 180): This is a more accurate measurement of renal function. It is a direct measurement of glomerular filtration rate.

Creatinine Clearance

Normal Findings

Adult (<20 years)
  Male: 90-139 ml/min or 0.87-1.34 ml/sec/m^2
  Female: 80-125 ml/min or 0.77-1.20 ml/sec/m^2
Values decrease 6.5 ml/min/decade of life after age 20 with decline in glomerular filtration rate (GFR).
Newborn: 40-65 ml/min

Indications

The creatinine clearance is used to measure the GFR of the kidney.

Test Explanation

Creatinine is a catabolic product of creatine phosphate, which is used in skeletal muscle contraction. The daily production of creatine, and subsequently creatinine, depends on muscle mass, which fluctuates very little. Creatinine is excreted entirely by the kidneys and therefore is directly proportional to the GFR (i.e., the number of milliliters of filtrate made by the kidneys per minute). The creatinine clearance (CC) is a measure of the GFR. Urine and serum creatinine levels are assessed and the clearance rate is calculated.

The amount of filtrate made in the kidney depends on the amount of blood to be filtered and on the ability of the glomeruli to act as a filter. The amount of blood present for filtration is decreased in renal artery atherosclerosis, dehydration, and shock. The ability of the glomeruli to act as a filter is decreased by diseases such as glomerulonephritis, acute tubular necrosis, and most other primary renal diseases. Significant bilateral obstruction to urinary outflow affects glomerular filtration (CC) only after it is long-standing.

When one kidney alone becomes diseased, the opposite kidney, if normal, has the ability to compensate by increasing its filtration rate. Therefore, with unilateral kidney disease or nephrectomy, a decrease in CC is not expected if the other kidney is normal.

Several nonrenal factors may influence CC. With each decade of age, the CC decreases 6.5 ml/min because of a decrease in the GFR. Because urine collections are timed, incomplete collections will falsely decrease CC. Muscle mass varies among people. Decreased muscle mass will give lower CC values. Likewise, ingestion of large amounts of meat will temporarily increase CC.

The CC test requires a 24-hour urine collection and a serum creatinine level. CC is then computed using the following formula:

$$\text{Creatinine clearance} = UV/P$$

where

U = number of milligrams per deciliter of creatinine excreted in the urine over 24 hours

V = volume of urine in milliliters per minute

P = serum creatinine in milligrams per deciliter

A 24-hour urine collection for creatinine is often measured along with other urine collections to assess the completeness of other 24-hour collections. In patients with normal creatinine the CC should indicate whether all the urine has been collected for the full 24 hours.

Age-related concerns

- Adult values decrease 6.5 ml/min with each decade of life after age 20 because of a decrease in GFR.

Interfering Factors

- Exercise may cause increased creatinine values.
- Incomplete urine collection may give a falsely lowered value.
- Pregnancy increases CC. This is due in part to the increased load placed on the kidney by the growing fetus.
- A diet high in meat content can cause transient elevation of the serum creatinine and CC. When the creatinine is high, its clearance is increased. Therefore the CC overestimates the GFR.
- Drugs that may cause *increased* levels include aminoglycosides (e.g., gentamicin), cimetidine, heavy-metal chemotherapeutic agents (e.g., cisplatin), and nephrotoxic drugs such as cephalosporins (e.g., cefoxitin).

Procedure and Patient Care

Before

- Explain the procedure to the patient.
- Tell the patient that no special diet is usually required.
- Note that some laboratories instruct the patient to avoid cooked meat, tea, coffee, or drugs on the day of the test. Check with the laboratory.

During

- Instruct the patient to begin the 24-hour urine collection. Discard the initial specimen and start the 24-hour timing at that point.
- Collect all the urine passed during the next 24 hours.
- Show the patient where to store the urine specimen.
- Keep the specimen on ice or refrigerated during the 24 hours.
- Indicate the starting time on the urine container and laboratory slip.
- Post the hours for the urine collection in a noticeable place to prevent accidental discharge of a specimen.
- Instruct the patient to void before defecating so that urine is not contaminated by feces.
- Remind the patient not to put toilet paper in the collection container.
- Encourage the patient to drink fluids during the 24-hour collection unless this is contraindicated for medical purposes.
- Instruct the patient to avoid vigorous exercise during the 24 hours, because exercise may cause an increased CC.
- Collect the last specimen as close as possible to the end of the 24-hour period. Add this urine to the container.
- Make sure a venous blood sample is drawn in a red-top tube during the 24-hour collection.
- Mark the patient's age, weight, and height on the requisition sheet.

After

- Transport the urine specimen promptly to the laboratory.
- Apply pressure or a pressure dressing to the venipuncture site.
- Observe the venipuncture site for bleeding.

Test Results and Clinical Significance

Increased levels

Exercise
Pregnancy
High cardiac output syndromes.
As blood flow increases to the kidney, GFR and CC increase.

Decreased levels

Impaired kidney function (e.g., renal artery atherosclerosis, glomerulonephritis, acute tubular necrosis)
Conditions causing decreased GFR (e.g., congestive heart failure, cirrhosis with ascites, shock, dehydration)
Conditions that are associated with decreased blood flow to the kidney will decrease GFR.

Related Tests

- Blood urea nitrogen (BUN) (p. 443): This is a test of renal function. Unlike creatinine, there are many nonrenal factors that can alter this test result.
- Creatinine, blood (p. 178): The creatinine is used to diagnose impaired renal function.

Cryoglobulin

Normal Findings No cryoglobulins detected

Indications

This test is performed to identify cryoglobulins in patients with symptoms of purpura, arthralgia, or Raynaud's phenomenon. Cryoglobulin testing is used to support the diagnosis of the diseases that are known to be associated with cryoglobulins.

Test Explanation

Cryoglobulins are abnormal immunoglobulin protein complexes that exist within the blood of patients with various diseases. These proteins will precipitate reversibly at low temperatures and redissolve with rewarming. These cryoglobulins can precipitate within the blood vessels of the fingers when exposed to cold temperatures. This precipitation causes slugging of the blood within those blood vessels. These patients may have symptoms of purpura, arthralgia, or Raynaud's phenomenon (pain, cyanosis, coldness of the fingers).

These proteins exist in varying degrees depending on the disease entity with which they are associated. Serum levels greater than 5 mg/ml are associated with multiple myeloma, macroglobulinemia, and leukemia. Globulin levels between 1 and 5 mg/ml are associated with rheumatoid arthritis. Levels less than 1 mg/ml can be associated with systemic lupus erythematosus, rheumatoid arthritis, infectious mononucleosis, viral hepatitis, endocarditis, cirrhosis, and glomerulonephritis. Idiopathic or primary cryoglobulinemia is not associated with any primary disease.

For this test, the blood sample is taken to the chemistry laboratory, where it is allowed to clot. It is then refrigerated for 3 to 7 hours. After that time the specimen is evaluated for precipitation. If precipitation is identified, it is measured and recorded. The cryoglobulins are then identified by immunoelectrophoresis. The tube is then rewarmed, and the specimen is reexamined for dissolution of that precipitation. If precipitation of the refrigerated specimen is identified and dissolved on rewarming, cryoglobulins are present.

Procedure and Patient Care

Before

- Explain the procedure to the patient.
- Inform the patient that an 8-hour fast may be required. This will minimize turbidity of the serum caused by ingestion of a recent (especially fatty) meal. Turbidity may make the detection of precipitation rather difficult.

During

- Collect 10 ml of venous blood in a red-top tube that has been prewarmed to body temperature.

After

- Apply pressure or a pressure dressing to the venipuncture site.
- Observe the venipuncture site for bleeding.
- If cryoglobulins are present, warn the patient to avoid cold temperatures and contact with cold objects to minimize Raynaud's symptoms. Tell the patient to wear gloves in cold weather.

Test Results and Clinical Significance

The following is a list of diseases associated with the presence of cryoglobulins:

Connective tissue disease (e.g., lupus erythematosus, Sjögren's syndrome, rheumatoid arthritis)

Lymphoid malignancies (e.g., multiple myeloma, leukemia, Waldenström's macroglobulinemia, lymphoma)

Acute and chronic infections (e.g., infectious mononucleosis, endocarditis, poststreptoccocal glomerulonephritis)

Liver disease (e.g., hepatitis, cirrhosis)

Related Tests

- Agglutinin, febrile, cold (p. 28): These agglutinins are antibodies that cause RBCs to aggregate at high or low temperatures, respectively. They are believed to be due to infection by organisms having antigenic groups similar to some of those found on the RBCs.
- Rheumatoid factor (p. 389): This test is useful in the diagnosis of rheumatoid arthritis. Other diseases, such as SLE, may cause a positive result.

Cytomegalovirus (CMV)

Normal Findings

No virus isolated

Indications

This test is used to identify CMV in suspected patients.

Test Explanation

CMV belongs to the viral family that includes herpes simplex, Epstein-Barr, and varicella-zoster viruses. CMV infection is widespread. Infections usually occur in the fetus, during early childhood, and in the young adult. Certain populations are at increased risk. Male homosexuals, transplant patients, and AIDS patients are particularly susceptible. Infections are acquired by contact with body secretions or urine. Blood transfusions are commonly implicated in the spread of CMV. As many as 35% of patients receiving multiple transfusions become infected with CMV. Most patients with acute disease have no or very few (mononucleosis-like) symptoms. Others may have mononucleosis-like symptoms of fever, lethargy, and anorexia. After infection there is an asymptomatic incubation period of about 60 days. Acute symptoms then develop. This is followed by a latent phase. Reactivation can occur at any time.

CVM is the most common congenital infection. Pregnant mothers can get the disease during their pregnancy, or a previous CMV infection can become reactivated. Approximately 10% of infected newborns exhibit permanent damage, usually mental retardation and auditory damage. Fetal infection can cause microcephaly, hydrocephaly, cerebral palsy, mental retardation, or death.

The term "TORCH" (toxoplasmosis, other, rubella, CVM, herpes) has been applied to infections with recognized detrimental effects on the fetus. The effects on the fetus may be direct or indirect (e.g., precipitating abortion or premature labor). Included in the category of other are infections (e.g., syphilis). All of these tests are discussed separately.

Virus culture is the most definitive method of diagnosis. However, a culture cannot differentiate an acute infection from a chronic, inactive infection. Immunofluorescence, enzyme-linked immunosorbent assay, and latex agglutination methods of identifying anti-CMV antibodies reveal much more information about the activity of the infection. CMV IgG antibody levels persist for years after infection. Identification of IgM antibodies, however, indicates a relatively recent infection. Three different CMV antigens can be detected immunologically. They are called early, intermediate-early, and late antigens and indicate onset of infection. CVM inclusion bodies can be identified in the renal cells sloughed into the urine and are seen during a routine urinalysis.

No specific therapy is known for this infection. If the diagnosis is established early by viral culture or serology, abortion may be an option. A fourfold increase in CMV titer in paired sera drawn 10 to 14 days apart is usually indicative of an acute infection.

Procedure and Patient Care

Before

- Explain the procedure to the patient.

During

- For culture specimens, a urine, sputum, or mouth swab is the specimen of choice. Fresh specimens are essential.
- The specimens are cultured in a virus laboratory, which takes about 3 to 7 days.
- For an antibody or antigen titer, draw 4 to 7 ml of blood in a gold- or red-top tube.
- Collect a specimen from the mother with suspected acute infection as early as possible.
- Collect the convalescent specimen 2 to 4 weeks later.

After

- Apply pressure or a pressure dressing to the venipuncture site.
- Assess the venipuncture site for bleeding.

Test Results and Clinical Significance

CMV infection

D-Dimer (Fragment D-Dimer, Fibrin Degradation Product [FDP])

Normal Findings

Qualitative: negative (no D-dimer fragments present)
Quantitative: <250 ng/ml or <250 mg/L (SI units)

Indications

This is a very specific confirmatory test for disseminated intravascular coagulation (DIC).

Test Explanation

The fragment D-dimer assesses both thrombin and plasmin activity. D-dimer is a fibrin degradation fragment that is made through fibrinolysis. As plasmin acts on the fibrin polymer clot, FDPs and D-dimer are produced. D-dimer assay is a highly specific measurement of the amount of fibrin degradation that occurs. Normal plasma does not have detectable amounts of fragment D-dimer.

This test provides a simple and confirmatory test for DIC. Positive results of the D-dimer assay correlate with positive results of FDPs. Although the D-dimer assay is more specific than the FDP assay, it is less sensitive. Therefore combining the FDP and the D-dimer test provides a highly sensitive and specific test for DIC.

Levels of D-dimer can also increase when a fibrin clot is lysed by thrombolytic therapy. Thrombotic problems, such as deep-vein thrombosis, pulmonary embolism, sickle cell anemia, and thrombosis of malignancy, are also associated with high D-dimer levels.

Procedure and Patient Care

Before

- Explain the procedure to the patient.
- Tell the patient that no fasting is required.

During

- Collect a venous blood sample in a blue-top tube.

After

- Apply pressure or a pressure dressing to the venipuncture site.
- Assess the venipuncture site for bleeding. If the patient is receiving anticoagulants or has coagulopathies, remember that the bleeding time will be increased.

Test Results and Clinical Significance

Increased levels

Disseminated intravascular coagulation *This is a phenomenon of rapid intramicrovascular coagulation and synchronous fibrinolysis. D-dimer is produced by the action of plasmin on the fibrin polymer clot.*

Primary fibrinolysis
During thrombolytic or defibrination therapy
D-dimer is produced by the action of plasmin on the fibrin polymer clot.

Deep-vein thrombosis
Pulmonary embolism
Arterial thromboembolism
Vaso-occlusive crisis of sickle cell anemia
The body's natural reaction to clot development is fibrinolysis. D-dimer is produced by the action of plasmin on the fibrin polymer clot.

Pregnancy
Malignancy
Surgery
These clinical situations are associated with varying degrees of clotting and fibrinolysis. D-dimer is produced by the action of plasmin on the fibrin polymer clot.

Related Tests

The following are tests used to assist in the diagnosis of DIC:

- Bleeding time (p. 115): This test is used to evaluate the vascular and platelet factors associated with hemostasis.
- Thrombin time (p. 408): This is a test of the fibrinogen to fibrin reaction.
- Prothrombin time (p. 366): The PT is used to evaluate the adequacy of the extrinsic system and common pathway in the clotting mechanism.
- Coagulating factor concentration (p. 154): This is a quantitative measurement of specific coagulation factors.
- Partial thromboplastin time, activated (p. 319): This test is used to evaluate the intrinsic system and the common pathway of clot formation. It is most commonly used to monitor heparin therapy.
- Fibrin degradation product (p. 213): This is a more sensitive and less specific test used to confirm the diagnosis of DIC.
- Euglobulin lysis time (p. 207): This test is used to evaluate systemic fibrinolysis.

Dexamethasone Suppression
(DS, Prolonged/Rapid DS, Cortisol Suppression, Adrenocorticotropic Hormone [ACTH] Suppression)

Normal Findings

Prolonged method

Expected values (normal)
Low dose: >50% reduction of plasma cortisol and 17-hydroxycorticosteroid (17-OCHS) levels
High dose: >50% reduction of plasma cortisol and 17-OCHS levels

Rapid method

Normal: nearly zero cortisol levels

Indications

The DS test is important for diagnosing adrenal hyperfunction (Cushing's syndrome) and distinguishing its cause.

Test Explanation

An elaborate feedback mechanism for cortisol exists to coordinate the function of the hypothalamus, pituitary gland, and the adrenal glands. Corticotropin-releasing hormone (CRH) is made in the hypothalamus. This stimulates ACTH production in the anterior pituitary gland. ACTH stimulates the adrenal cortex to produce cortisol. The rising levels of cortisol act as a negative feedback and curtail further production of CRH and ACTH. Cortisol is a potent glucocorticoid released from the adrenal cortex. This hormone affects the metabolism of carbohydrates, proteins, and fats. It especially has a profound effect on glucose serum levels.

The DS test is based on pituitary ACTH secretion being dependent on the plasma cortisol feedback mechanism. As plasma cortisol levels increase, ACTH secretion is suppressed; as cortisol levels decrease, ACTH secretion is stimulated. Dexamethasone is a synthetic steroid (similar to cortisol) that will suppress ACTH secretion. Under normal circumstances this results in reduced stimulation to the adrenal glands and ultimately a drop of 50% or more in plasma cortisol and 17-OCHS levels. This important feedback system does not function properly in patients with Cushing's syndrome.

In Cushing's syndrome caused by bilateral adrenal hyperplasia (Cushing's disease), the pituitary gland is reset upward and responds only to high plasma levels of cortisone and steroids. In Cushing's syndrome caused by adrenal adenoma or cancer (which acts autonomously), cortisol secretion will continue despite a decrease in ACTH. When Cushing's syndrome is caused by an ectopic ACTH-producing tumor (as in lung cancer), that tumor is also considered autonomous and will continue to secrete ACTH despite high cortisol levels. Again, no decrease occurs in plasma cortisol. Knowledge of the following defects in the normal cortisol-ACTH feedback system is the basis for understanding the DST:

Cushing's Syndrome Caused by *Bilateral Adrenal Hyperplasia*

Low dose: no change
High dose: 50% reduction of plasma cortisol and 17-OCHS levels

Cushing's Syndrome Caused by *Adrenal Adenoma or Carcinoma*

Low dose: no change
High dose: no change

Cushing's Syndrome Caused by *Ectopic ACTH-Producing Tumor*

Low dose: no change
High dose: no change

The DS test also may identify depressed persons likely to respond to electroconvulsive therapy or antidepressants rather than to psychologic or social interventions. ACTH production will not be suppressed after administration of low-dose DS in these patients.

The *prolonged* DS test can be performed over a 6-day period on an outpatient basis.

The *rapid* DS test is easily and quickly performed and is used primarily as a screening test to diagnose Cushing's syndrome. It is less accurate and less informative than the prolonged DS test, but when its results are normal, the diagnosis of Cushing's syndrome can safely be excluded. The ease with which the rapid DS test can be performed makes it useful in clinical medicine.

Interfering Factors

- Physical and emotional stress can elevate ACTH release and obscure interpretation of test results. Stress is stimulatory to the pituitary, which thereby secretes ACTH.
- Drugs that can affect test results include barbiturates, estrogens, oral contraceptives, phenytoin (Dilantin), spironolactone (Aldactone), steroids, and tetracyclines.

Procedure and Patient Care

Before

- Explain the procedure (prolonged or rapid test) to the patient.
- Obtain the patient's weight as a baseline for evaluating side effects of steroids.

During

Prolonged Test

- Obtain a baseline 24-hour urine collection for corticosteroids (urine 17-OCHS [see p. 835] or urinary cortisol).
- Collect blood for determination of baseline plasma cortisol levels if indicated. Collect 24-hour urine specimens daily over a 6-day period. Because 6 continuous days of urine collections are needed, no urine specimens are discarded except for the first voided specimen on day 1, after which the collection begins.
- On day 3 administer a low dose (0.5 mg) of DS by mouth every 6 hours for a total of 2 mg.
- On day 5 administer a high dose (2.0 mg) of DS by mouth every 6 hours for a total of 8 mg.
- Administer the DS with milk or an antacid to prevent gastric irritation.
- The urine samples for cortisol and 17-OCHS do not need a preservative.
- Note that the creatinine content is measured in all the 24-hour urine collections to demonstrate their accuracy and adequacy.
- Keep the urine specimens refrigerated or on ice during the collection period.

Rapid Test

- Give the patient 1 mg of dexamethasone by mouth at 11 PM.
- Administer the DS with milk or an antacid to prevent gastric irritation.
- If ordered, administer a barbiturate to sedate the patient and to ensure a good night's sleep.
- At 8 AM the next morning, draw blood for determination of the plasma cortisol level before the patient arises.
- If no cortisol suppression occurs after 1 mg of dexamethasone, administer a higher dose (8 mg) to suppress ACTH production. This is referred to as the overnight 8-mg DS suppression test.

After

- Evaluate the patient for evidence of gastric irritation.
- Assess the patient for steroid-induced side effects by monitoring weight, glucose levels, and potassium levels.
- Send specimens to the laboratory promptly.

Test Results and Clinical Significance

Adrenal hyperfunction (Cushing's syndrome)

Cushing's disease
Ectopic ACTH-producing tumors
In these illnesses, ACTH is produced without regard to the inhibitory feedback mechanism that normally exists. This is a result of neoplastic overproduction of ACTH in the pituitary or elsewhere in the body by an ACTH-producing cancer. ACTH is not suppressed. As a result, cortisol is not suppressed.

Adrenal adenoma or carcinoma *Neoplasms of the adrenal glands are not sensitive to the inhibitory feedback mechanism that normally exists. Therefore ACTH will be suppressed by the DS, but cortisol production (the end point of the test) is not.*
Bilateral adrenal hyperplasia *The inhibitory feedback mechanism that normally exists in the pituitary-adrenal system is blunted. Therefore at low dose no change in cortisol production is seen. At high dose, however, the ACTH and subsequently cortisol are suppressed.*
Mental depression *ACTH is not suppressed in individuals likely to require electroconvulsive or medicinal therapy for their depression.*

Related Tests

- Adrenocorticotropic hormone (ACTH) stimulation (p. 26): This test is used to evaluate the differential diagnosis of Cushing's syndrome or Addison's disease.
- Adrenocorticotropic hormone (ACTH) (p. 23): The serum ACTH study is a test of anterior pituitary gland function that affords the greatest insight into the causes of either Cushing's syndrome (overproduction of cortisol) or Addison's disease (underproduction of cortisol).
- Cortisol, blood (p. 167): This is a direct measurement of the cortisol blood level.
- Urinary cortisol (p. 827): This test is a measure of urinary cortisol. It is performed on patients who are suspected to have hyper- or hypofunctioning of the adrenal gland.

2,3-Diphosphoglycerate (2,3-DPG in Erythrocytes)

Normal Findings

12.3 ± 1.87 mmol/g of hemoglobin
4.2 ± 0.64 mmol/ml of erythrocytes
Levels are lower in newborns and even lower in premature infants.

Indications

This test is used in the evaluation of nonspherocytic anemia.

Test Explanation

2,3-DPG is a by-product of the glycolytic respiratory pathway of the RBC. A congenital enzyme deficiency in this vital pathway alters the RBC shape and survival significantly. Nonspherocytic anemia is the result. Another result of the enzyme deficiency is reduced synthesis of 2,3-DPG. 2,3-DPG controls O_2 transport from the RBCs to the tissues. Deficiencies of this enzyme result in alterations of the RBC O_2 dissociation curve that controls release of O_2 to the tissues. Many anemias not due to 2,3-DPG deficiency are associated with increased levels of 2,3-DPG as a compensatory mechanism.

Usually, 2,3-DPG levels increase in response to anemia or hypoxic conditions (e.g., obstructive lung disease, congenital cyanotic heart disease, after vigorous exercise). Increases in 2,3-DPG decrease the O_2 binding to hemoglobin so that O_2 is more easily released to the tissues when needed (lower arterial Po_2). Levels of 2,3-DPG are decreased as a result of inherited genetic defects. This genetic defect parallels sickle cell anemia and hemoglobin C diseases.

Interfering Factors

- Levels may be increased after vigorous exercise.
- High altitudes may increase 2,3-DPG levels.
- Banked blood has decreased amounts of 2,3-DPG.
- Acidosis decreases 2,3-DPG levels.

Procedure and Patient Care

Before

- Explain the procedure to the patient.
- Tell the patient that no fasting is required.

During

- Collect a venous blood sample in a red-top tube.

After

- Apply pressure or a pressure dressing to the venipuncture site.
- Assess the venipuncture site for bleeding.

Test Results and Clinical Significance

Increased levels

Anemia *Increased 2,3-DPG levels are compensatory to provide adequate O_2 to the tissues.*

Hypoxic heart and lung diseases (e.g., obstructive lung disease, cystic fibrosis, congenital cyanotic heart disease) *Hypoxemia stimulates the production of 2,3-DPG.*

Hyperthyroidism *Increased metabolic processes increase O_2 requirements. This need is met by increased 2,3-DPG.*

Chronic renal failure *Erythropoietin deficiency as a result of chronic renal failure causes anemia. Increased 2,3-DPG levels are compensatory to provide adequate O_2 to the tissues.*
Pyruvate kinase deficiency *This enzyme is important in the glycolytic respiratory pathway of the RBC. Its function is to metabolize 2,3-DPG by-products. In the absence of this enzyme, 2,3-DPG is not metabolized and increased levels result.*

Decreased levels

Polycythemia *2,3-DPG is made in the RBC as a result of its glycolytic respiratory process. Increased numbers of RBCs will cause compensatory decreased 2,3-DPG.*
Acidosis *Decreased 2,3-DPG is associated with metabolic or respiratory acidosis.*
After massive blood transfusion *Banked RBCs lose their 2,3-DPG during storage.*
2,3-DPG disease *The enzymes required for synthesis of 2,3-DPG are reduced. As a result, 2,3-DPG is reduced.*
Respiratory distress syndrome *The pathophysiology of this observation is unknow.*

Related Tests

- Complete blood cell count (p. 162): This is a series of tests that provide information about the hematologic system and many other organ systems.

Disseminated Intravascular Coagulation Screening (DIC Screening)

Normal Findings

No evidence of DIC

Indications

This group of tests is indicated for patients who are suspected of having acute DIC (demonstrate a coagulopathy), for patients who have chronic DIC (chronic microembolic processes), and for patients who are at great risk for DIC (patients with sepsis or advanced cancer).

Test Explanation

This is a group of tests used to detect DIC. Many pathologic conditions can instigate or are associated with DIC. The more common ones include bacterial septicemia, amniotic fluid embolism, retention of a dead fetus, malignant neoplasia, liver cirrhosis, extensive surgery (especially on the prostate or liver), extracorporeal heart bypass, extensive trauma, severe burns, and transfusion reactions.

In DIC the entire clotting mechanism is triggered inappropriately. This results in significant systemic or localized intravascular formation of fibrin clots. Consequences of this futile clotting are intravascular slugging and excessive bleeding caused by consumption of the platelets and clotting factors that have been used in intravascular clotting. The fibrinolytic system is also activated to break down the clot formation and the fibrin involved in the intravascular coagulation. This fibrinolysis results in the formation of fibrin degradation products (FDPs), which, by themselves, act as anticoagulants; these FDPs only serve to enhance the bleeding tendency.

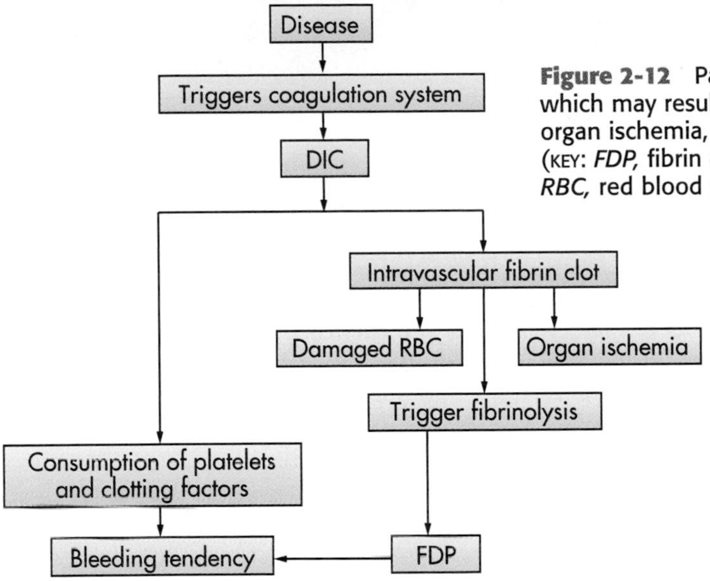

Figure 2-12 Pathophysiology of DIC, which may result in bleeding tendency, organ ischemia, and hemolytic anemia. (KEY: *FDP,* fibrin degradation products; *RBC,* red blood cells.)

Organ injury can occur as a result of the intravascular clots, which cause microvascular occlusion in various organs. This may cause serious anoxic injury in affected organs. Also, RBCs passing through partly plugged vessels are injured and subsequently hemolyzed. The result may be ongoing hemolytic anemia. Figure 2-12 summarizes DIC pathophysiology and effects. Heparin is sometimes used to treat DIC, because it inhibits the ongoing futile thrombin formation. This decreases the use of clotting factors and platelets, and bleeding ceases.

When a patient with a bleeding tendency is suspected of having DIC, a series of routinely performed laboratory tests are done (prothrombin time [PT], partial thromboplastin time [PTT] bleeding time, and platelet count). If they are abnormal, further testing should be performed (Table 2-19). With these tests, the hematologist can make the appropriate diagnosis confidently. All of these tests are discussed separately.

Table 2-19 DIC blood tests

Test	Result	Reference page
Bleeding time	Prolonged	115
Platelet count	Decreased	337
Prothrombin time	Prolonged	366
Partial thromboplastin time	Prolonged	319
Coagulation factors	I, II, V, VIII, X, XIII decreased	154
Fibrin degradation products	Increased	213
Red blood smear	Damaged RBC	
Euglobulin lysis time	Normal or prolonged	207
D-dimer	Increased	186
Thrombin time	Prolonged	408

Drug Monitoring
(Therapeutic Drug Monitoring [TDM])

Normal Findings (Table 2-20)

Indications This test is done to monitor drug levels.

Test Explanation

TDM entails measuring blood drug levels to determine effective drug dosages and to prevent toxicity. It is also used to identify noncompliant patients. Patient age and size, extent and rate of drug absorption or excretion, and metabolic rate can all affect drug levels. Measurement of drug levels is very important in patients who are beyond the normal range in these variables or who have other diseases that can affect drug levels. Drug monitoring is helpful in patients who take other medicines that may affect drug levels or act in a synergistic or antagonistic manner with the drug to be tested. There are some medi-

Table 2-20 ***Therapeutic drug monitoring data***

Drug	Use	Therapeutic level*	Toxic level*
Acetaminophen	Analgesic, antipyretic	Depends on use	>250 μg/ml
Amikacin	Antibiotic	15-25 μg/ml	>25 μg/ml
Aminophylline	Bronchodilator	10-20 μg/ml	>20 μg/ml
Amitriptyline	Antidepressant	120-150 ng/ml	>500 ng/ml
Carbamazepine	Anticonvulsant	5-12 μg/ml	>12 μg/ml
Chloramphenicol	Antiinfective	10-20 μg/ml	>25 μg/ml
Desipramine	Antidepressant	150-300 ng/ml	>500 ng/ml
Digitoxin	Cardiac glycoside	15-25 ng/ml	>25 ng/ml
Digoxin	Cardiac glycoside	0.8-2.0 ng/ml	>2.4 ng/ml
Disopyramide	Antiarrhythmic	2-5 μg/ml	>5 μg/ml
Ethosuximide	Anticonvulsant	40-100 μg/ml	>100 μg/ml
Gentamicin	Antibiotic	5-10 μg/ml	>12 μg/ml
Imipramine	Antidepressant	150-300 ng/ml	>500 ng/ml
Kanamycin	Antibiotic	20-25 μg/ml	>35 μg/ml
Lidocaine	Antiarrhythmic	1.5-5.0 μg/ml	>5 μg/ml
Lithium	Manic episodes of manic-depression psychosis	0.8-1.2 mEq/L	>2.0 mEq/L
Methrotrexate	Antitumor agent	>0.01 μmol	>10 μmol/24 hr
Nortriptyline	Antidepressant	50-150 ng/ml	>500 ng/ml
Phenobarbital	Anticonvulsant	10-30 μg/ml	>40 μg/ml
Phenytoin	Anticonvulsant	10-20 μg/ml	>30 μg/ml
Primidone	Anticonvulsant	5-12 μg/ml	>15 μg/ml
Procainamide	Antiarrhythmic	4-10 μg/ml	>16 μg/ml
Propranolol	Antiarrhythmic	50-100 ng/ml	>150 ng/ml
Quinidine	Antiarrhythmic	2-5 μg/ml	>10 μg/ml
Salicylate	Antipyretic, antiinflammatory, analgesic	100-250 μg/ml	>300 μg/ml
Theophylline	Bronchodilator	10-20 μg/ml	>20 μg/ml
Tobramycin	Antibiotic	5-10 μg/ml	>12 μg/ml
Valproic acid	Anticonvulsant	50-100 μg/ml	>100 μg/ml

*Levels vary according to the laboratory performing the test.

Box 2-4	Factors influencing blood drug levels	
Route of administration	Drug absorption	Drug delivery (cardiovascular function)
Drug metabolism	Drug excretion	Dosage
Age	Weight	Other medications
Other disease	Laboratory methods	Patient compliance

cines (e.g., antiarrhythmics, bronchodilators, antibiotics, anticonvulsants, cardiotonics) that have a very narrow therapeutic margin (i.e., the difference between therapeutic and toxic drug levels is small).

TDM is helpful if the desired therapeutic effect of the drug is not observed as expected. Dosages beyond normal may have to be prescribed. Likewise, if toxic symptoms appear with standard doses, TDM can be used to determine further dosing.

Table 2-20 lists the therapeutic and toxic ranges for the average patient. These ranges may not apply to all patients, because clinical response is influenced by many factors (Box 2-4). Also, note that different laboratories use different units for reporting test results and normal ranges. It is important that sufficient time pass between the administration of the medication and the collection of the blood sample to allow for adequate absorption and therapeutic levels to occur.

Blood is routinely used for TDM, because results indicate what is presently going on with the drug at any one particular time. Urine drug levels reflect the presence of the drug over the last several days. Therefore, if data concerning drug levels at a particular time are necessary, blood testing is required. Gas chromatography, thin-layer chromatography, radioimmunoassay, fluorescent immunoassay, and other laboratory methods are used to determine drug levels.

Blood samples can be taken at the drug's *peak* level (highest concentration of drug) or at the *trough* level (lowest concentration of drug). Peak levels are useful when testing for toxicity, and trough levels are useful for demonstrating a satisfactory therapeutic level. Trough levels are often referred to as residual levels. The time when the sample should be drawn after the last dose of the medication varies according to whether a peak or trough level is requested and according to the half-life (the time required for the body to decrease the drug blood level by 50%) of the drug. Table 2-21 lists the peak drug times for some common drugs. Both peak and trough levels should be within the therapeutic range. If peak levels are higher than the therapeutic range, toxicity may be experienced. It trough levels are below the therapeutic range, drug therapy is inadequate.

Procedure and Patient Care

Before

- Explain the procedure to the patient.
- Tell the patient that no food or fluid restrictions are needed.
- For patients suspected of having symptoms of drug toxicity, the best time to draw the blood specimen is when the symptoms are occurring.
- If there is a concern as to whether an adequate dose of the drug is achieved, it is best to obtain trough levels.

Table 2-21 *Peak drug times for some common drugs*

Drug (given by routine route)	Peak (hr)
Phenytoin	4-8
Phenobarbitol	12
Lithium	1-3
Tricyclic antidepressants	2-6
Procainamide	1-2
Procainamide SR	4
Lidocaine	2
Quinidine	2
Digoxin	½-1 ½
Theophylline	2-3
Gentamicin	½
Vancomycin	¼-2

During

- Collect approximately 7 to 10 ml of venous blood in a tube designated by the laboratory. *Peak* levels are usually obtained 1 to 2 hours after oral intake, approximately 1 hour after IM administration, and approximately 30 minutes after IV administration. *Residual* (trough) levels are usually obtained shortly before (0 to 15 minutes) the next scheduled dose. Consult with the pharmacy for specific times.

After

- Apply pressure or a pressure dressing to the venipuncture site.
- Assess the venipuncture site for bleeding.
- Clearly mark all blood samples with the following information: patient's name, diagnosis, name of drug, time of last drug ingestion, time of sample, and any other medications the patient is currently taking.
- Promptly send the specimen to the laboratory.

Test Results and Clinical Significance

Nontherapeutic levels of drugs

Toxic levels of drugs

One must always be aware that TDM is only a guide to treatment. Therapy may be successful at drug levels below therapeutic range. Further levels above therapeutic range may be necessary in some patients to obtain adequate therapy.

Related Tests

- Toxicology testing (p. 854): This is generally a urine test to determine the toxic effect of prescribed and nonprescribed drugs often used and abused in criminal behavior.

Epstein-Barr Virus Titer (EBV)

Normal Findings

Titers ≤1:10 are nondiagnostic.
Titers of 1:10 to 1:60 indicate infection at some undetermined time.
Titers of ≥1:320 suggest active infection.
Fourfold increase in titer in paired sera drawn 10 to 14 days apart is usually indicative of an acute infection.

Indications

This test is used to diagnose a suspected EBV infection (infectious mononucleosis [IM])

Test Explanation

EBV infects 80% of the U.S. population. Once infection occurs, the virus becomes dormant but can be reactivated later. EBV infection can produce IM. Mononucleosis is seen most often in children, adolescents, and young adults. Clinical features include acute fatigue, fever, sore throat, lymphadenopathy, and splenomegaly. Laboratory findings of lymphocytosis, atypical lymphocytes, and transient serum heterophil antibodies are seen in patients with acute EBV infection. Most patients with IM recover uneventfully and return to normal activity within 4 to 6 weeks. In Africa, EBV has been associated with Burkitt's lymphoma. In China, EBV infection has been associated with nasopharyngeal carcinoma.

After recovery from primary EBV infection, patients are lifelong, latent EBV carriers. In the last several years, specific immunologic tests to identify EBV activity indicate that latent EBV can reactivate and become associated with a constellation of chronic signs and symptoms resembling IM. Clinical manifestations of chronic EBV are variable and include nonspecific symptoms, such as profound fatigue (chronic fatigue syndrome), pharyngitis, myalgia, arthralgia, low-grade fever, headache, paresthesia, and loss of abstract thinking.

Serologic tests are the only way to make the diagnosis of EBV. The heterophil agglutination slide test (mononucleosis [mono] spot test) helps support the diagnosis. Other, more specific immunologic tests indicate more precisely the timing of the infection (Table 2-22). The viral capsid antigen-antibodies (VCAs) can be IgG or IgM. The EBV nuclear antigen (EBNA) is located in the nuclei of the infected lymphocyte. Another EBV antigen is called the early antigen (EA). There are two EA antigens. One is spread diffusely about the cytoplasm of the lymphocyte (EA-D), and the other is restricted to only one area of the cytoplasm (EA-R). EA-D is commonly found in nasopharyngeal cancer. EA-R is commonly found in Burkitt's lymphoma.

The interpretation of EBV antibody tests is based on the following assumptions:

1. Once the person becomes infected with EBV, the anti-VCA antibodies appear first.
2. Anti-EA (EA-D or EA-R) antibodies appear next or are present with anti-VCA an-

Table 2-22 Serologic studies and the timing of infections

Serologic study	Appears/Disappears	Clinical significance
Mono spot heterophil	5 days/2 wk	Acute or convalescent infection
VCA-IgM	7 days/3 mos	Acute or convalescent infection
VCA-IgG	7 days/exists for life	Acute, convalescent, or old infection
EBNA-IgG	3 wk/exists for life	Old infection
EA-D	7 days/2 wk	Acute or convalescent infection

tibodies early in the course of illness. An anti-EA antibody titer greater than 80 in a patient 2 years after acute IM indicates chronic EBV syndrome.

3. As the patient recovers, anti-VCA and anti-EA antibodies decrease and anti-EBNA antibodies appear. Anti-EBNA antibody persists for life and reflects a past infection.
4. After the patient is well, anti-VCA and anti-EBNA antibodies are always present but at lower ranges. Occasionally anti-EA antibody also may be present after the patient recovers.

If an acute infection is suspected to have occurred more than a few weeks prior to testing, the mono spot test may be negative. Detecting anti-VCA IgG or EBNA will not be helpful, because they indicate that an EBV infection has occurred sometime in the patient's life but not necessarily recently. But detecting anti-VCA IgM would indicate that the syndrome of complaints the patient experienced a few weeks prior was due to EBV.

Procedure and Patient Care

Before

- Explain the procedure to the patient.
- Tell the patient that no fasting or special preparation is required.

During

- Collect 5 to 10 ml of venous blood in a red-top tube.
- Record the date of onset of illness on the laboratory slip.
- Obtain serum samples as soon as possible after the onset of illness.
- Obtain a second blood specimen 14 to 21 days later.

After

- Apply pressure or a pressure dressing to the venipuncture site.
- Observe the venipuncture site for bleeding.

Test Results and Clinical Significance

Increased levels

IM

Chronic EBV carrier state

To make this diagnosis, one of the antibodies should be found in abnormal titers.

Chronic fatigue syndrome *These EBV antibodies are not found in all cases.*
Burkitt's lymphoma
Nasopharyngeal cancer (only occasionally in the United States)
These cancers are frequently associated with EBV carrier states. However, a cause-and-effect relationship has not been determined.

Related Tests

- Mononucleosis spot (p. 309): This test is used to detect heterophil antibodies that can support the diagnosis of EBV infection (IM).

Erythrocyte Sedimentation Rate
(ESR, Sed Rate Test)

Normal Findings

Westergren Method
Male: up to 15 mm/hr
Female: up to 20 mm/hr
Child: up to 10 mm/hr
Newborn: 0-2 mm/hr

Indications

The ESR is a nonspecific test used to detect illnesses associated with acute and chronic infection, inflammation (collagen-vascular diseases), advanced neoplasm, and tissue necrosis or infarction.

Test Explanation

ESR is a measurement of the rate at which the RBCs settle in saline solution or plasma over a specified time period. It is nonspecific and therefore not diagnostic for any particular organ disease or injury. Because inflammatory, neoplastic, infectious, and necrotic diseases increase the protein (mainly fibrinogen) content of plasma, RBCs have a tendency to stack up on one another, increasing their weight and causing them to descend faster. Therefore in these diseases the ESR will be increased. ESR provides the same information as an acute-phase reactant protein. That is to say that it occurs as a reaction to acute illnesses as described above.

The test can be used to detect occult disease. Many physicians use the ESR test in this way for routine patient evaluation for vague symptoms. Other physicians regard this test as so nonspecific that it is useless as a routine study. The ESR test occasionally can be helpful in differentiating disease entities or complaints. For example, in a patient with chest pain the ESR will be increased with myocardial infarction but will be normal with angina.

The ESR is a fairly reliable indicator of the course of disease and therefore can be used to monitor disease therapy, especially for inflammatory autoimmune diseases (e.g., temporal arteritis, polymyalgia rheumatica). In general, as the disease worsens, the ESR increases; as the disease improves, the ESR decreases. If the results of the ESR are equivocal or inconsistent with clinical impressions, the C-reactive protein test is often performed.

ESR has several limitations:

1. As mentioned above, it is nonspecific.
2. It is sometimes not elevated in the face of active disease.
3. Many other factors may influence the results (see below).

ESR elevation may lag behind other indicators early in an infection. Likewise, in the convalescent stage of a disease or infection, the ESR may remain elevated longer than other disease indicators. ESR cannot be used as an indicator of tumor burden when it is associated with neoplastic diseases, such as myeloma or breast cancer.

Interfering Factors

- Artificially low results can occur when the collected specimen is allowed to stand longer than 3 hours before the test.
- Pregnancy (second and third trimester) can cause elevated levels.
- Menstruation can cause elevated levels.
- The sedimentation tube must be perfectly vertical. Any tilt can distort results.
- Some anemias can falsely increase the ESR. There are correction nomograms available for variations in RBC count.
- Polycythemia is associated with decreased ESR.
- Diseases associated with increased proteins (e.g., macroglobulinemia) can falsely increase the ESR.
- Drugs that may cause *increased* ESR levels include dextran, methyldopa (Aldomet), oral contraceptives, penicillamine, procainamide, theophylline, and vitamin A.
- Drugs that may cause *decreased* levels include aspirin, cortisone, and quinine.

Procedure and Patient Care

Before

- Explain the procedure to the patient.
- Hold medications that may affect test results, if indicated.

During

- Collect approximately 5 to 10 ml of venous blood in a lavender-top tube.
- In the laboratory, the blood is aspirated into a calibrated sedimentation tube and allowed to settle, usually for 60 minutes. The remaining clear area (plasma) is measured as the sedimentation rate.
- An alternate method is performed by measuring the distance (in millimeters) that RBCs descend (or settle) in normal saline solution in 1 hour.

After

- Transport the specimen immediately to the laboratory.
- Apply pressure or a pressure dressing to the venipuncture site.
- Assess the venipuncture site for bleeding.

Test Results and Clinical Significance

Increased levels

Chronic renal failure (e.g. nephritis, nephrosis) *The pathophysiology of this observation is not well defined.*

Malignant diseases (e.g., multiple myeloma, Hodgkin's disease, advanced carcinomas) *Malignant diseases are often associated with increased abnormal serum proteins. Diseases associated with increased serum proteins are associated with increased ESR.*

Bacterial infection (e.g., abdominal infections, acute pelvic inflammatory disease, syphilis, pneumonia).

Inflammatory diseases (e.g., temporal arteritis, polymyalgia rheumatica, rheumatoid arthritis, rheumatic fever, systemic lupus erythematosus).

Necrotic diseases (e.g., acute myocardial infarction, necrotic tumor, gangrene of an extremity

ESR is an acute-phase reactant protein and is elevated in the above-mentioned acute illnesses.

Diseases associated with increased proteins (e.g., hyperfibrinogenemia, macroglobulinemia) *Diseases associated with increased serum proteins are associated with increased ESR.*

Severe anemias (e.g., iron deficiency or B_{12} deficiency) *With lower RBC volumes, the RBCs settle faster than in blood containing normal RBC volume.*

Falsely decreased levels

Sickle cell anemia

Spherocytosis

Diseases that distort the RBC are associated with decreased ESR.

Hypofibrinogenemia *Disease associated with increased proteins inhibit the sedimentation of RBCs.*

Polycythemia vera *Increased cells in the blood will inhibit the sedimentation of RBCs.*

Related Tests

- Complement assay (p. 160): Some of the complement components are also acute-phase reactant proteins.
- Fibrinogen (p. 215): This is an important protein involved in the hemostatic mechanism. It is also an acute-phase reactant protein.
- C-reactive protein (p. 172): This is also an acute-phase reactant protein.

Estrogen Fraction
(Estriol Excretion, Estradiol, Estrone)

Normal Findings

	Serum	Urine μg/24 hr
Estradiol		
Child <10 years	<15 pg/ml	0-6
Adult male	10-50 pg/ml	0-6
Adult female		
Follicular phase	20-350 pg/ml	0-13
Midcycle peak	150-750 pg/ml	4-14
Luteal phase	30-450 pg/ml	4-10
Postmenopausal	<20 pg/ml	0-4
Estriol		
Male or child <10 years	N/A	1-11
Adult female		
Follicular phase	N/A	0-14
Ovulatory phase	N/A	13-54
Luteal phase	N/A	8-60
Postmenopausal	N/A	0-11
Pregnant		
1st trimester	<38 ng/ml	0-800
2nd trimester	38-140 ng/ml	800-12,000
3rd trimester	31-460 ng/ml	5000-12,000
Total estrogen		
Male or child <10 years	N/A	4-25
Female not pregnant	N/A	4-60
Female pregnant		
1st trimester	N/A	0-800
2nd trimester	N/A	800-5000
3rd trimester	N/A	5000-50,000

Rising estriol levels indicate normal fetal growth.

Critical Values

Estriol levels 40% below average of two previous values demand immediate evaluation of fetal well-being.

Indications

Estrogen measurements are used to evaluate sexual maturity, menstrual problems, and fertility problems in females. This test is also used in the evaluation of males with gynecomastia or feminization syndromes. In pregnant women it is used to indicate fetal-placental health. In patients with estrogen-producing tumors it can be used as a tumor marker.

Test Explanation

There are three major estrogens. E1 (estrone) is predominantly produced in the ovary. In females there is a feedback mechanism for the secretion of E1. Low levels of E1 stimulate the hypothalamus to produce gonadotropin-releasing factors. These hormone factors stimulate the pituitary to produce follicle-stimulating hormone (FSH) and luteinizing hormone (LH). These two hormones stimulate the ovary to produce E1, which peaks during the ovulatory phase of the menstrual cycle. This hormone is measured most often to evaluate menopausal status, sexual maturity, and gynecomastia or feminization syndromes or as a tumor marker for patients with certain ovarian tumors. E1 is the most active endogenous estrogen in the nonpregnant female. E2 (estradiol-17-beta) and estrone production and actions are similar to E1

E3 (estriol) is the major estrogen in the pregnant female. Serial urine and blood studies of estriol excretion provide an objective assessment of placental function and fetal normality in high-risk pregnancies. Excretion of estriol increases around the eighth week of gestation and continues to rise until shortly before delivery. Estriol is produced in the placenta from estrogen precursors, which are made by the fetal adrenal gland and liver. The measurement of excreted estriol is an important index of fetal well-being. Rising values indicate an adequately functioning fetoplacental unit. Decreasing values suggest fetoplacental deterioration (failing pregnancy, dysmaturity, preeclampsia/eclampsia, complicated diabetes mellitus, encephaly, fetal death) and require prompt reassessment of the pregnancy. If the estriol levels fall, early delivery of the fetus may be indicated.

Serial studies usually begin at approximately 28 to 30 weeks of gestation and are then repeated weekly. The frequency of these estriol determinations can be increased as needed to evaluate a high-risk pregnancy. Collection may be done daily. Although the first collection is the baseline value, all collection results are compared with previous ones, because decreasing values suggest fetal deterioration. Some physicians use an average of three previous values as a control value.

Estriol excretion studies can be done using 24-hour urine tests or blood studies. Because urinary creatinine excretion is relatively constant, creatinine clearance is often simultaneously tested to assess the adequacy of the 24-hour urine collection for estriol. A serially increasing estriol/creatinine ratio is a favorable sign in pregnancy. Plasma estriol determinations also can be used to evaluate the fetoplacental unit. These studies can conveniently and rapidly assess the quantity of free estriol in the plasma by radioimmunoassay (RIA). The plasma collected by venipuncture is an accurate reflection of the current status of the placenta and fetus. The advantage of the plasma estriol determination is that it is more easily obtained than a 24-hour urine specimen and less affected by medications. All the estrogens can be measured by gas chromatography. But RIA techniques are more accurate and less affected by drugs or birth control pills.

Unfortunately only severe placental distress will decrease urinary estriol sufficiently to reliably predict fetoplacental stress. Furthermore, plasma and urinary estriol levels are normally associated with a significant daily variation, which may confuse serial results. Maternal illnesses, such as hypertension, preeclampsia, anemia, and impaired renal function, can also factitiously decrease urinary estriol levels. Because these problems create a high number of false-positive and false-negative findings, most clinicians now use nonstress fetal monitoring to indicate fetal-placental health.

Interfering Factors

- Recent administration of radioisotopes may alter test results if RIA methods are used.
- Glycosuria and urinary tract infections can increase urine estriol levels.

- Drugs that may *elevate* levels include adrenocorticosteroids, ampicillin, estrogen-containing drugs, phenothiazines, and tetracyclines.
- Drugs that may *decrease* levels include clomiphene.

Procedure and Patient Care

Before

- Explain the procedure to the patient.
- If the patient is going to collect the 24-hour urine specimen at home, give her the collection bottle (with a preservative, usually 1 gr of boric acid) and instruct her to keep the urine refrigerated.
- Tell the patient that no food or fluid restrictions are needed.

During

Blood

- Collect approximately 5 ml of venous blood in a red-top tube.

24-hour Urine

- Instruct the patient to begin the 24-hour urine collection after voiding. Discard the initial specimen and start the 24-hour collection at that point.
- Collect all urine passed during the next 24 hours. Make sure the patient knows where to store the urine container.
- Keep the specimen on ice or refrigerated during the 24-hour collection period.
- Indicate the starting time on the urine container and laboratory slip.
- Post the hours for the urine collection in a prominent place to prevent accidentally discarding the specimen.
- Instruct the patient to void before defecating so that the urine is not contaminated by feces.
- Remind the patient not to put toilet paper in the collection container.
- Encourage the patient to drink fluids during the 24 hours.
- Collect the last specimen as close as possible to the end of the 24-hour period. Add this urine to the collection.
- List any drugs that may affect test results on the laboratory slip.

After

- Apply pressure or a pressure dressing to the venipuncture site.
- Observe the venipuncture site for bleeding.
- Transport the 24-hour urine specimen promptly to the laboratory.
- Inform the patient how and when to obtain the results of this study.

Test Results and Clinical Significance

Increased levels

Feminization syndromes *Estrogens are increased in these syndromes for a variety of reasons. The male begins to develop female secondary sex characteristics.*

Precocious puberty *Children who develop secondary sexual characteristics at an abnormally early age often have a genetic defect in adrenal cortisol metabolism. As a result, large amounts of sex steroid precursors accumulate and are converted to estrogens by the ovary. This causes precocious secondary sexual changes.*

Ovarian tumor
Testicular tumor
Adrenal tumor
Gonadal tumors (e.g., granulosa thecal cell tumors) secrete estrogens. The higher the levels, the greater the tumor burden. In these instances estrogen can act as a tumor marker that can be used to monitor the disease.

Normal pregnancy *E3 is the main estrogen elevated during pregnancy, although E1 and 2 are also elevated. Multiple pregnancies are associated with particularly high levels of E3.*

Hepatic cirrhosis
Liver necrosis
Estrogens are catabolized, in part, by the liver. If liver function is deficient, estrogens and their precursors accumulate. Adult feminization can result.

Hyperthyroidism *An estrogen-related increase in the production of thyroid-binding globulin produces an elevation of serum total T4.*

Decreased levels

A failing pregnancy is associated with reduced placental production of E3 *Any disease that causes fetal distress, dysmaturity, Rh isoimmunization, preclampsia/eclampsia, anencephaly, or fetal death will be associated with reduced E3 levels.*

Turner's syndrome *This syndrome is seen in females who are missing one X chromosome. They have gonadal dysgenesis to varying degrees.*

Hypopituitarism
Primary and secondary hypogonadism
Stein-Leventhal syndrome
Diseases affecting the organs involved in the synthesis of sex hormones anywhere in the hypothalamus/pituitary/gonadal axis will be associated with reduced estrogen levels.

Menopause *With normal age-related ovarian failure, estrogen (especially E1) levels decline.*

Anorexia nervosa *Reduction in fat intake reduces sterol precursors available for estrogen synthesis.*

Related Tests

- Luteinizing hormone assay (LH) and follicle-stimulating hormone (FSH) (p. 296): These are measurements of gonadal stimulatory hormones.
- Fetal nonstress (p. 504): This is a more accurate test of placental/fetal viability.

Ethanol (Ethyl Alcohol, Blood Alcohol, Blood EOH)

Normal Findings

None

Critical Values

>300 mg/dl

Indications

This test is a measurement of alcohol in the blood. It is used to diagnose alcohol intoxication and overdose.

Test Explanation

Ethanol depresses the CNS and may lead to coma and death. This test is usually performed to evaluate alcohol-impaired driving or overdose. Proper collection, handling, and storage of the blood alcohol are important for medical/legal cases involving sobriety. The blood test is the specimen of choice. Blood is taken from a peripheral vein in living patients and from the aorta in cadavers. Ethanol also can be detected in the urine, in gastric contents, or by breath analyzer. Conversion tables are available to calculate blood levels based on alcohol levels identified in the various nonblood specimens.

Blood alcohol levels between 50 to 100 mg/dl (0.05% to 0.10% weight/volume) may cause flushing, slowing of reflexes, and impaired visual activity. Most courts do not consider this level definite proof of intoxication. Persons with alcohol levels below 0.05% are not considered under the influence of alcohol. Levels over 0.10% are considered in most states to be illegal and definite evidence of intoxication. Depression of the CNS occurs with levels over 100 mg/dl, and fatalities are reported with levels over 400 mg/dl. Levels of blood alcohol greater than 100 mg/dl can cause hypotension. This is especially important to recognize in the trauma patient in shock.

Interfering Factors

- Elevated blood ketones (as with diabetic ketoacidosis) can cause false elevation of blood and breath test results.
- Alcohols other than ethanol, such as isopropyl (rubbing) alcohol or methanol (grain), will also be detected by this test.
- Use of large amounts of isopropyl alcohol in cleansing skin for a needlestick can falsely elevate the test results.

✓ CLINICAL PRIORITIES

- This test is used to diagnose alcohol intoxication and overdose.
- Proper collection, handling, and storage of the blood alcohol are important for medical/legal cases involving sobriety.
- Patients should be advised as to their legal rights.

Procedure and Patient Care

Before

- Explain the procedure to the patient.
- Follow the institution's protocol if the specimen will be used for legal purposes.
- Patients should be advised as to their legal rights. Sometimes this is best done by a law enforcement officer. The alcohol level may be used as evidence for later court proceedings.

During

- Use a povidone-iodine wipe or peroxide instead of an alcohol wipe for cleansing the venipuncture site.
- Collect a venous blood sample in a gray- or red-top tube according to the agency's protocol.
- If a gastric or urine specimen is indicated, approximately 20 to 50 ml of fluid is necessary.
- Breath analyzers are taken at the end of expiration after a deep inspiration.

After

- Apply pressure or a pressure dressing to the venipuncture site.
- Assess the venipuncture site for bleeding.
- Follow the agency's protocol regarding specimen collection.
- The exact time of specimen collection should be indicated. Also, signatures of the collector and a witness may be needed in some instances for legal evidence.

Test Results and Clinical Significance

Increased levels

Alcohol intoxication or overdose *Alcohol is rapidly absorbed from the stomach in about 1 hour. If the stomach is empty, absorption is faster. Alcohol is metabolized in the liver. A 70-kg person with normal liver function can metabolize about 15 mg of alcohol per hour.*

Euglobulin Lysis Time
(Euglobulin Clot Lysis, Fibrinolysis/Euglobulin Lysis)

Normal Findings

90 minutes-6 hours.

Critical Values

<1 hour, indicating excessive fibrinolytic activity (danger of bleeding)

Indications

Euglobulin lysis time is a measure of the activity of the fibrinolytic system. This is an old test used to identify abnormal fibrinolysis in patients with certain diseases or as a result of thrombolytic therapy.

Test Explanation

The euglobulin lysis test is used to identify systemic fibrinolysis. Fibrinolysis is an important component of normal hemostasis. Clots are constantly being formed and dissolved. The fibrinolytic system is responsible for clot dissolution. When this system is abnormally activated by drugs or abnormal proteins, any fibrin clot that is formed will be dissolved immediately, resulting in a bleeding tendency. Primary fibrinolysins are proteins that occur rarely and are most usually associated with advanced malignancies. These proteins attack fibrinogen to interrupt clot formation and only secondarily attack fibrin to create clot dissolution. Secondary fibrinolysins occur as a part of the normal response to blood clotting. Plasmin is the main secondary fibrinolysin normally active in clot dissolution (see Figure 2-10, p. 156). Drugs such as streptokinase and urokinase used in therapeutic clot lysis (thrombolytic therapy of coronary, cerebral, and other organ arterial/ venous blood clots) stimulate the conversion of plasminogen to plasmin and are therefore also considered secondary fibrinolysins. Secondary fibrinolysins are normally a response to intravascular clotting and therefore primarily work on fibrin. This fibrin dissolution creates fibrin degradation products (FDPs). No FDPs are associated with the action of primary fibrinolysins, because these proteins occur without the presence of clot formation. As mentioned above, the main action of primary fibrinolysins is to neutralize fibrinogen. Without activation of fibrinogen, no fibrin is formed. Without fibrin, no FDPs can be made. Although measurement of FDPs may be more sensitive than the euglobulin lysis time, FDPs are positive only with secondary fibrinolysis. Euglobulin lysis time can detect either primary or secondary fibrinolysis.

This test is performed by adding the patient's plasma to a blood clot from a normal person. The clot is observed for 6 to 24 hours. The time measured from clot formation to clot lysis is referred to as the euglobulin lysis time. Clot lysis before 1 hour is considered abnormal. This test takes a long time to perform, is not quantitative, and cannot identify weak or low-volume fibrinolysins.

Primary fibrinolysins can occur with malignancies (e.g., prostate, pancreas). They can also develop during shock or sepsis. Secondary fibrinolysis can be abnormally activated by disseminated intravascular coagulation (DIC) or recent surgery (especially pulmonary surgery). When combined with thrombin time and measurement of FDPs, euglobulin lysis time is very helpful in identifying and differentiating primary from secondary fibrinolysis. This test also may be used to monitor streptokinase or urokinase therapy in patients with acute myocardial infarction.

Interfering Factors

- Vigorous exercise, increasing age, and hyperventilation are associated with increased fibrinolysis.
- Postmenopausal women and newborns may have decreased fibrinolysis and therefore prolonged euglobulin lysis times.
- Decreased fibrinogen levels may result in a falsely shortened clot lysis time, because of the reduced amount of fibrin to be lysed.
- Obese patients may have decreased fibrinolysis.
- Drugs that may cause *increased* fibrinolysis include steroids and adrenocorticotropic hormone.

Procedure and Patient Care

Before

- Explain the procedure to the patient.
- Instruct the patient not to exercise before the blood sample is collected.
- Tell the patient that no fasting is required.

During

- Collect approximately 5 ml of blood in a blue-top tube.
- Avoid excessive agitation of the blood sample.
- Deliver the blood specimen to the laboratory on ice immediately.

After

- Apply pressure or a pressure dressing to the venipuncture site.
- Assess the venipuncture site for bleeding.

Test Results and Clinical Significance

Increased fibrinolysis (shortened euglobulin lysis time)

Incompatible blood transfusion
Cirrhosis
Obstetric complications (e.g., antepartum hemorrhage, septic abortion, hydatidiform mole, amniotic embolism)
Malignancies (e.g., leukemia, cancer of the prostate or pancreas)
Shock (hemorrhagic or septic)
Proteins that neutralize fibrinogen and dissolve fibrin clots directly are rarely seen in these conditions. These are considered primary fibrinolysins.

Streptokinase or urokinase administration for thrombolytic therapy *These drugs stimulate the conversion of plasminogen to plasmin. The increased plasmin causes increased fibrin clot dissolution.*

Extensive vascular trauma or surgery *Surgery is associated with increased clot formation. This in turn activates the fibrinolytic system and secondary fibrinolysis occurs. A few days after surgery, however, clot lysis times are prolonged, because plasminogen is consumed and levels diminish. Clot dissolution is therefore reduced.*

DIC *DIC is associated with an abnormal increased intravascular clot formation. This in turn activates the fibrinolytic system and secondary fibrinolysis occurs. Also FDPs interrupt the polymerization of fibrin and further inhibit coagulation.*

Decreased fibrinolysis (increased lysis time)

Prematurity *Plasminogen may be diminished.*
Diabetes *The pathophysiology of this observation is not well known.*

Related Tests

- Thrombin time (p. 408): This test is used to evaluate the fibrinogen portion of the hemostatic mechanism. Because fibrinogen levels are affected by primary fibrinolysins, this test is helpful in the evaluation of fibrinolysis.

- Fibrin degradation product (FDP) (p. 213): This test is a direct measurement of FDPs that occur as a result of fibrinolysis. It is also helpful in the evaluation of fibrinolysis.
- Plasminogen (p. 331): This is a direct measurement of the amount of plasminogen (fibrinolysin) present in the serum.

Ferritin

Normal Findings

Male: 12-300 ng/ml or 12-300 mg/L (SI units)
Female: 10-150 ng/ml or 10-150 mg/L (SI units)
Child/adolescent
  1 month: 50-200 ng/ml
  2-5 months: 50-200 ng/ml
  6 months-15 years: 7-142 ng/ml
  Newborn: 25-200 ng/ml

Indications

This is the most sensitive test to determine iron deficiency anemia.

Test Explanation

The serum ferritin study is a good indicator of available iron stores in the body. Ferritin, the major iron-storage protein, is normally present in the serum in concentrations directly related to iron storage. In normal patients, 1 ng/ml of serum ferritin corresponds to approximately 8 mg of stored iron. Ferritin levels rise persistently in males and postmenopausal females. In premenopausal females, levels stay about the same. Decreases in ferritin levels indicate a decrease in iron storage associated with iron deficiency anemia. A ferritin level of below 10 mg/100 ml is diagnostic of iron deficiency anemia. A decrease in serum ferritin level often precedes other signs of iron deficiency, such as decreased iron levels or changes in RBC size, chromasia, and number. Only when protein depletion is severe can ferritin be decreased by malnutrition. Pregnancy is also associated with decreased ferritin levels. Increased levels are a sign of iron excess, as seen in hemochromatosis, hemosiderosis, iron poisoning, or recent blood transfusions. Increases in ferritin are also noted in patients with megaloblastic anemia, hemolytic anemia, and chronic hepatitis. Furthermore, ferritin is factitiously elevated in patients with chronic disease states such as neoplasm, alcoholism, uremia, collagen diseases, or chronic liver diseases. The ferritin test is also used in patients with chronic renal failure to monitor iron stores.

A limitation of this study is that ferritin also can act as an acute-phase reactant protein and may be elevated in conditions not reflecting iron stores (e.g., acute inflammatory diseases, infections, metastatic cancer, lymphomas). Elevations in ferritin occur 1 to 2 days after onset of the acute illness and the level peaks at 3 to 5 days. If iron deficiency coexists in patients with these diseases, it may not be recognized because the levels of ferritin would be factitiously elevated by the concurrent disease.

Table 2-23 ***Iron studies in various clinical states***

	Ferritin	Iron	TIBC	TS
Chronic blood loss	L	L	E	L
Acute blood loss	N	L	N	L
Iron deficiency	L	L	E	L
Hemolytic anemia	E	E	L	E
Chronic disease	E	L	L	L
Hemochromatosis	E	E	L	E
Pregnancy	L	L	E	L
Estrogen therapy	N	E	E	L
Acute inflammation	E	N	L	E

L = low; E = elevated; N = normal; TS = transferrin saturation; TIBC = total iron binding capacity.

When combined with the serum iron level and total iron-binding capacity (TIBC), this test is useful in differentiating and classifying anemias. For example, in patients with iron deficiency anemia the ferritin, iron, and transferrin saturation levels are low, whereas the TIBC and transferrin levels are high (Table 2-23). Ferritin is measured by either radioimmunoassay or enzyme immunoassay.

Interfering Factors

- Recent transfusions or recent ingestion of a meal containing a high iron content (red meats) may cause elevated ferritin levels. The iron that is ingested stimulates ferritin production to store the increased serum iron.
- Recent administration of a radionuclide can cause abnormal levels if testing is performed by radioimmunoassay.
- Hemolytic diseases may be associated with an artificially high iron content. Iron is freed from the hemoglobin that is released from the hemolyzed RBCs. Ferritin synthesis is increased to store the increased serum iron.
- Disorders of excessive iron storage (e.g., hemochromatosis, hemosiderosis) are associated with high ferritin levels. Ferritin synthesis is increased to store the increased serum iron.
- Menstruating women may have decreased ferritin levels, because their iron stores are generally low as a result of monthly menses.
- Drugs that may *increase* ferritin levels include iron preparations. Ferritin synthesis is increased to store the increased serum iron.

Procedure and Patient Care

Before

- Explain the procedure to the patient.
- Tell the patient that no fasting is required.

During

- Collect approximately 5 to 7 ml of venous blood in a red-top tube.

After

- Apply pressure or a pressure dressing to the venipuncture site.
- Assess the venipuncture site for bleeding.

Test Results and Clinical Significance

Increased levels

Hemochromatosis
Hemosiderosis
Increased iron stores in the tissues stimulate ferritin production for storage.

Megaloblastic anemia
Hemolytic anemia
RBCs in patients with anemias lyse and release iron into the bloodstream. Ferritin production is stimulated to store the excess free iron.

Alcoholic/inflammatory hepatocellular disease
Inflammatory disease
Advanced cancers
Because ferritin is an acute-phase reactant protein, its production is increased with acute diseases.

Chronic illnesses such as leukemias, cirrhosis, chronic hepatitis, or collagen vascular diseases *The pathophysiology of this observation is not known.*

Decreased levels

Iron deficiency anemia *When iron stores are decreased, less ferritin is required. Levels diminish.*
Severe protein deficiency *Ferritin is a protein. In severely depleted persons, ferritin synthesis is reduced.*
Hemodialysis *Iron stores can be reduced by dialysis. Decreased iron stores require less ferritin. Levels diminish.*

Related Tests

- Iron level (p. 274): This is a direct measurement of bound iron in the blood.
- Total iron-binding capacity (p. 274): TIBC is a measurement of all proteins available for binding mobile iron. Transferrin represents the largest quantity of iron-binding proteins.
- Transferrin (p. 274): Transferrin represents the largest quantity of iron-binding proteins.
- Transferrin or total iron-binding (TIBC) saturation (p. 276): This is a calculation of the percentage of transferrin and other mobile iron-binding proteins saturated with iron.

Fibrin Degradation Product (FDP, Fibrin Split Product [FSP], Fibrin Breakdown Product)

Normal Findings <10 mg/ml or dilution <1:4

Critical Values >40 mg/ml

Indications

This test is a direct quantitative measurement of FDPs. It is most commonly used as a part of the evaluation of disseminated intravascular coagulation (DIC).

Test Explanation

Measurement of FDPs provides a direct indication of the activity of the fibrinolytic system. The fibrinolytic system plays an important role in balancing clot formation and clot dissolution. Clot formation stimulates the activation of three major activators of the fibrinolytic system. These in turn act on plasminogen, which was previously absorbed into the clot, to form plasmin. Plasmin degenerates the fibrin polymer of the clot into fragments called FDPs (X, D, E, Y). These degradation products are usually cleared by macrophages. If present in increased quantities, they can have an anticoagulant effect by inhibiting fibrinogen conversion to fibrin and by interrupting fibrin polymerization to tighten the clot.

When present in large amounts, FDPs indicate increased fibrinolysis, as occurs in DIC and other secondary fibrinolytic disorders. This test is one of the DIC screening tests. FDPs are also present in thrombotic states (e.g., venous thrombosis). The thrombosis stimulates the activation of the fibrinolytic system. Other diseases can potentially cause activation of the fibrinolytic system and elevate FDP levels. These may include extensive malignancy, tissue necrosis, and gram-negative sepsis. Thrombolytic therapy used, for example, in myocardial infarction is associated with increased FDPs. Streptokinase or urokinase stimulates the conversion of plasminogen to plasmin. The plasmin splits the fibrinogen polymer into FDPs, as discussed above.

Interfering Factors

- Traumatic venipuncture may alter test results.
- The presence of rheumatoid factor may give falsely high levels.
- Drugs that may cause *increased* levels include barbiturates, heparin, streptokinase, and urokinase.

Procedure and Patient Care

Before

- Explain the procedure to the patient.
- Tell the patient that no fasting is required.

During

- Draw the sample before initiating heparin therapy.
- Collect a venous blood sample (usually only 2 ml) in a small, blue-top tube or in the colored tube designated by the laboratory.
- Avoid excessive agitation of the blood sample.
- Note that it is best to place the blood on ice and take it immediately to the hematology laboratory.
- List on the laboratory slip any drugs that may cause elevated levels.

After

- Apply pressure or a pressure dressing to the venipuncture site. Patients with suspected fibrinolysis are very susceptible to coagulopathy and can bleed significantly from a venipuncture.
- Assess the venipuncture site for bleeding.

Test Results and Clinical Significance

Increased levels

DIC caused by liver disease, transplant rejection, renal disease, and obstetric complications (e.g., preeclampsia, abruptio placentae, intrauterine fetal death), infection, burns, hypoxia, trauma, massive blood transfusion, hemoglobinopathies, septicemia, and advanced malignancies *In DIC the entire clotting mechanism is triggered inappropriately. This results in significant intravascular formation of fibrin clots. The fibrinolytic system is activated to break down the fibrin clot. This results in the formation of FDPs.*

Heart/vascular surgery *Although all surgery is associated with increased fibrinolysis, heart, lung, and vascular surgery are especially associated with fibrinolysis. FDPs subsequently become elevated.*

Thromboembolic states (e.g., venous thrombosis, pulmonary embolism) *Non-DIC thrombotic states activate the fibrinolytic system. FDPs subsequently become elevated.*

Related Tests

- Euglobulin lysis time (p. 207): This is a measure of the activity of the fibrinolytic system. This is an older test used to identify abnormal fibrinolysis occurring in patients with certain diseases or who receive thrombolytic therapy.
- Thrombin time (p. 408): This test is used to evaluate the fibrinogen portion of the hemostatic mechanism. Because fibrinogen levels are affected by primary fibrinolysins, this test is helpful in the evaluation of fibrinolysis.
- Disseminated intravascular coagulation screening (p. 192): See this section for a discussion of the etiology and pathophysiology of DIC.

Fibrinogen (Factor I, Quantitative Fibrinogen)

Normal Findings

Adult: 200-400 mg/dl or 2.0-4.0 g/L (SI units)
Newborn: 125-300 mg/dl

Critical Values

Values of <100 mg/dl can be associated with spontaneous bleeding.

Indications

Fibrinogen is primarily used to aid in the diagnosis of suspected bleeding disorders.

Test Explanation

Fibrinogen is essential to the blood-clotting mechanism. It is part of the "common pathway" in the coagulation system. Fibrinogen is converted to fibrin by the action of thrombin during the coagulation process. Fibrinogen, which is produced by the liver, is also an acute-phase reactant protein. It rises sharply during tissue inflammation or tissue necrosis. High levels also may be a useful predictor of increased risk of coronary artery or cerebrovascular disease. Reduced levels can be seen in patients with liver disease, malnourished states, and consumptive coagulopathies (e.g., disseminated intravascular coagulation [DIC]). Large-volume blood transfusions are also associated with low levels, because banked blood does not contain fibrinogen. Reduced levels of fibrinogen will cause a prolonged prothrombin and partial thromboplastin time.

Interfering Factors

- Blood transfusions within the past month may affect test results.
- Fibrinolysins can attack fibrinogen and reduce the serum levels.
- Drugs that may cause *increased* levels include estrogens and oral contraceptives.
- Drugs that may cause *decreased* levels include anabolic steroids, androgens, asparaginase, phenobarbital, streptokinase, urokinase, and valproic acid.

Procedure and Patient Care

Before

- Explain the procedure to the patient.
- Tell the patient that no fasting is required.

During

- Collect one tube of venous blood in a blue-top tube.

After

- Apply pressure or a pressure dressing to the venipuncture site.
- Assess the venipuncture site for bleeding.

Test Results and Clinical Significance

Increased levels

Acute inflammatory reactions (e.g., rheumatoid arthritis, glomerulonephritis)
Trauma
Acute infection such as pneumonia
Fibrinogen is an acute-phase reactant protein.

Coronary heart disease
Cigarette smoking
Elevated fibrinogen levels are merely an observation with no known pathophysiology.

Pregnancy *Pregnancy is associated with increased serum proteins (including fibrinogen).*

Decreased levels

Liver disease (hepatitis, cirrhosis) *Fibrinogen is not made in adequate volume.*
Consumptive coagulopathy (DIC)
Fibrinolysins
Primary and secondary fibrinolysins act to destroy fibrinogen within the serum.

Congenital afibrinogenemia *A genetic defect precludes the synthesis of fibrinogen.*
Advanced carcinoma
Malnutrition
Severe protein depletion is associated with reduced levels of fibrinogen (a protein).

Large-volume blood transfusion *Fibrinogen does not exist in normal levels in banked blood. The more that is transfused, the more the native fibrinogen is diluted.*

Related Tests

- Thrombin time (p. 408): This is a test of the fibrinogen to fibrin reaction.
- Prothrombin time (p. 366): The PT is used to evaluate the adequacy of the extrinsic system and common pathway in the clotting mechanism.
- Partial thromboplastin time (p. 319): This test is used to evaluate the intrinsic system and the common pathway of clot formation. It is most commonly used to monitor heparin therapy.
- Coagulating factor concentration (p. 154): This is a quantitative measurement of specific coagulation factors.
- Fibrin degradation product (FDP) (p. 213): This is a direct measurement of FDPs that occur as a result of fibrinolysis.

Folic Acid (Folate)

Normal Findings

5-20 mg/ml or 14-34 mmol/L (SI units)

Indications

This test quantifies the folate level in the blood. It is used in patients who have megaloblastic anemia. It is also used to assess nutritional status, especially in alcoholics.

Test Explanation

Folic acid, one of the B vitamins, is necessary for normal function of RBCs and WBCs and for the adequate synthesis of certain purines and pyrimidines, which are precursors of deoxyribonucleic acid (DNA). It is also used in the synthesis of several amino acids. Vitamin B_{12} is necessary for conversion of inactive 5-methyltetrahydrofolate to the active tetrahydrofolate, the active form of folate. As with vitamin B_{12}, the folate level depends on adequate dietary ingestion and normal intestinal absorption of this vitamin. Folic acid blood levels are performed to evaluate hemolytic disorders and to detect anemia caused by folic acid deficiency (in which the RBCs are abnormally large, causing megaloblastic anemia). These RBCs have a shortened life span and impaired oxygen-carrying capacity.

The main causes of folic acid deficiency include dietary deficiency (usually in the alcoholic patient), malabsorption syndrome, pregnancy, and certain anticonvulsant drugs. Decreased folic acid levels are seen in patients with folic acid deficiency anemia (megaloblastic anemia), hemolytic anemia, malnutrition, malabsorption syndrome, malignancy, liver disease, sprue, and celiac disease. Some drugs (e.g., anticonvulsants, antimalarials, alcohol, aminopterin, methotrexate) are folic acid antagonists and interfere with nucleic acid synthesis.

Elevated levels of folic acid may be seen in patients with pernicious anemia. Because there is not an adequate amount of vitamin B_{12} in these patients to metabolize folic acid, levels of folate rise in pernicious anemia. The folic acid test should be done in conjunction with tests for vitamin B_{12} levels.

The folate test is often part of the workup in alcoholic patients to assess nutritional status. Folate must be depleted for at least 5 months before megaloblastic anemia occurs.

Radioimmunoassay or enzyme immunoassay (RIA) techniques are now the most common methods of folic acid measurement.

Interfering Factors

- Because radioimmunoassay is the method of choice for folic acid determination, radionuclide administration should be avoided for at least 24 hours.
- Drugs that may cause *decreased* folic acid levels include alcohol, aminopterin, aminosalicylic acid, ampicillin, antimalarials, chloramphenicol, erythromycin, estrogens, methotrexate, oral contraceptives, penicillin, phenobarbital, phenytoin, and tetracyclines.

Procedure and Patient Care

Before

- Explain the procedure to the patient.
- Tell the patient that no fasting is usually required. (However, some laboratories prefer an 8-hour fast.)
- Instruct the patient not to consume alcoholic beverages before the test.
- Draw the specimen before starting folate therapy.

During

- Collect approximately 7 to 10 ml of venous blood in a red-top tube.
- Avoid hemolysis. Folate in the RBCs can falsely raise serum folate levels when hemolysis of the RBC occurs.
- Indicate on the laboratory slip any medications that may affect test results.

After

- Apply pressure or a pressure dressing to the venipuncture site.
- Assess the venipuncture site for bleeding.
- Transport the blood to the laboratory immediately after collection.

Test Results and Clinical Significance

Increased levels

Pernicious anemia *When there is an inadequate amount of vitamin* B_{12} to metabolize folic acid, levels of folate rise.

Vegetarianism *Increased ingestion of folate-containing vegetables can lead to increased levels of folic acid.*

Recent massive blood transfusion *Folate in the hemolyzed RBCs of banked blood can falsely raise serum folate levels.*

Decreased levels

Malnutrition *Inadequate intake of folic acid is the most common cause of folate deficiency. This is most common in alcoholics. Alcohol also reduces folic acid absorption.*

Malabsorption syndrome (e.g., sprue, celiac disease) *Folic acid, like vitamin* B_{12}*, is absorbed in the small intestine. In malabsorption, folic acid is not absorbed. Serum and tissue levels decline.*

Pregnancy *Folic acid deficiency in pregnancy probably results from a combination of inadequate intake and increased demand placed by the fetus on the maternal source of folic acid.*

Folic acid deficiency (megaloblastic) anemia
Hemolytic anemia
These anemias are the result of folic acid deficiency. The large megaloblastic RBCs cannot conform to small capillaries. Instead, they fracture and hemolyze. The shortened life span ultimately leads to anemia.

Malignancy
Liver disease
Chronic renal disease
The pathophysiology for these observations is not known.

Related Tests

- Vitamin B_{12} (p. 451): This is a measurement of the level of vitamin B_{12} in the serum. This test should be performed with a folic acid test. The clinical presentation of either deficiency is similar.
- Schilling test (p. 750): This is a test to determine the cause of vitamin B_{12} deficiency.
- Complete blood count (CBC) (p. 162): This is performed routinely and can identify megaloblastic anemia.

Gamma-Glutamyl Transpeptidase
(GGTP, g-GTP, Gamma-Glutamyl Transferase [GGT])

Normal Findings

Male and female >45 years: 8-38 U/L
Female <45 years: 5-27 U/L
Elderly: slightly higher than adult
Child: similar to adult
Newborn: 5 times higher than adult

Indications

This is a sensitive indicator of hepatobiliary disease. It is also used as an indicator of heavy and chronic alcohol use.

Test Explanation

The enzyme GGTP participates in the transfer of amino acids and peptides across the cellular membrane and possibly participates in glutathione metabolism. The highest concentrations of this enzyme are found in the liver and biliary tract. Lesser concentrations are found in the kidney, spleen, heart, intestine, brain, and prostate gland. Men may have higher GGTP levels than women because of the additional levels in the prostate. Very small amounts have been detected in endothelial cells of capillaries. This test is used to detect liver cell dysfunction, and it is highly accurate in indicating even the slightest degree of cholestasis. This is the most sensitive liver enzyme for detecting biliary obstruction, cholangitis, or cholecystitis. As with leucine aminopeptidase and 5′-nucleotidase, the elevation of GGTP generally parallels that of alkaline phosphatase; however, GGTP is more sensitive. Also, as with 5′-nucleotidase and leucine aminopeptidase, GGTP is not increased in bone diseases as is alkaline phosphatase. A normal GGTP level with an elevated alkaline phosphatase level would imply skeletal disease. An elevated GGTP and elevated alkaline phosphatase level would imply hepatobiliary disease. GGTP is also not elevated in childhood or pregnancy as alkaline phosphatase (ALP) usually is.

Another important clinical value of GGTP is that it can detect chronic alcohol ingestion. It is therefore very useful in the screening and evaluation of alcoholic patients. GGTP is elevated in approximately 75% of patients who chronically drink alcohol.

Why this enzyme is elevated after an acute myocardial infarction is not clear. It may represent the associated hepatic insult (if elevation occurs in the first 7 days) or the proliferation of capillary endothelial cells in the granulation tissue that replaces the infarcted myocardium. The elevation usually occurs 1 to 2 weeks after infarction.

Interfering Factors

- Values may be decreased in late pregnancy.
- Drugs that may cause *increased* GGTP levels include alcohol, phenytoin (Dilantin), and phenobarbital.
- Drugs that may cause *decreased* levels include clofibrate and oral contraceptives.

Procedure and Patient Care

Before

- Explain the procedure to the patient.
- Tell the patient that an 8-hour fast is recommended. Only water is permitted.

During

- Collect approximately 7 to 10 ml of venous blood in a red-top tube.
- Indicate on the laboratory slip any medications the patient is taking that may affect test results.

After

- Apply pressure or a pressure dressing to the venipuncture site.
- Assess the venipuncture site for bleeding. Patients with liver dysfunction often have prolonged clotting times.

Test Results and Clinical Significance

Increased levels

Liver diseases (e.g., hepatitis, cirrhosis, hepatic necrosis, hepatic tumor or metastasis, hepatotoxic drugs, cholestasis, jaundice) *Liver and biliary cells contain GGTP. When injured or diseased, these cells lyse and the GGTP leaks into the bloodstream.*

Myocardial infarction *The pathophysiology is not clear. It may be associated with hepatic insult or the proliferation of capillary endothelial cells in the granulation tissue that replaces the infarcted myocardium.*

Alcohol ingestion *The pathophysiology is not clear. It may be associated with hepatic insult.*

Pancreatic diseases (e.g., pancreatitis, cancer of the pancreas) *Pancreatic cells contain GGTP. When injured or diseased, these cells lyse and the GGTP leaks into the bloodstream.*

Epstein-Barr virus (infectious mononucleosis), cytomegalovirus infections, and Reye's syndrome *The pathophysiology is not clear. It may be associated with subclinical hepatitis that can occur with these infections.*

Related Tests

- Alanine aminotransferase (ALT) (p. 33): This liver enzyme is elevated in hepatocellular disease.

- Aspartate aminotransferase (AST) (p. 105): This liver enzyme is elevated in hepatocellular disease.
- 5′-Nucleotidase (p. 312): This liver enzyme is elevated in diseases affecting the biliary tree.
- Creatine phosphokinsase (CPK) (p. 173): This enzyme is similar to AST and exists predominantly in heart, skeletal muscle.
- Lactic dehydrogenase (LDH) (p. 278): This intracellular enzyme is used to support the diagnosis of injury or disease involving the heart, liver, RBCs, kidneys, skeletal muscle, brain, and lungs.
- Leucine aminopeptidase (LAP) (p. 286): This enzyme is specific to the hepatobiliary system. Diseases affecting that system will cause elevation of this enzyme.

Gastrin

Normal Findings

Adult: <100-200 pg/ml or <200 ng/L (SI units)
Child: <10-125 pg/ml
Levels are higher in elderly patients.

Indications

This test is used in the evaluation of patients with peptic ulcers to diagnose Zollinger-Ellison (ZE) syndrome or G-cell hyperplasia.

Test Explanation

Gastrin is a hormone produced by the G cells located in the distal part of the stomach (antrum). Gastrin is a potent stimulator of gastric acid. In normal gastric physiology an alkaline environment (created by food or antacids) stimulates the release of gastrin. Gastrin then stimulates the parietal cells of the stomach to secrete gastric acid. The pH environment in the stomach is thereby reduced. By negative feedback, this low pH environment suppresses further gastrin secretion.

ZE syndrome (gastrin-producing pancreatic tumor) and G-cell hyperplasia (overfunctioning of G cells in the distal stomach) are associated with high serum gastrin levels. Patients with these tumors have aggressive peptic ulcer disease. Unlike the patient with routine peptic ulcers, the patient with ZE syndrome or G-cell hyperplasia has a high incidence of complicated and recurrent peptic ulcers. It is important to identify this latter group of patients to institute more appropriate, aggressive medical and surgical therapy. The serum gastrin level will be normal in patients with routine peptic ulcers and greatly elevated in patients with ZE syndrome or G-cell hyperplasia.

It is important to note, however, that patients who are taking antacid peptic ulcer medicines, have had peptic ulcer surgery, or have atrophic gastritis will have a high serum gastrin level. However, levels usually are not as high as in patients with ZE syndrome or G-cell hyperplasia.

Not all patients with ZE syndrome exhibit increased levels of serum gastrin. Some may have "top" normal gastrin levels, which makes these patients difficult to differentiate from patients with routine peptic ulcer disease. ZE syndrome or G-cell hyperplasia can be diagnosed in these "top" normal patients by gastrin stimulation tests using calcium or secretin. Patients with these diseases will have greatly increased serum gastrin levels associated with the infusion of these drugs.

Interfering Factors

- Peptic ulcer surgery creates a persistent alkaline environment, which is the strongest stimulant to gastrin.
- Ingestion of high-protein food can result in an increase in serum gastrin two to five times the normal level.
- Diabetic patients taking insulin may have falsely elevated levels in response to hypoglycemia.
- Drugs that may *increase* serum gastrin include antacids, H_2-blocking agents (e.g., Tagamet, Zantac), and hydrogen pump inhibitors (e.g., Prilosec). These medications create an alkaline environment, which is the strongest stimulant to gastrin.
- Calcium or insulin can *increase* gastrin levels by acting as a gastrin stimulant.
- Other drugs that may *increase* gastrin levels include catecholamines and coffee.
- Drugs that may *decrease* levels include anticholinergics and tricyclic antidepressants.

Procedure and Patient Care

Before

- Explain the procedure to the patient.
- Instruct the patient to fast for 12 hours. Water is permitted.
- Tell the patient to avoid alcohol for at least 24 hours.

During

- Collect approximately 5 to 7 ml of venous blood in a red-top tube.
- For the *calcium infusion test,* administer calcium gluconate intravenously for 3 hours. A preinfusion serum gastrin level is then compared with specimens taken every 30 minutes for 4 hours.
- For the *secretin test,* administer secretin intravenously. Preinjection and postinjection serum gastrin levels are taken at 15-minute intervals for 1 hour after injection.
- Indicate on the laboratory slip any drugs that may affect test results.

After

- Apply pressure or a pressure dressing to the venipuncture site.
- Observe the venipuncture site for bleeding.

Test Results and Clinical Significance

Increased levels

ZE syndrome *This syndrome is associated with a pancreatic islet cell gastrin-producing tumor.*

G-cell hyperplasia *The G cells in the antrum of the stomach are hyperplastic and produce increased amounts of gastrin.*

Pernicious anemia
Atrophic gastritis
An achlorhydric alkaline environment exists in these illnesses. This is a strong stimulant to gastrin secretion.

Gastric carcinoma *Cancer of the stomach usually exists in an achlorhydric alkaline environment. This is a strong stimulant to gastrin secretion.*
Chronic renal failure *Gastrin is metabolized by the kidney. Without adequate kidney function, gastrin levels increase.*
Pyloric obstruction or gastric outlet obstruction *The stomach becomes distended. Gastric distention is a potent stimulant to gastrin production.*
Retained antrum after gastric surgery *Antral tissue mistakenly left on the duodenal stump after gastric resection is constantly bathed in duodenal alkaline juices. This is a strong stimulant to gastrin secretion.*

Related Tests

- Gastric analysis (p. 575): This is an older test of gastric juices that is used to diagnose ZE syndrome and to determine the adequacy of antipeptic medical and surgical therapy.

Glucagon

Normal Findings

30-210 pg/ml or 30-210 ng/L (SI units)

Indications

This is a direct measurement of glucagon in the blood. It is used to diagnose a glucagonoma. It is also useful in the evaluation of some diabetic patients. Finally, pancreatic function can be investigated with the use of this test.

Test Explanation

Glucagon is a hormone secreted by the alpha cells of the pancreatic islets of Langerhans. Glucagon is secreted in response to hypoglycemia and increases the blood glucose by breaking down glycogen to glucose in the liver. It also increases glucose in other tissues by inhibiting passage of glucose into cells and by encouraging efflux of glucose from the cell. Glucagon also oxidizes fatty acids to their basic glycerol components to form glucose. As serum glucose levels rise in the blood, glucagon is inhibited by a negative feedback mechanism.

Elevated glucagon levels may indicate the diagnosis of a glucagonoma (i.e., an alpha islet cell neoplasm). Glucagon deficiency occurs with extensive pancreatic resection or with burned-out pancreatitis. Arginine is a potent stimulator of glucagon. If the glucagon levels fail to rise even with arginine infusion, the diagnosis of glucagon deficiency as a result of pancreatic insufficiency is confirmed.

Normally glucagon decreases after ingestion of a carbohydrate-loaded meal through an elaborate negative feedback mechanism. This doesn't occur in patients with diabetes. Furthermore, in the insulin-dependent diabetic, glucagon stimulation caused by hypoglycemia does not occur. Arginine stimulation is performed to differentiate pancreatic insufficiency and diabetes. The diabetic will have an exaggerated elevation of glucagon with arginine. In pancreatic insufficiency, glucagon is not stimulated with arginine. Furthermore, in diabetic patients, hypoglycemia fails to stimulate glucagon release, as occurs in a nondiabetic person.

Because glucagon is thought to be metabolized by the kidneys, renal failure is associated with high glucagon levels and, as a result, high glucose levels. When rejection of a transplanted kidney occurs, one of the first signs of rejection may be increased serum glucagon levels.

Interfering Factors

- Test results may be invalidated if a patient has undergone a radioactive scan within the previous 48 hours. Glucagon is measured by radioimmunoassay. Administration of radionuclides can affect results.
- Levels may be elevated after prolonged fasting, stress, or moderate to severe exercise.
- Drugs that may cause *increased* levels include some amino acids (e.g., arginine), danazol, glucocorticoids, gastrin, cholecystokinin, sympathomimetic amines, insulin, and nifedipine.
- Drugs that may cause *decreased* levels include atenolol, propranolol, and secretin.

Procedure and Patient Care

Before

- Explain the procedure to the patient.
- Tell the patient that fasting is necessary for 10 to 12 hours before the test. Only water is permitted.

During

- Collect a venous blood sample in a lavender-top tube.

After

- Apply pressure or a pressure dressing to the venipuncture site.
- Assess the venipuncture site for bleeding.
- Place the specimen on ice and send it to the laboratory immediately.

Test Results and Clinical Significance

Increased levels

Familial hyperglucagonemia *There is a genetic defect that causes a predominance of a glucagon precursor.*

Glucagonoma *There are several syndromes, including the more common multiple endocrine neoplasia, that are associated with glucagonomas.*

Diabetes mellitus *The pathophysiology of this observation is not known.*

Chronic renal failure *Glucagon is metabolized by the kidney. With loss of that function, glucagon and glucose levels rise.*
Severe stress, including infection, burns, surgery, and acute hypoglycemia *Stress stimulates catecholamine release. This in turn stimulates glucagon secretion.*
Acromegaly *Growth hormone is a stimulator of glucagon.*
Hyperlipidemia *The pathophysiology of this observation is not well established.*
Acute pancreatitis *The contents of the pancreatic cells (including glucagon) are spilled into the bloodstream as they are injured during the inflammation.*
Pheochromocytoma *Catecholamines are potent stimulators to glucagon secretion.*

Decreased levels

Idiopathic glucagon deficiency *The pathophysiology of this process is not well understood. An autoantibody process may be the cause.*
Cystic fibrosis
Chronic pancreatitis *Burned-out pancreas tissue cannot secrete glucagon.*
Postpancreatectomy *In the absence of pancreatic tissue, glucagon secretion will not occur.*
Cancer of pancreas *Pancreatic tissue destroyed by tumor will not secrete glucagon.*

Related Tests

- Glucose, blood (see below): This test is commonly used to diagnose diabetes. Glucose levels are affected by glucagon.

Glucose, Blood
(Blood Sugar, Fasting Blood Sugar [FBS])

Normal Findings

Cord: 45-96 mg/dl or 2.5-5.3 mmol/L (SI units)
Premature infant: 20-60 mg/dl or 1.1-3.3 mmol/L
Neonate: 30-60 mg/dl or 1.7-3.3 mmol/L
Infant: 40-90 mg/dl or 2.2-5.0 mmol/L
Child <2 years: 60-100 mg/dl or 3.3-5.5 mmol/L
Child >2 years to adult: 70-105 mg/dl or 3.9-5.8 mmol/L
Elderly: increase in normal range after age 50 years

Critical Values

Adult male: <50 and >400 mg/dl
Adult female: <40 and >400 mg/dl
Infant: <40 mg/dl
Newborn: <30 and >300 mg/dl

Indications

This test is a direct measurement of the blood glucose level. It is most commonly used in the evaluation of diabetic patients.

Test Explanation

Through an elaborate feedback mechanism, glucose levels are controlled by insulin and glucagon. Glucose levels are low in the fasting state. In response, glucagon, which is made in the alpha cells of the pancreatic islet of Langerhans, is secreted. Glucagon breaks glycogen down to glucose in the liver and glucose levels rise. If the fasting persists, protein and fatty acids are broken down under glucagon stimulation. Glucose levels continue to rise.

Glucose levels are elevated after eating. Insulin, which is made in the beta cells of the pancreatic islets of Langerhans, is secreted. Insulin attaches to insulin receptors in muscle, liver, and fatty cells, where it drives glucose into these target cells to be metabolized to glycogen, amino acids, and fatty acids. Blood glucose levels diminish. Many other hormones (e.g., adrenocorticosteroids, adrenocorticotropic hormone [ACTH], epinephrine, thyroxine) can also affect glucose metabolism.

The serum glucose test is helpful in diagnosing many metabolic diseases. Serum glucose levels must be evaluated according to the time of day they are performed. For example, a glucose level of 135 mg/dl may be abnormal if the patient is in the fasting state, but this level would be within normal limits if the patient had eaten a meal within the last hour.

In general, true glucose elevations indicate diabetes mellitus; however, there are many other possible causes of hyperglycemia. Similarly, hypoglycemia has many causes. The most common cause is inadvertent insulin overdose in patients with brittle diabetes. If diabetes is suspected based on elevated fasting blood levels, a glycosylated hemoglobin or glucose tolerance test can be performed.

Glucose determinations must be performed frequently in new diabetic patients to monitor closely the insulin dosage to be administered. Finger stick blood glucose determinations are often performed before meals and at bedtime. Results are compared with a sliding-scale insulin chart ordered by the physician to provide coverage with subcutaneous regular insulin.

Interfering Factors

- Many forms of stress (e.g., trauma, general anesthesia, infection, burns, myocardial infarction) can cause increased serum glucose levels.
- Caffeine may cause increased levels.
- Most IV fluids contain dextrose, which is quickly converted to glucose. Most patients receiving IV fluids will have increased glucose levels.
- Many pregnant women experience some degree of glucose intolerance. If significant, it is called gestational diabetes.
- Drugs that may cause *increased* levels include antidepressants (tricyclics), beta-adrenergic blocking agents, corticosteroids, IV dextrose infusion, dextrothyroxine, diazoxide, diuretics, epinephrine, estrogens, glucagon, isoniazid, lithium, phenothiazines, phenytoin, salicylates (acute toxicity), and triamterene.

CLINICAL PRIORITIES

- Serum glucose levels must be evaluated according to the time of day they are obtained. Increased levels follow a recent meal.
- Glucose determinations must be performed frequently in new diabetic patients to determine appropriate insulin therapy. Finger stick blood glucose determinations are often performed before meals and at bedtime.
- Many forms of stress can cause increased serum glucose levels.
- Many drugs affect glucose levels.

- Drugs that may cause *decreased* levels include acetaminophen, alcohol, anabolic steroids, clofibrate, disopyramide, gemfibrozil, insulin, monoamine oxidase inhibitors, pentamidine, propranolol, tolazamide, and tolbutamide.

Procedure and Patient Care

Before

- Explain the procedure to the patient.
- For fasting blood sugar determination, keep the patient fasting at least 8 hours. Water is permitted.
- To prevent starvation, which may artificially raise the glucose levels, the patient should not fast longer than 16 hours.
- Withhold insulin or oral hypoglycemics until after blood is obtained.

During

- Collect approximately 7 ml of venous blood in a red- or gray-top tube.
- Glucose levels can also be evaluated by a finger stick blood test using either a visually read or a reflectance meter. The advantage of the visually read test is that it does not require an expensive machine. However, the patient must be able to visually interpret the color of the reagent strip. Using reflectance meters (e.g., Glucometer, Accu Check bG, Stat Tek) improves the accuracy of the blood glucose determination. However, this method is more complex because it requires machine calibration and control testing.

After

- Apply pressure or a pressure dressing to the venipuncture site.
- Observe the venipuncture site for bleeding.
- Be certain that the patient receives a meal after fasting blood work.

Test Results and Clinical Significance

Increased levels (hyperglycemia)

Diabetes mellitus *This disease is defined by glucose intolerance and hyperglycemia. A discussion of the many possible etiologies is beyond the scope of this manual.*

Acute stress response *Severe stress, including infection, burns, and surgery, stimulates catecholamine release. This in turn stimulates glucagon secretion, which causes hyperglycemia.*
Cushing's syndrome *Blood cortisol levels are high. This in turn causes hyperglycemia.*
Pheochromocytoma *Catecholamine stimulates glucagon secretion, which causes hyperglycemia.*
Chronic renal failure *Glucagon is metabolized by the kidney. With loss of that function, glucagon and glucose levels rise.*
Glucagonoma *Glucagon is autonomously secreted, causing hyperglycemia.*
Acute pancreatitis *The contents of the pancreatic cells (including glucagon) are spilled into the bloodstream as they are injured during the inflammation. The glucagon causes hyperglycemia.*
Diuretic therapy *Certain diuretics cause hyperglycemia.*
Corticosteroid therapy *Cortisol causes hyperglycemia.*
Acromegaly *Growth hormone stimulates glucagon, which causes hyperglycemia.*

Decreased levels (hypoglycemia)

Insulinoma *Insulin is autonomously produced without regard to biofeedback mechanisms.*
Hypothyroidism *Thyroid hormones affect glucose metabolism. With diminished levels of this hormone, glucose levels fall.*
Hypopituitarism *Many pituitary hormones (ACTH, growth hormone) affect glucose metabolism. With diminished levels of these hormones, glucose levels fall.*
Addison's disease *Cortisol affects glucose metabolism. With diminished levels of this hormone, glucose levels fall.*
Extensive liver disease *Most glucose metabolism occurs in the liver. With decreased function of the liver, glucose levels decrease.*
Insulin overdose *This is the most common cause of hypoglycemia. Insulin is administered at too high of a dose (especially in brittle diabetes) and glucose levels fall.*
Starvation *With decreased carbohydrate ingestion, glucose levels diminish.*

Related Tests

- Glucose, urine (p. 833): Testing for glucose in the urine is a part of routine urinalysis. If present, it reflects the degree of glucose elevation in the blood. Urine glucose tests are also used to monitor the effectiveness of therapy for diabetes mellitus.
- Glycosylated hemoglobin (p. 238): This is an accurate method of indicating average glucose levels over the past 100 to 120 days before the test.
- Glucose tolerance (p. 233): This is a test of a patient's capability to handle a glucose load.
- Glucose, postprandial (p. 229): This is a timed glucose measurement after a carbohydrate meal.
- Glucagon (p. 223): This is a direct measurement of glucagon, which acts to increase glucose in the blood.
- Insulin assay (p. 272): This is a direct measurement of insulin, which acts to decrease glucose in the blood.

Glucose, Postprandial (2-Hour Postprandial Glucose [2-Hour PPG], 2-Hour Postprandial Blood Sugar, 1-Hour Glucose Screen for Gestational Diabetes Mellitus)

Normal Findings

2-hour PPG

0-50 years: <140 mg/dl or <7.8 mmol/L (SI units)
50-60 years: <150 mg/dl
60 years and older: <160 mg/dl

1-hour glucose screen for gestational diabetes: <140 mg/dl

Indications

The 2-hour PPG test is a measurement of the amount of glucose in the patient's blood 2 hours after a meal is ingested (postprandial). It is used to diagnose diabetes mellitus.

Test Explanation

For this study, a meal acts as a glucose challenge to the body's metabolism. Insulin is normally secreted immediately after a meal in response to the elevated blood glucose level, causing the level to return to the pre-meal range within 2 hours. In patients with diabetes the glucose level usually is still elevated 2 hours after the meal. The PPG is an easily performed screening test for diabetes mellitus. If the results are >140 and <200 mg/dl, a glucose tolerance test may be performed to confirm the diagnosis. If the 2-hour PPG is >200 mg/dl, the diagnosis of diabetes mellitus is confirmed. Also, a glucose tolerance or glycosylated hemoglobin test can be performed to corroborate and better evaluate the disease.

The 1-hour glucose screen is used to detect gestational diabetes mellitus, which is the most common medical complication of pregnancy. Gestational diabetes is a carbohydrate intolerance first recognized during pregnancy and affects 3% to 8% of pregnant women, with up to half of these women developing overt diabetes later in life. The detection and treatment of gestational diabetes may reduce the risk for several adverse perinatal outcomes (e.g., excessive fetal growth and birth trauma, fetal death, neonatal morbidity).

Screening for gestational diabetes is performed with a 50-g oral glucose load followed by a glucose level determination 1 hour later. Screening is done between 24 and 28 weeks of gestation. However, patients with risk factors such as a previous history of gestational diabetes may benefit from earlier screening. Patients whose serum glucose level equals or exceeds 140 mg/dl should be evaluated by a 3-hour glucose tolerance test.

Interfering Factors

- Smoking during the testing period may increase the blood glucose level.
- Stress can increase glucose levels through the catecholamine effect of increasing serum glucose.

- If the patient eats a small snack or eats candy during the 2-hour interval, glucose levels will be falsely elevated.
- If the patient is not able to eat the entire test meal or vomits some or all of the meal, levels will be falsely decreased.

Procedure and Patient Care

Before

- Explain the procedure to the patient.
- Usually a fasting blood glucose is done before the meal is given. This acts as a baseline glucose level (see p. 225).
- For the 2-hour PPG, instruct the patient to fast for 12 hours prior to testing. The patient is to eat the entire meal (with at least 75 g of carbohydrates) and then not to eat anything else until the blood is drawn 2 hours later.
- For the 1-hour glucose screen for gestational diabetes, give the fasting or nonfasting patient a 50-g oral glucose load.
- Instruct the patient not to smoke during the test.
- Inform the patient that he or she should rest during the 1- or 2-hour interval, because exercise can increase glucose levels.

During

- Collect approximately 5 to 7 ml of blood in a red- or gray-top tube 1 or 2 hours after the patient has eaten the test meal.

After

- Apply pressure or a pressure dressing to the venipuncture site.
- Observe the venipuncture site for bleeding.

Test Results and Clinical Significance

Increased levels

Diabetes mellitus *This disease is defined by glucose intolerance and hyperglycemia. A discussion of the many possible etiologies is beyond the scope of this manual.*

Gestational diabetes mellitus *This disease is defined by glucose intolerance and hyperglycemia during pregnancy.*

Malnutrition *Malnourished patients have very poor glucose tolerance when they start to eat. The pathophysiology and theories of this observation are not well defined and are multiple.*

Hyperthyroidism *Thyroid hormone is an ancillary hormone that affects glucose metabolism and acts to increase glucose levels.*

Acute stress response *Severe stress, including infection, burns, and surgery, stimulates catecholamine release. This in turn stimulates glucagon secretion, which causes hyperglycemia.*

Cushing's syndrome *Blood cortisol levels are high. This in turn causes hyperglycemia.*

Pheochromocytoma *Catecholamine stimulates glucagon secretion, which causes hyperglycemia.*

Chronic renal failure *Glucagon is metabolized by the kidney. With loss of that function, glucagon and glucose levels rise.*

Glucagonoma *Glucagon is autonomously secreted, causing hyperglycemia.*

Diuretic therapy *Certain diuretics cause hyperglycemia.*

Corticosteroid therapy *Cortisol causes hyperglycemia.*
Acromegaly *Growth hormone stimulates glucagon, which causes hyperglycemia.*
Extensive liver disease *Most glucose metabolism occurs in the liver. With decreased function of the liver, glucose levels decrease.*

Decreased levels

Insulinoma *Insulin is autonomously produced without regard to biofeedback mechanisms*
Hypothyroidism *Thyroid hormone affects glucose metabolism. With diminished levels of this hormone, glucose levels fall.*
Hypopituitarism *Many pituitary hormones (adrenocorticotropic hormone, growth hormone) affect glucose metabolism. With diminished levels of these hormones, glucose levels fall.*
Addison's disease *Cortisol affects glucose metabolism. With diminished levels of this hormone, glucose levels fall.*
Insulin overdose *This is the most common cause of hypoglycemia. Insulin is administered at too high of a dose (especially in brittle diabetes), and glucose levels fall.*
Malabsorption or maldigestion *The test meal is not absorbed and glucose levels do not increase.*

Related Tests

- Glucose, blood (p. 225): This test is a direct measurement of the blood glucose level. It is most commonly the initial test in the evaluation of diabetic patients.
- Glycosylated hemoglobin (p. 238): This is an accurate method of indicating glucose tolerance in the recent past.
- Glucose tolerance (p. 233): This is a test of a patient's capability to handle a glucose load.

Glucose-6-Phosphate Dehydrogenase
(G-6-PD Screen)

Normal Findings Negative (screening test) or 8.0-8.6 U/g of hemoglobin

Indications

This test is used to identify G-6-PD deficiency in patients who have developed hemolysis after taking certain oxidizing drugs. It is especially useful in males of certain ethnic populations who are susceptible to this genetic defect.

Test Explanation

G-6-PD is an enzyme used in glucose metabolism. G-6-PD deficiency causes precipitation of hemoglobin and cellular membrane changes in RBCs. This may result in hemolysis of variable severity. This disease is a sex-linked, recessive trait carried on the X chromosome. The full effect of this genetic defect is not seen if the normal gene is present on a second X chromosome to oppose the genetic defect. In males there is no second X gene and the genetic defect is unopposed. Affected males inherit this abnormal gene from their mothers, who are usually asymptomatic. In these males the disease is most severe.

In rare cases when females have the defective gene on both X chromosomes, the disease is equally severe. Most commonly, however, women act as a "carrier" of the gene in that they have the defective gene on one X chromosome and have a normal gene for G-6-PD on the other X chromosome. These women have variable expressions of the disease from no symptoms to moderate symptoms if under a significant degree of stimulation.

In the United States, G-6-PD is found mainly in African-Americans. About 10% to 15% of that population is affected by the disease. Also, those of Mediterranean descent (Italians, Greeks, Sephardic Jews) are at risk for the genetic defect.

G-6-PD is an important enzyme involved in the "pentose pathway" of glucose metabolism that produces NADPH for energy in the RBC. Most of the glucose in a "young" RBC is metabolized to produce NADPH by the Embden-Meyerhof pathway. As the RBC ages, the pentose pathway becomes the dominant pathway of glucose metabolism. NADPH protects the RBC against potentially destructive oxidizing agents to which it may become exposed. If NADPH is present through the action of G-6-PD, the RBC is not susceptible to oxidizing agents. However, in patients with G-6-PD deficiency, oxidizing drugs can cause RBC destruction and hemolysis. Susceptible persons do not have hemolysis before exposure to the oxidizing drugs. After the oxidizing drug is administered, hemolysis can start as early as the first day and usually by the fourth day. The most common oxidizing drugs known to precipitate hemolysis and anemia in G-6-PD deficiency are antimalarials, sulfa, nitrofurantoins, aspirin, and phenacetin (Box 2-5). Infections or acidosis can also precipitate a hemolytic process in these patients. Certain foods (e.g., fava beans) are oxidizing and are therefore harmful to the G-6-PD–deficient patient.

This test is used to diagnose G-6-PD deficiency in suspected individuals. There are several different testing methods available for G-6-PD screening and testing. G-6-PD enzyme assay direct quantitation is most definitive.

Interfering Factors

- With the dye reduction and glutathione screening testing, reticulocytosis associated with a hemolytic episode may be associated with falsely high levels of G-6-PD.

Box 2-5 Drugs that precipitate hemolysis in G-6-PD–deficient patients

Antimalarials	Sulfa
Aspirin	Phenacetin
Antipyretics	Primaquine
Acetanilid	Phenazopyridine
Ascorbic acid	Quinidine
Dapsone	Nalidixic acid
Vitamin K (water soluble)	Sulfonamides
Nitrofurantoin (Furadantin)	Thiazide diuretics
Methylene blue	Tolbutamide (Orinase)

Procedure and Patient Care

Before

- Explain the procedure to the patient.
- Tell the patient that no fasting is required.

During

- Collect approximately 5 ml of venous blood in a lavender- or green-top tube.
- Avoid hemolysis.

After

- Apply pressure or a pressure dressing to the venipuncture site.
- Assess the venipuncture site for bleeding.
- If the test indicates a G-6-PD deficiency, give the patient a list of drugs that may precipitate hemolysis. Instruct patients with the Mediterranean type of this disease not to eat fava beans. Teach patients to read labels on any over-the-counter drugs for the presence of agents (e.g., aspirin, phenacetin) that may cause hemolytic anemia.

Test Results and Clinical Significance

Increased levels

Pernicious anemia
Megaloblastic anemia
Chronic blood loss
With the dye reduction and glutathione screening testing, reticulocytosis associated with a hemolytic episode may be associated with falsely high levels of G-6-PD.

Myocardial infarction
Hepatic coma
Hyperthyroidism
The pathophysiology of these observations is not well known.

Decreased levels

G-6-PD deficiency
Hemolytic anemia
Unusual nonspherocytic anemias

Glucose Tolerance
(GT, Oral Glucose Tolerance [OGT])

Normal Findings

Serum

Fasting: 70-115 mg/dl or <6.4 mmol/L (SI units)
30 minutes: <200 mg/dl or <11.1 mmol/L
1 hour: <200 mg/dl or <11.1 mmol/L
2 hours: <140 mg/dl or <7.8 mmol/L
3 hours: 70-115 mg/dl or <6.4 mmol/L
4 hours: 70-115 mg/dl or <6.4 mmol/L

Urine
Negative

Indications

This test is used to assist in the diagnosis of diabetes mellitus. It is also used in the evaluation of patients with hypoglycemia.

Test Explanation

The National Diabetes Data Group (NDDG) has defined criteria sufficient for the diagnosis of diabetes mellitus (Table 2-24). These include the following:

1. Sufficient clinical symptoms (polydipsia, polyuria, ketonuria, weight loss) plus unequivocal elevation in fasting blood glucose (FBG) or a non-FBG of greater than 200 mg/100 ml.
2. Elevated FBG of greater than 140 mg/100 ml on more than one occasion.
3. A normal FBG but a GT peak and 2-hour value of greater than 200 mg/100 ml on more than one occasion.

The GT test, then, is used when diabetes is suspected (retinopathy, neuropathy, diabetic-type renal diseases), but the criteria for the diagnosis cannot be met without the data obtained by the GT test. The GT test is also suggested for the following:

Patients with a family history of diabetes
Patients who are massively obese
Patients with a history of recurrent infections
Patients with delayed healing of wounds (especially on the lower legs or feet)
Women who have a history of delivering large babies, stillbirths, or neonatal births
Patients who have transient glycosuria or hyperglycemia during pregnancy or following myocardial infarction, surgery, or stress

Table 2-24 National Diabetes Data Group's reclassification of diabetic patients

NDDG classification	Diagnosis*	Old classification
Diabetes mellitus (insulin and noninsulin dependent)	Unequivocal signs/symptoms	Overt diabetes
	FBG >140 more than once; GT peak or 2 hour >200 more than once	
Impaired GT test	FBG normal and *either* GT peak or 2 hour >200	Latent (chemical) diabetes
Previous abnormality of glucose tolerance	Normal GT test but previous abnormal GT test	Subclinical diabetes
Potential abnormality of GT test	Genetic predisposition to diabetes (family history)	Prediabetes
Gestational diabetes mellitus	Onset of unequivocal diabetes or GT test results exceeding pregnancy criteria†	Diabetes of pregnancy

*Glucose levels are recorded in mg/100 ml.
†Onset or recognition of criteria during pregnancy but not before.

In the GT test, the patient's ability to tolerate a standard oral glucose load is evaluated by obtaining serum and urine specimens for glucose level determinations before glucose administration and then at 30 minutes, 1 hour, 2 hours, 3 hours, and sometimes 4 hours after the administration. Normally there is a rapid insulin response to the ingestion of a large oral glucose load. This response peaks in 30 to 60 minutes and returns to normal in about 3 hours. Patients with an appropriate insulin response are able to tolerate the dose quite easily, with only a minimal and transient rise in serum glucose levels within 1 to 2 hours after ingestion. Glucose will not spill over into the urine in normal patients.

Patients with diabetes will not be able to tolerate this load. As a result, their serum glucose levels will be greatly elevated from 1 to 5 hours (Figure 2-13). Also, glucose can be detected in their urine.

Gestational diabetes also can be diagnosed by the GT test. Generally the diagnosis of diabetes can be made if two or more of the results exceed the following:

Fasting: 105 mg/dl
1 hour: 190 mg/dl
2 hours: 165 mg/dl
3 hours: 145 mg/dl

The American Diabetes Association recommends that pregnant women who have not previously had an abnormal GT result should be tested at 24 and 28 weeks of gestation with a 50-g dose of glucose. A glucose level of >140 mg/100 ml would suggest that they be retested with a nonpregnant GT test 6 weeks or more after delivery.

GI absorption can vary among individuals. For that reason, some centers prefer to administer an IV glucose load rather than depend on GI absorption. Also, occasionally a patient is unable to tolerate the oral glucose load (e.g., patients with prior gastrectomy, short-bowel syndrome, malabsorption). In these instances an IV GT (IV GT) test can be performed by administering the glucose load intravenously. The values for the IV GT test differ slightly from those of the oral GT test because IV glucose is absorbed faster.

Glucose intolerance also may exist in patients with oversecretion of hormones that have an ancillary affect on glucose, such as patients with Cushing's syndrome, pheochromocytoma, acromegaly, aldosteronism, or hyperthyroidism. Patients with chronic renal failure, acute pancreatitis, myxedema, type IV lipoproteinemia, infection, or cirrhosis can also have an abnormal GT test. Certain drugs, as mentioned below, can also cause abnormal GT results.

The GT test is also used to evaluate patients with hypoglycemia. This hypoglycemia may occur as late as 5 hours after the initial glucose load.

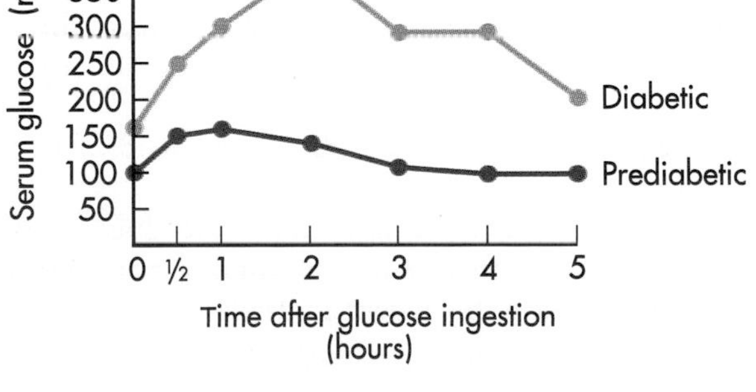

Figure 2-13 Glucose tolerance (GT) test curve for a diabetic and a prediabetic.

Contraindications

- Patients with serious concurrent infections or endocrine disorders, because glucose intolerance will be observed even though these patients may not be diabetic.
- Patient who vomit part or all of the glucose meal, which invalidates the test.

Potential Complications

- Dizziness, tremors, anxiety, sweating, euphoria, or fainting may occur during testing. If these symptoms occur, a blood specimen is obtained. If the glucose level is too high, the test may need to be stopped and insulin administered.

Interfering Factors

- Smoking during the testing period stimulates glucose because of the nicotine.
- Stress (e.g., from surgery, infection) can increase glucose levels.
- Exercise during the test can affect glucose levels.
- Fasting or reduced caloric intake prior to the GT test can cause glucose intolerance.
- Drugs that may cause glucose intolerance include antihypertensives, antiinflammatory drugs, aspirin, beta blockers, furosemide, nicotine, oral contraceptives, phenothiazines, psychiatric drugs, steroids, and thiazide diuretics.

Procedure and Patient Care

Before

- Explain the procedure to the patient.
- Educate the patient about the importance of having adequate food intake with adequate carbohydrates (150 g) for at least 3 days before the test.
- Instruct the patient to fast for 12 hours before the test.
- Instruct the patient to discontinue drugs (including tobacco) that could interfere with the test results.
- Give the patient written instructions explaining the pretest dietary requirement.
- Obtain the patient's weight to determine the appropriate glucose loading dose (especially in children).

During

- Obtain fasting blood and urine specimens.
- Administer the oral glucose solution, usually 75 g of glucose or dextrose for nonpregnant patients or 100 g for pregnant patients. There are several commercial preparations available. The glucose load may be diluted in as much as 300 ml of lemon juice/water mixture.
- Give pediatric patients a carbohydrate load of 1.75 g/kg body weight up to a maximum of 75 g.
- Instruct the patient to ingest the entire glucose load.
- Tell the patient that he or she cannot eat anything until the test is completed. However, encourage the patient to drink water. No other liquids should be taken during the testing period.

- Inform the patient that tobacco, coffee, and tea are not allowed, because they cause physiologic stimulation.
- Collect approximately 5 ml of venous blood in a gray-top tube at 30 and 60 minutes and at hourly periods.
- Collect urine specimens at hourly periods.
- During the testing period, assess the patient for reactions such as dizziness, sweating, weakness, and giddiness. (These are usually transient.) If the symptoms are persistent, obtain a serum glucose level.
- For the IV GT test, administer the glucose load intravenously over 3 to 4 minutes.
- Indicate on the laboratory slip any drugs that may affect test results.

After

- Apply pressure or a pressure dressing to the venipuncture sites.
- Mark on the tubes the time that the specimens are collected.
- Send all specimens promptly to the laboratory.
- Allow the patient to eat and drink normally.
- Administer insulin or oral hypoglycemics if ordered.
- Assess the venipuncture sites for bleeding.

Test Results and Clinical Significance

Increased levels

Diabetes mellitus *This disease is defined by glucose intolerance and hyperglycemia. A discussion of the many possible etiologies is beyond the scope of this manual.*

Acute stress response *Severe stress, including infection, burns, and surgery, stimulates catecholamine release. This in turn stimulates glucagon secretion, which causes hyperglycemia and glucose intolerance.*

Cushing's syndrome *Blood cortisol levels are high. This in turn causes hyperglycemia and glucose intolerance.*

Pheochromocytoma *Catecholamines stimulate glucagon secretion, which causes hyperglycemia and glucose intolerance.*

Chronic renal failure *Glucagon is metabolized by the kidney. With loss of that function, glucagon and glucose levels rise.*

Glucagonoma *Glucagon is autonomously secreted, causing hyperglycemia.*

Acute pancreatitis *The contents of the pancreatic cells (including glucagon) are spilled into the bloodstream as they are injured during the inflammation. The glucagon causes hyperglycemia.*

Diuretic therapy *Certain diuretics cause hyperglycemia.*

Corticosteroid therapy *Cortisol causes hyperglycemia and glucose intolerance.*

Acromegaly *Growth hormone stimulates glucagon, which causes hyperglycemia and glucose intolerance.*

Myxedema *Usually these patients have a flat GT curve, but they may have a "diabetic curve."*

Somogyi response to hypoglycemia *This is a reactive hyperglycemia following hypoglycemia that may occur from an exaggerated insulin response to the glucose load.*

After gastrectomy *These patients can dump most of the glucose load into the small intestines in just minutes because the normal pylorus is absent. This can cause rapid absorption of glucose into the bloodstream and cause a false elevation in glucose level during the early part of the test.*

Related Tests

- Glucose, blood (p. 225): This is the primary screening test to diagnose diabetes.
- Glucose, urine (p. 833): Testing for glucose in the urine is a part of routine urinanalysis. If present, it reflects the degree of glucose elevation in the blood. Urine glucose tests are also used to monitor the effectiveness of therapy for diabetes mellitus.
- Glycosylated hemoglobin (p. 238): This is an accurate method of indicating glucose tolerance in the recent past.
- Glucagon (p. 223): This is a direct measurement of glucagon, which acts to increase glucose in the blood.
- Insulin assay (p. 272): This is a direct measurement of insulin, which acts to decrease glucose in the blood.

Glycosylated Hemoglobin
(GHb, GHB, Glycohemoglobin, Hemoglobin A_{1c} [HbA_{1c}], Diabetic Control Index)

Normal Findings

Adult/elderly: 4%-8%
Child: usually <7%
Good diabetic control: 7–10%
Fair diabetic control: 11–13%
Poor diabetic control: 13%-20%
Values vary according to laboratory methods.

Indications

This test is used to monitor diabetes treatment. It measures the amount of HbA_{1c} in the blood. This test provides an accurate long-term index of the patient's average blood glucose level.

Test Explanation

In adults about 98% of the hemoglobin in the RBC is hemoglobin A. About 7% of hemoglobin A consists of a type of hemoglobin (HbA_1) that can combine strongly with glucose in a process called glycosylation. Once gylcosylation occurs, it is not easily reversible. HbA_1 is actually made up of three components (hemoglobin A_{1a}, A_{1b}, and A_{1c}). HbA_{1c} is the component that most strongly combines glucose. HbA_{1c} makes up the majority of the Hb_{A1}. About 70% of HbA_{1c} is glycosylated. Only 20% of A_{1a} and A_{1b} are glycosylated. HbA_{1c} is the most accurate measurement, because this is the majority of glycosylated hemoglobin. If total HbA_1 is measured, its value is always 2% to 4% higher than that of the glycosylated HA_{1c} component. Most often total HbA_1 is measured and reported as a percentage of total hemoglobin A. HbA_{1c} is fast becoming the most common component measured.

As the RBC circulates, it combines its HbA_1 with some of the glucose in the bloodstream to form glycohemoglobin (GHb). The amount of GHb depends on the amount of glucose available in the bloodstream over the RBCs' 120-day life span. Therefore determination of the GHb value reflects the average blood sugar level for the 100- to 120-day period before the test. The more glucose the RBC is exposed to, the greater the GHb percentage. One important advantage of this test is that the sample can be drawn at any time, because it is not affected by short-term variations (e.g., food intake, exercise, stress, hypoglycemic agents, patient cooperation). It is also possible for very high short-term blood glucose levels to cause an elevation of GHb. Usually, however, the degree of glucose elevation results not from a transient high level but from a persistent, moderate elevation over the entire life of the RBC.

The elevation in GHb occurs about 3 weeks after the sustained elevation in blood glucose. It takes at least 4 weeks for the GHb to decrease after a sustained reduction in blood glucose. Yet some effect of recent significantly high blood glucose elevation may be noted when measuring GHb.

The GHb test is particularly beneficial for:

1. Evaluating the success of diabetic treatment and patient compliance.
2. Comparing and contrasting the success of past and new forms of diabetic therapy.
3. Determining the duration of hyperglycemia in patients with newly diagnosed diabetes.
4. Providing a sensitive estimate of glucose imbalance in patients with mild diabetes.
5. Individualizing diabetic control regimens.
6. Providing a sense of reward for many patients when the test shows achievement of good diabetic control.
7. Evaluating the diabetic whose glucose levels change significantly day to day (brittle diabetes).
8. Differentiating short-term hyperglycemia in nondiabetics (e.g., recent stress or myocardial infarction) and diabetics (in whom the glucose has been persistently elevated).

Interfering Factors

- Hemoglobinopathies can affect results, because the quantity of hemoglobin A (and, as a result, HbA_1) varies considerably in these diseases.
- Falsely elevated values occur when the RBC life span is lengthened because the HbA_1 has a longer period available for glycosylation.

Procedure and Patient Care

Before

- Explain the procedure to the patient.
- Tell the patient that fasting is not indicated.

During

- Collect approximately 5 ml of venous blood in a gray- or lavender-top tube.

After

- Apply pressure or a pressure dressing to the venipuncture site.
- Assess the venipuncture site for bleeding.

Test Results and Clinical Significance

Increased levels

Newly diagnosed diabetic patient
Poorly controlled diabetic patient
Nondiabetic hyperglycemia (e.g., acute stress response, Cushing's syndrome, pheochromocytoma, glucagonoma, corticosteroid therapy, acromegaly)
Patients with the above illnesses tend to have persistently elevated glucose levels that cause an elevated GHb.

Splenectomized patients *In these patients RBC survival is prolonged. More time for hemoglobin glycosylation is available. GHb levels increase.*
Pregnancy *In some women with gestational diabetes or prediabetes, persistently high levels of glucose occur that cause elevated GHb levels.*

Decreased levels

Hemolytic anemia
Chronic blood loss
RBC survival is shortened. Therefore there is less time for glycosylation, and GHb levels decrease.

Chronic renal failure *These patients have reduced hemoglobin levels as a result of lack of erythropoietin, which is produced in the kidney. HbA_1* is also decreased.

Related Tests

- Glucose, blood (p. 225): This is the primary screening test for diabetes.
- Glucose, urine (p. 833): Testing for glucose in the urine is a part of routine urinalysis. If present, it reflects the degree of glucose elevation in the blood. Urine glucose tests are also used to monitor the effectiveness of therapy for diabetes mellitus.
- Glucose tolerance (p. 233): This is a test of a patient's capability to handle a glucose load.
- Glucose, postprandial (p. 229): This is a timed glucose measurement after a carbohydrate meal.
- Glucagon (p. 223): This is a direct measurement of glucagon, which acts to increase glucose in the blood.
- Insulin assay (p. 272): This is a direct measurement of insulin, which acts to decrease glucose in the blood.

Growth Hormone (GH, Human Growth Hormone [HGH], Somatotropin Hormone [SH])

Normal Findings

Men: <5 ng/ml or <5 μg/L (SI units)
Women: <10 ng/ml or <10 μg/L
Child: 0-10 ng/ml or 0-10 μg/L
Newborn: 10-40 ng/ml or 10-40 μg/L

Indications

This test is used to identify GH deficiency in adolescents with short stature, delayed sexual maturity, or other growth deficiencies. It is also used to document the diagnosis of GH excess in gigantic or acromegalic patients. Finally, it is often used as a screening test for pituitary hypofunction.

Test Explanation

GH, or somatotropin, is secreted by the acidophil cells in the anterior pituitary gland and plays a central role in modulating growth from birth until the end of puberty. There is an elaborate feedback mechanism associated with the secretion of GH. The hypothalamus secretes growth hormone–releasing hormone, which stimulates GH release from the pituitary. GH exerts its effects on many tissues through a group of peptides called somatomedins. The most commonly tested somatomedin is somatomedin C, which is produced by the liver and has a major effect on cartilage. High levels of somatomedins stimulate the production of somatostatin from the hypothalamus. Somatostatin inhibits further secretion of GH from the pituitary. GH is secreted during sleep, exercise, and ingestion of protein and in response to hypoglycemia.

In the total absence of GH, linear growth occurs at one half to one third of the normal rate. GH also plays a role in the control of body anabolism throughout life by increasing protein synthesis, increasing the breakdown of fatty acids in adipose tissue, and increasing the blood glucose level.

If GH secretion is insufficient during childhood, limited growth and dwarfism may result. Also, a delay in sexual maturity may occur in adolescents with reduced GH levels. Conversely, overproduction of GH during childhood results in gigantism, with the person reaching nearly 7 to 8 feet in height. An excess of GH during childhood (after closure of long bone end plates) results in acromegaly, which is characterized by an increase in bone thickness and width but no increase in height.

GH tests are also used to confirm hypopituitarism or hyperpituitarism. GH assay is the most widely used test for GH deficiency or excess. Because GH secretion is episodic, random assays for GH are not adequate determinants of GH deficiency. Normal GH levels overlap significantly with deficient levels. Low GH levels may indicate deficiency or may be normal for certain individuals at certain times of the day. To negate time variables in GH testing, GH should be drawn 1 to 1½ hours after deep sleep. Levels increase during sleep. Also, strenuous exercise can be performed for 30 minutes in an effort to stimulate GH production. GH levels drawn at the end of the exercise period are expected to be maximal. These two methods are helpful in evaluating GH deficiency.

To negate the common variations in GH secretion, screening for insulin-like growth factor (IGF-1) or somatomedin C provides a more accurate reflection of the mean plasma concentration of GH. These proteins are not affected by the time of day or food intake as is GH, because they circulate bound to proteins that are durable and long lasting. A GH stimulation test can be performed to evaluate the body's ability to produce GH.

Interfering Factors

- Random measurements of GH are not adequate determinants of GH deficiency, because hormone secretion is episodic.

- A radioactive scan performed within the week before the test may affect test results, because levels are determined by radioimmunoassay.
- GH secretion is increased by stress, exercise, diet, and low blood glucose levels.
- Drugs that may cause *increased* levels include amphetamines, arginine, dopamine, estrogens, glucagon, histamine, insulin, levodopa, methyldopa, and nicotinic acid.
- Drugs that may cause *decreased* levels include corticosteroids and phenothiazines.

Procedure and Patient Care

Before

- Explain the procedure to the patient.
- The patient should not be emotionally or physically stressed, because this can increase GH levels.
- It is preferred that patients have fasted and be well rested. Water is permitted.

During

- Collect one red-top tube of venous blood.
- Because approximately two thirds of the total production of GH occurs during sleep, its secretion also can be measured during hospitalization by obtaining blood samples while the patient is sleeping.

After

- Apply pressure or a pressure dressing to the venipuncture site.
- Assess the venipuncture site for bleeding.
- Indicate the patient's fasting status and the time the blood is collected on the laboratory slip. Include the patient's recent activity (e.g., sleeping, walking, eating).
- Because the half-life of GH is only 20 to 25 minutes, send the blood to the laboratory immediately after collection.

Test Results and Clinical Significance

Increased levels

Gigantism
Acromegaly
These two syndromes are caused by excess GH.

Anorexia nervosa *Starvation stimulates GH secretion.*
Stress
Major surgery
Hypoglycemia
Starvation
Deep-sleep state
Exercise
The above situations stimulate GH secretion.

Hypoglycemia *Hypoglycemia stimulates GH secretion.*

Decreased levels

GH deficiency
Pituitary insufficiency *GH is produced in the pituitary. Diseases, tumors, ischemia, or trauma to the pituitary or hypothalamus causes GH deficiency.*
Dwarfism *This is a result of GH deficiency in children.*
Hyperglycemia *Elevated glucose levels inhibit GH secretion.*
Failure to thrive *This is a result of GH deficiency in infants.*
Delayed sexual maturity *This is a result of GH deficiency in adolescents.*

Related Tests

- Growth hormone (GH) stimulation (p. 243): This is a test designed to stimulate the secretion of GH. It is required to accurately diagnose GH deficiency.
- Somatomedin C (p. 400): Somatomedin C levels parallel GH levels. However, they are not affected by the many factors that cause significant variations in GH results.

Growth Hormone Stimulation
(GH Provocation, Insulin Tolerance [IT], Arginine)

Normal Findings GH levels >10 ng/ml or 10 mg/L (SI units)

Indications

The GH stimulation test is used to identify patients who are suspected of having GH deficiency. A normal patient can have low GH levels, but if GH is still low after GH stimulation, the diagnosis can be more accurately made

Test Explanation

Because GH secretion is episodic, random measurement of plasma GH is not adequate to make the diagnosis of GH deficiency. To diagnose GH deficiency, GH stimulation tests are indicated. One of the most reliable GH stimulators is insulin-induced hypoglycemia, in which the blood glucose declines to less than 40 mg/dl. Other GH stimulants include vigorous exercise and drugs (e.g., arginine, glucagon, levodopa, clonidine).

Pituitary GH deficiency cannot be diagnosed by identifying a deficiency of GH to just one stimulant, because as many as 20% of normal patients will fail to respond to the stimulant. Therefore a double-stimulated test is usually performed after arginine infusion followed by insulin-induced hypoglycemia. Arginine is an amino acid that stimulates GH secretion; hypoglycemia also stimulates GH secretion. A GH concentration over 10 mg/L after stimulation effectively excludes GH deficiencies.

GH also can be stimulated by vigorous exercise. This entails running or stair-climbing for 20 minutes. Blood samples of GH are obtained at 0, 20, and 40 minutes. GH-releasing factor has recently been used to stimulate GH. This promises to be a much more accurate and specific test for a pituitary cause of GH deficiency. At present the best method of identifying patients deficient in GH is a positive stimulation test followed by a positive response to a therapeutic GH trial. GH deficiency is also suspected when bone age, as determined by x-ray films of the long bones (see p. 913), indicates retarded growth according to chronologic age.

Only minor discomfort is associated with this test and results from the insertion of the IV line and the hypoglycemic response induced by the insulin injection. This may include postural hypotension, somnolence, diaphoresis, and nervousness. This procedure is usually performed by a nurse under physician supervision. This test takes approximately 2 hours to perform.

Contraindications

- Patients with epilepsy, because seizures can be induced by the hypoglycemia
- Patients with cerebrovascular disease, because hypoglycemia may induce stroke
- Patients with myocardial infarction, because the stress associated with the hypoglycemia may cause angina or a myocardial infarction
- Patients with low basal plasma cortisol levels, because they cannot respond to or compensate for the hypoglycemia

Potential Complications

- Hypoglycemia may be so significant and severe as to cause ketosis, acidosis, and shock. With close observation, this is unlikely.

Interfering Factors

- A radioactive scan performed within 1 week before the test may affect test results, because radioimmunoassay of GH would be confounded by the previously administered radioisotope for the scan.

Procedure and Patient Care

Before

- Explain the procedure very carefully to the patient and, if appropriate, to the parents.
- Instruct the patient to remain on NPO status after midnight on the morning of the test. Water is permitted.

During

- Note the following procedural steps:
  1. A heparin lock IV line is inserted for the administration of medications and the withdrawal of frequent blood samples.
  2. Baseline blood levels are obtained for GH, glucose, and cortisol.
  3. Venous samples for GH are obtained 0, 60, and 90 minutes after injection of arginine and/or insulin.
  4. Blood glucose levels are monitored at 15- to 30-minute intervals with the glucometer. The blood sugar should drop to less than 40 mg/dl for effective measurement of GH reserve.

- Monitor the patient for signs of hypoglycemia, postural hypotension, somnolence, diaphoresis, and nervousness.
- Ice chips are often given during the test for patient comfort.

After

- Observe the venipuncture site for bleeding.
- Inform the patient and family that results may not be available for approximately 7 days. Many laboratories only run GH tests once a week.
- After the test give the patient cookies and punch or an IV glucose infusion.
- Send the blood to the laboratory immediately after collection, because the half-life of growth hormone is only 20 to 25 minutes.

Test Results and Clinical Significance

Decreased levels

Pituitary deficiency
GH deficiency
Diseases (e.g., tumor, infarction, trauma) of the pituitary can result in failure of the pituitary to secrete either GH or all the pituitary hormones. GH stimulation tests will fail to stimulate GH secretion.

Related Tests

- Somatomedin C (p. 400): Somatomedin C levels parallel GH levels. However, they are not affected by the many factors that cause significant variations in GH results.
- Growth hormone (p. 240): This test is a direct quantitative assay for GH.

Ham's Test (Acid Serum Test for Paroxysmal Nocturnal Hemoglobinuria [PNH])

Normal Findings

10%-50% hemolysis of RBCs

Indications

This test is used to diagnose PNH. It is the most accurate test for the diagnosis of this disease.

Test Explanation

PNH is an acquired bone marrow stem cell defect. It affects WBCs, RBCs, and platelets. The membrane of the affected blood cell has a defect that makes it unusually susceptible to cell lysis caused by antibody/complement complexes. These patients show signs of hemolysis (anemia, free hemoglobin in the urine, decreased haptoglobin levels). When the WBCs, RBCs, and platelets are affected, the patient can develop aplastic anemia.

Ham's test determines the specific susceptibility of the RBCs. In patients with PNH, intravascular hemolysis of RBCs occurs intermittently during sleep. The etiology is not known. The hemoglobinuria turns the urine red or brown as a result of large amounts of hemoglobin in the urine from RBC hemolysis.

The RBCs of patients with PNH are more likely to lyse in an acid pH than are the RBCs of normal patients, which is the basis for Ham's test. This test is performed by incubating the suspected patient's RBCs with fresh autologous or ABO-compatible homologous serum adjusted to a pH of 6.5 using dilute hydrochloric acid. The amount of hemolysis is then quantified photometrically. A positive test occurs when 10% to 80% hemolysis of RBCs is observed.

Another test for PNH is the sugar-water (or sucrose hemolysis) test. The basis for this test is that the RBCs of patients with PNH are more likely to lyse in a low ionic strength media than are the RBCs of normal patients. This is easier to perform than Ham's test and is more sensitive. This test is commonly used as a screening test for PNH and requires confirmation with Ham's test.

Contraindications

- Patients who have had recent blood transfusions.

Procedure and Patient Care

Before

- Explain the procedure to the patient.
- Tell the patient that no fasting is required.

During

- Collect approximately 5 to 7 ml of venous blood in a lavender-top tube.
- Indicate if the patient has had a recent blood transfusion.

After

- Apply pressure or a pressure dressing to the venipuncture site.
- Assess the venipuncture site for bleeding.

Test Results and Clinical Significance

Increased hemolysis

PNH

Type II congenital dyserythropoietic anemia

In both of these diseases, hemolysis is noted in an acid serum.

Related Tests

- Haptoglobin (p. 247): This is a test used to identify intravascular hemolysis. It does not indicate the specific type of hemolytic anemia, but just that hemolysis is occurring.

Haptoglobin

Normal Findings

Adult: 100-150 mg/dl or 16-31 mmol/L (SI units)
Newborn: 0-10 mg/dl

Critical Values <40 mg/dl

Indications

This test is used to identify the presence of intravascular hemolysis. This protein is decreased when significant hemolysis occurs. It is quite nonspecific for indicating the type of hemolytic anemia.

Test Explanation

The serum haptoglobin test is used to detect intravascular destruction (lysis) of RBCs. This is called hemolysis. Haptoglobins are glycoproteins produced by the liver. These haptoglobins are powerful, free hemoglobin-binding proteins. In hemolytic anemias associated with the hemolysis of RBCs, the released hemoglobin is quickly bound to haptoglobin and the new complex is rapidly catabolized. This results in a diminished amount of free haptoglobin in the serum; this decrease cannot be readily compensated for by normal liver production. As a result, the patient demonstrates a transient reduced level of haptoglobin in the serum.

Haptoglobins are also decreased in patients with primary liver disease not associated with hemolytic anemias. This occurs because the diseased liver is unable to produce these glycoproteins. Hematoma can reduce haptoglobin levels by the absorption of hemoglobin into the blood and by binding hemoglobin with haptoglobin.

Elevated haptoglobin concentrations are found in many inflammatory diseases, and therefore haptoglobin can be used as a nonspecific acute-phase reactant protein in much the same way as the erythrocyte sedimentation rate (see p. 199). That is, levels of haptoglobin increase with severe infection, inflammation, tissue destruction, acute myocardial infarction, burns, and some cancers.

Interfering Factors

- Ongoing infection can cause falsely elevated test results.
- Drugs that may cause *increased* haptoglobin levels include androgens and steroids.
- Drugs that may cause *decreased* levels include chlorpromazine, diphenhydramine, indomethacin, isoniazid, nitrofurantoin, oral contraceptives, quinidine, and streptomycin.

Procedure and Patient Care

Before

- Explain the procedure to the patient.
- Tell the patient that no fasting is required.

During

- Collect at least 2 ml of venous blood in a red-top tube.
- Avoid hemolysis, which may alter test results.

After

- Apply pressure or a pressure dressing to the venipuncture site.
- Assess the venipuncture site for bleeding.

Test Results and Clinical Significance

Increased levels

Collagen-rheumatic diseases
Infection (e.g., pyelonephritis, urinary tract infection, pneumonia)
Tissue destruction (e.g., myocardial infarction)
Nephritis
Ulcerative colitis
Neoplasia
The above and many other diseases can cause an elevation of haptoglobin, an acute-phase reactant protein.

Decreased levels

Hemolytic anemia (e.g., erythroblastosis fetalis, autoimmune hemolytic anemias, hemoglobinopathies [sickle cell], paroxysmal nocturnal hemoglobinuria, drug-induced hemolytic anemia, or uremia) *Hemolysis occurs, freeing hemoglobin in the plasma. The free hemoglobin is tightly bound to haptoglobin. The complex is catabolized and excreted. Haptoglobin cannot be replaced fast enough and levels in the blood fall.*

Transfusion reactions *ABO antibodies bind to ABO antigens on the RBC membrane and cause hemolysis. Hemoglobin is liberated from the RBC. The free hemoglobin is tightly bound to haptoglobin. The complex is catabolized and excreted. Haptoglobin cannot be replaced fast enough and levels in the blood fall.*

Prosthetic heart valves *The mechanical trauma of the valve on the RBC causes hemolysis, and hemoglobin is liberated from the RBC. The free hemoglobin is tightly bound to haptoglobin. The complex is catabolized and excreted. Haptoglobin cannot be replaced fast enough and levels in the blood fall.*

Primary liver disease *The diseased liver cannot make adequate amounts of haptoglobin. The liver is the sole source of haptoglobin.*

Hematoma
Tissue hemorrhage
The free hemoglobin in the hematoma binds the haptoglobin. The complex is catabolized and excreted. Haptoglobin cannot be replaced fast enough and levels in the blood fall.

Related Tests

- Ham's test (p. 245): This is a test to diagnose paroxysmal nocturnal hemoglobinuria, a form of hemolytic anemia.

Helicobacter pylori (*Campylobacter pylori,* Anti–*Helicobacter pylori* Immunoglobulin G [IgG] Antibody, *Campylobacter*-Like Organism [CLO])

Normal Findings

Not present

Indications

This test is used to detect *Helicobacter pylori* infections. It is indicated in patients who have recurrent or chronic gastric or duodenal ulceration or inflammation. When *H. pylori* is successfully treated, the ulcer or inflammation will heal.

Test Explanation

H. pylori, a bacterium that can be found in the mucus overlying the gastric mucosa and on the mucosal cells that line the stomach, is a risk factor for gastric diseases such as duodenal ulcers or chronic gastritis. This gram-negative bacillus may also be a possible cause of gastric carcinoma. Gastric colonization by this organism has been reported in about 90% to 95% of patients with a duodenal ulcer, in 60% to 70% of patients with a gastric ulcer, and in about 20% to 25% of patients with gastric cancer.

Approximately 10% of healthy persons under 30 years of age have gastric colonization with *H. pylori.* Gastric colonization increases with age, with people over 60 years having rates similar to their ages. Most patients with gastric colonization by *H. pylori* remain asymptomatic and never develop ulceration.

There are several methods of detecting the presence of this organism. The organism can be cultured from a specimen of mucus obtained through a gastroscope (see p. 536). The specimen is plated on an enriched medium such as chocolate or Skirrow's medium and incubated for 5 to 7 days at 37° C. Cultures are less accurate than the other tests. The organism can also be detected on a gastric mucosal biopsy. The organisms can be detected when the tissue is stained with Giemsa or Warthin-Starry silver stains. This is slightly more accurate than culture techniques.

Newer methods are available to detect this organism that are more easily performed and more accurate. Immunoassays of antibodies to *H. pylori* have been developed and are very accurate in detecting the presence of the organism. The IgG anti-*H. pylori* antibody is most commonly used. It becomes elevated 2 months after infection and stays elevated for over a year after treatment. The IgA anti-*H. pylori* antibody, like IgG, becomes elevated 2 months after infection but decreases 3 to 4 weeks after treatment. The IgM anti-*H. pylori* antibody is the first to become elevated (about 3 to 4 weeks) and is not detected 2 to 3 months after treatment. These antibody titers are fast becoming the "gold standard" for *H. pylori* detection.

There is also a breath test available for the detection of *H. pylori.* It is based on the capability of *H. pylori* to metabolize urea to CO_2. In the breath test, radioactive carbon is administered orally. Expired air is tested for radioactivity in the CO_2 ½ to 2 hours later. This test requires special equipment and storage capabilities for long-lived radioisotopes such as carbon.

Interfering Factors

- *H. pylori* can be transmitted by contaminated endoscopic equipment during endoscopic procedures.

Procedure and Patient Care

Before

- Explain the procedure to the patient.
- Tell the patient that no fasting is required for the blood test.
- If a biopsy or culture will be obtained by endoscopy, see discussion of esophagogastroduodenoscopy (EGD) on p. 536.

During

- Collect a venous blood sample according to the protocol of the laboratory performing the test.
- A gastric or duodenal biopsy can be obtained by endoscopy. Keep the specimen moist by the addition of approximately 2 to 5 ml of sterile saline solution placed in a sterile container.

After

- Apply pressure or a pressure dressing to the venipuncture site.
- Assess the venipuncture site for bleeding.
- If endoscopy was used to obtain a culture, see procedure for EGD on p. 536. The specimen should be transported to the laboratory within 30 minutes after collection.

Test Results and Clinical Significance

Increased levels

Acute and chronic gastritis
Recurrent duodenal ulcer
Gastric ulcer
Gastric carcinoma
The above-noted illnesses are associated with the presence of H. pylori. *Whether the infection is causative or contributive is not well known.*

Related Tests

- Gastrin (p. 221): This test is a measure of serum gastrin. This hormone stimulates gastric acid secretion. Oversecretion can cause recurrent peptic ulcers. The initial symptoms may be similar to chronic *H. pylori* infection.

Hematocrit (Hct, Packed Red Blood Cell Volume, Packed Cell Volume [PCV])

Normal Findings

Male: 42%-52% or 0.42-0.52 volume fraction (SI units)
Female: 37%-47% or 0.37-0.47 volume fraction (SI units)
  Pregnant female: >33%
Elderly: Values may be slightly decreased.
Child/adolescent (%)
  2-8 weeks: 39-59
  2-6 months: 35-50
  6 months-1 year: 29-43
  1-6 years: 30-40
  6-18 years: 32-44
Newborn: 44 to 64

Critical Values <15% or >60%

Indications

The Hct is an indirect measurement of RBC number and volume. It is used as a rapid measurement of RBC count. It is repeated serially in patients with ongoing bleeding or as a routine part of the complete blood count. It is an integral part of the evaluation of anemic patients.

Age-related concerns

- Values in children are age specific, with normal values varying throughout the first 18 years.
- Values are slightly decreased in the elderly.

Test Explanation

The Hct is a measure of the percentage of the total blood volume that is made up by the RBCs. The height of the RBC column is measured after centrifugation. It is compared to the height of the column of the total whole blood. The ratio of the height of the RBC column compared with the original total blood column is multiplied by 100%. This is the Hct value. It is routinely performed as part of a complete blood count. The Hct closely reflects the hemoglobin (Hgb) and RBC values. The Hct in percentage points usually is approximately three times the Hgb concentration in grams per deciliter when RBCs are of normal size and contain normal amounts of Hgb.

Normal values vary according to gender and age. Women tend to have lower values than men, and Hct values tend to decrease with age. Abnormal values indicate the same pathologic states as abnormal RBC counts and Hgb concentrations. Decreased levels indicate anemia (reduced number of RBCs). Increased levels can indicate erythrocytosis.

Like other RBC values, the Hct can be altered by many factors other than RBC production. For instance, in dehydrated patients the total blood volume is contracted. The RBCs make up a greater proportion of the total blood volume, and the Hct measurement is therefore falsely high. Likewise, if the RBC is morphologically increased in size, the RBCs will make up a greater proportion of the total blood volume, and Hct will again be falsely high.

The Hct can be measured in a capillary tube (by skin puncture) by placing the blood in the tube, which is then spun in a microcentrifuge. The percentage of the RBC portion of the column to the whole column is the Hct. This value is most often calculated by automated cell counting machines in hospital laboratories.

Decisions concerning the need for blood transfusion are usually based on the Hgb or the Hct. In an otherwise healthy person, transfusion is not considered as long as the Hgb is above 8 g/dl or the Hct is above 24. In younger people who can safely and significantly increase their cardiac output, a Hct of 18 may be acceptable. In an older individual with an already compromised oxygen-carrying capacity (cardiopulmonary diseases), transfusion may be recommended when the Hct level is below 30.

Interfering Factors

- Abnormalities in RBC size may alter Hct values. Larger RBCs are associated with higher Hct levels, because the larger RBCs take up a greater percentage of the total blood volume.
- Extremely elevated WBC counts decrease Hct, which would falsely indicate anemia.
- Hemodilution and dehydration may affect the Hct level (see above).
- Pregnancy usually causes slightly decreased values because of chronic hemodilution.
- Living in high altitudes causes increased Hct values as a result of a physiologic response to the decreased oxygen available at these high altitudes.
- Values may not be reliable immediately after hemorrhage because the percentage of total blood volume taken up by the RBC has not changed. Not until the total blood volume is replaced with fluids will the Hct decrease.
- Drugs that may cause *decreased* levels include chloramphenicol and penicillin.

✓ CLINICAL PRIORITIES

- Normal values vary according to gender and age.
- Pregnancy usually causes slightly decreased values because of chronic hemodilution.
- The Hct (in percentage points) is usually three times the Hgb concentration (in grams per deciliter) when RBCs are of normal size and contain normal amounts of Hgb.
- In dehydration the Hct is falsely elevated. In overhydration the value is decreased.

Procedure and Patient Care

Before

- Explain the procedure to the patient.
- Tell the patient that no fasting is required.

During

- Collect approximately 5 to 7 ml of venous blood in a lavender-top tube; however, only 0.5 ml is required when using capillary tubes.
- Avoid hemolysis.

After

- Apply pressure or a pressure dressing to the venipuncture site.
- Assess the venipuncture site for bleeding.

Test Results and Clinical Significance

Increased levels

Erythrocytosis *The number of RBCs is increased. This can result from illnesses or as a physiologic response to external situations.*

Congenital heart disease *Cyanotic heart diseases cause chronically low* Po_2 *levels. In response, the RBCs increase in number. Therefore the Hct increases.*

Polycythemia vera *This is a result of the bone marrow inappropriately producing great numbers of RBCs. Therefore the Hct increases.*

Severe dehydration (e.g., severe diarrhea, burns) *With depletion of extracellular fluid, the total blood volume decreases, but the number of RBCs stays the same. Therefore the percentage of total blood volume that is taken up by the RBCs increases and the Hct increases.*

Severe chronic obstructive pulmonary disease (COPD) *Chronic states of hypoxia cause stimulation of RBC production as a physiologic response to increased oxygen-carrying capacity. Therefore the Hct increases.*

Decreased levels

Anemia *This is a term given to the state associated with reduced RBC numbers. Because the Hct is an indirect reflection of RBC numbers, the Hct will also be reduced. Many different types of diseases are associated with anemia.*

Hemoglobinopathy *Patients with Hgb disorders or other blood dyscrasias have a reduced number and survival of RBCs. Therefore the Hct is decreased.*

Cirrhosis *This is a chronic state of fluid overload. The RBCs are diluted and make up a smaller percentage of the total blood volume. Therefore the Hct decreases.*

Hemolytic anemia (e.g., erythroblastosis fetalis, hemoglobinopathies, drug-induced hemolytic anemias, paroxysmal nocturnal hemoglobinuria) *The RBC survival is diminished in hemolytic anemia. The number of RBCs decreases and therefore the Hct is decreased.*

Hemorrhage *With active bleeding, the number of RBCs decreases and therefore the Hct is decreased. It takes time (several hours), however, for the Hct to fall. Only when the blood volume is replenished with fluid does the Hct diminish.*

Dietary deficiency *With certain vitamin or mineral deficiencies (e.g., iron), the RBC number or size is decreased. Therefore the Hct is decreased.*

Bone marrow failure *With reduced synthesis of the RBC, the Hct will decrease.*
Prosthetic valves *The prosthetic valve causes mechanical trauma to the RBC. The RBC survival is diminished. RBC numbers diminish and Hct decreases.*
Renal disease *Erythropoietin is made in the kidney and is a strong stimulant to RBC production. With a reduced level of erythropoietin, the RBC numbers diminish and the Hct is decreased.*
Normal pregnancy *In pregnancy, normally there is increased blood volume due to a chronic state of overhydration. Combined with a relative "malnourished" state, the Hct is diminished by a decrease in the number of RBCs and the percentage of total blood volume they make up.*
Rheumatoid/collagen vascular diseases (e.g., rheumatoid arthritis, lupus) *Chronic illnesses are associated with a reduced production of RBCs. Therefore the Hct is decreased.*
Lymphoma
Multiple myeloma
Leukemia
Hodgkin's disease
Hematologic cancers are often associated with bone marrow failure of RBC production. The number of RBCs diminishes and the Hct decreases.

Related Tests

- Hemoglobin (p. 254): This is a measurement of the concentration of Hgb in the blood. It is closely associated with the RBC count and Hct value.
- Red blood cell count (p. 372): This is a measurement of the number of RBCs per cubic millimeter of blood. It is closely associated with the Hgb and Hct values.
- Red blood cell indices (p. 375): These provide data about the size and Hgb content of the RBC.

Hemoglobin (Hgb, Hb)

Normal Findings

Male: 14-18 g/dl or 8.7-11.2 mmol/L (SI units)
Female: 12-16 g/dl or 7.4-9.9 mmol/L
Pregnant female: >11 g/dl
Elderly: Values are slightly decreased.
Child/adolescent
0-2 weeks: 12-20 g/dl
2-6 months: 10-17 g/dl
6 months-1 year: 9.5-14 g/dl
1-6 years: 9.5-14 g/dl
6-18 years: 10-15.5 g/dl
Newborn: 14-24 g/dl

Critical Values <5.0 g/dl or >20 g/dl

Indications

This test is a measure of the total amount of Hgb in the blood. It is used as a rapid indirect measurement of the RBC count. It is repeated serially in patients with ongoing bleeding or as a routine part of the complete blood count. It is an integral part of the evaluation of anemic patients.

Age-related concerns

- Values in children are age specific, with normal values varying throughout the first 18 years.
- Values are slightly decreased in the elderly.

Test Explanation

The Hgb concentration is a measure of the total amount of Hgb in the peripheral blood. The test is normally performed as part of a complete blood count. Hgb serves as a vehicle for oxygen and carbon dioxide transport. The oxygen-carrying capacity of the blood is determined by the Hgb concentration. Hgb also acts as an important acid-base buffer system.

As with the RBC count, normal values vary according to gender and age. Women tend to have lower values than men and Hgb values tend to decrease with age. The Hgb closely reflects the hematocrit (Hct) and RBC values. The Hct in percentage points usually is approximately three times the Hgb concentration in grams per deciliter when RBCs are of normal size and contain normal amounts of Hgb.

Abnormal values indicate the same pathologic states as abnormal RBC counts and Hct concentrations. Decreased levels indicate anemia (reduced number of RBCs). Increased levels can indicate erythrocytosis. In addition, however, changes in plasma volume are more accurately reflected by the Hgb concentration. Dilutional overhydration decreases the concentration, whereas dehydration tends to cause an artificially high value. Slight decreases in the values of Hgb and Hct during pregnancy reflect the expanded blood volume due to a chronic state of overhydration; the number of cells is actually increased during pregnancy. Hgb is usually measured by an automated cell counter. There is very little variability (2% to 3%) with most well-kept machines.

Hgb is made up of heme (iron surrounded by protoporphyrin) and globin consisting of an alpha- and beta-polypeptide chain. Abnormalities in the globin structure are called hemoglobinopathies (e.g., sickle cell disease, hemoglobin C disease). Some diseases are caused by abnormalities in globin chain synthesis (such as thalassemia). In these diseases the RBC counts can be low, the RBC survival can be diminished, and the RBC-carrying capacity can be reduced.

Too little Hgb puts a strain on the cardiopulmonary system to maintain good oxygen-carrying capacity. With critically low hemoglobin levels, patients are at great risk for angina, heart attack, congestive heart failure, and stroke. When Hgb levels are too high because of increased numbers of RBCs, intravascular sludging occurs, leading to stroke and other organ infarction. Decisions concerning the need for blood transfusion are usually based on the Hgb or the Hct. In an otherwise healthy person, transfusion is not considered as long as the Hgb is above 8 g/dl or the Hct is above 24. In younger people who can safely and significantly increase their cardiac output, an Hgb level of 6 g/dl may be acceptable. In an older individual with an already compromised oxygen-carrying capacity (cardiopulmonary diseases), transfusion may be recommended when the Hgb level is below 10.

Interfering Factors

- Slight Hgb decreases normally occur during pregnancy because of the dilution effect of the expanded blood volume.
- There is a slight diurnal variation in Hgb levels. Hgb levels are highest around 8 AM and are lowest around 8 PM. This may vary as much as 1 g/dl.
- Heavy smokers have higher Hgb levels than nonsmokers.
- Living in high altitudes causes increased Hgb values as a result of a physiologic response to the decreased oxygen available at these high altitudes.
- Drugs that may cause *increased* levels include gentamicin and methyldopa (Aldomet).
- Drugs that may cause *decreased* levels include antibiotics, antineoplastic drugs, aspirin, indomethacin (Indocin), rifampin, and sulfonamides.

✓ CLINICAL PRIORITIES

- Dilutional overhydration increases the Hgb concentration. Dehydration tends to cause an artificially high value.
- The Hct (in percentage points) is usually three times the Hgb concentration (in grams per deciliter) when RBCs are of normal size and contain a normal amount of Hgb.
- Living at high altitudes causes increased Hgb values as a result of a physiologic response to decreased oxygen levels.

Procedure and Patient Care

Before

- Explain the procedure to the patient.
- Tell the patient that no fasting is required.

During

- Collect approximately 5 to 7 ml of venous blood in a lavender-top tube.
- Avoid hemolysis.
- List on the laboratory slip any drugs that may affect test results.

After

- Apply pressure or a pressure dressing to the venipuncture site.
- Observe the venipuncture site for bleeding.

Test Results and Clinical Significance

Increased levels

Erythrocytosis *The number of RBCs is increased as a result of illnesses or as a physiologic response to external situations (e.g., high altitude).*

Congenital heart disease *Cyanotic heart diseases cause chronically low Po_2 levels. In response, the RBCs increase in number. Therefore the Hgb increases.*

Severe chronic obstructive pulmonary disease *Chronic states of hypoxia cause stimulation of RBC production as a physiologic response to increased oxygen-carrying capacity. Therefore the Hgb increases.*

Polycythemia vera *This is a result of the bone marrow inappropriately producing great numbers of RBCs. Therefore the Hgb increases.*

Severe dehydration (e.g., severe diarrhea, burns) *With depletion of extracellular fluid, the total blood volume decreases, but the number of RBCs stays the same. Therefore the percentage of total blood volume that is taken up by the RBCs increases and Hgb increases.*

Decreased levels

Anemia *This is a term given to the state associated with reduced RBC numbers. Because the Hgb is an indirect reflection of RBC numbers, the Hgb will also be reduced. Many different types of diseases are associated with anemia.*

Hemoglobinopathy *Patients with Hgb disorders or other blood dyscrasias have a reduced RBC number and survival. Therefore the Hgb is decreased.*

Cirrhosis *This is a chronic state of fluid overload. The RBCs are diluted and make up a smaller percentage of the total blood volume. Therefore the Hgb decreases.*

Hemolytic anemia (e.g., erythroblastosis fetalis, hemoglobinopathies, drug-induced hemolytic anemias, transfusion reactions, or paroxysmal nocturnal hemoglobinuria) *The RBC survival is diminished in hemolytic anemia. The number of RBCs decreases and the Hgb decreases.*

Hemorrhage *With active bleeding, the number of RBCs decreases and the Hgb decreases. It takes time (several hours), however, for the Hgb to fall. Only if the blood volume is replenished with fluid does the Hgb diminish.*

Dietary deficiency *With certain vitamin or mineral deficiencies (e.g., iron), the RBC number or size is decreased. Therefore the Hgb is decreased.*

Bone marrow failure *With reduced synthesis of the RBC, the Hgb will decrease.*

Prosthetic valves *The prosthetic valve causes mechanical trauma to the RBC. The RBC survival is diminished. RBC numbers diminish and Hgb decreases.*

Renal disease *Erythropoietin is made in the kidney and is a strong stimulant to RBC production. With a reduced level of erythropoietin, the RBC numbers diminish and the Hgb is decreased.*

Normal pregnancy *In pregnancy normally, there is increased blood volume due to a chronic state of overhydration. Combined with a relative "malnourished" state, the Hgb is diminished by a decrease in the number of RBCs and the percentage of total blood volume they make up.*

Rheumatoid/collagen vascular diseases (e.g., rheumatoid arthritis, lupus, sarcoidosis) *Chronic illnesses are associated with a reduced production of RBCs. Therefore the Hgb is decreased.*

Lymphoma
Multiple myeloma
Leukemia
Hodgkin's disease
Hematologic cancers are often associated with bone marrow failure of RBC production. The number of RBCs diminishes and the Hgb decreases.

Related Tests

- Hematocrit (p. 251): This is a measurement of the percentage of the total blood volume taken up by the RBCs. It is closely associated with Hgb values and RBC count.
- Red blood cell count (p. 372): This is a measurement of the number of RBCs per cubic millimeter of blood. It is closely associated with Hgb and Hct values
- Red blood cell indices (p. 375): These provide data about the size and Hgb content of the RBC.

Hemoglobin Electrophoresis
(Hgb Electrophoresis)

Normal Findings

Adult/elderly
- Hgb A_1: 95%-98%
- Hgb A_2: 2%-3%
- Hgb F: 0.8%-2%
- Hgb S: 0%
- Hgb C: 0%

Child (Hgb F)
- 6 months: 8%
- >6 months: 1%-2%

Newborn (Hgb F): 50%-80%

Indications

Hgb electrophoresis is a test that enables abnormal forms of Hgb (hemoglobinopathies) to be detected. This test is used to diagnose sickle cell anemia, thalassemia, and other hemoglobinopathies.

Test Explanation

Although many different Hgb variations have been described, the more common types are A_1, A_2, F, S, and C. Each major Hgb type is electrically charged to varying degrees. When the Hgb from lysed RBCs is placed on electrophoresis paper in an electromagnetic field, the Hgb variants migrate at different rates and therefore spread apart from each other. The migration of the various forms of Hgb make up a series of bands on the paper. The bands therefore correspond to the various forms of Hgb present. The pattern of bands is compared to normal and to other well-known abnormal patterns. A diagnosis can then be made. Furthermore, each band can be quantitated as a percentage of the total Hgb, indicating the severity of any recognized abnormality.

Hgb A_1 constitutes the major component of Hgb in the normal RBC. *Hgb A_2* is only a minor component (2% to 3%) of the normal Hgb total. *Hgb F* is the major Hgb component in the fetus but usually exists in only minimal quantities in the normal adult. Levels of Hgb F greater than 2% in patients over 3 years of age are considered abnormal. Hgb F is able to transport oxygen when only small amounts of oxygen are available (as in fetal life). In patients requiring compensation for prolonged chronic hypoxia (as in congenital cardiac abnormalities), Hgb F may be found in increased levels to assist in the transport of the available oxygen.

Hgb S is an abnormal form of Hgb associated with sickle cell anemia, which occurs predominantly in African-Americans. Hgb S is a relatively insoluble variant. When little oxygen is available, it assumes a crescent (sickle) shape that greatly distorts the RBC morphology. Vascular sludging is a consequence of the localized sickling and may lead to organ infarction. The duration of survival of the sickled RBC is diminished, and these patients also have anemia. *Hgb C* is another variant that exists in African-Americans. RBCs containing Hgb C have a decreased life span and are more readily lysed than normal RBCs. Mild to severe hemolytic anemia may result.

The Hgb content of some common hemoglobinopathies, as determined by electrophoresis, is as follows:

Sickle cell disease (homozygous SS)	**Sickle cell trait (heterozygous SA)**
Hgb S: 80%-100%	Hgb S: 20%-40%
Hgb A_1: 0%	Hgb A_1: 60%-80%
Hgb A_2: 2%-3%	Hgb A_2: 2%-3%
Hgb F: 2%	Hgb F: 2%

Hemoglobin C disease (homozygous)	**Hemoglobin H disease**
Hgb C: 90%-100%	Hgb A_1: 65%-90%
Hgb A_1: 0%	Hgb A_2: 2%-3%
Hgb A_2: 2%-3%	Hgb H: 5%-30%
Hgb F: 2%	

Thalassemia major (homozygous)	**Thalassemia minor (heterozygous)**
Hgb A_1: 5%-20%	Hgb A_1: 50%-85%
Hgb A_2: 2%-3%	Hgb A_2: 4%-6%
Hgb F: 65%-100%	Hgb F: 1%-3%

Interfering Factors

- Blood transfusions within the previous 12 weeks may alter test results.

Procedure and Patient Care

Before

- Explain the procedure to the patient.
- Tell the patient that no fasting is required.

During

- Collect approximately 7 ml of venous blood in a lavender-top tube.

After

- Apply pressure or a pressure dressing to the venipuncture site.
- Assess the venipuncture site for bleeding.

Test Results and Clinical Significance

Increased levels

Sickle cell disease
Hemoglobin H disease
Thalassemia major
Sickle cell trait
Thalassemia minor
Hemoglobin C disease
These hemoglobinopathies have a "classic" Hgb electrophoresis pattern that is diagnostic for the respective disease.

Related Tests

- Hemoglobin (p. 254): This is a direct measurement of the Hgb that exists in the "average" RBC.

Hepatitis Virus (Hepatitis-Associated Antigen [HAA], Australian Antigen)

Normal Findings Negative

Indications

This group of tests is used to diagnose and to identify the serologic type and current status of hepatitis. It is important to diagnose and identify the type of hepatitis as soon as possible so that the patient can be immediately treated and appropriately isolated.

Test Explanation

Hepatitis is an inflammation of the liver caused by viruses, alcohol ingestion, drugs, toxins, or overwhelming bacterial sepsis. The three common viruses now recognized to cause disease are hepatitis A, hepatitis B, and hepatitis non-A/non-B (also called hepatitis C) viruses. Hepatitis D and E viruses are much less common in the United States. Hepatitis D can only infect the liver by entering into a hepatitis B virus, which it uses as a carrying vehicle. Therefore hepatitis D cannot cause disease unless patients have hepatitis B virus in their bloodstream in the active, chronic, or carrier forms. The various types of hepatitis cannot be differentiated on the basis of their clinical presentation. The clinical presentations are quite similar in that they all may be manifested as low-grade fever, malaise, anorexia, and tiredness. Most often they are all associated with elevations of hepatocellular enzymes such as aspartate aminotransferase (AST), alanine aminotransferase (ALT), and lactic dehydrogenase (LDH).

Hepatitis A virus (HAV) was originally called infectious hepatitis. It has a short incubation period of 2 to 6 weeks and is highly contagious. During active infection, HAV is excreted in the stool and transmitted via oral-fecal contamination of food and drink. About half of those tested in United States have had this form of hepatitis. Most infections are not associated with symptoms severe enough to warrant medical evaluation. Although immunologic tests are not yet available to detect HAV antigen, two types of antibodies to HAV can be detected by the radioimmunoassay (RIA) and enzyme-linked immunosorbent assay (ELISA) methods.

The first type of antibody to HAV is IgM antibody (HAV-Ab/IgM), which appears approximately 3 to 4 weeks after exposure or just before hepatocellular enzyme elevations occur. These IgM levels usually return to normal in approximately 8 weeks.

The second type of antibody is IgG (HAV-Ab/IgG), which appears approximately 2 weeks after the the IgM begins to increase and slowly returns to normal levels. The IgG enzyme can remain detectable for more than 10 years after the infection. If the IgM antibody is elevated in the absence of the IgG antibody, acute hepatitis is suspected. If, however, IgG is elevated in the absence of IgM elevation, a convalescent or chronic stage of HAV viral infection is indicated.

Hepatitis B virus (HBV) is commonly known as serum hepatitis. It has a long incubation period of 5 weeks to 6 months. HBV is most frequently transmitted by blood transfusion; however, it also can be contracted via exposure to other body fluids. HBV may cause a severe and unrelenting form of hepatitis culminating in liver failure and death. The incidence is increased among blood transfusion recipients, male homosexuals, dialysis patients, transplant patients, IV drug abusers, and patients with leukemia or lymphoma. Hospital personnel are also at increased risk of infection mostly due to needlestick contamination. If a person is stuck by a contaminated needle, the risk of infection is about 10% to 30%. In addition to the acute phase of this disease, carrier and chronic states of this disease have been recognized.

HBV, also called the Dane particle, is made up of an inner core surrounded by an outer capsule. The outer capsule contains the hepatitis B surface antigen (HBsAg), formerly called Australian antigen. The inner core contains HBV core antigen (HBcAg). The hepatitis B e-antigen (HBeAg) is also found within the core. Antibodies to these antigens are called HBsAb, HBcAb, and HBeAb. The tests used to detect these antigens and antibodies are listed below and in Table 2-25.

1. *Hepatitis B surface antigen* (HBsAg). This is the most frequently and easily performed test for hepatitis B and the first test to become abnormal. HBsAg rises before the onset of clinical symptoms, peaks during the first week of symptoms, and returns to normal by the time jaundice subsides. HBsAg generally indicates active HBV infection. If the level of this antigen persists in the blood, the patient is considered to be a carrier.
2. *Hepatitis B surface antibody* (HBsAb). This antibody appears approximately 4 weeks after the disappearance of the surface antigen and signifies the end of the acute infection phase. HBsAb also signifies immunity to subsequent infection. Concentrated forms of this agent constitute the hyperimmunoglobulin given to patients who have come in contact with HBV-infected patients (e.g., contact by an inadvertent needle prick from a needle previously used on a patient with HBV infection). HBsAb is the antibody that denotes immunity after administration of hepatitis B vaccine.

Table 2-25 Hepatitis testing

Serology	Appearance/Disappearance	Application
HAV-Ab/IgM	4-6 wk/3-4 mo	Acute HAV infection
HAV-Ab/IgG	8-12 wk/10 yr	Previous HAV exposure/immunity
HBeAg	1-3 wk/6-8 wk	Acute HBV infection
HBeAb	4-6 wk/4-6 yr	Acute HBV infection ended
HBsAg	4-12 wk/1-3 mo	Acute HBV infection
HBsAb total	3-10 mo/6-10 yr	Previous HBV infection/immunity indicated
HBVc-Ab/IgM	2-12 wk/3-6 mo	Acute HBV infection
HBVc-Ab total	3-12 wk/life	Previous HBV infection/convalescent stage
HCV-Ab/IgG	3-4 mo/2 yr	Previous HCV infection
HDV Ag	1-3 days/3-5 days	Acute HDV infection
HDV-Ab/IgM	10 days/1-3 mo	Acute HDV infection
HDV-Ab total	2-3 mo/7-14 mo	Chronic HDV infection

3. *Hepatitis B core antigen* (HBcAg). No tests are currently available to detect this antigen.
4. *Hepatitis B core antibody* (HBcAb). This antibody appears approximately 1 month after infection with HBsAg and declines (although it remains elevated) over several years. HBcAb is also present in patients with chronic hepatitis. The HBcAb level is elevated during the time lag between the disappearance of HBsAg and the appearance of HBsAb. This interval is called the "core window." During this interval, HBcAb is the only detectable marker of a recent hepatitis infection.
5. *Hepatitis B e-antigen* (HBeAg). This antigen is generally not used for diagnostic purposes but rather as an index of infectivity. The presence of HBeAg correlates with early and active disease as well as with high infectivity in patients with acute HBV infection. The persistent presence of HBeAg in the blood predicts the development of chronic HBV infection.
6. *Hepatitis B e-antibody* (HBeAb). This antibody indicates that an acute phase of HBV infection is over, or almost over, and that the chance of infectivity is greatly reduced.

Non-A, non-B hepatitis (NANB), also called hepatitis C (HCV), is transmitted in a manner similar to HBV. Most cases of hepatitis are caused by blood transfusion. The incubation period is 2 to 12 weeks after exposure. The clinical manifestations of the illness parallel HBV. An HCV viral titer to detect HCV IgG antibodies is now available; however, no vaccine protection is available for this form of hepatitis.

Hepatitis D virus (HDV) is known to cause "delta hepatitis." As stated above, the HDV must enter the HBV to gain access to the liver and be infective. The patient must have HBV in the blood from a past or synchronously occurring infection. In the United States this is most commonly transmitted through tainted blood. The HDV antigen can be detected by immunoassay within a few days after infection. The IgM and total antibodies to HDV are detected early in the disease also. A persistent elevation of these antibodies indicates a chronic or carrier state.

Hepatitis E virus (HEV) was initially included in the NANB virus group but was isolated several years ago as an etiologic virus of short incubation. No antigen or antibody tests are currently widely available and accurate for the serologic identification of this infecting agent.

Procedure and Patient Care

Before

- Explain the procedure to the patient.
- Tell the patient that no fasting is required.

During

- Collect approximately 5 to 7 ml of venous blood in a red-top tube.
- Note that most of the testing for hepatitis is done by radioimmunoassay. Usually a hepatitis profile that includes several HBV antigens and antibodies is performed.

After

- Apply pressure or a pressure dressing to the venipuncture site.
- Assess the venipuncture site for bleeding.
- Handle the specimen as if it were capable of transmitting hepatitis.
- Immediately discard the needle in the appropriate receptacle.
- Send the specimen to the laboratory promptly.
- Advise any patient suspected of having hepatitis that they should refrain from intimate contact with another person. Until the serology indicates otherwise, the person should be considered infective.

Test Results and Clinical Significance

Increased levels

Hepatitis A
Hepatitis B
Hepatitis C (non-A, non-B hepatitis)
Hepatitis D
Hepatitis E
These serologic varieties of hepatitis can exist in an acute, chronic, carrier, or chronic active phase.

Related Tests

- Aspartate aminotransferase (AST) (p. 105), alanine aminotransferase (ALT) (p. 33), lactic dehydrogenase LDH (p. 278): These hepatocellular enzymes are elevated during the acute phase and chronic active phase of hepatitis.

HLA-B27 Antigen (Human Lymphocyte Antigen B27, Human Leukocyte A Antigen, White Blood Cell Antigens, Histocompatibility Leukocyte A Antigen)

Normal Findings Negative

Indications

HLA testing is used in histocompatibility testing for organ or other tissue transplantation. Because these antigens are present with certain diseases, it is used to support the diagnosis of these diseases. Finally, HLA testing is used in paternity investigations.

Test Explanation

The HLA antigens exist on the surface of WBCs and on the surface of all nucleated cells in other tissues. These antigens can be detected most easily on the cell surface of lymphocytes. The presence or absence of these antigens is determined by the genes on chromosome 6. There are four genes at this locus. Each gene controls the presence or absence of HLA A, B, C, and D. There is probably a fifth genetic locus that is closely related to D and is called DR.

The HLA system of antigens has been used to indicate tissue compatibility with tissue transplantation. If the HLA antigens of the donor are not compatible with the recipient, the recipient will make antibodies to those antigens and accelerate rejection. Transplant survival of the tissue is increased if HLA matching is good. Prior HLA sensitization causes antibodies to form in the blood of a transplant recipient and shortens the survival of RBCs or platelets when transfused.

The HLA system has also been used to assist in the diagnosis of certain other diseases. For example, HLA B27 is present in 80% of patients with Reiter's syndrome. When a patient presents with recurrent and multiple arthritic complaints, the presence of HLA-B27 supports the diagnosis of Reiter's syndrome. HLA-B27 is found in 5% to 7% of normal patients. Other HLA-disease associations are listed in Table 2-26.

Because HLA antigens are genetically determined, they are useful in paternity investigations. This is particularly helpful if the reputed father or child has an unusual HLA genotype. A common HLA genotype in either the father or child increases the likelihood that there are many potential "fathers" of that child.

For this test, lymphocytes from the patient are extracted and incubated with anti-HLA–specific cytotoxic antibody. If the patient has the particular HLA antigen, a complex will be formed on the cell surface. Serum complement is then added to the mixture, which kills the lymphocytes and aids in determining the titer of the HLA antigen.

Procedure and Patient Care

Before

- Explain the procedure to the patient.
- Tell the patient that no fasting or special preparation is required.

Table 2-26 HLA and diseases

HLA antigen	Disease
B27	Reiter's syndrome Ankylosing spondylitis *Yersinia enterocolitica* arthritis Anterior uveitis Graves' disease
B8	Celiac disease Chronic active hepatitis Multiple sclerosis Myasthenia gravis Dermatitis herpetiformis
B17	Psoriasis
Bw15 + B8	Juvenile diabetes
DR3 or DR4	Diabetes associated with beta cell autoantibodies
A3	Hemochromatosis
DR4	Rheumatoid arthritis
DR7, DRw3, B8	Gluten enteropathy

During

- Collect at least 10 ml of venous blood in a heparinized solution.

After

- Apply pressure or a pressure dressing to the venipuncture site.
- Assess the venipuncture site for bleeding.

Test Results and Clinical Significance

Positive for HLA antigens

Ankylosing spondylitis
Reiter's syndrome
Yersinia enterocolitica arthritis
Anterior uveitis
Graves' disease
Celiac disease/gluten enteropathy
Chronic active hepatitis
Multiple sclerosis
Myasthenia gravis
Dermatitis herpetiformis
Psoriasis
Juvenile diabetes/diabetes associated with beta cell autoantibodies
Hemochromatosis
Rheumatoid arthritis
Specific HLA antigens are present in these diseases in varying frequencies. The association of these HLA antigens with the pathophysiology of these diseases is not known.

Human T-cell Lymphotrophic Virus (HTLV) I/II Antibody

Normal Findings

Negative

Indications

Testing for this virus is helpful in the diagnosis of certain types of leukemias.

Test Explanation

Several forms of HTLV, a human retrovirus, affect humans. The virus is endemic in southern Japan, the Caribbean islands, South America, and portions of Africa. HTLV-I is associated with adult T-cell leukemia/lymphoma. HTLV-II is associated with adult hairy cell leukemia. Also, HTLV-I has been associated with neurologic disorders such as tropical spastic paraparesis. Humans can be infected with these viruses, however, and not develop any malignancy or diseases.

The human immunodeficiency viruses (HIVs), which are known to be the cause of acquired immunodeficiency syndrome (AIDS), are also retroviruses; however, HTLV infection is not associated with AIDS. HTLV transmission is similar, however, to HIV transmission (e.g., body fluid contamination, IV drug use, sexual contact, breast-feeding).

Most serologic tests for HTLV are performed using enzyme-linked immunosorbent assay (ELISA) techniques. Identification of antibodies to certain portions of the two viruses allows for specific diagnosis and differentiation of the two. Nucleic acid probes are also used at large testing laboratories.

Procedure and Patient Care

Before

- Explain the procedure to the patient.
- Tell the patient that no fasting is required.

During

- Collect approximately 7 ml of venous blood in a red-top tube.

After

- Apply pressure or a pressure dressing to the venipuncture site.
- Assess the venipuncture site for bleeding.

Test Results and Clinical Significance

Increased levels

Acute HTLV infection
Adult T-cell leukemia
Hairy cell leukemia
Tropical spastic paraparesis
The pathophysiology of the association of these illnesses with HTLV infection is not known.

Immunoglobulin Electrophoresis
(Gamma Globulin Electrophoresis)

Normal Findings

IgG	mg/dl
Adult	565-1765
Child	
1 mo	250-900
2-5 mo	200-700
6-9 mo	220-900
1 yr	340-1200
2-3 yr	420-1200
4-12 yr	460-1600

IgA	mg/dl
Adult	85-385
Child	
1 mo	1-4
2-5 mo	4-80
6-9 mo	8-80
1 yr	15-110
2-3 yr	18-150
4-12 yr	25-350

IgM	mg/dl
Adult	55-375
Child	
1 mo	20-80
2-5 mo	25-100
6-9 mo	35-125
1-8 yr	45-200
9-12 yr	50-250

IgD and IgE
Minimal

Indications

This test is used to assist in the diagnosis and monitoring of therapeutic response in many disease states. It is often ordered if a serum protein electrophoresis indicates a spike at the immunoglobulin level.

Test Explanation

Proteins within the blood are made up of albumin and globulin. Several types of globulin exist, one of which is gamma globulin. Antibodies are made up of gamma globulin protein and are called immunoglobulins. There are many classes of immunoglobulins (antibodies). *IgG* constitutes approximately 75% of the serum immunoglobulins; therefore it constitutes the majority of circulating blood antibodies. Maternal IgG can cross the placenta and is effective for the immune protection of the newborn in the first few months of life. *IgA* constitutes approximately 15% of the immunoglobulins within the body and is present primarily in the secretions of the respiratory and GI tract, in saliva, in colostrum, and in tears. IgA is also present to a smaller degree in the blood. *IgM* is an immunoglobulin primarily responsible for ABO blood grouping and rheumatoid factor, yet is involved in the immunologic reaction to many other infections (e.g., hepatitis, gram-negative sepsis). Since IgM does not cross the placenta, an elevation of IgM in the newborn indicates intrauterine infection such as rubella, cytomegalovirus (CMV), or a sexually transmitted disease (STD). *IgE* often mediates an allergic response and is measured to detect allergic diseases. *IgD,* which constitutes the smallest portion of the immunoglobulins, is rarely evaluated or detected.

Serum immunoelectrophoresis is used to detect and monitor the course of diseases including hypersensitivity diseases, immune deficiencies, autoimmune diseases, chronic infections, multiple myeloma, chronic viral infections, and intrauterine fetal infections. For this test, the serum is placed on a slide containing agar gel, and an electric current is passed through this gel. Immunoglobulins are separated out and electrophoresed according to the quantity and difference in electric charge. Specific antisera are placed alongside the slide to identify the specific type of immunoglobulin present.

Interfering Factors

- Drugs that may cause *increased* immunoglobulin levels include therapeutic gamma globulin, hydralazine, isoniazid (INH), phenytoin (Dilantin), procainamide, oral contraceptives, methadone, dextran, steroids, and tetanus toxoid and antitoxin.

Procedure and Patient Care

Before

- Explain the procedure to the patient.
- Tell the patient that no fasting or special preparation is required.

During

- Collect 7 to 10 ml of venous blood in a red-top tube.
- Indicate on the laboratory slip if the patient has received any vaccinations or immunizations within the past 6 months. Also list any drugs that may affect test results.

After

- Apply pressure or a pressure dressing to the venipuncture site.
- Observe the venipuncture site for bleeding.

Test Results and Clinical Significance

Increased IgA levels

Chronic liver diseases (e.g., primary biliary cirrhosis)
Chronic infections
Inflammatory bowel disease
The pathophysiology of these observations is not well known.

Decreased IgA levels

Ataxia
Telangiectasia
Congenital isolated deficiency
These illnesses are caused by isolated IgA or combined immunoglobulin deficiencies.

Hypoproteinemia (e.g., nephrotic syndrome, protein-losing enteropathies) *The hypoproteinemia that results from these diseases causes the IgA deficiency.*
Drug immunosuppression (steroids, dextran) *The production of IgA is diminished.*

Increased IgG levels

Chronic granulomatous infections (e.g., tuberculosis, Wegener's granulomatosis, sarcoidosis)
Hyperimmunization reactions
Chronic liver disease
Multiple myeloma (monoclonal IgG type)
Autoimmune diseases (e.g., rheumatoid arthritis, Sjögren's disease, systemic lupus erythromatosus)
All the above conditions stimulate IgG synthesis. The pathophysiology of this observation is not known.

Intrauterine devices *These devices work by creating a subclinical localized inflammatory reaction that is harmful to the sperm. Part of that reaction is the synthesis of IgG.*

Decreased IgG levels

Wiskott-Aldrich syndrome
Agammaglobulinemia
These diseases are a result of a genetic deficiency that results in inadequate synthesis of IgG and other immunoglobulins.

AIDS *This creates a deficiency throughout the entire immune system. IgG and other immunoglobins are diminished.*
Hypoproteinemia (e.g., nephrotic syndrome, protein-losing enteropathies) *The hypoproteinemia that results from these diseases causes the IgG deficiency.*

Drug immunosuppression (steroids, dextran) *The production of IgG is diminished.*
Non-IgG multiple myeloma
Leukemia
IgG production is diminished because the marrow is taken over by tumor cells.

Increased IgM levels

Waldenström's macroglobulinemia *This is a malignancy similar to myeloma in which IgM is secreted at high levels by the malignant lymphoplasma cells. It is very similar diagnostically to IgM myeloma.*
Chronic infections (e.g., hepatitis, mononucleosis, sarcoidosis) *These infections stimulate the humoral response and many of the immunoglobulins, including IgM.*
Autoimmune diseases (e.g., systemic lupus erythromatosus, rheumatoid arthritis) *The pathophysiology is not well known. It is assumed that these antibodies somehow contribute to the disease process.*

Acute infections *IgM is the first immunoglobulin to respond to an infectious agent (viral, bacterial, parasitic).*
Chronic liver disorders (e.g., biliary cirrhosis) *The pathophysiology is not well defined.*

Decreased IgM levels

Agammaglobulinemia *This disease is a result of a genetic deficiency in which the synthesis of IgM and other immunoglobulins is inadequate.*
AIDS *This creates a deficiency throughout the entire immune system. IgM and other immunoglobulins are diminished.*
Hypoproteinemia (e.g., nephrotic syndrome, protein-losing enteropathies) *The hypoproteinemia that results from these diseases causes the IgM deficiency.*
Drug immunosuppression (steroids, dextran) *The production of IgM is diminished.*
IgG or IgA multiple myeloma
Leukemia
IgM production is diminished because the marrow is taken over by tumor cells.

Increased IgE levels

Allergy reactions (e.g., hayfever, asthma, eczema, anaphylaxis) *Allergic reactions stimulate the production of IgE antibodies.*
Allergic infections (e.g., aspergillosis, parasites)

Decreased IgE levels

Agammaglobulinemia *This can be specific for IgE or may include the deficient production of all the immunglobulins.*

Related Tests

- Protein electrophoresis (p. 361): This is a quantification of all the components that make up the serum proteins, including albumin, alpha 1 and 2, beta 1 and 2, and gamma globulins. This test can also detect abnormal proteins created by neoplasms and infections.
- Protein, blood (p. 358): This is a measurement of albumin, globulin, or total protein together or separately.
- Prealbumin (p. 345): This is a quantification of prealbumin, which is a component of proteins. This test is used to assess a person's nutritional status. It is also used to indicate the status of liver function.

Insulin Antibody (Anti-Insulin Antibody)

Normal Findings

No antibody detected for bovine or porcine insulin

Indications

This test is used in the evaluation of insulin resistance. It is also used to identify type I diabetes and in patients suspected of having an allergy to insulin.

Test Explanation

Insulin antibodies are present in nearly all patients with diabetes treated with exogenous (human, bovine, porcine) insulin. These antibodies develop from impurities in animal insulin or from antigenic stimulation of the insulin molecule. With the increased use of human insulin, the frequency of anti-insulin antibodies has significantly decreased. Insulin antibodies may also be produced in patients who have never received exogenous insulin. These autoantibodies are present in nearly 50% of children at the time of diagnosis of juvenile diabetes.

The most common type of anti-insulin antibody is IgG, but IgA, IgM, IgD, and IgE also have been reported. Most of these insulin antibodies do not cause clinical problems, but they may complicate most insulin assays. Anti-insulin antibodies act as insulin-transporting proteins and bind the free insulin. This can reduce the amount of insulin available for glucose metabolism. They may also contribute to insulin resistance (daily insulin requirements exceeding 200 U/day for 2 days). IgM, especially, may cause insulin resistance. Insulin allergy (most common with animal insulin) may result from IgE antibodies to insulin.

These insulin antibodies are diagnostic of factitious hypoglycemia from surreptitious administration of insulin. In these cases, C-peptide studies may also determine whether hypoglycemia is caused by insulin abuse, because C-peptide is not produced when exogenous insulin is administered.

Interfering Factors

- Because anti-insulin antibodies are measured by radiobinding assay, radioactive scans within 7 days before the test may interfere with the test result.

Procedure and Patient Care

Before

- Explain the procedure to the patient.
- Tell the patient that no fasting is required.

During

- Collect a venous blood sample in a red-top tube.

After

- Apply pressure or a pressure dressing to the venipuncture site.
- Assess the venipuncture site for bleeding.
- In most hospitals or laboratories, the specimen is refrigerated and sent to a reference laboratory.

Test Results and Clinical Significance

Increased levels

Insulin resistance *The anti-insulin antibodies bind insulin and thereby diminish the amount of free insulin available for glucose metabolism.*

Allergies to insulin *Although allergies are most frequent with the use of animal-generated insulin, they can still occur with human insulin. A rash or lymphadenopathy may be the result of such an allergy.*

Factitious hypoglycemia *Because most patients develop anti-insulin antibodies to exogenous insulin, the identification of these antibodies supports the secretive self-administration of insulin in a patient who denies the use of insulin.*

Related Tests

- C-peptide (p. 169): This test is used to evaluate diabetic patients. It is also used to identify patients who secretly self-administer insulin.
- Insulin assay (see below): This test is used to diagnose insulinoma (tumor of the islets of Langerhans) and to evaluate abnormal lipid and carbohydrate metabolism. It is used in the evaluation of patients with fasting hypoglycemia.

Insulin Assay

Normal Findings

Adult: 5-24 mU/ml or 36-179 pmol/L (SI units)
Newborn: 3-20 mU/ml

Critical Values >30 mU/ml

Indications

This test is used to diagnose insulinoma (tumor of the islets of Langerhans) and to evaluate abnormal lipid and carbohydrate metabolism. It is used in the evaluation of patients with fasting hypoglycemia.

Test Explanation

The hormone insulin can be measured successfully by radioimmunoassay in most larger laboratories. Insulin regulates blood glucose levels by facilitating the movement of glucose out of the bloodstream and into the cells. Insulin secretion is primarily reactive to the blood glucose level. Normally, as the blood glucose level increases, the insulin level also increases; as the glucose level decreases, insulin release stops.

Some investigators believe that measuring the ratio of the blood sugar and insulin on the same specimen obtained during the oral glucose tolerance (GT) test is more reliable than measuring insulin levels alone. Combined with the oral GT test, the insulin assay can show characteristic curves. For example, patients with juvenile diabetes have low fasting insulin levels and display flat GT insulin curves, because there is little or no increase in insulin levels. Patients who are mildly diabetic have normal fasting insulin levels and display GT curves with a delayed rise.

When combined with a fasting blood sugar, insulin assay is very accurate in detecting insulinoma. After the patient fasts 12 to 14 hours, the insulin/glucose ratio should be less than 0.3. Patients with insulinoma have ratios greater than this. To increase the sensitivity and specificity of these combined tests for insulinoma, Turner and others have proposed the "amended" insulin/glucose ratios using variable mathematic "fudge" factors:

$$\frac{\text{Serum insulin level} \times 100}{\text{Serum glucose} - 30\text{ mg/100 ml}}$$

A Turner amended ratio of over 50 suggests insulinoma.

Interfering Factors

- Most patients treated with insulin for diabetes develop insulin antibodies within a few months. These antibodies can interfere with insulin radioimmunoassay results by competing with the insulin antibodies used in the insulin assay.
- Food intake and obesity may cause increased insulin levels.
- Recent administration of radioisotopes may affect test results by interfering with the radioimmunoassay method to detect insulin.
- Drugs that may cause *increased* insulin levels include corticosteroids, levodopa, and oral contraceptives.

Procedure and Patient Care

Before

- Explain the procedure to the patient.
- Keep the patient on NPO status for 8 hours.

During

- Collect approximately 5 ml of venous blood in a red-top tube and pack it in ice.
- Avoid hemolysis.
- If the serum insulin level will be measured during the GT test, collect the blood sample before oral ingestion of the glucose load and often at designated intervals after glucose ingestion.

After

- Apply pressure or a pressure dressing to the venipuncture site.
- Observe the venipuncture site for bleeding.
- Transport the specimen immediately to the laboratory.

Test Results and Clinical Significance

Increased levels

Insulinoma *This is a tumor of the beta cells in the islets of Langerhans of the pancreas. This is diagnosed in patients who have hyperinsulinemia despite hypoglycemia. These patients have persistently high C-peptide levels despite glucose levels of below 30 mg/dl. The amended Turner insulin/glucose ratio exceeds 50.*

Cushing's syndrome *The elevated glucose caused by the cortisol overproduction in the Cushingoid patient acts as a constant stimulant to insulin.*
Acromegaly *The elevated glucose caused by growth hormone overproduction in the acromegalic patient acts as a constant stimulant to insulin.*
Obesity *These patient have a persistently high insulin level.*
Fructose or galactose intolerance *These complex sugars cannot be metabolized normally and, like glucose, stimulate insulin production.*

Decreased levels

Diabetes *Insulin-dependent diabetes is, in part, due to lack of endogenous insulin.*
Hypopituitarism *This disease is associated with reduced thyroid and adrenal function along with reduced growth hormone levels. This leads to reduced glucose levels. Insulin production is diminished.*

Related Tests

- Glucose tolerance (p. 233): This is a test of a patient's capability to handle a glucose load.
- Glucose, postprandial (p. 229): This is a timed glucose measurement after a carbohydrate meal.
- C-peptide (p. 169): This test is used to evaluate diabetic patients. It is also used to identify patients who secretly self administer insulin.
- Insulin antibody (p. 270): This test is used in the evaluation of insulin resistance. It is also used to identify type I diabetes. It is used when allergy to insulin is suspected.

Iron Level (Fe), Total Iron-Binding Capacity (TIBC), Transferrin (Siderophilin) Saturation

Normal Findings

Iron: 13-31 mmol/L (SI units)
Male: 65-175 μg/dl or 11.6–31.3 μmol/L (SI units)
Female: 50-170 μg/dl or 9.0–30.4 μmol/L (SI units)
Newborn: 100-250 μg/dl
Child: 50-120 μg/dl
TIBC: 250-420 μg/dl or 45-73 mmol/L (SI units)
Transferrin
Adult male: 215-365 mg/dl
Adult female: 250-380 mg/dl
Child: 203-360 mg/dl
Newborn: 130-275 mg/dl
Transferrin saturation
Males: 20%-50%
Females: 15%-50%

Indications

These tests are used to evaluate iron metabolism in patients in whom iron deficiency, overload, or poisoning is suspected.

Test Explanation

Serum iron

Abnormal levels of iron are characteristic of many diseases, including iron deficiency anemia and hemochromatosis. As much as 70% of the iron in the body is found in the hemoglobin of the RBCs. The other 30% is stored iron in the form of ferritin and hemosiderin. Iron is supplied by the diet. About 10% of the ingested iron is absorbed in the small intestine and transported to the plasma. There the iron is bound to a globulin protein called transferrin and carried to the bone marrow for incorporation into hemoglobin. The serum iron determination is a measurement of the quantity of iron bound to transferrin.

Iron deficiency anemia is a result of reduced serum iron. It has many causes, including (1) insufficient iron intake, (2) inadequate gut absorption, (3) increased requirements (as in growing children and late pregnancy), and (4) loss of blood (as in menstruation, bleeding peptic ulcer, colon neoplasm). Iron deficiency results in a decreased production of hemoglobin, which in turn results in a small, pale (microcytic, hypochromic) RBC. A decrease in the mean corpuscular volume and mean corpuscular hemoglobin concentration (see p. 375) is also seen. A decreased serum iron level, elevated TIBC, and low transferrin saturation value are characteristic of iron deficiency anemia.

Iron overload or poisoning is called hemochromatosis or hemosiderosis. Excess iron is usually deposited in the brain, liver, and heart and causes severe dysfunction of these organs. Massive blood transfusions also may cause elevated serum iron levels, although only transiently. Transfusions should be avoided before serum iron level determinations.

Because serum iron levels may vary significantly during the day, the blood specimen should be drawn in the morning, especially when the results are used to monitor iron replacement therapy. The patient should refrain from eating for approximately 12 hours to avoid artificially high iron measurements caused by eating food with a high iron content.

TIBC and transferrin

TIBC is a measurement of all proteins available for binding mobile iron. Transferrin represents the largest quantity of iron-binding proteins. Therefore TIBC is an indirect, yet accurate measurement of transferrin. Ferritin is not included in TIBC, because it binds only stored iron. During iron overload, transferrin levels stay about the same or decrease, whereas the other less common iron-carrying proteins increase in number. In this situation, TIBC is less reflective of true transferrin levels. TIBC is increased in 70% of patients with iron deficiency.

Transferrin is a *negative* acute-phase reactant protein. That is, in various acute inflammatory reactions, transferrin levels diminish. Transferrin also is diminished in the face of chronic illnesses such as malignancy, collagen vascular diseases, or liver diseases. Hypoproteinemia is also associated with reduced transferrin levels. Pregnancy and estrogen therapy are associated with increased transferrin levels.

TIBC is usually measured by adding excess iron to the patient's serum. This saturates all the transferrin. Excess iron is removed. The iron that is left is measured and is a direct measurement of TIBC and an indirect measurement of transferrin. Many laboratories do not perform TIBC measurements. Transferrin is measured directly.

TIBC varies minimally with iron intake. TIBC is more a reflection of liver function (transferrin is produced by the liver) and nutrition than of iron metabolism. TIBC values often are used to monitor the course of patients receiving hyperalimentation.

TIBC and transferrin saturation

The percentage of transferrin and other mobile iron-binding proteins saturated with iron is calculated by dividing the serum iron level by the TIBC.

$$\text{Transferrin saturation (\%)} = \frac{\text{Serum iron level} \times 100\%}{\text{TIBC}}$$

The normal value for transferrin saturation is 20% to 50%. Calculation of transferrin saturation is helpful in determining the cause of abnormal iron and TIBC levels. Transferrin saturation is decreased to below 15% in patients with iron deficiency anemia. It is increased in patients with hemolytic, sideroblastic, or megaloblastic anemias and also in patients with iron overload or poisoning. Increased intake or absorption of iron (as in hemochromatosis) leads to elevated iron levels. In such cases the TIBC is unchanged; as a result, the percentage of transferrin saturation is very high.

Chronic illness (e.g., infections, neoplasia, cirrhosis) is characterized by a low serum iron level, decreased TIBC, and normal transferrin saturation. Pregnancy is marked by high levels of protein, including transferrin. Because iron requirements are high, it is not unusual to find low serum iron levels, high TIBC, and a low percentage of transferrin saturation in late pregnancy.

Contraindications

- Patients with hemolytic diseases, because they may have an artificially high iron content. The iron in the hemolyzed RBCs leaks out into the bloodstream.

Interfering Factors

- Recent blood transfusions may increase serum iron.
- Recent ingestion of a meal containing high iron content may increase serum iron.
- Hemolytic diseases may be associated with an artificially high iron content.
- Drugs that may cause *increased iron* levels include chloramphenicol, dextran, estrogens, ethanol, iron preparations, methyldopa, and oral contraceptives.
- Drugs that may cause *decreased iron* levels include adrenocorticotropic hormone (ACTH), chlolestyramine, chloramphenicol, colchicine, deferoxamine, methicillin, and testosterone.
- Drugs that may cause *increased TIBC* levels include fluorides and oral contraceptives.
- Drugs that may cause *decreased TIBC* levels include ACTH and chloramphenicol.

Procedure and Patient Care

Before

- Explain the procedure to the patient.

- Keep the patient fasting for 12 hours before the blood test. Water is permitted.
- Assess the patient for a history of recent blood transfusion and recent meals high in iron content. Both may affect test results.

During

- Collect approximately 5 to 7 ml of venous blood in a red-top tube. The specimen should always be obtained using a 20-gauge or larger needle.
- Avoid hemolysis, because the iron contained in the RBC will pour out into the serum and cause artificially high iron levels.
- Indicate on the laboratory slip any drugs that may affect test results.

After

- Apply pressure or a pressure dressing to the venipuncture site.
- Assess the venipuncture site for bleeding.

Test Results and Clinical Significance

Increased serum iron levels

Hemosiderosis or hemochromatosis *These two forms of iron deposits are created by serum iron excesses. They can be acquired or result from a genetic defect in iron metabolism.*

Iron poisoning *Increased iron intake increases serum iron levels.*

Hemolytic anemia *The iron in the hemoglobin of the hemolyzed RBCs leaks out into the bloodstream.*

Massive blood transfusions *There is about 1 mg of iron in each milliliter of packed RBCs.*

Hepatitis or hepatic necrosis *The pathophysiology of this observation is not well established.*

Lead toxicity *The lead overload may displace the iron stores.*

Decreased serum iron levels

Insufficient dietary iron *Because all body iron is from dietary intake, a persistently reduced intake will lead to reduced serum levels.*

Chronic blood loss (irregular menses, uterine cancer, GI cancer, inflammatory bowel disease, diverticulosis, urologic tract [hematuria] cancer, hemangioma, arteriovenous malformation) *Chronic blood loss depletes the iron because most of the iron in the body exists in the hemoglobin of the RBCs.*

Inadequate intestinal absorption of iron (e.g., malabsorption, short-bowel syndrome) *Because all body iron is from dietary intake, a persistently reduced intake will lead to reduced serum levels.*

Pregnancy (late) *Fetal requirements deplete the mother's body store of iron.*

Iron deficiency anemia *This anemia results when iron and iron stores become depleted.*

Neoplasia *Iron levels are depleted in these patient for several reasons.*

Increased TIBC or transferrin levels

Estrogen therapy
Pregnancy (late)
Polycythemia vera
Iron deficiency anemia
The pathophysiology of the observation in the above diseases is not clear.

Decreased TIBC or transferrin levels

Malnutrition
Hypoproteinemia
Transferrin is a protein. Its levels can be expected to decrease as protein is depleted from the body.

Inflammatory diseases
Cirrhosis
Transferrin is a negative acute-phase reactant protein. That is, in various acute inflammatory reactions, transferrin levels diminish.

Hemolytic anemia
Pernicious anemia
Sickle cell anemia
These anemias are associated with elevated iron levels and decreased TIBC. The pathophysiology of the latter is not clear.

Increased transferrin saturation or TIBC saturation

Hemochromatosis or hemosiderosis
Increased iron intake (oral or parenteral)
Increased iron levels saturate the TIBC.

Hemolytic anemias *The iron is increased (see above). Increased iron levels saturate the TIBC.*

Decreased transferrin saturation or TIBC saturation

Iron deficiency anemia
Chronic illnesses (e.g., malignancy, other chronic illnesses) *Iron levels are low, and transferrin levels are increased.*

Related Tests

- Ferritin (p. 210): This is a measure of iron stores and is the most accurate indicator of iron deficiency.

Lactic Dehydrogenase (LDH)

Normal Findings

Adult/elderly: 45-90 U/L (30° C), 115-225 IU/L, or 0.4-1.7 mmol/L (SI units)
Isoenzymes in adult/elderly
LDH-1: 17%-27%
LDH-2: 27%-37%
LDH-3: 18%-25%
LDH-4: 3%-8%
LDH-5: 0%-5%
Child: 60-170 U/L (30° C)
Infant: 100-250 U/L
Newborn: 160-450 U/L

Indications

This is an intracellular enzyme used to support the diagnosis of injury or disease involving the heart, liver, RBCs, kidneys, skeletal muscle, brain, and lungs.

Test Explanation

The enzyme LDH is found in the cells of many body tissues, especially the heart, liver, RBCs, kidneys, skeletal muscle, brain, and lungs. Because LDH is widely distributed through the body, the total LDH level is not a specific indicator of any one disease or indicative of injury to any one organ. When disease or injury affects the cells containing LDH, the cells lyse and LDH is spilled into the bloodstream where it is identified in higher than normal levels. The LDH is a measure of total LDH. Actually five separate fractions (isoenzymes) make up the total LDH. Each tissue contains a predominance of one or more LDH enzymes (Table 2-27).

The isoenzymes may be separated out by the use of electrophoresis or heat. When the blood specimen is heated to 60° C for 30 minutes, the heat-stable fractions 1 and 2 are separated out. Isoenzyme LDH-1 can also be detected by immunoassay, which is very accurate.

In general, isoenzyme LDH-1 comes mainly from the heart; LDH-2 comes primarily from the reticuloendothelial system; LDH-3 comes from the lungs and other tissues; LDH-4 comes from the kidney, placenta, and pancreas; and LDH-5 comes mainly from the liver and striated muscle. In normal persons, LDH-2 makes up the greatest percentage of total LDH.

Specific patterns of LDH isoenzymes are considered classic for certain diseases. For example:

Isolated elevation of LDH-1 (above LDH-2) indicates myocardial injury.

Isolated elevation of LDH-5 indicates hepatocellular injury or disease.

Elevation of LDH-2 and LDH-3 indicates pulmonary injury or disease.

Elevation of all LDH isoenzymes indicates multiorgan injury (e.g., myocardial infarction with congestive heart failure causing pulmonary and hepatic congestion along with decreased renal perfusion). Advanced malignancy and diffuse autoimmune inflammatory diseases such as lupus can also cause this pattern.

Table 2-27 ***LDH isoenzymes in tissue of origin***

Tissue	LDH isoenzyme
Heart	1, 2
RBC	1
Skeletal muscle	5
Lung	3, 2
Reticuloendothelial system	2
Kidney	1
Liver	5
Pancreas, placenta	4

With myocardial injury, the serum LDH level rises within 24 to 48 hours after a myocardial infarction (MI), peaks in 2 to 3 days, and returns to normal in approximately 5 to 10 days. This makes the serum LDH level especially useful for a delayed diagnosis of myocardial infarction (e.g., when the patient reports having had severe chest pain 4 days earlier). The LDH-1 level, of course, is a more sensitive and specific indicator of myocardial infarction than the total LDH level. Its sensitivity alone is over 95%. Normally the LDH-2 fraction is greater than the LDH-1 fraction. Therefore the normal LDH-1/LDH-2 ratio is less than 1. When the LDH-1 activity becomes greater than LDH-2, myocardial injury is strongly suspected. The reversal of the normal ratio is referred to as a "flipped LDH." That is, the LDH-1/LDH-2 ratio of less than 1 is reversed. In acute myocardial infarction the flipped LDH ratio usually appears in 12 to 24 hours and is present within 48 hours in approximately 80% of patients. When LDH-2 is greater than LDH-1 (a normal LDH-1/LDH-2 ratio), it is considered reliable evidence that myocardial infarction has not occurred. In the patient with chest pain due to angina only, the LDH probably will not be elevated.

It's important to note that two diseases causing elevated LDH may coexist and that one may obscure the other. For example, a patient who has one disease (e.g., pulmonary infarction or congestive heart failure) may also be having an acute myocardial infarction. The elevation in LDH-1 may be obscured by the elevation of LDH-2 or LDH-3. Some laboratories measure only the LDH-1 level by immunoassay. An elevated LDH level with greater than 40% LDH-1 is considered diagnostic of myocardial damage.

LDH is also measured in other body fluids. Elevated urine levels of total LDH indicate neoplasm or injury to the urologic system. When the LDH in an effusion (pleural, cardiac, peritoneal) is greater than 60% of the serum total LDH (i.e., effusion LDH/serum LDH ratio is greater than 0.6), the effusion is said to be an *exudate* and not a transudate.

Interfering Factors

- Hemolysis of blood will cause false-positive LDH levels since LDH exists in the RBC. Lysis of these cells causes the LDH to pour out into the specimen blood and falsely elevate the LDH level.
- Strenuous exercise may cause elevation of total LDH and specifically LDH-1, LDH-2, and LDH-5.
- Drugs that may cause *increased* LDH levels include alcohol, anesthetics, aspirin, clofibrate, fluorides, mithramycin, narcotics, and procainamide.
- Drugs that may cause *decreased* levels include ascorbic acid.

CLINICAL PRIORITIES

- Because LDH is widely distributed throughout the body, the total LDH level is not a specific indicator of any disease or organ injury. Isoenzymes are more specific and helpful diagnostically.
- When LDH-1 is greater than LDH-2, myocardial injury is strongly suspected. This may be referred to as a "flipped LDH."
- Isolated elevations of LDH-5 usually indicate hepatocellular injury or disease.
- Values vary markedly across the life span.

Procedure and Patient Care

Before

- Explain the procedure to the patient.
- Tell the patient that no fasting is required.
- Inform the patient if he or she will be receiving frequent venipuncture for the evaluation of a myocardial infarction.

During

- Collect approximately 7 to 10 ml of venous blood in a red-top tube.
- Because many diseases cause an increased LDH level, identify disease conditions on the laboratory slip.
- Record the date and time when blood was drawn on the laboratory slip for an accurate evaluation of the temporal pattern of enzyme elevations.

After

- Apply pressure or a pressure dressing to the venipuncture site.
- Assess the venipuncture site for bleeding.

Test Results and Clinical Significance

Increased levels

Myocardial infarction *These patients classically have significant elevations in LDH-1 and, to a lesser degree, LDH-2.*

Pulmonary disease (e.g., embolism, infarction, pneumonia, congestive heart failure) *These patients classically have significant elevations in LDH-2 and LDH-3.*

Hepatic disease (e.g., hepatitis, active cirrhosis, neoplasm) *These patients classically have significant elevations in LDH-5.*

RBC disease (e.g., hemolytic or megaloblastic anemia, RBC destruction from prosthetic heart valves) *These patients classically have significant elevations in LDH-1.*

Skeletal muscle disease and injury (e.g., muscular dystrophy, recent strenuous exercises, muscular trauma) *These patients classically have significant elevations in LDH-5.*

Renal parenchymal disease (e.g., infarction, glomerulonephritis, acute tubular necrosis, kidney transplantation rejection) *These patients classically have significant elevations in LDH-1.*

Intestinal ischemia and infarction *These patients classically have significant elevations in LDH-5.*

Neoplastic states

Testicular tumors (seminoma, dysgerminomas) *These patients classically have significant elevations in LDH-1.*

Lymphoma and other reticuloendothelial system (RES) tumors *These patients classically have significant elevations in LDH-3 and LDH-2.*

Advanced solid tumor malignancies *These patients classically have significant elevations in all LDH isoenzymes.*

Pancreatitis *These patients classically have significant elevations in LDH-4.*

Diffuse disease or injury (e.g., heat stroke, collagen disease, shock, hypotension) *These patients classically have significant elevations in all LDH isoenzymes.*

Related Tests

- Aspartate aminotransferase (AST) (p. 105): This is another enzyme predominantly existing in the liver.
- Gamma-glutamyl transpeptidase (GGTP) (p. 219): This is another enzyme predominantly existing in the liver.
- Alkaline phosphatase (p. 42): This is another enzyme predominantly existing in the liver.
- 5′-Nucleotidase- (p. 312): This is another enzyme predominantly existing in the liver.
- Creatine phosphokinase (CPK) (p. 173): This enzyme is used predominantly to evaluate heart and skeletal muscle.
- Alanine aminotransferase (ALT) (p. 33): This enzyme is used similarly to aspartate aminotransferase and exists predominantly in the liver.
- Leucine aminopeptidase (LAP) (p. 286): This enzyme is specific to the hepatobiliary system. Diseases affecting that system will cause elevation of this enzyme.

Lactose Tolerance

Normal Findings

Blood

Adult/elderly: rise in plasma glucose levels >20 mg/dl; no abdominal cramps or diarrhea

Breath

<50 ppm hydrogen increase over baseline

Indications

This test is used to identify patients who have lactose intolerance because of lactase insufficiency. This test is performed on adults who complain of diarrhea and in infants who have failure to thrive, persistent diarrhea, or vomiting.

Test Explanation

This test is performed to detect lactose intolerance. Lactose is a disaccharide typically found in dairy products; during digestion, lactose is broken down into glucose and galactose by the intestinal enzyme lactase. Because lactose-intolerant patients have an absence of lactase, lactose digestion will not occur. Thus the small bowel is flooded with a high lactose load. Bacterial metabolism of the lactose occurs within the intestine. This creates excess hydrogen ions and methane (flatus). It also has a strong cathartic effect. Symptoms of lactose intolerance include abdominal cramping, flatus, abdominal bloating, and diarrhea.

Although all adults have some degree of lactase reduction, severe lactose intolerance can occur in patients with inflammatory bowel disease, short-gut syndrome, and other malabsorption syndromes. Lactase deficiency can be congenital and become apparent in the newborn. These infants present with vomiting, diarrhea, malabsorption, and failure to thrive.

In this test a lactose load is given. If lactase is not present in sufficient quantities, lactose is not metabolized to glucose and galactose. Plasma levels of glucose do not rise as expected. Therefore lower-than-expected serum glucose levels suggest intestinal lactase deficiency. Patients who have malabsorption without lactase deficiency will also fail to elevate the blood glucose levels, not because the lactose was not broken down but because the glucose could not be absorbed. These patients can be excluded by following the lactose tolerance test with a glucose tolerance test. That is, after a positive lactose tolerance test, the patient returns and is given 25 g of a glucose/galactose preparation. A normal increase in glucose indicates that the patient can absorb glucose and that the problem is, indeed, lactase insufficiency.

There is also a breath test portion to this test in which the exhaled air is analyzed for hydrogen content. The hydrogen content is directly proportional to the amount of lactose not broken down and absorbed.

Age-related concerns

- This test can identify patients with lactose intolerance due to lactase deficiency.
- Lactase deficiency may be the cause of vomiting, diarrhea, malabsorption, and failure to thrive in *infants.*
- Although all *adults* have some degree of lactase reduction, severe lactose intolerance can occur in patients with inflammatory bowel diseases, short-gut syndrome, and other malabsorption syndromes.

Interfering Factors

- Enterogenous steatorrhea (i.e., malabsorption) will diminish absorption of glucose from the gut even if the lactose is broken down by normal levels of lactase.
- Strenuous exercise will reduce the glucose levels and possibly give a falsely positive test.
- Diabetics may have glucose levels that exceed 20 mg/dl despite lactase insufficiency.
- Smoking may increase blood glucose levels and cause false-positive results.

Procedure and Patient Care

Before

- Explain the procedure to the patient. Inform the patient that four blood samples will be needed.
- Instruct the patient to fast 8 hours before testing.
- Instruct the patient to avoid strenuous exercise for 8 hours before testing. This may factitiously affect the blood glucose level.
- Inform the patient that smoking is prohibited before testing. This may falsely increase the blood glucose level.

During

- Obtain 5 to 7 ml of venous blood in a gray-top tube from the fasting patient.
- Provide a specified dose of lactose for the patient. Usually 100 g of lactose is diluted with 200 ml of water for ingestion in adults.
- Note that pediatric doses of lactose are based on weight.
- Collect three more blood samples at 30, 60, and 120 minutes after the ingestion of lactose.
- Tell the patient that the only discomfort is the venipuncture; however, patients with lactase deficiency will have the symptoms previously described.
- If the breath test is being done, the exhaled air is evaluated for hydrogen content 30, 60, and 120 minutes after the ingestion of lactose.

After

- Apply pressure or a pressure dressing to the venipuncture site.
- Observe the venipuncture site for bleeding.
- Note that patients with abnormal test results may require a monosaccharide tolerance test (e.g., glucose or galactose tolerance test).

Test Results and Clinical Significance

Decreased levels

Lactase insufficiency *Lactase quantities are insufficient to break down the lactose load. Glucose is not absorbed, and serum glucose levels do not rise.*

Enterogenous diarrhea *Despite normal breakdown of lactose, the glucose is not absorbed because of malabsorption disease of the gut. Serum glucose levels do not rise.*

Related Test

- Glucose tolerance (p. 233): This test is used to assist in the diagnosis of diabetes mellitus. It is also used in the evaluation of patients with hypoglycemia. Since it differentiates the lactase-deficient patient from the patient with enterogenous malabsorption diarrhea, this test is helpful in the evaluation of patients suspected of having lactose intolerance.

Legionnaires' Disease Antibody

Normal Findings

No *Legionella* antibody titer

Indications

This test is indicated in patients suspected to have legionnaires' disease and who have negative cultures and smears identifying *Legionella.*

Test Explanation

Legionnaires' disease was originally described as a fulminating pneumonia caused by *Legionella pneumophila,* a tiny gram-negative, rod-shaped bacterium. Nearly half of the clinical cases have been caused by serogroup type 1. This organism can also cause an influenza type of illness called "Pontiac fever."

The diagnosis of legionnaires' disease can be made by culturing this organism from suspected infected fluid, such as blood, sputum, lung tissue, or pleural fluid. Sputum for this test is best obtained by transtracheal aspiration or from bronchial washings. However, growing this organism in culture is difficult. A negative culture does not mean that the patient does not have legionnaires' disease. Another method of diagnosis is by directly identifying the organism in a microscopic smear of infected fluid with the use of direct fluorescent antibody methods. If positive, this allows for rapid identification of *Legionella.* However, this is difficult also because the concentration may not be high enough to see the bacterium in the specimen.

The most common and easiest method for diagnosis is detection of the antibody directed against the legionnaires' bacterium in the patient's blood. This is done if the culture or direct fluorescent tests are negative. The indirect fluorescent antibody assay or enzyme-linked immunosorbent assay (ELISA) methods are commonly used. A presumptive diagnosis of legionnaires' disease can be made in a symptomatic person when a single antibody titer is 1:256 or greater. Another way to make the diagnosis is to perform the antibody test 1 and 3 weeks after the onset of symptoms. A fourfold rise in titer to at least 1:128 between the acute (1 week) and the convalescent (3 week) phases is diagnostic. Unfortunately it may take 4 to 6 weeks for serologic tests to be positive. The patient would be seriously ill by then. *Legionella* antigens in the urine may be identified a few days after the onset of the clinical symptoms. Unfortunately the sensitivity is very low (about 30%).

Procedure and Patient Care

Before

- Explain the procedure to the patient.
- Tell the patient that no fasting is required.

During

- Collect approximately 5 to 7 ml of blood in a red-top tube.

After

- Apply pressure or a pressure dressing to the venipuncture site.
- Observe the venipuncture site for bleeding.

Test Results and Clinical Significance

Increased levels

Legionnaires' disease

Leucine Aminopeptidase
(LAP, Aminopeptidase Cytosol)

Normal Findings

Blood
Male: 80-200 U/ml
Female: 75-185 U/ml
Urine: 2-18 U/24 hr

Indications

This test is used for diagnosing liver disorders. It aids in the differential diagnosis of patients with high levels of alkaline phosphatase.

Test Explanation

LAP is an intracellular enzyme that exists in the hepatobiliary system and, to a much smaller degree, in the pancreas and the small intestine. When disease or injury affects those organs, the cells lyse and LAP is spilled out into the bloodstream. Produced almost exclusively by the liver, LAP is used in diagnosing liver disorders and in the differential diagnosis of increased levels of alkaline phosphatase (ALP). LAP levels tend to parallel ALP levels in hepatic disease. LAP is a sensitive indicator of cholestasis; however, unlike ALP, LAP remains normal in bone disease. LAP can be detected in both the blood and the urine. Patients with elevated serum LAP levels will always show elevations in urine levels. When the urine LAP level is elevated, however, the blood level may have already returned to normal.

This enzyme was originally thought to be elevated during pregnancy and thus serve as an indication of the viability of the fetal-placental unit. However, it has been found that the enzyme found in pregnancy is immunochemically different from LAP.

Interfering Factors

- Pregnancy may cause increased values if tested by the enzyme method. Although there is not a quantitative increase in this "LAP-like" enzyme, its activity is increased. This causes a false increase in the LAP if tested by the enzyme method.
- Drugs that may cause *increased* LAP levels include estrogens and progesterones.

Procedure and Patient Care

Before

- Explain the procedure to the patient.
- Tell the patient that no fasting is required.

During

- Collect approximately 7 to 10 ml of venous blood in a red-top tube.
- If a urine sample is needed, follow the procedure for a 24-hour urine collection (see p. 815).

- Indicate on the laboratory slip any medications the patient is taking that may affect test results.

After

- Apply pressure or a pressure dressing to the venipuncture site.
- Assess the venipuncture site for bleeding. Patients with liver dysfunction often have prolonged clotting times.

Test Results and Clinical Significance

Increased levels

Hepatobiliary disease (e.g., hepatitis, cirrhosis, hepatic necrosis, hepatic ischemia, hepatic tumor, hepatotoxic drugs, cholestasis, gallstones) *LAP is an enzyme that exists in the liver and biliary cells. Disease or injury of these tissues will cause the cells to lyse. LAP will spill out into the bloodstream, and levels will rise.*

Related Tests

- Creatine phosphokinase (CPK) (p. 173): This enzyme is used similarly to aspartate aminotransferase (AST) and exists predominantly in heart and skeletal muscle.
- Alanine aminotransferase (ALT) (p. 33): This enzyme is used similarly to AST and exists predominantly in the liver.
- Lactic dehydrogenase (LDH) (p. 278): This is an intracellular enzyme used to support the diagnosis of injury or disease involving the heart, liver, RBCs, kidneys, skeletal muscle, brain, and lungs.
- Aspartate aminotransferase (AST) (p. 105): This is another enzyme predominantly existing in the liver.
- Gamma-glutamyl transpeptidase (GGTP) (p. 219): This is another enzyme predominantly existing in the liver.
- Alkaline phosphatase (p. 42): This is another enzyme predominantly existing in the liver.
- 5′-Nucleotidase- (p. 312): This is another enzyme predominantly existing in the liver.

Lipase

Normal Findings

0-110 U/L or 0-417 U/L (SI units) (values are method dependent)

Indications This test is used in the evaluation of pancreatic disease.

Test Explanation

The most common cause of an elevated serum lipase level is acute pancreatitis. Lipase is an enzyme secreted by the pancreas into the duodenum to break down triglycerides into fatty acids. As with amylase, lipase appears in the bloodstream following damage to or disease affecting the pancreatic acinar cells.

Because lipase was thought to be produced only in the pancreas, elevated serum levels were considered to be specific to pathologic pancreatic conditions. It is now apparent that other conditions can be associated with elevated lipase levels. Lipase is excreted through the kidneys. Therefore elevated lipase levels are often found in patients with renal failure. Intestinal infarction or obstruction also can be associated with lipase elevation. However, the lipase elevations in nonpancreatic diseases are less than three times the upper limit of normal as compared with pancreatitis, where they are often 5 to 10 times normal values. Still other conditions such as cholangitis, mumps, cholecystitis, or peptic ulcer are more rarely associated with elevated lipase levels.

In acute pancreatitis, elevated lipase levels usually parallel serum amylase levels. The lipase levels usually rise a little later than amylase (24 to 48 hours after the onset of pancreatitis) and remain elevated for 5 to 7 days. Because they peak later and remain elevated longer than the serum amylase levels, serum lipase levels are more useful in the late diagnosis of acute pancreatitis. Lipase levels are less useful in more chronic pancreatic diseases (e.g., chronic pancreatitis, pancreatic carcinoma).

Interfering Factors

- Drugs that may cause *increased* lipase levels include bethanechol, cholinergics, codeine, indomethacin, meperidine, methacholine, and morphine.
- Drugs that may cause *decreased* levels include calcium ions.

✓ CLINICAL PRIORITIES

- This test is useful in evaluating pancreatitis. Lipase elevations are often 5 to 10 times normal values in pancreatitis.
- In acute pancreatitis, elevated lipase levels usually parallel serum amylase levels. Because lipase levels peak later and remain elevated longer than amylase levels, they are more useful in the late diagnosis of acute pancreatitis.

Procedure and Patient Care

Before

- Explain the procedure to the patient.
- Instruct the patient to remain on NPO status, except for water, for 8 to 12 hours before the test.

During

- Collect 5 to 7 ml of venous blood in a red-top tube.
- Indicate on the laboratory slip drugs that may affect test results.

After

- Apply pressure or a pressure dressing to the venipuncture site.
- Observe the venipuncture site for bleeding.

Test Results and Clinical Significance

Increased levels

Pancreatic diseases (e.g., acute pancreatitis, chronic relapsing pancreatitis, pancreatic cancer, pancreatic pseudocyst) *Lipase exists in the pancreatic cell and is released into the bloodstream when disease or injury affects the pancreas.*

Biliary diseases (e.g., acute cholecystitis, cholangitis, extrahepatic duct obstruction) *Although the pathophysiology of these observations is not well known, it is suspected that lipase exists inside the cells of the hepatobiliary system. Disease or injury of these tissues would cause the lipase to leak into the bloodstream and cause levels to be elevated.*

Renal failure *Lipase is excreted by the kidney. If excretion is poor, as in renal failure, lipase levels will rise.*

Intestinal diseases (e.g., bowel obstruction, infarction) *Lipase exists in the mucosal cells lining the bowel (mostly in the duodenum). Injury through obstruction or ischemia will cause the cells to lyse. Lipase will leak into the bloodstream and cause levels to be elevated.*

Salivary gland inflammation or tumor *Like amylase, salivary glands contain lipase, although to a much smaller degree. Tumors, inflammation, or obstruction of salivary ducts will cause the cells to lyse. Lipase will leak into the bloodstream and cause levels to be elevated.*

Peptic ulcer disease *The pathophysiology of this observation is not well understood. Certainly, in perforated peptic disease the lipase in the GI contents leaks out into the peritoneum, where it is picked up by the bloodstream. Lipase levels rise.*

Related Test

- Amylase (p. 51): This is also an enzyme produced specifically in the pancreas. Disease affecting the pancreas also will cause elevations of this enzyme.

Lipoprotein (High-Density Lipoprotein [HDL], Low-Density Lipoprotein [LDL], Very-Low-Density Lipoprotein [VLDL])

Normal Findings

HDL

Male: >45 mg/dl or >0.75 mmol/L (SI units)

Female: >55 mg/dl or >0.91 mmol/L (SI units)

	HDL mg/dl (SI Units)	
Risk of Heart Disease	**Male**	**Female**
Low	60 (1.55)	70 (1.81)
Moderate	45 (1.17)	55 (1.42)
High	25 (0.65)	35 (0.90)

LDL: 60-180 mg/dl or <3.37 mmol/L (SI units)

VLDL: 25%-50%

Indications

Lipoproteins are considered to be an accurate predictor of heart disease. As part of the lipid profile, these tests are performed to indicate persons at risk for developing heart disease and to monitor therapy if abnormalities are found.

Test Explanation

Lipoproteins are proteins in the blood whose main purpose is to transport cholesterol, triglycerides, and other insoluble fats. They are used as markers indicating the levels of lipids within the bloodstream. With the use of electrophoresis, these lipoproteins can be grouped into:

Chylomicrons, which are primarily triglycerides
LDLs (beta lipoproteins), which are primarily cholesterol
VLDLs (prebeta lipoproteins), which are mainly triglycerides
HDLs (alpha lipoproteins), which are predominantly protein with a small amount of cholesterol

Lipids and cholesterol are used in the synthesis of sterol hormones (adrenal and gonadal). They are an important part of the structure of cellular membranes. Cholesterol is an integral part of bile. The lipid profile usually measures total cholesterol, triglycerides, HDL, LDL, and VLDL.

HDLs are carriers of cholesterol. They are produced in the liver and, to a smaller degree, in the intestines. The purpose of HDLs is believed to be removal of the cholesterol from the peripheral tissues and transport to the liver for excretion. Also, HDLs may have a protective effect by preventing cellular uptake of cholesterol and lipids. These potential actions may be the source of the protective cardiovascular characteristics associated with HDLs (*good cholesterol*) within the blood. Both HDL and total cholesterol are independent variables of risk of coronary heart disease (CHD). When combined in a ratio fashion, the accuracy of prediction is increased. The total cholesterol/HDL ratio should be at least 5:1, with 3:1 being ideal (Table 2-28).

LDLs are also cholesterol rich. Cholesterol carried by LDLs can be deposited into the peripheral tissues and is associated with an increased risk of arteriosclerotic heart and peripheral vascular disease. Therefore high levels of LDL (*bad cholesterol*) are atherogenic. The LDL level should be less than 160 mg/dl in persons with coronary artery disease and less than 180 mg/dl in those without disease (Table 2-29). LDL is very difficult to isolate

Table 2-28 Risk of CHD based on ratio of cholesterol to HDL

	Total cholesterol/HDL	
Risk of CHD	Male	Female
One half average	3.4	3.3
Average	5.0	4.4
Two times average (moderate)	10.0	7.0
Three times average (high)	24.0	11.0

Table 2-29 National Cholesterol Education Program Therapy Guidelines for LDL

Treatment	Risk factors present*	Initial level	Treatment goal
Dietary	No	>160	<160
Dietary	Yes	>130	<130
Drug†	No	>190	<160
Drug†	Yes	>160	<130

*Two or more risk factors, such as male sex, family history of premature CHD, smoking, hypertension, low HDL/cholesterol ratio, diabetes, cerebral or peripheral vascular disease, obesity.
†Cholesterol-lowering agents (such as Zocor, Mevacor)

and measure. Therefore the LDL is most usually derived by the Friedwald formula. In this formula, LDL is derived by subtracting the HDL plus one fifth of the triglycerides from the total cholesterol.

$$\text{LDL} = \text{Total cholesterol} - (\text{HDL} + \text{Triglycerides}/5)$$

There are other formulas for deriving LDL, which may account for different sets of normal values. The disadvantage of using any formula in determining LDL is that the end result is based on the accuracy of the testing for the components used to calculate the formula. Furthermore, the formula is inaccurate if the triglycerides exceed 400 mg/100 ml.

VLDLs, although carrying a small amount of cholesterol, are the predominant carriers of blood triglycerides. To a lesser degree, VLDLs are also associated with an increased risk of arteriosclerotic occlusive disease. The VLDL value is usually expressed as a percentage of total cholesterol. Levels in excess of 25% to 50% are associated with increased risk of coronary disease.

The HDL, LDL, and VLDL levels are a part of the lipid profile test that also evaluates cholesterol and triglycerides. The lipoprotein test is used to assess the risk of coronary artery disease. High levels of the "protective" HDL are associated with a decreased risk of coronary disease, whereas high levels of LDL and VLDL are associated with an increased risk of coronary occlusive disease.

To a large degree, levels of lipoproteins may be genetically determined. Levels of HDL can be increased in persons who engage in frequent physical activity or who use moderate doses of alcohol. On the other hand, LDL and VLDL are known to be increased in persons who have poor dietary habits associated with an increased intake of animal fats and snack foods. Genetic makeup, however, is probably the most important determinant of lipoprotein level.

Interfering Factors

- Smoking and alcohol ingestion decrease HDL levels.
- Binge eating can alter lipoprotein values.
- HDL values are age and sex dependent.
- HDL values, like cholesterol, tend to decrease significantly for as long as 3 months following myocardial infarction.

- HDL is elevated in hypothyroid patients and diminished in hyperthyroid patients.
- Drugs that may cause *increased* lipoprotein levels include aspirin, oral contraceptives, phenothiazines, steroids, thiazides, some beta blockers, and sulfonamides.

CLINICAL PRIORITIES

- Lipoproteins are considered to be predictors of heart disease. Blood levels should be collected after a 12 to 14-hour fast.
- HDL is often called *good cholesterol,* because it removes cholesterol from the tissues and transports it to the liver for excretion. High levels are associated with a decreased risk of coronary heart disease.
- LDL is often called *bad cholesterol,* because it carries cholesterol and deposits it into the peripheral tissues. High levels are associated with an increased risk of CHD.

Procedure and Patient Care

Before

- Instruct the patient to fast for 12 to 14 hours before testing. Only water is permitted.
- Inform the patient that dietary indiscretion within the previous few weeks may influence lipoprotein levels.

During

- Collect 5 to 10 ml of venous blood in a red-top tube.
- Indicate on the laboratory slip any drugs that may affect test results.

After

- Apply pressure or a pressure dressing to the venipuncture site.
- Observe the venipuncture site for bleeding.
- Instruct patients with high lipoprotein levels regarding diet, exercise, and appropriate body weight.

Test Results and Clinical Significance

Increased HDL

Familial HDL lipoproteinemia *Genetically, the patient is predetermined to have high HDL levels.*

Excessive exercise *HDL can rise with chronic exercise for 30 minutes three times a week. When the exercise greatly exceeds that minimum, HDL can become significantly elevated.*

Decreased HDL

Familial low HDL *Genetically, the patient is predetermined to have low HDL levels. As a result, these patients are at high risk for CHD.*

Hepatocellular disease (e.g., hepatitis, cirrhosis) *HDL is made in the liver. Without liver function, HDL is not made and levels fall.*

Hypoproteinemia (e.g., nephrotic syndrome, malnutrition) *With loss of proteins, HDL is not made and levels fall. When the hypoproteinemia is severe, however, and oncotic pressures fall, the production of lipoproteins could be stimulated and actually rise. Elevation of HDL, however, only occurs late in the disease.*

Increased LDL and VLDL

Familiar LDL lipoproteinemia *Genetically, the patient is predetermined to have high LDL levels.*

Nephrotic syndrome *The loss of proteins diminishes the plasma oncotic pressures. This appears to stimulate hepatic lipoprotein synthesis of LDL and possibly to diminish lipoprotein disposal of the same.*

Glycogen storage diseases (e.g., von Gierke's disease) *VLDL synthesis is increased and excretion is diminished. VLDL and LDL levels rise.*

Hypothyroidism *VLDL and LDL catabolism is diminished. VLDL and LDL levels rise.*

Alcohol consumption *Hyperlipidemias are known to occur in persons who drink excessive quantities of alcohol. However, there also may be a genetic factor associated with this observation.*

Chronic liver disease (e.g., hepatitis, cirrhosis) *The liver metabolizes LDL. Without that catabolism, blood levels increase.*

Hepatoma *The normal inhibition of LDL synthesis by eating dietary fats does not occur. LDL synthesis continues unabated. LDL levels rise.*

Gammopathies (e.g., multiple myeloma) *High levels of gamma globulins (IgG and IgM) attach to the VLDL and LDL molecule and thereby decrease their catabolism.*

Familial hypercholesterolemia type IIa *LDL receptors are altered, and LDL is produced at increased rates.*

Cushing's syndrome *VLDL synthesis is increased. VLDL is converted to LDL.*

Apoprotein CII deficiency *This genetic defect is associated with a deficiency of lipoprotein lipase. As a result, VLDL and other lipoproteins (chylomicrons) accumulate.*

Decreased LDL and VLDL

Familial hypolipoproteinemia *Genetically, the patient is predetermined to have low VLDL or LDL levels.*

Hypoproteinemia (e.g., malabsorption, severe burns, malnutrition) *Early in the course of this process, LDLs are low. However, later the LDL and VLDL levels can actually rise.*

Hyperthyroidism *Catabolism of LDL and VLDL is increased and levels fall.*

Related Tests

- Cholesterol (p. 143): This is a measure of total cholesterol in the blood. It is a part of the lipid profile.
- Triglyceride (p. 432): This is a measure of total triglyceride in the blood. It is a part of the lipid profile.

Long-Acting Thyroid Stimulator
(LATS, Thyroid-Stimulating Immunoglobulin [TSIG])

Normal Findings
Negative

Indications

LATS and other thyroid-stimulating immunoglobulins are used to support the diagnosis of Graves' disease, especially when the diagnosis is complex.

Test Explanation

The LATS antibody is an IgG immunoglobulin directed against the thyroid cell plasma membrane. LATS initially was thought to mimic the action of thyroid-stimulating hormone (TSH). LATS has recently been found to be a part of a group of IgG antibodies directed against the thyroid cell membrane. These immunoglobulins are all associated with Graves' disease and in some cases with Hashimoto's thyroiditis. They are helpful in the evaluation of patients in whom the diagnosis of Graves' disease is complicated by borderline data or conflicting data needed to support the diagnosis. Other components of this system include *thyroid-stimulating immunoglobulin (TSI)* and *TSH-binding inhibiting immunoglobulin (TBII).*

Like TSI and TBII, LATS can be found in 75% of patients with Graves' disease. It also can be found in some patients with Hashimoto's thyroiditis and hyperparathyroidism. LATS is found most frequently in patients with Graves' disease associated with exophthalmos and/or pretibial edema. Its effect on the thyroid is long lasting, and titers do not decrease until nearly 1 year after successful treatment of the thyroid disease. Because LATS crosses the placenta, it may be found in neonates whose mothers have Graves' disease.

Interfering Factors

- Recent administration of radioactive iodine may affect test results.

Procedure and Patient Care

Before

- Explain the procedure to the patient.
- Tell the patient that no fasting or special preparation is required.

During

- Collect approximately 5 ml of venous blood in a red-top tube.
- Notify the laboratory if the patient has received radioactive iodine in the preceding 2 days.
- Handle the blood sample gently. Hemolysis may interfere with interpretation of test results.

After

- Apply pressure or a pressure dressing to the venipuncture site.
- Observe the venipuncture site for bleeding.

Test Results and Clinical Significance

Increased levels

Hyperthyroidism
Malignant exophthalmos
Graves' disease
All of the thyroid-stimulating IgG immunoglobulins are elevated in these diseases.

Related Tests

- Triiodothyronine uptake (p. 438): This test is an indirect measurement of total T_4.
- Thyrotropin-releasing hormone (p. 415): This test assists in the evaluation of patients with hyper- and hypothyroidism. It is especially helpful in the differential diagnosis of hypothyroidism.
- Thyroid-stimulating hormone (p. 410): This test is used to diagnose primary hypothyroidism and to differentiate it from secondary (pituitary) and tertiary (hypothalamus) hypothyroidism.
- Thyroid-stimulating hormone (TSH) stimulation (p. 413): This test is also used to differentiate primary and secondary (and tertiary) hypothyroidism.
- Thyroid-binding globulin (p. 421): This is a measure of thyroid-binding globulin (TBG), the major thyroid hormone protein carrier. It is used in the evaluation of patients who have abnormal total T_4 and T_3 levels. When done concurrently with a T_4/T_3 test, one can more easily interpret the T_4 and T_3 levels.
- Thyroxine (p. 417): This is one of the first tests done in assessing thyroid function. It is used to diagnose thyroid function and to monitor replacement and suppressive therapy.
- Triiodothyronine (p. 435): T_3 is used to evaluate thyroid function. It is mostly used to diagnose hyperthyroidism. It is also used to monitor thyroid replacement and suppressive medical therapy.
- Thyroxine index, free (p. 426): This test is used to evaluate thyroid function. It corrects for changes in thyroid hormone–binding serum proteins that can affect total T_4 levels. It is used to diagnose hyper- and hypothyroidism.
- Thyroxine, free (p. 423): The FT_4 is used to evaluate thyroid function in patients who may have protein abnormalities that could affect total T_4 levels. It is used to diagnose thyroid function and to monitor replacement and suppressive therapy.
- Antithyroglobulin antibody (p. 89): This test is primarily used in the differential diagnosis of thyroid diseases such as Hashimoto's thyroiditis and chronic lymphocytic thyroiditis (in children).

Luteinizing Hormone Assay (LH Assay, Lutropin) and **Follicle-Stimulating Hormone** (FSH)

Normal Findings

Values may vary depending on assay method.

	LH (IU/L)	FSH (IU/L)
Adult		
Male	1.24-7.8	1.42-15.4
Female		
Follicular phase	1.68-15	1.37-9.9
Ovulatory peak	21.9-56.6	6.17-17.2
Luteal phase	0.61-16.3	1.09-9.2
Postmenopause	14.2-52.3	19.3-100.6
Child (age 1-10 years)		
Male	0.04-3.6	0.3-4.6
Female	0.03-3.9	0.68-6.7

Indications

LH/FSH levels are helpful in the determination of menopause. Furthermore, they are integral in the evaluation of suspected gonadal failure. Infertility evaluations must also include these tests.

Test Explanation

LH and FSH are glycoproteins produced in the anterior pituitary gland in response to stimulation by gonadotropin-releasing hormone (GNRH), previously called luteinizing-releasing hormone. GNRH is stimulated when circulating levels of estrogen (in females) or testosterone (in males) are low. Through a feedback mechanism, GNRH is stimulated by the hypothalamus, which in turn stimulates the production and release of LH and FSH. These two hormones then act on the ovary or testes. In the female, FSH stimulates the development of follicles in the ovary. In the male, FSH stimulates Sertoli cell development. In the female, LH stimulates follicular production of estrogen, ovulation, and formation of a corpus luteum. In the male, LH stimulates testosterone production from the Leydig cells. In the end, estrogen or testosterone is produced, which in turn inhibits FSH and LH. FSH is necessary for maturation of the ovaries and testes. FSH and LH are necessary for sperm production. In the female these hormones are secreted differently at different times in the menses cycle. The midcycle peak of FSH is necessary for follicle/ovum formation. LH also must peak about that same time to stimulate ovulation or corpus luteal formation that could potentially support an embryo if fertilization were to occur.

Earlier bioassays could not distinguish FSH from LH. Therefore they were often measured together. For that matter, early bioassays often included thyroid-stimulating hormone and human chorionic gonadotropin in the assay. Now, with the use of monoclonal antibodies and better immunoassays, these hormones can each be measured separately and accurately.

LH is secreted in a pulsatile manner. One specimen may not accurately indicate total body levels of this hormone. Often several specimens of blood are obtained 20 to 30 minutes apart, and the blood is pooled or results of each are averaged. The variable nature of LH can be diminished by measuring LH in a 24-hour urine sample. The disadvantage is that LH values can be falsely low because of dilution with large urine volumes. Spot urine tests have become very useful in the evaluation and treatment of infertility. Because LH is rapidly excreted into the urine, the plasma LH surge that precedes ovulation by 24 hours can be recognized quickly and easily. This is used to indicate the period when the women is most fertile. The best time to obtain a urine specimen is between 11 AM and 3 PM. Usually the woman begins to test her urine on the day following her menses and continues to do so daily. Home kits using a color change as an end point are now marketed to make this process even more convenient.

These hormones are used in the evaluation of infertility. Performing an LH assay is an easy way to determine if ovulation has occurred. An LH surge in blood levels indicates that ovulation has taken place. Under the influence of LH, the corpus luteum develops from the ruptured graafian follicle. Daily samples of serum LH around the woman's midcycle can detect the LH surge, which is believed to occur on the day of maximal fertility.

These assays also determine whether a gonadal insufficiency is primary (problem with the ovary/testicle) or secondary (caused by pituitary insufficiency resulting in reduced levels of FSH and LH). Elevated levels of FSH and LH in patients with gonadal insufficiency indicate primary gonadal failure, as may be seen in women with polycystic ovaries or during menopause. In secondary gonadal failure, LH and FSH levels are low as a result of pituitary failure or some other pituitary-hypothalamic impairment, stress, malnutrition, or physiologic delay in growth and sexual development.

FSH and LH assays are often done to diagnose menopause so that hormone replacement therapy can be instituted as soon as possible. LH hormones are also used to study testicular dysfunction in men and to evaluate endocrine problems related to precocious puberty in children. The use of these hormone assays can also help in the evaluation of disorders of sexual differentiation, such as Klinefelter's syndrome.

✓ CLINICAL PRIORITIES

- Levels of FSH and LH vary in the female patient according to phases in the menstrual cycle.
- These hormones are valuable in the evaluation of infertility. Daily samples of LH around a woman's midcycle can detect the LH surge, which is believed to occur on the day of maximum fertility.
- Spot urine tests have become useful in evaluating and treating infertility. Home test kits are now available for detecting LH in the urine.
- FSH and LH assays are often performed to diagnose menopause so hormone replacement can be started.

Interfering Factors

- Recent use of radioisotopes may affect test results if the testing method is performed by radioimmunoassay. The previously administered radioisotope may interfere with the results
- Human chorionic gonadotropin (HCG) and thyroid-stimulating hormone (TSH) may interfere with some immunoassay methods because of the similarities of part of the

hormone molecule. Therefore patients with HCG-producing tumors and hypothyroid patients should be expected to have falsely high LH levels.

- Drugs that may *increase* LH or FSH levels include cimetidine, digitalis, levodopa, anticonvulsants, clomiphene, naloxone, and spironolactone.
- Drugs that may *decrease* LH levels include estrogens, progesterones, testosterone, steroids, digoxin, oral contraceptives, and phenothiazines.

Procedure and Patient Care

Before

- Explain the procedure to the patient.
- Tell the patient that no food or fluid restrictions are needed.

During

Blood

- Collect approximately 7 to 10 ml of venous blood in a red-top tube.
- Indicate the date of the last menstrual period on the laboratory slip. Note if the woman is postmenopausal.

Urine

- Collect a 24-hour specimen, which may contain a preservative.
- Keep the specimen refrigerated during the collection period.
- Note that the patient may also perform LH assays at home using a home urine test or a 24-hour urine test.
- If a spot urine test is performed, follow the directions accompanying the kit.

After

- Apply pressure or a pressure dressing to the venipuncture site.
- Assess the venipuncture site for bleeding.

Test Results and Clinical Significance

Increased levels

Gonadal failure (e.g., physiologic menopause, ovarian dysgenesis [Turner's syndrome], testicular dysgenesis [Klinefelter's syndrome], castration, anorchia, hypogonadism, polycystic ovaries, complete testicular feminization syndrome) *Decreased levels of estrogen or testosterone occur with gonadal failure. Through a feedback mechanism, FSH and LH secretion is stimulated maximally.*

Precocious puberty *One cause of precocious puberty is oversecretion of FSH and LH.*

Pituitary adenoma *Some pituitary adenomas secrete FSH or LH without regard to any feedback mechanism.*

Decreased levels

Pituitary failure *FSH and LH are produced in the anterior pituitary. The first indication of pituitary failure is reduction of FSH/LH and the resulting gonadal failure.*

Hypothalamic failure *GNRH is produced in the hypothalamus and stimulates FSH/LH pro-*

duction. Failure of that portion of the brain to produce GNRH will cause reduced FSH/LH levels.

Stress
Anorexia nervosa
Malnutrition
The pathophysiology of these observations is not clear.

Lyme Disease

Normal Findings Negative (low titers of IgM and IgG antibodies)

Indications This test is used to diagnose Lyme disease.

Test Explanation

Lyme disease was first recognized in Lyme, Connecticut, in 1975. It is caused by a spirochete called *Borrelia burgdorferi*. The disease usually begins in the summer with a skin lesion called erythema chronicum migrans (ECM), which occurs at the site of a bite by a deer tick, usually *Ixodes dammini* or *pacificus*. Ticks are the best documented vectors of this spirochete, which is the causative agent for Lyme disease.

Weeks to months after the insect bite, some patients develop fatigue, meningoencephalitis, cranial or peripheral neuropathies, myocarditis, atrioventricular nodal block, or arthritis. The last manifestation is joint involvement, which often occurs intermittently in a few large joints for several years.

Cultures of the ECM can isolate the spirochete in half of the cases. However, it is difficult to culture and takes a long time to grow. Cultures of the blood or CSF are even less helpful. Currently serologic studies are the most sensitive and specific tests for the detection of Lyme disease. Enzyme-linked immunosorbent assay (ELISA) is the best diagnostic test for Lyme disease. This test determines titers of specific IgM and specific IgG antibodies to the *B. burgdorferi* spirochete. Levels of specific IgM antibody peak during the third to sixth week after disease onset and then gradually decline.

Titers of specific IgG antibodies are generally low during the first several weeks of illness, reach maximal levels 4 to 6 months later during arthritis attacks, and often remain elevated for years. Early in the illness the diagnosis usually can be determined from the gross appearance of ECM and known exposure to an endemic area (woods with large populations of deer). These patients do not require antibody determination. In the absence of ECM lesions, however, Lyme disease can be confused with various viral infections. In these patients a single titer of specific IgM antibody may suggest the correct diagnosis. Acute and convalescent sera can be tested to be certain. Later in the illness determination of specific IgG antibodies can differentiate Lyme disease from aseptic meningitis or unexplained cranial or peripheral nerve palsies.

Immunofluorescent testing is also done but is less specific, as other spirochete disease (such as syphilis or leptospirosis) confounds results. It is important to note that the diagnosis of Lyme disease can only be made with certainty when the clinical picture of the acute disease and the serologic results both support the diagnosis. Without the clinical picture, serologic tests are often falsely positive and the diagnosis is incorrectly made. The Centers for Disease Control requires the following for the diagnosis to made with certainty:

Isolation of *B. burgdorferi* from an infected tissue or specimen.

Identification of IgM and IgG antibodies to *B. burgdorferi* in the blood or CSF.

Acute and convalescent blood samples with significant positive antibody titers.

Because of the high incidence of false-positive ELISA tests for Lyme disease, it is now recommended that the diagnoses of all patients who have positive serologic tests for Lyme disease using the ELISA method be confirmed by a Western blot–specific Lyme disease test. (This is very similar to the situation with human immunodeficiency virus infection, wherein all positive ELISA tests are confirmed by the more specific and sensitive Western blot test.) Patients suspected of having Lyme disease should have the serologic test repeated if the initial test is negative.

Interfering Factors

- Previous infection with *B. burgdorferi* can cause positive serologic results. These patients no longer have Lyme disease.
- Other spirochete diseases (syphilis, leptospirosis) can cause false-positive results.

Procedure and Patient Care

Before

- Explain the procedure to the patient.
- Tell the patient that no fasting or special preparation is required.

During

- Collect approximately 7 to 10 ml of venous blood in a red-top tube.

After

- Apply pressure or a pressure dressing to the venipuncture site.
- Assess the venipuncture site for bleeding.

Test Results and Clinical Significance

Lyme disease

Lymphocyte Immunophenotyping
(AIDS T-Lymphocyte Cell Markers, CD4 Marker, CD4/CD8 Ratio, CD4 Percentage)

Normal Findings

Cells	%	No. of Cells/μL
T cells	60-95	800-2500
T-helper (CD4) cells	60-75	600-1500
T-suppressor (CD8) cells	25-30	300-1000
B cells	4-25	100-450
Natural killer cells	4-30	75-500
CD4/CD8 ratio	>1.0	

Indications

This test is used to detect the progressive depletion of CD4 T lymphocytes, which is associated with an increased likelihood of clinical complications from AIDS. Test results can indicate if an AIDS patient is at risk for developing opportunistic infections.

Test Explanation

All lymphocytes originate from reticulum cells in the bone marrow. One kind of lymphocyte that matures in the bone marrow is called a B lymphocyte. B lymphocytes provide humoral immunity (produce antibodies). A second type of lymphocyte matures in the thymus and is called a T lymphocyte. T lymphocytes are responsible for cellular immunity. CD4-helper cells and CD8-suppressor cells are examples of T lymphocytes. Finally, there is a group of lymphocytes that has neither T nor B markers. These are called "natural killer cells" and will chemically attack foreign or cancer cells without prior sensitization. Monoclonal antibodies against cell-surface markers are used to identify the various forms of lymphocytes. The absolute numbers and percentages are then counted by the use of flow cytometry. This can be performed on blood or on cell suspensions of tissue.

There are three related measurements of CD4 T lymphocytes. The first measurement is the *total CD4-cell count.* This is measured in whole blood and is the product of the WBC count, the lymphocyte differential count, and the percentage of lymphocytes that are CD4 T cells. The second measurement, the *CD4 percentage,* is a more accurate prognostic marker. It measures the percentage of CD4 lymphocytes in the whole blood sample by combining immunophenotyping with flow cytometry. This procedure relies on detecting specific antigenic determinants on the surface of the CD4 lymphocyte by antigen-specific monoclonal antibodies labeled with a fluorescent dye. The third prognostic marker, which is also more reliable than the total CD4 count, is the *ratio of CD4 cells to CD8 (T-suppressor) cells.*

Of the three T-cell measurements, the total CD4 count is the most variable. There is substantial diurnal variation in this count. Because it is a calculated measurement, the combination of laboratory error and personal fluctuation can result in wide variations in and laboratory error exist. The Multicenter AIDS Cohort Study suggests that the latter two measurements are more accurate than the total CD4 count. However, because the total CD4-cell count was originally thought to be the best marker, this test was used in many of the studies that now form the basis for practice recommendations. It will take time before the more accurate measurements find clinical pertinence in practice recommendations.

The pathogenesis of AIDS is largely attributed to a decrease in the T lymphocyte that bears the CD4 receptor. Progressive depletion of CD4 T lymphocytes is associated with an increased likelihood of clinical complications from AIDS. Therefore CD4 measurement is a prognostic marker that can indicate whether a patient infected with human immunodeficiency virus (HIV) is at risk for developing opportunistic infections. The measurement of CD4-cell levels is used to decide whether to initiate *Pneumocystis carinii* pneumonia prophylaxis and antiviral therapy and for determining the prognosis of patients with HIV infection.

Immunodeficiency associated with organ transplantation is also monitored by lymphocyte phenotyping. Lymphomas and other lymphoproliferative diseases are now classified and treated according to the predominant lymphocyte type identified. In some instances the prognosis of these diseases depends on lymphocyte phenotyping.

The U.S. Public Health Service has recommended that CD4 prognostic markers be monitored every 3 to 6 months in all persons infected with HIV. Because the CD4 counts gradually fall in virtually all such patients, periodic review of the count can be emotionally stressful for both the patient and physician. The patient confronts his or her mortality as the health care provider confronts his or her ultimate powerlessness against the relentlessly advancing infections.

As the CD4-cell measurements decrease, the percentage of persons developing AIDS increases. Forty-eight percent of patients can be expected to develop AIDS within 6 months when their CD4 count is 100 cells/mm^3. It is recommended that antiviral therapy be started in patients whose CD4 count is less than 500 to 600 cells/mm^3. *Pneumocystis carinii* pneumonia prophylaxis should be started when the CD4 count is less than 200 to 300 cells/mm^3.

CD4 prognostic markers also can be useful in guiding the approach to the patient's symptoms. Complaints such as cough and headache are common in most people; however, in patients infected with HIV, these symptoms often raise concerns about opportunistic infections. If the CD4 cell count exceeded 500 cells/mm^3 in the past 6 months, there is a very low probability that these symptoms result from opportunistic infections. Knowing this, the patient and physician can feel comfortable with routine care.

Contraindications

- Patients who are not emotionally prepared for the prognosis that the results may indicate

Interfering Factors

- Although diurnal variation is usually of no significance, it may have some impact when counts are low. Higher counts can be expected in the late morning hours.
- A recent viral illness can decrease total T-lymphocyte counts.

- Nicotine and very strenuous exercise have been shown to decrease lymphocyte counts. However, such data are now being questioned.
- Steroids can *increase* lymphocyte counts.
- Immunosuppressive drugs will *decrease* lymphocyte counts.

CLINICAL PRIORITIES

- Progressive depletion of CD4 T lymphocytes is associated with increased complications from AIDS.
- The CD4 percentage and CD4/CD8 ratio provide more accurate measurements of CD4 T lymphocytes than the total CD4 count.
- The US Public Health Service recommends monitoring CD4 counts every 3 to 6 months for all persons infected with HIV.

Procedure and Patient Care

Before

- Explain the procedure to the patient.
- Tell the patient that no fasting or preparation is required.
- Maintain a nonjudgmental attitude toward the patient's sexual practices.
- Allow the patient ample time to express his or her concerns regarding the results.

During

- Record the time of day when the blood specimen is obtained.
- Observe universal body and blood precautions. Wear gloves when handling blood products from all patients.
- Never recap needles. Dispose of needles and syringes required for obtaining the blood specimen in a puncture-proof container designed for this purpose.
- Obtain 10 ml of blood in a large green-top tube (containing sodium heparin).
- Obtain 5 ml of blood in a small purple-top tube (containing ethylene diaminetetraacetic acid).

After

- Keep the specimen at room temperature. Do not refrigerate.
- The specimen must be evaluated within 24 hours.
- Most specimens are sent to a central laboratory. Be sure to draw the blood immediately before the courier's departure to the reference laboratory.
- Apply pressure or a pressure dressing to the venipuncture site.
- Assess the puncture site for bleeding.
- Instruct the patient to observe the venipuncture site for infection. Patients with AIDS or organ recipients are immunocompromised and susceptible to infection.
- Encourage the patient to discuss his or her concerns regarding the prognostic information that may be obtained by these results.

Test Results and Clinical Significance

Increased counts

Chronic lymphocytic leukemia
B-cell lymphoma
These patients can be expected to have increased B-lymphocyte counts in their tumor tissue or in their peripheral blood.

T-cell lymphoma *These patients can be expected to have increased T-lymphocyte counts in their tumor tissue or in their peripheral blood (if their bone marrow is heavily involved with tumor).*

Decreased counts

Organ transplant patients *A decreased lymphocyte count is expected and desirable for immunosuppression of organ rejection.*
HIV-positive patients *When CD4 counts are below 200/mm^3, the patient is at increased risk for clinical symptoms from AIDS and the opportunistic infections that accompany this disease.*
Congenital immunodeficiency *Children with DiGeorge syndrome and thymic hypoplasia will have decreased or no B lymphocytes.*

Related Test

- AIDS serology (p. 30): This test is used to detect HIV antibody or antigen in high-risk persons.

Magnesium (Mg)

Normal Findings

Adult: 1.2-2.0 mEq/L
Newborn: 1.4-2.0 mEq/L
Child: 1.4-1.7 mEq/L

Critical Values

<0.5 or >3.0 mEq/L

Indications

This test is used to identify magnesium deficiency or overload.

Test Explanation

Most of the magnesium is found in the body intracellularly. About half is in the bone. Most of the magnesium is bound to an adenosine triphosphatase (ATP) molecule and is important in phosphorylation of ATP (main source of energy for the body). Therefore this electrolyte is critical in nearly all metabolic processes. Furthermore, magnesium acts as a cofactor that modifies the activity of many enzymes. Carbohydrate, protein, and nucleic acid synthesis and metabolism depend on magnesium.

Most organ functions, including neuromuscular tissue, also depend on magnesium. It is important to monitor magnesium levels in cardiac patients. Low magnesium levels may increase cardiac irritability and aggravate cardiac arrhythmias. Hypermagnesemia retards neuromuscular conduction and is demonstrated as cardiac conduction slowing (widened PR and Q-T intervals with wide QRS), diminished deep-tendon reflexes, and respiratory depression.

As intracellular elements, body levels of potassium, magnesium, and calcium (in order of quantity) are closely linked. The intracellular electrical charge must be maintained. When one of these positive electrically charged elements is low, another positive charged element is driven into the intracellular space to maintain electrical neutrality. Extracellular and blood levels therefore decrease. A total body reduction in one of those elements creates a comparable blood reduction in the others. Magnesium is especially closely related to calcium in that it increases the intestinal absorption of calcium. Magnesium is also important in calcium metabolism. Often hypocalcemia will respond to magnesium replacement.

Magnesium deficiency occurs in patients who are malnourished because of malabsorption or maldigestion or lack of food intake. This becomes especially significant in postoperative patients, who may not eat for 5 to 7 days and whose metabolism (and therefore the need for magnesium) is accelerated. Alcohol abuse increases magnesium loss in the urine. Moderate hypomagnesemia occurs with diabetes, hypoparathyroidism, hyperthyroidism, and hyperaldosteronism. Toxemia of pregnancy is also believed to be associated with reduced magnesium levels. Symptoms of magnesium depletion are mostly neuromuscular (i.e., weakness, irritability, tetany, EKG changes, delirium, and convulsions).

Increased magnesium levels most commonly are associated with ingestion of magnesium-containing antacids. Because most of the serum magnesium is excreted by the kidney, chronic renal diseases also cause elevated magnesium levels. Several drug interactions also can result in decreased or increased magnesium levels. Because magnesium is an intracellular cation, hemolysis of the collected blood sample should be avoided. Hemolysis will create falsely elevated levels of magnesium. Symptoms of increased magnesium include lethargy, nausea and vomiting, and slurred speech.

Interfering Factors

- Hemolysis should be avoided when collecting this specimen. Magnesium is an intracellular ion, and lysis of RBCs will release great quantities of magnesium into the blood and cause falsely high results
- Drugs that *increase* magnesium levels include thyroid medication, antacids, laxatives, calcium-containing medication, lithium, loop diuretics, and aminoglycoside antibiotics.
- Drugs that *decrease* magnesium levels include diuretics, some antibiotics, and insulin.

Procedure and Patient Care

Before

- Explain the procedure to the patient.
- Tell the patient that no special diet or fasting is required.

During

- Collect approximately 5 to 7 ml of venous blood in a red- or green-top tube.
- Avoid hemolysis.
- Indicate on the laboratory slip any drugs that may affect test results.

After

- Apply pressure or a pressure dressing to the venipuncture site.
- Assess the venipuncture site for bleeding.

Test Results and Clinical Significance

Increased levels

Renal insufficiency *Magnesium is excreted by the kidneys. With end-stage renal failure, excretion is reduced and magnesium accumulates in the blood. See discussion below regarding decreased magnesium levels in tubular diseases of the kidney.*

Addison's disease *Aldosterone enhances magnesium excretion. With reduced aldosterone, magnesium excretion is diminished.*

Ingestion of magnesium-containing antacids or salts *Magnesium is absorbed from the intestines. Blood levels rise.*

Hypothyroidism *The pathophysiology of this observation is not clear.*

Decreased levels

Malnutrition

Malabsorption

The major source of magnesium is dietary intake and absorption from the intestines. When either is inhibited, magnesium levels in the blood fall. Furthermore, in malabsorption all fat-soluble vitamins are lost. Vitamin D levels diminish, and hypocalcemia follows. Magnesium levels therefore fall in light of the low calcium (see above).

Hypoparathyroidism *In this disease, calcium is reduced. Because calcium enhances intestinal absorption of magnesium, it is not well absorbed, and blood levels diminish. In hyperparathyroidism, calcium levels are high and increase.*

Alcoholism *Ethanol increases magnesium losses in the urine.*

Chronic renal tubular disease *Magnesium is reabsorbed in the renal tubule. Diseases affecting this area of the kidney (e.g., tubular necrosis) or drugs that are toxic to the renal tubule (e.g., aminoglycosides) will allow increased losses of magnesium in the urine.*

Diabetic acidosis *With treatment of this disease, magnesium levels fall. As insulin is given to these patient to drive glucose into the cells, magnesium follows and blood levels drop.*

Metyrapone

Normal Findings

24-hour urine: baseline excretion of urinary 17-hydroxycorticosteroid (OCHS) more than doubled

Blood: 11-deoxycortisol increased to >7 mg/dl and cortisol <10 mg/dl

Indications

This test is useful in differentiating adrenal hyperplasia from a primary adrenal tumor by determining whether the pituitary-adrenal feedback mechanism is intact.

Test Explanation

Metyrapone (Metopirone) is a potent blocker of an enzyme involved in cortisol production. Cortisol production is therefore reduced. When this drug is given, the resulting decrease in cortisol production should stimulate pituitary secretion of adrenocorticotropic hormone (ACTH) by way of a negative feedback mechanism. Cortisol, itself, cannot be synthesized because of the metyrapone inhibition at the 11-beta-hydroxylation step, but an abundance of cortisol precursors (11-deoxycortisol and OCHS) will be formed. These cortisol precursors can be detected in the urine or in the blood. This test is similar to the ACTH stimulation test.

In patients with adrenal hyperplasia due to pituitary overproduction of ACTH, the cortisol precursors are greatly increased. This is because the normal adrenal-pituitary feedback response mechanism is still intact. No response to metyrapone occurs in patients with Cushing's syndrome resulting from adrenal adenoma or carcinoma, because the tumors are autonomous and therefore insensitive to changes in ACTH secretion. This test has no significant advantage over the ACTH stimulation test in the differential diagnosis of Cushing's disease.

This test is also used to evaluate the pituitary reserve capacity to produce ACTH. It can document that adrenal insufficiency exists as a result of pituitary disease (secondary adrenal insufficiency) rather than primary adrenal pathology. This test should not be performed if primary adrenal insufficiency is likely. A severe, life-threatening adrenal crisis could be precipitated. A normal response to ACTH should be demonstrated before metyrapone is given.

Contraindications

- Patients with possible primary adrenal insufficiency, because metyrapone could reduce the production of what little cortisol is produced and precipitate an adrenal crisis

Potential Complications

- Addison's disease and Addisonian crisis, because metyrapone inhibits cortisol production

Interfering Factors

- Recent administration of radioisotopes will interfere with test results performed by radioimmunoassay.
- Chlorpromazine (Thorazine) interferes with the response to metyrapone and should not be administered during the testing.

CLINICAL PRIORITIES

- This test evaluates the intactness of the pituitary-adrenal feedback mechanism.
- This test should not be performed on patients with adrenal insufficiency. A severe, life-threatening adrenal crisis could result.
- Patients should be carefully assessed for impending signs of addisonian crisis. This is a medical emergency and must be treated vigorously.

Procedure and Patient Care

Before

- Explain the procedure to the patient.
- Obtain a baseline 24-hour urine specimen for 17-OCHS level for the urine test.
- Obtain a baseline cortisol level (see p. 167) for the blood test.

During

Blood

- Administer 2 to 3 g of metyrapone at 11 PM the night before the blood specimen is to be collected. Collect a blood specimen in the morning.

Urine

- Obtain a 24-hour urine specimen for a 17-OCHS baseline level. Then collect a 24-hour urine specimen for the 17-OCHS level during and again 1 day after the oral administration of 500 to 750 mg of metyrapone, which is given every 4 hours for 24 hours.

After

- Assess the patient for impending signs of addisonian crisis (muscle weakness, mental and emotional changes, anorexia, nausea, vomiting, hypotension, hyperkalemia, vascular collapse).
- Note that addisonian crisis is a medical emergency that must be treated vigorously. Basically, the immediate treatment includes replenishing steroids, reversing shock, and restoring blood circulation.

Test Results and Clinical Significance

Increased levels

Adrenal hyperplasia *Cortisol precursors will be significantly increased as a result of accentuating the ACTH effect.*

Adrenal tumor *Tumors are autonomous and are not affected by inhibitory or stimulatory feedback. There is no apparent change in cortisol precursors.*

Ectopic ACTH syndrome *This syndrome occurs when neoplasms (usually lung cancer) produce ACTH without regard to regulatory mechanisms. There is no apparent change in cortisol precursors.*

Secondary adrenal insufficiency *There will be no significant change in cortisol precursors, because there is no pituitary function to stimulate the production of ACTH.*

Related Tests

- Adrenocorticotropic hormone (ACTH) (p. 23): This is a direct measurement of ACTH, which is used in the evaluation of Cushing's syndrome and Addison's disease.
- Adrenocorticotropic hormone (ACTH) stimulation (p. 26): This test is used similarly to the metyrapone test for evaluation of Addison's disease and Cushing's syndrome.

Mononucleosis Spot (Mononuclear Heterophil, Heterophil Antibody, Monospot)

Normal Findings

Negative (<1:28 titer)

Indications

This is a rapid slide test designed to assist in the diagnosis of infectious mononucleosis (IM)

Test Explanation

The mononucleosis test is performed to aid in the diagnosis of IM, a disease caused by the Epstein-Barr virus (EBV). Usually young adults are affected by mononucleosis. The clinical presentation is fever, pharyngitis, lymphadenopathy, and splenomegaly. Approximately 2 weeks after the onset of the disease, many patients are found to have IgM heterophil antibodies in their serum that react against warm RBCs. When these antibodies are present in serial dilutions of greater than 1:56, IM can be strongly considered. However, false-positive results can occur in patients who have other diseases that cause elevation of heterophil antibodies. Examples would include patients with lymphoma, systemic lupus erythematosus, Burkitt's lymphoma, leukemia, and some GI cancers. Burkitt's lymphoma is strongly associated with EBV.

Several heterophil agglutination tests are available, but the most frequently performed is the rapid slide spot test (monospot test). Heterophil antibodies, normally present in most individuals, are produced in increased quantities in patients with IM. These antibodies strongly and readily agglutinate horse RBCs. The spot slide test is performed by adding the patient's serum to horse RBCs on a slide. If agglutination occurs, heterophil antibodies are present in the patient's serum, indicating an EBV virus infection. About 30% of the cases of IM are "heterophil antibody negative." When the diagnosis of IM is still suspected, a repeat monospot test or EBV serologic test is done. The diagnosis of IM must include the following criteria:

Clinical presentation compatible with IM
Hematologic presentation compatible with IM (lymphocytosis)
Atypical lymphocytes in significant numbers
Positive serologic test for IM

Procedure and Patient Care

Before

- Explain the procedure to the patient.
- Tell the patient that no fasting or special preparation is required.

During

- Collect approximately 7 to 10 ml of venous blood in a red-top tube.

After

- Apply pressure or a pressure dressing to the venipuncture site.
- Observe the venipuncture site for bleeding.

Test Results and Clinical Significance

Increased levels

IM
Chronic EBV infection
Chronic fatigue syndrome
Burkitt's lymphoma
Some forms of chronic hepatitis
The above diseases are often associated with abnormal quantities of heterophil agglutinating antibodies similar to those formed in patients with IM.

Related Tests

- Epstein-Barr virus titer (p. 197): This is a more specific and sensitive test for EBV infections. It can also differentiate acute and chronic or old EBV infections.

Myoglobin

Normal Findings

0-85 ng/ml or 0-85 nmol/L (SI units)

Indications

This test is used in the early evaluation of a patient with suspected acute myocardial infarction (MI). It is also used to assist in the diagnosis of disease or injury of skeletal muscle.

Test Explanation

Myoglobin is an oxygen-binding protein found in cardiac and skeletal muscle. Measurement of myoglobin is an index of damage to the myocardium, such as occurs in MI or reinfarction. Increased levels, which indicate cardiac muscle injury or death, occur in about 3 hours. Although this test is more sensitive than creatine phosphokinase (CPK) isoenzymes, it is not as specific. Trauma, inflammation, or ischemic changes to the non-cardiac skeletal muscles can also cause elevated levels of myoglobin. The benefit of myoglobin over CPK-MB (see p. 174) is that it may become elevated earlier in some patients. This may prove beneficial since thrombolytic therapy should be started within the first 6 hours after an MI.

As already indicated, disease or trauma of the skeletal muscle also causes elevations in myoglobin. With sudden and severe muscle injury, myoglobin levels can reach very high levels. Because myoglobin is excreted in the urine and is nephrotoxic, the levels must be monitored in these types of patients. Myoglobin can also be measured in the urine. To screen for myoglobin, the routine urine dipstick for hemoglobin will also react for myoglobin.

Interfering Factors

- Recent administration of radioactive substances may affect test results determined by radioimmunoassay methods. The recently administered radioisotope may interfere with testing.
- Increased myoglobin levels can occur after IM injections. The injection can cause localized muscle injury and instigate an inflammatory response that could elevate myoglobin levels.

Procedure and Patient Care

Before

- Explain the procedure to the patient.
- Tell the patient that no fasting is required.

During

- Collect approximately 5 ml of venous blood in a red-top tube.

After

- Apply pressure or a pressure dressing to the venipuncture site.
- Observe the venipuncture site for bleeding.

Test Results and Clinical Significance

Increased levels

Myocardial infarction *Injury to cardiac muscle causes the cells to lyse and expel the myoglobin into the bloodstream.*

Skeletal muscle inflammation (myositis) *Injury to cardiac muscle causes the cells to lyse and expel the myoglobin into the bloodstream.*

Malignant hyperthermia
Muscular dystrophy
Skeletal muscle ischemia
Skeletal muscle trauma

Rhabdomyolysis
All of these diseases affect the skeletal muscles. This causes the muscle cells to lyse and expel the myoglobin into the bloodstream.

Seizures *Persistent seizure activity injures skeletal muscle tissue. This causes the muscle cells to lyse and expel the myoglobin into the bloodstream.*

Decreased levels

Polymyositis *In some cases, antimyoglobin antibodies exist and diminish myoglobin in the blood.*

Related Tests

- Creatine phosphokinase (CPK) (p. 173): This test is very useful in the evaluation of MI.
- Lactic dehyrogenase (LDH) (p. 278): This enzyme is also elevated when injury to muscle tissue occurs.

5′-Nucleotidase

Normal Findings

0.0-1.6 U or 27-233 nmol/sec/L (SI units)

Indications

5′-Nucleotidase is used to support the diagnosis of hepatobiliary obstructive disease. It is especially useful in helping confirm that an elevated alkaline phosphatase (ALP) is the result of liver pathology rather than pathology of another tissue origin.

Test Explanation

5′-Nucleotidase is an enzyme specific to the liver. The 5′-nucleotidase level is elevated in patients with liver diseases, especially those associated with cholestasis. It provides information similar to ALP. However, ALP is not specific to the liver. Diseases of the bone, sepsis, pregnancy, and other disease can produce ALP elevation. When there is doubt as to the cause of an elevated ALP, a 5′-nucleotidase test is recommended. If that enzyme is elevated along with the ALP, the pathologic source is certainly the liver. If the 5′-nucleotidase is normal in the face of an elevated ALP, the pathologic source is outside the liver (bone, kidney, spleen). Gamma-glutamyl transpeptidase (GGTP) is used similarly, as it is also specific to the liver.

Interfering Factors

- Drugs that may cause *increased* 5′-nucleotidase levels include hepatotoxic agents.

Procedure and Patient Care

Before

- Explain the procedure to the patient.
- Tell the patient that no fasting is required.

During

- Collect approximately 7 to 10 ml of venous blood in a red-top tube.
- Indicate on the laboratory slip any medication the patient is taking to aid in the interpretation of test results.

After

- Apply pressure or a pressure dressing to the venipuncture site.
- Assess the venipuncture site for bleeding. Patients with liver dysfunction often have prolonged clotting times.

Test Results and Clinical Significance

Increased levels

Bile duct obstruction
Cholestasis
The 5′-nucleotidase test is most specific for pathologic conditions that cause intra- or extrahepatic biliary obstruction.

Hepatitis
Cirrhosis
Hepatic necrosis
Hepatic ischemia
Hepatic tumor
Hepatotoxic drugs
To a lesser degree, hepatocellular disease is associated with elevations of this enzyme.

Related Tests

- Gamma-glutamyl transpeptidase (GGTP) (p. 219): This is another enzyme that, when elevated, specifically points to hepatic pathology.
- Alkaline phosphatase (ALP) (p. 42): This is an enzyme that exists in the liver and other organs. It is not specific to the liver, however.

Osmolality, Blood (Serum Osmolality)

Normal Findings

Adult/elderly: 285-295 mOsm/kg H_2O
Child: 275-290 mOsm/kg H_2O

Critical Values

<265 mOsm/kg H_2O
>320 mOsm/kg H_2O

Indications

This test is used to gain information about fluid status and electrolyte imbalance. It is also helpful in evaluating illnesses involving antidiuretic hormone (ADH).

Test Explanation

Osmolality measures the concentration of dissolved particles in blood. As the amount of free water in the blood increases or the amount of particles decreases, osmolality decreases. As the amount of water in the blood decreases or the amount of particles increases, osmolality increases. Osmolality increases with dehydration and decreases with overhydration.

There is an elaborate feedback mechanism that controls osmolality. Increased osmolality will stimulate secretion of ADH; this will result in increased water reabsorption in the kidney, more concentrated urine, and less concentrated serum. A low serum osmolality will suppress the release of ADH, resulting in decreased water reabsorption and large amounts of dilute urine. The simultaneous use of urine osmolality helps in the interpretation and evaluation of problems involving osmolality.

The serum osmolality test is useful in evaluating fluid and electrolyte imbalance. The test is very helpful in evaluating patients with seizures, ascites, hydration status, acid-base balance, and suspected ADH abnormalities. Osmolality is also helpful in identifying the presence of organic acids, sugars, or ethanol. In these cases there is an "osmolal gap." This gap represents the difference between what the osmolality should be based on calculations of serum sodium, glucose, and BUN (the three most important solutes in the blood) and the osmolality as truly measured. If the "gap" is large, solutes such as organic acids (ketones) or unusually high levels of glucose or ethanol by-products are suspected to be present. Finally, osmolality also plays an important role in toxicology and workups for coma patients. Values of 385 mOsm/kg H_2O are associated with stupor in patients with hyperglycemia. When values of 400 to 420 mOsm/kg H_2O are detected, grand mal seizures can occur. Values greater than 420 mOsm/kg H_2O can be lethal.

✓ CLINICAL PRIORITIES

- This test provides valuable information about fluid and electrolyte balance.
- Osmolality increases with dehydration and decreases with overhydration.
- The simultaneous measurement of urine osmolality helps in interpretating and evaluating problems with fluid balance.

Procedure and Patient Care

Before

- Explain the procedure to the patient.
- Tell the patient that no fasting is required.

During

- Collect approximately 5 to 10 ml of venous blood in a red-top tube.
- For pediatric patients, draw blood from a heel stick.

After

- Apply pressure or a pressure dressing to the venipuncture site.
- Observe the venipuncture site for bleeding.

Test Results and Clinical Significance

Increased levels

Hypernatremia
Hyperglycemia
Hyperosmolar nonketotic hyperglycemia
Ketosis
Azotemia
All of the above illnesses are associated with an increase in the number of particles dissolved in the blood.

Dehydration *Decreased replacement of ongoing water losses leads to dehydration and a rise in the serum osmolality.*

Mannitol therapy
Ingestion of ethanol, methanol, or ethylene glycol
These drugs stimulate free water loss from the kidneys and excretion in the urine. As a result, the serum osmolality is increased. Furthermore, their by-products cause an increase in the number of solutes in the blood and thereby increase the osmolality.

Uremia
Diabetes insipidus
Renal tubular necrosis
Severe pyelonephritis
The above illnesses are associated with poor urine concentration. Free water is lost and serum osmolality increases.

Decreased levels

Overhydration *The provision of free water above the ongoing losses creates a situation in which there is excess free water in the blood. Serum osmolality decreases.*

Syndrome of inappropriate ADH (SIADH) secretion *Several illnesses can create this syndrome. ADH is inappropriately secreted despite factors that normally would inhibit its secretion. As a result, large quantities of water are reabsorbed by the kidney. The serum becomes dilute and osmolality decreases.*

Paraneoplastic syndromes associated with carcinoma (lung, breast, colon) *These cancers act as an autonomous ectopic source for the secretion of ADH. The pathophysiology is the same as described above for SIADH.*

Related Tests

- Urine osmolality (p. 842): This is a measurement of the concentration of dissolved particles in the urine. When measured with the serum osmolality, greater insight is obtained about problems of fluid balance.
- Antidiuretic hormone (ADH) (p. 62): This is a direct measurement of ADH in the blood.
- Antidiuretic hormone (ADH) suppression (p. 65): This test is very helpful in the evaluation of ADH abnormalities.

Parathyroid Hormone (PTH, Parathormone)

Normal Findings

Assay	Assay Includes	Normal Values (pg/ml)
PTH intact (whole)	Intact PTH	10-65
PTH N-terminal	N-terminal Intact PTH	8-24
PTH C-terminal	C-terminal Intact PTH Midmolecule	50-330

Indications

PTH is measured to assist in the evaluation of hyper- or hypocalcemia. It is routinely monitored in patients with chronic renal failure (CRF).

Test Explanation

PTH is the only hormone secreted by the parathyroid gland in response to hypocalcemia. When calcium serum levels return to normal, PTH levels diminish. PTH, therefore, is one of the major factors affecting calcium metabolism. This test is useful in establishing a diagnosis of hyperparathyroidism and distinguishing nonparathyroid from parathyroid causes of hypercalcemia. Increased PTH levels are seen in patients with hyperparathyroidism (primary, secondary, or tertiary); in patients with nonparathyroid, ectopic PTH-producing tumors (pseudohyperparathyroidisim); or as a normal compensatory response to hypocalcemia in patients with malabsorption or vitamin D deficiency.

Primary hyperparathyroidism is most often caused by a parathyroid adenoma and only rarely from parathyroid cancer. These patients have high PTH and calcium levels. Secondary hyperparathyroidism is the exaggerated response of the parathyroid gland to kidney insensitivity to PTH in CRF patients. CRF patients have chronically low serum calcium levels in reaction to persistently high phosphate levels that the kidney fails to excrete. In response to this persistently low calcium, the parathyroid is constantly stimulated to produce PTH to attempt to maintain a normal calcium. This is called secondary hyperparathyroidism. These patients have high PTH and normal to slightly low calcium levels. Occasionally a patient with CRF overshoots the compensatory process and autonomously develops unnecessarily high PTH production that leads to hypercalcemia. This is called tertiary hyperparathyroidism. These patient have high PTH and high calcium levels.

It is important to measure serum calcium simultaneously with PTH. Most laboratories have a PTH/calcium nomogram already made up indicating what PTH level is considered normal for each calcium level.

Decreased PTH levels are seen in patients with hypoparathyroidism or as a compensatory response to hypercalcemia in patients with metastatic bone tumors, sarcoidosis, vitamin D intoxication, or milk-alkali syndrome. Of course, surgical ablation of the parathyroid glands is another cause of hypoparathyroidism.

Whole (intact) PTH is metabolized to several different fragments, including an amino acid or N-terminal, a midregion or midmolecule, and a carboxyl or C-terminal. The intact PTH and the N-terminal are metabolically active. These can all be measured by immunoassay. The intact PTH and all fragments generally provide accurate information concerning the level of PTH in the blood. The intact PTH is probably most often tested as it is most reliable.

Interfering Factors

- Recent injection of radioisotopes may interfere with this test if radioimmunoassay methods are used. However, radioimmunoassay is not a frequently used method of measuring PTH fragments.
- Drugs that *increase* PTH include phosphates, anticonvulsants, steroids, isoniazid, lithium, and rifampin.
- Drugs that *decrease* PTH include cimetidine, pindolol, and propranolol.

✓ CLINICAL PRIORITIES

- This test is routinely monitored in patients with CRF. These patients have chronically low serum calcium levels in reaction to persistently high phosphate levels that the kidney fails to excrete.
- It is important to measure serum PTH and serum calcium levels at the same time. These values are important for a differential diagnosis. Most laboratories have PTH/calcium nomograms indicating normal PTH levels for each calcium level.
- PTH levels are affected by a diurnal variation. Levels are highest around 2 AM and lowest around 2 PM. Usually an 8 AM blood specimen is drawn. If the patient works nights, the laboratory should be notified so that changes in the diurnal variation can be factored in.

Procedure and Patient Care

Before

- Explain the procedure to the patient.
- Keep the patient on NPO status except for water after midnight on the day of the test.

During

- Obtain an 8 AM blood specimen, because diurnal rhythm affects PTH levels. (Check with the laboratory if the patient works at night.) PTH levels are highest around 2 AM and lowest around 2 PM.
- Collect 5 to 10 ml of venous blood in a red-top tube. Note that some laboratories require 15 ml of blood in an iced plastic syringe.
- Obtain a serum calcium level determination at the same time if ordered. The serum PTH and serum calcium levels are important for a differential diagnosis.

After

- Indicate the time the blood was drawn on the laboratory slip, because a diurnal rhythm affects test results.
- Apply pressure or a pressure dressing to the venipuncture site.
- Check the venipuncture site for bleeding.
- Most PTH specimens are sent to a central laboratory. The specimen should be kept in cold temperatures and transported on dry ice.

Test Results and Clinical Significance

Increased levels

Hyperparathyroidism secondary to adenoma or carcinoma of the parathyroid gland *PTH is autonomously produced by the parathyroid gland. PTH levels are elevated.*

Non-PTH-producing tumors (paraneoplastic syndrome) commonly noted with lung, kidney, or breast carcinoma *These tumors produce a "PTH-related protein" that acts like PTH and increases serum calcium. Because it is structurally similar to PTH, it is measured with PTH testing and gives a falsely high PTH result.*

Congenital renal defect *These patients have a congenital kidney nonresponsiveness to "normal" quantities of PTH. As a result, calcium decreases despite normal quantities of PTH. The parathyroid is called on to produce even greater quantities of PTH. This is also called pseudohyperparathyroidism.*

Hypocalcemia *PTH elevation is the result of a physiologic compensation for low serum calcium.*

Chronic renal failure *These patients cannot excrete phosphates. As a result, serum calcium levels diminish. PTH elevation is the result of a physiologic compensation for low serum calcium. This is secondary hyperparathyroidism. Occasionally a CRF patient develops parathyroid hyperplasia that leads to PTH levels in excess of the amount physiologic homeostasis requires. This is called tertiary hyperparathyroidism.*

Malabsorption syndrome *These patients do not absorb calcium or fat-soluble vitamins such as vitamin D. Serum calcium falls. PTH elevation is the result of a physiologic compensation for low serum calcium.*

Vitamin D deficiency and rickets *Vitamin D is integral to the absorption of calcium from the gut. With inadequate levels, serum calcium decreases. PTH elevation is the result of a physiologic compensation for low serum calcium.*

Decreased levels

Hypoparathyroidism due to surgical ablation or immunoablation *PTH is not produced at levels necessary to maintain normal calcium levels.*

Hypercalcemia *Reduced PTH is a normal physiologic response to high serum calcium.*

Metastatic bone tumor *Tumor in the bone can mobilize large quantities of calcium. Reduced PTH is a normal physiologic response to high serum calcium.*

Hypercalcemia of malignancy (most often with lung, breast, or lymphoma cancer) *For unknown reasons, serum calcium levels become very high in these cancer patients. They do not have bone metastasis or PTH-related proteins. Reduced PTH is a normal physiologic response to high serum calcium.*

Sarcoidosis *These patients can develop elevated serum calcium levels. Reduced PTH is a normal physiologic response to high serum calcium.*

Vitamin D intoxication *These patients have high serum calcium levels as a result of vitamin D stimulating maximal calcium intestinal absorption. Reduced PTH is a normal physiologic response to high serum calcium.*

Milk-alkali syndrome *These infants are given cooked whole milk that is very high in calcium. They develop high serum calcium levels. Reduced PTH is a normal physiologic response to high serum calcium.*

DiGeorge syndrome *These immunodeficient children also have hypocalcemia that may be due to hypoparathyroidism.*

Related Tests

- Calcium, blood (p. 130): This is a direct measurement of serum calcium. This test should be done simultaneously with a PTH test to improve interpretation of PTH levels.
- Phosphate (p. 328): This is a direct measurement of the inorganic phosphate levels in the serum, which are affected by PTH.
- Tubular phosphate reabsorption (p. 441): This test provides an indirect measurement of PTH by estimating its effects on renal phosphate reabsorption.

Partial Thromboplastin Time, Activated
(APTT, Partial Thromboplastin Time [PTT])

Normal Findings

APTT: 30-40 seconds
PTT: 60-70 seconds
Patients receiving anticoagulant therapy: 1.5-2.5 times control value in seconds

Critical Values

APTT: >70 seconds
PTT: >100 seconds

Indications

The PTT test is used to assess the intrinsic system and the common pathway of clot formation. It is also used to monitor heparin therapy.

Test Explanation

Hemostasis and the coagulation system represent a homeostatic balance between factors encouraging clotting and factors encouraging clot dissolution. The first reaction of the body to active bleeding is blood vessel constriction. In small vessel injury this may be enough to stop bleeding. In large vessel injury, hemostasis is required to form a clot that will durably plug the hole until healing can occur. The primary phase of the hemostatic mechanism involves platelet aggregation to blood vessel (see Figure 2-10 on p. 156). Next, secondary hemostasis occurs. The first phase of reactions is called the intrinsic system. Factor XII and other proteins form a complex on the subendothelial collagen in the injured blood vessel. Through a series of reactions, activated factor XI (XIa) is formed and activates factor IX (IXa). In a complex formed by factors VIII, IX, and X, activated X (Xa) is formed.

At the same time the extrinsic system is activated and a complex is formed between tissue thromboplastin (factor III) and factor VII. Activated factor VII (VIIa) results. VIIa can directly activate factor X. Alternatively, VIIa can activate IX and X together.

The final step is a common pathway in which prothrombin is converted to thrombin on the surface of the aggregated platelets. The main purpose of thrombin is to convert fibrinogen to fibrin, which is then polymerized into a stable gel. Factor XIII crosslinks the fibrin polymers to form a stable clot.

Almost immediately three major activators of the fibrinolytic system act on plasminogen, which had previously been absorbed into the clot, to form plasmin. Plasmin degenerates the fibrin polymer into fragments that are cleared by macrophages.

The PTT evaluates factors I (fibrinogen), II (prothrombin), V, VIII, IX, X, XI, and XII. When the PTT is combined with the prothrombin time, nearly all of the hemostatic abnormalities can be recognized. When any of these factors exists in inadequate quantities, as in hemophilia A and B or consumptive coagulopathy, the PTT is prolonged. Because factors II, IX, and X are vitamin K–dependent factors, biliary obstruction, which precludes GI absorption of fat and fat-soluble vitamins (e.g., vitamin K), can reduce their concentration and thus prolong the PTT. Because coagulation factors are made in the liver, hepatocellular diseases will also prolong the PTT.

Heparin has been found to inactivate prothrombin (factor II) and to prevent the formation of thromboplastin. These actions prolong the intrinsic clotting pathway for approximately 4 to 6 hours after each dose of heparin. Therefore heparin is capable of providing therapeutic anticoagulation. The appropriate dose of heparin can be monitored by the PTT. PTT test results are given in seconds along with a control value. The control value may vary slightly from day to day because of the reagents used.

Recently activators have been added to the PTT test reagents to shorten normal clotting time and provide a narrow normal range. This shortened time is called the activated PTT. The normal APTT is 30 to 40 seconds. Desired ranges for therapeutic anticoagulation are 1.5 to 2.5 times normal (e.g., 70 seconds). The APTT specimen should be drawn 30 to 60 minutes before the patient's next heparin dose is given. If the APTT is less than 50 seconds, therapeutic anticoagulation may not have been achieved and more heparin is needed. An APTT greater than 100 seconds indicates that too much heparin is being given; the risk of serious spontaneous bleeding exists when the APTT is this high. The effects of heparin can be reversed by the administration of 1 mg of protamine sulfate for every 100 U of the heparin dose.

Heparin's effect, unlike that of warfarin, is immediate and short lived. When a thromboembolic episode (e.g., pulmonary embolism, arterial embolism, thrombophlebitis) occurs, immediate and complete anticoagulation is most rapidly and safely achieved by heparin administration. This drug is often given during cardiac and vascular surgery to prevent intravascular clotting during clamping of the vessels. Often small doses of heparin (5000 U subcutaneously every 12 hours) are given to prevent thromboembolism in high-risk patients. This dose alters the PTT very little, and the risk of spontaneous bleeding is minimal.

Interfering Factors

- Drugs that may prolong PTT test values include antihistamines, ascorbic acid, chlorpromazine, heparin, and salicylates.

✓ CLINICAL PRIORITIES

- The PTT is used to monitor heparin therapy. Heparin's effect is immediate and short lived.
- If too much heparin is given, its effects can be reversed by protamine sulfate.
- Patients receiving heparin need to be evaluated for bleeding tendencies. These include bruising, petechiae, low-back pain, and bleeding gums. Blood may be detected in the urine and stool.

Procedure and Patient Care

Before

- Explain the procedure to the patient.
- If the patient is receiving heparin by intermittent injection, plan to draw the blood specimen for the APTT 30 minutes to 1 hour before the next dose of heparin.
- If the patient is receiving continuous heparin, draw the blood at any time.

During

- Collect 5 to 14 ml of venous blood in one or two blue-top tubes.

After

- Apply pressure or a pressure dressing to the venipuncture site.
- Assess the venipuncture site for bleeding. Remember, if the patient is receiving anticoagulants or has coagulopathies, the bleeding time will be increased.
- Assess the patient to detect possible bleeding. Check for blood in the urine and all other excretions and assess the patient for bruises, petechiae, and bleeding gums.
- If severe bleeding occurs, note that the anticoagulant effect of heparin can be reversed by parenteral administration of protamine sulfate.

Test Results and Clinical Significance

Increased levels

Congenital clotting factor deficiencies (e.g., von Willebrand's disease, hemophilia, hypofibrinogenemia) *These hereditary illnesses are associated with very little, if any, of the respective clotting factors. As a result, the PTT is prolonged.*

Cirrhosis of liver
Vitamin K deficiency
The liver makes most of the clotting factors. For synthesis of some of those clotting factors, vitamin K is required. In the above illnesses the clotting factors of the intrinsic system and common pathways are inadequate in quantity. As a result, the PTT is prolonged.

Disseminated intravascular coagulation (DIC) *Key clotting factors involved in the intrinsic system are consumed.*

Heparin administration *Heparin inhibits the intrinsic system at several points. As a result, the PTT is prolonged.*

Coumarin administration *Although coumarin has a greater impact on the prothrombin time, it does inhibit the function of factors II, IX, and X. As a result, the PTT is prolonged.*

Decreased levels

Early stages of DIC *Circulating procoagulants exist in the early stages of DIC. These act to shorten or decrease the PTT.*

Extensive cancer (e.g., ovarian, pancreatic, colon) *The pathophysiology of this association is not well known.*

Related Tests

- Bleeding time (p. 115): This test is used to evaluate the vascular and platelet factors associated with hemostasis.
- Thrombin time (p. 408): This is a test of the fibrinogen to fibrin reaction.
- Prothrombin time (p. 366): This test is used to evaluate the adequacy of the extrinsic system and common pathway in the clotting mechanism.
- Coagulating factor concentration (p. 154): This is a quantitative measurement of specific coagulation factors.

Parvovirus B19 Antibody

Normal Findings

Negative for IgM- and IgG-specific antibodies to parvovirus B19

Indications

This test is performed on children who have vague symptoms of fever, arthralgias, and rash suggestive of erythema infectiosum. It is also becoming a part of routine testing for proposed organ donors.

Test Explanation

The parvovirus group includes several species-specific viruses of animals. Parvovirus B19 is known to be a human pathogen. Many of the severe manifestations of B19 viremia relate to the ability of the virus to infect and lyse RBC precursors in the bone marrow. The name "B19" was derived from the code number of the human serum in which the virus was discovered.

Erythema infectiosum is the most common manifestation of B19 infection and occurs predominantly in children. This pathogen is also referred to as "fifth disease," because it was classified in the late nineteenth century as the fifth in a series of six exanthems of childhood. This infection is also sometimes referred to as "academy rash." The typical presentation is a self-limiting, mild illness with a low-grade fever, malar rash, and occasionally arthralgia. Normally the rash begins on the face and may also develop on the arms and legs. Outbreaks of erythema infectiosum appear most often during the winter and spring months.

Recently parvovirus B19 has been associated with a number of other clinical problems, including:

Flu-like illness associated with joint inflammation, rash, and occasionally purpura in young adults

Hydrops fetalis and fetal loss in less than 10% of infected pregnant women

Transient aplastic crisis in patients with chronic hemolytic anemia. In immunocompromised patients (AIDS patients, organ donors), this virus can be so severe as to cause aplastic anemia and bone marrow failure. With increasing frequency, this antibody test is being required for all potential organ donors.

Chronic severe anemia in patients with immunodeficiency related to infection with human immunodeficiency virus (HIV), congenital immunodeficiency, acute lymphocytic leukemia during maintenance chemotherapy, and recipients of bone marrow transplants

Because of the recently discovered spectrum of diseases caused by parvovirus B19, laboratory diagnosis has come into great demand. Serologic testing for parvovirus B19-specific IgM and IgG antibodies can be detected by enzyme-linked immunosorbent assay and indirect fluorescent antibody immunofluorescence methods. Acute infections can be determined by B19-compatible symptoms and the presence of IgM antibodies that remain detectable up to a few months. Past infection or immunity is documented by IgG antibodies that persist indefinitely. Fetal infection may be recognized by hydrops fetalis and the presence of B19 DNA in amniotic fluid or fetal blood.

Procedure and Patient Care

Before

- Explain the procedure to the patient.
- Tell the patient that no fasting or special preparation is necessary.

During

- Collect a venous blood sample according to the laboratory protocol.

After

- Apply pressure or a pressure dressing to the venipuncture site.
- Assess the venipuncture site for bleeding.
- Inform the patient that it normally requires approximately 2 to 3 days to get test results.

Test Results and Clinical Significance

Increased levels

Erythema infectiosum (fifth disease)
Joint arthralgia and arthritis
These diseases are self-limiting and elevate antibodies through the course of viremia.

Hydrops fetalis
Fetal loss
These obstetric disasters could be due to maternal infection with parvovirus.

Transient aplastic anemia
Chronic anemia
Bone marrow failure
These problems occur mostly in patients who are immunocompromised. In such patients the viremia is much more significant. RBC precursors are target cells for the virus.

pH, Fetal Scalp

Normal Findings

pH: 7.25-7.35
O_2 saturation: 30%-50%
PO_2: 18-22 mm Hg
PCO_2: 40-50 mm Hg
Base excess: 0-10 mEq/L

Indications This test indicates fetal well-being or fetal distress.

Test Explanation

Measurement of fetal scalp blood pH provides valuable information on fetal acid-base status. This screening test is useful clinically for diagnosing fetal distress.

Although the oxygen partial pressure (PO_2), carbon dioxide partial pressure (PCO_2), and bicarbonate ion (HCO_3^-) concentration can be measured with the fetal scalp blood sample, the pH is the most useful clinically. The pH normally ranges from 7.25 to 7.35 during labor; a mild decline within the normal range is noted with contractions and as labor progresses.

Fetal hypoxia causes anaerobic glycolysis, resulting in excess production of lactic acid. This causes an increase in hydrogen ion concentration (acidosis) and a decrease in pH. Acidosis reflects the effect of hypoxia on cellular metabolism. A high correlation exists between low pH levels and low Apgar scores.

Contraindications

- Patients with premature membrane rupture, because infection can be instilled into the uterus
- Patients with active cervical infection (e.g., gonorrhea), because the active infection can be spread to the fetus

Potential Complications

- Continued bleeding from the puncture site
- Hematoma
- Ecchymosis
- Infection

✓ CLINICAL PRIORITIES

- The fetal scalp pH indicates fetal well-being or fetal distress.
- Fetal hypoxia causes anaerobic glycolysis, resulting in excess production of lactic acid. This causes a decrease in pH.
- A high correlation exists between a low pH and low Apgar scores.

Procedure and Patient Care

Before

- Explain the procedure to the patient.
- Obtain an informed consent for this procedure.
- Tell the patient that no fasting or sedation is required.

During

- Note the following procedural steps:
  1. Amnioscopy is performed with the mother in the lithotomy position.
  2. The cervix is dilated, and the endoscope (amnioscope) is introduced into the cervical canal.
  3. The fetal scalp is cleansed with an antiseptic and dried with a sterile cotton ball.
  4. A small amount of petroleum jelly is applied to the fetal scalp to cause droplets of fetal blood to bead.
  5. After the skin on the scalp is pierced with a small metal blade, beaded droplets of blood are collected in long, heparinized capillary tubes.
  6. The tube is sealed with wax and placed on ice to retard cellular respiration, which can alter the pH.
  7. The physician performing the procedure applies firm pressure to the puncture site to retard bleeding.
  8. Scalp blood sampling can be repeated as necessary.
- Note that this study is performed by a physician in approximately 10 to 15 minutes.
- Tell the patient that she may be uncomfortable during the cervical dilation.

After

- Inform the patient that she may have vaginal discomfort and menstrual-type cramping.
- After delivery assess the newborn and identify and document the puncture site(s).
- Cleanse the fetal scalp puncture site with an antiseptic solution and apply an antibiotic ointment.

Test Results and Clinical Significance

Increased levels

Fetal distress *Fetal hypoxia causes anaerobic glycolysis, resulting in excess production of lactic acid. This causes an increase in hydrogen ion concentration (acidosis) and a decrease in pH.*

Related Test

- Arterial blood gas (p. 97): This test provides valuable information in assessing and managing a patient's respiratory (ventilation) and metabolic (renal) acid-base and electrolyte homeostasis. It is also used to assess adequacy of oxygenation.

Phenylketonuria
(PKU, Guthrie Test, Phenylalanine Screening)

Normal Findings

Blood: negative (<2 mg/dl) (Guthrie technique)
Urine: no green coloration

Critical Values: >4 mg/dl (Guthrie technique)

Indications

This test is routinely performed on infants to exclude the diagnosis of PKU.

Test Explanation

An autosomal recessive inherited disease, PKU is characterized by deficiency of the enzyme called phenylalanine hydroxylase, which converts phenylalanine to tyrosine. Phenylalanine is an essential amino acid necessary for growth and metabolism; however, any excess must be degraded by conversion to tyrosine. An infant with PKU lacks the ability to make this necessary conversion. Thus phenylalanine accumulates in the blood. Its catabolic product, phenylpyruvic acid, builds up in the body and spills over into the urine. It is this metabolic product that is detected in the urine by color dipstick testing. If the amount of phenylalanine is not restricted in infants with PKU, progressive mental retardation results from the deposit of phenylalanine and its metabolic products in the brain. Dietary control must begin early to avoid brain damage; therefore diagnosis must be made early.

Routine screening of newborn infants for PKU is now mandatory in most of the United States. It is important to note that this test is not valid until the newborn has ingested an ample amount (for 2 or 3 days) of the amino acid phenylalanine, which is a constituent of both human and cow's milk. If the child is not eating well or does not weigh at least 5 pounds, the test should not be done, because results may be invalid. The urine PKU test is normally done after 6 weeks of age if, for some reason, a blood test was not done in the hospital. If the tests are positive, a blood phenylalanine test should be performed.

Interfering Factors

- Premature infants may have false-positive results as a result of delayed development of liver enzymes such as phenylalanine hydroxylase.
- Ketonuria can produce an altered urine color reaction.
- Infants tested before 24 hours of age may have false-negative results, because they have not ingested enough milk containing phenylalanine.
- Feeding problems (e.g., vomiting) may cause false-negative results, because the infant may not have tolerated enough milk containing phenylalanine.
- Drugs that may influence screening results include antibiotics, aspirin, and salicylates.

CLINICAL PRIORITIES

- PKU is an autosomal recessive inherited disease that results in mental retardation if not diagnosed and treated early. In infants with PKU, Lofenalac is substituted for milk.
- Routine screening for PKU is mandatory in most states. Screening is not valid if the newborn has not ingested an adequate amount of phenylalanine, which is a constituent of human's and cow's milk.
- If the PKU blood test was not done within several days of birth, a urine PKU test can be done after 6 weeks of age. This is usually done at the infant's first checkup.

Procedure and Patient Care

Before

- Inform the mother about the purpose and value of the test and the method of performance.
- Assess the infant's feeding patterns before performing the PKU test. An inadequate amount of protein ingested before performing the test can cause false-negative results.

During

- Place a few drops of blood from a heel stick onto a special piece of filter paper for the Guthrie test. This test is performed after the newborn has ingested an ample amount (for 2 to 3 days) of milk containing phenylalanine.

- Indicate on the laboratory slip the present date and time, date and time of birth, and time of first milk feeding.
- Note that *urine tests* also may be used to detect PKU in infants who are at least 6 weeks of age. These tests are usually done at the infant's first checkup:
  1. For the *diaper test,* drop 10% ferric chloride on a diaper that contains fresh urine. A green spot indicates probable PKU.
  2. For the *Phenistix test,* press a test stick against a diaper containing urine or dip the stick in the urine. A green color reaction indicates probable PKU.

After

- If test results are positive, inform the mother that dietary control must begin immediately to prevent brain damage to the infant. This is done by substituting Lofenalac for milk. Later, strained foods low in protein are added to the infant's diet. The dietary treatment is monitored by blood and urine testing.
- Instruct women with PKU who wish to have children to begin a low-phenylalanine diet before conception and continue throughout the pregnancy. The risk of producing a mentally retarded infant is very high if the mother remains on a general diet.

Test Results and Clinical Significance

Increased levels

PKU *Inadequate amounts of phenylalanine hydroxylase are present to break down phenylalanine.*
Low-birth-weight infants *These children may have inadequate liver enzyme synthesis, including phenylalanine hydroxylase.*
Hepatic encephalopathy *These children lack phenylalanine hydroxylase along with several other enzymes.*

Phosphate (P), Inorganic Phosphorus (PO_4)

Normal Findings

Adult: 3.0-4.5 mg/dl or 0.97-1.45 mmol/L (SI units)
Elderly: values slightly lower than adult
Child: 4.5-6.5 mg/dl or 1.45-2.10 mmol/L (SI units)
Newborn: 4.3-9.3 mg/dl or 1.4-3.0 mmol/L (SI units)

Critical Values: <1 mg/dl

Indications

This test is performed to assist in the interpretation of studies investigating parathyroid and calcium abnormalities. It is usually done to measure phosphate levels and ensure that adequate blood levels exist.

Test Explanation

Phosphorus in the body is in the form of a phosphate. Phosphorus and phosphate will be used interchangeably throughout this and other discussions. Most of the phosphate in the body is a part of organic compounds. Only a small part of total body phosphate is inorganic phosphate (i.e., not part of another organic compound). It is the *inorganic* phosphate that is measured when a "phosphate," "phosphorus," "inorganic phosphorus," or "inorganic phosphate" is requested. Most of the body's inorganic phosphorus is combined with calcium within the skeleton; however, approximately 15% of the phosphorus exists in the blood as a phosphate salt. The organic phosphate (not measured by this test) is used to synthesize part of the phospholipid compounds in the cell membrane, adenosine triphosphatase (ATP) for energy source in metabolism, nucleic acids, or enzymes (e.g., 2,3-diphoshoglycerate). The inorganic phosphate (measured in this test) contributes to electrical and acid-base homeostasis.

Dietary phosphorus is absorbed in the small bowel. The absorption is very efficient, and only rarely is hypophosphatemia caused by GI malabsorption. Antacids, however, can bind phosphorus and decrease intestinal absorption. Renal excretion of phosphorus should equal dietary intake to maintain a normal serum phosphate level. Phosphate levels vary significantly during the day, with lowest values occurring around 10 AM and highest values occurring 12 hours later.

Phosphorus levels are determined by calcium metabolism, parathormone (parathyroid hormone [PTH]), renal excretion, and, to a lesser degree, intestinal absorption. Because an inverse relationship exists between calcium and phosphorus, a decrease of one mineral results in an increase in the other. Therefore, serum phosphorus levels depend on calcium metabolism and vice versa. The regulation of phosphate by PTH is such that PTH tends to decrease phosphate reabsorption in the kidney. PTH and vitamin D, however, tend to stimulate phosphate absorption weakly within the gut.

Interfering Factors

- Laxatives or enemas containing sodium phosphate can *increase* phosphorus levels.
- Recent carbohydrate ingestion, including IV glucose administration, causes *decreased* phosphorus levels, because phosphorus enters the cell with glucose.
- Drugs that may cause *increased* levels include methicillin, steroids, some diuretics (furosemide and thiazides), and vitamin D (excessive).
- Drug that may cause *decreased* levels include antacids, albuterol, anesthesia agents, estrogens, insulin, oral contraceptives, and mannitol.

Procedure and Patient Care

Before

- Explain the procedure to the patient.
- Keep the patient on NPO status after midnight on the day of the test.
- If indicated, discontinue IV fluids with glucose for several hours before the test.

During

- Collect approximately 5 to 10 ml of venous blood in a red-top tube.

- Avoid hemolysis. Handle the tube carefully. Hemolysis can falsely elevate the phosphate level because phosphate is an intracellular ion. Cellular lysis of RBCs will cause the intracellular phosphate to spill into the blood.
- Use a heel stick to draw blood from infants.

After

- Take the specimen to the laboratory immediately.
- Indicate on the laboratory slip the time the blood was obtained.
- Apply pressure or a pressure dressing to the venipuncture site.
- Check the venipuncture site for bleeding.

Test Results and Clinical Significance

Increased levels (hyperphosphatemia)

Hypoparathyroidism *Renal reabsorption is enhanced.*

Renal failure *Renal excretion of phosphates is diminished.*

Increased dietary or IV intake of phosphorus *The increased intake obviously leads to transiently elevated phosphate levels.*

Acromegaly *Renal reabsorption is enhanced.*

Bone metastasis *The phosphate stores in the bones are mobilized by the destructive bone tumors.*

Sarcoidosis *Intestinal absorption of phosphates is increased because of the vitamin D effect produced by granulomatous infections.*

Hypocalcemia *Calcium and phosphates exist in an inverse relationship. When one is elevated, the other is low.*

Acidosis *When the pH is reduced, phosphates are driven out of the cell and into the bloodstream as part of a buffering system.*

Rhabdomyolysis
Advanced lymphoma or myeloma
Hemolytic anemia
Cell lysis associated with the above diseases causes intracellular phosphate to pour out into the bloodstream. Phosphate levels rise.

Decreased levels (hypophosphatemia)

Inadequate dietary ingestion of phosphorus *This is very rare, because phosphate reabsorption in the intestine is so efficient.*

Chronic antacid ingestion *Antacids bind the phosphate in the intestine and preclude absorption.*

Hyperparathyroidism *PTH increases urinary excretion of phosphates.*

Hypercalcemia *Calcium and phosphate levels have an inverse relationship. When one is elevated, the other is low.*

Chronic alcoholism *The pathophysiology of this observation is probably due to multiple causes. It may be, in part, nutritional and, in part, due to magnesium deficiency.*

Vitamin D deficiency (rickets) *Renal tubules fail to reabsorb phosphates.*

Treatment of hyperglycemia
Hyperinsulinism (childhood)
Insulin tends to drive phosphates into the cells.

Malnutrition *Rarely is malnutrition a cause of phosphate deficiency, because it is so efficiently absorbed through the intestine. However, when malnutrition is associated with a deficiency of fat-soluble vitamins such as vitamin D, phosphate renal reabsorption is diminished. Phosphate levels decrease.*

Alkalosis *Phosphate acts as a buffer. When pH increases, phosphate levels in the blood diminish because of an intracellular shift.*

Gram-negative sepsis

Related Tests

- Parathyroid hormone (p. 316): This is a measurement of parathyroid hormone, which raises serum phosphate and calcium levels.
- Calcium, blood (p. 130): This is a direct measurement of serum calcium. This test should be done simultaneously with phosphate measurements.

Plasminogen (Fibrinolysin)

Normal Findings

2.5-4.5 mmol/ml or 6.1 ± 2.3 Committee on Thrombolytic Agents (CTA) units

Indications

This test is used to diagnose suspected plasminogen deficiency in patients who present with multiple thromboembolic episodes.

Test Explanation

Plasminogen is a protein involved in the fibrinolytic process of intravascular blood clot dissolution (see Figure 2-10 on p. 156). Plasminogen is converted to plasmin by proteolytic cleavage. This reaction can be catalyzed by urokinase, streptokinase, or tissue plasminogen activator (t-PA). Plasmin can destroy fibrin and dissolve clots. This fibrinolytic system helps maintain a normal homeostatic balance between coagulation and anticoagulation.

Plasminogen levels are occasionally measured during fibrinolytic therapy (for coronary and peripheral arterial occlusion) and are diminished. Decreased levels of plasminogen are also found in hyperfibrinolytic states (e.g., disseminated intravascular coagulation [DIC], primary fibrinolysis), because the plasminogen is used up. Because plasminogen is made in the liver, patients with cirrhosis or other severe liver diseases can be expected to have decreased levels. There are also rare cases of hereditary deficiencies of this protein. Decreased plasminogen levels put a patient at great risk for arterial or venous thrombosis.

Pregnancy and especially eclampsia are associated with increased levels of plasminogen. Patients with inflammatory conditions that may be associated with increased levels of C-reactive protein also may have concomitant mild elevations of plasminogens, which are acute-phase reactant proteins.

Procedure and Patient Care

Before

- Explain the procedure to the patient.
- Tell the patient that no fasting is required.

During

- Collect a venous blood sample in a blue-top tube containing sodium citrate.
- Avoid excessive agitation of the blood sample.

After

- Apply pressure or a pressure dressing to the venipuncture site.
- Assess the venipuncture site for bleeding, especially if the patient is suspected of having a hyperfibrinolytic process (e.g., DIC).

Test Results and Clinical Significance

Increased levels

Pregnancy *The pathophysiology of this observation is not well known. It may relate to amniotic proteins gaining access to the maternal circulation.*

Decreased levels

Hyperfibrinolytic state (e.g., DIC, fibrinolysis)

Primary liver disease *Plasminogen is made in the liver. With severe liver disease, synthesis will not occur.*

Syndrome associated with hypercoagulation (e.g., venous and arterial clotting) *This syndrome can occur with many different types of diseases (e.g., colon cancer).*

Congenital deficiencies of plasminogen *Although rare, such deficiencies can occur and place the patient at great risk for thromboembolic episodes.*

Malnutrition *With severe malnutrition, protein depletion is so great as to interrupt plasminogen production.*

Related Tests

- Euglobulin lysis time (p. 207): This is a measure of the activity of the fibrinolytic system. It is an older test used to identify abnormal fibrinolysins that may be occurring in patients with certain diseases. It can also be used to monitor thrombolytic therapy.

Platelet Aggregation

Normal Findings Vary with platelet agonist used

Indications

This test is a measure of platelet function and aids in the evaluation of bleeding disorders.

Test Explanation

Platelet aggregation is important in hemostasis. A clump of platelets surrounds an area of acute blood vessel endothelial injury. Normal platelets adhere to this area of injury, and through a series of chemical reactions, they attract other platelets to the area. This is platelet aggregation, the first step in hemostasis. After this step the normal coagulation factor waterfall occurs. Certain diseases that affect either platelet number or function can inhibit platelet aggregation and thereby prolong bleeding times. Congenital syndromes, uremia, myeloproliferative disorders, and drugs are associated with abnormal platelet aggregation. If blood is passed through a heart-lung or dialysis pump, platelet injury can occur and aggregation capability can be reduced.

Many agonists are used to stimulate platelet aggregation in the laboratory. Platelet aggregation is measured by determining the turbidity of platelet-rich plasma. As platelet aggregation is stimulated in vitro, turbidity decreases and light transmission through the specimen increases. This test is performed with an optical device called an aggregometer. Usually the patient's blood specimen is spun to a platelet-rich component. Next, an agonist to platelet aggregation, such as adenosine diphosphate, collagen, epinephrine, or ristocetin, is added. Turbidity is then measured within the aggregometer, and a curve indicating light transmission per unit of time is plotted. Normal curves have been identified for any one agonist that is used.

This is a very sensitive test, and it can be significantly affected by a number of variables, including:

1. Concentration of sodium citrate
2. Platelet count
3. Storage temperature
4. Concentration of the agonist addition
5. Reaction temperature
6. Degrees of lipemia, hemoglobinemia, or bilirubinemia

Interfering Factors

- Factors that may cause *increased* platelet aggregation include blood storage temperature, hyperbilirubinemia, hemoglobinemia, hyperlipidemia, and platelet count.
- Drugs that may cause *decreased* platelet aggregation include aspirin, some antibiotics, beta blockers, clofibrate, dextran, ethanol, heparin, nonsteroidal antiinflammatory drugs (NSAIDs), phenothiazines, tricyclics, theophylline sodium warfarin (Coumadin), and heparin.

Procedure and Patient Care

Before

- Explain the procedure to the patient.
- Tell the patient that no fasting is required.

During

- Collect 5 to 7 ml of venous blood in a blue-top tube.
- If the patient is receiving any drugs that may interfere with platelet aggregation or has any diseases such as jaundice, hyperlipidemia, or hemolysis, this should be listed on the laboratory request slip.

After

- Apply pressure or a pressure dressing to the venipuncture site.
- Assess the venipuncture site for bleeding.
- Remember that abnormalities in platelet aggregation can prolong bleeding time, and a significant hematoma at the venipuncture site may occur.

Test Results and Clinical Significance

Prolonged platelet aggregation

Various congenital disorders (e.g., Glanzmann's, von Willebrand's disease) *Platelet aggregation is diminished in autosomal recessive diseases.*

Connective tissue disorder (e.g., lupus erythematosus) *The pathophysiology of these observations is not understood.*

Recent cardiopulmonary or dialysis bypass *Platelet injury develops as the platelets are passing through this machinery. The injured platelets are less likely to function normally in regard to aggregation.*

Uremia *Not only is there a reduced platelet number in uremic patients, but a reduced aggregation capability has also been observed.*

Various myeloproliferative diseases, including leukemia, myeloma, and dysproteinemia *The pathophysiology of these observations is not clear. It may be related to abnormal antibodies affecting the platelet membrane.*

Drugs (e.g., aspirin) *Drugs can have an immediate and in some cases long-lasting negative effect on platelet aggregation.*

Related Tests

- Clot retraction (p. 151): This is a qualitative assessment of platelet number and function.
- Platelet count (p. 337): This is a direct measurement of platelet number.
- Platelet antibody (p. 335): This test identifies antibodies directed against platelets.
- Bleeding time (p. 115): This test of coagulation is affected by platelet number and function.
- Platelet volume, mean (p. 340): This is a measurement of the size of the platelets. It is helpful in the evaluation of thrombocytopenia.

Platelet Antibody
(Antiplatelet Antibody Detection)

Normal Findings No antiplatelet antibodies identified

Indications

This test is used to evaluate thrombocytopenia and exclude an immune-associated etiology.

Test Explanation

Immune-mediated destruction of platelets may be caused by either autoantibodies directed against antigens located on the same person's platelets or alloantibodies that develop after exposure to transfused platelets received from a donor. These antibodies are usually directed to an antigen on the platelet membrane, such as human leukocyte antigen (HLA) (see p. 264) or platelet-specific antigen (e.g., PLA1, PLA2). Many different laboratory techniques can be used to demonstrate the antiplatelet antibodies. These tests can directly identify the immunoglobulin with the use of radioimmunoassay or immunofluorescence. Quantitative measurements are possible with cytofluorometry. Other tests identify complement binding on the affected platelet membrane. Most antiplatelet antibody testing is now performed using immunologic assays.

Antibodies directed to platelets will cause early destruction of the platelets and subsequent thrombocytopenia. Immunologic thrombocytopenia includes the following:

1. *Idiopathic thrombocytopenia purpura (ITP)* is a term that describes a group of disorders characterized by immune-mediated destruction of the platelets within the spleen or other reticuloendothelial organs. Platelet-associated IgG antibodies are detected in 90% of these patients.
2. *Posttransfusion purpura* is a rare syndrome characterized by the sudden onset of severe thrombocytopenia a few hours to a few days after transfusion of RBCs or platelets. This is usually associated with an antibody to ABO, HLA, or PLA antigens on the RBC. In most situations the blood recipient has previously been sensitized to a PLA1 antigen during previous transfusions or during previous pregnancy. Once these antibodies form, they destroy the donor's PLA1-positive platelets and the recipient's PLA-negative platelets.
3. *Maternal-fetal platelet antigen incompatibility* (neonatal thrombocytopenia) occurs when the fetal platelet contains a PLA1 antigen that is absent in the mother. Just like Rh RBC incompatibility, the mother creates anti-PLA1 antibodies that cross the placenta and destroy the fetal platelets. The mother is not thrombocytopenic. Neonatal thrombocytopenia can also occur if the mother has ITP autoantibodies that are passed through the placenta and destroy the fetal platelets also.
4. *Drug-induced thrombocytopenia* is usually caused by platelet-associated IgG antibodies. These antibodies are the result of a hypersensitivity to certain drugs. A host of drugs are known to induce autoimmune-mediated thrombocytopenia. They are *cimetidine,* analgesics (salicylates, acetaminophen), antibiotics (cephalosporins, penicillin, *sulfonamides*), *quinidine*-like drugs, hypnotics (phenobarbital), oral hypo-

glycemic agents (e.g., chlorpropamide), heavy metals (e.g., gold, organic arsenicals), diuretics (e.g., chlorothiazide), and others (e.g., digoxin, propylthiouracil, Antabuse, *heparin*). Those medications in italics are the most common offenders.

Procedure and Patient Care

Before

- Explain the procedure to the patient.
- Tell the patient that no fasting is required.

During

- Collect 10 to 30 ml of blood in a red-top tube. The amount of blood required depends on the initial platelet count.

After

- Apply pressure or a pressure dressing to the venipuncture site.
- Ensure adequate hemostasis in all patients who are suspected of having thrombocytopenia.
- A platelet count is usually done 1 to 2 hours after platelet transfusion. This not only documents the posttransfusion platelet count, but also eliminates a large proportion of posttransfusion immune thrombocytopenia reactions.

Test Results and Clinical Significance

Increased levels

Immune thrombocytopenia
  Idiopathic thrombocytopenia purpura
  Neonatal thrombocytopenia
  Posttransfusion purpura
  Drug-induced thrombocytopenia

The pathophysiology of these diseases is described in the section Test Explanation.

Related Tests

- Clot retraction (p. 151): This is a qualitative assessment of platelet number and function.
- Platelet count (p. 337): This is a direct measurement of platelet number.
- Platelet aggregation (p. 333): This is a test of platelet function.
- Bleeding time (p. 115): This test of coagulation is affected by platelet number and function.
- Platelet volume, mean (p. 340): This is a measurement of the size of the platelets. It is helpful in the evaluation of thrombocytopenia.

Platelet Count (Thrombocyte Count)

Normal Findings

Adult/elderly: 150,000-400,000/mm^3 or 150-400 $\times$ 10^9/L (SI units)
Child: 150,000-400,000/mm^3
Infant: 200,000-475,000 mm^3
Premature infant: 100,000-300,000/mm^3
Newborn: 150,000-300,000/mm^3

Critical Values

<50,000 or >1 million/mm^3

Indications

The platelet count is an actual count of the number of platelets (thrombocytes) per cubic milliliter of blood. It is performed on all patients who develop petechiae (small hemorrhages in the skin), spontaneous bleeding, increasingly heavy menses, or thrombocytopenia. It is used to monitor the course of the disease or therapy for thrombocytopenia or bone marrow failure.

Test Explanation

Platelets are formed in the bone marrow from megakaryocytes. They are small, round, nonnucleated cells whose main role is maintenance of vascular integrity. In blood vessel injury, hemostasis is required to form a clot that will durably plug the hole until healing can occur. The primary phase of the hemostatic mechanism involves platelet aggregation. From there, the platelets help initiate the coagulation factor waterfall. Most of the platelets exist in the bloodstream. A smaller percentage (25%) exists in the liver and spleen. Survival of platelets is measured in days (average of 7 to 9 days).

Platelet activity is essential to blood clotting. Counts of 150,000 to 400,000/mm^3 are considered normal. Counts of less than 100,000/mm^3 are considered to indicate *thrombocytopenia; thrombocytosis* is said to exist when counts are greater than 400,000/mm^3. *Thrombocythemia* is a term used to indicate a platelet count in excess of 1 million/mm^3. Vascular thrombosis with tissue or organ infarction is the major complication of thrombocythemia. The most common disease associated with spontaneous thrombocytosis is malignancy (leukemia, lymphoma, solid tumors such as colon). Thrombocytosis may also occur with polycythemia vera and postsplenectomy syndromes. It should be noted that even patients with elevated platelet counts can experience a bleeding tendency because the function (platelet aggregation) of those platelets may be abnormal. It is not at all uncommon for patients whose platelet counts exceed 1 million to experience spontaneous bleeding and thrombocytosis.

Spontaneous hemorrhage may occur with thrombocytopenia. If thrombocytopenia is severe, the platelets are often hand counted. Spontaneous bleeding is a serious danger when platelet counts fall below 20,000/mm^3. Petechiae and ecchymosis will also occur at that degree of thrombocytopenia. With counts above 40,000/mm^3, spontaneous bleeding rarely occurs, but prolonged bleeding from trauma or surgery may occur with counts at this level.

Causes of thrombocytopenia include:

1. Reduced production of platelets (secondary to bone marrow failure or infiltration of fibrosis, tumor, etc.)
2. Sequestration of platelets (secondary to hypersplenism)
3. Accelerated destruction of platelets (secondary to antibodies, infections, drugs, prosthetic heart valves)
4. Consumption of platelets (secondary to disseminated intravascular coagulation [DIC])
5. Platelet loss from hemorrhage
6. Dilution with large volumes of blood transfusions containing very few, if any, platelets

Interfering Factors

- Living in high altitudes may cause increased platelet levels.
- Because platelets can clump together, automated counting is subject to at least a 10% to 15% error.
- Strenuous exercise may cause increased levels.
- Decreased levels may be seen before menstruation.
- Drugs that may cause *increased* levels include estrogens and oral contraceptives.
- Drugs that may cause *decreased* levels include acetaminophen, aspirin, chemotherapeutic agents, chloramphenicol, colchicine, H_2-blocking agents (cimetidine, Zantac), hydralazine, indomethacin, isoniazid (INH), quinidine, streptomycin, sulfonamides, thiazide diuretics, and tolbutamide (Orinase).

Procedure and Patient Care

Before

- Explain the procedure to the patient.
- Tell the patient that no fasting is required.

During

- Collect approximately 5 to 7 ml of peripheral venous blood in a lavender-top tube.
- List on the laboratory slip any drugs or other factors that may affect test results.

After

- Apply pressure or a pressure dressing to the venipuncture site.
- Assess the venipuncture site for bleeding.
- If the results indicate that the patient has a serious platelet deficiency:
  1. Observe the patient for signs and symptoms of bleeding.
  2. Check for blood in the urine and all excretions.
  3. Assess the patient for bruises, petechiae, bleeding from the gums, epistaxis, and low-back pain.
  4. Reassess all venipuncture sites for sign of hematoma formation.

Test Results and Clinical Significance

Increased levels (thrombocytosis)

Malignant disorders (leukemia, lymphoma, solid tumors such as colon) *The pathophysiology of this observation is not known.*

Polycythemia vera *This is a hyperplasia of all the marrow cell lines, including platelets.*

Postsplenectomy syndrome *The spleen normally extracts aging platelets from the bloodstream. With surgical splenectomy, that job is less effectively done by other organs (liver, etc). As a result, the platelet count increases.*

Rheumatoid arthritis *The pathophysiology of this observation is not known.*

Iron deficiency anemia or following hemorrhagic anemia *Iron is not needed for platelet production. Anemia causes maximal stimulation of cellular production by the marrow. RBCs may not be so easily produced in light of iron deficiency. The platelet, however, can easily respond even in the presence of iron deficiency.*

Decreased levels (thrombocytopenia)

Hypersplenism *The spleen normally extracts aging platelets from the bloodstream. An enlarged spleen, however, extracts more platelets, both aging and new. The platelet count diminishes.*

Hemorrhage *The platelets are lost in the bleeding process. If not replaced by transfusion of platelets, it will take some time (hours to days) for the marrow to produce an adequate number of platelets. This problem is exacerbated with treatment that replenishes blood volume and RBC count. This treatment dilutes the remaining platelets and further decreases the platelet count.*

Immune thrombocytopenia (e.g., idiopathic thrombocytopenia, neonatal, posttransfusion, or drug-induced thrombocytopenia) *Antibodies directed against antigens on the platelet cell membrane destroy the platelet and the count decreases.*

Leukemia and other myelofibrosis disorders *The marrow is replaced by neoplastic or fibrotic tissue. Megakaryocyte function and numbers diminish. Platelets are not produced, and the count drops.*

Thrombotic thrombocytopenia *This disease and others such as HELLP (hemolysis [H], elevated liver enzymes [EL], low platelet count [LP]) syndrome are highlighted by thrombocytopenia, hemolytic anemia, and other hematologic abnormalities.*

Graves' disease *In a small number of these patient, thrombocytopenia occurs. The pathophysiology of this observation is not known.*

Inherited disorders (e.g., Wiskott Aldrich, Bernard-Soulier, Zieve syndromes) *The pathophysiology of this observation is not known.*

DIC *The pathophysiology of thrombocytopenia is not clear. In part, however, it is thought that ongoing thrombosis "consumes" the platelets much like coagulating factors are "consumed." DIC usually develops concurrently with other severe disease (e.g., gram-negative sepsis) that can also produce thrombocytopenia.*

Systemic lupus erythematosus *The pathophysiology of this observation is not known.*

Pernicious anemia *Unlike iron, vitamin* B_{12} is necessary for platelet production. A deficiency of this vitamin or folate will diminish the production of platelets.

Hemolytic anemia *Often the same disease process that produces the hemolysis (e.g., hemolytic-uremic syndrome) also destroys the platelets. The platelet count falls.*

Cancer chemotherapy *Cytotoxic drugs often affect the bone marrow. Platelets are not produced at adequate levels, and the count drops.*

Infection *Bacterial, viral, and rickettsial infections can cause thrombocytopenia, especially when the patient is immunocompromised (e.g., AIDS).*

Related Tests

- Platelet aggregation (p. 333): This is a test of platelet function.
- Platelet antibody (p. 335): This test identifies antibodies directed against platelets.
- Bleeding time (p. 115): This test of coagulation is affected by platelet number and function.
- Platelet volume, mean (p. 340): This is a measurement of the size of the platelets. It is helpful in the evaluation of thrombocytopenia.
- Clot retraction (p. 151): This is a qualitative assessment of platelet number and function.

Platelet Volume, Mean
(Mean Platelet Volume [MPV])

Normal Findings 25 μm in diameter

Indications

This test is helpful in the evaluation of platelet disorders, especially thrombocytopenia.

Test Explanation

The MPV is a measure of the volume of a large number of platelets determined by an automated analyzer. MPV is to platelets as mean corpuscular volume (see p. 376) is to the RBC.

The MPV varies with total platelet production. In cases of thrombocytopenia despite a normal reactive bone marrow (e.g., hypersplenism), the normal bone marrow releases immature platelets in an attempt to maintain a normal platelet count. These immature platelets are larger, and the MPV is increased. When bone marrow production of platelets is inadequate, the platelets that are released are small. This will be reflected as a low MPV; this makes the MPV very useful in the differential diagnosis of thrombocytopenic disorders.

Interfering Factors

- Blood collection tubes with ethylene diaminetetraacetic acid can create a variation of as much as 25% in the size of the platelets.

Procedure and Patient Care

Before

- Explain the procedure to the patient.
- Tell the patient that no fasting is required.

During

- Collect 5 to 7 ml of venous blood in a lavender-top tube.

After

- Apply pressure or a pressure dressing to the venipuncture site.
- Assess the venipuncture site for bleeding.
- If the patient is known to have a low platelet count:
  1. Observe the patient for signs and symptoms of bleeding.
  2. Check for blood in the urine and all excretions.
  3. Assess the patient for bruises, petechiae, bleeding of the gums, epistaxis, and low-back pain.

Test Results and Clinical Significance

Increased volume

Valvular heart disease
Immune thrombocytopenia (e.g., idiopathic thrombocytopenia, neonatal, posttransfusion, or drug induced-thrombocytopenia)
Massive hemorrhage
The above illness are all associated with thrombocytopenia and a normally reactive bone marrow that will produce a great number of immature platelets in an attempt to maintain a normal platelet count. These immature platelets are large and increase the MPV.

Vitamin B_{12} or folate deficiency *Megaloblastic changes affect the megakaryocyte just as the erythroid line is affected. The platelets that are produced are larger and may even be nucleated. The MPV is increased.*

Myelogenous leukemia *Large, abnormal platelets are formed by neoplastic megakaryocytes if they are involved in the leukemic process. The MPV will increase.*

Decreased volume

Aplastic anemia
Chemotherapy-induced myelosuppression
When bone marrow production of platelets is inadequate, the platelets that are released are small. MPV will be reduced.

Wiskott-Aldrich syndrome *This syndrome is characterized by eczema, immune deficiency, thrombocytopenia, and small platelets.*

Related Tests

- Platelet aggregation (p. 333): This is a test of platelet function.
- Platelet antibody (p. 335): This test identifies antibodies directed against platelets.
- Platelet count (p. 337): This is a direct measurement of the number of platelets.
- Clot retraction (p. 151): This is a qualitative assessment of platelet number and function.
- Bleeding time (p. 115): This test of coagulation is affected by platelet number and function.

Potassium, Blood (K)

Normal Findings

Adult/elderly: 3.5-5.0 mEq/L or 3.5-5.0 mmol/L (SI units)
Child: 3.4-4.7 mEq/L
Infant: 4.1-5.3 mEq/L
Newborn: 3.9-5.9 mEq/L

Critical Values

Adult: <2.5 or >6.5 mEq/L
Newborn: <2.5 or >8.0 mEq/L

Indications

This test is routinely performed in most patients investigated for any type of serious illness. Furthermore, because this electrolyte is so important to cardiac function, it is a part of all complete routine evaluations, especially in patients who take diuretics or heart medications.

Test Explanation

K is the major cation within the cell. The intracellular K concentration is approximately 150 mEq/L, whereas the normal serum K concentration is approximately 4 mEq/L. This ratio is the most important determinant in maintaining membrane electrical potential, especially in neuromuscular tissue. Because the serum concentration of potassium is so small, minor changes in concentration have significant consequences. K is excreted by the kidneys. There is no reabsorption of K from the kidneys. Therefore, if K is not adequately supplied in the diet (or by IV administration in the patient who is unable to eat), serum K levels can drop rapidly.

K is an important part of protein synthesis and maintenance of normal oncotic pressure and cellular electrical neutrality as indicated above. It contributes to the metabolic portion of acid-base balance in that the kidneys can shift K^+ for H^+ ions to maintain a physiologic pH.

Serum potassium concentration depends on many factors, including:

1. *Aldosterone* (and, to a lesser extent, glucocorticosteroids). This hormone tends to increase renal losses of K.
2. *Sodium reabsorption.* As sodium is reabsorbed, potassium is lost.
3. *Acid-base balance.* Alkalotic states tend to lower serum K levels by causing a shift of K into the cell. Acidotic states tend to raise serum K levels by reversing that shift.

Symptoms of *hyperkalemia* include irritability, nausea, vomiting, intestinal colic, and diarrhea. The electrocardiogram may demonstrate peaked T waves, a widened QRS complex, and a depressed ST segment. Signs of *hypokalemia* are related to a decrease in contractility of smooth, skeletal, and cardiac muscles, which results in weakness, paralysis, hyporeflexia, ileus, increased cardiac sensitivity to digoxin, cardiac arrhythmias (dysrhythmias), flattened T waves, and prominent U waves. This electrolyte has profound effects on the heart rate and contractility. The K level should be carefully followed in patients with uremia, Addison's disease, and vomiting and diarrhea and in patients taking steroid therapy and K-depleting diuretics. K must be closely monitored in patients taking digitalis-like drugs, because cardiac arrhythmias may be induced by hypokalemia and digoxin.

Interfering Factors

- Open and closing of the hand with a tourniquet in place may increase K levels.
- Hemolysis of blood during venipuncture or during laboratory processing causes increased levels.
- Drugs that may cause *increased* K levels include aminocaproic acid, antibiotics, antineoplastic drugs, captopril, epinephrine, heparin, histamine, isoniazid (INH), lithium, mannitol, K-sparing diuretics, K supplements, and succinylcholine.
- Drugs that may cause *decreased* levels include acetazolamide, aminosalicylic acid, glucose infusions, amphotericin B, carbenicillin, cisplatin, diuretics (K wasting), insulin, laxatives, lithium carbonate, penicillin G sodium (high doses), phenothiazines, salicylates (aspirin), and sodium polystyrene sulfonate (Kayexalate).

CLINICAL PRIORITIES

- This electrolyte has profound effects on the heart rate and contractility. K levels must be carefully monitored in patients taking digitalis-like drugs and diuretics, because cardiac arrhythmias may be induced by hypokalemia.
- Serum K levels are affected by acid-base balance. Alkalotic states lower K levels and acidotic levels raise levels.
- Hemolysis of blood during venipuncture or during laboratory processing can cause elevations.

Procedure and Patient Care

Before

- Explain the procedure to the patient.
- Tell the patient that no special diet or fasting is required.

During

- Instruct the patient to avoid opening and closing the hand after a tourniquet is applied.
- Collect approximately 5 to 7 ml of venous blood in a red- or green-top tube.
- Avoid hemolysis.
- Indicate on the laboratory slip any drugs that may affect test results.

After

- Apply pressure or a pressure dressing to the venipuncture site.
- Assess the venipuncture site for bleeding.
- Evaluate the patient with increased or decreased K levels for cardiac arrhythmias.
- Monitor patients taking digoxin and diuretics for hypokalemia.
- If indicated, administer resin exchanges (e.g., Kayexalate enema) to correct hyperkalemia.

Test Results and Clinical Significance

Increased levels (hyperkalemia)

Excessive dietary intake
Excessive IV intake
Because the amount of K in the serum is so small, minimal but significant increases in K intake can cause elevations in the serum level.

Acute or chronic renal failure *This is the most common cause of hyperkalemia. K excretion is diminished, and K levels rise.*

Addison's disease
Hypoaldosteronism
Aldosterone-inhibiting diuretics (e.g., spironolactone, triamterene)
Aldosterone excretion is absent. Aldosterone enhances K excretion. Without that effect, K excretion is diminished and K levels rise.

Crush injury to tissues
Hemolysis
Transfusion of hemolyzed blood
Infection
Potassium exists in high levels in the cell. With cellular injury and lysis, the K within the cell is released into the bloodstream.

Acidosis *To maintain physiologic pH during acidosis,* H^+ *ions are driven from the blood and into the cell. To maintain electrical neutrality,* K^+ *is expelled from the cell. K levels rise.*
Dehydration *The K becomes more concentrated in dehydrated patients, and serum levels appear to be elevated. When rehydrated, K levels may in fact be reduced.*

Decreased levels (hypokalemia)

Deficient dietary intake
Deficient IV intake
The kidneys cannot reabsorb K to compensate for the reduced K intake. K levels decline.

Burns
GI disorders (e.g., diarrhea, vomiting, villous adenomas)
Excessive K is lost because of ongoing fluid and electrolyte losses as indicated above.

Diuretics *These medications act to increase renal excretion of K. This is especially important for cardiac patients who take diuretics and digitalis preparations. Hypokalemia can exacerbate the ectopy that digoxin may instigate.*
Hyperaldosteronism *Aldosterone enhances K excretion.*
Cushing's syndrome *Glucocorticosteroids have an "aldosterone-like" effect.*

Renal tubular acidosis *Renal excretion of K is increased.*
Licorice ingestion *Licorice has an "aldosterone-like" effect.*
Alkalosis *To maintain physiologic pH during alkalosis, H^+ ions are driven out of the cell and into the blood. To maintain electrical neutrality, K^+ is driven into the cell. K levels fall.*
Insulin administration *In patients with hyperglycemia, insulin is administered. Glucose and K are driven into the cell. K levels drop.*
Glucose administration *In a normal person, insulin is secreted in response to glucose administration. Glucose and K are driven into the cell. K levels drop.*
Ascites *These patient have a decreased renal blood flow from reduced intravascular volume that results from the collection of fluid. The reduced blood flow stimulates the secretion of aldosterone, which increases K excretion. Furthermore, these patients are often taking K-wasting diuretics.*
Renal artery stenosis *These patients have a reduced renal blood flow. The pathophysiology is as described above.*
Cystic fibrosis *These patients have increased K loss in secretions and sweat.*
Trauma/surgery/burns *The body's response to trauma is mediated, in part, by aldosterone, which increases K excretion.*

Related Tests

- Sodium, blood, (p. 396), and chloride, blood (p. 141): These electrolytes are often measured with K. Metabolically, they are all intermingled.
- Potassium, urine (p. 847): This is used to identify increased K excretion.

Prealbumin (PAB, Thyroxine-Binding Prealbumin [TBPA], Thyretin, Transthyretin)

Normal Findings

Blood

Adult/elderly: 15-36 mg/dl or 150-360 mg/L (SI units)
Child
Cord: 13 mg/dl or 130 mg/L (SI units)
1 year: 10 mg/dl or 100 mg/L
2-36 months: 16-28 mg/dl or 160-280 mg/L

Urine (24-hour): 0.017-0.047 mg/day
CSF: approximately 2% of total CSF protein

Critical Values

Serum prealbumin levels <10.7 mg/dl indicate severe nutritional deficiency.

Indications

This test is used to indicate a person's nutritional status. It is also used to indicate liver function status.

Test Explanation

Prealbumin is one of the major plasma proteins. Because prealbumin can bind thyroxine, it is also called thyroxine-binding prealbumin. However, prealbumin is secondary to thyroxine-binding globulin in the transportation of triiodothyronine (T_3) and thyroxine (T_4). Prealbumin also plays a role in the transport and metabolism of vitamin A. Prealbumin is measured by immunoassay.

Since prealbumin levels in serum fluctuate more rapidly in response to alterations in synthetic rate than do those of other serum proteins, clinical interest in the quantification of serum prealbumin has centered on its usefulness as a marker of nutritional status. Its half-life of 1.9 days is much less than the 21-day half-life of albumin (see p. 358). Because of prealbumin's short half-life, it is a sensitive indicator of any change affecting protein synthesis and catabolism. Therefore, prealbumin is frequently ordered to monitor the effectiveness of total parenteral nutrition (TPN).

Prealbumin is significantly reduced in hepatobiliary disease because of impaired synthesis. Serum levels of prealbumin are better indicators of liver function than albumin levels. Prealbumin is also a negative acute-phase reactant protein; serum levels decrease in inflammation, malignancy, and protein-wasting diseases of the intestines or kidneys. Since zinc is required for synthesis of prealbumin, low levels occur with zinc deficiency. Increased levels of prealbumin occur in Hodgkin's disease and chronic kidney disease.

Because of the low level of prealbumin in the serum, this protein is not often visualized on serum protein electrophoresis. However, because prealbumin crosses the blood-brain barrier, it is found in the CSF and can be seen on CSF electrophoresis (see discussion of lumbar puncture on p. 579).

Interfering Factors

- Coexistent inflammation may make test result interpretation impossible.
- Drugs that may cause *increased* levels include estrogen, anabolic steroids, androgens, and prednisolone.
- Drugs that may cause *decreased* levels include amiodarone, estrogens, and oral contraceptives.

✓ CLINICAL PRIORITIES

- Clinical interest in prealbumin has centered on its usefulness as a marker of nutritional status. Its half-life of 1.9 days is much less than the 21-day half-life of albumin.
- Prealbumin is frequently indicated to monitor the effectiveness of TPN.
- Because prealbumin is a negative acute-phase reactant protein, serum levels may decrease with inflammatory processes and may make test result interpretation impossible.

Procedure and Patient Care

Before

- Explain the procedure to the patient.
- Tell the patient that no food or fluid restrictions are needed.
- If the patient is to collect a 24-hour urine specimen, provide a collection bottle.

During

- Collect a venous blood sample in a red-top tube.

After

- Apply pressure or a pressure dressing to the venipuncture site.
- Observe the venipuncture site for bleeding.
- Transport the 24-hour urine specimen to the laboratory promptly.
- Inform the patient how and when to obtain the results of this study.

Test Results and Clinical Significance

Increased levels

Some cases of nephrotic syndrome *The major characteristic of the nephrotic syndrome is proteinuria that causes hypoproteinemia. Because prealbumin is so rapidly made, a disproportionate percentage of prealbumin can exist in the blood when other proteins take somewhat longer to produce.*

Hodgkin's disease *The pathophysiology of this observation is not known.*

Chronic kidney disease *Protein in the blood is lost in the urine through the diseased kidney. Prealbumin also is lost.*

Pregnancy *The estrogen effect stimulates protein (prealbumin) synthesis.*

Decreased levels

Malnutrition

Liver damage

The synthesis of prealbumin is diminished.

Burns *There is acute loss of protein from the burn and chronically from the constant loss of serum through the burn.*

Inflammation *Prealbumin is a negative acute-phase reactant protein. That is, in the presence of inflammation, prealbumin levels diminish.*

Related Tests

- Protein, blood (p. 358): This is a measurement of albumin, globulin, and total protein together or separately.
- Protein electrophoresis (p. 361): This is a quantification of all the components that make up the serum proteins, including albumin, $alpha_1$, $alpha_2$, $beta_1$, $beta_2$, and gamma globulins. This test can also detect abnormal proteins created by neoplasms/infections.
- Immunoglobulin electrophoresis (p. 267): This is a quantification of the components that make up immunoglobulin, which is a gamma globulin.

Pregnancy Tests (Human Chorionic Gonadotropin [HCG], Beta Subunit)

Normal Findings

Qualitative: negative; positive in pregnancy
Quantitative
Whole HCG

Gestation (wk)	Whole HCG (mIU/ml)
<1	5-50
2	50-500
3	100-10,000
4	1,000-30,000
5	3,500-115,000
6-8	12,000-270,000
12	15,000-220,000
Males and nonpregnant females	<5

Beta subunit: depends on the method and test used

Indications

This test is used to diagnose pregnancy. It is also helpful in the monitoring of "high-risk" pregnancies. It can also be used as a tumor marker for certain cancers.

Test Explanation

All pregnancy tests are based on the detection of HCG, which is secreted by the placental trophoblast after the ovum is fertilized. HCG will appear in the blood and urine of pregnant women as early as 10 days after conception. In the first few weeks of pregnancy, HCG markedly rises and serum levels are higher than urine levels. After about a month HCG is about the same in either specimen.

HCG is a glycoprotein very similar to the pituitary proteins. These hormones are made up of two fractions, alpha and beta subunits. The alpha subunit is the same for all the glycoproteins. The beta subunit is unique to each. Therefore the beta subunit for HCG is specific for HCG. The whole HCG molecule is metabolized into the alpha and beta subunits in the blood. They are then excreted by the kidneys into the urine. Whole HCG will cross-react with pituitary hormones (especially luteinizing hormone [LH]). Therefore testing for whole HCG is less specific with a high incidence of false-positive results (cross-reactions with LH).

It is important to know that all of these pregnancy studies demonstrate the presence of HCG. Methods of pregnancy testing fall into four categories: biologic, immunologic, radioimmunologic, and radioreceptor assays.

Biologic tests (urine)

Biologic (animal) tests have been used since the 1920s and are primarily of historical interest today. Urine from the patient is injected into an animal (mice, rabbit, toad, frog). If HCG is present, a specific response (usually corpus luteum development in the ovaries) will occur in that animal. The exact response varies according to the animal used. The result is usually positive by the fortieth day after the last menses. These biologic tests have largely been replaced by less expensive, more accurate, and more rapidly performed immunologic tests.

Immunologic tests (agglutination inhibition test [AIT]) (blood and urine)

Immunologic tests are performed using commercially prepared antibodies against the whole HCG molecule and can be completed within 2 minutes or 2 hours, depending on the method used. These immunologic tests have a high false-positive rate and are usually not positive until about 28 days after the last menses. The high false-positive rate (lack of specificity) occurs because these antibodies were directed toward the whole HCG unit (alpha and beta subunits). The alpha subunit is the same for other pituitary hormones. This test would often detect LH, which would give a false-positive result.

Immunologic testing for the beta subunit of HCG, however, greatly improved accuracy and shortened the time for positive testing (18 days). Now, with the development of monoclonal antibodies, immunoassays can identify very small levels of HCG and pregnancy can be detected in 3 to 7 days after conception. Several immunologic tests are now commercially available for testing by the public. The patient's urine is tested and its color is compared to a standard containing a known small amount of HCG. If the color matches that standard, the woman is pregnant. These tests take from 5 to 120 minutes to perform.

Radioimmunoassay (RIA) (serum)

RIA is a highly sensitive and reliable blood test for detection of the beta unit of HCG. In this test, maternal serum HCG and "test" HCG that has been radioactively bound to an antibody (labeled) compete for binding sites on a resin form. The higher the concentration of maternal HCG, the fewer the number of binding sites available for the radiolabeled test HCG.

This study requires a blood sample in a red-top tube; however, RIA also may be performed with a urine test. The test can be done in 1 to 5 hours. This test is so sensitive that pregnancy can be diagnosed before the first missed menstrual period.

Radioreceptor assay (RRA) (serum)

The RRA for serum HCG is highly sensitive and accurate. This test can be performed in 1 hour. The major advantage of this study is its reliable diagnosis of early gestation in patients requesting termination of pregnancy and in cases where infertile couples are anxious to confirm pregnancy. This study is 90% to 95% accurate 6 to 8 days after conception. Even the minute amounts of HCG secreted in an ectopic pregnancy can be measured with this study. This test is also used in looking for early spontaneous abortion in patients who have difficulty maintaining early pregnancy. This test measures the ability of the patient's serum to inhibit the binding of radiolabeled HCG to receptors.

• • •

Normally HCG is not present in nonpregnant women, although in a very small number of women (<5%), HCG exists in very minute levels. The presence of HCG does not necessarily indicate a normal pregnancy. Ectopic pregnancy, hydatidiform mole of the uterus, and choriocarcinoma of the uterus can all produce HCG. Germ cell tumors (choriocarcinoma, embryonal cell cancers) of the testes or ovaries can produce HCG in men and nonpregnant women, respectively. Primary liver cell cancers (hepatoma) can also make HCG. Germ cell cancers and hepatomas can also produce alpha-fetoprotein (see p. 47). In these tumors, HCG is used as a valuable tumor marker to aid in tumor identification. For example, HCG and alpha-fetoprotein are serially measured in patients with cirrhosis, because they have a high chance of developing a hepatoma. If detected early enough, the tumor can be removed and cured. HCG is also used to monitor the therapy and disease progression/regression of these tumors. When HCG levels are elevated in these patients, tumor progression must be suspected. Decreasing HCG levels indicate effective antitumor treatment.

Interfering Factors

- Tests performed too early in the pregnancy, before there is a significant HCG level, may give false-negative results.
- Hematuria and proteinuria in the urine may cause false-positive results.
- Hemolysis of blood may interfere with test results.
- Urine pregnancy tests can vary according to the dilution of the urine. HCH levels may be undetectable on a dilute urine specimen but may be quite detectable on a concentrated urine specimen.
- Drugs that may cause *false-negative* urine results include diuretics (by causing dilute urine) and promethazine.
- Drugs that may cause *false-positive* results include anticonvulsants, antiparkinsonian drugs, hypnotics, and tranquilizers (especially promazine and its derivatives).

Procedure and Patient Care

Before

- Explain the procedure to the patient.
- If a urine specimen will be collected, give the patient a urine container the evening before so that she can provide a first-voided (most concentrated) morning specimen. This specimen generally contains the greatest concentration of HCG.

During

- Collect the first-voided urine specimen for urine testing.
- Collect approximately 7 to 10 ml of venous blood in a red-top tube for serum testing. Avoid hemolysis.

After

- Apply pressure or a pressure dressing to the venipuncture site.
- Assess the venipuncture site for bleeding.
- Emphasize to the patient the importance of antepartal health care.

Test Results and Clinical Significance

Increased levels

Pregnancy
Ectopic pregnancy
Highest beta HCG levels (>30,000 mIU/ml) are recorded in pregnancy. Lowest amounts are generally seen in ectopic pregnancy.

Hydatidiform mole of uterus
Choriocarcinoma of uterus
Germ cell (choriocarcinoma, teratomas, embryonal cell) tumors of testes or ovaries
Other tumors (poorly differentiated tumors, such as hepatoma and lymphoma)
HCG is produced in these patients in variable amounts. The extent of tumor burden and ability to secrete HCG affect HCG levels. The serial monitoring of HCG in these tumors is probably more important than the initial test result.

Decreased levels

Threatened abortion
Incomplete abortion
Dead fetus
These conditions are all associated with diminished viability of the placenta, which produces the HCG associated with pregnancy.

Progesterone Assay

Normal Findings (considerable variation according to method used and laboratory)

	Progesterone (ng/dl*)
<9 years	<20
10-15 years	20
Adult male	10-50
Female	
Follicular phase	<50
Luteal	300-2500
Postmenopausal	<40
Pregnancy (trimester)	
First	725-4400
Second	1950-8250
Third	6500-22,900

*Extraction/radioimmunoassay.

Indications

This test is used in the evaluation of women who are having difficulty becoming pregnant or maintaining a pregnancy. It is also used to monitor "high-risk" pregnancies.

Test Explanation

Progesterone acts primarily on the endometrium. It initiates the secretory phase of the endometrium in anticipation of implantation of a fertilized ovum. Normally progesterone is secreted by the ovarian corpus luteum following ovulation. In pregnancy, progesterone is produced by the corpus luteum for the first few weeks. After that the placenta begins to make progesterone. Both serum progesterone levels and the urine concentration of progesterone metabolites (pregnanediol) are significantly increased during the later half of a normal ovulatory cycle. Progesterone levels provide information about the occurrence and timing of ovulation. Because progesterone levels rise rapidly after ovulation, this study is useful in documenting whether ovulation has occurred and, if so, its exact time. This is very useful information in women who have difficulty becoming pregnant. A series of measurements can help define the day of ovulation. Plasma progesterone levels start to rise after ovulation along with luteinizing hormone (LH), and they continue to rise for approximately 6 to 10 days. The levels then fall and menses occurs. Blood samples drawn at days 8 and 21 of the menstrual cycle normally will show a large increase in progesterone levels in the latter specimen, indicating that ovulation has occurred. Serum progesterone levels can provide comparable information and are sometimes measured in lieu of endometrial biopsy (see p. 653) to determine the phase of the menstrual cycle.

During pregnancy, progesterone levels normally rise because of the placental production of progesterone. Repeated assays can be used to monitor the status of the placenta in cases of "high-risk" pregnancy. Hormone assay for progesterone is used today to monitor progesterone supplementation in patients with an inadequate luteal phase to maintain an early pregnancy.

Interfering Factors

- Recent use of radioisotopes may affect test results, because testing is done by radioimmunoassay. Prior administration of radionuclides can affect results.
- Hemolysis caused by rough handling of the sample may affect test results.
- Drugs that may interfere with test results include estrogen, clomiphene, and progesterone.

✓ CLINICAL PRIORITIES

- Progesterone levels provide information about the occurrence and timing of ovulation. This is useful information in women having difficulty becoming pregnant.
- Hormone assays for progesterone are used to monitor progesterone supplementation in women with an inadequate luteal phase to maintain an early pregnancy.
- During pregnancy, progesterone levels normally rise because of placental production of progesterone. Repeated assays can be used to monitor placental states in "high-risk" pregnancies. Decreasing values are seen when placental viability is threatened.

Procedure and Patient Care

Before

- Explain the procedure to the patient.
- Tell the patient that no fasting is required.

During

- Collect approximately 5 to 7 ml of venous blood in a red-top tube.
- Indicate the date of the last menstrual period on the laboratory slip.

After

- Apply pressure or a pressure dressing to the venipuncture site.
- Assess the venipuncture site for bleeding.

Test Results and Clinical Significance

Increased levels

Ovulation *This occurs with the normal development of a corpus luteum, which makes progesterone.*

Pregnancy *A healthy placenta produces progesterone to maintain the pregnancy.*

Luteal cysts of ovary *The corpus luteum produces progesterone in the nonpregnant female and in the early stages of pregnancy. Cysts can also produce progesterone for prolonged periods of time.*

Hyperadrenocorticalism
Adrenocortical hyperplasia
Adrenal cortical hormones are secreted at increased rates. 17-Hydroxyprogesterone is a precursor of these cortical hormones.

Choriocarcinoma of ovary *This tumor produces progesterone.*

Molar pregnancy *Hydatidiform mole can produce progesterone, although at lower levels than pregnancy.*

Decreased levels

Preeclampsia
Toxemia of pregnancy
Threatened abortion
Placental failure
Fetal death
All of the above obstetric emergencies are associated with decreased placental viability. Progesterone is made by the placenta during pregnancy. Decreasing values are seen when placental viability is threatened.

Ovarian neoplasm *Ovarian epithelial cancers can destroy the functional ovarian tissue. Progesterone levels may decrease.*

Amenorrhea
Ovarian hypofunction
Without ovulation, a corpus luteum will not develop. Progesterone will not be secreted and progesterone and pregnanediol levels will be lower than expected.

Related Tests

- Urine for pregnanediol (p. 849): Pregnanediol is a catabolic metabolite of progesterone that is excreted via the kidneys into the urine.

Prolactin Level (PRL)

Normal Findings

Adult male: 0-20 ng/ml
Adult female: 0-20 ng/ml
Pregnant female: 20-400 ng/ml

Indications

Prolactin levels are used to diagnose and monitor prolactin-secreting pituitary adenomas.

Test Explanation

Prolactin is a hormone secreted by the anterior pituitary gland (adenohypophysis). In females, prolactin promotes lactation. Its role in males has not been demonstrated. Prolactin secretion is controlled by prolactin-inhibiting and prolactin-releasing factors secreted by the hypothalamus. Thyroid-releasing hormone (TRH) can also stimulate prolactin production. During sleep, prolactin levels increase twofold to threefold, attaining circulating levels equaling those of pregnant women. With breast stimulation, pregnancy, nursing, stress, or exercise, a surge of this hormone occurs. Prolactin is elevated in patients with prolactin-secreting pituitary acidophilic or chromophobic adenomas. To a lesser extent, moderately high prolactin levels have been observed in women with secondary amenorrhea (i.e., postpubertal), galactorrhea, primary hypothyroidism, polycystic ovary syndrome, and anorexia. Paraneoplastic tumors (e.g., lung cancer) may cause ectopic secretion of prolactin as well. In general, very high prolactin levels are more likely to be due to pituitary adenoma than to other causes.

The prolactin level is helpful in diagnosing and monitoring pituitary adenomas. Successful treatment is associated with a reduction in serum prolactin levels. The success of treatment can be monitored by obtaining repeated prolactin levels. Several stimulation (with TRH or chlorpromazine) and suppression (with levodopa) prolactin tests have been designed to help differentiate pituitary adenoma from other causes of prolactin overproduction.

Interfering Factors

- Stress from illness, trauma, surgery, or even the fear of a blood test can elevate prolactin levels. In patients who are fearful of venipuncture, it is best to place a heparin lock and withdraw the blood specimen 2 hours later.
- Drugs that may cause *increased* values include phenothiazines, oral contraceptives, reserpine, opiates, verapamil, histamine antagonists, monoamine oxidase inhibitors, estrogens, and antihistamines.
- Drugs that may cause *decreased* values are ergot alkaloid derivatives, clonidine, levodopa, and dopamine.

Procedure and Patient Care

Before

- Explain the procedure to the patient.
- Tell the patient no fasting or special preparation is required.
- Inform the patient that this blood sample should be drawn in the morning.
- Record the use of any medication that may affect results.

During

- Obtain 5 to 7 ml of venous blood in a red-top tube.
- Transfer the specimen to the laboratory as soon as possible. If a delay occurs, the specimen should be placed on ice.

After

- Apply pressure or a pressure dressing to the venipuncture site.
- Assess the venipuncture site for bleeding.

Test Results and Clinical Significance

Increased levels

Galactorrhea *Voluminous galactorrhea can be caused by elevated prolactin levels. A small-volume nipple discharge is quite common and not pathologic unless it is bloody.*

Amenorrhea *Patients who have had normal menses and then stop having menses may be found to have elevated prolactin levels. Many are subsequently found to have prolactin-secreting pituitary adenomas.*

Prolactin-secreting pituitary tumor *Most of these are benign adenomas of the acidophilic type.*

Infiltrative diseases of hypothalamus and pituitary stalk (e.g., granuloma, sarcoidosis)
Metastatic cancer of pituitary gland
The pathologic destruction of the hypothalamus or pituitary can destroy the prolactin-inhibiting regulatory mechanisms.

Hypothyroidism *Patients with hypothyroidism due to thyroid failure have elevated TRH levels. TRH also stimulates prolactin production.*

Perineoplastic syndrome *These cancers are associated with ectopic production of prolactin.*

Stress (e.g., anorexia nervosa, surgery, strenuous exercise, trauma, severe illness) *The pathophysiology of these observations is not known.*

Empty sella syndrome *These patients have a large sella turcica noted on x-ray films but do not have a pituitary adenoma, yet they often have elevated prolactin levels.*

Polycystic ovary syndrome *The pathophysiology of this observation is not well known.*

Renal failure *These patients probably have a reduced clearance of prolactin.*

Decreased levels

Pituitary apoplexy (Sheehan's syndrome) *Women who have severe hemorrhage after obstetric delivery experience circulatory collapse. Their pituitary glands become infarcted. Prolactin levels are diminished along with other pituitary hormones.*

Pituitary destruction by tumor (craniopharyngioma) *Any disease that destroys the pituitary gland will, of course, be associated with reduced prolactin levels.*

Prostate-Specific Antigen (PSA)

Normal Findings <4 ng/ml

Indications

This test is used as a screening method for early detection of prostatic cancer. When combined with a rectal examination, nearly 90% of clinically significant cancers can be detected. This test is also used to monitor the disease after treatment.

Test Explanation

PSA is a glycoprotein (part carbohydrate, part protein) normally found in the cytoplasm of prostatic epithelial cells. This antigen can be detected in all males; however, levels are greatly increased in patients with prostatic cancer. Although PSA was originally measured by histochemical techniques, radioimmunoassay techniques have recently increased its accuracy.

Elevated PSA levels are associated with prostate cancer. The higher the levels, the greater the tumor burden. Furthermore, the PSA assay is a sensitive test for monitoring response to therapy. Successful surgery, radiation, or hormone therapy is associated with a marked reduction in the PSA blood level. Significant elevation in PSA subsequently indicates the recurrence of prostatic cancer.

PSA is more sensitive and specific than other prostatic tumor markers, such as prostatic acid phosphatase (PAP). Also, PSA is more accurate than PAP in monitoring response and recurrence of tumor after therapy.

PSA (and PAP) levels also may be minimally elevated in patients with benign prostatic hypertrophy (BPH) and prostatitis. PSA levels greater than 10 ng/ml indicate a high probability of prostate cancer. Lower values may be compatible with BPH or early prostate cancer. Several formulas have been created to partially correct for BPH, which normally occurs in elderly men. For example,

$$\text{Predicted PSA} = 0.12 \times \text{Gland volume (in cubic centimeters) as determined by ultrasound}$$

A PSA level greater than that predicted would indicate cancer. PSA levels have been age adjusted by some investigators. Levels above those predicted by age would be compatible with cancer. Another way to tell whether moderate elevations in PSA levels are due to cancer or BPH is to repeat the PSA test at 3- to 6-month intervals. A rising trend would indicate cancer.

PSA has been recommended for routine use in screening men over 50 years of age. When combined with direct digital rectal examination, it can detect almost 90% of prostate cancers.

PSA is also used to monitor therapy for prostatic cancer or BPH. Response to treatment is indicated by PSA reductions. This test is also used in the routine surveillance of patients who have been thought to be cured of prostate cancer or BPH. An elevation may indicate recurrence of the disease.

Interfering Factors

- Rectal examinations, well known to falsely elevate PAP levels, may also minimally elevate the PSA. To avoid this problem, the PSA should be drawn before rectal examination of the prostate or several hours afterward.
- Prostatic manipulation by biopsy or transurethral resection of the prostate (TURP) will significantly elevate the PSA levels. The blood test should be done before surgery or 6 weeks after manipulation.

Procedure and Patient Care

Before

- Explain the procedure to the patient.
- Tell the patient that no fasting is required.

During

- Collect approximately 5 ml of blood in a red-top tube.

After

- Apply pressure or a pressure dressing to the venipuncture site.
- Observe the venipuncture site for bleeding.

Test Results and Clinical Significance

Increased levels

Prostate cancer
BPH
Prostatitis
The PSA in the cytoplasm of the diseased prostate is expelled into the bloodstream, and PSA levels are elevated.

Related Tests

- Prostatic acid phosphatase (PAP) (p. 20): This is another tumor marker for prostate cancer. It is less specific and less sensitive than PSA, and its use is diminishing.

Protein, Blood (Albumin, Globulin, Total Protein)

Normal Findings

Adult/elderly	Total protein (children)	Albumin (children)
Total protein: 6.4-8.3 g/dl or 64.0-83.0 g/L (SI units)	Premature infant: 4.2-7.6 g/dl	Premature infant: 3.0-4.2 g/dl
Albumin: 3.5-5.0 g/dl or 35-50 g/L (SI units)	Newborn: 4.6-7.4 g/dl	Newborn: 3.5-5.4 g/dl
Globulin: 2.3-3.4 g/dl	Infant: 6.0-6.7 g/dl	Infant: 4.4-5.4 g/dl
	Child: 6.2-8.0 g/dl	Child: 4.0-5.9 g/dl

Indications

This test is used to assist in the diagnosis of many disease that affect proteins as a whole or one single fraction of proteins. More specifically, it is used to diagnose, evaluate, and monitor the disease course in patients with cancer (lymphoma, myeloma), intestinal/renal protein-wasting states, immune disorders, liver dysfunction, impaired nutrition, and chronic edematous states.

Test Explanation

Protein components can be separated out by chemical methods, ultracentrifuge, or electrophoresis. This discussion will be limited to the main groups of proteins (total protein, albumin, globulin). See the discussion on protein electrophoresis and immunoglobulin electrophoresis for more details about each specific subtype of albumin and globulin and the discussion on prealbumin for specifics concerning that subcategory of proteins.

Proteins are constituents of muscle, enzymes, hormones, transport proteins, hemoglobin, and several other key functional and structural entities within the body. Proteins are the most significant component contributing to the osmotic pressure within the vascular space. This osmotic pressure acts to keep fluid within the vascular space, minimizing extravasation of fluid.

Albumin and globulin (referring to nonalbumin protein) constitute most of the protein within the body and are measured in the total protein. *Albumin* is a protein that is formed within the liver. This makes up approximately 60% of the total protein. The major purpose of albumin in the blood is to maintain colloidal osmotic pressure. Furthermore, albumin transports important blood constituents, such as drugs, hormones, and enzymes. *Globulins* are the key building block of antibodies, glycoproteins, lipid proteins, clotting factors, complement, and acute-phase reactant proteins. Their role in maintaining osmotic pressure is far less significant than that of albumin. Globulins, to a lesser degree, also act as transport vehicles. Some globulins are made in the liver, but most are made in the reticuloendothelial system. Both albumin and globulins can be measured separately.

Albumin is synthesized within the liver and is therefore a measure of hepatic function. (Prealbumin may be a somewhat better test of liver function.) When disease affects the liver cell, the hepatocyte loses its ability to synthesize albumin, and the serum albumin level is diminished. Because the half-life of albumin is 12 to 18 days, however, severe impairment of hepatic albumin synthesis may not be recognized for several weeks or even months.

Serum albumin and globulin are also measures of nutrition. Malnourished patients, especially after surgery, have a greatly decreased level of serum proteins. Burn patients and patients who have protein-losing enteropathies and uropathies have low levels of protein despite normal synthesis. Pregnancy, especially the third trimester, is usually associated with reduced total proteins.

In some diseases, albumin is selectively diminished and globulins are normal or increased to maintain a normal total protein level. For example, in collagen-vascular diseases (e.g., systemic lupus erythematosus [SLE]), capillary permeability is increased. Albumin, a molecule much smaller than globulin, is selectively lost into the extravascular space. Therefore albumin levels will be low, but globulin levels will be normal or even high. Another group of diseases similarly associated with low-albumin, high-globulin, and normal total protein levels is chronic liver diseases. In these diseases the liver cannot produce albumin, but globulin is mostly made in the reticuloendothelial system. In both these types of diseases the albumin level is low, but the total protein level is normal because of increased globulin levels. These changes, however, can be detected if one measures the albumin/globulin (A/G) ratio or performs protein electrophoresis. Normally this ratio exceeds 1.0. In SLE or severe chronic hepatocellular dysfunction the ratios diminish. With the routine use of serum protein electrophoresis, the A/G ratio measurement is not as important.

The albumin fraction of the total protein can be factitiously elevated in dehydrated patients. Increased total protein levels, particularly the globulin fraction, occur with multiple myeloma and other gammopathies.

Interfering Factors

- Prolonged application of a tourniquet can increase both fractions of total proteins.
- Sampling of peripheral venous blood proximal to an IV administration site can result in an inaccurately low protein level, because of local dilution caused by the IV fluid. Likewise, massive IV infusion of crystalloid fluid can result in acute hypoproteinemia from dilution.
- Drugs that may cause *increased* protein levels include anabolic steroids, androgens, corticosteroids, dextran, growth hormone, insulin, phenazopyridine, and progesterone.
- Drugs that may cause *decreased* protein levels include ammonium ions, estrogens, hepatotoxic drugs, and oral contraceptives.

Procedure and Patient Care

Before

- Explain the procedure to the patient.
- Tell the patient that no fasting is usually required.

During

- Collect approximately 5 to 7 ml of blood in a red-top tube.

After

- Apply pressure or a pressure dressing to the venipuncture site.
- Observe the venipuncture site for bleeding. Patients with liver dysfunction often have prolonged clotting times.

Test Results and Clinical Significance

Increased albumin levels

Dehydration *As intravascular volume diminishes, albumin concentration measurements must increase mathematically.*

Decreased albumin levels

Liver disease (e.g., hepatitis, extensive metastatic tumor, cirrhosis, hepatocellular necrosis) *The liver is the site of synthesis of albumin. If production of albumin is inadequate, levels can be expected to fall.*

Protein-losing enteropathies (e.g., malabsorption syndromes, such as Crohn's disease, sprue, Whipple's disease) *Large volumes of protein are lost from the intestines, because absorption is inadequate. Albumin levels will fall.*

Protein-losing nephropathies (e.g., nephrotic syndrome, nephrosis) *Large volumes of albumin can be lost through the kidneys. This loss may be selective for albumin (lipoid nephrosis) or drain out all components of proteins (glomerulonephritis).*

Third-space losses (e.g., ascites, third-degree burns) *Large amounts of albumin can be lost in the serum that weeps from the chronic open burns. Albumin readily accumulates in the peritoneum of ascitic patients.*

Malnutrition *Lack of amino acids available for building proteins contributes to this observation.*

Increased capillary permeability (e.g., collagen-vascular diseases such as SLE) *Albumin can seep out of the microvascular spaces in the tissues and cause edema or in the kidneys and cause proteinuria. The serum albumin decreases.*

Overhydration *As the blood volume increases, albumin concentration measurements decrease mathematically.*

Inflammatory disease *Diseases associated with inflammation, necrosis, infarction, or burns cause an increase in acute-phase reactant proteins, mostly globulins. Therefore the globulin component of proteins increases and albumin decreases.*

Familial idiopathic dysproteinemia *This is a genetic disease in which albumin is significantly reduced (and globulins are increased).*

Increased globulin levels

Multiple myeloma and Waldenström's macroglobulinemia *These cancers are characterized by their production of gamma globulin from neoplastic plasma cells or lymphocytes. The total gamma globulin zone may not be increased, but a monoclonal spike in one portion is often seen.*

Chronic inflammatory disease (e.g., rheumatoid arthritis, SLE) *These disease are associated with autoantibodies, and patients may have an elevated globulin level.*

Cirrhosis *Most patients with this disease have elevated globulin levels. The pathophysiology is not well known.*

Acute and chronic infection *Infection is associated with an antibody response, and therefore an increase in globulins (gamma globulins) may occur.*

Decreased globulin levels

Genetic immune disorders *A host of immune deficiencies are associated with reduced or absent immunoglobulins, which decrease total globulin levels.*

Secondary immune deficiency *Several conditions (e.g., steroid use, nephrotic syndrome, severe gram-negative infection, lymphoma, leukemia) are associated with deficient levels of immunoglobulins. Total globulin levels may be reduced.*

Increased total protein levels

Dehydration *With a decrease in total blood volume, protein concentration will have to increase mathematically.*

Decreased total protein levels

See decreased albumin and globulin levels.

Related Tests

- Protein electrophoresis (see below): This is a quantification of all the components that make up the serum proteins, including albumin, $alpha_1$, $alpha_2$, beta, $beta_2$ and gamma globulins. This test can also detect abnormal proteins created by neoplasms or infections.
- Immunoglobulin electrophoresis (p. 267): This is a quantification of the components that make up immunoglobulins, which is a gamma globulin.
- Prealbumin (p. 345): This is a quantification of prealbumin, a component of proteins. This test is used to assess a person's nutritional status and the status of liver function.

Protein Electrophoresis (Serum Protein Electrophoresis [SPEP], Urine Protein Electrophoresis)

Normal Findings

Total protein: 6.4-8.3 g/dl or 64.0-83.0 g/L (SI units)
Albumin: 3.5-5.0 g/dl or 35-50 g/L (SI units)
$Alpha_1$ globulin: 0.1-0.3 g/dl or 1-3 g/L (SI units)
$Alpha_2$ globulin: 0.6-1.0 g/dl or 6-10 g/L (SI units)
Beta globulin: 0.7-1.1 g/dl or 7-11 g/L (SI units)

Indications

Evaluation and fractionation of serum proteins is used to diagnose, evaluate, and monitor the disease course in patients with cancer (lymphoma, myeloma), intestinal/renal protein-wasting states, immune disorders, liver dysfunction, impaired nutrition, and chronic edematous states.

Test Explanation

Proteins are constituents of muscle, enzymes, hormones, transport proteins, hemoglobin, and several other key functional and structural entities within the, body. Total serum protein is a combination of prealbumin, albumin, and globulins. See discussion on serum proteins.

Albumin is a small protein molecule that is most important in maintaining the oncotic pressure (the pressure that acts to keep water within the vascular space) of plasma. Albumin also acts as a carrier protein for drugs and hormones. The second type of protein in the blood, globulins, are larger molecules and are subclassified into three main groups: alpha, beta, and gamma. The globulins have very little effect on oncotic pressure. $Alpha_1$ globulins are mostly $alpha_1$-antitrypsin. Some transporting proteins such as thyroid and cortisol-binding globulin also contribute to this zone. $Alpha_2$ globulins include serum haptoglobins (bind hemoglobin during hemolysis), ceruloplasmin (carrier for copper), prothrombin, and cholinesterase (an enzyme used in the catabolism of acetylcholine). $Beta_1$ globulins include lipoproteins, transferrin, plasminogen, and complement proteins; $beta_2$ globulins include fibrinogen. Gamma globulins are the immune globulins (antibodies) (see p. 480).

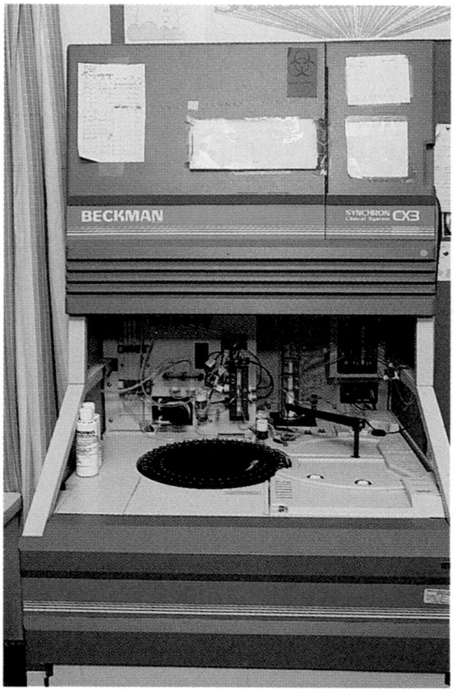

Figure 2-14 Equipment used to perform serum protein electrophoresis.

Serum protein electrophoresis can separate the various components of blood protein into bands or zones according to their electrical charge. A densitometer or similar instrument can quantify these bands (Figure 2-14). Several well-established electrophoretic patterns have been identified and can be associated with specific diseases (Table 2-30). Normally the pattern specific to immunoglobulins is *polyclonal* (i.e., there are many components that all make up the group of immunoglobulins). When the pattern of immunoglobulins changes to a large *monoclonal* spike (indicating an overabundance of one type of immunoglobulin), infection, allergy, or neoplasm such as myeloma is suspected.

Protein electrophoresis can also be done on urine to classify certain renal protein-losing nephropathies. Again, certain patterns may be specific for certain disease. Bence Jones proteins are associated with multiple myeloma. These patients have monoclonal spikes in the beta or gamma globulin zone. Lipoid nephrosis causes the kidneys to leak small protein particles, such as albumin. Therefore one would expect to see a spike in the albumin zone of the electrophoretic patten.

There are several different methods of electrophoresis. Each attempts to improve the

Table 2-30 Protein electrophoresis patterns in specific diseases

Pattern	Electrophoresis	Disease
Acute reaction	↓ Albumin ↑ $Alpha_2$ globulin	Acute infections, tissue necrosis, burns, surgery, stress, myocardial infarction
Chronic inflammatory	sl. ↓ Albumin sl. ↑ Gamma globulin N $Alpha_2$ globulin	Chronic infection, granulomatous diseases, cirrhosis, rheumatoid-collagen diseases
Nephrotic syndrome	↓↓ Albumin ↑↑ $Alpha_2$ globulin N ↑ Beta globulin	Nephrotic syndrome
Far-advanced cirrhosis	↓ Albumin ↑ Gamma globulin Incorporation of beta and gamma peaks	Far-advanced cirrhosis
Polyclonal gamma globulin elevation	↑↑ Gamma globulin with a broad peak	Cirrhosis, chronic infection, sarcoidosis, tuberculosis, endocarditis, rheumatoid-collagen disease
Hypogamma-globulinemia	↓ Gamma globulin with normal other globulin levels	Light-chain multiple myeloma
Monoclonal gammopathy	Thin spikes in gamma globulin	Myeloma, macroglobulinemia, gammopathies

↓ = decreased; ↑ = increased; sl.↓ = slightly decreased; sl.↑ = slightly increased; N= normal; ↓↓ = greatly decreased; ↑↑ = greatly increased.

specificity of the test. These various methods include radial immunodiffusion, immunonephelometry, immunofluorometry, and radioimmunoassay. These methods measure the exact quantity of each protein rather than providing a vague measurement quantity for each "type" of protein. Sensitivity and specificity can be even further improved with the use of immunoelectrophoresis or immunofixation, which can further separate out abnormal proteins that may contribute to each zone spike.

Interfering Factors

- Drugs that may alter normal serum electrophoretic patterns include aspirin, bicarbonates, chlorpromazine, corticosteroids, isoniazid, neomycin, phenacemide, salicylates, sulfonamides, and tolbutamide.

Procedure and Patient Care

Before

- Explain the procedure to the patient.
- Tell the patient that no fasting or preparation is required.

During

- Collect approximately 7 to 10 ml of venous blood in a red-top tube.
- Indicate on the laboratory slip any drugs that may affect test results.

- For a urine specimen, collect a first-voided morning specimen or a 24-hour specimen (preferred). No preservative is required as long as the specimen is kept refrigerated.

After

- Apply pressure or a pressure dressing to the venipuncture site.
- Observe the venipuncture site for bleeding.

Test Results and Clinical Significance

Increased albumin levels

Dehydration *As intravascular volume diminishes, albumin concentration measurements must increase mathematically.*

Decreased albumin levels

Malnutrition *Lack of amino acids available for building proteins contributes to this observation. Probably the liver dysfunction (albumin synthesis) associated with malnutrition also contributes to the low albumin levels.*

Pregnancy *Albumin levels progressively decrease until delivery.*

Liver disease (e.g., hepatitis, extensive metastatic tumor, cirrhosis, hepatocellular necrosis) *The liver is the site of synthesis of albumin. If production of albumin is inadequate, levels can be expected to fall.*

Protein-losing enteropathies (e.g., malabsorption syndromes, such as Crohn's disease, sprue, Whipple's disease) *Large volumes of protein are lost from the intestines because absorption is inadequate. Albumin levels will fall.*

Protein-losing nephropathies (e.g., nephrotic syndrome, nephrosis) *Large volumes of albumin can be lost through the kidneys. This loss may be selective for albumin (lipoid nephrosis) or drain out all components of proteins (glomerulonephritis).*

Third-space losses (e.g., ascites, third-degree burns) *Large amounts of albumin can be lost in the serum that weeps from the chronic open burns. Albumin readily accumulates in the peritoneum of ascitic patients.*

Overhydration *As the blood volume increases, albumin concentration measurements decrease mathematically.*

Increased capillary permeability (e.g., collagen-vascular diseases, such as lupus erythematosus) *Albumin can seep out of the microvascular spaces in the tissues and cause edema* **or** *in the kidneys and cause proteinuria. The serum albumin decreases.*

Inflammatory disease *Diseases associated with inflammation, necrosis, infarction, or burns cause an increase in acute-phase reactant proteins. These are mostly globulins. Therefore the globulin component of proteins increases and albumin decreases.*

Familial idiopathic dysproteinemia *This is a genetic disease in which albumin is significantly reduced (and globulins are increased).*

Increased alpha$_1$ globulin levels

Inflammatory disease *Alpha$_1$-antitrypsin is an acute-phase reactant protein that is increased with diseases associated with inflammation, necrosis, infarction, malignancy, or burns.*

Decreased alpha$_1$ globulin levels

Juvenile pulmonary emphysema *These patients have a genetic decrease or absence of this enzyme, which is important to normal pulmonary function.*

Increased alpha$_2$ globulin levels

Nephrotic syndrome *This probably represents a response to albumin reduction caused by protein-wasting nephropathies. However, the pathophysiology is not well defined.*

Inflammatory disease *Haptoglobin and ceruloplasmin are alpha$_2$ globulins. These proteins are acute-phase reactant proteins that are increased with diseases associated with inflammation, necrosis, infarction, malignancy, or burns.*

Decreased alpha$_2$ globulin levels

Hemolysis *Haptoglobin is an alpha$_2$ globulin and is decreased when hemolysis occurs (see p. 247).*

Wilson's disease *Ceruloplasmin is an alpha$_2$ globulin. It is decreased in Wilson's disease (see p. 139).*

Hyperthyroidism *The pathophysiology for this observation is not known.*

Severe liver dysfunction *Haptoglobulin is an alpha$_2$ globulin that is made in the liver. It is decreased when liver function is inadequate (see p. 247).*

Increased beta globulin levels

Hypercholesterolemia (which can occur by itself or in association with biliary cirrhosis, hypothyroidism, or nephrosis) *Beta lipoprotein is a beta globulin and is increased in hypercholesterolemia (see p. 289).*

Iron deficiency anemia *Transferrin is a beta globulin and is increased in this form of anemia (see p. 274).*

Decreased beta globulin levels

Malnutrition *Transferrin is a beta globulin and is decreased in malnutrition.*

Increased gamma globulin levels

Multiple myeloma and Waldenström's macroglobulinemia *These cancers are characterized by production of gamma globulin from neoplastic plasma cells or lymphocytes. The total gamma globulin zone may not be increased but a monoclonal spike in one portion is often seen.*

Chronic inflammatory disease (e.g., rheumatoid arthritis, systemic lupus erythematosus [SLE]). *These disease are associated with autoantibodies and patients will have a gamma globulin spike.*

Malignancy (e.g., Hodgkin's disease, lymphoma, leukemia) *These diseases may be associated with elevated gamma globulins.*

Hyperimmunization *A small spike can occur in the IgA portion of the gamma band.*

Cirrhosis *Most patients have gamma and some have beta globulin spikes associated with this disease. The pathophysiology is not well known.*

Acute and chronic infection *Infection is associated with an antibody response and therefore an increase in immunoglobulins (gamma globulins).*

Decreased gamma globulin levels

Genetic immune disorders *A host of immune deficiencies are associated with reduced or absent immunoglobulins.*

Secondary immune deficiency *Several conditions (e.g., steroid use, nephrotic syndrome, severe gram-negative infection, lymphoma, leukemia) are associated with deficient levels of immunoglobulins.*

Related Tests

- Protein, blood (p. 358): This is a measurement of albumin, globulin, and total protein together or separately.
- Immunoglobulin electrophoresis (p. 267): This is a quantification of the components that make up immunoglobulins, which are gamma globulins.
- Prealbumin (p. 345): This is a quantification of prealbumin, which is a component of proteins. This test is used to indicate the level of a person's nutritional status. It is also used to indicate the status of liver function.

Prothrombin Time (PT, Pro-time, International Normalized Ratio [INR])

Normal Findings

11.0-12.5 seconds; 85%-100%
Full anticoagulant therapy: >1.5-2.0 times control value; 20%-30%

Critical Values

>20 seconds
Full anticoagulant therapy: three times control value

Indications

The PT is used to evaluate the adequacy of the extrinsic system and common pathway in the clotting mechanism.

Test Explanation

The hemostasis and coagulation system is a homeostatic balance between factors encouraging clotting and the factors encouraging clot dissolution. The first reaction of the body to active bleeding is blood vessel constriction. In small vessel injury this may be enough to stop bleeding. In large vessel injury, hemostasis is required to form a clot that will durably plug the hole until healing can occur. The primary phase of the hemostatic mechanism involves platelet aggregation to blood vessel (Figure 2-10 on p. 156). Next, secondary hemostasis occurs. The first phase of reactions is called the intrinsic system. Factor XII and other proteins form a complex on the subendothelial collagen in the injured blood vessel. Through a series of reactions, activated factor XI (XIa) is formed and activates factor IX (IXa). In a complex formed by factors VIII, IX, and X, activated X (Xa) is formed.

At the same time the extrinsic system is activated and a complex is formed between tissue thromboplastin (factor III) and factor VII (which is exposed after cellular injury). Activated factor VII (VIIa) results. Factor VIIa can directly activate factor X. Alternatively, VIIa can activate IX and X together.

The final step is a common pathway in which prothrombin is converted to thrombin on the surface of the aggregated platelets. The main purpose of thrombin is to convert fibrinogen to fibrin, which is then polymerized into a stable gel. Factor XIII cross-links the fibrin polymers to form a stable clot.

Almost immediately three major activators of the fibrinolytic system act on plasminogen, which was previously absorbed into the clot, to form plasmin. Plasmin degenerates the fibrin polymer into fragments, which are cleared by macrophages.

The PT measures the clotting ability of factors I (fibrinogen), II (prothrombin), V, VII, and X (i.e., the extrinsic system and common pathway). When these clotting factors exist in deficient quantities, the PT is prolonged. Many diseases and drugs are associated with decreased levels of these factors. These include:

Hepatocellular liver disease (e.g., cirrhosis, hepatitis, neoplastic invasive processes). Factors I, II, V, VII, IX, and X are produced in the liver. With severe hepatocellular dysfunction, synthesis of these factors will not occur and serum concentrations of these factors will be decreased. Even a small decrease in factor VII will result in marked prolongation of the PT.

Obstructive biliary disease (e.g., bile duct obstruction secondary to tumor or gallstones, intrahepatic cholestasis secondary to sepsis or drugs). As a result of the biliary obstruction, the bile necessary for fat absorption fails to enter the gut and fat malabsorption results. Vitamins A, D, E, and K are fat soluble and also are not absorbed. Because the synthesis of factors II, VII, IX, and X depends on vitamin K, these factors will not be adequately produced and serum concentrations will fall. Factor VII is the first to decrease and will result in prolongation of the PT. Parenchymal (hepatocellular) liver disease can be differentiated from obstructive biliary disease by determination of the patient's response to parenteral vitamin K administration. If the PT returns to normal after 1 to 3 days of vitamin K administration (10 mg IM twice a day), it is safe to assume that the patient has obstructive biliary disease that is causing vitamin K malabsorption. If, on the other hand, the PT does not return to normal with the vitamin K injections, it can be assumed that severe hepatocellular disease exists and that the liver cells are incapable of synthesizing the clotting factors no matter how much vitamin K is available.

Coumarin ingestion The coumarin derivatives dicumarol and warfarin (Coumadin, Panwarfin) are used to prevent coagulation in patients with thromboembolic disease (e.g., pulmonary embolism, thrombophlebitis, arterial embolism). These drugs interfere with the production of vitamin K–dependent clotting factors, which results in a prolongation of PT, as already described. The adequacy of coumarin therapy can be monitored by following the patient's PT. Appropriate coumarin therapy for full anticoagulation should

Table 2-31 Preferred INR according to indication for anticoagulation

Indication	Preferred INR
Deep-vein thrombosis prophylaxis	1.5-2.0
Orthopedic surgery	2.0-3.0
Deep-vein thrombosis	2.0-3.0
Prevention of embolus in patients in atrial fibrillation*	2.0-3.0
Pulmonary embolism	3.0-4.0
Prosthetic valve prophylaxis	2.5-3.5

*Often not recommended.

prolong the PT by 1.5 to 2 times the control value (or 20% to 30% of the normal value if percentages are used).

To provide uniform PT results for physicians in different parts of the country and the world, the World Health Organization has recommended that PT results now include the use of the *international normalized ratio* (INR) value. The reported INR results are independent of the reagents or methods used, because the standard method of obtaining therapeutic anticoagulation by keeping PT ratios of 1.5 to 2 times the control value in certain clinical indications would be converted to a figure that takes the sensitivity of the thromboplastin used as reagent and the type of instrument into account. These international sensitivity indices are different for various thromboplastin levels and according to whether mechanical or photo-optical methods and instruments are used. Many hospitals are now reporting PT times in both absolute numbers and INR numbers. A therapeutic INR is usually considered to be 2.0 to 3.5 in most institutions, depending on the clinical situation (Table 2-31).

Coumarin derivatives are slow acting, but their action may persist for 7 to 14 days after discontinuation of the drug. The action of a coumarin drug can be reversed in 12 to 24 hours by slow parenteral administration of vitamin K (phytonadione). The administration of plasma will even more rapidly reverse the coumarin effect. The action of coumarin drugs can be enhanced by drugs such as aspirin, quinidine, sulfa, and indomethacin. Barbiturates, chloral hydrate, and oral contraceptives cause increased coumarin drug binding and therefore may decrease the effects of binding coumarin drugs.

PT test results may also be given in seconds along with a control value. The control value usually varies somewhat from day to day, because the reagents used may vary. The patient's PT should be approximately equal to the control value. Some laboratories report PT values as percentages of normal activity, because the patient's results are compared with a curve representing normal clotting time. Normally the patient's PT is 85% to 100%.

Interfering Factors

- Alcohol intake can prolong PT times. Alcohol diminishes liver function. Many factors are made in the liver. Lesser quantities of coagulation factors result in prolonged PT times.
- A diet high in fat or leafy vegetables may shorten PT times. Absorption of vitamin K

is enhanced. Vitamin K–dependent factors are made at increased levels, thereby shortening PT times.

- Diarrhea or malabsorption syndromes can prolong PT times. Vitamin K is malabsorbed, and as a result, factors II, VII, IX, and X are not made.
- Drugs that may cause *increased* levels include allopurinol, aminosalicylic acid, barbiturates, beta-lactam antibiotics, chloral hydrate, cephalothins, chloramphenicol, chlorpromazine (Thorazine), cholestyramine, cimetidine, clofibrate, colestipol, ethyl alcohol, glucagon, heparin, methyldopa (Aldomet), neomycin, oral anticoagulants, propylthiouracil, quinidine, quinine, salicylates, and sulfonamides.
- Drugs that may cause *decreased* levels include anabolic steroids, barbiturates, chloral hydrate, digitalis, diphenhydramine (Benadryl), estrogens, griseofulvin, oral contraceptives, and vitamin K.

Procedure and Patient Care

Before

- Explain the procedure to the patient.
- Tell the patient that no fasting is required.
- If the patient is receiving warfarin, obtain the blood specimen before the patient is given the daily dose of warfarin. The daily dose may be increased, decreased, or kept the same depending on the PT test results for that day.

During

- Collect approximately 5 to 7 ml of venous blood in a blue-top tube.
- List on the laboratory slip any drugs that may affect test results.

After

- Apply pressure or a pressure dressing to the venipuncture site.
- Assess the venipuncture site for bleeding. Remember, hemostasis will be delayed if the patient is taking warfarin or if the patient has any coagulopathies.
- If the PT is greatly prolonged, evaluate the patient for bleeding tendencies (i.e., check for blood in the urine and all excretions and assess the patient for bruises, petechiae, and low-back pain). Back pain may be a symptom of retroperitoneal bleeding.
- If severe bleeding occurs, the anticoagulant effect of warfarin can be reversed by the slow parenteral administration of vitamin K (phytonadione). If coagulation must be returned to near normal more quickly, plasma can be given.
- Because of drug interactions, instruct the patient not to take any medication unless specifically ordered by the physician.

Home Care Responsibilities

- Coumadin levels will be regulated by PT and INR values.
- Inform patients to evaluate themselves for bleeding tendencies. Patients should assess themselves for bruises, petechiae, low-back pain, and bleeding gums. Blood may be detected in the urine and stool.
- Because of many drug interactions, instruct patients on Coumadin therapy not to take any other medications unless approved by their physician.

Test Results and Clinical Significance

Increased levels (prolonged PT)

Liver disease (e.g., cirrhosis, hepatitis) *Coagulation factors are made in the liver. With liver disease, synthesis is inadequate and the PT is increased.*

Hereditary factor deficiency *A genetic defect causes a decrease in a coagulation factor. The PT is increased. Factors II, V, VII, or X could be similarly affected.*

Vitamin K deficiency *Vitamin K–dependent factors (II, VII, IX, X) are not made. The PT is increased.*

Bile duct obstruction *Fat-soluble vitamins, including vitamin K, are not absorbed. Vitamin K–dependent factors (II, VII, IX, X) are not made. The PT is increased.*

Coumarin ingestion *Synthesis of the vitamin K–dependent coagulation factors is inhibited. The PT is increased.*

Disseminated intravascular coagulation *Coagulation factors are consumed in the intravascular coagulation process. The PT is increased.*

Massive blood transfusion *Coagulation is inhibited by the anticoagulant in the banked blood. Furthermore, with massive bleeding, the factors are diluted out by the "factor-poor" banked blood.*

Salicylate intoxication

Related Tests

- Bleeding time (p. 115): This test is used to evaluate the vascular and platelet factors associated with hemostasis.
- Thrombin time (p. 408): This is a test of the fibrinogen to fibrin reaction.
- Partial thromboplastin time (p. 319): This test is used to evaluate the intrinsic system and the common pathway of clot formation. It is most commonly used to monitor heparin therapy.
- Coagulating factor concentration (p. 154): This is a quantitative measurement of specific coagulation factors.

Rabies-Neutralizing Antibody

Normal Findings <1:16

Indications

This test is performed after vaccination to document seroprotection in animal care workers. It is also used to determine exposure to rabies and in the diagnosis of rabies.

Test Explanation

Identification and documentation of the presence of rabies-neutralizing antibody is important for veterinary health care workers and others who are at risk or may have been exposed to the rabies virus. This test is performed on persons who are at great risk for animal bites (veterinarians and their staff, zoo workers, those who work with animals in laboratories) and on those who have received the human diploid cell rabies vaccine (HDCV). A rabies titer of greater than 1:16 is considered protective.

Rabies antibody is also used in diagnosing rabies in patients suspected of being exposed to the virus. A fourfold rise in antibody titer over several weeks in a person not previously exposed to the HDCV indicates rabies exposure. If the patient has received HDCV and has been bitten by an animal suspected of having rabies infection, a very high antibody titer may support the diagnosis. The presence of antibody in the CSF is also supportive of the diagnosis, because usually there are not antibodies in the CSF after the HDCV vaccine, but there are antibodies after a bite from a rabies-infected animal. In patients who may have been exposed to rabies the human rabies immunoglobulin (HRIG) is given after the antibody titers have been obtained. Half of the HRIG is given into the area of the bite, and half is administered as an IM injection into the gluteal region. At the same time the first of the HDCV shots are administered to begin vaccination. Four subsequent IM injections are administered over the next 28 days. One can expect to see increases in rabies antibody levels in about 10 days, but protective levels may not be present for several weeks. Postexposure protocols exist to determine the proper handling of the patient and animal, depending on the real risk of the animal's infection.

The rabies antibody is identified by the direct fluorescent antibody method. More recently immunofluorescence has been used.

Procedure and Patient Care

Before

- Explain the procedure to the patient.
- Tell the patient that no fasting or special preparation is required.

During

- Collect 7 to 10 ml of venous blood in a red-top tube.

After

- Apply pressure or a pressure dressing to the venipuncture site.
- Assess the venipuncture site for bleeding.

Test Results and Clinical Significance

Exposure to rabies vaccine *This causes a relatively low titer of 1:16 or greater.*

Recent bite exposure to rabies virus *This causes a progressive rise in titer to levels of 1:200 to 1:160,000.*

Active rabies in patient or animal *Antibody titers are extremely high in patients who present with encephalitis and brain stem dysfunction. These patients rarely recover from the disease.*

Red Blood Cell Count
(RBC Count, Erythrocyte Count)

Normal Findings (million/mm³)

Adult/elderly
 Male: 4.7-6.1
 Female: 4.2-5.4
Child
 2-8 weeks: 4.0-6.0
 2-6 months: 3.5-5.5
 6 months-1 year: 3.5-5.2
 1-6 years: 4.0-5.5
 6-18 years: 4.0-5.5
Newborn: 4.8-7.1

Indications

The RBC count is closely related to the hemoglobin (p. 254) and hematocrit (p. 251) levels and represents different ways of evaluating the number of RBCs in the peripheral blood. It is repeated serially in patients with ongoing bleeding or as a routine part of the complete blood count. It is an integral part of the evaluation of anemic patients.

Test Explanation

This test is a count of the number of circulating RBCs in 1 mm^3 of peripheral venous blood. The RBC count is routinely performed as part of a complete blood count. Within each RBC are molecules of hemoglobin that permit the transport and exchange of oxygen to the tissues and carbon dioxide from the tissues. The RBC is produced by the erythroid elements in the bone marrow. Under the stimulation of erythropoietin, RBC production is increased. Normally RBCs survive in the peripheral blood for approximately 120 days. During that time the RBC is transported through the bloodstream. In the smallest of capillaries the RBC must fold and bend to conform to the size of these tiny vessels. Toward the end of the RBC's life, the cell membrane becomes less pliable; the aged RBC is then lysed and extracted from the circulation by the spleen. Abnormal RBCs have a shorter life span and are extracted earlier (see RBC survival studies on p. 743). Intravascular RBC trauma, such as that caused by artificial heart valves or peripheral vascular atherosclerotic plaques, also shortens the RBC's life. An enlarged spleen, such as that caused by portal hypertension or leukemia, may inappropriately destroy and remove normal RBCs from the circulation.

Normal RBC values vary according to gender and age. Women tend to have lower values than men, and RBC counts tend to decrease with age. When the value is decreased by more than 10% of the expected normal value, the patient is said to be anemic. Low RBC values are caused by many factors, including:

1. Hemorrhage (as in GI bleeding or trauma)
2. Hemolysis (as in glucose-6-phosphate dehydrogenase deficiency, spherocytosis, or secondary splenomegaly)

3. Dietary deficiency (as of iron or vitamin B_{12})
4. Genetic aberrations (as in sickle cell anemia or thalassemia)
5. Drug ingestion (as of chloramphenicol, hydantoins, or quinidine)
6. Marrow failure (as in fibrosis, leukemia, or antineoplastic chemotherapy)
7. Chronic illness (as in tumor or sepsis)
8. Other organ failure (as in renal disease)

RBC counts greater than normal can be physiologically induced as a result of the body's requirements for greater oxygen-carrying capacity (e.g., at high altitudes). Diseases that produce chronic hypoxia (e.g., congenital heart disease) also provoke this physiologic increase in RBCs. Polycythemia vera is a neoplastic condition involving uncontrolled production of RBCs.

Like the hemoglobin and hematocrit values, the RBC count can be altered by many factors other than RBC production. For instance, in dehydrated patients the total blood volume is contracted. The RBCs will be more concentrated, and the RBC count will be falsely high. Likewise, in overhydrated patients the RBCs are diluted and the RBC count/mm^3 will be falsely low. In most hospitals and laboratories the RBC count is done by an automated counting machine with an error of about 4% to 5%.

Interfering Factors

- Normal RBC decreases are seen during pregnancy as a result of normal body fluid increases that dilute the RBCs. Also, there is an element of nutritional deficiency that is often associated with pregnancy that may play a role in the anemia of pregnancy.
- Living in high altitudes causes increased RBC counts as a result of a physiologic response to the decreased oxygen available at these high altitudes.
- Hydration status: As stated above, dehydration factitiously increases the RBC count, and overhydration decreases the RBC count.
- Drugs that may cause *increased* RBC levels include gentamicin and methyldopa.
- Drugs that may cause *decreased* RBC levels include chloramphenicol, hydantoins, and quinidine.

Procedure and Patient Care

Before

- Explain the procedure to the patient.
- Tell the patient that no fasting is required.

During

- Collect approximately 5 to 7 ml of blood in a lavender-top tube.
- Thoroughly mix the blood with the anticoagulant by tilting the tube.
- Avoid hemolysis.
- List on the laboratory slip any drugs or other patient factors that may affect RBC levels.

After

- Apply pressure or a pressure dressing to the venipuncture site.
- Observe the venipuncture site for bleeding.

Test Results and Clinical Significance

Increased levels

Erythrocytosis *The number of RBCs increases as a result of illnesses or as a physiologic response to external situations (e.g., high altitude).*

Congenital heart disease *Cyanotic heart diseases cause chronically low* PO_2 *levels. In response, the RBCs increase in number.*

Severe chronic obstructive pulmonary disease (COPD) *Chronic states of hypoxia cause stimulation of RBC production as a physiologic response to increase oxygen-carrying capacity.*

Polycythemia vera *This is a result of the bone marrow inappropriately producing great numbers of RBCs.*

Severe dehydration (e.g., severe diarrhea or burns) *With depletion of extracellular fluid, the total blood volume decreases, but the number of RBCs stays the same. Because they are more concentrated, the number of RBCs per cubic millimeter is increased.*

Hemoglobinopathies *In response to the decreased oxygen-carrying capacity of abnormal hemoglobin, more RBCs may be produced to provide adequate oxygen-carrying capacity.*

Decreased levels

Anemia *This is a state associated with reduced RBC numbers. Many different types of diseases are associated with anemia.*

Hemoglobinopathy *Patients with hemoglobin disorders or other blood dyscrasias may have a reduced RBC number and survival.*

Cirrhosis *This is a chronic state of fluid overload. The RBCs are diluted, and the number of RBCs per cubic millimeter is reduced.*

Hemolytic anemia (e.g., erythroblastosis fetalis, hemoglobinopathies, drug-induced hemolytic anemias, transfusion reactions, paroxysmal nocturnal hemoglobinuria) *The RBC survival is diminished in hemolytic anemia. The number of RBCs decreases.*

Hemorrhage *With active bleeding, the number of RBCs decreases. It takes time (several hours), however, for the RBC count to fall. Only if the blood volume is replenished with fluid will the RBC count diminish.*

Dietary deficiency *With certain vitamin or mineral deficiencies (e.g., iron, vitamin* B_{12}*), the RBC size or number is decreased.*

Bone marrow failure *This results in reduced synthesis of RBC.*

Prosthetic valves *Prosthetic valves cause mechanical trauma to the RBC. The RBC survival is diminished and numbers diminish.*

Renal disease *Erythropoietin is made in the kidney and is a strong stimulant to RBC production. With reduced levels of erythropoietin, the RBC numbers diminish.*

Normal pregnancy *Normally there is increased blood volume during pregnancy due to a chronic state of overhydration. Combined with a relative "malnourished" state, the RBC count per cubic millimeter of blood is diminished.*

Rheumatoid/collagen-vascular diseases (e.g., rheumatoid arthritis, lupus, sarcoidosis) *Chronic illnesses are associated with reduced production of RBCs.*

Lymphoma
Multiple myeloma
Leukemia
Hodgkin's disease
Hematologic cancers are often associated with bone marrow failure of RBC production.

Related Tests

- Hematocrit (p. 251): This is a measurement of the percentage of the total blood volume taken up by the RBCs. It is closely associated with the hemoglobin value and the RBC count.
- Hemoglobin (p. 254): This is a measurement of the concentration of hemoglobin in the blood. It is closely associated with the RBC count and hematocrit value.
- Red blood cell indices (see below): These indices provide information about the size and hemoglobin content of the RBC.

Red Blood Cell Indices (RBC Indices, MCV, MCH, MCHC, Blood Indices, Erythrocyte Indices, Red Cell Distribution Width [RDW])

Normal Findings

Mean corpuscular volume (MCV)
Adult/elderly/child: 80-95 mm^3
Newborn: 96-108 mm^3
Mean corpuscular hemoglobin (MCH)
Adult/elderly/child: 27-31 pg
Newborn: 32-34 pg
Mean corpuscular hemoglobin concentration (MCHC)
Adult/elderly/child: 32-36 g/dl (or 32%-36%)
Newborn: 32-33 g/dl (or 32%-33%)
Red blood cell distribution (RDW)
Adult: variation of 11%-14.5%

Indications

The RBC indices provide information about the size (MCV and RDW), weight (MCH), and hemoglobin concentration (MCHC) of RBCs. This test is useful in classifying anemias.

Test Explanation

This test is routinely performed as part of an automated complete blood count. The results of the RBC, hematocrit, and hemoglobin tests are necessary to calculate the RBC indices. When investigating anemia, it is helpful to categorize the anemia according to the RBC indices, as shown in Table 2-32. Cell size is indicated by the terms "normocytic," "microcytic," and "macrocytic." Hemoglobin content is indicated by the terms "normochromic," "hypochromic," and "hyperchromic." Additional information about the RBC size, shape, color, and intracellular structure is described in the blood smear study (see p. 641).

Table 2-32	Categorization of anemia according to RBC indices
	NORMOCYTIC,[1] NORMOCHROMIC[2] ANEMIA
	Iron deficiency (detected early)
	Chronic illness (e.g., sepsis, tumor)
	Acute blood loss
	Aplastic anemia (e.g., chloramphenicol toxicosis)
	Acquired hemolytic anemias (e.g., from a prosthetic cardiac valve)
	MICROCYTIC,[3] HYPOCHROMIC[4] ANEMIA
	Iron deficiency (detected late)
	Thalassemia
	Lead poisoning
	MICROCYTIC, NORMOCHROMIC ANEMIA
	Renal disease (because of the loss of erythropoietin)
	MACROCYTIC,[5] NORMOCHROMIC ANEMIA
	Vitamin B_{12} or folic acid deficiency
	Hydantoin ingestion
	Chemotherapy

[1] Normal RBC size.
[2] Normal color (normal hemoglobin content).
[3] Smaller than normal RBC size.
[4] Less than normal color (decreased hemoglobin content).
[5] Larger than normal RBC size.

Mean corpuscular volume

The MCV is a measure of the average volume, or size, of a single RBC and is therefore used in classifying anemias. MCV is derived by dividing the hematocrit by the total RBC count:

$$MCV = \frac{\text{Hematocrit (\%)} \times 10}{\text{RBC (million/mm}^3\text{)}}$$

Normal values vary according to age and gender. When the MCV value is increased, the RBC is said to be abnormally large, or *macrocytic.* This is most frequently seen in megaloblastic anemias (e.g., vitamin B_{12} or folic acid deficiency). When the MCV value is decreased, the RBC is said to be abnormally small, or *microcytic.* This is associated with iron deficiency anemia or thalassemia. It is important to recognize that a significant number of patients with disorders associated with a variation in MCV may, in fact, not have an abnormality in MCV. For example, only 65% of patients with iron deficiency anemia will have a reduced MCV. Furthermore, the normal values for MCV and, for that matter, all the RBC indices vary considerably. Each laboratory must develop its own normal indices values.

Mean corpuscular hemoglobin

The MCH is a measure of the average amount (weight) of hemoglobin within an RBC. MCH is derived by dividing the total hemoglobin concentration by the number of RBCs:

$$\text{MCH} = \frac{\text{Hemoglobin (g/dl)} \times 10}{\text{RBC (million/mm}^3\text{)}}$$

Because macrocytic cells generally have more hemoglobin and microcytic cells have less hemoglobin, the causes for these values closely resemble those for the MCV value. This has been documented with the use of automated counting instruments. The MCH adds very little information to the other indices.

Mean corpuscular hemoglobin concentration

The MCHC is a measure of the average concentration or percentage of hemoglobin within a single RBC. MCHC is derived by dividing the total hemoglobin concentration by the hematocrit:

$$\text{MCHC} = \frac{\text{Hemoglobin (g/dl)} \times 100}{\text{Hematocrit (\%)}}$$

When values are decreased, the cell has a deficiency of hemoglobin and is said to be *hypochromic* (frequently seen in iron deficiency anemia and thalassemia). When values are normal, the anemia is said to be *normocytic* (e.g., hemolytic anemia). RBCs cannot be considered *hyper*chromic. Only 37 g/dl of hemoglobin can fit into the RBC. Alteration in RBC shape (spherocytosis, acute transfusion reactions, erythroblastosis fetalis) may cause automated counting machines to indicate MCHC levels above normal.

Red blood cell distribution width

The RDW is an indication of the variation in RBC size. It is calculated by a machine using the MCV and RBC values. Variations in the width of the RBCs may be helpful when classifying certain types of anemia. The RDW is essentially an indicator of the degree of anisocytosis, a blood condition characterized by RBCs of variable and abnormal size.

The newer electronic cell counting machines are able to sort out RBCs according to size and compare those sizes to a histogram. Normally all the RBCs are about the same size with very little variation. This creates a histogram with a single narrowed peak. Certain diseases change the size of some of the RBCs, whereas the less abnormal RBCs are less affected. For example, with folic acid deficiency or iron deficiency, the newer RBCs are more significantly affected than the older cells and therefore will be of significantly different size. This creates a histogram with multiple peaks indicating large numbers of cells at variable sizes.

Interfering Factors

- Abnormal RBC size may affect the MCH and MCHC.
- Extremely elevated WBC counts (>50,000) may increase the MCV and MCH indices when performed by automated counters.
- Large RBC precursors, for example, reticulocytes (see p. 387), cause an abnormally high MCV. This commonly occurs in response to anemias when the bone marrow is not pathologic.
- Marked elevation in lipid levels (>2000 mg/dl) causes automated cell counters to indicate high hemoglobin levels. MCV, MCHC, and MCH will be calculated falsely high.

- The presence of cold agglutinins also falsely elevates MCHC, MCH, and MCV.
- Drugs that may *increase* MCV results include zidovudine, phenytoin, and azathioprine.

Procedure and Patient Care

Before

- Explain the procedure to the patient.
- Tell the patient that no fasting is required.

During

- Collect approximately 5 to 7 ml of venous blood in a lavender-top tube.
- Avoid hemolysis.
- Transport the specimen to the hematology laboratory, where the blood is passed through automated machines that calculate the RBC indices.

After

- Apply pressure or a pressure dressing to the venipuncture site.
- Assess the venipuncture site for bleeding.

Test Results and Clinical Significance

Increased MCV

Pernicious anemia (vitamin B_{12} deficiency)
Folic acid deficiency
These are the most common causes of macrocytic anemia. These vitamin deficiencies may be caused by malnutrition, malabsorption, competitive parasites, or enzyme deficiencies that impair utilization of these vitamins.

Antimetabolite therapy *This form of chemotherapy for cancer treatment and, in lesser doses, for arthritis treatment acts as vitamin B_{12} and folate inhibitors and can cause a macrocytic anemia.*
Alcoholism *This is probably more nutritionally related to malnutrition.*
Chronic liver disease *The pathophysiology of this observation is multifactorial and includes poor nutrition, erythropoietin alterations, and the effects of chronic illness.*

Decreased MCV

Iron deficiency anemia
Thalassemia
Anemia of chronic illness
These are the most common diseases associated with microcytosis.

Increased MCH

Macrocytic anemias *The MCH is increased if the size of the RBC is large.*

Decreased MCH

Microcytic anemia
Hypochromic anemia
The MCH is decreased if the size of the RBC is small or the hemoglobin is diminished.

Increased MCHC

Spherocytosis *This is caused by the automated cell counter's false perception of an elevation in the MCHC caused by a variation in the shape of the RBC. The RBC can only hold 37 g/dl of hemoglobin. There can be no "real" hyperchromatism.*
Intravascular hemolysis *This is caused by free hemoglobin in the blood. The automated counter sees the free hemoglobin and incorporates that into its calculations.*
Cold agglutinins *Cold agglutinins cause the misperception of increased MCV and decreased hematocrit. The automated machine calculates a falsely high MCHC.*

Decreased MCHC

Iron deficiency anemia
Thalassemia
These are the most common causes of hypochromatism. Thalassemia minor (heterozygous) may not be clinically evident except by measurement of RBC count, MCV, and MCHC.

Increased RDW

Iron deficiency anemia
B_{12} vitamin or folate deficiency anemia
Increased variation in RDW is caused by a combination of factors in these diseases. RBC fragmentation alters RBC size and shape. Furthermore, new cells produced when the deficiency was greatest will be markedly different in size and shape than the older RBCs that were produced before the deficiencies were as severe.

Hemoglobinopathies (e.g., sickle cell or C disease) *Fragmentation increases RDW variation. Furthermore, different RBCs have different amounts of pathologic hemoglobin and therefore will be affected by fragmentation to varying degrees.*
Hemolytic anemias *Fragmentation increases RDW variation.*
Posthemorrhagic anemias *The marrow's response to bleeding is to release premature RBCs into the bloodstream. These are larger than mature RBCs and contribute to RDW variation.*

Related Tests

- Hematocrit (p. 251): This is a measurement of the percentage of the total blood volume taken up by the RBCs. It is closely associated with the hemoglobin value and the RBC count.
- Hemoglobin (p. 254): This is a measurement of the concentration of hemoglobin in the blood. It is closely associated with the RBC count and hematocrit value.
- Red blood cell (RBC) count (p. 372): This is a measurement of the number of RBCs per cubic millimeter of blood. It is closely associated with the hemoglobin and hematocrit values.

Renin Assay, Plasma (Plasma Renin Activity [PRA], Plasma Renin Concentration [PRC])

Normal Findings

Adult/elderly
- Upright position, sodium depleted (sodium-restricted diet)
  - Ages 20-39 years: 2.9-24.0 ng/ml/hr
  - >40 years: 2.9-10.8 ng/ml/hr
- Upright position, sodium replaced (normal sodium diet)
  - Ages 20-39 years: 0.1-4.3 ng/ml/hr
  - >40 years: 0.1-3.0 ng/ml/hr

Child
- 0-3 years: <16.6 ng/ml/hr
- 3-6 years: <6.7 ng/ml/hr
- 6-9 years: <4.4 ng/ml/hr
- 9-12 years: <5.9 ng/ml/hr
- 12-15 years: <4.2 ng/ml/hr
- 15-18 years: <4.3 ng/ml/hr

Indications

PRA is used to evaluate hypertension. It is helpful in the differential diagnosis of aldosteronism.

Test Explanation

Renin is an enzyme released by the juxtaglomerular apparatus of the kidney into the renal veins in response to hyperkalemia, sodium depletion, decreased renal blood perfusion, or hypovolemia. Renin activates the renin-angiotensin system, which produces angiotensin II, a powerful vasoconstrictor that also stimulates aldosterone production from the adrenal cortex. Angiotensin and aldosterone increase the blood volume, blood pressure, and serum sodium (Figure 2-15). After release of renin from the kidney into the bloodstream, angiotensinogen, an alpha$_2$ globulin that is made in the liver, is converted into angiotensin I. This is then converted into angiotensin II in the lung.

Renin is not actually measured in this test. (In research laboratories, renin can be directly measured with great difficulty.) The PRA test actually measures, by radioimmunoassay, the rate of angiotensin I generation per unit time. This is the most commonly used renin assay. The PRC is used to measure the maximum renin effect. This is useful in patients who are pregnant or have estrogen-induced increased protein levels. The PRA and the PRC are very difficult to perform. Most assays are performed at central laboratories. The specimen must be drawn under ideal circumstances, handled by the local laboratory correctly, and transferred to the central laboratory in a timely manner. Even then, results may vary significantly.

The PRA is a screening procedure for the detection of essential, renal, or renovascular hypertension. The PRA may be supplemented by other tests, such as the renal vein renin

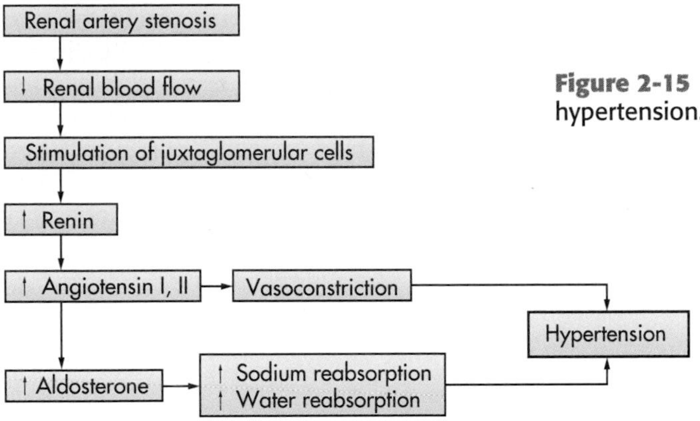

Figure 2-15 Physiology of renovascular hypertension.

assay. A determination of the PRA and a measurement of the plasma aldosterone level are used in the differential diagnosis of primary vs. secondary hyperaldosteronism (Table 2-33). Patients with primary hyperaldosteronism (adrenal adenoma overproducing aldosterone or Conn's syndrome) will have increased aldosterone production associated with decreased renin activity. Patients with secondary hyperaldosteronism (caused by renovascular occlusive disease or primary renal disease) will have increased levels of plasma renin.

The *renin stimulation test* can be performed to more clearly diagnose and distinguish primary and secondary hyperaldosteronism. In this test, PRA is obtained while the patient is in the recumbent position and on a low-salt diet. The PRA is then repeated with the patient on the same diet while the patient is standing erect. In primary hyperaldosteronism the blood volume is greatly expanded. A change in position or reduced salt intake will not result in decreased renal perfusion or sodium level. Therefore renin levels do not increase. In secondary hyperaldosteronism (or normal persons with essential hypertension), the renal perfusion decreases while in the upright position and sodium levels do decrease with decreased intake. Therefore renin levels increase.

The PRA is assessed as part of the *captopril test* (a new screening test for renovascular hypertension). Patients with renovascular hypertension have greater falls in blood pres-

Table 2-33 ***Differential diagnosis using renin and aldosterone levels***

Disease	Renin (PRA)	Aldosterone
Conn's syndrome	Low	High
Renal artery stenosis (or occlusion)	High	High
Primary renal disease	High	High
Increased salt intake	Low	Low
Salt restriction	High	High
Hypokalemia	Low	Low
Sodium-losing diuretic therapy	High	High
Addison's disease	High	Low
Cushing's syndrome	Low	High
Essential hypertension	Low	Normal

sure and increases in PRA after administration of angiotensin-converting enzyme (ACE) inhibitors than do those with essential hypertension. For the captopril test, the patient receives an oral dose of captopril (ACE inhibitor) after a baseline PRA test, and blood pressure measurements are then taken. Subsequent blood pressure measurements and a repeat PRA test at 60 minutes are used for test interpretation. This is an excellent screening procedure to determine the need for a more invasive radiographic evaluation (such as digital subtraction renal arteriography (p. 884) or bilateral renal arteriography; see p. 892).

Interfering Factors

- Renin is increased during pregnancy by virtue of increased substrate proteins concomitantly present in the serum during testing.
- Renin is increased with reduced salt intake. Reduced sodium acts as a direct stimulant to renin production.
- Renin is increased by high licorice ingestion. Licorice has an aldosterone-like effect. This increases sodium reabsorption in the kidney and raises blood pressure, which in turn inhibits renin production.
- There is a diurnal variation in renin production. Values are higher early in the day.
- Renin levels are increased when the patient is in an upright position. Normally the upright position decreases renal perfusion because the blood pools in the veins of the lower extremities. This decreased renal perfusion is a strong stimulant to renin production. Renin levels are decreased in the recumbent position for the same reason (i.e., renal perfusion is increased in the recumbent position and renin levels diminish).
- Drugs that *increase* levels of renin include antihypertensives, ACE inhibitors, diuretics, estrogens, oral contraceptives, and vasodilators.
- Drugs that *decrease* renin levels include beta blockers, clonidine, potassium, licorice, and reserpine.

CLINICAL PRIORITIES

- There is a diurnal variation in renin production. Renin levels are higher in the morning. A morning blood sample is usually drawn.
- Renin levels are affected by body position. Levels are higher in the upright position and decreased in the recumbent position.
- Renin levels are increased with reduced salt intake, because reduced sodium levels are a stimulus to renin production.

Procedure and Patient Care

Before

- Explain the procedure to the patient.
- Instruct the patient to maintain a normal diet with a restricted amount of sodium (approximately 3 g/day) for 3 days before the test.

- Instruct the patient to discontinue medications (e.g., diuretics, steroids, antihypertensives, vasodilators, oral contraceptives) and licorice for 2 to 4 weeks before the test.
- Draw a morning sample usually, because renin values are higher in the morning.
- For stimulation tests, instruct the patient to significantly reduce sodium intake (supplemented with potassium) for 3 days prior to testing.

During

- Usually perform the test with the patient in an upright position.
- For the stimulation test, the blood is drawn in the recumbent and upright position.
- Ensure that the patient stands or sits upright for 2 hours before the blood is drawn.
- If a recumbent sample is ordered, have the patient remain in bed in the morning until the blood sample has been obtained.
- It is best to release the tourniquet immediately prior to obtaining the blood specimen, because stasis can lower renin levels.
- Collect approximately 7 to 12 ml of venous blood and place it in a chilled lavender-top tube with ethylene diaminetetraacetic acid (EDTA) as an anticoagulant. Heparin can falsely decrease results.
- Gently invert the blood tube to allow adequate mixing of the blood sample and the anticoagulant.
- Record the patient's position, dietary status, and time of day on the laboratory slip. Also, note any medication that the patient is currently taking.
- Place the tube of blood on ice, and immediately send it to the laboratory.
- In the laboratory, the blood will be centrifuged and the serum frozen.

After

- Apply pressure or a pressure dressing to the venipuncture site.
- Observe the venipuncture site for bleeding.
- Tell the patient that usually a normal diet and medications may be resumed.

Test Results and Clinical Significance

Increased levels

Essential hypertension *A small percentage of these patients have renin hypertension.*

Malignant hypertension *A large percentage of these patients with aggressive hypertensive episodes have secondary hyperaldosteronism (usually due to renal vascular occlusion or stenosis).*

Renovascular hypertension *Renal artery stenosis or occlusion decreases the renal blood flow, which is a strong stimulant to renin production.*

Chronic renal failure *Of and by itself, diseases of the kidney can stimulate the production of renin.*

Salt-losing GI disease (vomiting or diarrhea) *These patients develop hyponatremia, which is a strong stimulant to renin production.*

Addison's disease *These patients are hyponatremic, which is a strong stimulant to renin production.*

Renin-producing renal tumor *Tumors of the juxtaglomerular apparatus are rare. They can produce renin.*

Bartter's syndrome *This syndrome is associated with potassium wasting in the kidney, high renin levels, and high aldosterone levels. This is caused by a tubular defect in sodium reabsorption.*

Cirrhosis *These patients have increased total body water, which dilutes sodium. Sodium levels are chronically low, which is a stimulant for renin production.*

Hyperkalemia *This is a direct stimulant for renin production.*

Hemorrhage *Any form of hypotension (including cardiogenic or septic shock) is associated with a reduction in the renal blood flow, which is a strong stimulant to renin production.*

Decreased levels

Primary hyperaldosteronism *This is usually caused by an adrenal adenoma, and aldosterone levels are high. Aldosterone inhibits further renin production.*

Steroid therapy *Glucocorticosteroids also have an aldosterone effect, which acts to increase serum sodium levels, decrease potassium levels, and increase blood volume. These responses all tend to diminish renin levels.*

Congenital adrenal hyperplasia *An enzyme defect in cortisol synthesis causes an accumulation of cortisol precursors, some of which have strong aldosterone-like activity. These act to increase serum sodium levels, decrease potassium levels, and increase blood volume, which tend to diminish renin levels.*

Related Tests

- Aldosterone (p. 37): This is a direct measurement of aldosterone level. It is used to evaluate hypertension and aldosteronism.
- Renin assay, renal vein (see below): This is a test whereby the blood specimen for the renin assay is obtained from the renal veins. It is helpful in indicating which kidney is the cause of renin elevation.

Renin Assay, Renal Vein

Normal Findings Renin ratio of involved kidney to uninvolved kidney <1.4

Indications

This test is used to document unilateral renal production of elevated levels of renin (renovascular hypertension).

Test Explanation

Renin is an enzyme released by the juxtaglomerular apparatus of the kidney into the renal veins in response to hyperkalemia, sodium depletion, decreased renal blood perfusion, or hypovolemia. Renin activates the renin-angiotensin system, which produces angiotensin II, a powerful vasoconstrictor that also stimulates aldosterone production from the adrenal cortex. Angiotensin and aldosterone increase the blood volume, blood pressure, and serum sodium (see Figure 2-15 on p. 381).

Renal vein assays for renin are used to diagnose renovascular hypertension, that is, hypertension that is due to inappropriately high renin levels from a diseased kidney or a hypoperfused kidney. By injection of a radiopaque dye into the inferior vena cava, the renal veins can be identified. A catheter is placed into each renal vein, and blood is withdrawn from each vein. Radioimmunoassay is used to determine the renin quantity in each sample. If hypertension is caused by renal artery stenosis or renal pathology, the renal vein renin level of the affected kidney should be 1.4 or more times greater than that of the unaffected kidney. If the levels are the same, the hypertension is not caused by a renovascular source. This is very helpful in determining whether a stenosis seen on a renal angiogram is significantly contributing to hypertension. Any stenosis identified on an arteriogram would not be considered severe enough to cause renin-related hypertension if renin levels from that renal vein were not at least 1.4 times that from the opposite kidney. Another cause for the patient's elevated blood pressure should be considered.

Contraindications

- Patients who are allergic to shellfish or iodinated dye can have an allergic reaction to the radiopaque dye that can vary from mild hives to anaphylaxis.

Potential Complications

- Allergic reactions to iodinated dye may vary from mild flushing, itching, and urticaria to severe, life-threatening anaphylaxis (evidenced by respiratory distress, drop in blood pressure, shock). In the unusual event of anaphylaxis the patient may be treated with diphenhydramine (Benadryl), steroids, and epinephrine. Oxygen and endotracheal equipment should be on hand for immediate use.

Procedure and Patient Care

Before

- Explain the procedure to the patient.
- Ensure that written and informed consent for this procedure is obtained by the physician.
- Assess the patient for allergies to iodine.
- Inform the radiologist if an allergy to iodinated contrast media is suspected. The radiologist may prescribe a diphenhydramine/steroid preparation to be administered before testing. Usually a hypoallergenic, nonionic contrast medium will be used during the test.
- Place the patient on a "no added salt" diet and diuretics for 3 days before the examination to maximize renin levels.
- Keep the patient on NPO status after midnight on the day of the study.
- Instruct the patient to remain in the upright position for 2 hours before the test.
- Premedicate the fasting patient as ordered. Meperidine and atropine are typically used.

During

- Note the following procedural steps:

1. The patient is taken to the radiology department and placed on the fluoroscopy table in a supine position.
2. The patient's groin is prepared and draped in a sterile manner and then anesthetized.
3. The femoral vein is punctured, and a catheter is placed into the vein and advanced into the inferior vena cava.
4. Fluoroscopy is used to monitor the catheter placement.
5. Dye is injected, and the renal veins are identified.
6. The catheter is placed into one renal vein at a time, and separate blood specimens are withdrawn and labeled.
7. The catheter is removed, and a pressure dressing is applied to the puncture site.

- Note that this procedure is usually performed by a radiologist in less than 1 hour.
- Inform the patient that the groin puncture needed for this study is uncomfortable.

After

- Usually place the patient on bed rest for several hours.
- Monitor the patient's vital signs.
- Usually send the blood to a commercial laboratory for analysis.
- Assess the patient for renal vein thrombosis, which may occur 1 to 7 days after the procedure. This will be manifested by costovertebral tenderness, hematuria, and elevated creatinine levels.
- Observe the venous puncture site frequently for hematoma or hemorrhage.
- Apply cold compresses to the puncture site if needed to reduce discomfort and swelling.
- Evaluate the patient for delayed reaction to the dye (dyspnea, rashes, tachycardia, hives). This usually occurs within the first 2 to 6 hours after the test. Treat the patient with antihistamines or steroids.

Test Results and Clinical Significance

Increased levels

Renal artery stenosis
Renal artery occlusion
Renal artery stenosis or occlusion decreases the renal blood flow, which is a strong stimulant to unilateral renin production.

Renin-producing renal tumor *Tumors of the juxtaglomerular apparatus are rare. They can produce unilateral renin elevation.*

Related Tests

- Aldosterone (p. 37): This is a direct measurement of aldosterone level. It is used to evaluate hypertension and patients with aldosteronism.
- Renin assay, plasma (p. 380): Renin assay is used to evaluate hypertension. It is helpful in the differential diagnosis of aldosteronism.

Reticulocyte Count (Retic Count)

Normal Findings

Reticulocyte count
  Adult/elderly/child: 0.5%-2% of total number of RBCs
  Infant: 0.5%-3.1% of total number of RBCs
  Newborn: 2.5%-6.5% of total number of RBCs
Reticulocyte index: 1.0

Indications

The reticulocyte count is an indication of the ability of the bone marrow to respond to anemia and make RBCs. It is used to classify and monitor therapy of anemias.

Test Explanation

The reticulocyte count is a test for determining bone marrow function and evaluating erythropoietic activity. This test is also useful in classifying anemias. A reticulocyte is an immature RBC that can be readily identified under a microscope by staining the peripheral blood smear with Wright's or Giemsa stain. It is an RBC that still has some microsomal and ribosomal material left in the cytoplasm. It sometimes takes a few days for that material to be cleared from the cell. Normally there are a small number of reticulocytes in the bloodstream.

The reticulocyte count gives an indication of RBC production by the bone marrow. Increased reticulocyte counts indicate the marrow is releasing an increased number of RBCs into the bloodstream, usually in response to anemia. A normal or low reticulocyte count in a patient with anemia indicates that the marrow response to the anemia by way of production of RBCs is inadequate and perhaps contributing to or is the cause of the anemia (as in aplastic anemia, iron deficiency, vitamin B_{12} deficiency, depletion of iron stores). An elevated reticulocyte count found in patients with a normal hemogram indicates increased RBC production compensating for an ongoing loss of RBCs (hemolysis or hemorrhage).

Because the reticulocyte count is a percentage of the total number of RBCs, a normal to low number of reticulocytes can appear high in the anemic patient, because the total number of mature RBCs is low. To determine if a reticulocyte count indicates an appropriate erythropoietic (RBC marrow) response in patients with anemia and a decreased hematocrit, the reticulocyte index is calculated as follows:

$$\text{Reticulocyte index} = \text{Reticulocyte count (\%)} \times \frac{\text{Patient's hematocrit}}{\text{Normal hematocrit}}$$

The reticulocyte index in a patient with a good marrow response to the anemia should be 1.0. If it is below 1.0, even though the reticulocyte count is elevated, the bone marrow response is inadequate in its ability to compensate (as seen in iron deficiency, vitamin B_{12} deficiency, marrow failure). In these clinical situations, if iron or vitamin B_{12} is administered, the reticulocyte count will rise significantly to the point that the index equals or exceeds 1.0.

Interfering Factors

- Pregnancy may cause an increased reticulocyte count.
- Howell-Jolly bodies are blue stippling material in the RBC that occurs in severe anemia or hemolytic anemia. The RBCs containing these Howell-Jolly bodies look like reticulocytes and are miscounted by the automated counter machines to be reticulocytes and give a falsely high number of reticulocytes.

Procedure and Patient Care

Before

- Explain the procedure to the patient.
- Tell the patient that no fasting is required.

During

- Collect approximately 5 to 7 ml of venous blood in a lavender-top tube.

After

- Apply pressure or a pressure dressing to the venipuncture site.
- Observe the venipuncture site for bleeding.

Test Results and Clinical Significance

Increased levels

Hemolytic anemia (e.g., immune hemolytic anemia, hemoglobinopathies, hypersplenism, trauma from a prosthetic heart valve) *The RBC survival is decreased and RBCs are destroyed at a faster rate than normal. The marrow attempts to compensate for the shortened RBC survival by producing large numbers of RBCs, some of which are immature RBCs called reticulocytes.*

Hemorrhage (3 to 4 days later) *In response to significant blood loss, the marrow attempts to compensate by producing large numbers of RBCs, some of which are immature RBCs called reticulocytes.*

Erythroblastosis fetalis *Immune-mediated destruction of RBCs reduces RBC survival. The marrow attempts to compensate for the shortened RBC survival by producing large numbers of RBCs, some of which are immature RBCs called reticulocytes.*

Treatment for iron, vitamin B_{12}, or folate deficiency *After replacement treatment for anemia caused by nutritional deficiency, the marrow responds by increasing production of RBCs, some of which are immature RBCs called reticulocytes.*

Decreased levels

Pernicious anemia and folic acid deficiency
Iron deficiency anemia
These nutritional deficiencies suppress marrow production of RBCs, including reticulocytes.

Aplastic anemia
Radiation therapy
Marrow failure
The marrow fails to produce RBCs and reticulocytes.

Chronic diseases *In patients with chronic diseases, marrow production of RBCs and reticulocytes is reduced.*

Related Tests

- Hemoglobin (p. 254) and hematocrit (p. 251): These are indirect measurements of the RBC.
- Red blood cell (RBC) count (p. 372): This is a direct count of the total number of RBCs.

Rheumatoid Factor
(RF, Rheumatoid Arthritis [RA] Factor)

Normal Findings

Negative (<60 U/ml by nephelometric testing); elderly patients may have slightly increased values.

Indications The RF test is useful in the diagnosis of rheumatoid arthritis.

Test Explanation

RA is a chronic inflammatory disease that affects most joints, especially the metacarpal and phalangeal joints, the proximal interphalangeal joints, and the wrists; however, any synovial joint can be involved. The American College of Rheumatology has defined criteria for the diagnosis of RA. They include:

Morning stiffness for at least 6 weeks
Pain in at least one joint for the preceding 6 weeks
Swelling in at least one joint for the preceding 6 weeks
Symmetric bilateral joint swelling
Presence of subcutaneous nodules
X-ray changes compatible with RA

In this disease, abnormal IgG antibodies produced by lymphocytes in the synovial membranes act as "antigens." Other IgG and IgM antibodies in the patient's serum react with the fc component of the abnormal synovial antigenic IgG to produce immune complexes. These immune complexes activate the complement system and other inflammatory systems to cause joint damage. The reactive IgM and sometimes IgG and IgA make up what is called the RF. IgG and IgA can also react to the synovial IgG antigen. Tissues other than the joints, including blood vessels, lungs, nerves, and heart, may also be involved in the autoimmune inflammation.

Tests for RF are directed toward identification of the IgM antibodies. The exact role, if any, that RF plays in the pathophysiology of the disease is not well known. Approximately 80% of patients with RA have positive RF titers. To be considered positive, RF must be found in a dilution of greater than 1:80; when RF is found in titers of less than 1:80, diseases such as systemic lupus erythematosus (SLE), scleroderma, and other autoimmune conditions should be considered. Although the normal value is "no rheumatoid factor identifiable at low titers," a small number of normal patients will have RF present in a very low titer. Furthermore, a negative RF does not exclude the diagnosis of RA. When the nephelometric testing procedure is used, the normal value is considered to be less than 60 U/ml. RF is not a useful disease marker, because it does not disappear in patients who are experiencing a remission of symptoms.

There are many serologic methods for detecting RF. The sheep cell agglutination test or the latex fixation test was most easily performed in the past. Better quantitation is now obtained by nephelometry. In the sheep cell agglutination test, rabbit IgG is placed on the sheep RBCs. When this is mixed with the patient's serum (which has been serially diluted), visual agglutination occurs if any RF is present. In the latex fixation test, human IgG is placed on a synthetic latex particle and mixed with the patient's serum. Visual agglutination is then detected if RF is present (Figure 2-16).

Other autoimmune diseases (see Table 2-5 on p. 77), such as SLE or Sjögren's syndrome, also may cause a positive RF test. RF is occasionally seen in patients with tuberculosis, chronic hepatitis, infectious mononucleosis, and subacute bacterial endocarditis as well. Elderly patients often have false-positive results.

Interfering Factors

- Elderly patients often have false-positive results.

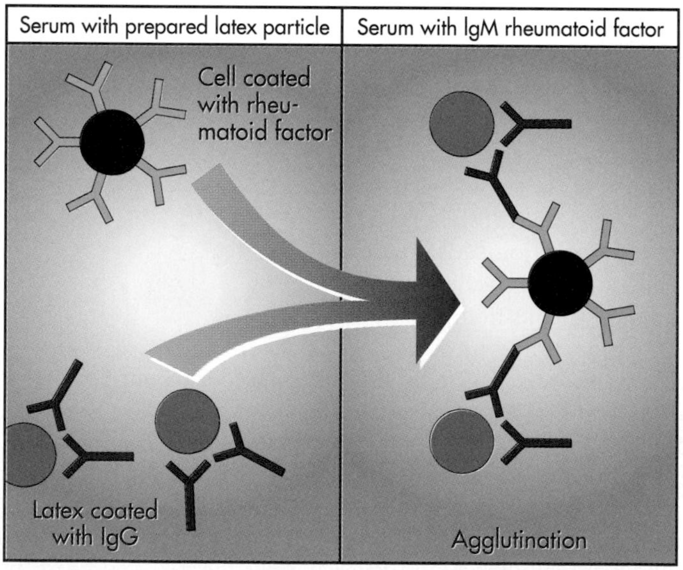

Figure 2-16 Example of rheumatoid factor test by agglutination.

Procedure and Patient Care

Before

- Explain the procedure to the patient.
- Tell the patient that no fasting or other preparation is required.

During

- Collect approximately 7 ml of venous blood in a red-top tube.

After

- Apply pressure or a pressure dressing to the venipuncture site.
- Observe the venipuncture site for bleeding.

Test Results and Clinical Significance

Increased levels

RA
Other autoimmune disease (e.g., SLE, Sjögren's syndrome, scleroderma)
Chronic viral infection
Subacute bacterial endocarditis
Tuberculosis
Chronic active hepatitis
Dermatomyositis
Infectious mononucleosis
Leukemia
Biliary cirrhosis
Syphilis
Renal disease
The pathophysiology of these observations is not known.

Related Tests

- Antibodies–Anti-DNA (p. 68), Anti-SS (p. 84), anti-ENA (p. 69), and antinuclear (p. 76): These antibodies are also present in some cases of RA.

Rubella Antibody
(German Measles, Hemagglutination Inhibition [HAI])

Normal Findings

Method	Result	Interpretation
HAI	<1:8	No immunity to rubella
HAI	>1:20	Immune to rubella
Latex agglutination (LA)	Negative	No immunity to rubella
Enzyme-linked immunosorbent assay (ELISA) IgM	<0.9 IU/ml	No infection
ELISA IgM	>1.1	Active infection
ELISA IgG	<7 IU/ml	No immunity to rubella
ELISA IgG	>10 IU/ml	Immune to rubella

Critical Values

Evidence of susceptibility in pregnant women with recent exposure to rubella

Indications

Screening for rubella antibodies is performed to detect immunity to rubella. This is important for pregnant women or health care workers working with pregnant women. It is also used to diagnose rubella in newborns, children, and adults.

Test Explanation

These tests detect the presence of IgG and/or IgM antibodies to rubella. They become elevated a few days to a few weeks (depending on the method of testing) after the onset of the rash. IgM tends to disappear after about 6 weeks. IgG, however, persists at low, but detectable levels for years. These antibodies become elevated in patients with active rubella infection or with past infections. This test is very accurate, therefore, in determining a patient's susceptibility or immunity to the rubella virus, the causative agent for German measles. It is vitally important to identify exposure to rubella infection and susceptibility status in pregnant women, because congenital rubella infection in the first trimester of pregnancy is associated with congenital abnormalities (heart defects, brain damage, deafness), abortion, or stillbirth. All pregnant women should be screened for rubella during the first prenatal test. This test is sometimes used before pregnancy if a women is not sure if she has had rubella. If antibodies are not present, she can be immunized prior to pregnancy. The term "TORCH" (toxoplasmosis, other, rubella, cytomegalovirus, herpes) has been applied to infections with recognized detrimental effects on the fetus. The effects on the fetus may be direct or indirect (e.g., precipitating abortion or premature labor). Included in the category of "other" are infections (e.g., syphilis). All of these tests are discussed separately.

If the woman's titer is greater than 1:10 to 1:20, she is not susceptible to rubella. If the woman's titer is 1:8 or less, she has little or no immunity to rubella. Pregnant women should be strongly advised to stay away from any small children, especially those with symptoms of an upper respiratory tract infection (prodromal symptoms of rubella) during pregnancy. In addition, all health care personnel associated with maternal and child care should be screened for rubella. Immunization, if required, is not done during pregnancy but should be done before or after delivery for nonimmune women.

A change in the HAI titer (measures IgG and IgM) from the acute to the chronic phase in a patient with a rash is the most useful method of demonstrating that the rash was due to a rubella infection. With a rubella rash, diagnosis of rubella is confirmed by obtaining an acute sample (approximately 3 days after the onset of the rash) and a convalescent sample (approximately 2 to 3 weeks later). A fourfold increase in the acute to the convalescent titer indicates that the rash was caused by an active rubella infection. Alternatively, in a pregnant woman with a rash suspected to be from rubella, an IgM antibody titer can be measured. If the titer is positive, recent infection has occurred. IgM titers appear 1 to 2 days after onset of the rash and disappear 5 to 6 weeks after infection.

Antirubella antibody testing is also used to diagnose rubella in infants (congenital rubella). Rubella is suspected in low-birth-weight infants. Although IgG antibodies can be passed from mother to fetus, IgM antirubella antibodies cannot pass through the placenta. If an infant has IgM antibodies, acute congenital or newborn rubella is suspected. Antibody testing is often used in children with congenital abnormalities that may have resulted from congenital rubella infection. This test is also recommended for anyone with a rash that may be due to rubella.

The HAI method tests for IgG and IgM. LA detects IgG only and is often used as a simple screen for immunity. ELISA methods for detecting IgG and IgM are now the standard for antirubella testing. They provide a more accurate testing method and antibody quantities can be determined.

Procedure and Patient Care

Before

- Explain the purpose of the test to the patient.

During

- Collect approximately 7 ml of venous blood in a red-top tube.

After

- Apply pressure or a pressure dressing to the venipuncture site.
- Assess the venipuncture site for bleeding.
- Inform the patient when to return for a follow-up HAI titer if indicated.

Test Results and Clinical Significance (Table 2-34)

Table 2-34 ***Rubella antibody testing***

Indication	Antibody
Evaluate immune status	IgG
Identify active infection	IgM or IgG, acute and convalescent
Congenital infection	IgM

Sickle Cell
(Sickle Cell Prep, Sickledex, Hemoglobin [Hgb]S)

Normal Findings Negative

Indications This test is used to screen for sickle cell disease or trait.

Test Explanation

Both sickle cell disease (homozygous for Hgb S) and sickle cell trait (heterozygous for Hgb S) can be detected by this study. Sickle cell anemia results from a genetic homozygous defect and is caused by the presence of Hgb S instead of Hgb A (Figure 2-17). In the United States 5% to 10% of African-Americans have sickle cell trait and less than 1% have sickle cell anemia.

When Hgb S becomes deoxygenated, it tends to precipitate in such a way that the RBC assumes a sickle shape. These sickled RBCs cannot pass freely through the capillaries, and thus they cause plugging of the microvascular tree. This may compromise the blood supply to various organs. Hgb S is found in varying quantities (8% to 10%) of the black population.

The routine peripheral blood smear of patients with sickle cell disease does not contain sickled RBCs unless hypoxemia is present. In the sickle cell prep a deoxygenating agent (e.g., 2% sodium metabisulfite) is added to the patient's blood. If 25% or more of the patient's Hgb is of the S variation, the cells will assume the crescent (sickle) shape and the test is positive. If no sickling occurs, the test is negative. In the solubility tests (e.g., Sickledex) a dithionate is added to the patient's blood. Hgb S will precipitate out. A negative test indicates that the patient has no or very little Hgb S levels. These tests cannot differentiate between sickle cell disease and trait. With sickle cell disease, 80% to 100% of the Hgb is the S variation. With the trait, 20% to 40% of the Hgb is the S variation. Other less common Hgb variants (Hgb C-Harlem) also may cause sickling.

This test is only a screening test, and its sensitivity varies according to the method used by the laboratory. The definitive diagnosis of sickle cell disease or trait is made by Hgb electrophoresis, in which Hgb S can be identified and quantified.

Interfering Factors

- Any blood transfusions within 3 to 4 months before the sickle cell test may cause false-negative results, because the donor's normal Hgb may dilute the recipient's abnormal Hgb S.
- Polycythemia may cause false-negative results.
- Infants less than 3 months of age may have false-negative results, because even infants with sickle cell disease have a significant amount of Hgb F in their RBCs at that age. Hgb F will not cause sickling. After 6 months of age the Hgb S variant increases in numbers in these infants. It is then that the test will be positive.
- Drugs that may cause false-negative results include phenothiazines.

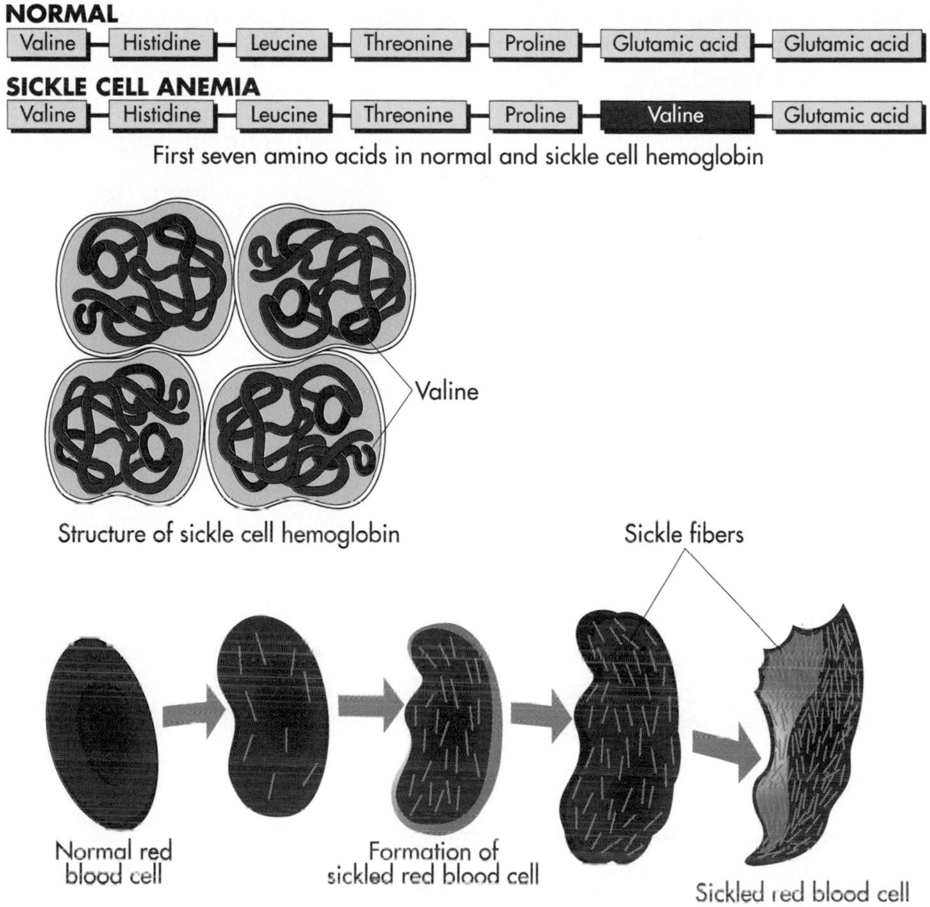

Figure 2-17 Sickle cell anemia. Sickle cell Hgb is produced by a recessive allele of the gene encoding the beta chain of Hgb. It represents a single amino acid change from a glutamic acid to valine at the sixth position in the chain. In the folded beta chain the sixth position contacts the alpha chain, and the amino acid change causes the Hgbs to aggregate into long chains, altering the shape of the cell.

Procedure and Patient Care

Before

- Explain the procedure to the patient.
- Tell the patient that no fasting is required.

During

- Collect approximately 7 ml of venous blood in a lavender-top tube.

After

- Apply pressure or a pressure dressing to the venipuncture site.
- Check the venipuncture site for bleeding.
- If the test is positive, Hgb electrophoresis should be performed.

- If the test is positive, offer the family genetic counseling. A patient with one recessive gene (heterozygous) is said to have sickle cell trait. A patient with two recessive genes (homozygous) has sickle cell anemia.
- Inform patients with sickle cell anemia that they should avoid situations in which hypoxia may occur (e.g., strenuous exercise, air travel in unpressurized aircraft, travel to high-altitude regions).

Test Results and Clinical Significance

Increased levels

Sickle cell trait
Sickle cell anemia
In these clinical situations more than 25% of the Hgb is of the S variation. Sickling will occur.

Related Tests

- Hemoglobin electrophoresis (p. 258): This test can identify and measure Hgb S. Sickle cell disease can be differentiated from the trait.

Sodium, Blood (Na)

Normal Findings

Adult/elderly: 136-145 mEq/L or 136/145 mmol/L (SI units)
Child: 136-145 mEq/L
Infant: 134-150 mEq/L
Newborn: 134-144 mEq/L

Critical Values

$<$120 or $>$160 mEq/L

Indications

This test is a part of a routine laboratory evaluation of all patients. It is one of the tests automatically performed when "serum electrolytes" are requested. This test is used to evaluate and monitor fluid and electrolyte balance and therapy.

Test Explanation

Sodium is the major cation in the extracellular space, where there are serum levels of approximately 140 mEq/L. The concentration of sodium intracellularly is only 5 mEq/L. Therefore sodium salts are the major determinants of extracellular osmolality. The sodium content in the blood is a result of a balance between dietary sodium intake and renal excretion. Nonrenal (e.g., sweat) sodium losses normally are minimal.

Many factors regulate sodium balance. Aldosterone causes conservation of sodium by stimulating the kidneys to reabsorb sodium and decreasing renal losses. Natriuretic hormone, or third factor, is stimulated by increased sodium levels. This hormone decreases renal absorption and increases renal losses of sodium. Antidiuretic hormone (ADH), which controls the reabsorption of water at the distal tubules of the kidney, affects sodium serum levels by dilution or concentration.

Physiologically, water and sodium are closely interrelated. As free body water is increased, serum sodium is diluted and the concentration may decrease. The kidney compensates by conserving sodium and excreting water. If free body water were to decrease, the serum sodium concentration would rise; the kidney would then respond by conserving free water. Aldosterone, ADH (vasopressin), and natriuretic factor all assist in these compensatory actions of the kidney to maintain appropriate levels of free water.

An average dietary intake of approximately 90 to 250 mEq/day is needed to maintain sodium balance in adults. Symptoms of *hyponatremia* may begin when sodium levels are below 125 mEq/L. The first symptom is weakness. When sodium levels fall below 115 mEq/L, confusion and lethargy occur and may progress to stupor and coma if levels continue to decline. Symptoms of *hypernatremia* include dry mucous membranes, thirst, agitation, restlessness, hyperreflexia, mania, and convulsions.

Interfering Factors

- Recent trauma, surgery, or shock may cause increased levels because renal blood flow is decreased. Renin and angiotensin (see p. 381) stimulate the secretion of aldosterone, which stimulates increased renal absorption of sodium.
- Drugs that may cause *increased* levels include anabolic steroids, antibiotics, clonidine, corticosteroids, cough medicines, laxatives, methyldopa, carbenicillin, estrogens, and oral contraceptives.
- Drugs that may cause *decreased* levels include carbamazepine, diuretics, sodium-free IV fluids, sulfonylureas, triamterene, angiotensin-converting enzyme inhibitors, captopril, haloperidol, heparin, nonsteroidal antiinflammatory drugs, tricyclic antidepressants, and vasopressin.

Procedure and Patient Care

Before

- Explain the procedure to the patient.
- Tell the patient that food or fluid is not restricted.

During

- Collect 5 to 10 ml of venous blood in a red- or green-top tube.
- If the patient is receiving an IV infusion, obtain the blood from the opposite arm.
- List on the laboratory slip any drugs that may affect test results.

After

- Apply pressure or a pressure dressing to the venipuncture site.
- Assess the venipuncture site for bleeding.

Test Results and Clinical Significance

Increased levels (hypernatremia)

INCREASED SODIUM INTAKE

Increased dietary intake *If sodium (usually in the form of salt) is ingested at high quantities without adequate free water, hypernatremia will occur.*

Excessive sodium in IV fluids *The normal kidney can excrete about 450 to 500 mEq of sodium per day. If intake of sodium exceeds that amount in a patient without ongoing losses or a prior sodium deficit, sodium levels can be expected to rise.*

DECREASED SODIUM LOSS

Cushing's syndrome *Corticosteroids have an "aldosterone-like" effect. See below.*

Hyperaldosteronism *Aldosterone stimulates the kidneys to absorb sodium at the level of the renal tubule.*

EXCESSIVE FREE BODY WATER LOSS

GI loss (without rehydration) *If free water is lost, residual sodium becomes more concentrated.*

Excessive sweating *Although sweat does contain some sodium, most is free water. This causes the serum sodium to become more concentrated. If the water loss is replaced without any sodium, sodium dilution and hyponatremia can occur.*

Extensive thermal burns *If the burn is extensive, serum and a great amount of free water is lost through the open wounds. Sodium becomes more concentrated. As fluid is replaced and the body physiologically responds by stimulating ADH, sodium can be diluted and hyponatremia may occur.*

Diabetes insipidus *The deficiency of ADH and the inability of the kidney to respond to ADH causes large free water losses. Sodium becomes concentrated.*

Osmotic diuresis *With osmotic diuresis (excluding hyperglycemia, see below), water may be lost at a rate that exceeds sodium loss. In those situations, sodium levels increase as a result of greater concentration. If, however, free water is therapeutically provided, sodium levels may become dilute and hyponatremia may occur.*

Decreased levels (hyponatremia)

DECREASED SODIUM INTAKE

Deficient dietary intake *Sodium intestinal absorption is highly efficient. Salt deficiency is rare.*

Deficient sodium in IV fluids *If IV replacement therapy provides sodium at a level less than minimal physiologic losses or less than ongoing losses, residual sodium will become diluted.*

INCREASED SODIUM LOSS

Addison's disease *Aldosterone and corticosteroid hormone levels are inadequate. Sodium is not reabsorbed by the kidneys and is lost in the urine.*

Diarrhea, vomiting, or nasogastric aspiration *Sodium in the GI contents is lost with the fluid. Hyponatremia is magnified if IV fluid replacement does not contain adequate amounts of sodium.*

Intraluminal bowel loss (ileus, mechanical obstruction) *Great amounts of extracellular fluid are "third spaced" into the lumen of the dilated bowel. This fluid contains sodium. Hyponatremia is magnified if IV fluid replacement does not contain adequate amounts of sodium.*

Diuretic administration *Many diuretics work by inhibiting sodium reabsorption by the kidney. Sodium levels can diminish.*

Chronic renal insufficiency *The kidney loses its reabsorptive capabilities. There are large sodium losses in the urine.*

Large-volume aspiration of pleural or peritoneal fluid *Sodium concentration is the same as serum in these fluids. The aspiration of these fluids is compensated by secretion of ADH, which acts to increase renal absorption of free water. Sodium becomes diluted.*

INCREASED FREE BODY WATER

Excessive oral water intake *Psychogenic polydypsia can dilute sodium.*

Hyperglycemia *Each 60 mg/100 ml increase of glucose above normal decreases the sodium 1 mEq/L, because the osmotic effect of the glucose pulls in free water from the extracellular space and dilutes sodium. Also, sodium ketotic salts are lost in the urine. Sodium levels diminish further.*

Excessive IV water intake *When IV therapy provides less sodium than maintenance and ongoing losses, sodium will be diluted. If sodium-free IV therapy is given to a patient who has a significant sodium deficit, sodium dilution will occur with rehydration.*

Congestive heart failure
Ascites
Peripheral edema
These conditions are associated with increased free water retention. Sodium is diluted.

Syndrome of inappropriate or ectopic secretion of ADH *Oversecretion of ADH stimulates the kidney to reabsorb free water. Sodium is diluted.*

Related Tests

- Sodium, urine (p. 851): This measurement of sodium in the urine is helpful in assessing sodium and water balance.
- Aldosterone (p. 37): More than any other hormone, aldosterone has a significant effect on sodium blood levels.
- Antidiuretic hormone (ADH) (p. 62): By affecting free body water excretion, sodium levels become diluted or concentrated.

Somatomedin C
(Insulin-like Growth Factors I, IGF-1)

Normal Findings

Adult: 42-110 ng/ml
Child

Age (yr)	Girls (ng/ml)	Boys (ng/ml)
0-8	7-110	4-87
9-10	39-186	26-98
11-13	66-215	44-207
14-16	96-256	48-255

Indications

Somatomedin C is a screening test to identify patients with growth hormone (GH) deficiency, pituitary insufficiency, and acromegaly. These levels depend on the levels of GH.

Test Explanation

GH, or somatotropin, is secreted by the acidophil cells in the anterior pituitary gland and plays a central role in modulating growth from birth until the end of puberty. There is an elaborate feedback mechanism associated with the secretion of GH. The hypothalamus secretes growth hormone–releasing hormone (GHRH), which stimulates GH release from the pituitary. GH exerts its effects on many tissues through a group of peptides called somatomedins. The most commonly tested somatomedin is somatomedin C, which is produced by the liver and has its major effect on cartilage. High levels of somatomedins stimulate the production of somatostatin from the hypothalamus. Somatostatin inhibits further secretion of GH from the pituitary.

GH is secreted during sleep and is stimulated by exercise and ingestion of protein and in response to hypoglycemia. As a result of these and other factors that can cause great variation in GH secretion, a significant overlap between normal and abnormal results may be seen on random GH assays. To negate the common variations in GH secretion,

Box 2-6 Causes of short stature

- GH deficiency
- Gonadal dysgenesis
- Russell-Silver dwarfism
- Hypothyroidism
- Pseudohypoparathyroidism
- Laron dwarfism
- Cushing's syndrome
- Bone/cartilage dysplasia
- Idiopathic

Table 2-35 Initial tests for patients with short stature

Test	Reason for test
Thyroxine	r/o hypothyroidism
Somatomedin C	r/o GH deficiency
GH	r/o GH deficiency
GH stimulation	r/o GH deficiency
X-ray films of wrists	Document growth retardation
Calcium (serum levels)	r/o pseudohypoparathyroidism
Phosphate (serum levels)	r/o rickets
Bicarbonate (serum levels)	r/o renal tubular acidosis
BUN	r/o renal failure
Complete blood count	r/o anemia or nutritional or chronic disorders
Sedimentation rate	r/o inflammatory bowel diseases
Chromosomal karyotype	r/o chromosomal abnormalities (gonadal dysgenesis)

r/o = rule out.

screening for insulin-like GH (IGF-1) or somatomedin C provides a more accurate reflection of the mean plasma concentration of GH. Somatomedins are not affected by the time of day, food intake, or exercise as is GH, because they circulate bound to proteins that are durable and long lasting. As a result, there is no overlap of somatomedin C normal and abnormal results.

Somatomedin C is produced by the liver. Values in females are higher (by about 15%). Values are higher in children than in adults. Normally there is a large increase during the pubertal growth spurt.

Levels of somatomedin C depend on levels of GH. As a result, somatomedin levels are low when GH levels are deficient. (See discussion of GH for causes of and diseases associated with GH deficiency.) Nonpituitary causes of reduced somatomedin C include malnutrition, severe chronic illnesses, severe liver disease, hypothyroidism and Laron's dwarfism. The test methodology used is radioimmunoassay, immunochemiluminometric, or radioreceptor assay. Abnormally low test results require an abnormally reduced or absent GH during a GH stimulation test to make the diagnosis of GH deficiency. The causes of short stature and the initial tests for patients with short stature are listed in Box 2-6 and Table 2-35.

Interfering Factors

- A radioactive scan performed a week before the test may affect test results, because somatomedin C is often measured by radioimmunoassay. Results may be confounded by the prior administration of radioisotopes.
- Estrogens may cause *decreased* levels.

Procedure and Patient Care

Before

- Explain the procedure to the patient.
- Tell the patient that an overnight fast is preferred.

During

- Collect one red-top tube of venous blood.

After

- Apply pressure or a pressure dressing to the venipuncture site.
- Assess the venipuncture site for bleeding.

Test Results and Clinical Significance

Increased levels

Gigantism
Acromegaly
These two syndromes are caused by excess GH levels, which increase somatomedin C.

Stress
Major surgery
Hypoglycemia
Starvation
Deep-sleep state
Exercise
The above conditions stimulate GH secretion, which increases somatomedin C.

Hypoglycemia *Hypoglycemia stimulates GH, which stimulates somatomedin C.*

Decreased levels

GH deficiency *Somatomedin C is dependent on GH levels.*
Pituitary insufficiency *GH is produced in the pituitary. Diseases, tumors, ischemia, or trauma to the pituitary or hypothalamus causes GH deficiency. Somatomedin C is dependent on GH levels.*
Dwarfism *This is a result of GH and somatomedin C deficiency in children.*
Laron dwarfism *This syndrome is associated with GH receptor resistance. Somatomedin C secretion does not occur.*
Hyperglycemia *Elevated glucose levels inhibit GH and somatomedin C secretion.*
Failure-to-thrive *This is a result of GH and somatomedin C deficiency in infants.*
Delayed sexual maturity *This is a result of GH and somatomedin C deficiency in adolescents.*

Malnutrition
Malabsorption
Anorexia nervosa
These diseases lead to hypoproteinemia. Since somatomedin C is a protein, levels will be reduced with hypoproteinemia.

Severe liver disease *Somatomedin C is made in the liver. With severe liver disease, somatomedin levels fall.*
Hypothyroidism *Somatomedin C levels fall in hypothyroid patients.*

Related Tests

- Growth hormone stimulation (p. 243): This is a test designed to stimulate the secretion of GH. It is required to accurately make the diagnosis of GH deficiency.
- Growth hormone (p. 240): This is a direct quantitative assay for GH.

Syphilis Detection (Serologic Test for Syphilis [STS], Venereal Disease Research Laboratory [VDRL], Rapid Plasma Reagin [RPR], Fluorescent Treponemal Antibody [FTA])

Normal Findings

Negative or nonreactive

Indications

These serologic tests are used to diagnose and to document successful therapy of syphilis.

Test Explanation

Syphilis is caused by a spirochete *Treponema pallidum.* The disease is divided into four stages: acute, secondary, latent, and tertiary. The acute stage is marked by the development of a chancre on the skin near the infection (usually the genitalia). The chancre develops about 3 to 6 weeks after inoculation and lasts for about 4 to 6 weeks. The secondary stage is highlighted by a rash (often on the soles and palms) and generalized lymphadenopathy. This stage lasts for about 3 months. The latent stage represents a period of disease inactivity and can last for 5 years. Some patients are cured of the infection during this stage. Most go into the tertiary stage marked by CNS, cardiovascular, and ocular signs and symptoms.

The immunologic tests for syphilis detect antibodies to *T. pallidum.* There are two groups of antibodies. The first group of tests detects the presence of a nontreponemal antibody called reagin, which reacts to phospholipids in the body (which are probably similar to lipids in the membrane of *T. pallidum*). The second group of tests detects antibodies directed against the *Treponema* organism itself. The nontreponemal antibody tests are grouped as serologic screening tests for syphilis and are relatively nonspecific. These antibodies are most often detected by the Wassermann test or the VDRL test. A newer, more sensitive nontreponemal test is the RPR test. The VDRL and RPR tests, by virtue of their testing for a nonspecific antibody, have a high false-positive (or cross-reactive) rate. The VDRL test becomes positive approximately 2 weeks after the patient's inoculation with *Treponema* and returns to normal after adequate treatment. The test is positive in nearly all primary and secondary stages of syphilis and in two thirds of patients with tertiary syphilis.

If the VDRL or RPR test is positive, the diagnosis must be confirmed by the more specific *Treponema* test, such as the fluorescent treponemal antibody absorption test (FTA-ABS). The FTA test, which tests for a specific treponemal antibody, is more accurate than the VDRL and RPR tests and becomes positive about 4 to 6 weeks after inoculation. To improve its specificity, non-*pallidum* antibodies are absorbed out of the patient's serum before the serum is added to the *T. pallidum*–impregnated slide. Anti–gamma globulin antibodies that are fluorescent are then added to the slide. If anti–*T. pallidum* antibodies exist in the patient's serum, they will react to the *T. pallidum* on the slide and the fluorescent anti–gamma globulin antibodies that were subsequently added will attach to the patient's serum antibody–*T. palladium* complex and make it visible under the fluorescent microscope. The FTA test is required before the diagnosis of syphilis can be made with certainty. A microhemagglutination test (MHA-TP) test is also available and is comparable in accuracy to the "gold standard" FTA-ABS test. Enzyme-linked immunosorbent assay (ELISA) methods are also available for serologic testing for syphilis.

If the VDRL or RPR test is positive and the FTA-ABS is negative, other diseases that can cause positive screening serologic syphilis tests must be sought (Box 2-7).

Screening for syphilis is usually done during the first prenatal checkup of pregnant women using the VDRL test. Syphilis, if untreated, may cause abortion, stillbirth, or premature labor. The effect on the fetus can be CNS damage, hearing loss, or possible death. In patients who have symptoms compatible with primary syphilis, an FTA-ABS test is recommended. Congenital syphilis is difficult to distinguish from the passive immunity provided by a mother who has syphilis. However, the FTA-ABS result of the infant is usually much higher than the mother's in congenital syphilis. The term "TORCH" (toxoplasmosis, other, rubella, cytomegalovirus, herpes) has been applied to infections with recognized detrimental effects on the fetus. The effects on the fetus may be direct or indirect (e.g., precipitating abortion, premature labor). Included in the category of "other" are infections (e.g., syphilis). All of these tests are discussed separately.

In general, serologic tests return to normal after successful treatment for syphilis. The earlier the disease is treated, the sooner the serologic tests return to normal. In the early primary stage the serologic tests may become negative in 2 to 4 months after successful antibiotic treatment. When treating later stages of the disease, it may take longer than 1 year for the patient to convert to a seronegative result. In the tertiary stage the patient may never convert to negative. Testing should be routinely performed to document successful therapy.

Interfering Factors

- Excessive hemolysis and gross lipemia may cause false-positive STS test results.
- Excess chyle in the blood may cause false-positive STS test results. Testing should be performed after at least an 8-hour fast.
- Recent ingestion of alcohol may cause false-positive STS test results. Alcohol should be avoided for 24 hours prior to testing.
- Many conditions cause false-positive results when VDRL and RPR tests are used (Box 2-7).
- If the patient is tested too soon after inoculation and before antibodies have developed, the tests may be falsely negative. The test should be repeated in 2 months or the patient should be treated despite the negative test results (if clinical suspicion is high).

Box 2-7 Diseases that can cause false-positive VDRL/RPR

Malaria	Typhus
Leptospirosis	Cat-scratch fever
Leprosy	Hepatitis
Mononucleosis	Periarteritis nodosa
Systemic lupus erythematosus	Acute viral or bacterial infections
Lymphogranuloma venereum	Hypersensitivity reactions
Mycoplasmal pneumonia	Recent vaccinations

✓ CLINICAL PRIORITIES

- If the patient is tested too soon after inoculation and before antibodies have developed, the tests may be falsely negative.
- Because the FTA tests for a specific treponemal antibody, it is more accurate than the VDRL and RPR tests. The FTA test becomes positive about 4 to 6 weeks after inoculation.
- Screening for syphilis is usually performed during the first prenatal checkup of pregnant women using the VDRL test.

Procedure and Patient Care

Before

- Explain the procedure to the patient.
- Check with the laboratory regarding food and alcohol fasting requirements.

During

- Collect approximately 7 ml of blood in a red-top tube.

After

- Apply pressure or a pressure dressing to the venipuncture site.
- Check the venipuncture site for bleeding.
- If the test is positive, instruct the patient to inform recent sexual contacts so they can be evaluated.
- If the test is positive, be sure the patient receives the appropriate antibiotic therapy.
- If a screening serology test is positive, a more specific antitreponemal test is required to make the diagnosis.

Test Results and Clinical Significance

Positive results

Syphilis

Testosterone (Total Testosterone Serum Level)

Normal Findings

Age	Male (ng/dl)	Female (ng/dl)
Newborn	75-400	20-64
1-5 months	1-177	1-5
6-12 months	2-7	2-5
1-5 years	2-25	2-10
6-9 years	3-30	2-20
Puberty	5-800	2-40
Adult	280-1100	15-70

Indications

Testosterone levels are used to evaluate ambiguous sex characteristics, precocious puberty, virilizing syndromes in the female, and infertility in the male. This test can also be used as a tumor marker for rare tumors of the ovary and testicle.

Test Explanation

Androgens include dehydroepiandrosterone (DHEA), androstenedione, and testosterone. In the adrenal glands, DHEA is produced in the process of making cortisol and aldosterone. DHEA is also produced de novo by the testes or the ovaries. DHEA is the precursor of androstenedione, which is the precursor of testosterone (and estrogen).

In the male most of the testosterone is made by the Leydig cells in the testicle; this accounts for 95% of the circulating testosterone in men. In the female about half of the testosterone is made by the conversion of DHEA to testosterone in the peripheral fat tissue. Another 30% is made by the same conversion of DHEA in the adrenal gland, and 20% is directly made by the ovaries.

Approximately 60% of circulating testosterone binds strongly to sex hormone–binding globulin (SHBG), which is also called testosterone-binding globulin. Most of the remaining testosterone is bound loosely to albumin, and approximately 2% is free or unbound. The unbound portion is the active component. Most assays for testosterone measure the total testosterone (i.e., bound and unbound portions). The free testosterone can be measured if necessary.

In males a biofeedback mechanism exists that starts in the hypothalamus. Gonadotropin-releasing hormone (GnRH) induces the pituitary to produce luteinizing hormone (LH) (called interstitial cell–stimulating hormone in the male) and follicule-stimulating hormone (FSH). LH stimulates the Leydig cells to produce testosterone. FSH stimulates the Sertoli cells to produce sperm. Testosterone then acts to inhibit further secretion of GnRH.

Physiologically, testosterone stimulates spermatogenesis and influences the development of male secondary sexual characteristics. Overproduction of this hormone in the young male may cause precocious puberty. This can be caused by testicular, adrenal, or pituitary tumors. Overproduction of this hormone in females causes masculinization, which is manifested as amenorrhea and excessive growth of body hair (hirsutism). Ovarian and adrenal tumors/hyperplasia and medications (e.g., danazol) are all potential causes of masculinization in the female. Reduced levels of testosterone in the male suggest hypogonadism or Klinefelter's syndrome.

There are several *testosterone stimulation tests* that can be performed to more accurately evaluate hypogonadism. Human chorionic gonadotropin, clomiphene, and GnRH can be used to stimulate testosterone secretion.

Methods used for the measurement of testosterone include radioimmunoassay and extraction chromatography. There is a slight diurnal variation in the secretion of testosterone. Levels are maximal around 7 AM and minimal around 8 PM.

Interfering Factors

- Drugs that may cause *increased* testosterone levels include alcohol, anticonvulsants, barbiturates, estrogens, and oral contraceptives.

- Drugs that may cause *decreased* testosterone levels include androgens, dexamethasone, diethylstilbestrol, digoxin, alcohol, steroids, ketoconazole, phenothiazine, and spironolactone.

Procedure and Patient Care

Before

- Explain the procedure to the patient.
- Tell the patient that no fasting is required.
- Because testosterone levels are highest in the early morning hours, blood should be drawn in the morning.

During

- Collect 7 ml of peripheral venous blood in a red-top tube.

After

- Apply pressure or a pressure dressing to the venipuncture site.
- Assess the venipuncture site for bleeding.

Test Results and Clinical Significance

Increased levels (male)

Idiopathic sexual precocity *This is usually due to oversecretion of LH, which stimulates the testicles to produce testosterone.*

Pinealoma *This is a hypothalamic tumor that produces an increased quantity of GnRH, which stimulates the pituitary to produce LH, which in turn stimulates the testicles to produce testosterone.*

Encephalitis *This viral infection of the CNS can stimulate the hypothalamus to produce an increased quantity of GnRH, which stimulates the pituitary to produce LH, which in turn stimulates the testicles to produce testosterone.*

Congenital adrenal hyperplasia *An enzyme deficiency in the production of cortisol causes an accumulation of large amounts of DHEA. DHEA is a precursor of androstenedione, which is a precursor of testosterone.*

Adrenocortical tumor *Neoplasm involving the adrenal gland can produce large amounts of testosterone or DHEA. DHEA is a precursor of androstenedione, which is a precursor of testosterone.*

Testicular or extragonadal tumor *Leydig cell tumors can produce testosterone, which can cause precocious puberty in males. However, no spermatogenesis occurs because gonadotropin hormones are not produced and are, in fact, inhibited.*

Hyperthyroidism *These patients have elevated bound testosterone because of elevated SHBG proteins. This causes elevation of the total testosterone levels.*

Testosterone resistance syndromes *These patients resist the effect of testosterone on tissue. In response, higher levels of testosterone are secreted.*

Decreased levels (male)

Klinefelter's syndrome *These patients have an extra X chromosome (XXY). This syndrome is associated with primary testicular failure.*

Cryptorchidism *These patients usually have normal testosterone levels, but occasionally testicles that fail to descend into the scrotum can be atrophic.*
Primary and secondary hypogonadism *Infection, tumor, or congenital abnormalities are all possible causes of primary (testicular) or secondary (pituitary) failure.*
Down syndrome *The pathophysiology of this genetic defect is not defined.*
Orchidectomy *The testicles must both be removed. Surgical removal of just one testicle does not cause deficient testosterone levels.*
Hepatic cirrhosis *These patients have reduced proteins and therefore have reduced amounts of bound testosterone, which makes up most of the total testosterone that is measured.*

Increased levels (female)

Ovarian tumor *Arrhenoblastoma is an uncommon ovarian tumor that can produce testosterone.*
Adrenal tumor *Neoplasms involving the adrenal gland can produce large amounts of testosterone or DHEA. DHEA is a precursor of androstenedione, which is a precursor of testosterone. Hirsutism in females is common with these tumors.*
Congenital adrenocortical hyperplasia *An enzyme deficiency in the production of cortisol causes an accumulation of large amounts of DHEA. DHEA is a precursor of androstenedione, which is a precursor of testosterone. In females this can result in pseudohermaphroditism (ambiguous sex genitalia).*
Trophoblastic tumor *These tumors (hydatiform mole, choriocarcinoma) produce HCG, which can stimulate the production of testosterone.*
Polycystic ovaries *This syndrome is associated with obesity, hirsutism, and amenorrhea. Patients have increased testosterone levels. The pathophysiology is not well defined.*
Idiopathic hirsutism *The pathophysiology of this observation is not known.*

Related Tests

- Androstenedione (p. 53): Androstenedione is used in the diagnosis of virilizing syndromes, especially in the female.

Thrombin Time
(TT, Thrombin Clotting Time [TCT])

Normal Findings 8-12 seconds

Indications

This test is used to evaluate the fibrinogen portion of the hemostatic mechanism. (See discussion of partial thromboplastin time for details.)

Test Explanation

This test is used infrequently today to evaluate the fibrinogen-to-fibrin reaction, one of the final reactions in the common pathway of hemostasis. Direct measurements of fibrinogen and the increasing use of other tests have decreased the usefulness of TT. This test is significantly affected by the antithrombin effect of heparin but is not affected by coumarin products. Its use in monitoring heparin therapy has been supplanted by the activated partial thromboplastin time (APTT).

The TT is performed by adding equal aliquots of the patient's serum and commercially available thrombin. It can detect hypofibrinogenemia and is still used to monitor streptokinase clot dissolution therapy.

Interfering Factors

- Drugs that *prolong* TT include streptokinase, urokinase, and heparin.

Procedure and Patient Care

Before

- Explain the procedure to the patient.
- If the patient is receiving heparin by intermittent injection, plan to draw the blood specimen for the TT 30 minutes to 1 hour before the next dose of heparin.
- If the patient is receiving continuous heparin, draw the blood at any time.

During

- Collect 5 to 14 ml of venous blood in a blue-top tube.

After

- Apply pressure or a pressure dressing to the venipuncture site.
- Assess the venipuncture site for bleeding. Remember, if the patient is receiving anticoagulants or has coagulopathies, the bleeding time will be increased.
- Assess the patient to detect possible bleeding. Check for blood in the urine and all other excretions, and assess the patient for bruises, petechiae, and bleeding gums.
- If severe bleeding occurs, note that the anticoagulant effect of heparin can be reversed by parenteral administration of protamine sulfate.

Test Results and Clinical Significance

Increased TT time

Severe liver disease *Fibrinogen is made in the liver. With impaired liver function, fibrinogen is reduced and the TT is prolonged.*

Congenital hypofibrinogenemia
Acquired hypofibrinogenemia
Severe liver disease
Levels of fibrinogen are reduced and the TT is prolonged.

Fibrinolysis *The fibrin clot that forms is immediately denigrated and clotting does not occur.*
Disseminated intravascular coagulation (DIC) *Fibrin is consumed in this syndrome. Also, fibrin degradation products that are formed during this disease destroy any fibrin clots that may occur.*

Related Tests

- Bleeding time (p. 115): This test is used to evaluate the vascular and platelet factors associated with hemostasis.

- Partial thromboplastin time, activated (p. 319): This test is used to evaluate the intrinsic system and the common pathway of clot formation. It is most commonly used to monitor heparin therapy.
- Prothrombin time (p. 366): This test is used to evaluate the adequacy of the extrinsic system and common pathway in the clotting mechanism. It is most commonly used to monitor warfarin therapy.
- Coagulating factor concentration (p. 154): This is a quantitative measurement of specific coagulation factors.

Thyroid-Stimulating Hormone
(TSH, Thyrotropin)

Normal Findings

Adult: 2-10 μU/ml or 2-10 mU/L (SI units)
Newborn: 3-18 μU/ml or 3-18 mU/L
Cord: 3-12 μU/ml or 3-12 mU/L
Values vary among laboratories.

Indications

This test is used to diagnose primary hypothyroidism and to differentiate it from secondary (pituitary) and tertiary (hypothalamus) hypothyroidism.

Test Explanation

The TSH (also called thyrotropin) concentration aids in differentiating primary and secondary hypothyroidism. Pituitary TSH secretion is stimulated by hypothalamic thyroid-releasing hormone (TRH). Low levels of triiodothyronine (T_3) and thyroxine (T_4) are the underlying stimuli for TRH and TSH. Therefore a compensatory elevation of TRH and TSH occurs in patients with primary hypothyroid states, such as surgical or radioactive thyroid ablation; in patients with burned-out thyroiditis, thyroid agenesis, idiopathic hypothyroidism, or congenital cretinism; or in patients taking antithyroid medications.

In secondary or tertiary hypothyroidism the function of the pituitary or hypothalamus gland, respectively, is faulty as a result of tumor, trauma, or infarction. Therefore TRH and TSH cannot be secreted, and plasma levels of these hormones are near zero despite the stimulation that occurs with low T_3 and T_4 levels.

The TSH test is used to monitor exogenous thyroid replacement or suppression as well. The goal of thyroid replacement therapy is to provide an adequate amount of thyroid medication so that TSH secretion is minimal, indicating a euthyroid state. The goal of thyroid suppression is to completely suppress the thyroid gland and TSH secretion by providing excessive thyroid medication. This treatment is used to diminish the size of a thyroid goiter. The dose of medication is given to keep the TSH level less than 2.0 for replacement. Even lower TSH levels are preferred if thyroid suppression is the clinical goal.

This test is also used to detect primary hypothyroidism in newborns with low screening T_4 levels. TSH and T_4 levels are frequently measured to differentiate pituitary and thyroid dysfunction. A decreased T_4 and normal or elevated TSH level can indicate a thyroid disorder. A decreased T_4 with a decreased TSH level can indicate a pituitary disorder.

Interfering Factors

- Recent radioisotope administration may affect test results.
- Severe illness may cause decreased TSH levels.
- There is a diurnal variation in TSH levels. Basal levels occur around 10 AM and highest levels (about two to three times basal levels) occur around 10 PM.
- Drugs that may cause *increased* levels include antithyroid medications, lithium, potassium iodide, and TSH injection.
- Drugs that may cause *decreased* levels include aspirin, dopamine, heparin, steroids, and T_3.

✓ CLINICAL PRIORITIES

- This test is useful for differentiating primary hypothyroidism and secondary (pituitary) and tertiary (hypothalamus) hypothyroidism. Elevations of TSH occur in patients with primary hypothyroid states. In contrast, plasma levels of TSH are near zero in patients with secondary and tertiary hypothyroidism.
- This test may be used to detect primary hypothyroidism in newborns with low screening T_4 levels.
- TSH levels are subject to a diurnal variation. Basal levels occur around 10 AM and highest levels occur around 10 PM.

Procedure and Patient Care

Before

- Explain the procedure to the patient.
- Tell the patient that no food or drink restrictions are necessary.

During

- Collect approximately 5 ml of venous blood in a red-top tube.
- Use a heel stick to obtain blood from newborns.

After

- Apply pressure or a pressure dressing to the venipuncture site.
- Assess the venipuncture site for bleeding.

Test Results and Clinical Significance

Increased levels

Primary hypothyroidism (thyroid dysfunction)
Thyroiditis

Thyroid agenesis
Congenital cretinism
Large doses of iodine
Radioactive iodine injection
Surgical ablation of thyroid
Severe and chronic illnesses
In these diseases, inadequate thyroid hormone levels act as a potent stimulant for the release of TSH from the anterior pituitary. TSH levels rise. In some cases, however, TSH may be diminished.

Pituitary TSH-secreting tumor *This is very rare, but when it occurs, TSH levels, of course, are increased.*

Decreased levels

Secondary hypothyroidism (pituitary or hypothalamus dysfunction) *Diseases of the hypothalamus diminish the capability of the hypothalamus to secrete TRH, which is the major factor that determines TSH production and secretion. Diseases of the pituitary diminish pituitary production of TSH.*
Hyperthyroidism *Increased levels of thyroid hormones inhibit the release of TSH.*
Suppressive doses of thyroid medication *When thyroid medication (e.g., Synthroid) is administered (usually to shrink a goiter), TSH levels fall due to inhibition by the thyroid medication.*
Factitious hyperthyroidism *These patient take thyroid medication without prescription. These medications act to inhibit TSH production.*

Related Tests

- Long-acting thyroid stimulator (p. 294): LATS and other thyroid-stimulating immunoglobulins are used to support the diagnosis of Graves' disease, especially when the diagnosis is complex.
- Thyrotropin-releasing hormone (p. 415): This test assists in the evaluation of patients with hyper- and hypothyroidism. It is especially helpful in the differential diagnosis of hypothyroidism.
- Triiodothyronine uptake (p. 438): This test is an indirect measurement of total T_4.
- Thyroid-stimulating hormone stimulation (p. 413): This test is also used to differentiate primary from secondary (and tertiary) hypothyroidism.
- Thyroxine-binding globulin (p. 421): This is a measure of TBG, the major thyroid hormone protein carrier. It is used in the evaluation of patients who have abnormal total T_4 and T_3 levels. When performed concurrently with the T_4/T_3 test, T_4 and T_3 levels can more easily be interpreted.
- Thyroxine (p. 417): This is one of the first tests done for assessing thyroid function. It is used to diagnose thyroid function and to monitor replacement and suppressive therapy.
- Triiodothyronine (p. 435): T_3 is used to evaluate thyroid function. It is mostly used to diagnose hyperthyroidism. It is also used to monitor thyroid replacement and suppressive therapy.
- Thyroxine index, free (p. 426): This test is used to evaluate thyroid function. It corrects for changes in thyroid hormone–binding serum proteins that can affect total T_4 levels. It is used to diagnose hyper- and hypothyroidism.

- Thyroxine, free (p. 423): The FT_4 is used to evaluate thyroid function in patients who may have protein abnormalities that could affect total T_4 levels. It is used to diagnose thyroid function and to monitor replacement and suppressive therapy.
- Antithyroglobulin antibody (p. 89): This test is primarily used in the differential diagnosis of thyroid diseases, such as Hashimoto's thyroiditis and chronic lymphocytic thyroiditis (in children).

Thyroid-Stimulating Hormone Stimulation
(TSH Stimulation)

Normal Findings

Increased thyroid function with administration of exogenous TSH

Indications

This test is used to differentiate primary and secondary (and tertiary) hypothyroidism.

Test Explanation

The TSH stimulation test is used to differentiate primary (thyroid) hypothyroidism and secondary (hypothalamic-pituitary) hypothyroidism. Normal people and patients with hypothalamic-pituitary hypothyroidism are capable of increasing thyroid function when exogenous TSH is given. Patients with primary hypothyroidism due to disease in the thyroid, however, are not; their thyroid gland is inadequate and cannot function no matter how much stimulation it receives. Patients with less than a 10% increase in radioactive iodine uptake (RAIU) or less than a 1.5 mg/dl rise in thyroxine (T_4) are considered to have primary hypothyroidism. If the hypothyroidism is caused by inadequate pituitary secretion of TSH or hypothalamic secretion of thyroid-releasing hormone (TRH), the RAIU should increase at least 10% and the T_4 level should rise 1.5 μg/dl or more. This is characteristic of secondary hypothyroidism.

Procedure and Patient Care

Before

- Explain the procedure to the patient.
- Obtain baseline levels of RAIU (see p. 740) or T_4 as indicated.
- Tell the patient that no fasting is required.

During

- Administer 5 to 10 U of TSH intramuscularly for 3 days.
- Repeat the measurement of RAIU or T_4 as indicated.

After

- Apply pressure or a pressure dressing to the venipuncture site.
- Assess the venipuncture site for bleeding.

Test Results and Clinical Significance

Increased levels

Primary hypothyroidism (thyroid dysfunction)
Thyroiditis
Thyroid agenesis
Congenital cretinism
Large doses of iodine
Radioactive iodine injection
Surgical ablation of thyroid
Severe and chronic illnesses
In these diseases the thyroid is unable to increase T_4 levels or RAIU no matter how significant the stimulation, because the disease involves the thyroid itself.

Secondary hypothyroidism (pituitary or hypothalamus dysfunction) *The thyroid is capable of producing T_4 and RAIU, but the pituitary/hypothalamic stimulation is inadequate for appropriate stimulation of those functions. When TSH is administered, T_4 and RAIU increase significantly.*

Related Tests

- Long-acting thyroid stimulator (p. 294): LATS and other thyroid-stimulating immunoglobulins are used to support the diagnosis of Graves' disease, especially when the diagnosis is complex.
- Thyrotropin-releasing hormone (p. 415): This test assists in the evaluation of patients with hyper- and hypothyroidism. It is especially helpful in the differential diagnosis of hypothyroidism.
- Thyroid-stimulating hormone (p. 410): This test is used to diagnose primary hypothyroidism and to differentiate it from secondary (pituitary) and tertiary (hypothalamus) hypothyroidism.
- Triiodothyronine uptake (p. 438): This test is an indirect measurement of total T_4.
- Thyroxine-binding globulin (p. 421): This is a measure of TBG, the major thyroid hormone protein carrier. It is used in the evaluation of patients who have abnormal total T_4 and T_3 levels. When performed concurrently with a T_4/T_3 test, the T_4 and T_3 levels can more easily be interpreted.
- Thyroxine (p. 417): This is one of the first tests done for assessing thyroid function. It is used to diagnose thyroid function and to monitor replacement and suppressive therapy.
- Triiodothyronine (p. 435): T_3 is used to evaluate thyroid function. It is primarily used to diagnose hyperthyroidism. It is also used to monitor thyroid replacement and suppressive therapy.
- Thyroxine index, free (p. 426): This test is used to evaluate thyroid function. It corrects for changes in thyroid hormone–binding serum proteins that can affect total T_4 levels. It is used to diagnose hyper- and hypothyroidism.
- Thyroxine, free (p. 423): The FT_4 is used to evaluate thyroid function in patients who may have protein abnormalities that could affect total T_4 levels. It is used to diagnose thyroid function and to monitor replacement and suppressive therapy.

- Antithyroglobulin antibody (p. 89): This test is primarily used in the differential diagnosis of thyroid diseases, such as Hashimoto's thyroiditis and chronic lymphocytic thyroiditis (in children).

Thyrotropin-Releasing Hormone (TRH, Thyrotropin-Releasing Factor [TRF])

Normal Findings

Prompt rise in serum thyroid-stimulating hormone (TSH) level to approximately twice the baseline value in 30 minutes after an IV bolus of TRH

Clinical Disease	Baseline TSH μU/ml	Stimulated TSH*
Euthyroid	<10	>2
Hyperthyroid	<10	<2
Primary hypothyroid (thyroid)	>10	>2
Secondary hypothyroid (pituitary)	<10	<2
Tertiary hypothyroid (hypothalamus)	<10	>2

*Stimulated TSH (times the baseline) is measured 30 minutes after the IV injection of 500 μg of TRH.

Indications

This test assists in the evaluation of patients with hyper- and hypothyroidism. It is especially helpful in the differential diagnosis of hypothyroidism.

Test Explanation

The TRH test assesses the responsiveness of the anterior pituitary gland via its secretion of TSH to an IV injection of TRH. After the TRH injection the normally functioning pituitary gland should secrete TSH (and prolactin). In hyperthyroidism, either a slight or no increase in the TSH level is seen, because pituitary TSH production is suppressed by the inhibitory effect of excess circulating thyroxine (T_4) and triiodothyronine (T_3) on the pituitary gland. A normal result is considered reliable evidence for excluding the diagnosis of thyrotoxicosis. The TRH test is one of the most reliable confirmatory procedures for hyperthyroidism; other tests are often compared with it to determine their accuracy.

In addition to assessing the responsiveness of the anterior pituitary gland, this test aids in the detection of primary, secondary, and tertiary hypothyroidism. In primary hypothyroidism (thyroid gland failure) the increase in the TSH level is two or more times the normal result. With secondary hypothyroidism (anterior pituitary failure), no TSH response occurs. Tertiary hypothyroidism (hypothalamic failure) may be diagnosed by a delayed rise in the TSH level. Multiple injections of TRH may be needed to induce the appropriate TSH response in this case.

The TRH test also may be useful in differentiating primary depression, manic-depressive psychiatric illness, and secondary types of depression. In primary depression the TSH response is blunted in most patients, whereas patients with other types of depression have a normal TRH-induced TSH response.

Interfering Factors

- The normal response may be exaggerated in women.
- The normal response may be less than expected in the elderly.
- Pregnancy may increase the TSH response to TRH.
- Drugs that may modify the TSH response include antithyroid drugs, aspirin, corticosteroids, estrogens, levodopa, and T_4.

Procedure and Patient Care

Before

- Explain the procedure to the patient.
- Instruct the patient to discontinue thyroid preparations for 3 to 4 weeks before the TRH test.
- Assess the patient for medications currently being taken.
- Tell the patient that no fasting or sedation is required.

During

- Administer a 500-μg IV bolus of TRH.
- Obtain venous blood samples at intervals and measure TSH levels.

After

- Apply pressure or a pressure dressing to the venipuncture site.
- Assess the venipuncture site for bleeding.
- Indicate on the laboratory slip if the patient is pregnant.
- List any medications that the patient is taking.

Test Results and Clinical Significance

Increased levels

Hyperthyroidism *Because the pituitary is already maximally suppressed by the high levels of T_3 and T_4, pituitary response to TRH will be blunted and baseline levels will be less than double.*

Primary hypothyroidism (thyroid disease) *Because the TSH is already stimulated by the lack of T_3 and T_4, stimulation will be maximized by the TRH and stimulated TSH will be more than double the baseline.*

Secondary hypothyroidism (pituitary disease) *Because the diseased pituitary is unable to produce TSH, no matter how significant the stimulation, TSH will not double after TRH stimulation.*

Tertiary hypothyroidism (hypothalamus) *The pituitary is functioning normally. If TRH is provided exogenously, the pituitary will respond normally and produce twice the TSH level.*

Psychiatric primary depression *In primary depression the TSH response is blunted in most patients, whereas patients with other types of depression have a normal TRH-induced TSH response.*

Related Tests

- Long-acting thyroid stimulator (p. 294): LATS and other thyroid-stimulating immunoglobulins are used to support the diagnosis of Graves' disease, especially when the diagnosis is complex.
- Thyroid-stimulating hormone (p. 410): This test is used to diagnose primary hypothyroidism and to differentiate it from secondary (pituitary) and tertiary (hypothalamus) hypothyroidism.
- Thyroid-stimulating hormone stimulation (p. 413): This test is also used to differentiate primary and secondary (and tertiary) hypothyroidism.
- Thyroxine-binding globulin (p. 421): This is a measure of TBG, the major thyroid hormone protein carrier. It is used in the evaluation of patients who have abnormal total T_4 and T_3 levels. When performed concurrently with a T_4/T_3 test, the T_4 and T_3 levels can be more easily interpreted.
- Thyroxine (see below): This is one of the first tests done for assessing thyroid function. It is used to diagnose thyroid function and to monitor replacement and suppressive therapy.
- Triiodothyronine (p. 435): T_3 is used to evaluate thyroid function. It is primarily used to diagnose hyperthyroidism. It is also used to monitor thyroid replacement and suppressive therapy.
- Thyroxine index, free (p. 426): This test is used to evaluate thyroid function. It corrects for changes in thyroid hormone–binding serum proteins that can affect total T_4 levels. It is used to diagnose hyper- and hypothyroidism.
- Thyroxine, free (p. 423): The FT_4 is used to evaluate thyroid function in patients who may have protein abnormalities that could affect total T_4 levels. It is used to diagnose thyroid function and to monitor replacement and suppressive therapy.
- Antithyroglobulin antibody (p. 89): This test is primarily used in the differential diagnosis of thyroid diseases, such as Hashimoto's thyroiditis and chronic lymphocytic thyroiditis (in children).
- Triiodothyronine uptake (p. 438): This test is an indirect measurement of total T_4.

Thyroxine (T_4, Thyroxine Screen)

Normal Findings

Age	µg/dl
1-3 days	11-22
1-2 weeks	10-16
1-4 months	8-16
1-5 years	7-15
5-10 years	6-13
10-15 years	5-12
Adult male	4-12
Adult female	5-12
Adult >60 years	5-11

Critical Values

Adult: <2.0 μg/dl if myxedema coma possible; >20 μg/dl if thyroid storm possible
Newborn: <7.0 μg/dl

Indications

This is one of the first tests done for assessing thyroid function. It is used to diagnose thyroid function and to monitor replacement and suppressive therapy.

Test Explanation

Thyroid hormones are produced when tyrosine incorporates organic iodine to form monoiodotyrosine. This complex picks up another iodine and becomes diiodotyrosine. Two diiodotyrosines combine to form tetraiodothyronine (also called T_4 thyroid hormone). If a diiodotyrosine combines with a monoiodotyrosine, triiodothyronine (also called T_3 thyroid hormone) is formed. T_4 makes up nearly all of what we call thyroid hormone. T_3 makes up less than 10% of thyroid hormone. Nearly all of T_4 and T_3 is bound to protein. Thyroxine-binding globulin (TBG) binds most of T_3 and T_4. Albumin and prealbumin bind the rest. It is the unbound or "free" hormone that is metabolically active. T_4 can be measured by radioimmunoassay or enzyme-linked immunosorbent assay techniques. The serum T_4 test is a measure of total T4 (i.e., bound and free T_4).

Thyrotropin-releasing hormone (TRH) is secreted in the hypothalamus. This stimulates the anterior pituitary to secrete thyrotropin (thyroid-stimulating hormone [TSH]). TSH stimulates the thyroid to secrete thyroid hormone. The increased levels of T_3 and T_4 inhibit further production of TRH.

The serum T_4 study is a direct measurement of the total amount of T_4 present in the patient's blood. Greater than normal levels indicate hyperthyroid states, and subnormal values are seen in hypothyroid states. Newborns are screened by T_4 tests to detect hypothyroidism. Mental retardation can be prevented by early diagnosis.

This is a very reliable test of thyroid function; however, results are affected by TBG. Because T_4 is bound by serum proteins such as TBG, any increase in these proteins (as in pregnant women and patients taking oral contraceptives) will cause factitiously elevated levels of T_4 (and T_3). Therefore levels of these carrier proteins (e.g., TBG) are concomitantly measured (by T_3 resin uptake studies). Furthermore, T_3 resin results must be considered in interpreting the T_4 test results.

Interfering Factors

- T_4 levels may be increased after iodinated contrast x-ray studies.
- Pregnancy will cause increased levels.
- Drugs that may cause *increased* levels include iodine, iodinated contrast media, clofibrate, estrogens, heroin, amphetamines, methadone, and oral contraceptives.
- Drugs that may cause *decreased* levels include anabolic steroids, propylthiouracil, barbiturates, furosemide, nonsteroidal antiinflammatory agents, androgens, antithyroid drugs (e.g., propylthiouracil), lithium, phenytoin (Dilantin), and propranolol (Inderal).

CLINICAL PRIORITIES

- This test is used to diagnose thyroid function and to monitor replacement or suppressive therapy.
- This is a very reliable test of thyroid function. However, because T_4 is bound to serum proteins (such as TBG), T_4 levels are affected by levels of carrier proteins. Carrier proteins can be measured by the T_3 resin uptake test. This helps in interpreting results.
- Newborns are screened by T_4 tests to detect hypothyroidism. A heel stick is used to collect the blood. Mental retardation can be prevented by early diagnosis.

Procedure and Patient Care

Before

- Explain the procedure to the patient.
- Evaluate the patient's medication history.
- If indicated, instruct the patient to stop taking exogenous T_4 medication 1 month before testing.
- Tell the patient that no fasting is required.

During

Adult

- Collect a venous blood specimen in a red-top tube.
- List on the laboratory slip any drugs that may affect test results.

Newborn

- Perform a heel stick to obtain blood.
- Thoroughly saturate the circles on the filter paper with blood.
- Note that prompt collection and processing are crucial to the early detection of hypothyroidism.
- Note that the optimal collection time is 2 to 4 days after birth.
- All newborns should be screened before discharge (regardless of age), however, because of the consequences of delayed diagnosis.

After

- Apply pressure or a pressure dressing to the venipuncture site.
- Assess the venipuncture site for bleeding.

Test Results and Clinical Significance

Increased levels

Primary hyperthyroid states (e.g., Graves' disease, Plummer's disease, toxic thyroid adenoma) *The thyroid produces increased T_4 despite lack of TSH stimulation.*

Acute thyroiditis *The thyroid secretes increased T_4 during the acute inflammatory stages of thyroiditis (e.g. Hashimoto's thyroiditis). However, in the latter stages the thyroid may become burned out and the patient may become hypothyroid.*

Familial dysalbuminemic hyperthyroxinemia *These patients have a genetically defective form of albumin that binds T_4 unusually tightly. As a result, the bound portion of T_4 increases. The patient is not hyperthyroid, because the protein-bound T_4 is not metabolically active.*

Factitious hyperthyroidism *Patients who self-administer T_4 will have elevated levels. Many patients believe they will feel more energetic or will lose weight faster if they take T_4.*

Struma ovarii *Ectopic thyroid tissue in the ovary or anywhere can produce excess T_4.*

TBG increase (e.g., as occurs in pregnancy, hepatitis, congenital hyperproteinemia) *Because the T_4 assay measures total bound and unbound T_4, any condition associated with elevated TBG will cause an elevation of T_4.*

Decreased levels

Hypothyroid states (e.g., cretinism, surgical ablation, myxedema) *The thyroid in these diseases cannot produce an adequate amount of T_4 despite the stimulation provided.*

Pituitary insufficiency *The pituitary produces an insufficient amount of thyrotropin. As a result, the thyroid is not stimulated to produce T_4.*

Hypothalamic failure *The hypothalamus produces an insufficient amount of TRH. As a result, the pituitary does not produce thyrotropin, and the thyroid is not stimulated to produce T_4.*

Protein malnutrition and other protein-depleted states (e.g., nephrotic syndrome) *With a reduced protein source, TBG and albumin decrease. Because T_4 assay measures hormone bound to these proteins, T_4 can be expected to be reduced.*

Iodine insufficiency *Iodine is the basic raw material for T_4. Without iodine, T_4 cannot be produced. With the introduction of iodide in most table salts, iodine insufficiency is rare in the United States.*

Nonthyroid illnesses (e.g., renal failure, Cushing's disease, cirrhosis, surgery, advanced cancer. *The pathophysiology of these observations is not well known. It may be, in part due to a depletion of thyroid-binding proteins associated with severe medical illnesses.*

Related Tests

- Long-acting thyroid stimulator (p. 294): LATS and other thyroid-stimulating immunoglobulins are used to support the diagnosis of Graves' disease, especially when the diagnosis is complex.
- Thyroid-releasing hormone (p. 415): This test assists in the evaluation of patients with hyper- and hypothyroidism. It is especially helpful in the differential diagnosis of hypothyroidism.
- Thyroid-stimulating hormone (p. 410): This test is used to diagnose primary hypothyroidism and to differentiate it from secondary (pituitary) and tertiary (hypothalamus) hypothyroidism.
- Thyroid-stimulating hormone stimulation (p. 413): This test is also used to differentiate primary and secondary (and tertiary) hypothyroidism.
- Thyroxine-binding globulin (p. 421): This is a measure of TBG, the major thyroid hormone protein carrier. It is used in the evaluation of patients who have abnormal total T_4 and T_3 levels. When performed concurrently with a T_4/T_3 test, the T_4 and T_3 levels can be more easily interpreted.
- Triiodothyronine uptake (p. 438): This test is an indirect measurement of total T_4.
- Triiodothyronine (p. 435): T_3 is used to evaluate thyroid function. It is primarily used to diagnose hyperthyroidism. It is also used to monitor thyroid replacement and suppressive therapy.

- Thyroxine index, free (p. 426): This test is used to evaluate thyroid function. It corrects for changes in thyroid hormone–binding serum proteins that can affect total T_4 levels. It is used to diagnose hyper- and hypothyroidism.
- Thyroxine, free (p. 423): The FT_4 is used to evaluate thyroid function in patients who may have protein abnormalities that could affect total T_4 levels. It is used to diagnose thyroid function and to monitor replacement and suppressive therapy.
- Antithyroglobulin antibody (p. 89): This test is primarily used in the differential diagnosis of thyroid diseases, such as Hashimoto's thyroiditis and chronic lymphocytic thyroiditis (in children).

Thyroxine-Binding Globulin
(TBG, Thyroid-Binding Globulin)

Normal Findings

Age	Males (mg/dl)	Females (mg/dl)
1-5 days	2.2-4.2	2.2-4.2
1-11 months	1.6-3.6	1.7-3.7
1-9 years	1.2-2.8	1.5-2.7
10-19 years	1.4-2.6	1.4-3.0
>20 years	1.7-3.6	1.7-3.6
Oral contraceptives	–	1.5-5.5
Pregnancy (third trimester)	–	4.7-5.9

Indications

This is a measure of TBG, the major thyroid hormone protein carrier. It is used in the evaluation of patients who have abnormal total T_4 and T_3 levels. When performed concurrently with a T_4/T_3 test, the T_4 and T_3 levels can be more easily interpreted.

Test Explanation

Assays of T_4 and T_3 are a measure of total T_4/T_3 levels. That is, they are a measure of bound and unbound thyroid hormones. Most of these hormones are bound to TBG. The unbound or "free T_4/T_3" is the metabolically active hormone. Certain illnesses are associated with elevated or decreased TBG levels. With increased TBG levels, more T_4 and T_3 is bound to that protein. Less free, metabolically active T_4/T_3 is available. TSH is stimulated to produce higher levels of T_4 and T_3 to compensate. T_4 and T_3 levels increase but do not cause hyperthyroidism, because the increase is merely a compensation for the increased TBG. When total T_4 is elevated, one must ascertain whether that elevation is due to an elevation in TBG or a real elevation in T_4 alone associated with hyperthyroidism. There are other indirect measurements of TBG, including thyroid hormone–binding ratio (THBR) (see p. 438).

The most common causes of elevated TBG are pregnancy, hormone replacement therapy, or use of oral contraceptives. Elevated TBG is also present in some cases of porphyria and in infectious hepatitis. Decreased TBG is commonly associated with other causes of hypoproteinemia (e.g., nephrotic syndrome, GI malabsorption, malnutrition).

Interfering Factors

- Previous administration of diagnostic radioisotopes may confound test results, because TBG is measured by radioimmunoassay.
- Drugs that *increase* TBG include estrogens, methadone, tamoxifen, and oral contraceptives.
- Drugs that *decrease* TBG include steroids, androgens, danazol, phenytoin, and propanolol.

Procedure and Patient Care

Before

- Explain the procedure to the patient.
- Tell the patient that no fasting is required.

During

- Collect approximately 5 to 7 ml of venous blood in a red-top tube.
- List on the laboratory slip any drugs that may affect test results.

After

- Apply pressure or a pressure dressing to the venipuncture site.
- Assess the venipuncture site for bleeding.

Test Results and Clinical Significance

Increased levels

Pregnancy (and estrogen replacement therapy, estrogen-producing tumors) *All proteins, including TBG, are increased with increased estrogen levels.*
Infectious hepatitis *The pathophysiology of this observation is not well known.*
Genetic increase of TBG *Rarely a patient will have a genetic variation that causes elevated TBG.*
Acute intermittent porphyria *The pathophysiology of this observation is not well known.*

Decreased levels

Protein-losing enteropathy
Protein-losing nephropathy
Malnutrition
Decreased protein levels include decreased TBG.

Testosterone-producing tumors *Testosterone decreases TBG levels.*
Ovarian failure *With reduced estrogens (e.g., menopause), TBG is reduced.*
Major stress *Major stress is often associated with low proteins, including TBG.*

Related Tests

- Long-acting thyroid stimulator (p. 294): LATS and other thyroid-stimulating immunoglobulins are used to support the diagnosis of Graves' disease, especially when the diagnosis is complex.

- Thyrotropin-releasing hormone (p. 415): This test assists in the evaluation of patients with hyper- and hypothyroidism. It is especially helpful in the differential diagnosis of hypothyroidism.
- Thyroid-stimulating hormone (p. 410): This test is used to diagnose primary hypothyroidism and to differentiate it from secondary (pituitary) and tertiary (hypothalamus) hypothyroidism.
- Thyroid-stimulating hormone stimulation (p. 413): This test is also used to differentiate primary and secondary (and tertiary) hypothyroidism.
- Triiodothyronine uptake (p. 438): This test is an indirect measurement of total T_4.
- Thyroxine (p. 417): This is one of the first tests done for assessing thyroid function. It is used to diagnose thyroid function and to monitor replacement and suppressive therapy.
- Triiodothyronine (p. 435): T_3 is used to evaluate thyroid function. It is mostly used to diagnose hyperthyroidism. It is also used to monitor thyroid replacement and suppressive medical therapy.
- Thyroxine index, free (p. 426): This test is used to evaluate thyroid function. It corrects for changes in thyroid hormone–binding serum proteins that can affect total T_4 levels. It is used to diagnose hyper- and hypothyroidism.
- Thyroxine, free (see below): The FT_4 is used to evaluate thyroid function in patients who may have protein abnormalities that could affect total T_4 levels. It is used to diagnose thyroid function and to monitor replacement and suppressive therapy.
- Antithyroglobulin antibody (p. 89): This test is primarily used in the differential diagnosis of thyroid diseases, such as Hashimoto's thyroiditis and chronic lymphocytic thyroiditis (in children).

Thyroxine, Free (FT_4)

Normal Findings

Age	ng/dl
0-4 days	2-6
2 weeks-20 years	0.8-2
Adult	0.8-2.7

Indications

The FT_4 is used to evaluate thyroid function in patients who may have protein abnormalities that could affect total T_4 levels. It is used to diagnose thyroid function and to monitor replacement and suppressive therapy.

Test Explanation

Thyroid hormone is made up of thyroxine (T_4) and triiodothyronine (T_3). Over 90% of thyroid hormone is made up of T_4. As much as 99% of T_4 is bound to proteins (thyroxine-binding globulin [TBG] and albumin). Only 1% to 5% of total T_4 is unbound or "free."

The free T_4 is the metabolically active thyroid hormone. When measuring total T_4, the bound and the unbound portion is measured. Abnormalities in protein levels can have a significant effect on the total T_4 results. Pregnancy and hormone replacement therapy increase TBG and will cause T_4 to be falsely elevated, suggesting that hyperthyroidism exists when, in fact, the patient is euthyroid. If the free T_4 is measured in these patients, it will be normal, indicating that free T_4 is a more accurate indicator of thyroid function than total T_4. Likewise, when TBG is reduced (e.g., hypoproteinemia), the total T_4 is also reduced, suggesting hypothyroidism. Measurement of free T_4 would indicate normal levels and thereby discount the abnormal total T_4 as merely a result of the reduced TBG and not as a result of hypothyroidism.

This test is used to determine thyroid function, especially when the patient has concurrent clinical problems that may alter protein blood levels. Greater than normal levels indicate hyperthyroid states, and subnormal values are seen in hypothyroid states. This test is performed by direct dialysis extraction of free T_4 and measured by radioimmunoassay. There are significant laboratory variations in results and testing quality. The FT_4 index may be a better indication of true thyroid function.

Interfering Factors

- Neonates have higher levels than older children and adults.
- Prior use of radioisotopes can alter test results, because the method used to determine free T_4 levels is radioimmunoassay.
- Drugs that *increase* FT_4 levels include heparin, aspirin, danazol, and propanolol.
- Drugs that *decrease* FT_4 levels include furosemide, phenytoins, methadone, and rifampicin.
- Exogenously administered thyroxine will cause elevated FT_4 results.

CLINICAL PRIORITIES

- This test is used to evaluate thyroid function in patients who may have protein abnormalities that could affect total T_4 levels.
- High levels indicate hyperthyroidism and low levels indicate hypothyroidism.

Procedure and Patient Care

Before

- Explain the procedure to the patient.
- Evaluate the patient's medication history.
- If indicated, instruct the patient to stop taking exogenous T_4 medication 1 month before testing.
- Tell the patient that no fasting is required.

During

- Collect a venous blood specimen in a red-top tube.
- List on the laboratory slip any drugs that may affect test results.

After

- Apply pressure or a pressure dressing to the venipuncture site.
- Assess the venipuncture site for bleeding.

Test Results and Clinical Significance

Increased levels

Primary hyperthyroid states (e.g., Graves' disease, Plummer's disease, toxic thyroid adenoma) *The thyroid produces increased T_4 despite lack of TSH stimulation.*

Acute thyroiditis *The thyroid secretes increased T_4 during the acute inflammatory stages of thyroiditis (e.g., Hashimoto's thyroiditis). However, in the latter stages the thyroid may become burned out and the patient may become hypothyroid.*

Factitious hyperthyroidism *Patients who self-administer thyroxine will have elevated levels. Many patients believe they will feel more energetic or will lose weight faster if they take T_4.*

Struma ovarii *Ectopic thyroid tissue in the ovary or anywhere can produce excess T_4.*

Decreased levels

Hypothyroid states (e.g., cretinism, surgical ablation, myxedema) *The thyroid in these diseases cannot produce an adequate amount of T_4 despite the stimulation provided.*

Pituitary insufficiency *The pituitary produces an insufficient amount of thyrotropin. As a result, the thyroid is not stimulated to produce T_4.*

Hypothalamic failure *The hypothalamus produces an insufficient amount of TRH. As a result, the pituitary does not produce thyrotropin, and the thyroid is not stimulated to produce T_4.*

Iodine insufficiency *Iodine is the basic raw material for T_4. Without iodine, T_4 cannot be produced. With the introduction of iodide in most table salts, iodine insufficiency has become rare in the United States.*

Nonthyroid illnesses (e.g., renal failure, Cushing's disease, cirrhosis, surgery, advanced cancer) *The pathophysiology of these observations is not well known.*

Related Tests

- Long-acting thyroid stimulator (p. 294): LATS and other thyroid-stimulating immunoglobulins are used to support the diagnosis of Graves' disease, especially when the diagnosis is complex.
- Thyrotropin-releasing hormone (p. 415): This test assists in the evaluation of patients with hyper- and hypothyroidism. It is especially helpful in the differential diagnosis of hypothyroidism.
- Thyroid-stimulating hormone (p. 410): This test is used to diagnose primary hypothyroidism and to differentiate it from secondary (pituitary) and tertiary (hypothalamus) hypothyroidism.
- Thyroid-stimulating hormone stimulation (p. 413): This test is also used to differentiate primary and secondary (and tertiary) hypothyroidism.
- Thyroxine-binding globulin (p. 421): This is a measure of TBG, the major thyroid hormone protein carrier. It is used in the evaluation of patients who have abnormal total T_4 and T_3 levels. When performed concurrently with a T_4/T_3 test, the T_4 and T_3 levels can be more easily interpreted.
- Thyroxine (p. 417): This is one of the first tests done for assessing thyroid function. It

is used to diagnose thyroid function and to monitor replacement and suppressive therapy.

- Triiodothyronine (p. 435): T_3 is used to evaluate thyroid function. It is primarily used to diagnose hyperthyroidism. It is also used to monitor thyroid replacement and suppressive therapy.
- Triiodothyronine uptake (p. 438): This test is an indirect measurement of total T_4.
- Thyroxine index, free (see below): This test is used to evaluate thyroid function. It correcrs for changes in thyroid hormone–binding serum proteins that can affect total T_4 levels. It is used to diagnose hyper- and hypothyroidism.
- Antithyroglobulin antibody (p. 89): This test is primarily used in the differential diagnosis of thyroid diseases, such as Hashimoto's thyroiditis and chronic lymphocytic thyroiditis (in children).

Thyroxine Index, Free (FTI, T_7, FT_4 Index, FT_4I)

Normal Findings

0.8-2.4 ng/dl or 10-31 pmol/L (SI units)
Adult index: 1.5 to 4.5 if units are eliminated

Indications

This test is used to evaluate thyroid function. It corrects for changes in thyroid hormone–binding serum proteins that can affect total T_4 levels. It is used to diagnose hyper- and hypothyroidism.

Test Explanation

The FT_4I study measures the amount of free thyroxine (T_4), which is only 1% of the total T_4. Free T_4 is the unbound T_4 that enters the cell and is metabolically active. The diagnostic value of measuring the FT_4I is that it is not affected by thyroxine-binding globulin (TBG) abnormalities; therefore it correlates more closely with the true hormonal status than total T_4 or triiodothyronine (T_3) determinations. To determine the FT_4I, T_3 uptake is measured and multiplied by the measured T_4. This simple mathematical computation corrects the estimated total T_4 assay for the effects of TBG protein alterations. If TBG is increased, the T_3 uptake decreases and corrects for the increased T_4 associated with the increased TBG. However, when the TBG is normal and the T_4 is elevated, the FT_4 will be increased, indicating true hyperthyroidism. Therefore the FT_4I yields the same information as the free T_4 radioimmunoassay.

This index is useful in diagnosing hyperthyroidism and hypothyroidism, especially in patients with abnormalities in TBG levels. High FT_4I calculations suggest hyperthyroidism; low FT_4I values suggest hypothyroidism. The FT_4I study also aids in the evaluation of the thyroid status of pregnant women and patients who have abnormal TBG levels as a result of being treated with certain drugs (e.g., estrogen, phenytoin, salicylates).

CLINICAL PRIORITIES

- The diagnostic value of measuring the FT_4I is that it is not affected by TBG abnormalities. Therefore it correlates more closely with hormonal states than the T_4 or T_3 tests.
- The FT_4I is determined by a mathematical calculation using the T_3 uptake and the T_4 values. This calculation corrects the estimated total T_4 assay for the effects of TBG protein abnormalities.
- A high FT_4I calculation suggests hyperthyroidism. Low levels suggest hypothyroidism.

Interfering Factors

(See factors affecting T_4 on p. 418 and T_3 uptake on p. 439).

Procedure and Patient Care

Before

- Explain the procedure to the patient.
- Obtain the T_4 value and T_3 uptake ratio.

During

- Multiply the T_3 uptake value by the T_4 value to obtain the FT_4I:

$$FT_4I = \frac{T_4\text{ (total)} \times T_3\text{ uptake (THBR) (\%)}}{100}$$

After

- Apply pressure or a pressure dressing to the venipuncture site.
- Check the venipuncture site for bleeding.

Test Results and Clinical Significance

Increased levels

Primary hyperthyroid states (e.g., Graves' disease, Plummer's disease, toxic thyroid adenoma) *The thyroid produces increased T_4 despite lack of TSH stimulation.*

Acute thyroiditis *The thyroid secretes increased T_4 during the acute inflammatory stages of thyroiditis (e.g., Hashimoto's thyroiditis). However, in the latter stages the thyroid may become burned out and the patient may become hypothyroid.*

Factitious hyperthyroidism *Patients who self-administer T_4 will have elevated levels. Many patients believe they will feel more energetic or will lose weight faster if they take T_4.*

Struma ovarii *Ectopic thyroid tissue in the ovary or anywhere can produce excess T_4.*

Decreased levels

Hypothyroid states (e.g., cretinism, surgical ablation, myxedema) *The thyroid in these diseases cannot produce an adequate amount of T_4 despite the stimulation provided.*

Pituitary insufficiency *The pituitary produces an insufficient amount of thyrotropin. As a result, the thyroid is not stimulated to produce T_4.*

Hypothalamic failure *The hypothalamus produces an insufficient amount of thyrotropin-releasing hormone. As a result, the pituitary does not produce thyrotropin, and the thyroid is not stimulated to produce T_4.*
Iodine insufficiency *Iodine is the basic raw material for T_4. Without iodine, T_4 cannot be produced. With the introduction of iodide in most table salts, iodine insufficiency has become rare in the United States.*

Related Tests

- Long-acting thyroid stimulator (p. 294): LATS and other thyroid-stimulating immunoglobulins are used to support the diagnosis of Graves' disease, especially when the diagnosis is complex.
- Thyrotropin-releasing hormone (p. 415): This test assists in the evaluation of patients with hyper- and hypothyroidism. It is especially helpful in the differential diagnosis of hypothyroidism.
- Thyroid-stimulating hormone (p. 410): This test is used to diagnose primary hypothyroidism and to differentiate it from secondary (pituitary) and tertiary (hypothalamus) hypothyroidism.
- Thyroid-stimulating hormone stimulation (p. 413): This test is also used to differentiate primary and secondary (and tertiary) hypothyroidism.
- Thyroxine-binding globulin (p. 421): This is a measure of TBG, the major thyroid hormone protein carrier. It is used in the evaluation of patients who have abnormal total T_4 and T_3 levels. When performed concurrently with a T_4/T_3 test, the T_4 and T_3 levels can be more easily interpreted.
- Thyroxine (p. 417): This is one of the first tests done for assessing thyroid function. It is used to diagnose thyroid function and to monitor replacement and suppressive therapy.
- Triiodothyronine (p. 435): T_3 is used to evaluate thyroid function. It is primarily used to diagnose hyperthyroidism. It is also used to monitor thyroid replacement and suppressive therapy.
- Thyroxine, free (p. 423): This test is used to evaluate thyroid function in patients who may have protein abnormalities that could affect total T_4 levels. It is used to diagnose thyroid function and to monitor replacement and suppressive therapy.
- Triiodothyronine uptake (p. 438): This test is an indirect measurement of total T_4.
- Antithyroglobulin antibody (p. 89): This test is primarily used in the differential diagnosis of thyroid diseases, such as Hashimoto's thyroiditis and chronic lymphocytic thyroiditis (in children).

Tourniquet (Capillary Fragility)

Normal Findings

<2 petechiae

Indications

This test evaluates capillary integrity and platelet number and function.

Test Explanation

Petechiae occur as a result of increased capillary fragility (microvessels easily rupture and a small amount of bleeding occurs in the skin) or from thrombocytopenia (causing spontaneous bleeding in the skin). Petechiae are small, round nonraised red spots in the skin.

Production of petechiae can be induced in patients who have increased capillary fragility or thrombocytopenia. There are two methods of inducing petechiae. The most common is with positive pressure where a blood pressure cuff is applied to an extremity and inflated above venous pressure. The second way is with negative pressure where a suction cup is applied to an area of skin for a particular period of time. Patients with thrombocytopenia, poor platelet function, or purpura will develop petechiae. The number of petechiae in the study are graded as follows:

1 + Few petechiae present
2 + Many petechiae present
3 + Multiple petechiae present over a broader area
4 + Confluent petechiae present

The number of petechiae generally is proportional to the severity of the disease. This test is rarely used today since platelet counts are so easily available. It is helpful, however, in identifying those patients with increased capillary fragility. The size of petechiae, if uniform, may indicate the source of the positive test. Large petechiae are associated with thrombocytopenia. Small pinpoint petechiae are more likely related to increased capillary fragility.

Interfering Factors

- Premenstrual women experience transient episodes of increased capillary fragility.
- Postmenopausal women who do not use hormones experience increased capillary fragility.
- Prolonged use of steroids increases capillary fragility.
- Women, especially those with sun-damaged skin, can have increased capillary fragility

Procedure and Patient Care

Before

- Explain the procedure to the patient.
- Obtain an informed consent if required by the institution.
- Tell the patient that no fasting is required.
- Examine the extremity for preexisting petechiae or ecchymoses.

During

For Positive Pressure Test

- Place a blood pressure cuff on the upper arm and inflate it to a level above venous pressure (around 70 mm Hg) for 5 minutes.
- Relieve the cuff pressure.
- Inspect the distal extremity for petechiae.

For Negative Pressure Test

- Place a lubricated suction cup (2 cm in diameter) on the upper arm skin.
- Remove the suction after 1 minute.
- Examine the site for petechiae.

After

- Explain the results to the patient.
- If the test is positive, explain to the patient that appropriate precautions should be taken to avoid soft tissue injury.

Test Results and Clinical Significance

Positive: >2 petechiae

Immunologic thrombocytopenia (e.g., idiopathic thrombocytopenic purpura)
Drug-induced thrombocytopenia
Thromboasthenia (poor platelet function)
Reduced platelets cause spontaneous microbleeding. Interestingly, nonimmunologic thrombocytopenia is rarely associated with a positive tourniquet test.

Herediatry telangiectasia
Vascular purpura (autoimmune diseases)
Senile purpura
Allergic purpura
Scurvy
Increased capillary permeability causes petechiae.

Hemophilia *Spontaneous bleeding causes petechiae.*

Related Tests

- Platelet count (p. 337): This is a direct measurement of platelet number.
- Platelet volume, mean (p. 340): This is a direct measurement of platelet volume.
- Platelet aggregation (p. 333): This is a direct measurement of platelet function.
- Platelet antibody (p. 335): This test identifies platelet antibodies that destroy the platelet.
- Bleeding time (p. 115): This is an indirect measurement of bleeding tendency. It is abnormal in patients with low platelet counts or in patients with increased permeability.

Toxoplasmosis Antibody Titer

Normal Findings

IgG titers: <1:16 indicate no previous infection.
IgG titers: 1:16-1:256 are usually prevalent in the general population.
IgG titers: >1:256 suggest recent infection.
IgM titers: >1:256 indicate acute infection.

Indications

These serologic tests are used to diagnose acute toxoplasmosis infection in immunosupressed patients, pregnant women, and newborn infants. Immunity obtained from prior infection (e.g., fetal infection) is also determined by this test.

Test Explanation

Toxoplasmosis is a protozoan disease caused by *Toxoplasma gondii,* which is found in humans and many animals (especially cats). Humans become infected by eating poorly cooked or raw meat. Exposure to feces of cats or other infected material can cause infection. Most often infected humans are asymptomatic. When symptoms occur, this disease is characterized by CNS lesions, which may lead to blindness, brain damage, and death. The condition may occur congenitally or sometime after birth. Because approximately 25% to 70% of the adult population have been exposed to toxoplasmosis as determined by positive antibody titers, the Centers for Disease Control recommends that pregnant women be serologically tested for this disease. Again, most acutely infected pregnant women are asymptomatic, and the best way to diagnose infection is by antibody testing.

The presence of antibodies before pregnancy indicates prior exposure and chronic asymptomatic infection. The presence of these antibodies probably ensures protection against congenital toxoplasmosis in the child. Fetal infection occurs if the mother acquires toxoplasmosis after conception and passes it to the fetus through the placenta. Repeat testing of pregnant patients with low or negative titers may be done before the twentieth week and before delivery to identify antibody converters and determine appropriate therapy (e.g., therapeutic abortion at 20 weeks, treatment during the remainder of the pregnancy, or treatment of the newborn).

Hydrocephaly, microcephaly, chronic retinitis, and convulsions are complications of congenital toxoplasmosis. Congenital toxoplasmosis is diagnosed when the antibody levels are persistently elevated or a rising titer is found in the infant 2 to 3 months after birth.

The term "TORCH" (toxoplasmosis, other, rubella, cytomegalovirus, herpes) has been applied to infections with recognized detrimental effects on the fetus. The effects on the fetus may be direct or indirect (e.g., precipitating abortion or premature labor). Included in the category of "other" are infections (e.g., syphilis). All of these tests are discussed separately.

Because of the difficulty in growing toxoplasmosis in culture, the best way to diagnose this disease is by serologic testing. The most commonly used test is the indirect fluorescent antibody test. With this technique, IgM and IgG can be detected in sum or separately. IgM rises about 1 week after inoculation, peaks in about 2 to 3 months, and declines to undetectable levels in about 1 year. IgG begins to rise about 2 weeks after inoculation, peaks in about 2 to 3 months, and declines to low but persistent levels in about 6 months. Low titers of IgG especially indicate past infections and protection from passing acute infection to an unborn child. High or rapidly rising titers of either IgM or IgG indicate acute infection in the adult or newborn infant. Hemagglutination is another more easily performed method of detecting IgG antibodies to toxoplasmosis. This is often used to screen new mothers. Enzyme-linked immunosorbent assay (ELISA) and radioimmunoassay are other techniques to identify antibodies.

Elevated IgM antibodies, IgG titers greater than 1:1000, or a fourfold rise in IgG antibodies indicates an acute toxoplasmosis infection. Low, but significant titers of IgG indicate past infection. High, nonrising titers indicate acute infection more than 3 to 12 months prior to testing.

Interfering Factors

- Rheumatoid factor or antinuclear antibodies can cause false-positive results.
- Other active congenital infections can cause false-positive results.

Procedure and Patient Care

Before

- Explain the procedure to the patient.

During

- Collect approximately 5 ml of blood in a red-top tube.
- Indicate on the laboratory slip if the patient is pregnant or has been exposed to cats.

After

- Apply pressure or a pressure dressing to the venipuncture site.
- Assess the venipuncture site for bleeding.

Test Results and Clinical Significance

Increased levels

Toxoplasmosis infection

Triglyceride (TG)

Normal Findings

Adult/elderly
Male: 40-160 mg/dl or 0.45-1.81 mmol (SI units)
Female: 35-135 mg/dl or 0.40-1.52 mmol/L (SI units)

Children	Male	Female
0-5 years	30-86 mg/dl	32-99 mg/dl
6-11 years	31-108 mg/dl	35-114 mg/dl
12-15 years	36-138 mg/dl	41-138 mg/dl
16-19 years	40-163 mg/dl	40-128 mg/dl

Critical Values >400 mg/dl

Indications

TGs identify the risk of developing coronary heart disease. This test is part of a lipid profile that includes the measurement of cholesterol and lipoproteins. This test is also performed on patients suspected of having fat metabolism disorders.

Test Explanation

TGs are a form of fat in the bloodstream. They are transported by very-low-density lipoproteins (VLDLs) and low-density lipoproteins (LDLs). TGs are produced in the liver using glycerol and other fatty acids as building blocks. TGs act as a storage source for energy. When TG levels in the blood are high, TGs are deposited in the fatty tissues. TGs constitute most of the fat in the body and are a part of a lipid profile that also evaluates cholesterol and lipoprotein. A lipid profile is performed to assess the risk of coronary and vascular disease.

Interfering Factors

- Ingestion of fatty meals may cause elevated TG levels.
- Ingestion of alcohol may cause elevated levels of TG by increasing the production of VLDL.
- Pregnancy may cause increased levels.
- Drugs that may cause *increased* TG levels include cholestyramine, estrogens, and oral contraceptives.
- Drugs that may cause *decreased* levels include ascorbic acid, asparaginase, clofibrate, and colestipol.

Procedure and Patient Care

Before

- Explain the procedure to the patient.
- Instruct the patient to fast for 12 to 14 hours before the test. Only water is permitted.
- Tell the patient not to drink alcohol for 24 hours before the test.
- Inform the patient that dietary indiscretion for as much as 2 weeks before this test will influence results.

During

- Collect 5 to 10 ml of venous blood in a red-top tube.

After

- Apply pressure or a pressure dressing to the venipuncture site.
- Assess the venipuncture site for bleeding.
- Mark the patient's age and gender on the laboratory slip.
- Instruct patients with increased TG levels regarding diet, exercise, and appropriate weight.

Test Results and Clinical Significance

Increased levels

Glycogen storage disease (von Gierke's disease) *VLDL (TG-carrying proteins) synthesis is increased, whereas catabolism is decreased. TG levels in the blood increase.*

Familial hypertriglyceridemia *This is a genetic predisposition to elevated TGs.*

Apoprotein C-II deficiency *This congenital disease is associated with lipoprotein lipase deficiency. TGs accumulate.*

Hyperlipidemias *As lipids in the blood increase, so does TG, the major blood lipid.*

Hypothyroidism *Catabolism of TG is diminished.*

High-carbohydrate diet *Excess carbohydrates are converted into TG and blood levels of TG rise.*

Poorly controlled diabetes *Diabetics have an increased synthesis of TG-carrying VLDL and a decreased catabolism of the same. Therefore TG blood levels increase.*

Nephrotic syndrome *The loss of proteins diminishes the plasma oncotic pressures. This appears to stimulate hepatic lipoprotein synthesis of VLDL and LDL. Also, lipoprotein disposal is possibly diminished.*

Chronic renal failure *Insulin levels are high in these patients, because insulin is excreted by the kidney. Insulin increases lipogenesis and causes TG levels to increase. Also, these patients have a deficiency in lipoprotein lipase that clears the blood of TG.*

Decreased levels

Malabsorption syndrome *These patients have a malabsorption of fat from the diet. As TG is the major component of dietary fat, TG levels can be expected to fall in light of poor GI absorption.*

Abetalipoproteinemia *Not only do these patients have a malabsorption of fat, but they also have a defective synthesis of apoprotein B (TG-carrying lipoproteins). TG blood levels are low.*

Malnutrition *These patient have diminished fat in the diet. As TG is the major component of dietary fat, TG levels can be expected to fall.*

Hyperthyroidism *The catabolism of VLDL, the main TG-carrying lipoprotein, is increased. Therefore, TG blood levels diminish.*

Related Tests

- Cholesterol (p. 143): This is a measure of total cholesterol in the blood. It is a part of the lipid profile.
- Lipoprotein (HDL, VLDL, and LDL) (p. 289): These proteins play an important role in the transport of lipids in the bloodstream. They, too, have been used in the assessment of risk for coronary heart disease.

Triiodothyronine
(Total T_3 Radioimmunoassay [T_3 by RIA], Free T_3)

Normal Findings

Age	ng/dl
1-3 days	100-740
1-11 months	105-245
1-5 years	105-270
6-10 years	95-240
11-15 years	80-215
16-20 years	80-210
20-50 years	70-205
>50 years	40-180

Indications

T_3 is used to evaluate thyroid function. It is primarily used to diagnose hyperthyroidism. It is also used to monitor thyroid replacement and suppressive therapy.

Test Explanation

Thyroid hormones are produced when tyrosine incorporates organic iodine to form a monoiodotyrosine. This complex picks up another iodine and becomes diiodotyrosine. Two diiodotyrosines combine to form tetraiodothyronine (also called T_4 thyroid hormone). If a diiodotyrosine combines with a monoiodotyrosine, triiodothyronine (also called T_3 thyroid hormone) is formed. A large proportion of T_3 is formed in the liver by conversion of T_4 to T_3. As with the T_4 test, the serum T_3 test is an accurate indicator of thyroid function. T_3 is less stable than T_4 as it is much less tightly bound to serum proteins than T_4. Only about 7% to 10% of thyroid hormone is composed of T_3. And 70% of that T_3 is bound to proteins (thyroxine-binding globulin [TBG] and albumin). Only minute quantities are unbound or "free." It is the *free T_3* that is metabolically active. Furthermore, measurement of free T_3 is not subject to the effects that alterations of serum proteins have on the total T_3, which is described in this test. This test measures the total bound and unbound (free) T_3. Generally, when the T_3 level is below normal, the patient is in a hypothyroid state.

Other severe nonthyroidal diseases can decrease T_3 levels by diminishing the conversion of T_4 to T_3 in the liver. This makes T_3 levels less useful in indicating hypothyroid states. Furthermore, there is considerable overlap between hypothyroid states and normal thyroid function. Because of this, T_3 levels are primarily used to assist in the diagnosis of hyperthyroid states. An elevated T_3 indicates hyperthyroidism, especially when T_4 is also elevated. In a rare form of hyperthyroidism called "T_3 toxicosis," T_4 is normal and T_3 is elevated.

In the hypothalamus, thyrotropin-releasing hormone (TRH) is secreted. This stimulates the anterior pituitary to secrete thyrotropin (thyroid-stimulating hormone [TSH]). TSH stimulates the thyroid to secrete thyroid hormone. The increased levels of T_3 and T_4 inhibit further production of TRH.

This test is performed by direct dialysis extraction of both bound T_3 and free T_3 and is measured by radioimmunoassay. This test is not the same as the T_3 uptake test and should not be confused with it.

Interfering Factors

- Radioisotope administration before the test may alter the results, because this test is performed by radioimmunoassay methods.
- Total T_3 values are increased in pregnancy, because serum proteins are increased at that time. Free T_3, however, is not affected by protein levels.
- Drugs that may cause *increased* levels include estrogen, methadone, and oral contraceptives.
- Drugs that may cause *decreased* levels include anabolic steroids, androgens, phenytoin (Dilantin), propranolol (Inderal), reserpine, and salicylates (high dose).

CLINICAL PRIORITIES

- The T_3 test is primarily used to diagnose hyperthyroidism.
- T_3 is less useful in the diagnosis of hypothyroidism since other nonthyroidal diseases can decrease T_3 levels by decreasing the conversion of T_4 to T_3 in the liver.
- This test in *not* the same as the T_3 resin uptake test.

Procedure and Patient Care

Before

- Explain the procedure to the patient.
- Determine whether the patient is taking any exogenous T_3 medication, because this will affect test results.
- Withhold drugs that may affect results (with physician's approval).
- Tell the patient that no fasting is required.

During

- Collect approximately 5 to 10 ml of venous blood in a red-top tube.
- List on the laboratory slip any medications the patient is currently taking.

After

- Apply pressure or a pressure dressing to the venipuncture site.
- Observe the venipuncture site for bleeding.

Test Results and Clinical Significance

Increased levels

Primary hyperthyroid states (e.g., Graves' disease, Plummer's disease, toxic thyroid adenoma) *The thyroid produces increased T_3 despite lack of TSH stimulation.*

Acute thyroiditis *The thyroid secretes increased T_3 during the acute inflammatory stages of thyroiditis (e.g., Hashimoto's thyroiditis). However, in the latter stages the thyroid may become burned out and the patient may become hypothyroid.*

Factitious hyperthyroidism *Patients who self-administer T_3 will have elevated levels. Many patients believe they will feel more energetic or will lose weight faster if they take T_3.*

Struma ovarii *Ectopic thyroid tissue in the ovary or anywhere can produce excess T_3.*

TBG increase (e.g., as occurs in pregnancy, hepatitis, congenital hyperproteinemia) *Because T_3 assay measures total bound and unbound T_3, any condition associated with elevated TBG will cause elevation of T_3. Free T_3 will not be elevated, however.*

Decreased levels

Hypothyroid states (e.g., cretinism, surgical ablation, myxedema) *The thyroid in these diseases cannot produce an adequate amount of T_3 despite the stimulation provided.*

Pituitary insufficiency *The pituitary produces an insufficient amount of thyrotropin. As a result, the thyroid is not stimulated to produce T_3.*

Hypothalamic failure *The hypothalamus produces an insufficient amount of TRH. As a result, the pituitary does not produce thyrotropin, and the thyroid is not stimulated to produce T_3.*

Protein malnutrition and other protein-depleted states (e.g., nephrotic syndrome) *With a reduced protein source, TBG and albumin decrease. Because the T_3 assay measures hormones bound to these proteins, T_3 can be expected to be reduced. Free T_3 levels will be unaffected by serum protein changes.*

Iodine insufficiency *Iodine is the basic raw material for T_3. Without iodine, T_4 cannot be produced. With the introduction of iodide in most table salts, iodine insufficiency has become rare in the United States.*

Nonthyroid illnesses (e.g., renal failure, Cushing's disease, cirrhosis, surgery, advanced cancer) *The pathophysiology of these observations is not well known. It may be, in part, due to a depletion of thyroxine-binding proteins, which is associated with severe medical illnesses. T_3 is more significantly affected by these diseases than is T_4.*

Hepatic diseases *Because a large proportion of T_3 is made by conversion of T_4 in the liver, severe liver dysfunction may affect T_3 levels. Often, however, other peripheral tissues take over T_3 synthesis by T_4 conversion.*

Related Tests

- Long-acting thyroid stimulator (LATS) (p. 294): LATS and other thyroid-stimulating immunoglobulins are used to support the diagnosis of Graves' disease, especially when the diagnosis is complex.
- Thyrotropin-releasing hormone (p. 415): This test assists in the evaluation of patients with hyper- and hypothyroidism. It is especially helpful in the differential diagnosis of hypothyroidism.
- Thyroid-stimulating hormone (p. 410): This test is used to diagnose primary hypothyroidism and to differentiate it from secondary (pituitary) and tertiary (hypothalamus) hypothyroidism.
- Thyroid-stimulating hormone (TSH) stimulation (p. 413): This test is also used to differentiate primary and secondary (and tertiary) hypothyroidism.
- Thyroxine-binding globulin (p. 421): This is a measure of TBG, the major thyroid hormone protein carrier. It is used in the evaluation of patients who have abnormal total

T_4 and T_3 levels. When performed concurrently with a T_4/T_3 test, the T_4 and T_3 levels can be more easily interpreted.

- Thyroxine (p. 417): This is one of the first tests done for assessing thyroid function. It is used to diagnose thyroid function and to monitor replacement and suppressive therapy.
- Triiodothyronine uptake (see below): This test is an indirect measurement of total T_4.
- Thyroxine index, free (p. 426): This test is used to evaluate thyroid function. It corrects for changes in thyroid hormone–binding serum proteins that can affect total T_4 levels. It is used to diagnose hyper- and hypothyroidism.
- Thyroxine, free (p. 423): The FT_4 is used to evaluate thyroid function in patients who may have protein abnormalities that could affect total T_4 levels. It is used to diagnose thyroid function and to monitor replacement and suppressive therapy.
- Antithyroglobulin antibody (p. 89): This test is primarily used for the differential diagnosis of thyroid diseases, such as Hashimoto's thyroiditis and chronic lymphocytic thyroiditis (in children).

Triiodothyronine Uptake (T_3 Resin Uptake, Resin Triiodothyronine Uptake Test [RT_3U, T_3RU], Thyroid Hormone-Binding Ratio [THBR])

Normal Findings 24%-34% or 24-34 AU (arbitrary units; SI units)

Indications

Along with T_4, this is a helpful test to evaluate thyroid function. Prior to direct T_4 assay this was used as an indirect measurement of T_4. It is also an indirect measurement of the quantity of thyroid hormone–binding proteins.

Test Explanation

This test was formerly called the T_3 uptake. Because it is not a measurement of T_3, but rather a measurement of the amount of unsaturated thyroid-binding sites on protein (thyroxine-binding globulin [TBG] and thyroid-binding prealbumin [TBPA]), the term "thyroid hormone–binding ratio" (THBR) has been recommended.

This test is actually an indirect measurement of total T_4. In this test, radioactive T_3 (RT_3) is added to the patient's serum along with a hormone-binding resin. The number of protein-binding sites available for the RT_3 depends primarily on the amount of T_4 already occupying those sites, since T_4 represents most of the thyroid hormone that is bound to protein. The lower the T_4 levels are, the more RT_3 binds on the serum proteins and less on the hormone-binding resin. The higher the T_4 levels are, the less RT_3 can bind to serum proteins and the more that is available to bind to the resin. Therefore the higher the resin uptake, the higher the T_4 level and vice versa. As one may expect, the THBR not only depends on the T_4 level but also on the amount of thyroid hormone–binding proteins, specifically TBG. As TBG increases, the THBR will decrease. Likewise, as TBG decreases, THBR increases, assuming T_4 stays the same. Therefore it is important to measure the T_4 and the THBR together, as shown in Table 2-36.

Table 2-36	Results of THBR and T_4 with clinical diagnoses	
THBR	T_4	Clinical diagnosis
Increased	Increased	Hyperproteinemia (e.g., pregnancy, estrogen)
Increased	Decreased	Hypothyroidism
Decreased	Increased	Hyperthyroidism
Decreased	Decreased	Hypoproteinemia (e.g., protein wasting)

Pregnancy, oral contraceptives, and some genetic disorders tend to inappropriately increase the quantity of these carrying proteins. As a result, T_4 and T_3 levels may be artificially elevated, but the patient may be euthyroid. Similarly, androgenic hormones, intercurrent serious illness, and nephrotic syndromes tend to lower the quantity of these proteins, causing falsely low T_3 and T_4 levels in euthyroid patients.

The T_3 uptake test is useful for the diagnosis of hypothyroidism or hyperthyroidism. This test is also used with the T_4 test to provide the free T_4 index. It is important to note that the RT_3U test is not a measurement of serum T_3. With the increasing availability of direct assay for T_3, T_4, and TBG, this test is used less frequently.

THBR levels consistent with hypothyroidism are not too different from low normal levels. This test is less than 60% accurate in indicating hypothyroidism.

Interfering Factors

- Recent radioisotope scans before the blood collection may affect test results, because radioactive-labeled T_3 is used in this test method.
- Severe acidosis may increase THBR. The pathophysiology is not known.
- Drugs that may cause *increased* TBG and TBPA levels include anabolic steroids, heparin, phenytoin (Dilantin), salicylates (high dose), thyroid agents, and warfarin (Coumadin).
- Drugs that may cause *decreased* levels include antithyroid agents, clofibrate, estrogen, oral contraceptives, and thiazides.

Procedure and Patient Care

Before

- Explain the procedure to the patient.
- Tell the patient that no fasting is required.

During

- Collect approximately 5 to 7 ml of venous blood in a red-top tube.
- List on the laboratory slip any drugs that may affect test results.

After

- Apply pressure or a pressure dressing to the venipuncture site.
- Assess the venipuncture site for bleeding.

Test Results and Clinical Significance

Increased levels

Hyperthyroidism *With increased production of T_4 and T_3, blood levels rise. Fewer TBG-binding sites are available for the RT_3, which will then bind an increased percentage of resin sites.*

Hypoproteinemia (e.g., protein malnutrition, protein-losing enteropathy, nephropathy) *Fewer TBG-binding sites are available for the RT_3, which will then bind an increased percentage of resin sites.*

Familial dysalbuminemic hyperthyroxinemia *These patients have a genetically defective form of albumin that binds T_4 unusually tightly. Fewer binding sites are available for the RT_3, which will then bind an increased percentage of resin sites.*

Nonthyroid illnesses (e.g., renal failure, Cushing's disease, cirrhosis, surgery, advanced cancer) *The pathophysiology of these observations is not well known. It may be, in part, due to a depletion of thyroid-binding proteins, which is associated with severe medical illnesses. Fewer protein binding sites are available for RT_3, which will then bind an increased percentage of resin sites.*

Factitious hyperthyroidism *Patients who self-administer T_4 will have elevated levels. Fewer TBG-binding sites are available for the RT_3, which will then bind an increased percentage of resin sites.*

Struma ovarii *Ectopic thyroid tissue in the ovary or anywhere can produce excess T_4. Fewer TBG-binding sites are available for the RT_3, which will then bind an increased percentage of resin sites.*

Decreased levels

An increase in TBG (e.g., as occurs in pregnancy, hepatitis, congenital hyperproteinemia) *There are more protein-binding sites available for RT_3, and therefore less RT_3 is bound to the resin.*

Hypothyroid states (e.g., cretinism, surgical ablation, pituitary insufficiency, hypothalamic failure, myxedema) *The thyroid in these diseases does not produce an adequate amount of T_4. T_4 levels are decreased. More protein-binding sites are available for RT_3 binding and less is bound to the resin.*

Hepatitis and cirrhosis *These illnesses are associated with elevated TBG. Therefore there are more protein-binding sites available for RT_3 and less RT_3 is bound to the resin.*

Related Tests

- Long-acting thyroid stimulator (LATS) (p. 294): LATS and other thyroid-stimulating immunoglobulins are used to support the diagnosis of Graves' disease, especially when the diagnosis is complex.
- Thyrotropin-releasing hormone (p. 415): This test assists in the evaluation of patients with hyper- and hypothyroidism. It is especially helpful in the differential diagnosis of hypothyroidism.
- Thyroid-stimulating hormone (p. 410): This test is used to diagnose primary hypothyroidism and to differentiate it from secondary (pituitary) and tertiary (hypothalamus) hypothyroidism.
- Thyroid-stimulating hormone (TSH) stimulation (p. 413): This test is also used to differentiate primary and secondary (and tertiary) hypothyroidism.

- Thyroxine-binding globulin (p. 421): This is a measure of TBG, the major thyroid hormone protein carrier. It is used in the evaluation of patients who have abnormal total T_4 and T_3 levels. When performed concurrently with a T_4/T_3 test, the T_4 and T_3 levels can be more easily interpreted.
- Thyroxine (p. 417): This is one of the first tests done for assessing thyroid function. It is used to diagnose thyroid function and to monitor replacement and suppressive therapy.
- Triiodothyronine (p. 435): T_3 is used to evaluate thyroid function. It is mostly used to diagnose hyperthyroidism. It is also used to monitor thyroid replacement and suppressive therapy.
- Thyroxine index, free (p. 426): This test is used to evaluate thyroid function. It corrects for changes in thyroid hormone–binding serum proteins that can affect total T_4 levels. It is used to diagnose hyper- and hypothyroidism.
- Thyroxine, free (p. 423): The FT_4 is used to evaluate thyroid function in patients who may have protein abnormalities that could affect total T_4 levels. It is used to diagnose thyroid function and to monitor replacement and suppressive therapy.
- Antithyroglobulin antibody (p. 89): This test is primarily used for the differential diagnosis of thyroid diseases, such as Hashimoto's thyroiditis and chronic lymphocytic thyroiditis (in children).

Tubular Phosphate Reabsorption
(TPR, Tubular Reabsorption of Phosphate [TRP])

Normal Findings 80%-90%

Indications

This test is used to estimate parathyroid hormone function. It is used to assist in the diagnosis of hyperparathyroidism. Since the development of direct parathyroid hormone (PTH) assay, this test is rarely used.

Test Explanation

The TPR test provides an indirect measurement of PTH by estimating its effects on renal phosphate reabsorption. PTH decreases phosphate reabsorption at the level of the renal tubule and increases phosphate excretion. TPR is generally done to detect primary hyperparathyroidism. This test value is calculated using the serum creatinine level (see p. 178), the serum phosphate concentration (see p. 328), and the creatinine clearance rate (see p. 180). Results are based on the ratio of phosphate clearance to creatinine clearance:

$$\% \text{ TPR} = 1 - \left(\frac{\text{Urine } PO_4 \times \text{Serum creatinine}}{\text{Urine creatinine} \times \text{Serum } PO_4} \right) \times 100$$

Values less than 80% indicate diminished renal tubular reabsorption of phosphate and suggest primary hyperparathyroidism. Decreased values also may be associated with sarcoidosis, myeloma, and hypercalcemia caused by malignancy.

Interfering Factors

- Low-phosphate diets raise TPR values.
- High-phosphate diets lower TPR values.

Procedure and Patient Care

Before

- Explain the procedure to the patient.
- Instruct the patient concerning the method that will be used (24-hour urine or hourly samples).
- Instruct the patient that he or she should have a normal phosphate diet (500 mg/day and 3000 mg/week).

During

24-hour Urine Test

- Keep the patient on NPO status except for water for 8 hours before drawing the blood sample.
- Collect the 24-hour urine sample using a preservative.
- Draw the blood early in the urine collection.

Hourly Urine Test

- Instruct the patient to drink several 8-ounce glasses of water and empty the bladder. (This marks the beginning of the test.)
- One hour later draw a blood specimen for phosphorous and creatinine measurements.
- One hour later (2 hours after beginning the test) instruct the patient to void for determination of the urine volume and urine concentration of creatinine and phosphorus.
- Note that urine may be collected again 1 hour later.

After

- Mark each specimen with the time it was collected.
- Send the specimen to the laboratory as soon as it is collected.

Test Results and Clinical Significance

Increased levels

Hypoparathyroidism (primary or secondary) *These patients have a reduced PTH. Therefore TPR levels are increased because of a lack of PTH effect on reducing TPR.*

Decreased levels

Primary hyperparathyroidism *PTH decreases phosphate tubular reabsorption.*
Sarcoidosis
Myeloma
These patients have hypercalcemia and reduced TPR. The pathophysiology of this observation is not well defined.

Hypercalcemia caused by malignancy *PTH-like hormone can be excreted by such cancers as lung, kidney, and breast cancer. PTH decreases TPR. In most cases of hypercalcemia of malignancy, no evidence of increases in PTH is found. Nevertheless, these patients develop hypercalcemia and hypophosphatemia due to reduced TPR.*

Related Tests

- Parathyroid hormone (PTH) (p. 316): This is a direct and more accurate method of determining PTH levels.

Urea Nitrogen, Blood (Blood Urea Nitrogen [BUN], Serum Urea Nitrogen)

Normal Findings

Adult: 10-20 mg/dl or 3.6-7.1 mmol/L (SI units)
Elderly: may be slightly higher than adult
Child: 5-18 mg/dl
Infant: 5-18 mg/dl
Newborn: 3-12 mg/dl
Cord: 21-40 mg/dl

Critical Values >100 mg/dl (indicates serious impairment of renal function)

Indications

BUN is an indirect and rough measurement of renal function and glomerular filtration rate (if normal liver function exists). It is also a measurement of liver function. It is performed on patients undergoing routine laboratory testing. It is usually performed as a part of a multiphasic automated testing process.

Test Explanation

The BUN measures the amount of urea nitrogen in the blood. Urea is formed in the liver as the end product of protein metabolism and digestion. During ingestion, protein is broken down into amino acids. In the liver these amino acids are catabolized and free ammonia is formed. The ammonia molecules are combined to form urea, which is then deposited in the blood and transported to the kidneys for excretion. Therefore the BUN is directly related to the metabolic function of the liver and the excretory function of the kidney. It serves as an index of the function of these organs. Patients who have elevated BUN levels are said to have azotemia or be azotemic.

Nearly all renal diseases cause an inadequate excretion of urea, which causes the blood concentration to rise above normal. If the disease is unilateral, however, the unaffected kidney can compensate for the diseased kidney and the BUN may not become elevated. The BUN also increases in conditions other than primary renal disease. Prerenal azotemia refers to elevation of the BUN as a result of pathologic conditions that affect urea nitrogen accumulation before it gets to the kidney. Examples of prerenal azotemia include shock, dehydration, congestive heart failure, and excessive protein catabolism. Postrenal azotemia refers to pathologic conditions that affect urea nitrogen accumulation after it gets to the kidney. Examples of this include ureteral and urethral obstruction.

Finally, the synthesis of urea depends on the liver. Patients with severe primary liver disease will have a decreased BUN. With combined liver and renal disease (as in hepatorenal syndrome), the BUN can be normal because poor hepatic functioning results in decreased formation of urea and is not an indicator that renal excretory function is adequate.

The BUN is interpreted in conjunction with the creatinine test. These tests are referred to as "renal function studies." The BUN is less accurate than creatinine as an indicator of renal disease.

Interfering Factors

- Changes in protein intake may affect BUN levels. Low-protein diets will decrease BUN if caloric intake is maintained with carbohydrates. High-protein diets or alimentary tube feeding is associated with elevated BUN levels.
- To some degree, muscle mass determines BUN levels. Women and children tend to have lower BUN levels than men.
- Advanced pregnancy may cause increased levels as a result of high protein metabolism.
- Overhydration and underhydration will affect levels. Overhydrated patients tend to dilute the BUN and have lower levels. Dehydrated patients tend to concentrate BUN and have higher levels.
- Drugs that may cause *increased* BUN levels include allopurinol, aminoglycosides, cephalosporins, chloral hydrate, cisplatin, furosemide, guanethidine, indomethacin, methotrexate, methyldopa, nephrotoxic drugs (e.g., aspirin, amphotericin B, bacitracin, carbamazepine, colistin, gentamicin, methicillin, neomycin, penicillamine, polymyxin B, probenecid, vancomycin), propranolol, rifampin, spironolactone, tetracyclines, thiazide diuretics, and triamterene.
- Drugs that may cause *decreased* levels include chloramphenicol and streptomycin.

✓ CLINICAL PRIORITIES

- Almost all renal diseases cause an inadequate excretion of urea, which causes the BUN to rise. Since the synthesis of urea depends on the liver, severe liver disease can cause a decreased BUN. Therefore the BUN is directly related to the metabolic function of the liver and the excretory function of the kidney.
- Changes in protein intake can affect BUN levels. Low-protein diets can decrease the BUN and high-protein diets can increase the BUN levels.
- Hydration status can also affect levels. Overhydration will dilute the BUN and cause lower levels. Dehydration tends to concentrate the BUN and cause higher levels.

Procedure and Patient Care

Before

- Explain the procedure to the patient.
- Tell the patient that no fasting is required.

During

- Collect approximately 5 ml of blood in a red-top tube.
- Avoid hemolysis.

After

- Apply pressure or a pressure dressing to the venipuncture site.
- Observe the venipuncture site for bleeding.

Test Results and Clinical Significance

Increased levels

PRERENAL CAUSES

Hypovolemia
Shock
Burns
Dehydration
With reduced blood volume, renal blood flow is diminished. Therefore renal excretion of BUN is decreased and BUN levels rise.

Congestive heart failure
Myocardial infarction
With reduced cardiac function, renal blood flow is diminished. Therefore renal excretion of BUN is decreased and BUN levels rise.

GI bleeding
Excessive protein ingestion (alimentary tube feeding)
Blood or feeding supplements overload the gut with protein. Urea is formed at a higher rate and BUN accumulates.

Excessive protein catabolism
Starvation
As protein is broken down to amino acids at an accelerated rate, urea is formed at a higher rate and BUN accumulates.

Sepsis *For a host of reasons, renal blood flow and primary renal function are reduced. BUN levels rise.*

RENAL CAUSES

Renal disease (e.g., glomerulonephritis, pyelonephritis, acute tubular necrosis)
Renal failure
Nephrotoxic drugs
Primary renal diseases are all associated with reduced excretion of BUN.

POSTRENAL AZOTEMIA

Ureteral obstruction from stones, tumor, or congenital anomalies
Bladder outlet obstruction from prostatic hypertrophy or cancer or bladder/urethral congenital anomalies.
Obstruction of the flow of urine causes reduced excretion and BUN levels rise.

Decreased levels

Liver failure *BUN is made in the liver from urea. Reduced liver function is associated with reduced BUN levels.*
Overhydration due to fluid overload syndrome of inappropriate antidiuretic hormone secretion (SIADH) *BUN is diluted by fluid overload.*
Negative nitrogen balance (e.g., malnutrition, malabsorption) *With protein depletion, urea production is reduced and therefore BUN is reduced.*
Pregnancy *Early pregnancy is associated with increased water retention and BUN dilution.*
Nephrotic syndrome *This syndrome is associated with protein loss in the urine. With protein depletion, BUN is reduced.*

Related Tests

- Creatinine, blood (p. 178): This is a more accurate test of renal function that is not dependent on liver function.
- Creatinine clearance (p. 180): Like creatinine, this is a more accurate test of renal function.

Uric Acid, Blood

Normal Findings

Adult
Male: 2.1-8.5 mg/dl or 0.15-0.48 mmol/L (SI units)
Female: 2.0-6.6 mg/dl or 0.09-0.36 mmol/L (SI units)
Elderly: Values may be slightly increased.
Child: 2.5-5.5 mg/dl or 0.12-0.32 mmol/L (SI units)
Newborn: 2.0-6.2 mg/dl

Critical Values >12 mg/dl

Indications

This test is used in the evaluation of gout or recurrent urinary calculus.

Test Explanation

Uric acid is a nitrogenous compound that is the final breakdown product of purine (a deoxyribonucleic acid [DNA] building block) catabolism. Seventy-five percent of uric acid is excreted by the kidney and 25% by the intestinal tract. When uric acid levels are elevated (hyperuricemia), the patient may have gout. Gout is a form of arthritis caused by deposition of uric acid crystals in periarticular tissue. Soft tissue deposits of uric acid can also occur and are called tophi. Uric acid can become supersaturated in the urine and crystalize to form kidney stones that can block the ureters.

Uric acid is made primarily in the liver. The blood level is determined by the rate of synthesis by the liver and the rate of excretion by the kidney. There is some variation of uric acid with age and sex.

Causes of hyperuricemia can be overproduction or decreased excretion of uric acid (e.g., kidney failure). Overproduction of uric acid may occur in patients with a catabolic enzyme deficiency that stimulates purine metabolism or in patients with cancer, in whom purine and DNA turnover is great. Many causes of hyperuricemia are undefined and therefore labeled as idiopathic.

Interfering Factors

- Stress may cause increased uric acid levels.
- X-ray contrast agents increase uric acid excretion and may cause decreased levels.
- High-protein infusion (especially glycine), as in total parental nutrition, may cause increased uric acid, which is a breakdown product of glycine.
- Drugs that may cause *increased* levels include alcohol, ascorbic acid, aspirin (low dose), caffeine, cisplatin, diazoxide, epinephrine, ethambutol, levodopa, methyldopa (Aldomet), nicotinic acid, phenothiazines, and theophylline.
- Drugs that may cause *decreased* levels include allopurinol, aspirin (high dose), azathioprine (Imuran), clofibrate, corticosteroids, estrogens, diuretics, glucose infusions, guaifenesin, mannitol, probenecid, and warfarin.

Procedure and Patient Care

Before

- Explain the procedure to the patient.
- Follow the institution's requirements regarding fasting. (Some recommend that the patient fast.)

During

- Collect approximately 5 to 7 ml of venous blood in a red-top tube.
- List on the laboratory slip any drugs that may affect test results.

After

- Apply pressure or a pressure dressing to the venipuncture site.
- Assess the venipuncture site for bleeding.

Test Results and Clinical Significance

Increased levels (hyperuricemia)

INCREASED PRODUCTION OF URIC ACID

Increased ingestion of purines *Nucleic acid content is high in such foods as liver, sweetbreads, kidney, and anchovies.*

Genetic inborn error in purine metabolism *The most common is an X-linked disorder that causes an increase in an enzyme that produces increased synthesis of purines and therefore an increased amount of purine breakdown products, including uric acid. A second type of genetic error is a deficiency of an enzyme that produces ribonucleic acid (RNA) and DNA from building blocks of those substances. With a deficiency of these enzymes, these building blocks accumulate and are broken down to uric acid, which is then present in high levels in the blood.*

Metastatic cancer
Multiple myeloma
Leukemias
Cancer chemotherapy
Rapid cell destruction associated with rapidly growing cancers (with high cell turnover) and especially after chemotherapy for those rapidly growing tumors causes the cells to lyse and spill their nucleic acids into the bloodstream. These free nucleic acids are converted to uric acid in the liver. Levels of uric acid increase.

Hemolysis *The nucleic acid in the RBC and adenosine triphosphate (ATP) in the RBC are spilled into the bloodstream when hemolysis occurs. These free nucleic acids are converted to uric acid in the liver. Levels of uric acid increase.*

Rhabdomyolysis (e.g., heavy exercise, burns, crush injury, epileptic seizure, myocardial infarction) *Muscle cell lysis leads to excessive muscle ATP (uric acid is a breakdown product of adenosine) in the blood. Uric acid levels increase*

DECREASED EXCRETION OF URIC ACID

Idiopathic *This is the most common cause of hyperuricemia. These patients, for unknown reasons, have reduced uric acid clearance in the kidney. As a result, uric acid accumulates in the blood. Patients with gout excrete less than half the uric acid in their urine as normal persons.*

Chronic renal disease *The pathophysiology as to why these individuals cannot excrete uric acid in appropriate quantities is not known for sure. It may be due to decreased glomerular filtration only, but other mechanisms seem to be at work here.*

Acidosis (ketotic [diabetic or starvation] or lactic) *Decreased renal tubular secretion of uric acid in the urine causes reduced excretion of uric acid. Furthermore, ketoacids (as occur in diabetic or alcoholic ketoacidosis) may compete with uric acid for tubular excretion and may cause decreased uric acid excretion. Uric acid levels increase in the blood.*

Hypothyroidism
Toxemia of pregnancy
Hyperlipoproteinemia
The pathophysiology of these observations is not well defined.

Alcoholism *Alcohol consumption causes accelerated breakdown of ATP in the liver, which increases uric acid production. The chronic acidosis from excessive alcohol ingestion decreases renal tubular secretion of uric acid into the urine. Both lead to hyperuricemia.*

Shock or chronic blood volume depletion states *The increased tubular reabsorption of water and electrolytes causes increased tubular reabsorption of uric acid.*

Decreased levels

- Wilson's disease
- Fanconi's syndrome

- Lead poisoning

Wilson's disease and accompanying Fanconi's syndrome are associated with increased uric acid renal excretion. Heavy metal poisoning is also associated with this observation.

Yellow atrophy of liver *With severe liver dysfunction, uric acid will not be made and levels in the blood will be low.*

Related Tests

- Uric acid, urine (p. 857): This test is used to evaluate uric acid levels in the urine and is used in the evaluation of patients with nephrolithiasis.

Uroporphyrinogen-I-Synthase

Normal Findings 1.27-2.00 mU/g of hemoglobin or 81.9-129.6 U/mol (SI units)

Indications

This test is used to identify persons at risk for porphyria. It is also used to diagnose porphyria in the acute and latent stages.

Test Explanation

Porphyria is a group of genetic disorders characterized by an accumulation of porphyrin products in the liver or RBC. Liver porphyrias are much more common. Symptoms of liver porphyrias include abdominal pain, neuromuscular signs and symptoms, constipation, and occasionally psychotic behavior. This group of disorders results from enzymatic deficiencies in the synthesis of heme (a portion of hemoglobin). Acute intermittent porphyria (AIP) is the most common form of liver porphyrias; this is caused by a deficiency

Box 2-8 Factors that precipitate acute porphyrias

SURGERY

INFECTION

LOW CALORIC DIET

DRUGS:

Barbiturates	Sulfonamides	Meprobamate	Glutethimide
Methyprylon	Phenytoins	Succinimides	Carbamazepine
Valproic acid	Griseofulvin	Ergots	Estrogens/progestins
Danazol	Alcohol	Methyldopa	Theophylline
Amphetamines	Arsenic	Chlordiazepoxide	Phenylbutazone

in uroporphyrinogen-I-synthase (also called porphobilinogen deaminase). This enzyme is necessary for erythroid cells to make heme.

Most patients with AIP have no symptoms (latent phase) until the acute phase is precipitated by medication or some other factor (Box 2-8). The acute phase is highlighted by symptoms of abdominal and muscular pain, nausea, vomiting, hypertension, mental symptoms (anxiety, insomnia, hallucinations, paranoia), sensory loss, and urinary retention. Hemolytic anemia also may occur with these acute attacks. These acute symptoms are associated with increased serum and urine levels of porphyrin precursors (see urine tests for aminoleuvulinic acid, porphyrins, and porphobilinogens).

This enzyme is significantly reduced during the acute and latent phases of this disorder. It is important to identify this disease process, because acute bouts of porphyria occasionally may be fatal. The acute phase can be avoided by controlling factors that can precipitate the acute symptoms.

Procedure and Patient Care

Before

- Explain the procedure to the patient.
- Tell the patient that no fasting is required.

During

- Collect 7 ml of peripheral venous blood in a purple-top tube.
- Because this test is based on the hemoglobin measurement, measure the hemoglobin level on the patient at the same time.

After

- Blood samples should be stored frozen during laboratory transfer to avoid a false decrease in enzyme level.
- Indicate on the laboratory slip if the patient is having symptoms of acute porphyria.
- Apply pressure or a pressure dressing to the venipuncture site.
- Assess the venipuncture site for bleeding.

Test Results and Clinical Significance

Decreased levels

Acute intermittent porphyria

Related Tests

- Aminolevulinic acid, urine (p. 831): This test is used to diagnose porphyria. It is also used in the evaluation of children with subclinical lead poisoning.
- Porphyrins and porphobilinogens, urine (p. 844): This is a quantitative measurement of porphyrins and porphobilinogen in the urine. This test helps define the porphyrin pattern that can classify the type of porphyria.

Vitamin B_{12} (Cyanocobalamin)

Normal Findings

100-700 pg/ml or 72-517 pmol/L

Indications

This test measures the amount of vitamin B_{12} in the blood. It is used to identify the cause of megaloblastic anemia and to evaluate malnourished patients.

Test Explanation

Vitamin B_{12} is necessary for conversion of the inactive form of folate to the active form. This reaction is vital for the synthesis of nucleic acids and amino acids. This is most notable in the formation and function of RBCs. Vitamin B_{12} deficiency, like folic acid deficiency, causes anemia. The RBCs formed in light of these deficiencies become large megaloblastic RBCs. These RBCs cannot conform to the size of small capillaries. Instead they fracture and hemolyze. The shortened life span ultimately leads to anemia. RBCs are not the only blood cells affected. Other marrow cells are also affected, causing giant segmented neutrophils, large nucleated platelets, etc. It may take 6 to 18 months of vitamin B_{12} depletion before anemia develops.

Meats, eggs, and dairy products are the main source of vitamin B_{12}. In the stomach, gastric acid detaches vitamin B_{12} from its binding proteins. Intrinsic factor (IF), necessary for vitamin B_{12} absorption in the small intestine, is made in the stomach mucosa. Without IF, vitamin B_{12} cannot be absorbed. Deficiency of IF is the most common cause of vitamin B_{12} deficiency (pernicious anemia [PA]). The next most common cause of vitamin B_{12} deficiency is lack of gastric acid to separate the ingested vitamin B_{12} from its binding proteins. A third cause of vitamin B_{12} deficiency is malabsorption caused by diseases of the small terminal ileum.

Interfering Factors

- Chloral hydrate is known to *increase* vitamin B_{12} levels.
- Drugs known to *decrease* vitamin B_{12} levels include alcohol, aminoglycosides, aminosalicyclic acid, anticonvulsants, colchicine, and oral contraceptives.

Procedure and Patient Care

Before

- Explain the procedure to the patient.
- Tell the patient that no fasting is usually required. (However, some laboratories prefer an 8-hour fast.)
- Instruct the patient not to consume alcoholic beverages before the test.
- Draw the specimen before starting vitamin B_{12} therapy.

During

- Collect approximately 5 to 10 ml of venous blood in a red-top tube.
- Indicate on the laboratory slip any medications that may affect test results.

After

- Apply pressure or a pressure dressing to the venipuncture site.
- Assess the venipuncture site for bleeding.
- Transport the blood immediately to the laboratory after collection.

Test Results and Clinical Significance

Increased levels

Leukemia
Polycythemia vera
The pathophysiology of these observations is not well known.

Severe liver dysfunction
Myeloproliferative disease
In the above-noted illnesses, transcobalamin (a vitamin B12 carrier protein) is increased, giving a falsely high vitamin B12 level.

Decreased levels

Pernicious anemia *Intrinsic factor, necessary for vitamin B_{12} absorption, is deficient.*
Malabsorption syndromes (e.g., inflammatory bowel disease, sprue, Crohn's disease) *Absorption of vitamin B_{12} is inadequate.*
Intestinal worm infestation *There is competition for vitamin B_{12} in the gut. Very little vitamin B_{12} is left for absorption.*

Atrophic gastritis
Zollinger-Ellison syndrome
Large proximal gastrectomy
Intrinsic factor, necessary for vitamin B_{12} absorption, is deficient, because the mucosal gastric cells necessary for production of IF are absent.

Resection of terminal ileum *Vitamin B_{12} is absorbed at the terminal portion of the ileum. Without that piece of intestine, vitamin B_{12} cannot be absorbed.*
Achlorhydria *Gastric acid is necessary to separate vitamin B_{12} from binding proteins. Without gastric acid, vitamin B_{12} stays bound and cannot be absorbed from the intestine.*
Pregnancy *Vitamin B_{12} deficiency in pregnancy is probably due to a combination of inadequate intake and increased demand placed by the fetus on the maternal source of folic acid.*

Vitamin C deficiency
Folic acid deficiency
The pathophysiology of these observations is not clear.

Related Tests

- Folic acid (p. 217): This is a measurement of serum folic acid level. Folic acid should always be determined when vitamin B_{12} levels are measured. The clinical symptoms of either deficiency are the same.

- Schilling test (p. 750): This is a test to assist in the determination of the cause of vitamin B_{12} deficiency.
- Complete blood count (CBC) (p. 162): This is performed routinely and can identify megaloblastic anemia.

Water Deprivation
(Antidiuretic Hormone [ADH] Stimulation)

Normal Findings

Neurogenic diabetes insipidus: >9% rise in urine osmolality
Nephrogenic diabetes insipidus: <9% rise in urine osmolality
Psychogenic polydipsia: <9% rise in urine osmolality

Indications

This test is used to aid in the differential diagnosis of polyuria. Polyuria can occur as a result of neurogenic diabetes insipidus (DI), nephrogenic DI, or psychogenic polydipsia.

Test Explanation

In this test the patient is deprived of fluids. Patients who have DI will dehydrate quickly as indicated by a rise in urine and serum osmolality. Patients with primary psychogenic polydipsia take a longer time to dehydrate. Next, ADH is administered. Neurogenic DI patients have no endogenous ADH but can concentrate their urine and raise urine osmolality if ADH is provided exogenously. Patients with nephrogenic DI have kidneys that are insensitive to ADH. They will experience little or no rise in urine osmolality. Patients who have psychogenic polydipsia will experience a less than 9% rise in urine osmolality.

Potential Complications

- Severe dehydration may occur in patients with neurogenic DI. If their urine output is high, they should be watched closely during the period of dehydration.

Interfering Factors

- Diuretics can confuse the results and increase the danger of fluid restriction.

Procedure and Patient Care

Before

- Explain the procedure to the patient.
- Explain the recommended fluid restriction.
  Patients with a urine output of less than 4000/24 hr undergo fluid restriction after midnight prior to the test.

Patients with a urine output of greater than 4000/24 hr begin fluid restriction at the time the test starts, because they may get dangerously dehydrated if asked to restrict water from midnight.

- The test starts at 6 AM and stops at noon.

During

- Obtain and record the patient's body weight hourly for the duration of the procedure.
- Obtain urine osmolality hourly from 6 AM to noon or until three consecutive hourly determinations show a urine osmolality increase of less than 30 mOsm/kg.
- At that point obtain a serum osmolality. It must be greater than 288 mOsm/kg for the patient to be considered adequately dehydrated and water deprived.
- If the body weight drops more than 2 kg, discontinue the test and rehydrate the patient.
- Administer 5 U of vasopressin (or 1 μg of desmopressin, an analog of ADH) subcutaneously.
- Obtain urine osmolality 30 to 60 minutes after the injection.

After

- Rehydrate the patient with oral fluids.
- Record vital signs in both the recumbent and erect position to be sure that no orthostasis exists from inadequate rehydration.
- Observe the venipuncture sites for bleeding.

Test Results and Clinical Significance

Rise in urine osmolality of more than 9%

Neurogenic (or central) DI caused by CNS trauma, tumor, or infection
Surgical ablation of pituitary gland
ADH is not produced in these patients, but the kidneys can respond to exogenously administered ADH by concentrating the urine.

Little or no increase in urine osmolality during deprivation portion of test or after injection

Nephrogenic DI caused by primary renal diseases *Patients with nephrogenic DI due to chronic kidney diseases will experience little or no rise in urine osmolality during the dehydration phase of the test, because the kidney has lost its concentrating abilities. Furthermore, their kidneys are insensitive to the urine-concentrating effect of ADH.*

Hypokalemia *These patients have the same lack of response as do patients with nephrogenic DI.*

Psychogenic polydipsia *These patients frequently take longer than usual to dehydrate to a serum osmolality of 288, and the urine osmolality rises less than 9% after vasopressin injection.*

Related Tests

- Antidiuretic hormone (ADH) (p. 62): This is a serum assay for direct measurement of ADH. This test is used in the differential diagnosis of neurogenic DI, nephrogenic DI, or psychogenic polydipsia.

- Osmolality, serum (p. 313): This test is a measurement of solute load in the serum.
- Osmolality, urine (p. 842): This test is a measurement of solute load in the urine.
- Sodium, blood (p. 396): This is a direct measurement of sodium level in the blood.
- Sodium, urine (p. 851): This is a direct measurement of sodium level in the urine.

White Blood Cell Count and Differential Count (WBC and Differential, Leukocyte Count, Neutrophil Count, Lymphocyte Count, Monocyte Count, Eosinophil Count, Basophil Count)

Normal Findings

Total WBCs

Adult/child >2 years: 5000-10,000/mm^3 or 5-10.0 × 10^9/L (SI units)
Child <2 years: 6200-17,000/mm^3
Newborn: 9000-30,000/mm^3

Differential Count

	(%)	Absolute (per mm^3)
Neutrophils	55-70	2500-8000
Lymphocytes	20-40	1000-4000
Monocytes	2-8	100-700
Eosinophils	1-4	50-500
Basophils	0.5-1.0	25-100

Critical Values WBCs <2500 or >30,000/mm^3

Indications

The measurement of the total and differential WBC count is a part of all routine laboratory diagnostic evaluations. It is especially helpful in the evaluation of the patient with infection, neoplasm, allergy, or immunosuppression (Box 2-9).

Age-related concerns

- The WBC values tend to be age related.
- Normal newborns and infants tend to have higher WBC values than adults.
- It is not uncommon for the elderly to fail to respond to infection by the absence of leukocytosis. The elderly may not develop an increased WBC count even in the presence of a severe bacterial infection.

Box 2-9 Precautions for immunocompromised patients

Observe protective isolation.
- Wash hands before entering room.
- Wear mask, gown, and gloves.
- Restrict visitors.
- Prohibit visitation by people with infections (viral, fungal, bacterial).

Avoid bacteremia from patient's own bacterial flora.
- Do not take rectal temperatures.
- Do not perform rectal examinations or enemas.
- Do not allow patient to floss teeth.

Avoid bacterial contamination from foods.
- Serve only foods from newly opened packages.
- Avoid fresh fruits and vegetables.
- All foods should be cooked.

Avoid infection by administration of IM injections, if possible.

Observe closely for infections or fever.

Test Explanation

The WBC count has two components. The first is a count of the *total number of WBCs* (leukocytes) in 1 mm^3 of peripheral venous blood. The other component, the *differential count,* measures the percentage of each type of leukocyte present in the same specimen. An increase in the percentage of one type of leukocyte means a decrease in the percentage of another. Neutrophils and lymphocytes make up 75% to 90% of the total leukocytes. These leukocyte types can be identified easily by their morphology on a peripheral blood smear (see p. 641) or by automated counters. The total leukocyte count has a wide range of normal values, but many diseases may induce abnormal values. An increased total WBC count (leukocytosis, WBC count greater than 10,000) usually indicates infection, inflammation, tissue necrosis, or leukemic neoplasia. Trauma or stress, either emotional or physical, may increase the WBC count. In some infections, especially sepsis, the WBC count may be extremely high and reach levels associated with leukemia. This is called a "leukemoid" reaction and quickly resolves as the infection is successfully treated.

A decreased total WBC count (leukopenia; WBC count less than 4000) occurs in many forms of bone marrow failure (e.g., following antineoplastic chemotherapy or radiation therapy, marrow infiltrative diseases, overwhelming infections, dietary deficiencies, autoimmune diseases).

The major function of WBCs is to fight infection and react against foreign bodies or tissues. Five types of WBCs may easily be identified on a routine blood smear. These cells, in order of frequency, include neutrophils, lymphocytes, monocytes, eosinophils, and basophils. All of these WBCs arise from the same "pluripotent" stem cell within the bone marrow as the RBC (Figure 2-18). Beyond this origin, however, each cell line differentiates separately. Most mature WBCs are then deposited into the circulating blood.

WBCs are divided into granulocytes and nongranulocytes. Granulocytes have granules in their cytoplasm when stained and examined on a routine smear. Granulocytes include

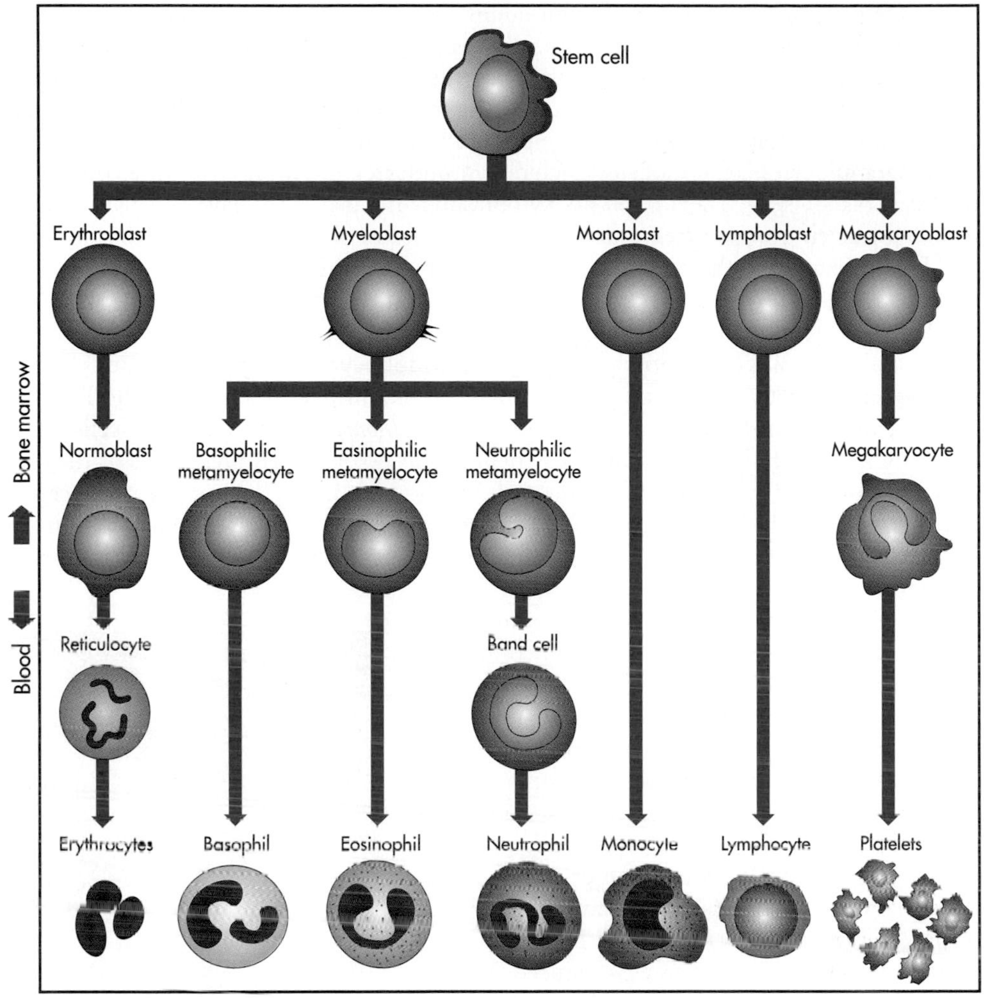

Figure 2-18 Development of blood cells.

neutrophils, basophils, and eosinophils. Granulocytes have multilobed nuclei and are sometimes referred to as polymorphonuclear leukocytes (PMNs or "polys").

Neutrophils are the most common PMN and are produced in 7 to 14 days and remain in the circulation for only 6 hours. The primary function of the neutrophil is phagocytosis (killing and digestion of bacterial microorganisms). Acute bacterial infections and trauma stimulate neutrophil production, resulting in an increased WBC count. When neutrophil production is significantly stimulated, early immature forms of neutrophils often enter the circulation. These immature forms are called *band* or *stab cells.* This occurrence, referred to as a "shift to the left" in WBC production, is indicative of an ongoing acute bacterial infection.

Basophils (also called mast cells) and especially *eosinophils* are involved in the allergic reaction. They are capable of phagocytosis of antigen-antibody complexes. As the allergic response diminishes, the eosinophil count decreases. Eosinophils and basophils do not respond to bacterial or viral infections. The cytoplasm of basophils contains heparin, histamine, and serotonin. These cells infiltrate the tissue (e.g., hive in the skin) involved in the allergic reaction and serve to further the inflammatory reaction. Parasitic infestations also are capable of stimulating the production of these cells.

Nongranulocytes (agranulocytes) include lymphocytes and monocytes (the count also includes histiocytes). They have no cytoplasmic granules and have a small, single, rounded nuclei. *Lymphocytes* are divided into two types: T cells (mature in the thymus) and B cells (mature in the bone marrow). T cells are primarily involved with cellular-type immune reactions, whereas B cells participate in humoral immunity (antibody production). T cells are the killer cells, suppressor cells, and the T4 helper cells (see lymphocyte immunophenotyping). The primary function of lymphocytes is to fight chronic bacterial infection and acute viral infections. The differential count does not separate the T and B cells but rather counts the combination of the two. *Monocytes* are phagocytic cells capable of fighting bacteria similar to the way neutrophils do. Through phagocytosis, they remove necrotic debris and microorganisms from the blood. The monocytes produce interferon, which is the body's endogenous immunostimulant. Monocytes can be produced more rapidly, however, and can spend a longer time in the circulation than the neutrophils.

The WBC and differential count are routinely measured as part of the complete blood count (see p. 162) (Figure 2-19). Serial WBC counts and differential counts have both diagnostic and prognostic value. For example, a persistent increase in the WBC count may indicate worsening of an infectious process (e.g., appendicitis). A reduction in WBC count to the normal range from a previously elevated range indicates resolution of an infection. A dramatic decrease in the WBC count below the normal range may indicate marrow failure. In patients receiving chemotherapy a reduced WBC count may contraindicate further chemotherapy.

The absolute count is calculated by multiplying the differential count (%) by the total WBC count. For example, the *absolute neutrophil count* (ANC) is helpful in determining the patient's real risk for infection. It is calculated by multiplying the WBC count by the percent of neutrophils and percent of bands, that is:

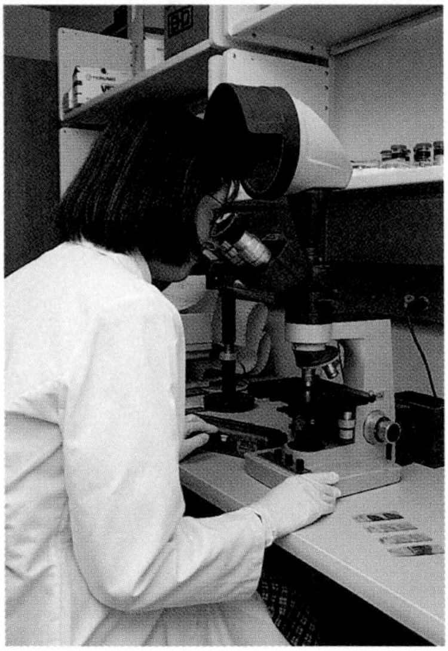

Figure 2-19 Medical technologist conducting a microscopic examination of WBCs.

ANC = WBC × (% Neutrophils + % Bands)

If the ANC is below 1000, the patient should be placed in protective isolation as he or she is severely immunocompromised and is at great risk for infection.

Interfering Factors

- Eating, physical activity, and stress may cause an increased WBC count and alter the differential values.

- Pregnancy (final month) and labor may be associated with increased WBC levels.
- Patients who have had a splenectomy have a persistent mild to moderate elevation of WBC counts.
- The WBC count tends to be lower in the morning and higher in the late afternoon.
- The WBC count tends to be age related. Normal newborns and infants tend to have higher WBC counts than adults. It is not uncommon for the elderly to fail to respond to infection by the absence of leukocytosis. In fact, the elderly may not develop an increased WBC count even in the face of a severe bacterial infection.
- Drugs that may cause *increased* WBC levels include adrenaline, allopurinol, aspirin, chloroform, epinephrine, heparin, quinine, steroids, and triamterene (Dyrenium).
- Drugs that may cause *decreased* WBC levels include antibiotics, anticonvulsants, antihistamines, antimetabolites, antithyroid drugs, arsenicals, barbiturates, chemotherapeutic agents, diuretics, and sulfonamides.

CLINICAL PRIORITIES

- An increased WBC count (leukocytosis) usually indicates infection, inflammation, tissue necrosis, or leukemic neoplasia.
- Serial WBC and differential counts have both diagnostic and prognostic value. For example, a persistent increase in the WBC count may indicate a worsening of an infectious process (e.g., appendicitis).
- A drastic decrease in WBCs below the normal range may indicate bone marrow failure.

Procedure and Patient Care

Before

- Explain the procedure to the patient.
- Tell the patient that no fasting is required.

During

- Collect approximately 5 to 7 ml of venous blood in a lavender-top tube.

After

- Apply pressure or a pressure dressing to the venipuncture site.
- Check the venipuncture site for bleeding.

Test Results and Clinical Significance

Increased WBC count (leukocytosis)

Infection *WBCs are integral to initiating and maintaining the body's defense mechanism against infection.*

Leukemic neoplasia or other myeloproliferative disorders *These neoplastic cells are produced by the marrow and are released into the bloodstream.*

Other malignancy *Advanced nonmarrow cancers (e.g., lung) are associated with leukocytosis. The pathophysiology of this observation is not defined.*

Trauma, stress, or hemorrhage *The WBC count is probably under hormonal influence (e.g., epinephrine). However, the pathophysiology of this observation is not defined.*

Tissue necrosis
Inflammation
The pathophysiology of these observations is complex, including the recognition of necrotic or normal tissue as "foreign" so that a WBC response is instituted.

Dehydration *Not only is dehydration a stress that, by itself, increases the WBC count, but also by virtue of hemoconcentration, the WBC count increases.*

Table 2-37 Causes of abnormalities in the WBC differential count

Type of WBC	Elevated	Decreased
Neutrophils	*Neutrophilia* Physical or emotional stress Acute suppurative infection Myelocytic leukemia Trauma Cushing's syndrome Inflammatory disorders (e.g., rheumatic fever, thyroiditis, rheumatoid arthritis) Metabolic disorders (e.g., ketoacidosis, gout, eclampsia)	*Neutropenia* Aplastic anemia Dietary deficiency Overwhelming bacterial infection (especially in the elderly) Viral infections (e.g., hepatitis, influenza, measles) Radiation therapy Addison's disease Drug therapy: myelotoxic drugs (as in chemotherapy)
Lymphocytes	*Lymphocytosis* Chronic bacterial infection Viral infection (e.g., mumps, rubella) Lymphocytic leukemia Multiple myeloma Infectious mononucleosis Radiation Infectious hepatitis	*Lymphocytopenia* Leukemia Sepsis Immunodeficiency diseases Lupus erythematosus Later stages of human immunodeficiency virus infection Drug therapy: adrenocorticosteroids, antineoplastics Radiation therapy
Monocytes	*Monocytosis* Chronic inflammatory disorders Viral infections (e.g., infectious mononucleosis) Tuberculosis Chronic ulcerative colitis Parasites (e.g., malaria)	*Monocytopenia* Drug therapy: prednisone
Eosinophils	*Eosinophilia* Parasitic infections Allergic reactions Eczema Leukemia Autoimmune diseases	*Eosinopenia* Increased adrenosteroid production
Basophils	*Basophilia* Myeloproliferative disease (e.g., myelofibrosis, polycythemia rubra vera) Leukemia	*Basopenia* Acute allergic reactions Hyperthyroidism Stress reactions

Thyroid storm *The WBC count is probably influenced by thyroid hormones. Marked increases in these hormones could be associated with an increased WBC count.*
Steroid use *Glucocorticosteroids stimulate WBC production.*

Decreased WBC count (leukopenia)

Drug toxicity (e.g., cytotoxic chemotherapy; see also drugs that decrease the WBC count)
Bone marrow failure
Overwhelming infections
Dietary deficiency (e.g., vitamin B_{12}, iron deficiency)
Congenital marrow aplasia
Bone marrow infiltration (e.g., myelofibrosis)
The above are associated with all different forms of bone marrow failure whereby WBC production is reduced.

Autoimmune disease *The pathophysiology of this observation is not known.*
Hypersplenism *The spleen more aggressively extracts WBCs from the bloodstream.*

Increased/decreased differential count

See Table 2-37.

Related Tests

- Lymphocyte immunophenotyping (p. 301): This test is used to detect the progressive depletion of CD4 T lymphocytes, which is associated with an increased likelihood of clinical complications from AIDS. Test results can indicate if an AIDS patient is at risk for developing opportunistic infections.
- Peripheral blood smear (p. 641): This is a direct microscopic analysis of the cellular components of the blood.

D-Xylose Absorption (Xylose Tolerance)

Normal Findings

Age	60-min Plasma (mg/dl)	120-min Plasma (mg/dl)	Urine (g/5 hr) (%)
Child	>15-20	>20	>4.0 [16-32%]
Adult	20-57	30-58	>3.5-4.0 [>14%]

Indications

This test is used to evaluate the absorptive capability of the intestines. It is used in the evaluation of patients suspected of having malabsorption.

BLOOD STUDIES 2

Test Explanation

D-Xylose is a monosaccharide that is easily absorbed by the normal intestine. In patients with malabsorption, intestinal D-xylose absorption is diminished, and as a result, blood levels and urine excretion will be reduced. D-Xylose is the monosaccharide chosen for the test, because it is not metabolized by the body. Serum levels directly reflect intestinal absorption.

Also, this monosaccharide is used because absorption does not require pancreatic or biliary exocrine function. Its absorption is directly determined by the absorptive function of the small intestine. This test is used to differentiate diarrhea caused by maldigestion (pancreatic/biliary dysfunction) and diarrhea caused by malabsorption (sprue, Whipple's disease, Crohn's disease). It is also used to quantitate the degree of malabsorption to monitor therapy.

In this test the patient is asked to drink a fluid containing a prescribed amount of D-xylose. Blood and urine levels are subsequently evaluated. Excellent GI absorption is documented by high blood levels and good urine excretion of D-xylose. Poor intestinal absorption is marked by low blood levels and urine excretion.

Contraindications

- Patients who are dehydrated, because the 25-g dose can cause diarrhea and may precipitate hypovolemia in these patients

Interfering Factors

- Patients with abnormal kidney function, because they may not be able to excrete the xylose. The urine measurement for D-xylose should not be performed, and the interpretation should be based on the blood results only.
- Drugs that may affect test results include aspirin, atropine, and indomethacin.

Procedure and Patient Care

Before

- Explain the procedure to the patient.
- Instruct the adult patient to fast for 8 hours before testing. Water should be encouraged, however.
- Tell the pediatric patient or the parents that the patient should fast for at least 4 hours before testing.

During

- Collect approximately 7 ml of venous blood in a red-top tube before the patient ingests the D-xylose.
- Collect a first-voided morning urine specimen and send it to the laboratory.
- Ask the patient to drink 25 g of D-xylose dissolved in 8 ounces of water. Record the time of ingestion. A 5-g dose can be given instead of the 25-g dose to avoid diarrhea. However, the test results will be less accurate.

- Calibrate pediatric doses according to the patient's body weight (0.5 g/pound of body weight in children).
- Repeat venipunctures to obtain blood in exactly 2 hours for an adult and 1 hour for a child.
- Collect urine for a designated time, usually 5 hours, in a dark bottle. Refrigerate the urine during the collection period.
- Observe the patient for nausea, vomiting, and diarrhea, which may occur as side effects of D-xylose.
- Instruct the patient to remain in a restful position. Intense physical activity may alter the digestive process and affect the test results.

After

- Observe the venipuncture site for bleeding.
- Provide the patient with food or drink and inform the patient that normal activity may be resumed after completion of the study.

Test Results and Clinical Significance

Decreased levels

Malabsorption caused by sprue, lymphatic obstruction, enteropathy (e.g., radiation), Crohn's disease, or Whipple's disease *The D-xylose is not absorbed in these patients; therefore blood and urine levels are not as normally expected.*

Short-bowel syndrome *Because of the lack of absorptive surface, absorption of D-xylose does not occur. Therefore blood and urine levels are not as normally expected.*

Related Tests

- Small bowel series (p. 991): This is an x ray test that visualizes the mucosa of the small intestine. Patients with Crohn's disease and other malabsorption syndromes may have obvious abnormal findings.

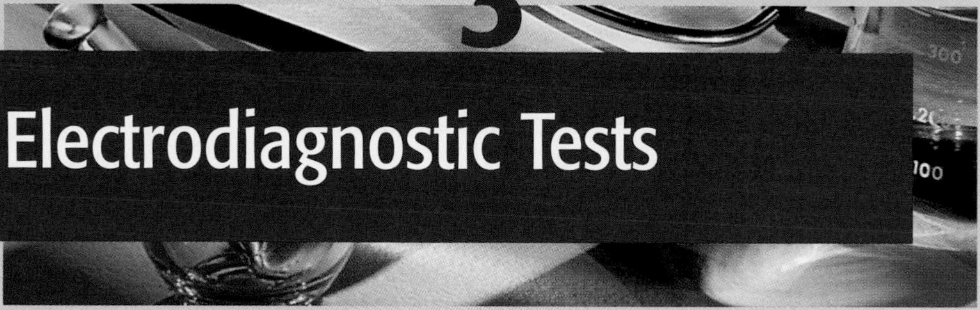

3

Electrodiagnostic Tests

TESTS

Overview

Reason for Performing Electrodiagnostic Studies

Most electrodiagnostic studies use electrical activity and electronic devices to evaluate disease or injury to a specified area of the body. The electrical impulses can be generated spontaneously or can be stimulated. For example, electrocardiography records spontaneous electrical impulses generated by the heart during the cardiac cycle. In electromyography the electrical impulses are stimulated by an electrical shock applied to the body. For the caloric study, nystagmus is induced by irrigating the ear canal with water. The electrical activity is usually detected by electrodes placed on the body. The electrodes are attached to instruments for receiving and recording electrical impulses. Table 3-1 lists the various areas of the body that can be evaluated by electrodiagnostic studies.

Procedural Care for Electrodiagnostic Studies

Before

- Explain the procedure to the patient.
- Obtain baseline values for comparison during and after the test.
- Explain food restrictions, if indicated. For example, caloric studies require fasting to reduce the possibility of nausea and vomiting. On the other hand, fasting would affect electroencephalography results by causing hypoglycemia.
- Determine if there are any drug restrictions. Sedatives may adversely affect most test results.
- Because of its stimulating effect, caffeine is restricted before most studies.
- Most of these studies are considered noninvasive and do not require a consent form.

During

- For most tests, some type of electrode is applied to the patient to record electrical activity.

Table 3-1 ***Body areas evaluated by electrodiagnostic studies***

Name of test	Evaluation
Caloric study	Cranial nerve VIII
Cardiac stress	Cardiac muscle
Electrocardiography	Cardiac muscle and conduction system
Electroencephalography	Brain
Electromyography	Neuromuscular system
Electroneurography	Peripheral nerves
Electronystagmography	Oculo-vestibular reflex pathway
Electrophysiologic studies	Cardiac conduction system
Evoked potential studies	Sensory pathways of the eyes, ears, and peripheral nerves
Contraction stress (fetal)	Fetal viability
Nonstress (fetal)	Fetal viability
Holter monitoring	Cardiac rhythm
Pelvic floor sphincter electromyography	Urinary or fecal continence

- Some tests (such as electromyography) require some type of stimulation. Slight discomfort is felt if electrical stimulation is applied.
- The patient needs to remain still during testing. Any movement can alter test results.

After

- Monitor the patient for a return to pretest baseline activity.
- Some studies may cause nausea and vomiting. The patient should rest until these symptoms subside.
- If any sedation was given, safety precautions should be in effect.

Potential Complications of Electrodiagnostic Testing

Most tests in this category have few potential complications. Those mentioned below apply to specific tests and are grouped accordingly.

Cardiac Stress Testing

- Cardiac arrhythmias
- Severe angina
- Fainting
- Myocardial infarction

Contraction Stress Test

- Premature labor

Reporting of Results

Many of these tests are performed by technicians. Test results are available after interpretation by a physician.

Caloric Study (Oculovestibular Reflex Study)

Normal Findings Nystagmus with irrigation

Indications

This test is used to evaluate the function of cranial nerve VIII. It also can indicate disease in the temporal portion of the cerebrum.

Test Explanation

Caloric studies are used to evaluate the vestibular portion of the eighth cranial nerve (CN VIII) by irrigating the external auditory canal with hot or cold water. Stimulation with cold water normally causes rotary nystagmus (involuntary rapid eye movement) away from the ear being irrigated; hot water induces nystagmus toward the side of the ear being irrigated. If the labyrinth is diseased or the CN VIII is not functioning (e.g., from tumor compression), no nystagmus is induced. This study aids in the differential diagnosis of abnormalities that may occur in the vestibular system, brainstem, or cerebellum. When results are inconclusive, electronystagmography (p. 492) may be performed.

Contraindications

- Patients with a perforated eardrum
  Cold air may be substituted for the fluid.
- Patients with an acute disease of the labyrinth (e.g., Meniere's syndrome)
  The test can be performed when the acute attack subsides.

Interfering Factors

- Drugs such as sedatives and antivertigo agents can alter test results.

CLINICAL PRIORITIES

- This study aids in evaluating the vestibular portion of the eighth cranial nerve.
- During this test, the external auditory canal is irrigated with hot or cold water to induce nystagmus.
- Most patients will experience nausea and dizziness during this test.

Procedure and Patient Care

Before

- Explain the procedure to the patient.
- Hold solid foods before the test to reduce the incidence of vomiting.

During

- Although the exact procedures for caloric studies vary, note the following steps in a typical test:
  1. Before the test, the patient is examined for the presence of nystagmus, postural deviation (Romberg's sign), and past-pointing. This examination provides the baseline values for comparison during the test.
  2. The ear canal should be examined and cleaned by a physician before testing to ensure that the water will flow freely to the middle ear area.
  3. The ear on the suspected side is irrigated first because the patient's response may be minimal.
  4. After an emesis basin is placed under the ear, the irrigation solution is directed into the external auditory canal until the patient complains of nausea and dizziness, or nystagmus is observed. This usually occurs in 20 to 30 seconds.
  5. If after 3 minutes no symptoms occur, the irrigation is stopped.
  6. The patient is tested again for nystagmus, past-pointing, and Romberg's sign.
  7. After approximately 5 minutes, the procedure is repeated on the other side.
- Note that this procedure is usually performed by a physician or technician in approximately 15 minutes.

- Tell the patient that he or she will probably experience nausea and dizziness during the test.

After

- Usually, place the patient on bed rest for approximately 30 to 60 minutes until nausea or vomiting subsides.
- Ensure patient safety related to dizziness.

Test Results and Clinical Significance

Brainstem inflammation, infarction, or tumor
Cerebellar inflammation, infarction, or tumor
Vestibular or cochlear inflammation or tumor
Acoustic neuroma
Eighth nerve neuritis or neuropathy
The above-noted diseases involve the CNS from the vestibular/cochlear end organ to the temporal area of the cerebrum.

Related Tests

- Electronystagmography (p. 492): During this test, nystagmus is stimulated in a manner similar to that described for caloric studies. The direction, velocity, and amplitude of the nystagmus are recorded through the use of electrodes.

Cardiac Stress Testing (Stress Testing, Exercise Testing, Electrocardiograph [EKG] Stress Testing, Exercise Testing, Nuclear Stress Testing, Echo Stress Testing)

Normal Findings

Patient able to obtain and maintain maximal heart rate of 85% for predicted age and gender with no cardiac symptoms or EKG change
No cardiac muscle wall dysfunction

Indications

Stress testing is used in the following situations:

1. To evaluate chest pain in a patient suspected of having coronary disease (Occasionally a person may have significant coronary stenosis that is not apparent during normal physical activity. If, however, the pain can be reproduced with exercise, one may infer that coronary occlusion is present.)
2. To determine the limits of safe exercise during a cardiac rehabilitation program or to assist patients with cardiac disease in maintaining good physical fitness
3. To detect labile or exercise-related hypertension

4. To detect intermittent claudication in patients with suspected vascular occlusive disease in the extremities (In this situation, the patient may experience leg muscle cramping while performing the exercise.)
5. To evaluate the effectiveness of treatment in patients who take antianginal or antiarrhythmic medications
6. To evaluate the effectiveness of cardiac intervention (such as bypass grafting or angioplasty)

Test Explanation

Stress testing is a noninvasive study that provides information about the patient's cardiac function. In stress testing the heart is stressed in some way. The heart is then evaluated during the stress. Changes indicating ischemia indicate coronary occlusive disease. By far the most commonly used method of stress is exercise (bike or treadmill). Chemical stress methods are becoming more common due to their safety and increased accuracy. A third method, less frequently used, is pacer stress (Box 3-1).

During *exercise stress testing,* the EKG, heart rate, and blood pressure are monitored while the patient engages in some type of physical activity (stress). Two methods of stress testing are pedaling a stationary bike and walking on a treadmill. With the stationary bicycle the pedaling tension is slowly increased to increase the heart rate. With the treadmill test the speed and grade of incline are increased. The treadmill test is the most frequently used because it is the most easily standardized and reproducible (Figures 3-1 and 3-2). The various grades of exercise are determined by the cardiologist in attendance based on estimation of cardiac function capabilities.

The usual goal of the exercise stress testing is to increase the heart rate to just below maximal levels or to the "target heart rate." This target heart rate is usually 80% to 90% of the maximal heart rate. The test is usually discontinued if the patient reaches that target heart rate or develops any symptoms or EKG changes. The maximal heart rate is determined by a chart that takes into account the patient's age (about 230 minus the patient's age) and gender. The normal maximal heart rate for adults varies from 150 to 200 beats/min; patients taking calcium channel blockers and sympathetic blockers have a lower-than-expected maximal heart rate.

Exercise stress testing is based on the principle that occluded arteries will be unable to meet the heart's increased demand for blood during the testing. This may become obvious with symptoms (e.g., chest pain, fatigue, dyspnea, tachycardia, cardiac arrhythmias

Box 3-1 Commonly used methods of stressing the heart

EXERCISE	CHEMICAL	PACING
Treadmill	Vascular dilation drugs	
Bicycle	Dipyridamole	
	Adenosine	
	Stimulatory drugs	
	Dobutamine	

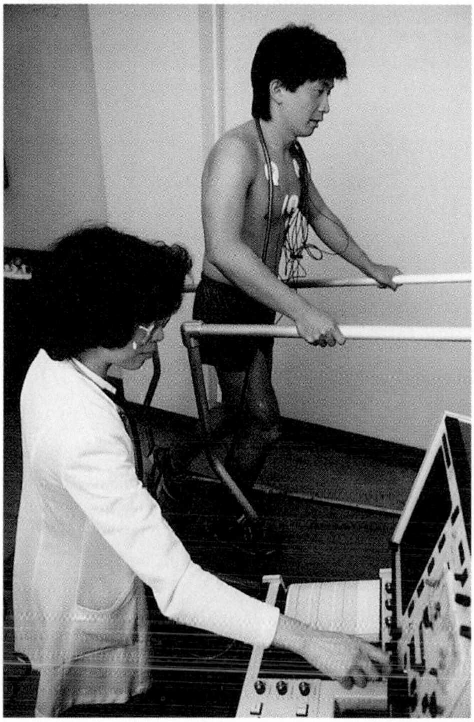

Figure 3-1 Patient taking exercise stress test while nurse monitors the EKG response.

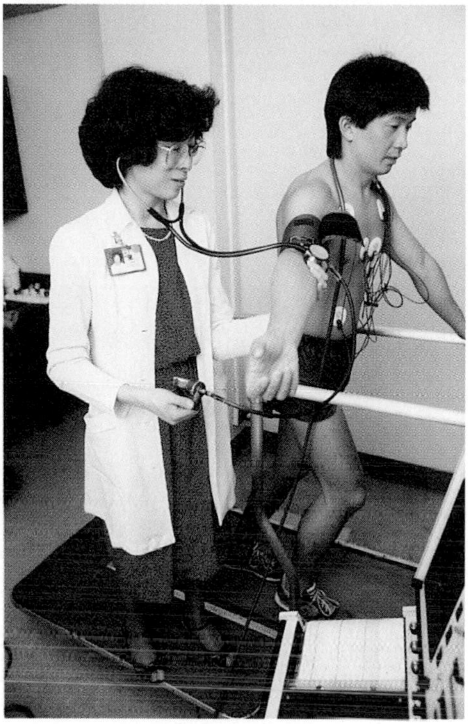

Figure 3-2 Nurse monitoring blood pressure response during exercise stress testing.

[dysrhythmias], fall in blood pressure) or EKG changes (e.g., ST-segment variance greater than 1 mm, increasing premature ventricular contractions, other rhythm disturbances). An advantage of stress testing is that these symptoms can be stimulated and identified in a safe environment. Besides the electrodiagnostic method of cardiac evaluation, the stressed heart also can be evaluated by nuclear scanning or echocardiography. Findings of ischemia are discussed in "Test Results and Clinical Significance."

When exercise testing is not advisable or the patient is unable to exercise to a level adequate to stress the heart (patients with an orthopedic, arthritic, neurologic, or pulmonary limitation), *chemical stress testing* is recommended. Chemical stress testing is being increasingly used because of its accuracy and ease of performance. Although chemical stress testing is less physiologic than exercise testing, it is safer and more controllable. *Dipyridamole (Persantine)* is a coronary vasodilator. If one coronary artery is significantly occluded, the coronary blood flow is diverted to the opened vessels. This causes a "steal syndrome" away from the stenotic or occluded coronary vessel. That is, the dipyridamole-induced vascular dilation "steals" the blood from the ischemic areas and diverts it to the open, dilated coronary vessels. Caution must be taken, however, because this can precipitate angina or myocardial infarction. This test should be performed only with a cardiologist

Box 3-2 Commonly used methods of cardiac evaluation during stress testing

Electrophysiologic parameters: EKG, blood pressure, and heart rate
Cardiac nuclear scanning (p. 704)
Echocardiography (p. 787)

Box 3-3 Criteria for discontinuation of an exercise stress test

Attainment of maximal performance
Abnormal EKG changes
- Ectopy
- Flipped T waves
- ST changes

Excessive heart rate changes: tachycardia or bradycardia
Chest pain
Syncope
Excessive hypertension or hypotension
Severe shortness of breath
Leg claudication
Cyanosis

in attendance. IV aminophylline can reverse the effect of dipyridamole. *Adenosine* works similarly to dipyridamole.

Dobutamine is another chemical that can stress the heart. Dobutamine stimulates the heart function. This entails administration of progressively greater amounts of dobutamine over 3-minute intervals. The normal heart muscle increases (augments) its contractility (wall motion). Ischemic muscle has no augmentation. In fact, in time the ischemic area becomes hypokinetic. Infarcted tissue is akinetic. In chemical stress testing the stressed heart is evaluated by nuclear scanning or echocardiography.

Pacing is another method of stress testing. In patients with permanent pacemakers, the rate of capture can be increased to a rate that would be considered a cardiac stress. The heart is then evaluated electrodiagnostically or with nuclear scanning or echocardiography.

As indicated in Box 3-2, the methods of evaluating the heart are electrophysiologic parameters, nuclear scanning, and echocardiography. Echocardiography is fast becoming the method of choice for urgent and elective cardiac evaluation with or without stress testing.

Stress testing is discontinued with any of the criteria noted in Box 3-3.

Contraindications

- Patients with unstable angina, because stress may induce an infarction
- Patients with severe aortic valvular heart disease, because their stress tolerance is easily reached and is quite low

- Patients who cannot participate in an exercise program because of their impaired lung or motor function
  However, they can be stressed chemically.
- Patients who have recently had a myocardial infarction
  In this case, however, limited stress testing can be done.
- Patients with severe congestive heart failure
- Patients who have severe claudication and cannot walk adequately to stress their hearts
  However, they can be stressed chemically.

Potential Complications

- Fatal cardiac arrhythmias
- Severe angina
- Myocardial infarction
- Fainting

Interfering Factors

- Heavy meals before testing can divert blood to the GI tract.
- Nicotine from smoking can cause coronary artery spasm.
- Medical problems such as hypertension, valvular heart disease (especially of the aortic valve), severe anemia, hypoxemia, and chronic pulmonary disease can affect results.
- Left ventricular hypertrophy may affect test results.
- The EKG is not a reliable indicator of ischemia in patients with left bundle branch block.
- Drugs that can affect test results include beta blockers (e.g., propranolol [Inderal]), calcium channel blockers, digoxin, and nitroglycerin.

Procedure and Patient Care (for Exercise Stress Testing and Electrodiagnostic Monitoring)

Before

- Explain the procedure to the patient.
- Instruct the patient to abstain from eating, drinking, and smoking for 4 hours.
- Inform the patient about the risks of the test and obtain informed consent.
- Instruct the patient to bring comfortable clothing and shoes in which to exercise. Slippers are not acceptable.
- Inform the patient if any medications should be discontinued before testing.
- Obtain a pretest EKG.
- Record the patient's vital signs for baseline values.
- Apply and secure appropriate EKG electrodes.

During

- Note that a physician usually is present during stress testing.
- After the patient begins to exercise, adjust the treadmill machine settings to apply increasing levels of stress at specific intervals. It is helpful to encourage and support the patient at each level of increased stress.

- Encourage patients to verbalize any symptoms.
- Note that during the test the EKG tracing and vital signs are monitored continuously.
- Terminate the test if the patient complains of chest pain, exhaustion, dyspnea, fatigue, or dizziness.
- Note that testing usually takes approximately 45 minutes.
- Inform the patient that the physician in attendance usually interprets the results and will explain them to the patient.

After

- Place the patient in the supine position to rest after the test.
- Monitor the EKG tracing and record vital signs at poststress intervals until recordings and values return to pretest levels.
- Remove electrodes and paste.

Test Results and Clinical Significance

Coronary artery occlusive disease *Subclinical coronary artery occlusive disease often becomes evident with stress testing.*

Exercise-related hypertension *In this form of hypertension the blood pressure is in excess of what is considered normal for the level of exercise.*

Intermittent claudication *As with the coronary system, peripheral vascular stenosis or occlusion may not become evident until the legs are stressed as in an exercise stress test.*

Abnormal cardiac rhythms–stress induced *Ectopy may not occur or become symptomatic until the person is stressed.*

Related Tests

- Cardiac nuclear scanning (p. 704): This test is used to evaluate the heart during stress testing.
- Echocardiography (p. 478): This test is also used to evaluate the heart during stress testing.

Contraction Stress, Fetal
(CST, Oxytocin Challenge [OCT])

Normal Findings Negative

Indications

The CST is a method to evaluate the viability of a fetus. It documents the ability of the placenta to provide an adequate blood supply to the fetus. The CST can be used to evaluate any high-risk pregnancy in which fetal well-being may be threatened. These pregnancies include those marked by diabetes, hypertensive disease of pregnancy (toxemia), intrauterine growth retardation, Rh-factor sensitization, history of stillbirth, postmaturity, or low estriol levels.

Test Explanation

The CST, frequently called the oxytocin challenge test (OCT), is a relatively noninvasive test of fetoplacental adequacy used in the assessment of high-risk pregnancy. (Other tests used to evaluate the fetoplacental unit are listed in Box 3-4.) For this study a temporary stress in the form of uterine contractions is applied to the fetus after the IV administration of oxytocin. The reaction of the fetus to the contractions is assessed by an external fetal heart monitor. Uterine contractions cause transient impediment of placental blood flow. If the placental reserve is adequate, the maternal-fetal oxygen transfer is not significantly compromised during the contractions and the fetal heart rate (FHR) remains normal (a *negative* test). The fetoplacental unit can then be considered adequate for the next 7 days.

If the placental reserve is inadequate, the fetus does not receive enough oxygen during the contraction. This results in intrauterine hypoxia and late deceleration of the FHR. The test is considered to be *positive* if consistent, persistent, late decelerations of the FHR occur with two or more uterine contractions. False-positive results caused by uterine hyperstimulation can occur in 10% to 30% of patients. Thus positive test results warrant a complete review of other studies (e.g., amniocentesis) before the pregnancy is terminated by delivery.

The test is considered to be *unsatisfactory* if the results cannot be interpreted (e.g., because of hyperstimulation of the uterus, excessive movement of the mother, or deceleration of unknown meaning [not associated with contractions]). In the case of unsatisfactory results, other means of evaluation should be considered (ultrasound or amniocentesis).

Two advantages of the CST are that it can be done at any time and that its results are available shortly afterward. Although this test can be performed reliably at 32 weeks of gestation, it usually is done after 34 weeks. The CST can induce labor, and a fetus at 34 weeks is more likely to survive an unexpectedly induced delivery than a fetus at 32 weeks. The nonstress test (p. 504) of the fetus is the preferred test in almost every instance and can be performed more safely at 32 weeks; it can then be followed 2 weeks later by the CST if necessary. The CST may be performed weekly until delivery terminates pregnancy.

A noninvasive, alternative method of performing the CST is called the *breast stimulation* or *nipple stimulation technique*. Stimulation of the nipple causes nerve impulses to the

Box 3-4 Tests used in the evaluation of the fetoplacental unit

Contraction stress test
Nonstress test
Obstetric ultrasound
Amniocentesis
Fetoscopy
Biophysical profile
Alpha-fetoprotein
Estriol excretion
Pregnanediol

hypothalamus that trigger the release of oxytocin into the mother's bloodstream. This causes uterine contractions and may eliminate the need for IV administration of oxytocin. Uterine contractions are usually satisfactory after 15 minutes of nipple stimulation (gentle twisting of the nipples). Advantages of this technique include the ease of performing the test, shorter duration of the study, and elimination of the need to start, monitor, and stop IV infusions. If sufficient contractions do not result from nipple stimulation, the standard CST procedure is followed.

The CST is performed safely on an outpatient basis in the labor and delivery unit, where qualified nurses and necessary equipment are available. The test is performed by a nurse with a physician available. The duration of this study is approximately 2 hours. The discomfort associated with the CST may consist of mild labor contractions. Breathing exercises are usually sufficient to control any discomfort.

Contraindications

- Patients with multiple pregnancy, because the myometrium is under greater tension and is more likely to be stimulated to premature labor
- Patients with a prematurely ruptured membrane, because labor may be stimulated by the CST
- Patients with placenta previa, because vaginal delivery may be induced
- Patients with abruptio placentae, because the placenta may separate from the uterus as a result of the oxytocin-induced uterine contractions
- Patients with a previous hysterotomy, because the strong uterine contractions may cause uterine rupture
- Patients with a previous vertical or classic cesarean section, because the strong uterine contractions may cause uterine rupture (The test can be performed, however, if it is carefully monitored and controlled.)
- Patients with pregnancies of less than 32 weeks, because early delivery may be induced by the procedure

Potential Complications

- Premature labor

Interfering Factors

- Hypotension may cause false-positive results.

✓ CLINICAL PRIORITIES

- The blood pressure needs to be carefully monitored during this test to avoid hypotension, which may cause diminished placental blood flow and a false-positive test result.
- This test is usually performed after 34 weeks' gestation since it could induce labor.
- The breast stimulation technique is an alternative method of performing the CST that eliminates the need for IV administration of oxytocin.

Procedure and Patient Care

Before

- Explain the procedure to the patient.
- Obtain informed consent for the procedure.
- Teach the patient breathing and relaxation techniques.
- Record the patient's blood pressure and the FHR before the test as baseline values.
- If the CST is performed on an elective basis, the patient may be kept on NPO status in case labor occurs.

During

- Note the following procedural steps:
  1. After the patient empties her bladder, place her in a semi-Fowler's position and tilted slightly to one side to avoid vena caval compression by the enlarged uterus.
  2. Check her blood pressure every 10 minutes to avoid hypotension, which may cause diminished placental blood flow and a false-positive test result.
  3. Place an external fetal monitor over the patient's abdomen to record the fetal heart tones. Attach an external tokodynamometer to the abdomen at the fundal region to monitor uterine contractions.
  4. Record the output of the fetal heart tones and uterine contractions on a two-channel strip recorder.
  5. Monitor baseline FHR and uterine activity for 20 minutes.
  6. If uterine contractions are detected during this pretest period, withhold oxytocin and monitor the response of the fetal heart tone to spontaneous uterine contractions.
  7. If no spontaneous uterine contractions occur, administer oxytocin (Pitocin) by IV infusion pump.
  8. Increase the rate of oxytocin infusion until the patient is having moderate contractions, then record the FHR pattern.
  9. After the oxytocin infusion is discontinued, continue FHR monitoring for another 30 minutes until the uterine activity has returned to its preoxytocin state. The body metabolizes oxytocin in approximately 20 to 25 minutes.

After

- Monitor the patient's blood pressure and the FHR.
- Discontinue the IV line and assess the site for bleeding.

Test Results and Clinical Significance

Fetoplacental inadequacy *Any disease, trauma, or alteration in the fetoplacental unit will cause deceleration of the FHR. This would include maternal causes, placental causes, or fetal diseases (or severe genetic defects).*

Related Tests

- Nonstress, fetal (p. 504): This is a preferred method to evaluate the fetoplacental unit. This test is performed in a manner similar to that described for the CST except that oxytocin is not used.

Electrocardiography
(Electrocardiogram [ECG, EKG])

Normal Findings

Normal heart rate (60-100 beats/min), rhythm, and wave deflections

Indications

This electrodiagnostic test records the electrical impulses that stimulate the heart to contract. It is used to evaluate arrhythmias, conduction defects, myocardial injury and damage, hypertrophy–both left and right, and pericardial diseases. It is also used to assist in the diagnosis of other noncardiac diseases such as electrolyte abnormalities, drug level abnormalities, and pulmonary diseases.

Test Explanation

The EKG is a graphic representation of the electrical impulses that the heart generates during the cardiac cycle. These electrical impulses are conducted to the body's surface, where they are detected by electrodes placed on the patient's limbs and chest. The monitoring electrodes detect the electrical activity of the heart from a variety of spatial perspectives. The EKG lead system is composed of several electrodes that are placed on each of the four extremities and at varying sites on the chest. Each combination of electrodes is called a *lead.*

A 12-lead EKG provides a comprehensive view of the flow of the heart's electrical currents in two different planes. There are six limb leads (combination of electrodes on the extremities) and six chest leads (corresponding to six sites on the chest). Leads I, II, and III are considered the *standard limb leads.* Lead I records the difference in electrical potential between the left arm (LA) and the right arm (RA). Lead II records the electrical potential between the RA and the left leg (LL). Lead III reflects the difference between the LA and the LL. The right leg (RL) electrode is an inactive ground in all leads. There are three *augmented limb leads:* aV_R, aV_L, and aV_F (*a,* augmented; *V,* vector [unipolar]; *R,* right arm; *L,* left arm; *F,* left foot or leg). The augmented leads measure the electrical potential between the center of the heart and the right arm (aV_R), the left arm (aV_L), and the left leg (aV_F). The six standard *chest, or precordial, leads* (V_1, V_2, V_3, V_4, V_5, V_6) are recorded by placing electrodes at six different positions on the chest, surrounding the heart. (The exact locations of the leads are indicated in "Procedure and Patient Care.")

In general, it is said that leads II, III, and aV_F look at the inferior portion of the heart. Leads aV_L and I look at the lateral portion of the heart. Leads V_2 to V_4 look at the anterior portion of the heart.

The EKG is recorded on special paper with a graphic background of horizontal and vertical lines for rapid measurement of time intervals (*X* coordinate) and voltages (*Y* coordinate). Time duration is measured by vertical lines 1 mm apart, each representing 0.04 second. Voltage is measured by horizontal lines 1 mm apart. Five 1-mm squares equal 0.5 mV.

The normal EKG pattern is composed of waves arbitrarily designated by the letters *P,*

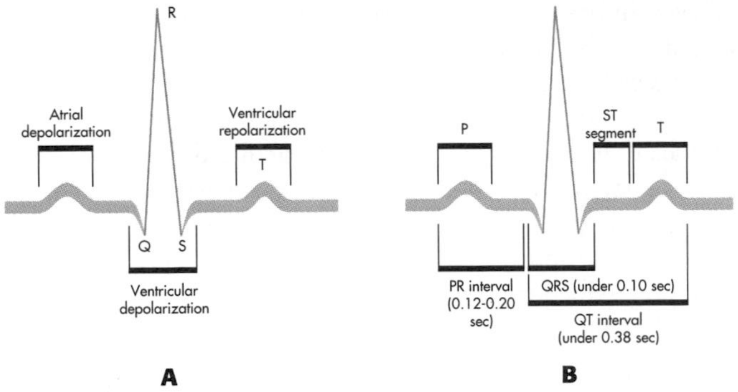

Figure 3-3 **A,** Normal EKG deflections during depolarization and repolarization of the atrium and ventricles. **B,** Principal EKG intervals between P, QRS, and T waves.

Q, R, S, and *T.* The Q, R, and S waves are grouped together and described as the QRS complex. The significance of the waves and the time intervals are as follows (Figure 3-3):

P wave. This represents atrial electrical depolarization associated with atrial contraction. It represents electrical activity associated with the spread of the original impulse from the sinoatrial (SA) node through the atria. If the P waves are absent or altered, the cardiac impulse originates outside the SA node.

PR interval. This represents the time required for the impulse to travel from the SA node to the atrioventricular node. If this interval is prolonged, a conduction delay exists in the atrioventricular node (e.g., a first-degree heart block). If the PR interval is shortened, the impulse must have reached the ventricle through a "shortcut" (as in Wolff-Parkinson-White syndrome).

QRS complex. This represents ventricular electrical depolarization associated with ventricular contraction. This complex consists of an initial downward (negative) deflection (Q wave), a large upward (positive) deflection (R wave), and a small downward deflection (S wave). A widened QRS complex indicates abnormal or prolonged ventricular depolarization time (as in a bundle branch block).

ST segment. This represents the period between the completion of depolarization and the beginning of repolarization of the ventricular muscle. This segment may be elevated or depressed in transient muscle ischemia (e.g., angina) or in muscle injury (as in the early stages of myocardial infarction).

T wave. This represents ventricular repolarization (i.e., return to neutral electrical activity).

U wave. This deflection follows the T wave and is usually quite small. It represents repolarization of the Purkinje fibers within the ventricles.

Through the analysis of these wave forms and time intervals, valuable information about the heart may be obtained. The EKG is used primarily to identify abnormal heart rhythms (arrhythmias, or dysrhythmias) and to diagnose acute myocardial infarction, conduction defects, and ventricular hypertrophy. It is important to note that the EKG may be normal, even in the presence of heart disease, if the heart disorder does not affect the electrical activity of the heart.

For some patients at high risk for malignant ventricular dysrhythmias, a *signal-averaged EKG* (SAEKG) can be performed. This test averages several hundred QRS waveforms to detect late potentials that are likely to lead to ventricular dysrhythmias. SAEKG has been a useful precursor to electrophysiologic studies (EPS) (p. 494) because it can identify ventricular tachycardia in patients with unexplained syncope. SAEKGs can be performed at the bedside in 15 to 20 minutes and must be ordered separately from a standard EKG.

Vectorcardiography, which was once considered to have great potential in the diagnosis of heart disease, has proven to be difficult to evaluate and to use routinely. Vectorcardiography is very similar to EKG except that it looks at the heart as a three-dimensional picture. Echocardiography (p. 787) and EPS (p. 494) have replaced the acute need for vectorcardiography.

Interfering Factors

- Inaccurate placement of the electrodes
- Electrolyte imbalances
- Poor contact between the skin and the electrodes
- Movement or muscle tremors (twitching) during the test
- Drugs that can affect results include digitalis, quinidine, and barbiturates

Procedure and Patient Care

Before

- Explain the procedure to the patient.
- Tell the patient that no food or fluid restriction is necessary.
- Assure the patient that the flow of electric current is *from* the patient. He or she will feel nothing during this procedure.
- Expose only the patient's chest and arms. Keep the abdomen and thighs adequately covered.

During

- Note the following procedural steps:
  1. The skin areas designated for electrode placement are prepared by using alcohol swabs or sandpaper to remove skin oil or debris. Sometimes the skin is shaved if the patient has a large amount of hair.
  2. Electrode paste is applied to ensure electrical conduction between the skin and the electrodes.
  3. The four limb leads are usually held in place by straps that encircle the extremity. Newer machines have clamps that can easily be opened and applied to the extremity.
  4. Many cardiologists recommend that arm electrodes be placed on the upper arm, because fewer muscle tremors are detected there.
  5. The chest leads are applied one at a time, three at a time, or six at a time, depending on the type of EKG machine. These leads are positioned as follows:

     V_1: in the fourth intercostal space (4ICS) at the right sternal border

V_2: in 4ICS at the left sternal border
V_3: midway between V_2 and V_4
V_4: in 5ICS at the midclavicular line
V_5: at the left anterior axillary line at the level of V_4 horizontally
V_6: at the left midaxillary line at the level of V_4 horizontally

- List medications the patient is taking on the EKG request form.
- Note that cardiac technicians, nurses, or physicians perform this procedure in less than 5 minutes at the bedside or in the cardiology clinic.
- Tell the patient that although this procedure carries no discomfort, he or she must lie still in the supine position without talking while the EKG is recorded.

After

- Remove the electrodes from the patient's skin and wipe off the electrode gel.
- Indicate on the EKG strip or request slip if the patient was experiencing chest pain during the study. The pain may be correlated to an arrhythmia on the EKG.

Test Results and Clinical Significance

Arrhythmia (dysrhythmia) *Arrhythmias can start in the atrium or the ventricle. They can cause the heart to speed up (tachyarrhythmias) or to slow down (bradyarrhythmias). With serious arrhythmias, cardiac output can fall significantly, causing the patient to lose consciousness (syncope). Often the patient may experience palpitations during some arrhythmias. Most arrhythmias are asymptomatic, however.*

Acute myocardial infarction
Myocardial ischemia
Old myocardial infarction
Acute myocardial muscle damage is often seen as elevations in the ST segment or as inverted T waves. Old myocardial infarctions (or areas of dead muscle tissue) appear as deep Q waves on the EKG. The EKG should be one of the first tests to be performed on an adult patient who complains of chest pain.

Conduction defects
Conduction system disease
Wolff-Parkinson-White syndrome
The number and type of conduction defects are too great to discuss within the planned scope of this book. Some conduction defects slow the normal conduction of electrical voltage through the heart (e.g., bundle branch block). Some (e.g., Wolff-Parkinson-White syndrome) speed up the electrical conduction.

Ventricular hypertrophy *As a result of prolonged strain on the left ventricle (e.g., aortic stenosis), the thickened myocardium produces large R waves in V_5 and V_6 and large S waves in V_1.*

Cor pulmonale
Pulmonary embolus
The right heart strain associated with acute pulmonary diseases (e.g., embolism) is called acute cor pulmonale. The classic EKG findings are "$S_1Q_3T_3$," which means the presence of an S wave in lead I, a Q wave in lead III, and T wave inversion in lead III. Many times, however, there may be no changes other than tachycardia associated with pulmonary emboli.

Table 3-2 Electrolyte abnormalities and associated EKG abnormalities

Electrolyte abnormality	EKG abnormality
Increased calcium	Prolonged PR interval Shortened QT interval
Decreased calcium	Prolonged QT interval
Increased potassium	Narrowed, elevated T waves AV conduction changes Widened QRS complex
Decreased potassium	Prolonged U wave Prolonged QT interval

Electrolyte imbalance *Each electrolyte abnormality is associated with different EKG changes (Table 3-2).*

Pericarditis *The EKG findings of pericarditis are classic for that disease. There are widespread elevations of the ST segments involving most of the leads (except aVR). The QRS complexes are normal. When effusion is associated with the pericarditis, the voltages are diminished throughout.*

Related Tests

- Echocardiography (p. 478): This is another method of imaging the heart with the use of ultrasound.
- Cardiac nuclear scanning (p. 704): This is a nuclear method of cardiac imaging.

Electroencephalography
(Electroencephalogram [EEG])

Normal Findings

Normal frequency, amplitude, and characteristics of brain waves

Indications

This electrodiagnostic test is performed to identify and evaluate patients with seizures. Pathologic conditions involving the brain cortex (such as tumors, infarction) can also be detected. Finally, the EEG is a confirmatory test for determination of brain death.

Test Explanation

The EEG is a graphic recording of the electrical activity of the brain. EEG electrodes are placed on the scalp overlying multiple areas of the brain to detect and record electrical impulses within the brain. This study is invaluable in the investigation of epileptic states, where the focus of seizure activity is characterized by rapid, spiking waves seen on the graph. Patients with cerebral lesions (e.g., tumors, infarctions) will have abnormally slow EEG waves, depending on the size and location of the lesion. Because this study determines the overall electrical activity of the brain, it can be used to evaluate trauma and drug intoxication and also to determine cerebral death in comatose patients.

The EEG also can be used to monitor cerebral blood flow during surgical procedures. For example, during carotid endarterectomy, the carotid vessel must be temporarily occluded. When this surgery is performed with the patient under general anesthesia, the EEG can be used for the early detection of cerebral tissue ischemia, which would indicate that continued carotid occlusion will result in a cerebrovascular accident (stroke) syndrome. Temporary shunting of the blood during the surgery is then required.

Interfering Factors

- Fasting may cause hypoglycemia, which could modify the EEG pattern.
- Drinks containing caffeine (e.g., coffee, tea, cocoa, cola) interfere with the test results.
- Body and eye movements during the test can cause changes in the brain wave patterns.
- Lights (especially bright or flashing) can alter test results.
- ✗ Drugs that may affect test results include sedatives.

✓ CLINICAL PRIORITIES

- The patient should not be in the fasting state during this test. Hypoglycemia could modify the EEG pattern.
- Stimulants (such as coffee, tea, cola) should not be taken prior to testing because of their stimulating effects.
- Sleep may need to be shortened if a sleep EEG will be attempted.

Procedure and Patient Care

Before

- Explain the procedure to the patient.
- Assure the patient that this test cannot "read the mind" or detect senility.
- Assure the patient that the flow of electrical activity is *from* the patient. He or she will not feel anything during the test.
- Instruct the patient to wash his or her hair the night before the test. No oils, sprays, or lotion should be used.
- Check if the physician wants the patient to discontinue any medications before the study. (Anticonvulsants should be taken unless contraindicated by the physician.)
- Instruct the patient if sleeping time should be shortened the night before the test. Adults may not be allowed to sleep more than 4 or 5 hours, and children not more than 5 to 7 hours, if a sleep EEG will be attempted at the time of testing.
- Do not administer any sedatives or hypnotics before the test because they will cause abnormal waves on the EEG.

- Tell the patient not to fast before the study. Fasting may cause hypoglycemia, which could alter test results.
- Instruct the patient not to drink any coffee, tea, cocoa, or cola on the morning of the test because of their stimulating effect.
- Tell the patient that he or she needs to remain still during the test. Any movement, including opening the eyes, will create interference and alter the EEG recording.

During

- Note the following procedural steps:
  1. The EEG is usually performed in a specially constructed room that is shielded from outside disturbances.
  2. The patient is placed in a supine position on a bed or reclining on a chair.
  3. Sixteen or more electrodes are applied to the scalp with electrode paste in a specified pattern (as determined by the *10-20 system*) over both sides of the head, covering the prefrontal, frontal, temporal, parietal, and occipital areas (Figures 3-4, *A*, 3-4, *B*, and 3-5). In some laboratories the electrodes are tiny needles superficially placed in the skin of the scalp.
  4. One electrode may be applied to each earlobe for grounding.
  5. After the electrodes are applied, the patient is instructed to lie still with his or her eyes closed.
  6. The technician continuously observes the patient during the EEG recording for any movements that could alter results.
  7. Approximately every 5 minutes the recording is interrupted to permit the client to move if desired.
- In addition to the resting EEG, note that the following *activating procedures* can be performed:
  1. The patient is *hyperventilated* (asked to breathe deeply 20 times a minute for 3 min-

A

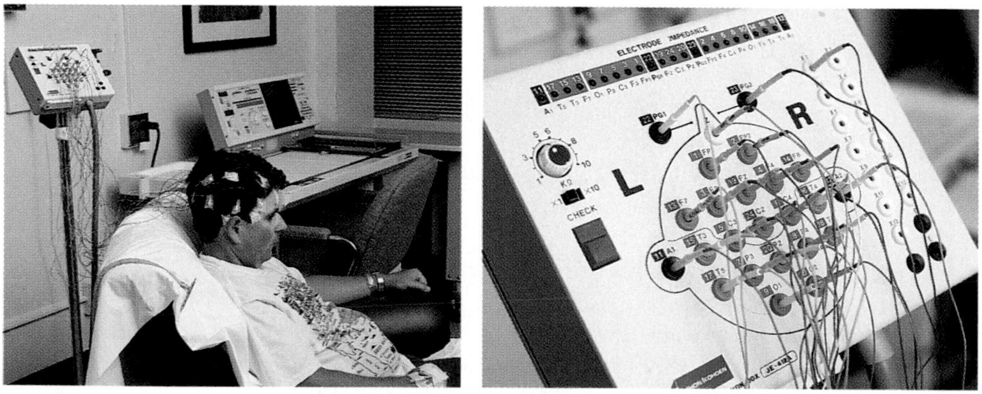

B

Figure 3-4 Electroencephalography (EEG). A routine EEG takes approximately 1 1/4 hours. The actual test lasts approximately 30 minutes. Electrodes are attached to the patient's head **(A)** with the wires leading to corresponding areas on the equipment **(B)** for recording brain wave activity.

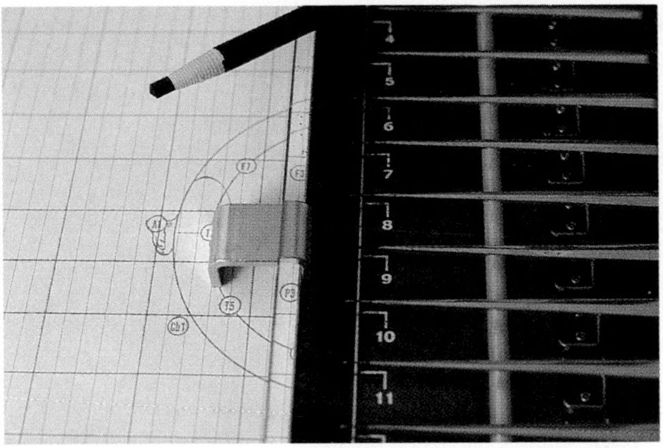

Figure 3-5 Equipment used to record brain waves during an EEG.

utes) to induce alkalosis and cerebral vasoconstriction, which can activate otherwise hidden abnormalities.

2. *Photostimulation* is performed by flashing a light at variable speeds over the patient's face with the eyes opened or closed. Photostimulated seizure activity may be seen on the EEG.
3. A *sleep EEG* may be performed to aid in the detection of some abnormal brain waves that are seen only if the patient is sleeping (e.g., frontal lobe epilepsy). The sleep EEG is performed after orally administering a sedative or hypnotic. A recording is performed while the patient is falling asleep, while the patient is asleep, and while the patient is waking.

- Note that this study is performed by an EEG technician in approximately 45 minutes to 2 hours.
- Tell the patient that no discomfort is associated with this study, other than possibly missing sleep.

After

- Help the patient to remove the electrode paste. The paste may be removed with acetone or witch hazel.
- Instruct the patient to shampoo the hair.
- Ensure safety precautions until the effects of any sedatives have worn off. Keep the bed's siderails up.
- Tell the patient who has had a sleep EEG not to drive home alone.

Test Results and Clinical Significance

Seizure disorders (e.g., epilepsy) *Major, minor, and focal motor seizures can be detected by the EEG only when they are occurring. Between seizures the EEG may be normal.*

Brain tumor
Brain abscess
Intracranial hemorrhage
Cerebral infarct
Most pathologic areas of the brain exhibit localized slowing of brain waves.

Box 3-5 Criteria for brain death

- Absence of hypothermia (temperature greater than 32.2° C)
- Absence of possibility of drug- or metabolic-induced coma
- Absence of neuromuscular blockade administration
- Absence of response to painful or other noxious stimuli
- No attempt at respiration with a Pco_2 of >50 mm Hg
- No brainstem reflexes
  - Fixed pupils
  - No corneal reflexes
- Confirmatory tests (not necessary, but helpful)
  - Isoelectric EEG (may be repeated in 6 hours)
  - Cerebral flow study indicating no blood flow to the brain

Cerebral death *Cerebral death is total cessation of brain blood flow and function while the patient is being ventilated. The EEG is flat, that is, there is no electrical activity. Box 3-5 lists the criteria for brain death.*

Encephalitis *Diffuse global slowing of the EEG waves may be noted.*

Narcolepsy *Sleep waves are noted during what are normally waking hours.*

Metabolic encephalopathy *This may be drug induced or may occur with hypoxia (e.g., after a cardiac arrest), hypoglycemia, etc. The EEG usually shows diffuse slowing of electrical activity.*

Related Test

- Evoked potential studies (p. 497): These tests are used to evaluate specific areas of the cortex that receive incoming stimulus from the eyes, ears, and lower or upper extremity sensory nerves.

Electromyography (EMG)

Normal Findings

No evidence of neuromuscular abnormalities

Indications

This test is used in the evaluation of patients with diffuse or localized muscle weakness. Combined with electroneurography, EMG can identify primary muscle diseases and differentiate them from primary neurologic pathologic conditions.

Test Explanation

By placing a recording electrode into a skeletal muscle, one can monitor the electrical activity of a skeletal muscle in a way very similar to electrocardiography. The electrical activity is displayed on an oscilloscope as an electrical waveform. An audio electrical amplifier can be added to the system so that both the appearance and sound of the electrical potentials can be analyzed and compared simultaneously. EMG is used to detect primary muscular disorders as well as muscular abnormalities caused by other system diseases (e.g., nerve dysfunction, sarcoidosis, paraneoplastic syndrome).

Spontaneous muscle movement, such as fibrillation and fasciculation, can be detected during EMG. When evident, these rapid waveforms indicate injury or disease of the nerve innervating that muscle or spastic myotonic muscle disease. Reduced amplitude (size) of the electrical waveform is indicative of a primary muscle disorder (e.g., polymyositis, muscular dystrophies, various myopathies). A progressive decrease in amplitude of the electrical waveform during contraction is a classic sign of myasthenia gravis. A decrease in the number of muscle fibers able to contract is observed with peripheral nerve damage. This study is usually done in conjunction with electroneurography (p. 490) and also may be called electromyoneurography.

The EMG is performed by a physical therapist, physiatrist, or neurologist in approximately 30 to 60 minutes. This test is moderately uncomfortable. Slight pain may occur with the insertion of the needle electrode.

Contraindications

- Patients receiving anticoagulant therapy, because the electrodes may induce intramuscular bleeding
- Patients with extensive skin infection, because the electrodes may penetrate the infected skin and spread the infection to the muscle

Potential Complications

- Rarely, hematoma at the needle insertion site

Interfering Factors

- Edema, hemorrhage, or thick subcutaneous fat can interfere with the transmission of electrical waves to the electrodes and alter test results.
- Patients with excessive pain may have false results.

✓ CLINICAL PRIORITIES

- This test cannot be done on patients receiving anticoagulation therapy because the electrodes may induce bleeding.
- Slight pain may occur with insertion of the needle electrodes into the muscle for EMG.
- If ordered, serum enzyme tests (such as aspartate aminotransferase [AST], lactic dehydrogenase [LDH], creatine phosphokinase [CPK]) should be done 5 to 10 days after EMG because penetration of the muscle may cause misleading elevations of the enzymes.

Procedure and Patient Care

Before

- Explain the procedure to the patient. Allay any fears and allow the patient to express concerns.
- Obtain informed consent if required by the institution.
- Tell the patient that fasting is not usually required; however, some facilities may restrict stimulants (coffee, tea, cocoa, cola, cigarettes) for 2 to 3 hours before the test.
- If serum enzyme tests (e.g., aspartate aminotransferase [AST], creatine phosphokinase [CPK], lactic dehydrogenase [LDH]) are ordered, the specimen should be drawn before EMG or 5 to 10 days afterward because the penetration of the muscle by the electrodes may cause misleading elevations of these enzymes, which can be produced by the muscle tissue.
- Premedication or sedation is usually avoided because of the need for patient cooperation.

During

- Note the following procedural steps:
  1. This study is usually done in an EMG laboratory. This may be specially designed (with copper-lined walls) to minimize extraneous electrical activity.
  2. The patient's position and the position of the electrode depend on the muscle being studied.
  3. A needle that acts as a recording electrode is inserted into the muscle being examined (Figure 3-6).
  4. A reference electrode is placed nearby on the skin surface.
  5. The patient is asked to keep the muscle at rest.
  6. The oscilloscope display is viewed for any evidence of spontaneous electrical activity, such as fasciculation or fibrillation.
  7. The patient is asked to contract the muscle slowly and progressively.
  8. The electrical waves produced are examined for their number, form, and amplitude. This evaluates the muscular component of the test.
  9. Next, a nerve enervating a particular muscle group is stimulated, and the resulting muscle contraction is evaluated as described in step 8. This evaluates the nerve portion of the neuromuscular component.

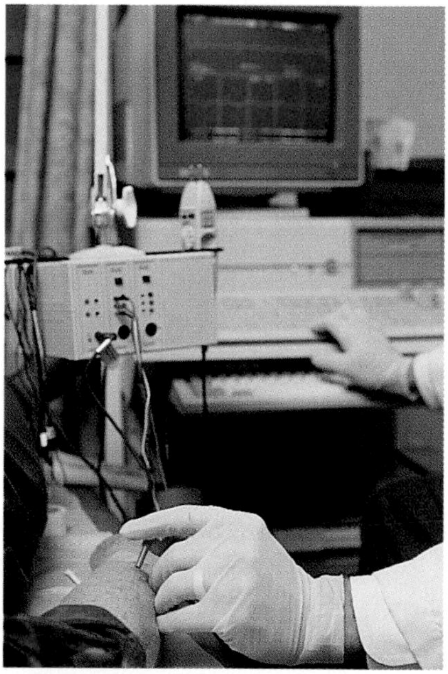

Figure 3-6 Patient having electromyogram (EMG) of forearm. Small needle size makes procedure virtually painless.

After

- Observe the needle site for hematoma or inflammation.
- Provide pain medication if needed.

Test Results and Clinical Significance

Polymyositis *This disease is evident by fast small spontaneous waveforms (myotonia), caused by hyperirritibility of the muscle membrane.*

Muscular dystrophy
Myopathy
Traumatic injury
These primary muscle diseases are evident by decreased electrical activity and amplitude. Even with nerve stimulation, little or no activity is seen. This indicates weakened muscle tissue.

Hyperadrenalism
Hypothyroidism
These endocrine diseases are noted by decreased electrical activity in both amplitude and frequency. This indicates weakened muscle tissue.

Paraneoplastic syndrome (e.g., lung cancer)
Sarcoidosis
These two diseases can be associated with ectopic production of adrenocorticotropic hormone. As in hyperadrenalism, decreased electrical activity in both amplitude and frequency are noted. This indicates weakened muscle tissue.

Guillain-Barré syndrome
Myasthenia gravis
Peripheral nerve injury, entrapment, or compression
Spinal cord injury or disease
Acetylcholine blockers (e.g., curare, snake venom)
Multiple sclerosis
Diabetic neuropathy
Anterior poliomyelitis
Muscle denervation
Amyotrophic lateral sclerosis
These neurologic diseases and injuries are evident as reduced muscle electrical activity with spontaneous contraction. With electrical stimulation, the electrical activity within the muscle is more normal.

Related Tests

- Electroneurography (p. 490): This is similar to EMG except that it evaluates the integrity of the peripheral nerves. This test is often performed with EMG.

Electroneurography
(Nerve Conduction Studies)

Normal Findings

No evidence of peripheral nerve injury or disease
(Conduction velocity is usually decreased in the elderly.)

Indications

This test is performed to identify peripheral nerve injury in patients with localized or diffuse weakness, to differentiate primary peripheral nerve disease from muscular injury, and to document the severity of injury in legal cases. It also is used to monitor the nerve injury and response to treatment.

Test Explanation

Electroneurography, or nerve conduction studies, allows the detection and location of peripheral nerve injury or disease. By initiating an electrical impulse at one site (proximal) of a nerve and recording the time required for that impulse to travel to a second site (distal) of the same nerve, the conduction velocity of any impulse in that nerve can be determined. This study is usually done in conjunction with electromyography (EMG) (p. 486) and also may be called *electromyoneurography.*

The normal value for conduction velocity varies from one nerve to another. Individual variation also exists. It is always best to compare the conduction velocity of the suspected side with the contralateral nerve conduction velocity. In general, a range of normal conduction velocity will be approximately 50 to 60 m/sec.

Traumatic transection or contusion of a nerve will usually cause maximal slowing of conduction velocity in the affected side compared with the normal side. Neuropathies, both local and generalized, also will cause a slowing of conduction velocity. A velocity greater than normal does not indicate a pathologic condition.

Because conduction velocity may require contraction of a muscle as an indication of an impulse arriving at the recording electrode, primary muscular disorders may cause a falsely slow nerve conduction velocity. This "muscular" variable is eliminated if one evaluates the suspected pathologic muscle group before performing nerve conduction studies. This muscular factor can be evaluated by measuring *distal latency* (i.e., the time required for stimulation of the distal end of the nerve to cause muscular contraction). Once the distal latency is calculated, the nerve conduction study is then performed normally by stimulating the proximal portion of the nerve bundle. Conduction velocity can then be determined by the following equation:

$$\text{Conduction velocity (in meters per second)} = \frac{\text{Distance (in meters)}}{\text{Total latency} - \text{Distal latency}}$$

This test takes approximately 15 minutes and is performed by a physiatrist or a neurologist. This test is uncomfortable in that a mild shock is required for nerve impulse stimulation.

Interfering Factors

- Patients in severe pain may have false results.

Procedure and Patient Care

Before

- Explain the procedure to the patient. Allay any fears and allow the patient to express concerns.
- Obtain informed consent if required by the institution.
- Tell the patient that no fasting or sedation is usually required.

During

- Note the following procedural steps:
  1. This test can be performed in a nerve conduction laboratory or at the patient's bedside.
  2. The patient's position depends on the area of suspected peripheral nerve injury or disease.
  3. A recording electrode is placed on the skin overlying a muscle innervated solely by the relevant nerve.
  4. A reference electrode is placed nearby.
  5. All skin-to-electrode connections are ensured by using electrical paste.
  6. The nerve is stimulated by a shock-emitting device at an adjacent location.
  7. The time between nerve impulse and muscular contraction (distal latency) is measured in milliseconds on an EMG machine.
  8. The nerve is similarly stimulated at a location proximal to the area of suspected injury or disease.
  9. The time required for the impulse to travel from the site of initiation to muscle contraction (total latency) is recorded in milliseconds.
  10. The distance between the site of stimulation and the recording electrode is measured in centimeters.
  11. Conduction velocity is converted to meters per second and is computed as in the previous equation.

After

- Remove the electrode gel from the patient's skin.

Test Results and Clinical Significance

Peripheral nerve injury or disease
Carpal tunnel syndrome
Herniated disk disease
Poliomyelitis
Diabetic neuropathy
With peripheral nerve injury, nerve conduction is reduced. Treatment of the nerve entrapment can improve the nerve function and conduction.

Myasthenia gravis
Guillain-Barré syndrome
These diseases affect the spinal cord and to a lesser degree, the peripheral nerves. The extent to which the peripheral nerve is diseased will determine the extent of abnormality of the nerve conduction velocity.

Related Tests

- Electromyography (EMG) (p. 486): This test is often performed simultaneously with electroneurography to determine distal latency (muscular contraction) and to identify muscular disorder as a contributing cause of weakness.

Electronystagmography (ENG)

Normal Findings

Normal nystagmus response
Normal oculovestibular reflex

Indications

This electrodiagnostic test is used to evaluate patients with vertigo and to differentiate organic from psychogenic vertigo. With this test, central (cerebellum, brainstem, eighth cranial nerve) pathologic conditions can be differentiated from peripheral (vestibular-cochlear) pathologic conditions. If a known lesion exists, ENG can identify the site of the lesion. This test is also used to evaluate unilateral deafness.

Test Explanation

ENG is used to evaluate nystagmus (involuntary rapid eye movement) and the muscles controlling eye movement. By measuring changes in the electrical field around the eye, this study can make a permanent recording of eye movement at rest, with a change in head position, and in response to various stimuli. The test delineates the presence or absence of nystagmus, which is caused by the initiation of the oculovestibular reflex. Nystagmus should occur when initiated by positional, visual, or caloric (p. 467) stimuli. Unlike caloric studies, where nystagmus is usually determined visually, with ENG, the direction, velocity, and degree of nystagmus can be recorded. If nystagmus does not occur with stimulation, the vestibular-cochlear apparatus, cerebral cortex (temporal lobe), auditory nerve, or brainstem is abnormal. Tumors, infection, ischemia, and degeneration can cause such abnormalities. The pattern of nystagmus when put together with the entire clinical picture helps in the differentiation between central and peripheral vertigo. This test is used in the differential diagnosis of lesions in the vestibular system, brainstem, and cerebellum.

It also may help evaluate unilateral hearing loss and vertigo. Unilateral hearing loss may be due to middle ear problems or nerve injury. If the patient experiences nystagmus with stimulation, the auditory nerve is working and hearing loss can be blamed on the middle ear.

Contraindications

- Patients with perforated eardrums, who should not have water irrigation
- Patients with pacemakers

Interfering Factors

- Blinking of the eyes can alter test results.
- Drugs that can alter results include sedatives, stimulants, and antivertigo agents.

CLINICAL PRIORITIES

- Various procedures are used to stimulate nystagmus, such as pendulum tracking, changing head position, and changing gaze position.
- Sedatives, stimulants, and antivertigo drugs can alter test results.
- Food should not be eaten before this test to reduce the possibility of vomiting.

Procedure and Patient Care

Before

- Explain the procedure to the patient.
- Instruct the patient not to apply facial makeup before the test because electrodes will be taped to the skin around the eyes.
- Hold solid food before the test to reduce the likelihood of vomiting.
- Instruct the patient not to drink caffeine or alcoholic beverages for approximately 24 to 48 hours (as ordered) before the test.
- Check with the physician regarding withholding any medications that could interfere with the test results.

During

- Note the following procedural steps:
  1. This procedure is usually performed in a darkened room with the patient seated or lying down on an examining table.
  2. If there is any wax in the ear, it is removed.
  3. Electrodes are taped to the skin around the eyes (Figure 3-7).
  4. Various procedures are used to stimulate nystagmus, such as pendulum tracking, changing head position, changing gaze position, and caloric studies (p. 467).
  5. Several recordings are made with the patient at rest and to demonstrate patient response to various procedures (e.g., blowing air into the ear, irrigating the ear with water).
  6. Nystagmus response is compared with the expected ranges, and the results are recorded as normal, borderline, or abnormal.

- Note that this procedure is performed by a physician or audiologist in approximately 1 hour.
- Tell the patient that nausea and vomiting may occur during the test.

After

- Consider prescribing bed rest until nausea, vertigo, or weakness subsides.

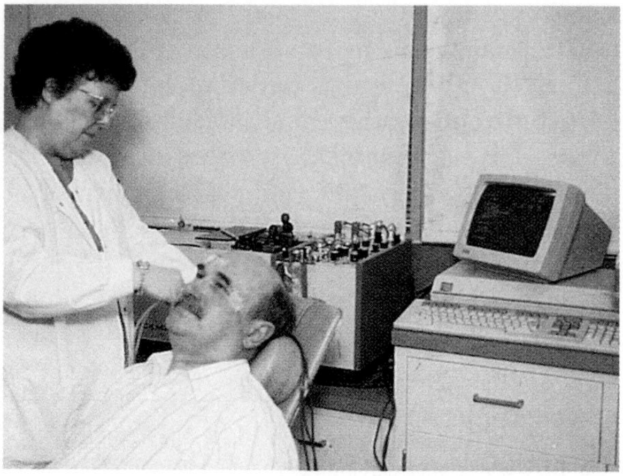

Figure 3-7 Electrodes are applied to a patient in preparation for electronystagmography (ENG).

Test Results and Clinical Significance

Brainstem lesions
Cerebellum lesions
Eighth cranial nerve injury
Tumors, infection, or degeneration of the CNS can be diagnosed, localized, and differentiated from peripheral vestibular diseases.

Vestibular system lesions *Infection is the most common pathologic condition affecting the peripheral vestibular system.*

Congenital disorder
Demyelinating disease
The demyelinating disorders (such as multiple sclerosis) are usually central, whereas the congenital disorders are usually peripheral.

Related Tests

- Caloric study (p. 467): This is a test in which nystagmus is stimulated by warm or cold water (or air) and the presence or absence of nystagmus is observed.

Electrophysiologic Study
(EPS, Cardiac Mapping)

Normal Findings

Normal conduction intervals, refractive periods, and recovery times

Indications

EPS is a method of studying evoked potentials within the heart. It is used to evaluate patients with syncope, palpitations, or arrhythmias. It is used to identify the location of conduction defects that cause abnormal electroconduction and arrhythmias. It can also be used to monitor antiarrhythmic therapy. Through EPS the area known to induce arrhythmias can be obliterated by radiofrequency waves.

Test Explanation

In this invasive procedure, multiple electrode catheters are fluoroscopically placed through a peripheral vein and into the right atrium and/or ventricle or, less often, through an artery into the left atrium and/or ventricle. With close cardiac monitoring the electrode catheters are used to pace the heart and potentially induce arrhythmias (dysrhythmia). Defects in the heart conduction system can then be identified; arrhythmias that are otherwise unapparent also can be induced, identified, and treated. The effectiveness of the antiarrhythmic drugs (e.g., lidocaine, phenytoin, quinidine) can be assessed by determining the electrical threshold required to induce arrhythmias.

EPS can also be therapeutic. With the use of radiofrequency, sites with documented low thresholds for inducing arrhythmias can be obliterated to stop the arrhythmias.

Contraindications

- Patients who are uncooperative
- Patients with acute myocardial infarction

Potential Complications

- Cardiac arrhythmias (dysrhythmias) leading to ventricular tachycardia or fibrillation
- Perforation of the myocardium
- Catheter-induced embolic cerebrovascular accident (stroke) or myocardial infarction
- Peripheral vascular problems
- Hemorrhage
- Phlebitis at the venipuncture site

Interfering Factors

✓ Drugs that may interfere with test results include analgesics, sedatives, and tranquilizers.

✓ CLINICAL PRIORITIES

- In this procedure, electrode catheters are fluoroscopically placed into the heart to pace the heart and to induce arrhythmias. The effectiveness of antiarrhythmic drugs can be evaluated.
- After this procedure, the patient is kept on bed rest for about 6 to 8 hours to allow the blood vessel access site to seal.
- After this test the patient is carefully monitored for arrhythmias and hypotension.

Procedure and Patient Care

Before

- Instruct the patient to fast for 6 to 8 hours before the procedure. Fluids are usually permitted until 3 hours before the test.
- Obtain an informed consent from the patient.
- Encourage the patient to verbalize any fears regarding this test.
- Shave and prepare the catheter insertion site.
- Collect a blood sample for potassium or drug levels, if indicated.
- Obtain peripheral IV access for the administration of drugs.

During

- Note the following procedural steps:
  1. After being transported to the cardiac catheterization laboratory, the patient has electrocardiographic (EKG) leads attached.
  2. The catheter insertion site, usually the femoral artery or vein, is prepared and draped in a sterile manner.
  3. Under fluoroscopic guidance the catheter is passed to the atrium and ventricle.
  4. Baseline surface intracardiac EKGs are recorded.
  5. Various parts of the cardiac electroconduction system are stimulated by atrial or ventricular pacing.
  6. Mapping of the electroconduction system and its defects is performed by measuring evoked potentials.
  7. Arrhythmias (dysrhythmias) are identified.
  8. Drugs may be administered to assess their efficacy in preventing EPS-induced arrhythmias.
  9. Because dangerous arrhythmias can be prolonged, cardioversion must be immediately available.
  10. Not only are vital signs and the heart monitored, but also the patient is constantly engaged in light conversation to assess mental status and consciousness.
- Note that this procedure is performed by a cardiologist within a darkened cardiac catheterization laboratory in approximately 1 to 4 hours.
- Tell the patient that he or she may experience palpitations, light-headedness, or dizziness when arrhythmias are induced. Report these sensations to the physician. For most patients, this is an anxiety-producing experience.
- Inform the patient that discomfort from catheter insertion is minimal.

After

- Keep the patient on bed rest for approximately 6 to 8 hours.
- Evaluate the venous access site for swelling and bleeding.
- Monitor the patient's vital signs for at least 2 to 4 hours for hypotension and arrhythmias (dysrhythmias). Additional monitoring is especially important for certain medications that the patient received during the test. For example, if the patient received quinidine, he or she should be monitored for hypotension and abdominal cramping.
- Continue cardiac monitoring to identify arrhythmias. Transfer arrangements to a monitored unit may be necessary.
- Cover the area with sterile dressings if the electrical catheter is left in place for subsequent studies.

Test Results and Clinical Significance

Electroconduction defects
Cardiac arrhythmia (dysrhythmia)
Sinoatrial node defects (e.g., sick sinus syndrome)
Atrioventricular node defects and heart blocks
These arrhythmias and others can be determined by EPS. The site and actual presence could only be guessed before EPS. Furthermore, areas of arrhythmia inducement can be obliterated by burning the tissue with radiofrequency.

Related Test

- Electrocardiography (EKG) (p. 478): This is the only other mechanism available to identify and locate the source of arrhythmia.

Evoked Potential Studies (EP Studies, Evoked Brain Potentials, Evoked Responses, Visual-Evoked Potentials [VER], Auditory Brainstem-Evoked Potentials [ABEP], Somatosensory-Evoked Responses [SER])

Normal Findings No neural conduction delay

Indications

EP studies are indicated for patients who are suspected of having a sensory deficit but are unable to indicate or are unreliable in indicating recognition of a stimulus. These may include infants, comatose patients, or patients who are unable to communicate. These tests are used to evaluate specific areas of the cortex that receive incoming stimulus from the eyes, ears, and lower or upper extremities sensory nerves. They are used to monitor natural progression or treatment of deteriorating neurologic diseases. Finally, they are also used to identify histrionic or malingering patients who have sensory deficit complaints.

Test Explanation

EP studies focus on changes and responses in brain waves that are evoked from stimulation of a sensory pathway. The study of EPs grew out of early work with the electroencephalogram (EEG) (p. 482). Although the EEG measures "spontaneous" brain electrical activity, the sensory EP study measures minute voltage changes produced in response to a specific stimulus, such as a light pattern, a click, or a shock. In contrast to the EEG, which records signals that reach amplitudes of up to 50 to 100 mV, EP signals are usually less than 5 mV. Because of this, they can be detected only with an averaging computer. The computer averages out (or cancels) unwanted random waves to sum the evoked response that occurs at a specific time after a given stimulus.

EP studies allow one to measure and assess the entire sensory pathway from the peripheral sensory organ all the way to the brain cortex (recognition of the stimulus). They are useful in studying patients who cannot or will not reliably indicate recognition of the stimulus. Such patients may include infants or comatose, histrionic, or malingering patients. These tests are also used to monitor progressive neurologic diseases (e.g., multiple sclerosis).

Clinical abnormalities are usually detected by an increase in *latency,* which refers to the delay between the stimulus and the wave response. Normal latency times are calculated depending on body size, position of the body where the stimulus is applied, conduction velocity of axons in the neural pathways, number of synapses in the system, location of nerve generators of EP components (brainstem or cortex), and presence of CNS pathologic conditions. Conduction delays indicate damage or disease anywhere along the neural pathway from the sensory organ to the cortex.

Sensory stimuli used for the EP study can be visual, auditory, or somatosensory. The sensory stimulus chosen depends on what sensory system is suspected to be pathologic (e.g., questionable blindness, deafness, or numbness). Also, the sensory stimulus chosen may depend on the area of brain where abnormality is suspected. (Auditory stimuli check the brainstem and temporal lobes of the brain; visual stimuli test the optic nerve, central neural visual pathway, and occipital portions of the brain; somatosensory stimuli check the peripheral nerves, spinal cord, and parietal lobe of the brain.) Increased latency (i.e., abnormally prolonged time from the time of stimulus to the time of brain EEG recognition) indicates a pathologic condition of the sensory organ or the specific neural pathway as described previously.

Visual-evoked responses (VERs) are usually stimulated by a strobe light flash, reversible checkerboard pattern, or retinal stimuli (Figure 3-8). A visual stimulus to the eye causes

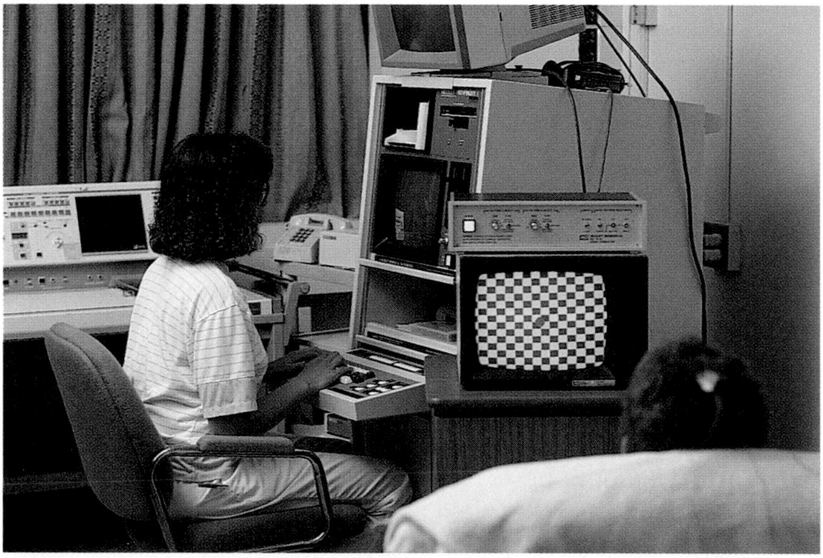

Figure 3-8 Patient undergoing test for visual-evoked potentials diagnostic study. The patient is asked to concentrate on the yellow dot in the middle of the screen while the checkerboard pattern moves. Usually a patch is placed over one eye at a time. The room is darkened for the actual procedure.

an electrical response in the occipital area that can be recorded with "EEG-like" electrodes placed on the scalp overlying the vertex and on the occipital lobes. Ninety percent of patients with multiple sclerosis show abnormal latencies in VERs, a phenomenon attributed to demyelination of nerve fibers. In addition, patients with other neurologic disorders (e.g., Parkinson's disease) show an abnormal latency with VERs. The degree of latency seems to correlate with the disease severity. Abnormal results also may be seen in patients with lesions of the optic nerve, optic tract, visual center, and the eye itself. Absence of binocularity, which is a neurologic developmental disorder in infants, can be detected and evaluated by VERs. Eyesight problems or blindness can be detected in infants through VERs or *electroretinography.* This test also can be used during eye surgery to provide a warning of possible damage to the optic nerve. Infants' gross visual acuity can even be checked via VERs.

Auditory brainstem-evoked potentials (ABEPs) are usually stimulated by clicking sounds to evaluate the central auditory pathways of the brainstem (Figure 3-9). Either ear can be evoked to detect lesions in the brainstem that involve the auditory pathway without affecting hearing. One of the most successful applications of ABEPs has been screening low-birth-weight newborns and other infants for hearing disorders. Recognition of deafness enables infants to be fitted with corrective devices as soon as possible before learning to speak (to prevent speech abnormalities). ABEPs also have great therapeutic implications in the early detection of posterior fossa brain tumors.

Somatosensory-evoked responses (SERs) are usually stimulated by sensory stimulus to an area of the body. The time is then measured for the current of the stimulus to travel along the nerve to the cortex of the brain. SERs are used to evaluate patients with spinal cord injuries and to monitor spinal cord functioning during spinal surgery. They are also used to monitor treatment of diseases (e.g., multiple sclerosis), to evaluate the location and extent of areas of brain dysfunction after head injury, and to pinpoint tumors at an early stage. These tests can also be used to identify malingering or hysterical numbness. The latency is normal in these patients despite the fact that they indicated numbness, etc.

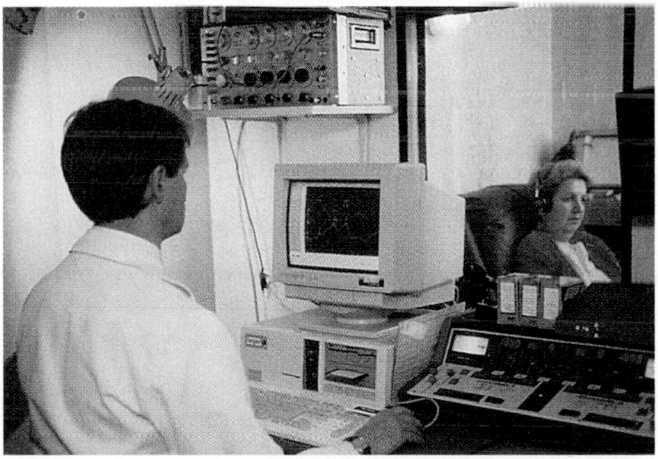

Figure 3-9 Patient undergoing test for auditory brainstem-evoked potentials (ABEPs).

One of the main benefits of EPs is their objectivity, because voluntary patient response is not needed. This makes EPs useful with nonverbal and uncooperative patients. This objectivity permits the distinction of organic from psychogenic problems. This is invaluable in settling lawsuits concerning workers' compensation insurance. The projected future of EPs is that they will aid in diagnosing and monitoring mental disorders and child learning disabilities and in detecting adult mental disorders (e.g., alcoholic brain damage).

Procedure and Patient Care

Before

- Explain the procedure to the patient.
- Instruct the patient to shampoo his or her hair before the test.
- Tell the patient that no fasting or sedation is required.

During

- Note that the position of the electrode depends on the type of EP study to be done:
  1. For *VERs,* electrodes are placed on the scalp along the vertex and the cortex lobes. Stimulation occurs by using a strobe light, checkerboard pattern, or retinal stimuli.
  2. *ABEPs* are stimulated with clicking noises or tone bursts delivered via earphones. The responses are detected by scalp electrodes placed along the vertex and on each earlobe.
  3. *SER*s are stimulated using electrical stimuli applied to nerves at the wrist (medial nerve) or the knee (peroneal nerve). The response is detected by electrodes placed over the sensory cortex of the opposite hemisphere on the scalp.
- Note that this study is performed by a physician in less than 30 minutes.
- Tell the patient that little discomfort is associated with this study.

After

- Remove the gel used for the adherence of the electrodes.

Test Results and Clinical Significance

Prolonged latency for ABEP

Demyelinating diseases (e.g., multiple sclerosis) *Demyelinating diseases destroy the function and integrity of the peripheral and central nervous system. Latency is prolonged.*

Tumor–acoustic neuroma *These tumors grow where the eighth cranial nerve passes under the temporal lobe. Destruction by compression prolongs latency.*

Cerebrovascular accident (CVA) (stroke)
Temporal lobe cortex
Brainstem

Infarctions of either portion of the brain will prolong ABEP latency. The brainstem is an important part of the reflex auditory mechanism.

Auditory nerve damage *Without a functioning auditory nerve, the stimulus cannot reach the cortex. ABEP latency will be prolonged or absent.*

Deafness *Without auditory sensory functioning, the stimulus cannot reach the cortex. Stimulus recognition will not occur. The test can be performed with vibratory stimuli, however. This bypasses the function of the inner ear.*

Prolonged latency for VER

Parkinson's disease
Demyelinating diseases (e.g., multiple sclerosis)
Diseases affecting the peripheral and central nervous system prolong VER latency.

Optic nerve damage *Without a functioning optic nerve, the stimulus cannot reach the cortex. VER latency will be prolonged or absent.*
Ocular disease or injury
Blindness
Without visual sensory functioning, the stimulus cannot reach the cortex. Stimulus recognition will not occur.

Optic tract disease
Occipital lobe tumor or CVA
Unilateral or bilateral latency may be noted in diseases that compress or destroy occipital cortical tissue.

Absence of binocularity
Visual field defects
These defects are caused by congenital or acquired diseases, infections, tumors, etc.

Abnormal latency for SER

Spinal cord injury
Cervical disk disease
Spinal cord demyelinating diseases
Because the spinal cord is the path by which stimulus reaches the cortex, diseases affecting the spinal cord will prolong latency.

Peripheral nerve injury, transection, or disease *The somatic stimulus must travel by way of sensory peripheral nerves to the spinal cord. Diseases that affect the function of these nerves will prolong latency.*
Parietal cortical tumor or CVA *Unilateral or bilateral latency may be noted in diseases that compress or destroy parietal cortical tissue.*

Related Tests

- Electroencephalography (EEG) (p. 482): This electrodiagnostic test is used to detect large electrical waves generated by the cortical structures of the brain and to identify areas of seizure activity or wave slowing compatible with specific pathologic conditions.

Holter Monitoring (Ambulatory Monitoring, Ambulatory Electrocardiography, Event Recorder)

Normal Findings Normal sinus rhythm

Indications

Holter monitoring is used to record a patient's heart rate and rhythm for 1 or more days. It is indicated in patients who experience syncope, palpitations, atypical chest pains, or unexplained dyspnea.

Test Explanation

Holter monitoring is a continuous recording of the electrical activity of the heart. This can be performed for periods up to 72 hours. With this technique, an electrocardiogram (EKG) is recorded continuously on magnetic tape during unrestricted activity, rest, and sleep. The Holter monitor is equipped with a clock that permits accurate time monitoring on the EKG tape. The patient is asked to carry a diary and record daily activities, as well as any cardiac symptoms that may develop during the period of monitoring (Figure 3-10).

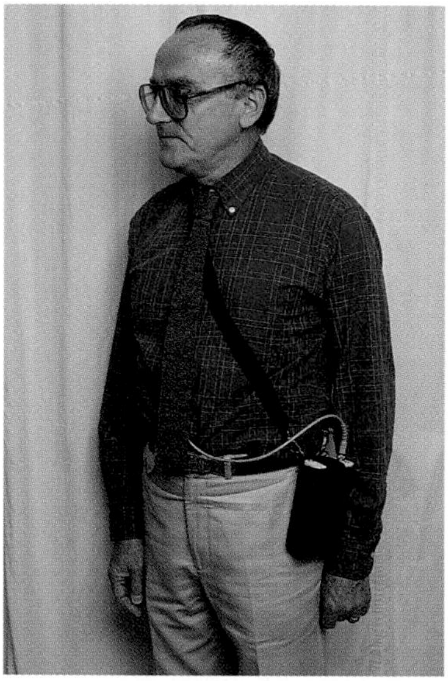

Figure 3-10 Patient wearing Holter monitor.

Most units in present use are equipped with an "event marker." This is a button the patient can push when symptoms such as chest pain, syncope, or palpitations are experienced. This type of monitor is referred to as an *event recorder.* Many recorders store the rhythm immediately preceding activation of the recorder. Stored information can be transmitted by telephone to a recording station.

The Holter monitor is used primarily to identify suspected cardiac rhythm disturbances and to correlate these disturbances with symptoms such as dizziness, syncope, palpitations, or chest pain. The monitor is also used to assess pacemaker function and the effectiveness of antiarrhythmic medications.

After completion of the determined time period, usually 24 to 72 hours, the Holter monitor is removed from the patient and the record tape is played back at high speed. The EKG tracing is usually interpreted by computer, which can detect any significant abnormal waveform patterns that occurred during the testing. Two different computer printouts can be generated. The first is generated from an "event recording," in which representative tracings during noted events are printed out. Tracings demonstrating maximum and minimum heart rates are also printed. A report then can be generated as to the frequency and severity of abnormal cardiac events, especially in relation to the patient's symptoms. The second type of report is generated from a "full disclosure recording," in which all the beats are printed out and are scanned by a technologist, who looks for aberrant waveforms. These aberrancies are then provided to the cardiologist for review.

Contraindications

- Patients who are unable to cooperate with maintaining the lead placement
- Patients who are unable to maintain an accurate diary of significant activities or events

Interfering Factors

- Interruption in the electrode contact with the skin

Procedure and Patient Care

Before

- Explain the procedure to the patient.
- Instruct the patient about care of the Holter monitor.
- Inform the patient about the necessity of ensuring good contact between the electrodes and the skin.
- Teach the patient how to maintain an accurate diary. Stress the need to record significant symptoms.
- Instruct the patient to note in the diary if any interruption in Holter monitoring occurs.
- Assure the patient that the electrical flow is coming from the patient and that he or she will not experience any electrical stimulation from the machine.
- Instruct the patient not to bathe during the period of cardiac monitoring.
- Tell the patient to minimize the use of electrical devices (e.g., electric toothbrushes, shavers), which may cause artificial changes in the EKG tracing.

During

- Prepare the sites for electrode placement with alcohol. (This is usually done in the cardiology department by a technologist.) (See equipment in Figure 3-11.)
- Securely place the gel and electrodes at the appropriate sites. The chest and abdomen are usually the most appropriate locations for limb-lead electrode placement. The precordial leads also may be placed.
- Usually, do not use the extremities for electrode placement to minimize alterations in tracing that occur with normal physical activity.
- Encourage the patient to call if he or she has any difficulties.
- Use a tight undershirt or netlike dressing to hold the leads in place.

After

- Gently remove the tape and other paraphernalia securing the electrodes.
- Wipe the patient clean of electrode gel.
- Inform the patient that the Holter monitoring interpretation will be available in a few days.

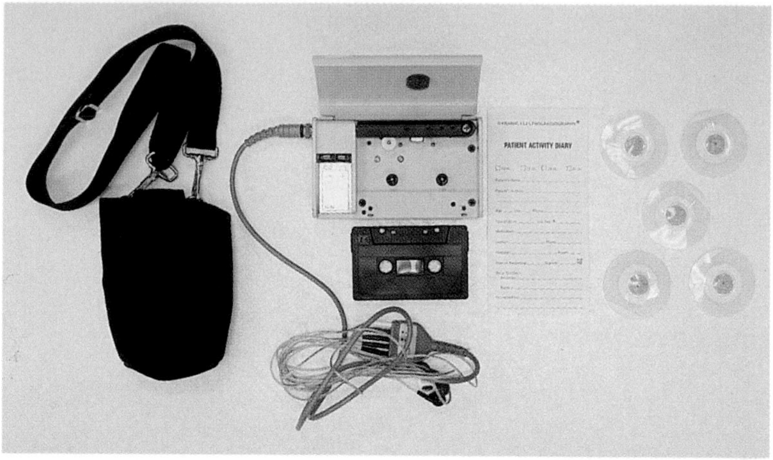

Figure 3-11 Equipment for ambulatory electrocardiography (Holter monitoring).

Test Results and Clinical Significance

Cardiac arrhythmia (dysrhythmia) *Tachycardia or bradycardia may be noted and may be a cause of syncope for the patient. Frequent premature beats may be identified.*

Ischemic changes *If a patient experiences unusual pain symptoms during a particular exercise, a monitor can be applied and that particular exercise performed. If the pain occurs and associated EKG ischemic changes are noted on the monitor, the diagnosis of angina can be made even though the pain is atypical.*

Related Tests

- Electrocardiography (EKG) (p. 478): This is an electrodiagnostic test of the heart taken at one point in time, whereas Holter monitoring continually records EKG data during the entire time of monitoring.

Nonstress, Fetal (NST, Fetal Activity Determination)

Normal Findings

"Reactive" fetus (heart rate acceleration associated with fetal movement)

Indications

The NST is a method to evaluate the viability of a fetus. It documents the placenta's ability to provide an adequate blood supply to the fetus. The NST can be used to evaluate any high-risk pregnancy in which fetal well-being may be threatened. These pregnancies include those marked by diabetes, hypertensive disease of pregnancy (toxemia), intrauterine growth retardation, Rh-factor sensitization, history of stillbirth, postmaturity, or low estriol levels.

Test Explanation

The NST is a noninvasive study that monitors acceleration of the fetal heart rate (FHR) in response to fetal movement. This FHR acceleration reflects the integrity of the CNS and fetal well-being. Fetal activity may be spontaneous, induced by uterine contraction, or induced by external manipulation. Oxytocin stimulation is not used. Fetal response is characterized as "reactive" or "nonreactive." The NST indicates a *reactive* fetus when, with fetal movement, two or more FHR accelerations are detected, each of which must be at least 15 beats/min for 15 seconds or more within any 10-minute period. The test is 99% reliable in indicating fetal viability and negates the need for the contraction stress test (CST, p. 474). If the test detects a *nonreactive* fetus (i.e., no FHR acceleration with fetal movement) within 40 minutes, the patient is a candidate for the CST. A 40-minute test period is used because this is the average duration of the sleep-wake cycle of the fetus. The cycle may vary considerably, however.

The NST is useful in screening high-risk pregnancies and in selecting those patients who may require the CST. An NST is now routinely performed before the CST to avoid the complications associated with oxytocin administration. No complications are associated with the NST.

✓ CLINICAL PRIORITIES

- An NST is routinely performed before the CST to avoid the complications associated with oxytocin administration.
- Fetal activity is enhanced by a high maternal serum glucose level. Therefore the mother should eat prior to this study.
- If this test indicates a nonreactive fetus, further testing (such as the CST) is indicated to evaluate fetal health.

Procedure and Patient Care

Before

- Explain the procedure to the patient.
- Encourage verbalization of the patient's fears. The necessity for the study usually raises realistic fears in the expectant mother.
- If the patient is hungry, instruct her to eat before the NST is begun. Fetal activity is enhanced with a high maternal serum glucose level.

During

- After the patient empties her bladder, place her in the Sims' position.
- Place an external fetal monitor on the patient's abdomen to record the FHR. The

mother can indicate fetal movement by pressing a button on the fetal monitor whenever she feels the fetus move. The FHR and fetal movement are concomitantly recorded on a two-channel strip graph.
- Observe the fetal monitor for FHR accelerations associated with fetal movement.
- If the fetus is quiet for 20 minutes, stimulate fetal activity by external methods, such as rubbing or compressing the mother's abdomen, ringing a bell near the abdomen, or placing a pan on the abdomen and hitting the pan.
- Note that a nurse performs the NST in approximately 20 to 40 minutes in the physician's office or a hospital unit.
- Tell the patient that no discomfort is associated with the NST.

After

- If the results detect a nonreactive fetus, calmly inform the patient that she is a candidate for the CST.

Test Results and Clinical Significance

Nonreactive fetus *This result alone does not indicate fetal distress. But when combined with other noninvasive tests such as CST, biophysical profile, alpha-fetoprotein, pregnanediol, and obstetric ultrasound, fetal health can be accurately determined.*

Related Tests

- Contraction stress test (p. 474): This test is frequently called the oxytocin challenge test. It is a relatively noninvasive test of fetoplacental adequacy used in the assessment of high-risk pregnancy.

Pelvic Floor Sphincter Electromyography
(Pelvic Floor Sphincter EMG, Rectal EMG Procedure)

Normal Findings

Increased EMG signal during bladder filling
Silent EMG signal on voluntary micturition
Increased EMG signal at the end of voiding
Increased EMG signal with voluntary contraction of the anal sphincter

Indications

This test is used to document pelvic diaphragm muscle weakness or paralysis. It is performed most often in patients who have urinary or fecal incontinence. The pathologic condition causing the muscle weakness can be muscular or neurologic.

Test Explanation

This urodynamic test uses the placement of electrodes on or in the pelvic floor musculature to evaluate the neuromuscular function of the urinary or anal sphincter. The main benefit of this study is to evaluate the external sphincter (skeletal muscle) activity during voiding. This test is also used to evaluate the bulbocavernosus reflex and voluntary control of external sphincter or pelvic floor muscles. The pelvic floor sphincter EMG also aids in the investigation of "functional" or "psychologic" disturbances of voiding. Fecal incontinence caused by muscular dysfunction can also be identified by rectal sphincter EMG.

Three electrodes are used for this procedure. Recordings may be made from surface electrodes or needle electrodes within the muscle; surface electrodes are most often used. These electrodes allow for observation of and change in the muscle activity before and during voiding.

Patient cooperation is essential. If the patient does not cooperate, the interpretation of the test results will be difficult. A urologist, physiatrist, or neurologist performs this study in less than 30 minutes. This study is slightly more uncomfortable than urethral catheterization.

Contraindications

- Patients who cannot cooperate during the procedure

Procedure and Patient Care

Before

- Explain the procedure to the patient.
- Inform the patient that cooperation is essential.

During

- Note the following procedural steps:
  1. Two electrodes are placed at the 2 o'clock and 10 o'clock positions on the perianal skin to monitor the pelvic floor musculature during voiding.
  2. The third electrode is usually placed on the thigh and serves as a ground.
  3. Electrical activity is recorded with the bladder empty and the patient relaxed.
  4. Reflex activity is evaluated by asking the patient to cough and by stimulating the urethra and trigone by gently tugging on an inserted Foley catheter (bulbocavernosus reflex).
  5. Voluntary activity is evaluated by asking the patient to contract and relax the sphincter muscle.
  6. The bladder is filled with sterile water at room temperature at a rate of 100 ml/min.
  7. The EMG responses to filling and detrusor hyperreflexia (if present) are recorded.
  8. Finally, when the bladder is full and with the patient in a voiding position, the filling catheter is removed and the patient is asked to urinate. In the normal patient, the EMG signals build during bladder filling and cease promptly on voluntary micturition, remaining silent until the pelvic floor contracts at the end of voiding.

9. The electrical waves produced are examined for their number, amplitude, and form.

After

- If needle electrodes were used, observe the needle site for hematoma or inflammation.

Test Results and Clinical Significance

Neuromuscular dysfunction of the lower urinary sphincter
Pelvic floor muscle dysfunction of the anal sphincter
With overly relaxed pelvic musculature, the frequency and amplitude of the electrical waveform are diminished. This is most commonly seen in elderly women who have had significant muscle stretching during childbirth. It is also seen in patients who have neurologic injury to the nerves innervating the pelvic muscles. The resultant weakness can affect the posterior portion of the pelvic sling and cause anal incontinence. It can affect the anterior portion of the pelvic muscle and cause cystocele, uterine prolapse, and/or urinary incontinence.

Related Tests

- Electromyography (EMG) (p. 486): This test is used to diagnose peripheral muscle pathologic conditions. Theoretically these two studies are similar.
- Urine flow studies (p. 631): This test is often performed at the same time to evaluate incontinent patients.

4

Endoscopic Studies

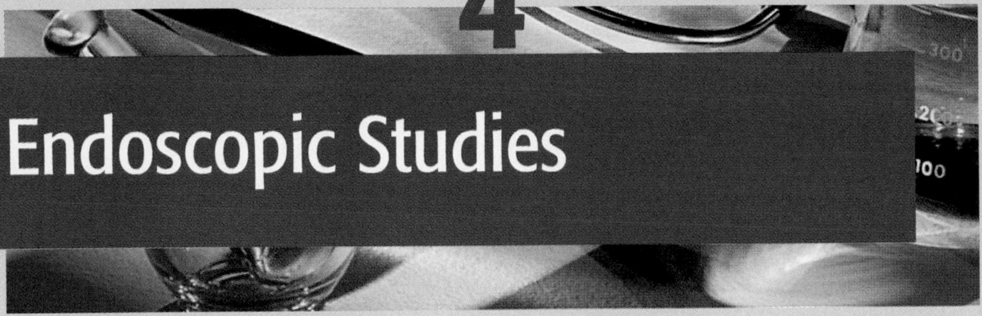

TESTS

Overview

Indications for Endoscopy

Endoscopy is a general term referring to the inspection of the internal body organs and cavities by using an endoscope. Endoscopic procedures are named for the organ or body area to be visualized and/or treated. Table 4-1 provides an overview of body areas viewed by endoscopy.

In addition to direct observation, endoscopy permits biopsy of suspicious tissue, removal of polyps, injection of variceal blood vessels, and the performance of many surgical procedures as indicated in Box 4-1. Furthermore, areas of stricture within a lumen of a hollow viscus can be dilated and stented during endoscopy (Box 4-1).

Instrumentation

Endoscopes are tubular instruments with a light source and a viewing lens for observation. The endoscope can be inserted through a body orifice (e.g., rectum) or through a small incision (e.g., arthroscopy). There are two basic types of endoscopes: rigid and flexible. *Rigid metal scopes* were the first type available and are still used in operative endoscopy. *Flexible fiberoptic scopes* are most often used in pulmonary and GI endoscopy. An example of a flexible fiberoptic endoscope used in esophagogastroduodenoscopy (EGD) is shown in Figure 4-1. These scopes allow the transmission of images over flexible, light-carrying bundles of glass wires. Since flexible fiberoptic scopes can transmit light around corners, they can provide views of the body structures beyond the reach of the older, rigid GI endoscopes. These scopes contain accessory lumens for the insertion of water or med-

Table 4-1 Types of endoscopies and areas of visualization

Type	Area of visualization
Arthroscopy	Joints
Bronchoscopy	Larynx, trachea, bronchi, and alveoli
Colonoscopy	Rectum and colon
Colposcopy	Vagina and cervix
Cystoscopy	Urethra, bladder, ureters, and prostate (males)
Enteroscopy	Upper colon and small intestines
Endourology	Bladder and urethra
Endoscopic retrograde cholangiopancreatography (ERCP)	Pancreatic and biliary ducts
Esophagogastroduodenoscopy (EGD)	Esophagus, stomach, duodenum
Fetoscopy	Fetus
Gastroscopy (part of EGD)	Stomach
Hysteroscopy	Uterus
Laparoscopy	Abdominal cavity
Mediastinoscopy	Mediastinal lymph nodes
Sigmoidoscopy	Anus, rectum, sigmoid colon
Sinus endoscopy	Sinus cavities
Thoracoscopy	Pleura and lung
Transesophageal echocardiography (TEE)	Heart

ication or the suctioning of debris. Also, instruments can be inserted through these lumens to do the following:

Obtain biopsy specimens (with forceps or brushes)
Coagulate blood vessels
Provide laser beams to coagulate vessels or remove tissue

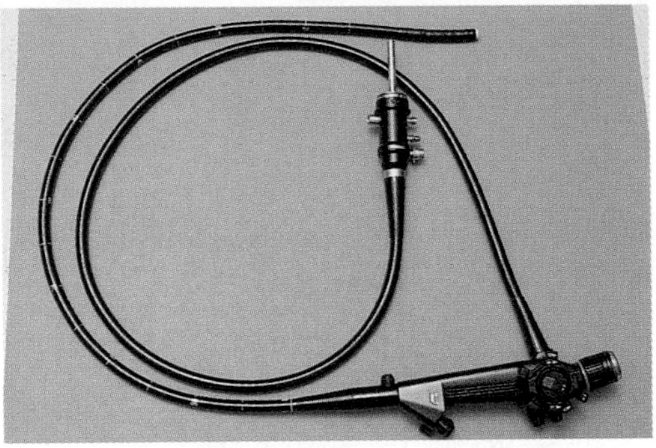

Figure 4-1 Endoscope used to perform esophagogastroduodenoscopy (EGD).

The *rigid endoscopes* are usually metal and are usually used for operative endoscopy (e.g., laparoscopy) or endourology. Their size varies. In general, the larger they are, the greater the width of view. These rigid scopes are lighted by fiberoptic light cords that shine a bright beam through the scope.

Many endoscopic procedures are now performed via a video chip in the tip of a camera that is placed over the viewing lens. The image is then transmitted in color to a nearby television monitor (Figure 4-2). This permits others in the room to observe the procedure and more actively participate in assistance. In many situations, endoscopy eliminates the need for open surgery.

Box 4-1 Endoscopic surgical procedures (exclusive of those mentioned in the text)

LAPAROSCOPY
Cholecystectomy
Hiatal hernia repair
Inguinal hernia repair
Video-assisted colectomy

PELVISCOPY
Oophorectomy
Video-assisted hysterectomy
Tubal ligation
Oophoropexy
Ovarian cystectomy

THORACOSCOPY
Wedge lung resection
Video-assisted lung resection

ARTHROSCOPY
Meniscus removal or repair
Ligamentous repair
Tendon repair
Tendon release (carpal tunnel)

SINUS ENDOSCOPY
Drainage of sinuses

CYSTOSCOPY
Transurethral resection of prostate (TURP)
Transurethral resection of superficial bladder tumors
Removal of ureteral and bladder calculi
Retrograde cystoscopy
Ureteral stent placement

ESOPHAGOGASTRODUODENOSCOPY (EGD)
Dilation of lumen strictures
Placement of esophageal stents

ENDOSCOPIC RETROGRADE CHOLANGIOPANCREATOGRAPHY (ERCP)
Stent placement in the pancreatobiliary tree

FETOSCOPY
Placement of CNS shunts

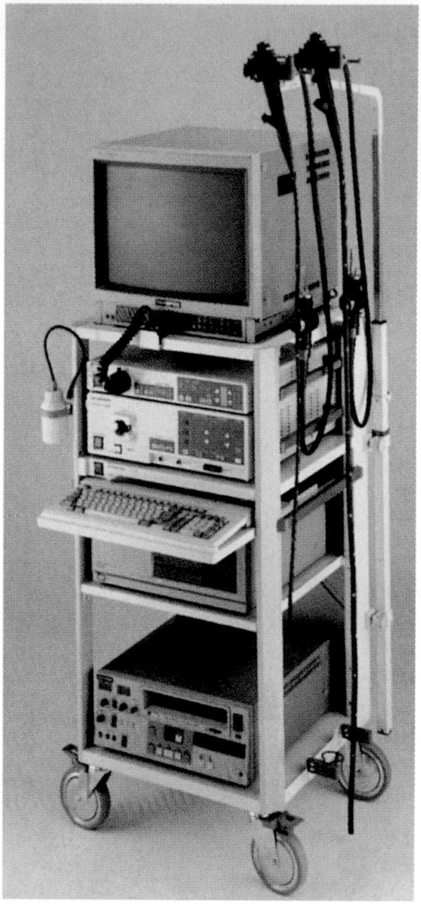

Figure 4-2 Video endoscopy equipment.

Procedural Care for the Endoscopic Patient

Pulmonary and Gastrointestinal Endoscopy

Endoscopic procedures are generally considered invasive. Client preparation and care are similar to those for most minor surgical procedures. General principles are described in this section. Detailed descriptions are included in this chapter with each individual test.

Before

- Explain the test preparation.
- Preparation varies with the endoscopy to be performed. For example, gastroscopy requires that the patient be kept on NPO status for 8 to 12 hours before the procedure to prevent vomiting and aspiration.
- Dentures should be removed, and loose teeth should be noted and recorded.
- For colonoscopy the bowel must be cleansed and free of fecal material to allow adequate visualization of the mucosa.
- GI endoscopy should precede barium contrast studies. Barium can coat the GI mucosa and preclude adequate visualization of the mucosa.
- Baseline laboratory tests (e.g., measurement of hemoglobin, hematocrit, electrolyte levels) should be performed, especially if a surgical procedure or biopsy is possible.
- A good history concerning bleeding tendencies and allergies should be obtained before the procedure.
- Because GI endoscopy is considered "dirty," IV antibiotics are recommended for patients who have cardiac valvular disease (to prevent endocarditis) or patients who have prosthetic joints (to prevent seeding of the joint).

During

- Endoscopic procedures are preferably performed in a specially equipped endoscopy room or in the operating room. However, in cases of emergency, endoscopy can be performed at the bedside.
- Because heavy sedation is provided, resuscitative equipment should be available.
- Air is instilled into the bowel during GI endoscopy to maintain patency of the bowel lumen and to allow better visualization of the mucosa. If cautery is to be used, the air is exchanged for CO_2 to prevent ignition of O_2 or methane inside the bowel.
- Because air insufflation is used, the patient may experience gas pains during the procedure.
- Any surgical or biopsy procedures can be performed.

After

- Specific postprocedure interventions are determined by the type of endoscopic examination performed. All GI procedures have the potential complication of perforation and bleeding. See the discussion of potential complications.
- These procedures use sedation. Safety precautions should be observed until the effects of the sedatives have worn off. A family member or friend should drive the patient home after the test.
- After lower GI tract endoscopy, the patient may complain of rectal discomfort. A warm tub bath may be soothing.
- Usually the patient is kept on NPO status for 2 hours after pulmonary endoscopy or upper GI tract endoscopy. Be certain that the swallowing mechanism and cough reflex have returned to normal before allowing fluids or food.

Operative Endoscopy and Endourology

Before

- These procedures usually require general anesthesia. Furthermore, complications of operative endoscopy may require open surgery to treat them. Therefore the patient must be prepared for general anesthesia and the possibility of open surgery. Routine preoperative care and teaching must be performed.
- The area to be examined should be shaved to remove hair if preferred by the surgeon.
- Because genitourinary (GU) endoscopy is considered potentially "dirty," IV antibiotics are recommended for patients who have cardiac valvular disease (to prevent endocarditis) or patients who have prosthetic joints (to prevent seeding of the joint).

During

- During laparoscopy, CO_2 is instilled into the peritoneal cavity. This may cause significant gas pains and shoulder pain postoperatively if not all the CO_2 is allowed to escape.
- During cystoscopy, water is used to distend the bladder to allow visualization of the bladder mucosa. Accurate measurement of intake and output is difficult.
- The appropriate surgical procedure is performed as indicated in each test.

After

- Patients undergoing endoscopic surgical procedures should be monitored in the same way as any postsurgical patient.

Potential Complications of Endoscopy

Specific complications depend on the type of endoscopic procedure performed. The following guidelines apply to most types of endoscopies.

- Perforation of organ or cavity
  Examine the abdomen for evidence of colon perforation. Assess for abdominal distention, tenderness, and pain.
- Persistent bleeding from a biopsy site
  Assess the vital signs. Watch for a decrease in blood pressure and an increase in pulse rate. Inspect body secretions (such as stool, urine, sputum) for blood.

- Respiratory depression as a result of oversedation
  Carefully assess the patient for respiratory depression. Naloxone (Narcan) may be used to reverse opiates, such as meperidine (Demerol). Flumazenil (Ronazicon) may be used to reverse the effects of benzodiazepines, such as diazepam (Valium) and midazolam (Versed).
- Infections and transient bacteremia
  This is a special concern with cystoscopy. Patients need to be encouraged to drink lots of fluids to maintain a constant flow of urine to prevent stasis and accumulation of bacteria in the bladder. Observe also for signs and symptoms of sepsis, which include elevated temperature, flushing, chills, hypotension, and tachycardia.
- Aspiration when upper airway or upper GI tract was evaluated
  Instruct the patient not to eat or drink anything until tracheal anesthesia has worn off and the gag reflex has returned, usually in 2 hours.
- Cardiovascular problems
  Arrhythmias and even myocardial infarctions can result. Vasovagal-induced bradycardia can be treated with atropine.

Reporting of Results

Most results are directly observed by the physician performing the procedure. Tissues for biopsy or culture need to be sent to the laboratory for evaluation. Results are discussed with the patient as soon as the effect of any sedation has worn off. However, because the sedation has an amnesic effect, the patient may not recall the results of the test. If possible a written reminder of the physician's findings and instructions should be provided to the patient.

Arthroscopy

Normal Findings

Normal ligaments, menisci, and articular surfaces of the joint

Indications

Arthroscopy is an endoscopic procedure that allows examination of a joint interior with a specially designed endoscope.

Test Explanation

Arthroscopy is a highly accurate test because it allows direct visualization of an anatomic site (Figure 4-3). Although this technique can visualize many joints of the body, it is most often used to evaluate the knee for meniscus cartilage or ligament injury. It is also used in the differential diagnosis of acute and chronic disorders of the knee (e.g., arthritic inflammation versus injury).

Physicians can now perform corrective surgery on the knee through the endoscope. Meniscus removal, spur removal, ligamentous repair, and biopsy are but a few of the procedures that are done through the arthroscope. Arthroscopy provides a safe, convenient alternative to open surgery (arthrotomy) because surgery is done through small trocars that are placed into the joint. Surgical maneuvers are carried out under direct vision of the camera that is attached to the arthroscope. Because a large incision is avoided, recovery is faster and more comfortable.

Arthroscopy is also used to monitor the progression of disease and the effectiveness of therapy. Visual findings may be recorded by attaching a video camera to the arthroscope. Joints that can be evaluated by the arthroscope include the tarsal, ankle, knee, hip, carpal, wrist, shoulder, and temporomandibular joints.

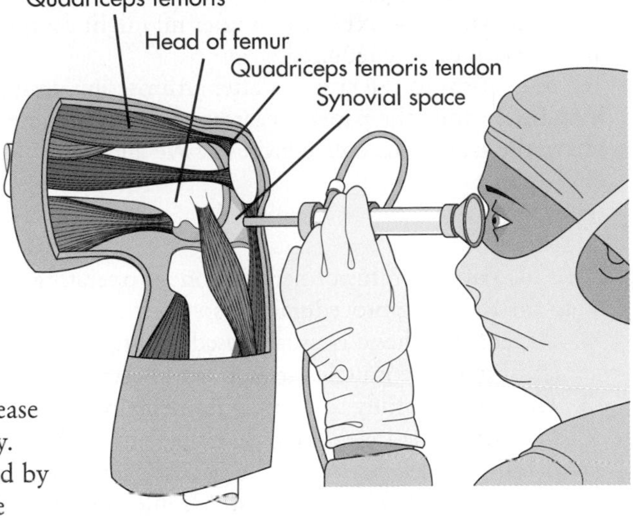

Figure 4-3 Arthroscopy.

This procedure is performed in the operating room by an orthopedic surgeon in approximately 1/2 to 2 hours. Patients receiving local anesthesia have transient discomfort from the injection of the local anesthetic and the pressure of the tourniquet on the leg. A thumping sensation may be felt as the arthroscope is inserted into the joint. The joint may be painful and slightly swollen for several days or weeks, depending on the amount of surgery performed.

Contraindications

- Patients with ankylosis, because it is almost impossible to maneuver the instrument into a joint stiffened by adhesions
- Patients with local skin or wound infections, because of the risk of sepsis
- Patients who have recently had an arthrogram, because they will have some residual inflammation subsequent to the injection of the contrast dye

Potential Complications

- Infection
- Hemarthrosis
- Swelling
- Thrombophlebitis
- Joint injury
- Synovial rupture

Procedure and Patient Care

Before

- Explain the procedure to the patient.
- Ensure that the physician has obtained written consent for this procedure.

- Follow the routine preoperative procedure of the institution.
- Keep the patient on NPO status after midnight on the day of the test because general anesthesia is usually required.
- Tell the patient to use crutches after arthroscopy until he or she can walk without limping. Instruct the patient regarding the appropriate crutch gait.
- Shave the hair in the area 6 inches above and below the joint before the test (as ordered).

During

- Place the patient on his or her back on an operating room table.
- Note the following procedural steps:
    1. General anesthesia is usually used to diminish pain and to allow for complete relaxation of the muscles around the knee.
    2. The leg is carefully scrubbed, elevated, and wrapped with an elastic bandage from the toes to the lower thigh to drain as much blood from the leg as possible.
    3. A tourniquet is placed on the patient's leg. If the tourniquet is not used, a fluid solution (usually saline) is instilled into the patient's knee immediately before insertion of the arthroscope to distend the knee and to help reduce bleeding.
    4. The foot of the table is lowered so that the patient's knee is at a 45° angle.
    5. A small incision is made in the skin around the knee.
    6. The arthroscope (a lighted instrument) is inserted into the joint space to visualize the inside of the knee joint.
    7. Although the entire joint can be viewed from one puncture site, additional punctures for better visualization and surgical maneuvers are often necessary.
    8. After the area is examined, biopsy or appropriate surgery can be performed.
    9. Before removing the arthroscope, the joint is irrigated. Steroids are sometimes injected to diminish inflammation. Pressure is then applied to the knee to remove the irrigating solution.
    10. After a few stitches are placed into the skin, a pressure dressing is applied over the incision site.

After

- Assess the patient's neurologic and circulatory status.
- Assess vital signs and observe the patient for signs of infection, including fever, swelling, increased pain, and redness or drainage at the incision site.
- Instruct the patient to elevate the knee when sitting and to avoid overbending the knee so that swelling is minimized.
- Inform the patient that he or she can usually walk with the assistance of crutches; however, this depends on the extent of the procedure and the physician's protocol.
- Tell the patient to minimize use of the joint for several days.
- Examine the incision site for bleeding.
- Apply ice to reduce pain and swelling.
- Inform the patient that the sutures will be removed in approximately 7 to 10 days.

Home Care Responsibilities

- Teach the patient to walk on crutches.
- Educate the patient to observe for signs of bleeding into the joint (significant swelling, increasing pain, or joint weakness).
- Teach the patient to observe for signs of infection of the joint (fever, swelling, redness about the joint, and increasing pain).
- Educate the patient to observe for signs of phlebitis. This is not uncommon in a person immobilized by joint pain. The involved leg may become swollen, painful, and edematous.
- Instruct the patient not to drive until approved by the physician.
- Ice should be applied at home to minimize the normal swelling that may occur around the involved joint.

Test Results and Clinical Significance

Torn cartilage *Either meniscus (in the knee) is fractured. It may further injure the underlying joint surface.*

Torn ligament *Ligaments support the joint. Injury to this structure weakens joint stability.*

Patellar disease
Patellar fracture
Fracture, inflammation, and malformation can be seen with knee arthroscopy.

Chondromalacia *Disease or structural damage to the cartilaginous joint surfaces can cause joint pain and dysfunction.*

Osteochondritis dissecans *Injury to the joint surfaces can occur as a result of joint fragments in the joint space.*

Cyst (e.g., Baker's) *This is a synovial cyst behind the knee as a result of synovial fluid herniating into the soft tissue surrounding the knee.*

Synovitis inflammation of the lining of the joint
Osteoarthritis
Rheumatoid arthritis
Degenerative arthritis
Destruction of the articular surfaces causes inflammation in the joint.

Trapped synovium *Synovial tissue can become trapped between two bones of the joint and cause pain and inflammation.*

Related Tests

- Arthrocentesis (p. 568): This procedure is performed by inserting a needle into the joint space to obtain synovial fluid for analysis.
- Arthrography (p. 898): This x-ray test of the joint space provides information about anatomic and disease abnormalities affecting the joint.
- MRI of the knee (p. 1009): This scanning technique provides valuable information by placing the patient in a magnetic field.

Bronchoscopy

Normal Findings Normal larynx, trachea, bronchi, and alveoli

Indications

Bronchoscopy permits endoscopic visualization of the larynx, trachea, and bronchi by either a flexible fiberoptic bronchoscope or a rigid bronchoscope.

Test Explanation

There are many diagnostic and therapeutic uses for bronchoscopy. *Diagnostic* uses of bronchoscopy include the following:

1. Direct visualization of the tracheobronchial tree for abnormalities (e.g., tumors, inflammation, strictures)
2. Biopsy of tissue from observed lesions
3. Aspiration of "deep" sputum for culture and sensitivity and for cytologic determinations
4. Direct visualization of the larynx for identification of vocal cord paralysis, if present. With pronunciation of "eeee" the cords should move towards the midline.

Therapeutic uses of bronchoscopy include the following:

1. Aspiration of retained secretions in patients with airway obstruction or postoperative atelectasis
2. Control of bleeding within the bronchus
3. Removal of foreign bodies that have been aspirated
4. Brachytherapy, which is endobronchial radiation therapy using an iridium wire placed via the bronchoscope
5. Palliative laser obliteration of bronchial neoplastic obstruction

The rigid bronchoscope is a wide-bore metal tube that permits visualization of only the larger airways. It is used mainly for the removal of large foreign bodies. Its use has radically diminished since the advent of the newer flexible fiberoptic bronchoscope.

Because of its smaller size and its flexibility, the flexible fiberoptic bronchoscope has increased the diagnostic reach to the smaller bronchi. It also has accessory lumens through which cable-activated instruments can be used for removing biopsy specimens of pathologic lesions (Figure 4-4). In addition, the collection of bronchial washings (obtained by flushing the airways with saline solution), pulmonary toilet, and the instillation of anesthetic agents can be carried out through these extra lumens. Double-sheathed, plugged-protected brushes also can be passed through this accessory lumen. Specimens for cytologic and bacteriologic study can be obtained with these brushes. This allows more accurate determination of pulmonary infectious agents. Needles can be placed through the scope to obtain biopsy specimens from tissue immediately adjacent to the bronchi. Laser therapy can now be performed through the bronchoscope to burn out endotracheal lesions.

This procedure is performed by a physician, usually a pulmonary specialist or a surgeon, in approximately 30 to 45 minutes. No discomfort is usually felt. This test is performed at the bedside or in an appropriately equipped endoscopy room.

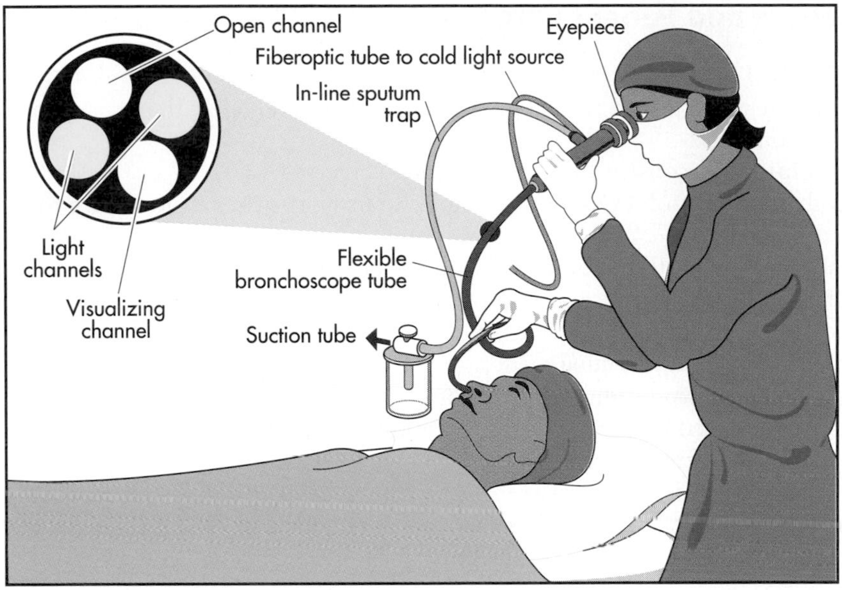

Figure 4-4 Flexible fiberoptic bronchoscope. The four channels consist of two that provide a light source, one vision channel, and one open channel that accommodates instruments or allows administration of an anesthetic or oxygen.

Contraindications

- Patients with hypercapnia and severe shortness of breath who cannot tolerate interruption of high-flow oxygen
  Bronchoscopy, however, can be performed through a special oxygen mask or an endotracheal tube so that the patient can receive oxygen if required.
- Patients with severe tracheal stenosis, which may make it difficult to pass the scope

Potential Complications

- Fever
- Hypoxemia
- Laryngospasm
- Bronchospasm
- Pneumothorax
- Aspiration
- Hemorrhage (after biopsy)
- Infection
- Cardiac arrest

Age-related concerns

- Children have a smaller bronchus. The bronchoscope can significantly decrease the available space for them to breathe. They are at higher risk of hypoxemia than adults.

Procedure and Patient Care

Before

- Explain the procedure to the patient. Allay any fears and allow the patient to verbalize any concerns.
- Obtain informed consent for this procedure.
- Keep the patient on NPO status for 4 to 8 hours before the test to reduce the risk of aspiration.
- Instruct the patient to perform good mouth care to minimize the risk of introducing bacteria into the lungs during the procedure.
- Remove and safely store the patient's dentures, glasses, or contact lenses before administering the preprocedural medications.
- Administer the preprocedural medications as ordered. Atropine may be used to prevent vagal-induced bradycardia and to minimize secretions. Meperidine may be used to sedate the patient and relieve anxiety.
- Reassure the patient that he or she will be able to breathe during this procedure.
- Instruct the patient not to swallow the local anesthetic sprayed into the throat. Provide a basin for expectoration of the lidocaine.

During

- Note the following procedural steps for *fiberoptic bronchoscopy:*
  1. The patient's nasopharynx and oropharynx are anesthetized topically with lidocaine spray before the insertion of the bronchoscope.
  2. The patient is placed in the sitting or supine position, and the scope is inserted through the nose or mouth and into the pharynx (Figure 4-5).
  3. After the scope passes into the larynx and through the glottis, more lidocaine is sprayed into the trachea to prevent the cough reflex.
  4. The scope is passed farther, well into the trachea, bronchi, and the first- and second-generation bronchioles, for systematic examination of the bronchial tree.
  5. Biopsy specimens and washings are taken if a pathologic condition is suspected.
  6. If bronchoscopy is performed for pulmonary toilet (removal of mucus), each bronchus is aspirated until clear.

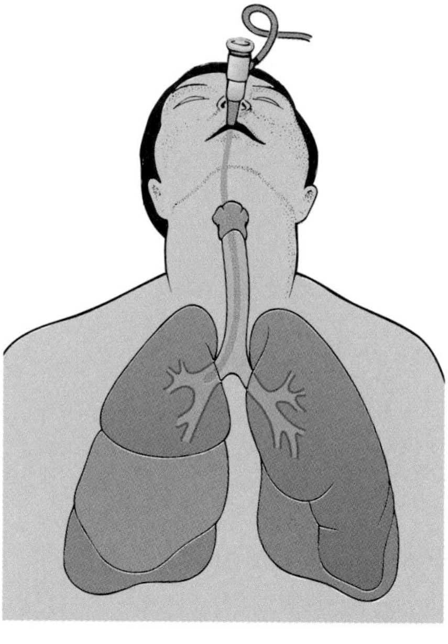

Figure 4-5 Bronchoscopy. A bronchoscope is inserted through the trachea and into the bronchus.

- Note the following procedural steps for *rigid bronchoscopy:*
  1. This test is usually performed in the operating room with the patient under heavy sedation or general anesthesia.
  2. The patient is placed in the supine position with the neck hyperextended.

3. The tube is inserted through the mouth and larynx and then into the trachea.
- Monitor the patient's oxygen saturation to be sure that the patient is oxygenating well. These patients often have pulmonary diseases that already compromise their oxygenation. When a scope is placed, breathing may be further impaired.

After

- Instruct the patient not to eat or drink anything until the tracheobronchial anesthesia has worn off and the gag reflex has returned, usually in approximately 2 hours.
- Observe the patient's sputum for hemorrhage if biopsy specimens were removed. A small amount of blood streaking may be expected and is normal for several hours. Large amounts of bleeding can cause a chemical pneumonitis.
- Observe the patient closely for evidence of impaired respiration or laryngospasm. The vocal cords may go into spasms after intubation. Emergency resuscitation equipment should be readily available.
- Inform the patient that postbronchoscopy fever often develops within the first 24 hours.
- If a tumor is suspected, collect a postbronchoscopy sputum sample for a cytologic determination.
- Inform the patient that warm saline gargles and lozenges may be helpful if a sore throat develops.
- Note that a chest x-ray film may be ordered to identify a pneumothorax if a deep biopsy was obtained.

Home Care Responsibilities

- Suggest that the patient gargle with saline or soothing mouthwash to minimize a sore throat.
- Fever is not uncommon after bronchoscopy. High persistent fever should be reported immediately.
- Bronchospasm or laryngospasm should be reported immediately to emergency personnel.
- Inform the patient that biopsy or culture reports will be available in 2 to 7 days.

Test Results and Clinical Significance

Inflammation *Bronchitis is readily obvious with this method. Cultures can be obtained to identify infections.*

Strictures *Strictures can be identified and sometimes dilated with this technique.*

Cancer *Neoplasm of the larynx, bronchus, or lung can be identified, and a biopsy can be performed. The extent of the tumor and its resectability can sometimes be determined. The amount of lung that is required to be removed can be estimated at bronchoscopy. Laser energy can be delivered to diminish the intraluminal size of the tumor. Iridium radiation strips can be positioned accurately at bronchoscopy.*

Hemorrhage *Hemorrhage can be identified and sometimes controlled by this technique. The source of the hemorrhage can be determined.*

Foreign body *Often foreign bodies can be removed by fiberoptic flexible bronchoscopy. Large-bore rigid bronchoscopy may be required.*

Abscess *Pockets of infection can be diagnosed and drained by bronchoscopy. Good cultures can be obtained.*

Infection *Infections can be identified and cultures can be obtained to provide information for treatment. Difficult-to-grow organisms can be better cultured by this technique. This is especially helpful for tuberculosis, fungal infections, and* Pneumocystis carinii.

Related Tests

- Computed tomography of the chest (p. 942): This test can visualize the mediastinal structure but cannot be specific about a disease process.
- Chest radiography (p. 924): This test is important in the complete evaluation of the pulmonary and cardiac systems.

Colonoscopy

Normal Findings

Normal rectum, colon, and distal small bowel

Indications

This test allows for direct visualization of the rectum, colon, and small bowel. It is used to diagnose suspected pathologic conditions of these organs. It is recommended for patients who have had a change in bowel habits or obvious or occult blood in the stool or who have abdominal pain. It is also used as a surveillance tool for patients who have had colorectal cancer, inflammatory bowel disease, or polyposis.

Test Explanation

With fiberoptic colonoscopy the entire colon from anus to cecum (and often a portion of terminal ileum) can be examined in most patients. (Table 4-2 lists types of GI endoscopies.) As with sigmoidoscopy (p. 550), benign and malignant neoplasms, polyps, mucosal inflammation, ulceration, and sites of active hemorrhage can be visualized. Diseases such as cancer, polyps, ulcers, and arteriovenous (AV) malformations also can be visualized. Biopsy specimens of cancers, polyps, and inflammatory bowel diseases can be taken through the colonoscope with cable-activated instruments. Sites of active bleeding can be

Table 4-2 Types of GI endoscopies

Endoscopy	Portion of bowel examined
Anoscopy	Anus and distal rectum
Proctoscopy	Rectum
Sigmoidoscopy	
Rigid	Anus, rectum, and sigmoid colon to 25 cm
Flexible	Anus, rectum, and sigmoid colon to 60 cm
Colonoscopy	Anus, rectum, and entire colon

coagulated with the use of laser, electrocoagulation, and injection of sclerosing agents.

This test is recommended for patients who have Hemoccult-positive stools, lower GI tract bleeding, or a change in bowel habits. This test is also recommended for patients who are at high risk for colon cancer. They include patients with a strong personal or family history of colon cancer, polyps, or ulcerative colitis.

The test is performed by a physician trained in GI endoscopy in approximately 30 to 60 minutes. It is usually performed in an endoscopy suite or the operating room. Since the patient is heavily sedated, he or she experiences very little discomfort.

Contraindications

- Patients who are uncooperative
  As in all studies that require technical finesse, patient cooperation is essential to successful completion of the test.
- Patients whose medical conditions are not stable
  This test requires sedation, which may induce hypotension in medically unstable patients.
- Patients who are bleeding profusely from the rectum
  The viewing lens will become covered with blood clots, preventing visualization of the lower intestinal tract.
- Patients with a suspected perforation of the colon
  The air insufflated during colonoscopy may worsen the fecal peritoneal soilage.
- Patient with toxic megacolon
  These patients may worsen with the test preparation.
- Patients with a recent colon anastomosis (within the past 14 to 21 days)
  The anastomosis may break down with significant insufflation of CO_2.

Age-related concerns

- The elderly should be cautious due to the dehydration and exhaustion that may result from the test preparation. It may be helpful for someone to stay with the elderly patient if this is done on an outpatient basis.

Potential Complications

- Bowel perforation
- Persistent bleeding from a biopsy site
- Respiratory depression as a result of oversedation

Interfering Factors

- Poor bowel preparation may result in the stool immediately obstructing the lens and precluding adequate visualization of the colon.
- Active bleeding may obstruct the lens system and preclude adequate visualization of the colon.

CLINICAL PRIORITIES

- Patients need to drink lots of fluid to preclude dehydration from the test preparation.
- It is recommended that the patient drink the entire gallon of the glycol preparation within 4 hours.
- Nausea and vomiting should indicate immediate cessation of the preparation procedure.
- Patients with valvular heart disease should receive prophylactic antibiotics before the test.

Procedure and Patient Care

Before

- Explain the procedure to the patient.
- Fully inform the patient about the risks of the procedure and obtain an informed consent.
- Instruct the patient in the appropriate bowel preparation. One type is the *2-day bowel preparation,* which uses clear liquids for 2 days, along with a strong cathartic such as magnesium citrate and bisacodyl (Dulcolax). On the day of examination, an enema is given. A *1-day preparation* using a glycol bowel preparation (Colyte) has become more widely used. After the patient ingests a gallon of Colyte, enemas are not usually needed.
- The gallon should be consumed within 4 hours if possible.
- Lemonade powder may be added to the glycol cathartic.
- Avoid an oral bowel preparation in patients with upper GI tract obstruction, suspected acute diverticulitis, or recent bowel resectional surgery.
- Assure patients that they will be appropriately draped to avoid unnecessary embarrassment.
- Administer appropriate preendoscopy sedation, usually meperidine (Demerol) and diazepam (Valium). Atropine is often ordered to minimize patient secretions.

During

- Note the following procedural steps:
  1. IV access is obtained.
  2. After a rectal examination indicates adequate bowel preparation, the patient is sedated.
  3. The patient is placed in the lateral decubitus position, and the colonoscope is placed into the rectum.
  4. Under direct visualization, the colonoscope is directed to the cecum. Often a significant amount of manipulation is required to obtain this position.
  5. As in all endoscopy, air is insufflated to distend the bowel for better visualization.
  6. Complete examination of the large bowel is carried out.
  7. Polypectomy, biopsy, and other endoscopic surgery is performed after appropriate visualization.
  8. When the laser or coagulator is used, the air is removed and CO_2 is used as an insufflating agent to avoid explosion.

After

- Explain to patients that air has been insufflated into the bowel. They may experience flatulence or gas pains.
- Examine the abdomen for evidence of colon perforation (abdominal distention and tenderness).
- Assess the patient's vital signs. Watch for a decrease in blood pressure and an increase in pulse rate as an indication of hemorrhage.
- Inspect the stools for gross blood.
- Notify the physician if the patient develops increased pain or significant GI bleeding.
- Allow the patient to eat when fully alert if no evidence of bowel perforation exists.
- Encourage the patient to drink a lot of fluids when intake is allowed. This will make up for the dehydration associated with the bowel preparation.

Home Care Responsibilities

- Observe for increasing abdominal pain, which may indicate bowel perforation.
- Inform the patient that frequent, bloody bowel movements may indicate poor hemostasis if biopsy or polypectomy was performed.
- Observe for abdominal bloating and inability to pass flatus, which may indicate colon obstruction if a neoplasm was identified.
- Assess for weakness and dizziness, which may indicate orthostasis and hypovolemia due to dehydration.
- Evaluate for fever and chills, which may indicate a bowel perforation.

Test Results and Clinical Significance

Colon cancer *This is seen as a red, friable, fleshy tumor concentrically involving the mucosa of the bowel.*

Colon polyp *This is a tumor that protrudes from only one part of the mucosa of the bowel. Some cancers and most polyps can be removed with the colonoscope. A biopsy specimen can be obtained from neoplasms.*

Inflammatory bowel disease (e.g., ulcerative or Crohn's colitis) *The mucosa of the bowel is red, friable, and thickened. Patients with ulcerative colitis are at great risk for the development of cancer over time. These patients should frequently undergo colonoscopy to identify any cancer or precancerous conditions.*

AV malformations *These are small red dots on the mucosa of the bowel. They are a common form of bleeding in the adult, especially those with aortic sclerosis and valvular disease. These lesions can be fulgurated by electrocautery through the colonoscope.*

Hemorrhoids *These are excess fleshy tissue immediately inside the anus.*

Diverticulosis *This is the presence of diverticuli, which are outpouchings in the wall of the colon. Recognition of these abnormalities is important but usually does not require surgical therapy.*

Ischemic or postinflammatory stricture *This is a fibrotic narrowing of the bowel lumen. Stricture may follow any injury to the bowel. It is a result of fibrosis and scarring that follows an acute insult to the bowel.*

Related Tests

- Barium enema (p. 900): This is another form of visualization of the bowel. It is not as accurate as colonoscopy. Noninvasive diagnostic or therapeutic procedures cannot be performed without colonoscopy.

Colposcopy

Normal Findings

Normal vagina and cervix

Indications

Colposcopy is used to identify malignant and premalignant lesions of the vagina and cervix. It is helpful in the more thorough evaluation of abnormal Papanicolaou (Pap) smears.

Test Explanation

Colposcopy provides an in situ macroscopic examination of the vagina and the cervix with a colposcope, which is a macroscope with a light source and a magnifying lens. With this procedure, tiny areas of dysplasia, carcinoma in situ, and invasive cancer that would be missed by the naked eye can be visualized, and biopsy specimens can be obtained. The study is performed on patients with abnormal vaginal epithelial patterns, cervical lesions, or suspicious Pap smear results and on those women who were exposed to diethylstilbestrol in utero. It may be a sufficient substitute for cone biopsy (removal and examination of a cone of tissue from the cervix) in evaluating the cause of abnormal cervical cytologic findings (Table 4-3).

It is important to realize that colposcopy is useful only in identifying a suspicious lesion. Definitive diagnosis requires biopsy of the tissue. One of the major advantages of

Table 4-3 ***Gynecologic procedures***

Test	Advantage	Disadvantages
Colposcopy	Evaluates the vagina and cervix	Cannot evaluate the endocervix High false positive rate
Hysteroscopy	Evaluates the endometrium	Cannot evaluate the cervix and endocervix
Cone biopsy of the cervix	Evaluates the cervix and endocervix	Cannot evaluate the endometrium
Pap smear	Evaluates the cervix, endocervix, and endometrium	Misses important pathologic conditions of those tissues and may overread inflammation Cannot localize the lesion

this procedure is that of directing the biopsy to the area most likely to be truly representative of the lesion. A biopsy performed without colposcopy may not necessarily be representative of the lesion's true pathologic condition, resulting in a significant risk of missing a serious lesion.

The patient will need to have diagnostic conization in the following instances:

1. Colposcopy and endocervical curettage do not explain the problem or match the cytologic findings of the Pap smear within one grade.
2. The entire transformation zone (between squamous and columnar epithelium) is not seen. This area is also called the endocervix, where many cancers can initiate.
3. The lesion extends up the cervical canal beyond the vision of the colposcope.

The need for up to 90% of cone biopsies is eliminated by an experienced colposcopist. Endocervical curettage may routinely accompany colposcopy to detect unseen lesions in the endocervical canal.

Colposcopy is performed by a physician in approximately 5 to 10 minutes. Some women complain of pressure pains from the vaginal speculum, and momentary discomfort may be felt if biopsy specimens are obtained. If the discomfort exceeds that which mild sedation treats, a paracervical block can be performed.

Contraindications

- Patients with heavy menstrual flow

Potential Complications

- Infectious cervicitis
- Hemorrhage
- Vasovagal reaction

Interfering Factors

- Failure to cleanse the cervix of foreign materials (e.g., creams, medications) may impair visualization.

Procedure and Patient Care

Before

- Explain the procedure to the patient.
- Obtain informed consent if required by the institution.

During

- Note the following procedural steps:
  1. The patient is placed in the lithotomy position, and a vaginal speculum is used to expose the vagina and cervix. An endocervical curettage is performed to minimize any dropping of endocervical cells onto the external surface of the cervix.
  2. After the cervix is sampled for cytologic findings, it is cleansed with a 3% acetic acid solution to remove excess mucus and cellular debris. The acetic acid also accentuates the difference between normal and abnormal epithelial tissues.

3. The colposcope is focused on the cervix, which is then carefully examined. Photographs and rough sketches of the cervix may be created.
4. Usually the entire lesion can be outlined, and the most atypical areas can be selected for biopsy specimen removal.
5. A biopsy can be performed at this time on any abnormality.

After

- The cervix is cleaned with normal saline solution, and hemostasis is ensured.
- Inform the patient that she may have vaginal bleeding if biopsy specimens were taken. Suggest that she wear a sanitary pad.
- Instruct the patient to abstain from intercourse and not to insert anything (except a tampon) into the vagina until healing of the biopsy is confirmed.
- Inform the patient when and how to obtain the results of this study.

Test Results and Clinical Significance

Dysplasia *This is visible as a white sharply bordered lesion after acetic acid is applied.*
Carcinoma in situ *This is visible as a pink or reddened well-circumscribed punctate lesion.*
Invasive cancer *This lesion is noted by its disarray of blood vessels and a mass effect in the cervix.*

Related Tests

- Papanicolaou (PAP) smear (p. 666): This is a smear of the cells that have been shed by the cervix and uterus. Early detection of cancer of the uterus and cervix can be accomplished by routine use of this test.
- Conization/cytology (p. 526): A concentric piece of cervix and endocervix is obtained for microscopic evaluation.

Cystoscopy (Endourology)

Normal Findings

Normal structure and function of the urethra, bladder, ureters, and prostate (in males)

Indications

This endoscopic test is used to evaluate patients with suspected pathologic conditions involving the urethra, bladder, and lower ureters. It is also used to perform a biopsy on and to treat pathologic conditions related to those structures. This procedure is commonly performed for patients with the following problems:

Hematuria
Recurrent or resistant urinary tract infections
Urinary symptoms of dysuria, frequency, urinary retention, inadequate urinary stream, urgency, and incontinence

Test Explanation

Cystoscopy provides direct visualization of the urethra and bladder through the transurethral insertion of a cystoscope into the bladder (Figure 4-6). Cystoscopy is used *diagnostically* to allow the following:

1. Direct inspection and biopsy of the prostate, bladder, and urethra
2. Collection of a separate urine specimen directly from each ureter by the placement of ureteral catheters
3. Measurement of bladder capacity and determination of ureteral reflux
4. Identification of bladder and ureteral calculi
5. Placement of ureteral catheters (Figure 4-7) for retrograde pyelography (p. 982)
6. Identification of the source of hematuria

Cystoscopy is used *therapeutically* to provide the following:

1. Resection of small, superficial bladder tumors (transurethral resection of the bladder)
2. Removal of foreign bodies and stones
3. Dilation of the urethra and ureters
4. Placement of catheters to drain urine from the renal pelvis

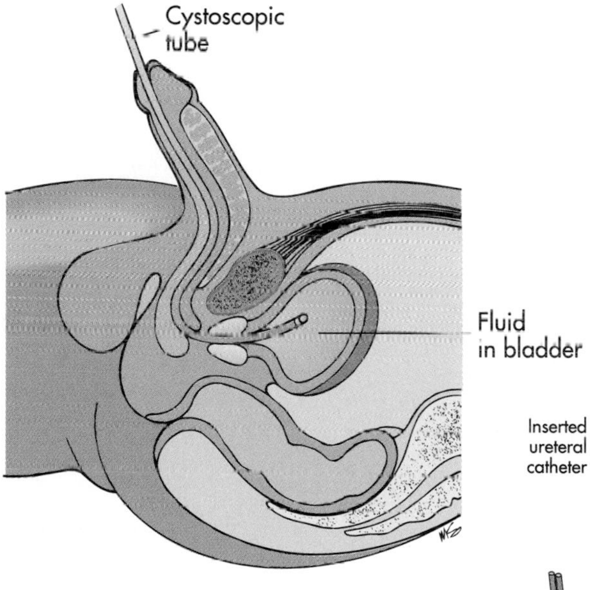

Figure 4-6 Cystoscopic examination of the male bladder.

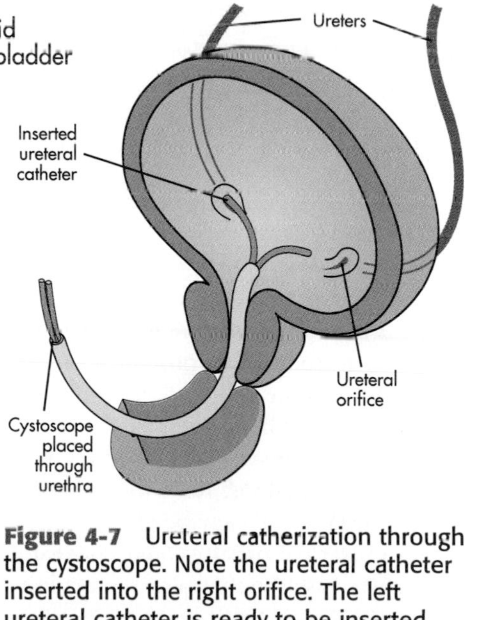

Figure 4-7 Ureteral catherization through the cystoscope. Note the ureteral catheter inserted into the right orifice. The left ureteral catheter is ready to be inserted.

5. Coagulation of bleeding areas
6. Implantation of radium seeds into a tumor
7. Resection of hypertrophied or malignant prostate gland overgrowth (transurethral resection of the prostate [TURP])
8. Placement of ureteral stents for identification of ureters during pelvic surgery

The cystoscope consists primarily of an obturator and a telescope. The obturator is used to insert the cystoscope atraumatically. After the cystoscope is within the bladder, the obturator is removed and the telescope is passed through the cystoscope. The lens and lighting system of the telescope permit adequate visualization of the lower genitourinary tract. Transendoscopic instruments, such as forceps, scissors, needles, and electrodes, are used when needed.

Endourology is an endoscopic procedure that visualizes the bladder and urethra. It is more comprehensive than cystoscopy because it includes a detailed visualization of the urethra. This test is important in the evaluation of hematuria, chronic infection, suspected stones, and radiographic filling defects. On inspection the urethra may show inflammation or structural causes of obstruction (e.g., stricture, neoplasia, prostatic hypertrophy). If the obstruction is functional rather than structural (e.g., detrusor–bladder neck dyssynergia), no site of obstruction will be demonstrated by endoscopy.

Diagnostic cystoscopy can be done in the urologist's office in about 15 minutes. There is very little discomfort associated with the procedure. An anesthetic gel is used on the urethra. If diagnostic or therapeutic instrumentation is required, the procedure is usually done in the operating room under general or spinal anesthesia.

Potential Complications

- Perforation of the bladder
- Sepsis by seeding the bloodstream with bacteria from infected urine
- Hematuria
- Urinary retention

Procedure and Patient Care

Before

- Explain the procedure to the patient.
- Ensure that an informed consent is obtained.
- If enemas are ordered to clear the bowel, assist the patient as needed and record the results.
- Encourage the patient to drink fluids the night before the procedure to maintain a continuous flow of urine for collection and to prevent multiplication of bacteria that may be introduced during this technique.
- If the procedure will be done with the patient under local anesthesia, small volumes of liquids may be acceptable.
- If the procedure will be performed with the patient under general anesthesia, follow routine precautions. Keep the patient on NPO status after midnight on the day of the test. IV fluids may be given.
- Administer the preprocedural medications as ordered 1 hour before the study. Sedatives decrease the spasm of the bladder sphincter, decreasing the patient's discomfort.

During

- Note the following procedural steps:
  1. Cystoscopy is usually performed in the operating room but also can be done in the urologist's office.
  2. The patient is placed in the lithotomy position with his or her feet in stirrups.
  3. The external genitalia are cleansed with an antiseptic solution such as povidone-iodine (Betadine).
  4. A local anesthetic gel is instilled into the urethra if general anesthesia has not been used.
  5. The cystoscope is inserted, and the bladder is distended with saline.
  6. The desired diagnostic or therapeutic studies are performed.
- Instruct the patient to lie very still during the entire procedure to prevent trauma to the urinary tract.
- Tell the patient that he or she will have the desire to void as the cystoscope passes the bladder neck and with bladder distention.
- When the procedure is completed, bed rest should be prescribed for a short time.
- Note that if endourology is performed, the urethra will also be evaluated.
- Note that this procedure is performed by a urologist in approximately 25 minutes.
- When local anesthesia is used, inform the patient of the associated discomfort (much more than with urethral catheterization).

After

- Instruct the patient not to walk or stand alone immediately after the legs have been removed from the stirrups. The orthostasis that may result from standing erect may cause dizziness and fainting.
- Assess the patient's ability to void for at least 24 hours after the procedure. Urinary retention may be secondary to edema caused by instrumentation.
- Note the urine color. Pink-tinged urine is common. The presence of bright-red blood or clots should be reported to the physician.
- Monitor the patient for complaints of back pain, bladder spasms, urinary frequency, and burning on urination. Warm sitz baths and mild analgesics may be ordered and given. Sometimes belladonna and opium (B&O) suppositories are given to relieve bladder spasms. Warm, moist heat to the lower abdomen may help to relieve pain and to promote muscle relaxation.
- Encourage increased intake of fluids. A dilute urine decreases dysuria. Fluids also maintain a constant flow of urine to prevent stasis and the accumulation of bacteria in the bladder.
- Check and record the patient's vital signs as ordered. Watch for a decrease in blood pressure and an increase in pulse rate as an indication of hemorrhage.
- Observe for signs and symptoms of sepsis (elevated temperature, flushing, chills, decreased blood pressure, increased pulse rate).
- Note that antibiotics are occasionally ordered 1 day before and continuing through 3 days following the procedure to reduce the incidence of bacteremia that may occur with instrumentation of the urethra and bladder.
- Encourage the patient to use cathartics, especially after cystoscopic surgery. Increases in intraabdominal pressure caused by constipation may initiate severe lower urologic bleeding.

- If postprocedure irrigation is ordered, use an isotonic solution containing mannitol, glycine, or sorbitol to prevent fluid overhydration in the event any of the irrigation is absorbed through opened venous sinuses in the bladder.
- If a catheter is left in after the procedure, provide catheter care instructions.

Home Care Responsibilities

- Watch for signs of urinary retention for 24 to 48 hours.
- Watch for signs of bleeding. Pink urine is normal; clots are not.
- Report symptoms of increasing lower abdominal pain immediately.
- Use warm sitz baths or B&O suppositories to reduce bladder spasms.
- Encourage the patient to drink lots of fluids.
- Watch for fever, shaking chills, or prolonged dysuria as possible signs of urinary tract infection.
- If ordered, stress the importance of postprocedure antibiotics.

Test Results and Clinical Significance

Lower urologic tract tumor *Bladder cancers or polyps are seen as red friable tumors arising from the mucosa. Sometimes noninvasive tumors can be completely removed by the cystoscope.*

Stones in the ureter or bladder *These can be retrieved through endourologic surgery. If the stones are too large for retrieval, they can be fractured mechanically or with laser or ultrasound.*

Prostatic hypertrophy *This is a benign lesion that occludes the urethra. Removal of the portion of the prostate blocking the urethra (by TURP) resolves the obstruction.*

Prostate cancer *This malignant lesion can obstruct the urethra. Removal of the portion of the prostate cancer that is blocking the urethra (by TURP) resolves the obstruction. In the elderly, this is not an aggressive tumor.*

Inflammation of the bladder and urethra *A red, thickened bladder mucosa indicates chronic infection. This may be due to urethral stricture, bladder diverticula, or inadequate bladder function.*

Urethral, ureteral, or vesical stricture *A fibrous obstruction of the urethra or ureteral opening into the bladder indicates stricture, which is usually benign.*

Related Tests

- Cystometry (p. 615): This is a test of bladder function and capacity.
- Cystography (p. 948): This is an x-ray study of the bladder. It is used to identify bladder tumors, leaks, or fistulas.

Endoscopic Retrograde Cholangiopancreatography
(ERCP, ERCP of the Biliary and Pancreatic Ducts)

Normal Findings

Normal size of biliary and pancreatic ducts
No obstruction or filling defects within the biliary or pancreatic ducts

Indications

This test is used in the evaluation of the jaundiced patient. It is also used to evaluate patients with unexplained upper abdominal pain or pancreatitis.

Test Explanation

With the use of a fiberoptic endoscope, ERCP provides radiographic visualization of the bile and pancreatic ducts. This is especially useful in patients with jaundice. If a partial or total obstruction of those ducts exists, characteristics of the obstructing lesion can be demonstrated. Stones, benign strictures, cysts, ampullary stenosis, anatomic variations, and malignant tumors can be identified. Only ERCP and percutaneous transhepatic cholangiography (PTHC) can provide direct radiographic visualization of the biliary and pancreatic ducts. PTHC (p. 976) is an invasive procedure with significant morbidity; ERCP is associated with much less morbidity but must be performed by an experienced endoscopist.

In contrast to an oral cholecystogram or an IV cholangiogram, which does not visualize the biliary tree when high levels of bilirubin are present, the biliary ducts of jaundiced patients can be visualized by ERCP. As a result, this test is extremely important in the evaluation of patients with jaundice.

Incision of the papillary muscle in the ampulla of Vater can be performed through the scope at the time of ERCP. This incision widens the distal common duct so that common bile duct gallstones can be removed. Stents can be placed through strictured bile ducts during ERCP, allowing the bile of jaundiced patients to be internally drained. Pieces of tissue and brushings of the common bile duct can be obtained by ERCP for pathologic review.

Manometric studies of the sphincter of Oddi and pancreatobiliary ducts can be performed at the time of ERCP. These are used to investigate unusual functional abnormalities of these structures.

Contraindications

- Patients who are uncooperative
  Cannulation of the ampulla of Vater requires that the patient lie very still.
- Patients whose ampulla of Vater is not accessible endoscopically because of previous upper GI tract surgery (e.g., gastrectomy patients whose duodenum containing the ampulla is surgically separated from the stomach)
- Patients with esophageal diverticula
  The scope can fall into a diverticulum and perforate its wall.
- Patients with known acute pancreatitis, because ERCP can worsen this inflammation

Potential Complications

- Perforation of the esophagus, stomach, or duodenum
- Gram-negative sepsis
  This results from introducing bacteria through the biliary system and into the blood. Usually this occurs in patients who have obstructive jaundice.

- Pancreatitis
  This results from pressure of the dye injection.
- Aspiration of gastric contents into the lungs
- Respiratory arrest as a result of oversedation

Interfering Factors

- Barium within the abdomen as a result of a previous upper GI series or barium enema x-ray studies precludes adequate visualization of the biliary and pancreatic ducts.

Procedure and Patient Care

Before

- Explain the procedure to the patient.
- Obtain informed consent from the patient.
- Inform the patient that breathing will not be compromised by the insertion of the endoscope.
- Keep the patient on NPO status as of midnight the day of the test.
- Administer appropriate premedication (e.g., midazolam [Versed] and atropine), if ordered.

During

- Note the following procedural steps:
  1. A flat plate of the abdomen is taken to ensure that any barium from previous studies will not obscure visualization of the bile duct.
  2. The patient is placed in the supine position or on the left side.
  3. The patient is usually sedated with a narcotic and a sedative/hypnotic.
  4. The pharynx is sprayed with a local anesthetic (lidocaine [Xylocaine]) to inactivate the gag reflex and to lessen the discomfort caused by the passage of the scope.
  5. A side-viewing fiberoptic duodenoscope is inserted through the oral pharynx and passed through the esophagus and stomach and into the duodenum (Figure 4-8).
  6. Glucagon is often administered intravenously to minimize the spasm of the duodenum and to improve visualization of the ampulla of Vater. Simethicone may be instilled to diminish any bubbles present that may inhibit visualization of the ampulla.
  7. Through the accessory lumen within the scope, a small

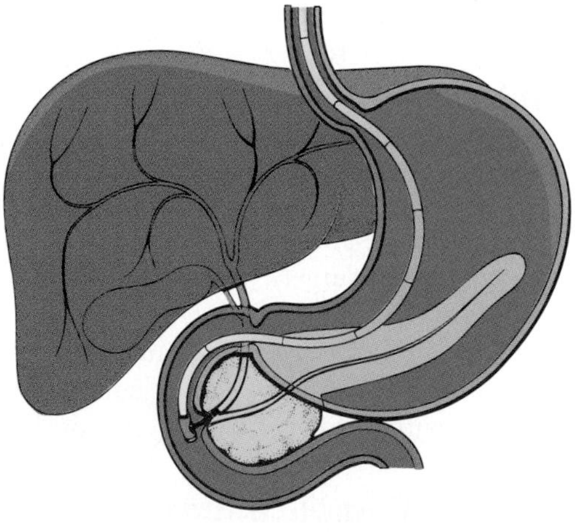

Figure 4-8 Endoscopic retrograde cholangiopancreatography (ERCP). The fiberoptic scope is passed into the duodenum. Note the small catheter being advanced into the biliary duct.

catheter is passed through the ampulla and into the common bile or pancreatic ducts.

8. Radiographic dye is injected, and x-ray films are taken.

- Note that the test usually takes approximately 1 hour and is performed by a physician trained in endoscopy. The x-ray films are interpreted by the radiologist.
- Tell the patient that no discomfort is associated with the dye injection but that minimal gagging may occur during the initial introduction of the scope into the oral pharynx.

After

- Do not allow the patient to eat or drink until the gag reflex returns.
- Observe the patient closely for development of abdominal pain, nausea, and vomiting. This may herald the onset of ERCP-induced pancreatitis.
- Observe safety precautions until the effects of the sedatives have worn off.
- Monitor the patient for signs of respiratory depression. Medication (e.g., naloxone [Narcan]) should be available to counteract serious respiratory depression. Resuscitative equipment should also be present.
- Assess the patient for signs and symptoms of septicemia, which may indicate the onset of ERCP-induced cholangitis.
- Inform the patient that he or she may be hoarse and have a sore throat for several days. Drinking cool fluids and gargling will help to relieve some of this soreness.

Home Care Responsibilities

- A sore throat is expected. A soothing mouthwash gargle may help.
- Notify the doctor immediately if increasing abdominal pain, nausea, or vomiting occurs. These may be the early signs of pancreatitis or gastroduodenal perforation.
- Notify the physician immediately of fever or shaking chills. These may indicate possible cholangitis.
- Encourage the patient to eat lightly for the next 12 to 24 hours.

Test Results and Clinical Significance

Tumor, strictures, or gallstones of the common bile duct *This is obvious in the presence and character of the filling defect noted in the dye-filled duct.*

Sclerosing cholangitis
Biliary sclerosis
These are apparent as a long area of strictures involving, but not limited to, the extrahepatic ducts.

Cysts of the common bile duct *These congenital cysts are seen as large balloonlike dilations of any portion of the extrahepatic ducts.*

Tumor, strictures, or inflammation of the pancreatic duct *Some tumors of the pancreas present as large cystic structures involving and leading from the pancreatic duct. Most pancreatic tumors, however, appear as a localized narrowing of the pancreatic duct with a dilated duct distal to the narrowing. Strictures and inflammation usually involve the entire duct with very little duct dilation beyond the narrowing.*

Pseudocyst of the pancreatic duct *This results from pancreatic duct injury (usually following severe pancreatitis). The pancreatic juices leak out of the duct and into the peripancreatic tissue. A cyst is formed that communicates with the main pancreatic duct.*

Chronic pancreatitis *This may be seen as multiple small partial strictures involving multiple short segments of the pancreatic duct with dilation of the duct in between the strictures. This gives the appearance of "beading" along the duct.*

Anatomic biliary or pancreatic duct variations *Variable pathologic and nonpathologic anomalies can occur. Usually no symptoms are caused by these abnormalities.*

Cancer of the duodenum or ampulla *These cancers are quite obvious as friable tumor masses emanating from the mucosa of those regions.*

Related Tests

- Intravenous cholangiography: Dye is injected IV and concentrated in the bile. The biliary ducts can be visualized with plain film and tomography x-rays. This is rarely performed because ERCP, when possible, visualizes the ducts much better.
- Percutaneous transhepatic cholangiography (p. 976): The liver is percutaneously punctured with a needle, and a catheter is threaded into the biliary duct radical. Dye is injected, and the biliary tree can be visualized radiographically.

Esophagogastroduodenoscopy (EGD, Upper Gastrointestinal [UGI] Endoscopy, Gastroscopy)

Normal Findings Normal esophagus, stomach, and duodenum

Indications

This test is used to visualize the lumen of the esophagus, stomach, and duodenum. It is used to evaluate patients with the following:

Dysphagia
Weight loss
Early satiety
Upper abdominal pain
"Ulcer symptoms" or dyspepsia
Alcoholism and suspected varices
Results of barium swallow or upper GI x-ray study that are suggestive of a pathologic condition

Test Explanation

Endoscopy enables direct visualization of the upper GI tract by means of a long, flexible, fiberoptic-lighted scope. The lumen of the esophagus, stomach, and duodenum are examined for tumors, varices, mucosal inflammations, hiatal hernias, polyps, ulcers, and obstructions. The endoscope has one to three channels. The first channel is used for viewing, the second for insufflation of air and aspiration of fluid, and the third for passing

Table 4-4	GI tract endoscopy
Endoscopy	Area evaluated
Esophagoscopy	Esophagus
Gastroscopy	Esophagus and stomach
EGD	Esophagus, stomach, and duodenum
Enteroscopy	Esophagus, stomach, duodenum, and upper jejunum
Panendoscopy	Esophagus, stomach, duodenum, upper jejunum and colon (per colonoscopy)
ERCP	Duodenum, ampulla, and pancreatobiliary ducts

cable-activated instruments to perform a biopsy of suspected pathologic tissue. Probes also can be passed through the third channel to allow coagulation or injection of sclerosing agents to areas of active GI bleeding. A laser beam can pass through the endoscope to perform endoscopic surgery (e.g., obliteration of tumors or polyps, control of bleeding), and the fiberoptics of endoscopy are so refined that video images and "still pictures" can be taken.

With endoscopy, one can not only evaluate the esophagus, stomach, and duodenum, but with the use of an extra-long fiberoptic endoscope, one can also visualize and perform a biopsy of tissue in the upper small intestinal tract. This procedure is referred to as *enteroscopy* (Table 4-4). Abnormalities of the small intestine, such as arteriovenous (AV) malformations, tumors, enteropathies (e.g., celiac disease), and ulcerations, can be diagnosed with enteroscopy.

Besides being much more sensitive and specific than an upper GI series in diagnosing diseases of the esophagus, stomach, and duodenum, EGD also can be used therapeutically. An experienced endoscopist often can control active GI tract bleeding by electrocoagulation, laser coagulation, or the injection of sclerosing agents, such as alcohol. Also, with the endoscope, benign and malignant strictures can be dilated to reestablish patency of the upper GI tract. Biliary stents and a percutaneous gastrostomy can be placed with the use of EGD. The role of endoscopic surgery is expanding in light of its dramatic success and minimal morbidity.

Contraindications

- Patients who cannot cooperate fully
  As in all studies that require technical finesse, patient cooperation is essential for successful, safe, and accurate test completion.
- Patients with severe upper GI tract bleeding
  The viewing lens will become covered with blood clots, preventing adequate visualization. However, if the stomach can be lavaged and aspirated to clear the blood clots, EGD can be performed.
- Patients with esophageal diverticula
  The scope can easily fall into the diverticulum and perforate the wall of the esophagus.

- Patients with suspected perforation
  The perforation can be worsened by the insufflation of pressurized air into the GI tract.
- Patients who have had recent upper GI tract surgery
  The anastomosis may not be able to withstand the pressure of the required air insufflation. This may lead to anastomotic disruption.

Potential Complications

- Perforation of the esophagus, stomach, and duodenum
- Bleeding from a biopsy site
- Pulmonary aspiration of gastric contents
- Oversedation from the medication administered during the test
- Hypotension induced by the sedative medication
  Usually the patient already has some significant element of hypovolemia or dehydration.
- Local IV phlebitic reaction to the injection of sclerosing sedative medication

Interfering Factors

- Food in the stomach
- Excessive GI tract bleeding

Procedure and Patient Care

Before

- Explain the procedure to the patient.
- Obtain informed consent if required by the institution.
- Instruct the patient to abstain from eating as of midnight the day of the test.
- Reassure the patient that this test is not painful. Tell the patient that the throat will be anesthetized with a spray to depress the gag reflex.
- Encourage the patient to verbalize fears. Provide support.
- Remove the patient's dentures and eyewear before testing.
- Remind the patient that he or she will not be able to speak during the test but that respiration will not be affected.
- Instruct the patient not to bite down on the endoscope.
- Instruct the patient in appropriate oral hygiene because the tube will be passed through the mouth.

During

- Note the following procedural steps:
  1. The patient is placed on the endoscopy table in the left lateral decubitus position.
  2. The throat is topically anesthetized with viscous lidocaine (Xylocaine) or another anesthetic spray. This is to decrease the gag reflex caused by passage of the endoscope.
  3. The patient is usually sedated. This minimizes anxiety and allows the patient to experience a "light" sleep.

4. The endoscope is gently passed through the mouth and finally into the esophagus; once in the esophagus, visualization can be performed.
5. Air is insufflated to distend the upper GI tract for adequate visualization.
6. The esophagus, stomach, and duodenum are evaluated.
7. During enteroscopy, the upper small bowel is visualized and a biopsy is performed if needed.
8. Biopsy or any endoscopic surgery is performed with direct visualization.
9. At the completion of direct inspection and surgery, the excess air and GI tract secretions are aspirated through the scope.

- Note that the test is performed in the endoscopy laboratory by a physician trained in GI endoscopy and takes approximately 20 to 30 minutes.
- Tell the patient that the test is mildly uncomfortable.

After

- Inform the patient that he or she may have hoarseness or a sore throat after the test.
- Withhold any fluids until the patient is completely alert and the swallowing reflex returns to normal, usually 2 to 4 hours.
- Observe the patient's vital signs. Evaluate the patient for bleeding, fever, abdominal pain, dyspnea, or dysphagia.
- Inform the patient that he or she may experience some postendoscopic bloating, belching, and flatulence.
- Observe safety precautions until the effects of the sedatives have worn off.
- Inform the patient that the sedation may cause some retrograde and antegrade amnesia for a few hours.

Home Care Responsibilities

- A sore throat is expected after EGD. A soothing mouthwash may help.
- Notify the doctor immediately if bleeding, fever, abdominal pain, dyspnea, or dysphagia occurs.
- Inform the patient that is is normal to have some bloating, belching, and flatulence after the procedure.

Test Results and Clinical Significance

Tumors (benign or malignant) of the esophagus, stomach, or duodenum *These appear as red, friable ulcers or masses in the mucosa of the respective organ. These tumors can obstruct, bleed, or perforate.*

Esophageal diverticula *These are outpouchings of the esophagus at the level of the cricopharyngeal muscle or the diaphragm.*

Hiatal hernia *A hiatal hernia exists when a portion of the stomach is above the diaphragm (seen as an extrinsic compression of the lower esophagus).*

Esophagitis, gastritis, duodenitis *A reddened friable mucosa without ulcer or mass is classic for inflammation.*

Gastroesophageal varices *Submucosal vessels that protrude into the lumen of the distal esophagus and stomach are called varices and indicate a reversal of portal blood flow due to hepatic cirrhosis.*
Peptic ulcer *This benign, acid-induced ulcer usually occurs in the duodenum but may occur in the distal stomach. It is a small to moderate-sized ulcer seen in the mucosa of the organ.*
Peptic stricture and subsequent scarring *Following healing of an ulcer or inflammation, scarring and stricture can form and partially obstruct the lumen of the organ involved (usually the esophagus).*
Extrinsic compression by a cyst or tumor outside the upper GI tract *Tumors, cysts, or enlarged organs can compress the upper GI tract. This is noted by a convex narrowing involving the organ being evaluated.*
Source of upper GI tract bleeding *Ulcers, tumors, varices, AV malformations, inflammation, and bleeding can be identified and often treated by EGD.*

Related Tests

- Barium swallow and upper GI series (pp. 906 and 998): These x-ray contrast studies also evaluate the upper GI tract. They are not as accurate as EGD. Furthermore, biopsy and therapy cannot be performed by the x-ray studies, but they can be performed by EGD.

Fetoscopy

Normal Findings

No fetal distress or diseases seen
No hematologic abnormalities noted

Indications

Fetoscopy is indicated for any woman who is at risk for delivery of a baby with a significant birth defect. It is used also to perform corrective surgery on the fetus when possible.

Test Explanation

Fetoscopy is an endoscopic procedure that allows direct visualization of the fetus via the insertion of a tiny, telescope-like instrument through the abdominal wall and into the uterine cavity (Figure 4-9). Direct visualization may lead to diagnosis of a severe malformation, such as a neural tube defect. During the procedure, fetal blood samples to detect congenital blood disorders (e.g., hemophilia, sickle cell anemia) can be drawn from a blood vessel in the umbilical cord for biochemical analysis. Fetal skin biopsies also can be done to detect primary skin disorders. Fetoscopic surgery (placement of CNS shunts, etc.) is becoming more and more a reality.

Fetoscopy is performed at approximately 18 weeks of gestation. At this time the vessels of the placental surface are of adequate size and the fetal parts are readily identifiable. A therapeutic abortion would not be as hazardous at this time as it would be if it were done later in the pregnancy. An ultrasound examination is usually performed the day after the procedure to confirm the adequacy of the amniotic fluid and fetal viability.

Potential Complications

- Spontaneous abortion
- Premature delivery
- Amniotic fluid leak
- Intrauterine fetal death
- Amnionitis

CLINICAL PRIORITIES

- Ultrasound examination is performed prior to the procedure to identify a safe area to enter the uterine cavity.
- After the test, mothers who are Rh negative should receive RhoGAM unless the fetal blood is also Rh negative.
- Ultrasound examination is usually performed the day after the procedure to confirm the adequacy of the amniotic fluid and to assess fetal viability.

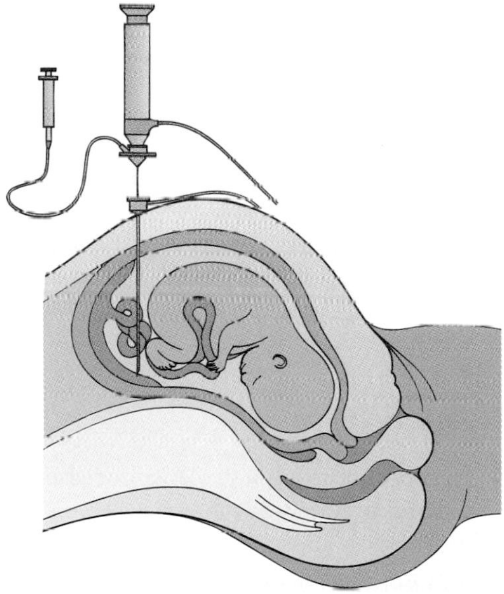

Figure 4-9 Fetoscopy for fetal blood sampling.

Procedure and Patient Care

Before

- Explain the procedure to the patient.
- Obtain informed consent for this procedure.
- Assess the fetal heart rate (FHR) before the test to serve as a baseline value.
- Administer meperidine (Demerol), if ordered, before the test because it crosses the placenta and quiets the fetus. This prevents excessive fetal movement, which would make the procedure more difficult.

During

- Note the following procedural steps:
  1. The woman is placed in the supine position on an examining table.
  2. The abdominal wall is anesthetized locally.
  3. Ultrasonography is performed to locate the fetus and the placenta and to identify a safe area to penetrate the uterus.
  4. The endoscope is inserted.
  5. Biopsy specimens and blood samples may be obtained.
- Note that this procedure is performed by a physician in 1 to 2 hours.
- Tell the patient that the only discomfort associated with this study is the injection of the local anesthetic.

After

- Assess the FHR and compare with the baseline value to detect any side effects related to the procedure.
- Monitor the mother and fetus carefully for alterations in blood pressure, pulse rate, uterine activity, and fetal activity; vaginal bleeding; and loss of amniotic fluid.
- Administer RhoGAM to mothers who are Rh negative unless the fetal blood is found to be Rh negative.
- Instruct the mother to avoid strenuous activity for 1 to 2 weeks following the procedure and to report any pain, bleeding, amniotic fluid loss, or fever.
- At times, if ordered, administer antibiotics prophylactically after the test to prevent amnionitis.

Test Results and Clinical Significance

Developmental defects (e.g., neural tube defects) *These defects are visible on a fetus exceeding 20 weeks in age.*

Congenital blood disorders (e.g., hemophilia, sickle cell anemia) *These congenital abnormalities are identified by evaluation of the fetal blood.*

Primary skin disorders *These may be obvious at the time of fetoscopy. Skin biopsies can be performed.*

Related Tests

- Amniocentesis (p. 560): This procedure involves placing a needle through the abdominal and uterine walls into the amniotic cavity to withdraw fluid for analysis. Valuable information about fetal status is obtained.
- Chorionic villus sampling (p. 1006): This is a test whereby the chorionic placental tissue (which has the same genetic material as the fetus) is tested for genetic analysis and karyotyping. This is a rapid and accurate method of determining genetic defects. CVS can be performed earlier in pregnancy than can amniocentesis.

Hysteroscopy

Normal Findings Normal structure and function of the uterus

Indications

This test allows direct visualization of the endometrial cavity. It is indicated for women with an abnormal Papanicolaou smear, dysfunctional uterine bleeding, or postmenopausal bleeding.

Test Explanation

Hysteroscopy is an endoscopic procedure that provides direct visualization of the uterine cavity by inserting a hysteroscope (a thin, telescope-like instrument) through the vagina and cervix and into the uterus. Hysteroscopy can be used to identify the cause of abnormal uterine bleeding, infertility, and repeated miscarriages. It is also used to evaluate and diagnose uterine adhesions (Asherman's syndrome), polyps, fibroids, and displaced intrauterine devices (IUDs).

In addition to diagnosing and evaluating uterine problems, hysteroscopy can also correct uterine problems. For example, uterine adhesions and small fibroids can be removed through the hysteroscope, thus avoiding open abdominal surgery. Hysteroscopy can also be used to perform endometrial ablation, which destroys the uterine lining in order to treat some cases of heavy uterine bleeding.

The hysteroscope can be used with many other instruments. For example, hysteroscopy may be done before a dilation and curettage or concurrently with a laparoscopy. Hysteroscopy may also confirm the results of other tests, such as hysterosalpingography (p. 950). Depending on the amount of surgery and time associated with hysteroscopy, general, spinal, or light sedative anesthesia is used. It takes only about 30 minutes for simple hysteroscopy. This test is usually performed by a gynecologist in the operating room. The patient receiving local anesthesia or only light sedation may feel some cramping during the procedure. In general, it is not a painful procedure.

Contraindications

- Patients with pelvic inflammatory disease
- Patients with vaginal discharge

Potential Complications

- Uterine perforation
- Infection

Procedure and Patient Care

Before

- Explain the procedure to the patient.
- Obtain informed consent for this procedure.

- Schedule the procedure after menstrual bleeding has ceased and before ovulation. This allows better visualization of the inside of the uterus and avoids damage to a newly formed pregnancy.
- Inform the patient that hysteroscopy may be performed with local, regional, or general anesthesia. If general anesthesia will be given, the patient should be on NPO status for at least 8 hours before the test. This test may also be performed without anesthesia.
- Tell the patient to void before the procedure because a distended bladder can be more easily perforated.

During

- Note the following procedural steps:
  1. Hysteroscopy may be performed in the operating room or in the doctor's office. Local, regional, general, or no anesthesia may be used. (The type of anesthesia depends on other procedures that may be done at the same time.)
  2. The patient is placed in the lithotomy position. The vaginal area is cleansed with an antiseptic solution.
  3. The cervix may be dilated before this procedure.
  4. The hysteroscope is inserted through the vagina and cervix and into the uterus.
  5. A liquid or gas is released through the hysteroscope to expand the uterus for better visualization.
  6. If minor surgery will be performed, small instruments will be inserted through the hysteroscope.
  7. For more detailed or complicated procedures, a laparoscope may be used (p. 545) to concurrently view the outside of the uterus.
  8. After the desired procedure is performed, the hysteroscope is removed.

After

- Tell the patient that it is normal to have slight vaginal bleeding and cramps for a day or two after the procedure.
- Inform the patient that signs of fever, severe abdominal pain, or heavy vaginal discharge or bleeding should be reported to her physician.
- If the patient has any discomfort from the gas inserted during the hysteroscopy or laparoscopy, assure her that this usually lasts less than 24 hours.

Test Results and Clinical Significance

Endometrial cancer, polyps, or hyperplasia *Cancer appears as thickened endometrium in one or multiple portions of the uterus. Hyperplasia looks similar but is not as isolated and seems more diffuse. Polyps appear as pedunculated mucosal tissue protruding from the endometrium.*

Uterine fibroids *Small fibroids are easily seen because they distort the endometrium.*

Asherman's syndrome *Intrauterine adhesions may be associated with previous uterine infections and can be lysed through hysteroscopy.*

Septate uterus *This and other developmental abnormalities can be visualized by hysteroscopy.*

Displaced IUD *The location of a displaced IUD is easily seen.*

Related Tests

- Dilation and curettage (D&C) (p. 653): This is another procedure that allows one to examine scrapings of the endometrium under a microscope. This test has nearly the same indications as hysteroscopy. However, sampling is random, and serious lesions may be missed.

Laparoscopy (Pelvic Endoscopy, Gynecologic Video Laparoscopy, Peritoneoscopy)

Normal Findings

Normal-appearing female reproductive organs

Indications

Laparoscopy is used to directly visualize the abdominal and pelvic organs when a pathologic condition is suspected. It is used to evaluate patients with the following:

Acute abdominal or pelvic pain
Chronic abdominal or pelvic pain
Suspected advanced cancer
Abdominal mass of uncertain cause
Diseases that will improve with laparoscopic surgery (oophorectomy, appendectomy, cholecystectomy, colectomy, hernia repair, hiatal hernia repair, etc.)

Test Explanation

During laparoscopy the abdominal organs can be visualized by inserting a scope through the abdominal wall and into the peritoneum (Figure 4-10). Usually a television camera is applied to the scope, and the scope's view is seen on color monitors. This is particularly helpful in diagnosing abdominal and pelvic adhesions, tumors and cysts affecting any ab-

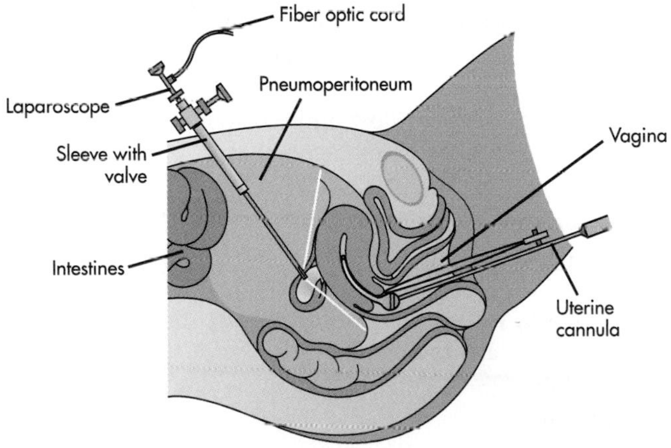

Figure 4-10 Gynecologic laparoscopy.

Table 4-5 Differences between laparotomy and laparoscopy

	Laparotomy	Laparoscopy
Difficulty in technique	Moderate	High
Size of incision	One large	Multiple and small
Expense of equipment in the operating room	Moderate	High
Expense of postoperative care	High	Low
Postoperative mobility	Low	High
Postoperative pain	High	Minimal to moderate
Postoperative hospitalization	4-10 days	1-2 days
Duration of postoperative recovery	Weeks	Days
Return to work	6 weeks	1 week

dominal organ, and tubal and uterine causes of infertility. In addition, endometriosis, ectopic pregnancy, ruptured ovarian cyst, and salpingitis can be detected during an evaluation for pelvic pain. This procedure is also used to stage cancers and determine their resectability. Surgical procedures (e.g., cholecystectomy, appendectomy, hernia repair, tubal ligation, oophorectomy, hiatal hernia repair, bowel resection, and many more) can be performed with the laparoscope. As noted in Table 4-5, laparoscopy affords many advantages to the patient in comparison with an open laparotomy.

Laparoscopy is performed by a surgeon. The patient is under general anesthesia so that no pain or discomfort is experienced during the procedure. Most patients have mild to moderate incisional pain. However, the patient may complain of shoulder or subcostal discomfort from diaphragmatic irritation caused by pneumoperitoneum.

Contraindications

- Patients who have had multiple surgical procedures, because adhesions may have formed between the viscera and the abdominal wall, making safe access to the abdomen impossible
  There are techniques described to allow limited laparoscopy in these situations.
- Patients with suspected intraabdominal hemorrhage, because visualization through the scope will be obscured by the blood

Potential Complications

- Perforation of the bowel, with spilling of intestinal contents into the peritoneum
- Hemorrhage from the trocar site or surgical site

Interfering Factors

- Adhesions may obstruct the field of vision.

CLINICAL PRIORITIES

- During the procedure the peritoneal cavity is filled with 3 to 4 L of CO_2 to separate the abdominal wall from the intraabdominal viscera.
- After the procedure, patients may have shoulder or subcostal discomfort from pneumoperitoneum. This usually lasts only 24 hours.
- After the procedure, patients should be assessed for bleeding (increased pulse rate, decreased blood pressure) and perforated viscus (abdominal tenderness, guarding, decreased bowel sounds).

Procedure and Patient Care

Before

- Explain the procedure to the patient.
- Ensure that an informed consent for this procedure is obtained. Because of the possibility of intraabdominal injury, an open laparotomy may be required. Be sure the patient is aware of that.
- If enemas are ordered to clear the bowel, assist the patient as needed and record the results.
- Because the procedure is usually performed with the patient under general anesthesia, follow the routine general anesthesia precautions.
- Shave and prepare the patient's abdomen as ordered.
- Keep the patient on NPO status after midnight on the day of the test. IV fluids may be given.
- Instruct the patient to void before going to the operating room because a distended bladder can be easily penetrated.

During

- After general anesthesia is induced, a catheter and nasogastric tube are inserted to minimize the risk of penetrating a distended stomach or bladder with the initial needle placement.
- Note the following procedural steps:
  1. Laparoscopy is performed in the operating room. The patient is initially placed in supine position. Other positions may be assumed in order to maximize visibility.
  2. After the abdominal skin is cleansed, a blunt-tipped (Verres) needle is inserted through a small incision in the periumbilical area and into the peritoneal cavity. Alternatively, a slightly larger incision is placed in the skin and the abdominal wall is separated under direct vision. The peritoneal cavity is entered directly. Adhesions can be lysed under direct vision.
  3. The peritoneal cavity is filled with approximately 3 to 4 L of CO_2 to separate the abdominal wall from the intraabdominal viscera, enhancing visualization of pelvic and abdominal structures.
  4. A laparoscope is inserted through a trocar to examine the abdomen (see Figure 4-10). Other trocars can be placed as conduits for other instrumentation.

5. After the desired procedure is completed, the laparoscope is removed and the CO_2 is allowed to escape.
6. The incision(s) is closed with a few skin stitches and covered with an adhesive bandage.

After

- Assess the patient frequently for signs of bleeding (increased pulse rate, decreased blood pressure) and perforated viscus (abdominal tenderness, guarding, decreased bowel sounds). Report any significant findings to the physician.
- If patients have shoulder or subcostal discomfort from pneumoperitoneum, assure them that this usually lasts only 24 hours. Minor analgesics usually relieve this discomfort.
- If a surgical procedure has been performed laparoscopically, provide appropriate specific postsurgical care.

Test Results and Clinical Significance

Abdominal adhesions *Occasionally these can be the source of chronic abdominal pain.*

Ovarian tumor or cyst *These are obvious as masses affecting the ovaries.*

Endometriosis *Endometriosis varies from small white wispy scars on the peritoneal surface to large inflammatory masses distorting normal anatomy.*

Ectopic pregnancy *This usually appears to be a large mass with or without a surrounding inflammation involving just one fallopian tube.*

Pelvic inflammatory disease (salpingitis) *The pelvic structures are red and inflamed.*

Uterine fibroids *Large soft masses are seen on and in the uterus.*

Abscess or infection *This can come from any number of abdominal or pelvic causes, including appendicitis, infection of fallopian tubes, diverticulitis, or acute cholecystitis.*

Cancer *A large primary or metastatic cancer in the abdomen is usually obvious. The extent of tumor spread can be assessed.*

Ascites *Fluid within the abdomen can be aspirated and tested to indicate its source if not apparent at laparoscopy.*

Other abdominal pathologic conditions *Every abdominal abnormality cannot be mentioned here. Suffice it to say that nearly every significant abdominal pathologic process that affects the visceral or parietal peritoneal surface can usually be seen.*

Mediastinoscopy

Normal Findings

No mediastinal tumors or abnormal lymph nodes

Indications

This procedure provides direct visualization of the mediastinum and the lymph nodes contained within. It is used most commonly to determine the cancer stage of a person with known lung cancer. It is also used to evaluate patients with mediastinal masses of uncertain causes.

Test Explanation

Mediastinoscopy is a surgical procedure in which a mediastinoscope (a lighted instrument scope) is inserted through a small incision made at the suprasternal notch. The scope is passed into the superior mediastinum to inspect the mediastinal lymph nodes and to remove biopsy specimens. Because these lymph nodes receive lymphatic drainage from the lungs, assessment of them can provide information on intrathoracic diseases such as carcinoma, granulomatous infections, and sarcoidosis; therefore mediastinoscopy is used in establishing the diagnosis of various intrathoracic diseases. This procedure is also employed to "stage" patients with lung cancer and to assess whether they are candidates for surgery. Evidence of metastasis to the mediastinal lymph nodes is usually a contraindication to thoracotomy because the tumor is considered inoperable. Biopsies of tumors occurring in the mediastinum (e.g., thymoma or lymphoma) can also be performed through the mediastinoscope.

Contraindications

- Patients who have superior vena cava obstruction
  These patient have tremendous venous collateralization in the mediastinum. Mediastinoscopy in this group of patients is fraught with danger from hemorrhage.

Potential Complications

- Puncture of the esophagus, trachea, or great blood vessels
- Pneumothorax

Procedure and Patient Care

Before

- Explain the procedure to the patient.
- Ensure that the physician has obtained an informed consent for this procedure.
- Check whether the patient's blood needs to be typed and crossmatched.
- Provide preoperative care as with any other surgical procedure.
- Keep the patient on NPO status after midnight on the day of the test.
- Administer preprocedural medication approximately 1 hour before the test, as ordered.

During

- Note the following procedural steps:
  1. The patient is taken to the operating room for this surgical procedure.
  2. The patient is placed under general anesthesia.
  3. An incision is made in the suprasternal notch.
  4. The mediastinoscope is passed through this neck incision and into the superior mediastinum.
  5. Biopsies of the lymph nodes are performed.
  6. The scope is withdrawn, and the incision is sutured closed.
- Note that this procedure is performed by a surgeon in approximately 1 hour.
- Inform the patient that he or she will be asleep during the procedure.

Home Care Responsibilities

- Assess for cough or shortness of breath, which may indicate a pneumothorax.
- Note that subcutaneous emphysema may indicate a pneumothorax.
- Assess for mediastinal crepitus on auscultation, which may indicate mediastinal air from a pneumothorax or the bronchus or esophagus.
- Note that distended neck veins and pulsus paradoxus may indicate lack of cardiac filling due to a large mediastinal hematoma.
- Observe for hypotension and tachycardia, which may indicate bleeding from the biopsy site or the great vessels.
- Evaluate for hoarseness, which may indicate injury to the recurrent laryngeal nerve.
- Assess for fever, chills, and sepsis, which may indicate mediastinitis from infection.

After

- Provide postoperative care as with any other surgical procedure.

Test Results and Clinical Significance

Lung cancer–primary into the mediastinum or metastatic to the lymph nodes *It is routine to stage lung cancers with mediastinoscopy prior to thoracotomy.*

Thymoma *These tumors of the anterior superior mediastinum can be easily seen by this technique.*

Tuberculosis or sarcoidosis *Granulomatous inflammations can involve the mediastinal lymph nodes.*

Lymphoma or Hodgkin's disease *Lymphomas routinely involve the mediastinum. In a patient with previously established lymphoma, this procedure is not needed. However, mediastinoscopy may be the least invasive method of diagnosis if lymphoma has not yet been diagnosed.*

Infection (fungal, mycoplasma, etc.) *Coccidioidomycosis, histoplasmosis, and* Pnuemocystis carinii *can be diagnosed by this technique if the mediastinum is involved.*

Related Tests

- Computed tomography of the chest (p. 942): This test can visualize the mediastinal structure but cannot be specific about a disease process.

Sigmoidoscopy (Proctoscopy, Anoscopy)

Normal Findings Normal anus, rectum, and sigmoid colon

Indications

This test allows for direct visualization of the rectum and sigmoid colon. It is used to diagnose suspected pathologic conditions of these organs. It is recommended for patients who have had a change in bowel habits or obvious or occult blood in the stool or who have abdominal pain. It is part of routine screening for colorectal cancer in people over the age of 50.

Test Explanation

Endoscopy of the lower GI tract allows one to visualize and perform biopsies of tumors, polyps, hemorrhoids, or ulcers of the anus, rectum, and sigmoid colon. *Anoscopy* refers to examination of the anus; *proctoscopy* to examination of the anus and rectum; and *sigmoidoscopy* (the most frequent procedure) to examination of the anus, rectum, and sigmoid colon. This test can be performed with a rigid (to 25 cm from the anus) or flexible (to 60 cm from the anus) sigmoidoscope. Because the lower GI tract is difficult to visualize radiographically, direct visualization by sigmoidoscopy is diagnostically helpful.

Furthermore, sigmoidoscopy, like colonoscopy, can be therapeutic. Reduction of sigmoid volvulus, removal of polyps, and obliteration of hemorrhoids can be performed through the sigmoidoscope. The American Cancer Society recommends a sigmoidoscopy every 3 to 5 years after the age of 50. If a neoplastic abnormality (benign or malignant) is found, a total colonoscopy (p. 522) should be performed.

Note that a physician trained in GI endoscopy usually performs this procedure in the GI laboratory, operating room, or outpatient clinic or at the patient's bedside in approximately 15 to 20 minutes. Very little discomfort is associated with the test. A sense of having to defecate during the procedure is uncomfortable. It is caused by the scope within the rectum.

Contraindications

- Patients who are uncooperative
- Patients with diverticulitis
  The insufflation of air needed to distend the rectum and colon for passage of the scope may cause a perforation of the diverticulitis.
- Patients with painful anorectal conditions (e.g., fissures, fistulas, hemorrhoids), because of the anal pain associated with passage of the scope
- Patients with severe bleeding
  Blood clots obstruct the view of the scope.
- Patients suspected of having perforated colon lesions

Potential Complications

- Perforation of the colon
- Bleeding from biopsy sites

Interfering Factors

- Poor bowel preparation may obscure visualization of the bowel mucosa.
- Rectal bleeding may obstruct the lens system and preclude adequate visualization.

Procedure and Patient Care

Before

- Explain the procedure to the patient.
- Obtain informed consent for this procedure.
- Assist the patient with the bowel preparation. In most cases, two Fleet enemas are sufficient for examining the lower sigmoid colon and rectum. An oral cathartic is usually required to examine as far as 60 cm.
- Instruct the patient to ingest only a light breakfast on the morning of the endoscopy.
- Assure patients that they will be properly draped to avoid unnecessary embarrassment.

During

- Note the following procedural steps:
  1. The patient is placed on the endoscopy table or bed in the left lateral decubitus position. Some physicians prefer the knee-chest position; many operating and examining tables are easily converted to make the knee-chest position more comfortable. This procedure also can be performed with the patient in the lithotomy position.
  2. Usually no sedation is required.
  3. The anus is mildly dilated with a well-lubricated finger.
  4. The rigid or flexible sigmoidoscope is placed into the rectum and advanced to its point of maximal penetration.
  5. Air is insufflated during the procedure to distend more fully the lower intestinal tract.
  6. The sigmoid, rectum, and anus are visualized.
  7. Biopsy specimens can be obtained and polypectomy can be performed at the time of sigmoidoscopy.

After

- Inform the patient that because air has been insufflated into the bowel during the procedure, he or she may have flatulence or gas pains. Ambulation may help.
- Observe the patient for signs of abdominal distention, increased tenderness, or rectal bleeding.
- Tell the patient that slight rectal bleeding may occur if biopsy specimens have been taken.

Home Care Responsibilities

- Observe for increasing abdominal pain, which may indicate bowel perforation.
- Note that fever and chills may indicate a bowel perforation.
- Inform the patient that frequent bloody bowel movements may indicate poor hemostasis if biopsy or polypectomy was performed.
- Observe for abdominal bloating and inability to pass flatus, which may indicate colon obstruction if a neoplasm was identified.

Test Results and Clinical Significance

Colorectal cancer *This is seen as a red friable fleshy tumor concentrically involving the mucosa of the bowel.*

Colorectal polyp *This is a tumor that protrudes from only one part of the mucosa of the bowel. Some cancers and most polyps can be removed with the sigmoidoscope. Biopsy specimens can be obtained from neoplasms.*

Ulcerative proctitis *Ulcerative colitis (UC) frequently involves the rectum. That is one characteristic that separates UC from Crohn's disease.*

Pseudomembranous colitis *The rectum is the best location to most easily make the diagnosis of this disease. Usually this inflammation is the result of* Clostridium *overgrowth caused by prolonged use of clindamycin.*

Intestinal ischemia *This usually is apparent by seeing dark mucosa in the sigmoid colon. The sigmoid colon is the portion of colon most vulnerable if ischemia occurs. Ischemia always shows up in the mucosa first.*

Related Tests

- Barium enema (p. 900): This is an x-ray contrast study of the colon and rectum. The rectum, however, is not well evaluated by this study.
- Colonoscopy (p. 522): This is a direct visualization of the entire colon and rectum. It is more extensive and invasive than sigmoidoscopy. The required preparation is more complete.

Sinus Endoscopy

Normal Findings

Normal sinuses

Indications

This procedure is used to evaluate and treat patients with recurrent or resistant sinus infections.

Test Explanation

Patients with recurrent or resistant sinus infections often require surgical drainage. However, with the advent of sinus endoscopy, the sinus cavities can be accessed and drained without surgery. Cultures can be obtained, and antibiotic therapy can be more appropriately provided. The treatment of sinusitis is important to prevent the development of complications, such as mucoceles, cysts, or sinus bone destruction. The most accessible sinuses include the anterior ethmoid, middle turbinate, and middle meatus areas.

This procedure can also be used to visualize suspected neoplasms involving the sinuses. The test is usually performed by a surgeon trained in ear, nose, and throat (ENT) diseases. There is usually little postoperative pain associated with this procedure.

Potential Complications

- Bleeding
- CSF leak (occurs only with ethmoid sinus endoscopy)

Procedure and Patient Care

Before

- Explain the procedure to the patient.
- Ensure that an informed consent for this procedure is obtained.
- If the procedure is to be performed under general anesthesia, keep the patient on NPO status after midnight on the day of the test. IV fluids may be given. This procedure can also be done under local anesthesia, depending on the amount of endoscopic surgery that will be required.

During

- Note the following procedural steps:
  1. Sinus endoscopy is performed in the operating room if general anesthesia is required; otherwise it can be done in the office. The patient is initially placed in the supine position.
  2. After the skin near the nose and mouth is cleansed, the nose is sprayed with a Xylocaine/epinephrine solution to diminish any bleeding.
  3. The sinuses are viewed with an endoscope preformed at various angles to permit optimal viewing.
  4. Sinus contents are examined and aspirated for culture testing.

After

- Place a small 4 × 4 gauze pad under the nose to collect any fluid or blood that may further drain from the nose.
- Assess the patient frequently for signs of bleeding. Report any significant findings to the physician.
- Allow the patient to have oral fluids.

Test Results and Clinical Significance

Chronic or resistant sinusitis *These diseases usually come from inadequate drainage of the sinuses. Endoscopy should hasten cure.*

Sinus tumors *These can be visualized and cells obtained to assist in the diagnosis of these tumors.*

Sinus cysts
Sinus mucoceles
These usually occur after years of chronic sinus infections.

Thoracoscopy

Normal Findings Normal pleura and lung

Indications

This procedure is used to directly visualize the pleura, lung, and mediastinum. Tissue can be obtained for testing. It is also helpful in assisting in the staging and dissection of lung cancers.

Test Explanation

Thoracoscopy is experiencing a renewal as a result of the development of instrumentation for operative laparoscopy. With this technique the parietal pleura, visceral pleura, and mediastinum can be directly visualized. Tumors involving the chest cavity can be staged by direct visualization. A biopsy of any abnormality can be performed. Collections of fluid can be drained and aspirated for testing. Dissection for lung resection can be carried out with the thoracoscope (*video-assisted thoracotomy* [VAT]), thereby minimizing the extent of a thoracotomy incision. VAT is especially helpful for lung biopsy in patients with pulmonary nodules of uncertain cause or for suspected *Pneumocystis* infections in immunocompromised patients.

The patient must be aware of the possibility of requiring an open thoracotomy if the procedure cannot be performed thoracoscopically or if bleeding occurs that cannot be controlled any other way. Any patient who can have an open thoracotomy can have a thoracoscopy.

Contraindications

- Patients with previous lung surgery, because it is difficult to obtain access to the free pleural space

Potential Complications

- Bleeding
- Infection or empyema
- Prolonged pneumothorax

Procedure and Patient Care

Before

- Explain the procedure to the patient.
- Ensure that an informed consent for this procedure is obtained. Because of the possibility of intrathoracic injury, an open thoracotomy may be required. Be sure the patient is aware of that.

- Because the procedure is usually performed with the patient under general anesthesia, follow the routine general anesthesia precautions.
- Shave and prepare the patient's chest as ordered.
- Keep the patient on NPO status after midnight on the day of the test. IV fluids may be given.

During

- Note the following procedural steps:
  1. Thoracoscopy is performed in the operating room. The patient is initially placed in the lateral decubitus position.
  2. After the thorax is cleansed, a blunt-tipped (Verres) needle is inserted through a small incision and the lung is collapsed.
  3. A thoracoscope is inserted through a trocar to examine the chest cavity. Other trocars can be placed as conduits for other instrumentation.
  4. After the desired procedure is completed, the scope and trocars are removed.
  5. Usually a small chest tube is placed to assure full reexpansion of the lung.
  6. The incision(s) is closed with a few skin stitches and covered with an adhesive bandage.

After

- Assess the patient frequently for signs of bleeding (increased pulse rate, decreased blood pressure). Report any significant findings to the physician.
- Provide analgesics to relieve the minor to moderate pain that may be experienced.
- If a surgical procedure has been performed thoracoscopically, provide appropriate specific postsurgical care.
- Note that a chest x-ray examination is performed after the procedure to ensure complete reexpansion of the lung.

Test Results and Clinical Significance

Primary lung cancer
Metastatic cancer to the lung or pleura
Often these tumors can be easily seen and biopsies performed, or the tumors can be removed through or with the help of thoracoscopy.

Empyema *The infected fluid can be drained directly and good specimens obtained for cultures.*
Pleural diseases such as tumor, infection, or inflammation *Biopsies of either the parietal or visceral pleura can be performed during this procedure.*
Pulmonary infection *Thoracoscopy is particularly helpful in obtaining lung tissue for suspected infections such as tuberculosis,* Pneumocystis carinii, *coccidioidomycosis, or histoplasmosis.*

Related Tests

- Laparoscopy (p. 545): This test is to the abdomen as thoracoscopy is to the chest. Most of the instruments are the same.

5

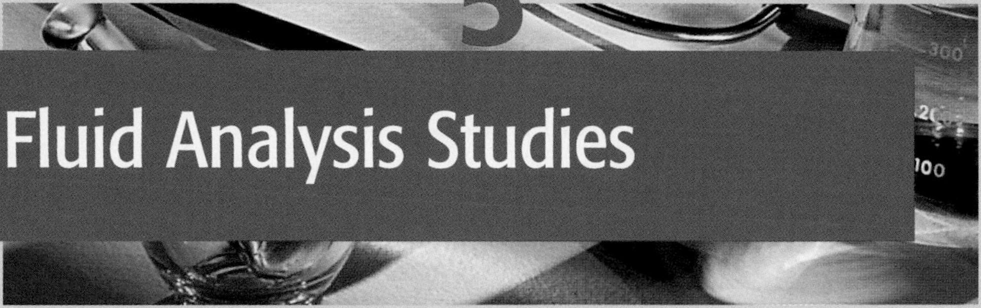

Fluid Analysis Studies

TESTS

Overview

Reasons for Performing Fluid Analysis

Body fluid analysis can provide a significant amount of information concerning diseases that affect a patient. Normal body fluids can provide information concerning the body's hormonal status (cervical mucus test) and fertility (semen analysis, Sims-Huhner test). CSF analysis (obtained by lumbar puncture) can provide significant data concerning diseases involving the CNS (brain and spinal cord). The normal collection of fluid that surrounds a fetus during pregnancy can be aspirated to gain information about the present and future health of the child and mother.

Abnormal accumulations of fluid *(effusions)* can be aspirated from the body in order to gain information about the disease process that caused the fluid to develop. Effusions can occur nearly anywhere in the body. Their presence is abnormal. In this chapter we discuss effusions within the pericardium, pleura, peritoneum, and joints. Effusions are classified as to whether they are considered a transudate or an exudate. The purpose of this classification is to categorize possible diagnoses. In general, exudates are caused by inflammatory, infectious, or neoplastic diseases. Transudates are generally caused by venous engorgement, hypoproteinemia, or fluid overload.

Other body fluids are analyzed to indicate specific disease such as cystic fibrosis (sweat electrolytes or pancreatic enzymes). The secretion of these body fluids is stimulated to obtain enough fluid for analysis.

Most body fluids are not easily obtained. Usually a cavity of the body must be invaded to obtain the fluids for analysis. A needle is used for aspiration of fluid from the subarachnoid space of the CNS (lumbar puncture), uterus (amniocentesis), pericardium (pericardiocentesis), pleura (thoracentesis), peritoneum (paracentesis), or joint (arthrocentesis). This aspiration must be done under complete and assured sterile technique to avoid the introduction of infection to the body cavity. The quantity aspirated can vary from 20 cc to 5 L, depending on the location and original volume of the fluid. Testing of the fluid should be performed immediately to prevent inaccurate results due to cellular or chemical deterioration. If testing cannot be done immediately, guidelines for preservation should be closely followed. Usually the fluid is evaluated for gross appearance, color, odor, red and white cell counts and differential, albumen and protein content, glucose and lactic dehydrogenase (LDH) levels, cytology, fungi, tuberculosis, and bacteria (culture or Gram stain). Other tests may be performed, depending on the specifics of the fluid or the suspected disease.

Not only is the aspiration of fluid helpful diagnostically, but it is often helpful therapeutically. The aspiration of fluid from the pleura often improves ventilation and oxygenation. Aspiration of fluid from the peritoneum often relieves pressure and allows the patient to breathe more easily and eat more comfortably. Joint fluid aspiration may improve joint function. Pericardial fluid aspiration improves diastolic filling and cardiac output. Furthermore, therapeutic drugs (steroids or antibiotics) or diagnostic contrast materials (for x-ray evaluation) can be injected through the aspirating needle.

Although some other body fluids do not require aspiration, care must still be applied to obtaining and transporting the fluid properly (semen analysis, cervical mucus, sweat electrolytes, and pancreatic enzymes). One must be aware that the evaluation of some body fluids may be very important as criminal legal evidence (Sims-Huhner test in rape cases).

Procedural Care for Fluid Analysis

Before

- Explain the procedure to the patient.
- Obtain informed consent for this procedure.
- Tell the patient that no fasting is necessary unless heavy sedation or an operative procedure is used to obtain the fluid.
- Have the patient urinate or empty the bladder before the test to avoid inadvertent puncture of the bladder during paracentesis or hip joint aspiration.
- Obtain the patient's weight.
- Obtain baseline vital signs.

During

- The patient is positioned in a manner designed to make the fluid most accessible to the aspirating needle.
- Aspirating techniques are always performed under sterile techniques.
- When obtaining semen or cervical mucus, penile or vaginal preparation is contraindicated.
- With aspiration techniques a variable amount of fluid is aspirated. Small volumes are aspirated into a syringe. For larger volumes the aspirating needle is attached to a plastic tubing. The other end of the tubing is placed in the collection receptacle (usually a container with a pressurized vacuum).
- If medications are to be administered, a syringe containing the preparation is attached to the needle and the drug is injected.
- To compare fluid levels to blood level and to calculate ratios, blood is simultaneously drawn for glucose, albumin, total protein, LDH, etc.

After

- All tests performed on fluid should be performed immediately to avoid false results due to chemical or cellular deterioration.
- Place a small bandage over the needle site when aspiration is performed.
- Label the specimen with the patient's name, date, source of fluid, and diagnosis.
- Send the specimen promptly to the laboratory.
- Observe the puncture site for bleeding, continued drainage, or signs of infection if aspiration is performed.
- Monitor vital signs for evidence of hemodynamic changes if large volumes of fluid are withdrawn.
- Write any recent antibiotic therapy on the microbiology laboratory requisition slip.
- Place the patient is a position designed to minimize further leakage of fluid from an aspiration site.
- Monitor the patient and educate the patient about signs of potential complications.

Potential Complications of Fluid Analysis Testing

The complications associated with fluid analysis are those of aspirating fluid for analysis. In general, they include the following:

- Injury to an organ by penetration with the aspirating needle
- Bleeding into the fluid space as a result of blood vessel penetration during aspiration
- Reflex bradycardia and hypotension due to the patient's anxiety about the procedure
- Infection of the soft tissue around the needle aspiration site
- Infection of the remaining fluid within the fluid space
- Seeding of the aspirating needle tract with tumor when malignant effusion exists
- Persistent leakage of effusion fluid after withdrawal of the aspirating needle

Other specific complications are discussed with each test.

Reporting Results

In most instances, fluid is obtained by a physician. The laboratory tests are performed by technologists and are usually reported the same day. Cytologic study results are interpreted by a pathologist and are reported after several days. Culture and sensitivity reports also take several days.

Amniocentesis (Amniotic Fluid Analysis)

Normal Findings

Weeks' gestation	Amniotic fluid volume (ml)
15	450
25	750
30-35	1500
Full term	<1500

Amniotic fluid appearance: clear; pale to straw yellow
Lecithin/sphingomyelin (L/S) ratio: ≥2:1
Bilirubin: <0.2 mg/dl
No chromosomal or genetic abnormalities
Phosphatidylglycerol (PG): positive for PG
Lamellar body count: >30,000
Alpha-fetoprotein: 2.0 μg/ml

Indications

Amniocentesis is performed on women to gather information about the fetus. Fetal maturity, fetal distress, and risk of respiratory distress syndrome can be assessed. Genetic and chromosomal abnormalities can be identified. Maternal-fetal Rh incompatibility can be diagnosed. The sex of the child can be ascertained. This is important for a mother carrying a sex-linked gene. Neural tube defects can also be recognized. The test is performed on mothers whose pregnancies are considered to be high risk. These may include diabetic mothers, very obese mothers, aged mothers (over 35 to 40 years) especially if there is a family history of trisomy 21, mothers with repeated spontaneous abortions, mothers whose prior children have genetic defects, and mothers in a couple in which either the mother or the father is a carrier for genetic defects. This test is also done on women who have an abnormal obstetric ultrasound.

Test Explanation

Amniocentesis involves the placement of a needle through the patient's abdominal and uterine walls into the amniotic cavity to withdraw fluid for analysis. Studying amniotic fluid is vitally important in assessing the following:

1. **Fetal maturity status,** especially pulmonary maturity (when early delivery is preferred). Fetal maturity is determined by analysis of the amniotic fluid in the following manner:
   a. *L/S ratio.* The L/S ratio is a measure of fetal lung maturity, which is determined by measuring the phospholipids in amniotic fluid. Lecithin is the major constituent of surfactant, an important substance required for alveolar ventilation. If surfactant is insufficient, the alveoli collapse during expiration. This results in atelectasis and respiratory distress syndrome (RDS), which is a major cause of death in immature babies. In the immature fetal lung, the sphingomyelin concentration in amniotic fluid is higher than the lecithin concentration. At 35 weeks of gestation, the concentration of lecithin rapidly increases, whereas sphingomyelin concentration decreases. An L/S ratio of 2:1 (3:1 in mothers with diabetes) or greater is a highly reliable indication that the fetal lung, and therefore the fetus, is mature. In such a case the infant would be unlikely to develop RDS after birth. As the L/S ratio decreases, the risk of RDS increases.

   b. *Phosphatidylglycerol (PG).* This is a minor component (about 10%) of lung surfactant phospholipids. However, since PG is synthesized almost entirely by mature lung alveolar cells, it is a good indicator of lung maturity. Since PG appears late in gestation, this test indicates a more mature surfactant than that found in the L/S ratio described previously. In healthy pregnant women, PG appears in amniotic fluid after 35 weeks of gestation, and levels gradually increase until term. An advantage of the PG assay is that it is not affected by contamination of amniotic fluid by blood or meconium. These two contaminants cause false-positive and false-negative results for the L/S ratio evaluation. In addition, the presence of PG in the amniotic fluid in the vagina after the membranes are ruptured indicates a low risk for RDS of the newborn. The simultaneous determination of the L/S ratio and the presence of PG is an excellent method of assessing fetal maturity based on pulmonary surfactant.

   c. *Lamellar body count.* This new test to determine fetal maturity is also based on the presence of surfactant. Lamellar bodies are concentrically layered structures produced by type II pneumocytes. On cross section, these small (about 3 μm) structures look like an onion. These lamellar bodies represent the storage form of pulmonary surfactant. Because lamellar bodies and platelets are indistinguishable to cell counters, the lamellar body count is obtained by analyzing the amniotic fluid with a cell counter and recording the platelet count. Lamellar body results are calculated in units of particle density per microliter of amniotic fluid. Some researchers have recommended cutoffs of 30,000/μl and 10,000/μl to predict low and high risk for RDS, respectively. If the count is greater than 30,000/μl, the negative predictive value for RDS is 100% (that is, there is a 100% chance that the infant's lungs are mature enough to not experience RDS). If the lamellar body count is less than 10,000/μl, the probability of RDS is high (67%). Values between 10,000/μl and 30,000/μl represent intermediate risk for RDS. At this time, not enough information is available on lamellar body count in diabetics to advocate its use in this high-risk group. There are several advantages of lamellar body counts. First, they are faster, more precise, and more objective, and they require less amniotic fluid than phospholipid analysis. Second, test results are not invalidated by the presence of blood or meconium. Third, the instrumentation required for this test is readily available, thus allowing it to be performed in all laboratories. (Some laboratories cannot perform phospholipid analysis.)

2. **Sex of the fetus.** Sons of mothers who are known to be carriers of X-linked recessive traits have a 50:50 risk of inheritance. It is important to note that amniocentesis is not done to determine the sex of the child just out of interest.
3. **Genetic and chromosomal aberrations,** such as hemophilia, Down's syndrome, and galactosemia. Genetic and chromosomal studies performed on cells aspirated within the amniotic fluid can indicate the gender of the fetus (important in sex-linked diseases such as hemophilia) or any of the described genetic and chromosomal aberrations (e.g., trisomy 21).
4. **Fetal status affected by Rh isoimmunization.** Mothers with Rh isoimmunization have a series of amniocentesis procedures during the second half of pregnancy to assess the level of bilirubin pigment in the amniotic fluid. The quantity of bilirubin is used to assess the severity of hemolytic anemia in Rh-sensitized pregnancy. The higher the amount of bilirubin, the lower the amount of fetal hemoglobin. Amniocentesis is usually initiated at 24 to 25 weeks. This allows assessment of the severity of the disease and the status of the fetus. Early delivery or blood transfusion may be indicated. It is important to take into consideration the volume of amniotic fluid because bilirubin concentration will be affected by total fluid volume.
5. **Hereditary metabolic disorders,** such as cystic fibrosis.
6. **Anatomic abnormalities,** such as neural tube closure defects (myelomeningocele, anencephaly, spina bifida). Increased levels of alpha-fetoprotein (AFP) in the amniotic fluid may indicate a neural crest abnormality (p. 47). Decreased levels of AFP may be associated with increased risk of trisomy 21.
7. **Fetal distress,** detected by meconium staining of the amniotic fluid. This is caused by relaxation of the anal sphincter. In this case the normally colorless and pale, straw-colored amniotic fluid may be tinged with green. Other color changes may also indicate fetal distress. For example, a yellow discoloration may indicate a blood incompatibility. A yellow-brown opaque appearance may indicate intrauterine death. A red color indicates blood contamination from either the mother or the fetus.

In the past, other tests were performed on the amniotic fluid. Most of these are no longer done. The shake test (also called foam stability or rapid surfactant test) was a crude way of determining fetal maturity by identifying surfactant as an agent that prolongs the stability of an emulsifier. Measurement of creatinine level was another test to determine fetal maturity based on muscle mass of the fetus. Again, this test is too inaccurate to be very useful. Staining fetal cells with Nile blue for identification of fat as a determinant of fetal maturity has also lost favor because of its inaccuracy.

Amniocentesis may be done on the premise that elective abortion should be performed if the fetus is severely defective. Chorionic villus sampling (CVS) may be even better than amniocentesis for karyotyping and genetic analysis. The cells obtained from amniocentesis take several weeks to grow in culture. Cell samples from CVS take less than half that time to grow and test. Furthermore, CVS can be performed earlier in the pregnancy than can amniocentesis. (The earliest one can obtain amniotic fluid for CVS is at about 12 to 14 weeks.) Thus with CVS a decision can be made concerning abortion much earlier in the pregnancy than with amniocentesis.

The timing of the amniocentesis varies according to the clinical circumstances. With advanced maternal age and if chromosomal or genetic aberrations are suspected, the test should be done early enough to allow a safe abortion. (At 14 to 16 weeks of gestation at least 150 ml of fluid exists.) This timing is essential because of the 2 weeks necessary for cell growth to determine the study's results. If information on fetal maturity is sought, performing the study during or after the thirty-fifth week of gestation is best. Placental localization by ultrasonography should be done before amniocentesis to avoid the needle passing into the placenta, possibly interrupting the placenta, and inducing bleeding or abortion.

Contraindications

- Patients with abruptio placentae
- Patients with placenta previa
- Patients with a history of premature labor (before 34 weeks of gestation, unless the patient is receiving antilabor medication)
- Patients with an incompetent cervix

Potential Complications

- Miscarriage
- Fetal injury
- Leak of amniotic fluid
- Infection (amnionitis)
- Abortion
- Premature labor
- Maternal hemorrhage with possible maternal Rh isoimmunization
- Amniotic fluid embolism
- Abruptio placentae
- Inadvertent damage to the bladder or intestines

Interfering Factors

- Fetal blood contamination can cause falsely elevated AFP levels.
- Hemolysis of the specimen can alter results.
- Contamination of the specimen with meconium or blood may result in inaccurate L/S ratios.

CLINICAL PRIORITIES

- Instructions regarding emptying the bladder vary according to gestational age. Before 20 weeks, the bladder should be kept full to support the uterus. After 20 weeks, the bladder must be emptied to minimize the chance of puncture.
- Prior to this procedure the placenta should be localized by ultrasonography to select a site to avoid placental puncture.
- Women who have Rh-negative blood should receive RhoGAM because of the risk of immunization from fetal blood.

Procedure and Patient Care

Before

- Explain the procedure to the patient. Allay any fears and allow the patient to verbalize her concerns.
- Obtain an informed consent from the patient and her spouse.
- Tell the patient that no food or fluid is restricted.
- Evaluate the mother's blood pressure and the fetal heart rate.
- Follow instructions regarding emptying the bladder, which depend on gestational age. Before 20 weeks of gestation, the bladder may be kept full to support the uterus. After 20 weeks, the bladder may be emptied to minimize the chance of puncture.
- Localize the placenta by ultrasound examination before the study to permit selection of a site that will avoid placental puncture.

During

- Place the patient in the supine position.
- Note the following procedural steps:
  1. The skin overlying the chosen site (often determined by obstetric ultrasonography) is prepared and usually anesthetized locally.
  2. A long needle with a stylet is inserted through the midabdominal wall and directed at an angle toward the middle of the uterine cavity (Figure 5-1).
  3. The stylet is then removed and a sterile plastic syringe attached.
  4. After 5 to 10 ml of amniotic fluid is withdrawn, the needle is removed. (This fluid volume is replaced by newly formed amniotic fluid within 3 to 4 hours after the procedure.)
  5. The specimen is placed in a light-resistant container to prevent breakdown of bilirubin.
  6. The site is covered with an adhesive bandage.
  7. If the amniotic fluid is bloody, the physician must determine whether the blood is maternal or fetal in origin. Kleinhauer-Böetke stain will stain fetal cells pink. Meconium in the fluid is usually associated with a compromised fetus.
- Amniotic fluid volume is calculated by injecting a known concentration of solute (such as para-aminohippuric acid [PAH]) into the amniotic fluid to distribute throughout the amniotic fluid. Amniotic fluid is then withdrawn, and the PAH concentration is determined.

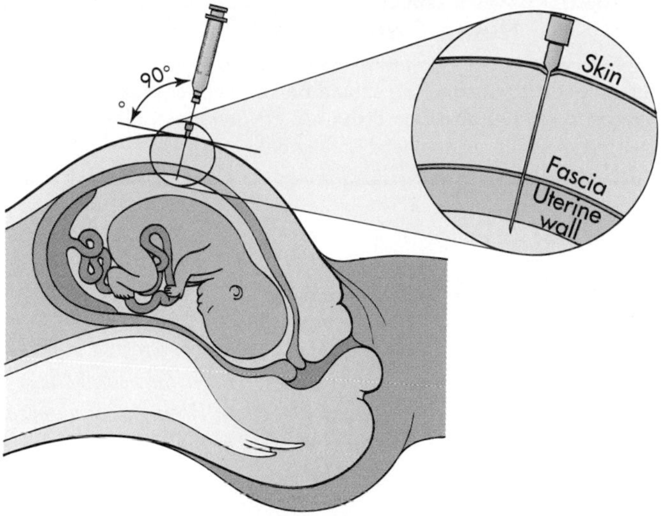

Figure 5-1 Amniocentesis. Ultrasound scanning is usually used to determine the placental site and to locate a pocket of amniotic fluid. The needle is then inserted. Three levels of resistance are felt as the needle penetrates the skin, fascia, and uterine wall. When the needle is placed within the uterine cavity, amniotic fluid is withdrawn.

- Note that this procedure takes approximately 20 to 30 minutes.
- Tell the patient that the discomfort associated with amniocentesis is usually described as a mild uterine cramping that occurs when the needle contacts the uterus. Some women may complain of a "pulling" sensation as the amniotic fluid is withdrawn.
- Remember that many women are extremely anxious during this procedure.

After

- Place amniotic fluid in a sterile, siliconized glass container and transport it to a special chemistry laboratory for analysis. Sometimes the specimen may be sent by air mail to another commercial laboratory for genetic and other testing.
- Inform the patient that the results of this study are usually not available for at least 2 weeks.
- For women who have Rh-negative blood, administer RhoGAM because of the risk of immunization from the fetal blood.
- Assess the fetal heart rate after the test to detect any ill effects related to the procedure. Compare this value with the preprocedural baseline value.
- If the patient felt dizzy or nauseated during the procedure, instruct her to lie on her left side for several minutes before leaving the examining room.
- Observe the puncture site for bleeding or other drainage.
- Instruct the patient to call her physician if she has any fluid loss, bleeding, temperature elevation, abdominal pain or cramping, fetal hyperactivity, or unusual fetal lethargy.

Home Care Responsibilities

- Inform the patient that the puncture site should be checked for bleeding or amniotic fluid loss.
- Instruct the patient to call her physician if she has any fluid loss, bleeding, temperature elevation, abdominal cramping, or unusual fetal movement.

Test Results and Clinical Significance

Hemolytic disease of the newborn *This may be apparent as increased bilirubin in the amniotic fluid. The fetal hemolysis causes free heme to form. This is then catabolized to bilirubin.*
Rh isoimmunization *A rising anti-Rh antibody titer in an Rh-negative woman would indicate potential for erythroblastosis fetalis (Rh-positive fetus). The higher the bilirubin in the amniotic fluid, the greater the risk to the fetus.*

Neural tube closure defects (e.g., myelomeningocele, anencephaly, spina bifida)
Abdominal wall closure defects (e.g., gastroschisis, omphalocele)
Sacrococcygeal teratoma.
An elevated AFP level most commonly indicates neural tube defects. However, other closing defects (e.g., abdominal wall) can occur. Neoplasms associated with neural tube defects may also be associated with increased AFP levels. Blood levels of AFP are also increased with these abnormalities.

Meconium staining *This is evidence of fetal distress and is noted as greenish staining of the amniotic fluid.*
Immature fetal lungs *This may occur with premature labor, maternal hypertension, or placental injuries. The risk of RDS increases as evidence of fetal lung immaturity increases. Fetal lung maturity is diminished in diabetic mothers. This is also noted in hydrops fetalis.*

Hereditary metabolic disorders (e.g., cystic fibrosis, Tay-Sachs disease, galactosemia)
Genetic or chromosomal aberrations (e.g., sickle cell anemia, thalassemia, Down's syndrome)
Sex-linked disorders (e.g., hemophilia)
The genetic defects of many diseases can be recognized through gene recognition and karyotyping. Other genetic defects causing metabolic disorders can be recognized by the results of protein analysis of the amniotic fluid.

Polyhydramnios *This occurs in patients who have diabetes. When polyhydramnios (>2000 ml) is present, the risk of congenital aberrations increases significantly.*
Oligohydramnios *This is recognized as less than 300 ml of amniotic fluid at 25 weeks' gestation. It is associated with fetal renal diseases. Near term, it is associated with early membrane rupture, intrauterine growth retardation, or significant postterm pregnancy.*

Related Tests

- Chorionic villus sampling (CVS) (p. 1006): This is a test whereby the chorionic placental tissue (which has the same genetic material as the fetus) is tested for genetic analysis and karyotyping. This is a rapid and accurate method of determining genetic defects. CVS can be performed earlier in pregnancy than can amniocentesis.

- Alpha-fetoprotein (p. 47): This is a blood test in which elevated levels indicate neural tube defects.
- Fetoscopy (p. 540): This is another method of obtaining fetal tissue for genetic and maturity testing.
- Obstetric ultrasound (p. 792): Significant fetal disease and evidence of fetal distress can be evident on ultrasound examination. If findings are abnormal, amniocentesis is indicated.

Amyloid Beta Protein Precursor, Soluble
(sBPP)

Normal Findings
> 450 U/L

Indications

This test is used to support the clinical diagnosis of Alzheimer's disease and other senile dementias.

Test Explanation

Alzheimer's disease is one of the most important of all degenerative neurologic diseases because of its devastating nature and its frequency of occurrence. It has recently been confirmed that the histologic lesions of the brain known as senile plaques (which contain amyloid) and the amyloid in the meningeal blood vessels of patients with Alzheimer's disease consist of this newly described protein. Recent evidence suggests that it may be this protein that exerts neurotoxic effects. The amyloid peptide (beta or A4 peptide) gene is on chromosome 21. This is the same chromosome on which the familial Alzheimer's disease gene has been localized in some families. In some families with familial Alzheimer's disease, there are mutations in the amyloid precursor protein gene.

This test is used in the diagnosis of Alzheimer's disease. A CSF sample is obtained by lumbar puncture (p. 579). The sBPP is normally found in the CSF of healthy individuals. Low levels may be found in some elderly patients suffering from dementia. Low levels may indicate an alteration in the formation of the amyloid beta protein or its precursors, which is characteristic of Alzheimer's disease.

Procedure and Patient Care

Before

- Explain the procedure to the patient.
- Refer to the instructions for a lumbar puncture and CSF examination (p. 579).

During

- Collect a CSF specimen as indicated in the lumbar puncture discussion.

After

- Follow the postprocedure guidelines for a lumbar puncture.

Test Results and Clinical Significance

Decreased levels

- Alzheimer's disease *The diagnosis of this disease is still clinical. Chemical tests are continually being evaluated in order to assist in the diagnosis of Alzheimer's disease.*

Arthrocentesis with Synovial Fluid Analysis (Synovial Fluid Analysis, Joint Aspiration)

Normal Findings

Synovial fluid: clear and straw colored with few WBCs, no crystals, and a good mucin clot
Chemical test values (e.g., glucose determination): approximating those found in the bloodstream

Indications

Arthrocentesis is performed to establish the diagnosis of joint infection, arthritis, crystal-induced arthritis (gout and pseudogout), synovitis, or neoplasms involving the joint. This procedure is also used to identify the cause of joint inflammation or effusion, to monitor chronic arthritic diseases, and to inject antiinflammatory medications (usually corticosteroids) into a joint space.

Test Explanation

Arthrocentesis is performed by inserting a sterile needle into the joint space of the involved joint in order to obtain synovial fluid for analysis. Synovial fluid is a liquid found in small amounts within the joints. Aspiration (withdrawal of the fluid) may be performed on any major joint, such as the knee, shoulder, hip, elbow, wrist, or ankle.

The fluid sample is examined microscopically and chemically. A culture of the fluid is usually performed. Normal joint fluid is clear, straw colored, and quite viscous due to the hyaluronic acid, which acts as a lubricant. Viscosity is reduced in patients with inflammatory arthritis. Viscosity can be roughly estimated by forcing some synovial fluid from a syringe. Fluid of high viscosity forms a "string" several inches long; fluid of low viscosity drips in a manner similar to water.

The *mucin clot test* correlates with the viscosity. This test is performed by adding acetic acid to joint fluid. The formation of a tight, ropy clot indicates qualitatively good mucin and the presence of adequate molecules of intact hyaluronic acid. The mucin clot is poor in quality and quantity in the presence of an inflammatory joint disease, such as rheumatoid arthritis. By itself, synovial fluid should not spontaneously form a fibrin clot (clot without the addition of acetic acid) because normal joint fluid does not contain fibrinogen. If, however, bleeding into the joint (from trauma or injury) has occurred, the synovial fluid will clot.

The synovial fluid glucose value is usually within 10 ml/dl of the serum glucose value. For proper interpretation the synovial fluid glucose and serum glucose samples should be drawn simultaneously after the patient has fasted for 6 hours. The synovial fluid glucose level falls with increasing severity of inflammation. Although lowest in septic arthritis (the synovial fluid glucose value may be less than 50% of the serum glucose value), a low synovial glucose level also may be seen in patients with rheumatoid arthritis. The synovial fluid is also tested for protein, uric acid, and lactate levels. Increased uric acid levels indicate gout. Increased protein and lactate levels indicate bacterial infection.

Cell counts are also performed on the synovial fluid. Normally the joint fluid contains less than 200 WBCs/mm^3 and 2000 RBCs/ml. An increased WBC count with a high percentage of neutrophils (over 75%) supports the diagnosis of acute bacterial infectious arthritis. Leukocytes can also occur in other conditions, such as acute gouty arthritis and rheumatoid arthritis. The differential white cell count, however, will indicate monocytosis or lymphocytosis with these later-mentioned diseases.

Bacterial and fungal cultures are usually requested and performed when infection is suspected. Gonococci are a cause of joint infection. The administration of antibiotics prior to arthrocentesis may diminish growth of bacteria from synovial fluid cultures and confound results. Smears for acid-fast stains for tubercle bacilli are also performed on the synovial fluid. Synovial fluid is also examined under polarized light for the presence of crystals, which permits differential diagnosis between gout and pseudogout. (The calcium pyrophosphate dihydrate crystals of pseudogout are birefringent [blue on red background] when examined with a polarized light microscope.)

The synovial fluid is also analyzed for complement levels (p. 160). Complement levels are decreased in patients with systemic lupus erythematosus, rheumatoid arthritis, or other immunologic arthritis. These decreased joint complement levels are due to consumption of the complement induced by the antigen-antibody immune complexes within the joint cavity.

One of the most important tests routinely performed on synovial fluid is the microscopic examination for crystals. For example, urate crystals indicate gouty arthritis. Calcium pyrophosphate crystals are found in pseudogout. Cholesterol crystals occur in rheumatoid arthritis.

A physician performs this procedure in an office or at the patient's bedside in approximately 10 minutes. The only discomfort associated with this test is from the injection of the local anesthetic. The joint-space pain may worsen after fluid aspiration, especially in patients with acute arthritis. The administration of steroids is also associated with pain for as much as 2 days after the injection.

Contraindications

- Patients with skin or wound infections in the area of the needle puncture, because of the risk of sepsis

Potential Complications

- Joint infection
- Hemorrhage in the joint area

Procedure and Patient Care

Before

- Explain the procedure to the patient.
- Obtain an informed consent if this is the institution's policy.
- Keep the patient on NPO status after midnight on the day of the test. This is done to prevent alterations of the chemical determinations (e.g., glucose) that may be performed with the study. However, this study may be done more conveniently in a physician's office without the patient fasting.

During

- Have the patient lie on his or her back with the joint fully extended.
- Note the following procedural steps:
  1. The skin is locally anesthetized to minimize pain.
  2. The area is aseptically cleansed, and a needle is inserted through the skin and into the joint space.
  3. Fluid is obtained for analysis. The joint area sometimes may be wrapped with an elastic bandage to compress free fluid within a certain area, thereby ensuring maximal collection of fluid.
  4. If a corticosteroid or other medications (for example, antibiotics) are to be administered, a syringe containing the steroid preparation is attached to the needle and the drug is injected.
  5. The needle is removed, and a pressure dressing may be applied to the site.
  6. Sometimes a peripheral venous blood sample is taken to compare chemical tests on the blood with chemical studies on the synovial fluid.

After

- Assess the joint for any pain, fever, or swelling, which may indicate infection.
- Apply ice to decrease pain and swelling.
- Keep a pressure dressing on the joint to avoid re-collection of joint fluid or development of a hematoma.
- Tell the patient to avoid strenuous use of the joint for the next several days.

Test Results and Clinical Significance

Infection

Septic arthritis

This can be the result of penetrating trauma or blood-borne infection resulting from bacteremia. One would expect to see a red, warm, swollen, and painful joint. The joint fluid would be expected to have a reduced glucose level, increased levels of WBCs, protein, and lactate (due to the lactate produced by the bacteria). Gram stains and cultures (p. 681) would be expected to grow the offending organism.

Degenerative arthritis (osteoarthritis) *Degenerative changes involving the joint space may be due to excess nongouty crystals within the joint space and cartilage. The course is usually chronic and without acute flare-up. Nonsteroidal antiinflammatory drugs are usually helpful.*

Synovitis *This can be inflammatory or infectious. The synovial membrane is the tissue surrounding the joint space.*

Neoplasm *Synovial, cartilaginous, and bony tumors (benign and malignant) can begin in the joint. Protein levels can be expected to be elevated. Microscopy may reveal malignant cells.*
Joint effusion *Joint effusion (fluid in the joint) causes the joint to be swollen. The fluid is obtained to determine the source of the effusion.*

Systemic lupus erythematosus
Rheumatoid arthritis
Autoimmune or collagen vascular diseases can be associated with immunogenic arthritis. One may expect a reduced complement level and increased levels of WBCs, and protein.

Gout
Pseudogout
Crystal-induced arthritis occurs when urate (gout) or calcium pyrophosphate (pseudogout) is deposited into the joint-surrounding structures and joint surface cartilage. Inflammation follows, and arthritis occurs. In time, cartilage destruction occurs.

Related Tests

- Arthroscopy (p. 514): This is an endoscopic procedure designed to directly view the joint space and to provide access to the joint for surgical treatment of disease and injury.
- Arthrography (p. 898): This x-ray test of the joint space provides information about anatomic and disease abnormalities affecting the joint.

Breast Cyst and Nipple Discharge Fluid Analysis

Normal Findings No evidence of atypical or neoplastic cells

Indications

These two tests are used to attempt to make the diagnosis of cancer within breast cysts or to exclude the diagnosis of breast cancer as a cause of persistent nipple discharge.

Test Explanation

Fluid from breast cysts or nipple discharge can be examined cytologically for evidence of cancer cells. These two tests are very much overused in view of the accuracy and information they provide the physician about either a breast cyst or nipple discharge. It is important to recognize that all simple cysts (as recognized by ultrasound, p. 783) are benign. It is very, very unusual even for a complex cyst to be a cancer (cystic adenocarcinoma of the breast). As a result, cyst aspiration for cytologic examination is not useful. The only exceptions to that generality are if the aspirated fluid is bloody or if the cyst does not completely collapse after aspiration. Furthermore, results may even be misleading. It can be difficult to differentiate malignancy from severe inflammatory ductal cells. Often the report indicates atypical or suspicious changes due to deterioration of the normal cells. This report often leads to unnecessary breast biopsies. Cytology of cyst aspiration fluid should be reserved for cysts that repeatedly recur after multiple (more than three) aspirations.

Cytologic examination of nipple discharge is nearly as inaccurate as what has been described for cyst aspiration and for the same reasons. It is extremely rare for a nonbloody nipple discharge to be caused by cancer. Only 10% to 12% of bloody discharges are due to breast cancer. Of that small percentage, less than half have cytologic changes. Therefore, cytologic study of nipple discharge is not very helpful in the diagnosis of breast cancer. As with cyst aspiration, cellular deterioration can be misinterpreted as atypical or suspicious cytologic changes. This, too, may cause an unnecessary breast biopsy.

Potential Complications

- Infection in the breast as a result of the needle aspiration
- Pneumothorax as a result of the needle penetrating a thin chest wall in attempting to aspirate a cyst in the posterior portion of the breast
- Hematoma in the breast as a result of intraglandular bleeding from a blood vessel penetrated by the aspirating needle

Interfering Factors

- The use of hormone replacement therapy can cause either nipple discharge or cystic development within the breast.

Procedure and Patient Care

Before

- Because cyst aspiration may cause intraglandular bleeding that may temporarily distort mammography, a bilateral mammogram may be performed prior to cyst aspiration.
- Inform the patient of the proposed procedure.
- Allay the patient's concern about anticipated pain related to cyst aspiration. Only a very small bore needle is used. If a larger bore needle is required, local anesthesia is used first.

During

Nipple Discharge

- Note the following procedure:
  1. Express the nipple discharge from the breast.
  2. Smear the discharge onto a clean microscope slide as one would for a Pap smear.
  3. The cells are immediately fixed either by immersing the slide in equal parts of 95% alcohol and ether or by using a commercial spray (e.g., Aqua Net hair spray). The secretions must be fixed before drying because drying will distort the cells and make interpretation difficult. Furthermore, this fixing process kills any infectious organisms so that the specimen is less infectious to the personnel who handle the specimen.
  4. The slide is labeled with the patient's name, date of birth, date of test, and site of the lesion.

Cyst Aspiration

- Note the following procedure:
  1. While the patient is in the supine position, the cyst is identified palpably or by ultrasound guidance.
  2. The skin overlying the cyst is prepared in a sterile manner.
  3. If a 25-gauge needle is to be used for aspiration, no local anesthesia is required. If, however, the fluid is suspected to be thick, a 20-gauge needle is used. In this circumstance, local anesthesia is infiltrated into the skin.
  4. The needle is inserted through the skin and into the cyst. Fluid is aspirated until the cyst is completely collapsed.
  5. The fluid is injected into a fixative solution (Carbowax) and appropriately labeled as described above.

After

- Pressure is applied to the aspiration site. An adhesive bandage is applied.
- The patient should be informed that it is not uncommon to develop an ecchymosis in the area of the breast where the aspiration was performed.
- Allay the patient's fears, stating that if clear cyst fluid was obtained, the lesion is most certainly benign.

Test Results and Clinical Significance

Cancer

Benign cyst

As indicated previously, cystic adenocarcinoma of the breast is very rare. When clear fluid is obtained and the cyst collapses completely, the cyst is considered to be benign.

Intraductal papilloma *This is a common cause of breast discharge. Intraductal papillomas are benign, and no treatment is required unless the discharge is copious.*

Related Tests

- Ultrasound of the breast (p. 783): This method of cyst visualization can be used to direct cyst aspiration.
- Stereotaxic mammography (p. 965): This method of cyst visualization can also be used to direct cyst aspiration.

Cervical Mucus (Fern)

Normal Findings

Arborization, or ferning, of cervical mucus during midcycle

Indications

This inexpensive test is used to indicate the timing of ovulation in ovulating women who are being evaluated for infertility. It can also be used to determine ovarian function in women approaching menopause. There are several more accurate tests to determine ovarian function and time of ovulation. This test, however, is cheap and easily performed.

Test Explanation

The cervical mucus can be examined near midcycle and just before menstruation to detect ovulation. Because pregnancy is impossible without ovulation, this study is used in the evaluation of infertility to predict the day of ovulation and to determine whether ovulation occurs.

At ovulation the cervical mucus is clear, abundant, watery, and elastic. This elasticity, or spinnbarkeit (Figure 5-2), increases at ovulation. Excellent spinnbarkeit occurs when the mucus can be stretched at least 5 to 6 cm.

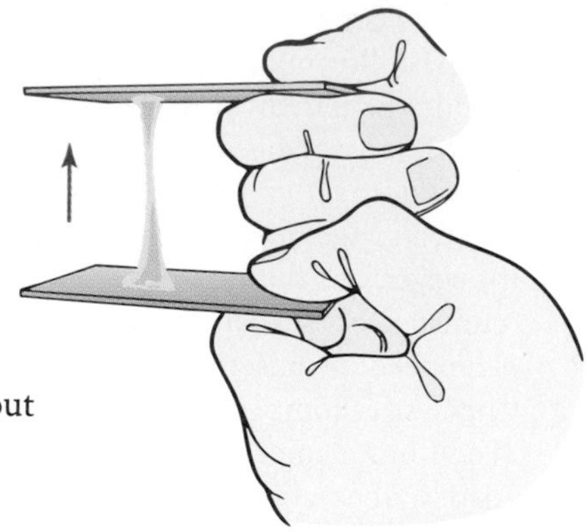

Figure 5-2 Spinnbarkeit (elasticity) of the cervical mucus increases at ovulation.

When the cervical mucus is spread on a clean glass slide and allowed to dry, a pattern of "arborization," or "ferning," occurs. This is caused by the increased levels of salt and water interacting with the glycoproteins in the mucus during ovulation. This pattern is correlated with estrogen activity and is therefore present in all ovulatory women at midcycle. When the cervical mucus is checked again immediately before menstruation, no ferning is found due to progesterone activity. Therefore, during a normal ovulatory cycle, the ferning of cervical mucus will occur at midcycle and no ferning will occur before menstruation.

Besides its absence in anovulatory premenopausal patients, ferning of the cervical mucus is also absent in postmenopausal, castrated, or normally pregnant women. This is due to the presence of fern-inhibiting progesterone.

Interfering Factors

- Slides cleaned with tap water may produce false ferning. The slides used for the mucus must be washed in distilled water.
- Cervical trauma during this procedure may cause blood to mix with the mucus and inhibit ferning.

Procedure and Patient Care

Before

- Explain the procedure to the patient.
- Tell the patient that no fasting or sedation is required.

During

- Note that this procedure is performed at midcycle to detect estrogen-induced ferning and is repeated approximately 7 days later to detect the progesterone inhibition of ferning.

- Note the following procedural steps:
  1. The patient is placed in the lithotomy position.
  2. A nonlubricated speculum is inserted into the vagina to expose the cervix.
  3. A cotton-tipped applicator is gently inserted into the cervical canal and rotated.
  4. The mucus that adheres to the cotton swab is spread on the clean glass slide and allowed to dry at room temperature. No staining is used.
  5. The dried spread of mucus is examined under the low-power lens of a microscope for the presence of ferning.
- Note that this procedure is performed by a physician in approximately 15 minutes.
- Tell the patient that the only discomfort associated with this study is the insertion of the speculum.

After

- Inform the patient that she is usually given the results immediately after the test.

Test Results and Clinical Significance

Infertility *Evaluation of the cervical mucus can indicate lack of ovulation, inadequate corpus luteum function, or inadequate ovarian function. Any one of these abnormalities can lead to infertility. The identification of antispermatozoal antibodies (p. 82) in the cervical mucus can also be performed.*

Pregnancy
Menopause
During menopause or pregnancy, cervical elasticity is reduced and ferning is absent.

Related Tests

- Progesterone assay (p. 351): This test is used in the evaluation and decision making of women who are having difficulty becoming pregnant or maintaining a pregnancy. It is also used to monitor "high-risk" pregnancies.
- Pregnanediol (p. 849): This urine test measures pregnanediol, a metabolite of progesterone. Like progesterone, it is used in the evaluation and decision making of women who are having difficulty becoming or maintaining a pregnancy.
- Estrogen fraction (p. 202): Measurement of estrogens in the blood is used to evaluate sexual maturity, menstrual problems, and fertility problems in females.

Gastric Analysis (Tube Gastric Analysis, Tubeless Gastric Analysis, Diagnex Blue Test)

Normal Findings

Tube gastric analysis
  Basal acid output: 2-5 mEq/hr
  Maximal acid output: 10-20 mEq/hr
Tubeless gastric analysis: detectable dye in urine

Indications

This test is used in the evaluation of patients with unusually aggressive peptic ulcer disease or Zollinger-Ellison syndrome. Its usefulness has declined markedly since the development of newer tests to diagnose these diseases. It is still used for monitoring antipeptic surgical and medical treatment.

Test Explanation

In gastric analysis the contents of the stomach are aspirated to determine the amount of acid produced by the parietal cells within the stomach lining during the resting or basal state (basal acid output [BAO]) and during the stimulated state (maximal acid output [MAO]). This information is useful in the following clinical settings:

1. To differentiate causes of hypergastrinemia. Patients who have high gastrin levels because of antacid ingestion, previous antipeptic surgery, or atrophic gastritis will have reduced values of BAO and MAO. Patients who have high gastrin levels resulting from Zollinger-Ellison (ZE) syndrome or G-cell hyperplasia will have elevated levels of BAO and MAO.
2. To determine whether a gastric ulcer is benign or malignant. Because a benign peptic ulcer requires the presence of acid, ulcerations that occur in the absence of acid (as determined by gastric analysis) are usually malignant. Differentiation between benign and malignant, however, can be better determined by biopsy directed by esophagogastroduodenoscopy (p. 536).
3. To determine the presence of ZE syndrome. In this disease a pancreatic islet cell tumor secretes high levels of gastrin, which constantly and maximally stimulates the stomach to secrete acid. Therefore the stomach is always in the stimulated state and never in the resting state. This causes the value of the BAO to approach that of the MAO. The BAO/MAO ratio would then be greater than 0.6 in ZE syndrome. Because of the development of direct measurement of serum gastrin levels, however, gastric analysis is no longer used for this purpose.
4. To determine the efficacy of medical or surgical antiulcer therapy. To be therapeutic, medical or surgical treatment of peptic ulcer disease must substantially decrease the acid output of the stomach. Baseline values are determined by a pretreatment gastric analysis. The study is repeated during treatment. Effective therapy is indicated by a 50% reduction in the quantity of acid produced. This last indication is probably the only present use for gastric analysis.

Gastric analysis is usually performed by a nurse or physician in approximately 3 hours. It can be performed in a laboratory or at the patient's bedside. Except for the initial gagging usually associated with insertion of the nasogastric (NG) tube, this test is not uncomfortable. (No NG tube insertion is needed for the tubeless test.)

Contraindications

- Patients with carcinoid syndrome

Potential Complications

- Because histamine is the drug most frequently used to stimulate gastric acid, patients with congestive heart failure, carcinoid syndrome, or hypertension may have their conditions exacerbated.

Interfering Factors

- Surgical vagotomy may alter test results.
- Smoking stimulates secretion of the gastric cells.
- Food or fluid alters gastric acid secretion.
- Drugs that may *increase* gastric acid secretion include adrenergic blockers, caffeine, calcium salts, cholinergics, corticosteroids, ethanol, and reserpine.
- Drugs that may *decrease* gastric acid secretion include antacids, anticholinergics, H_2-blocking agents (e.g., Tagamet, Pepcid, Zantac), and tricyclic antidepressants.

CLINICAL PRIORITIES

- Inform the patient that smoking should be avoided before gastric analysis because smoking may stimulate gastric acid secretion and alter test results.
- During this test, carefully observe patients with congestive heart failure, carcinoid syndrome, and hypertension because the histamine injection may exacerbate these conditions.
- After this test, observe the patient for histamine-induced uterine, intestinal, and bronchial spasms.

Procedure and Patient Care

Before

- Explain the procedure to the patient. Most patients are very apprehensive about this study.
- Instruct the patient to be on NPO status after midnight on the day of the test.
- Instruct the patient to abstain from anticholinergic medications, which may inhibit the stimulating action of the histamine.
- Instruct the patient to abstain from smoking, which stimulates gastric acid secretion.

During

- Note the following procedural steps:

Tube Gastric Analysis

1. To assess the gastric acid secretion reliably, an NG tube must be inserted into the dependent portion of the stomach.
2. A syringe is attached to the tube while initial gastric acid is aspirated and discarded.

3. Four subsequent samples are aspirated at 15-minute intervals. These are marked as BAO. The BAO is determined by multiplying the number of milliequivalents in the highest basal sample by 4. Then histamine, 0.04 mg/kg body weight, is administered subcutaneously to the patient. (Occasionally, betazole hydrochloride is administered.)
4. Eight subsequent specimens are taken at 15-minute intervals. These are the MAO specimens. The MAO is determined by multiplying the number of milliequivalents of the highest measurement by 4.

Tubeless Gastric Analysis

1. In this type of test, which uses Diagnex blue (Diagnex blue test), the patient is asked to ingest a gastric stimulant (e.g., a tablet of caffeine).
2. A resin dye, such as Diagnex blue, is then ingested. If the gastric contents contain hydrochloric acid (HCl), the stomach acid displaces the dye from the Diagnex resin.
3. The dye is absorbed by the bowel and excreted in the urine in approximately 2 hours. The urine will be changed to blue. The absence of blue in the urine usually indicates the absence of HCl in the stomach.

After

- Observe the patient for side effects of the histamine injection. They may include uterine, intestinal, or bronchial spasm.
- Observe the patient for capillary dilation, which may be evidenced by increased pulse rate and mildly decreased blood pressure.
- If the tubeless gastric analysis uses Diagnex, inform the patient that the urine may stay blue or blue-green for several days.

Test Results and Clinical Significance

Zollinger-Ellison syndrome *In these patients the BAO nearly equals the MAO because they are already maximally stimulated by the overproduction of gastrin secreted by the pancreatic tumor that exists in them.*

Peptic ulceration *These patients may have elevated BAO levels, but MAO levels will be significantly increased.*

Inadequate therapeutic effect from surgical vagotomy
Inadequate therapeutic antipeptic ulcer medication
Normally BAO and MAO levels of acid should be minimal in these treated patients. Abnormal BAO and MAO indicates inadequate treatment.

Pernicious anemia *These patients have atrophic gastric mucosa and therefore cannot make acid. BAO and MAO levels are reduced.*

Related Tests

- Upper GI series and esophagogastroduodenoscopy (pp. 536 and 999): These are the most commonly used tests to identify peptic ulcers.
- Gastrin (p. 221): This is a much more accurate test to identify and monitor therapy for Zollinger-Ellison syndrome.

Lumbar Puncture and Cerebrospinal Fluid Examination

(LP and CSF Examination, Spinal Tap, Spinal Puncture, Cerebrospinal Fluid Analysis, Cisternal Puncture)

Normal Findings

Pressure: <200 cm H_2O
Color: clear and colorless
Blood: none
Cells:
- RBC: 0
- WBC
  - Total
    - Neonate: 0-30 cells/μl
    - 1-5 years: 0-20 cells/μl
    - 6-18 years: 0-10 cells/μl
    - Adult: 0-5 cells/μl
  - Differential
    - Neutrophils: 0%-6%
    - Lymphocytes: 40%-80%
    - Monocytes: 15%-45%

Culture and sensitivity: no organisms present
Protein: 15-45 mg/dl CSF (up to 70 mg/dl in elderly adults and children)
Protein electrophoresis
- Prealbumin: 2%-7%
- Albumin: 56%-76%
- $Alpha_1$ globulin: 2%-7%
- $Alpha_2$ globulin: 4%-12%
- Beta globulin: 8%-18%
- Gamma globulin: 3%-12%
- Oligoclonal bands: none
- IgG: 0.0-4.5 mg/dl

Glucose: 50-75 mg/dl CSF or 60%-70% of blood glucose level
Chloride: 700-750 mg/dl
Lactic dehydrogenase (LDH): <2.0-7.2 U/ml
Lactic acid: 10-25 mg/dl
Cytology: no malignant cells
Serology for syphilis: negative
Glutamine: 6-15 mg/dl

Indications

This examination may assist in the diagnosis of primary or metastatic brain or spinal cord neoplasm, cerebral hemorrhage, meningitis, encephalitis, degenerative brain disease, autoimmune diseases involving the CNS, neurosyphilis, and demyelinating disorders (e.g., multiple sclerosis, acute demyelinating polyneuropathy).

Test Explanation

By placing a needle in the subarachnoid space of the spinal column (Fig. 5-3), one can measure the pressure of that space and obtain CSF for examination and diagnosis. Lumbar puncture may also be used to inject therapeutic or diagnostic agents and to administer spinal anesthetics.

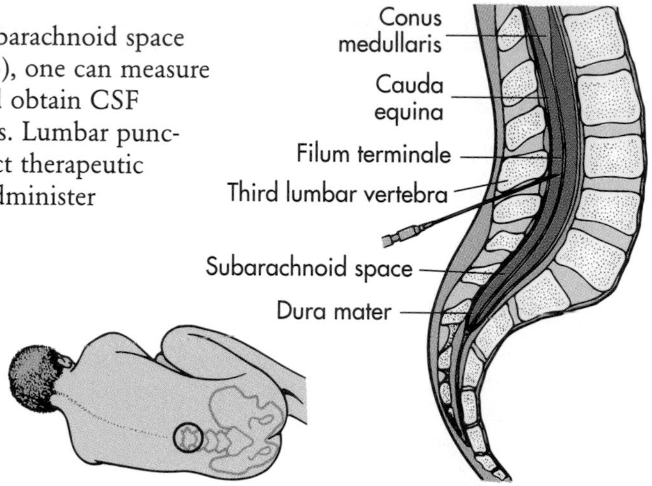

Figure 5-3 Patient position for a lumbar puncture (LP).

CSF is made by selective secretion from the plasma by the choroid plexus (a group of small blood vessels) in the ventricles of the brain. There are three membranes surrounding the brain and spinal cord. From inner to outer, they are the pia mater, arachnoid, and dura mater. The CSF exists within the space between the pia mater and the arachnoid (called the subarachnoid space). This fluid (about 150 to 200 cc) bathes and protects the brain and spinal cord. The fluids acts as a shock absorber when head or back trauma or sudden change in position occurs. The CSF transports nutrients and clears metabolic wastes. Because the CSF is made from plasma, its constituents are about the same as plasma. Chloride levels are higher, however. Blood constituents of larger molecular size cannot be secreted by the choroid plexus (blood-brain barrier).

Examination of the CSF includes evaluation for the presence of blood, bacteria, and malignant cells, as well as quantification of the amount of glucose and protein present. Color is noted, and various other tests, such as a serologic test for syphilis (p. 584), are performed.

Occasionally, lumbar puncture is contraindicated because of nearby infection or suspected spinal canal CSF blockage. In these cases, cisternal puncture (placement of the aspirating needle through the cisterna magna) (Figure 5-4) is performed.

Pressure

By attaching a sterile manometer to the needle used for LP, the pressure within the subarachnoid space can be measured. A pressure of 200 cm H_2O or above is considered abnormal and indicative of increased spinal pressure. Because the subarachnoid space surrounding the brain is freely connected to the subarachnoid space of the spinal cord, any increase in intracranial pressure will be directly reflected as an increase at the lumbar site. Tumors, infection, hydrocephalus, and intracranial bleeding can cause increased intracranial and spinal pressure. If it is suspected that this normal connection is obstructed by tumor or postinfection scarring, a Queckenstedt-Stookey test is performed (see "Procedure and Patient Care") to document that. Intracranial pressure is related to the volume of

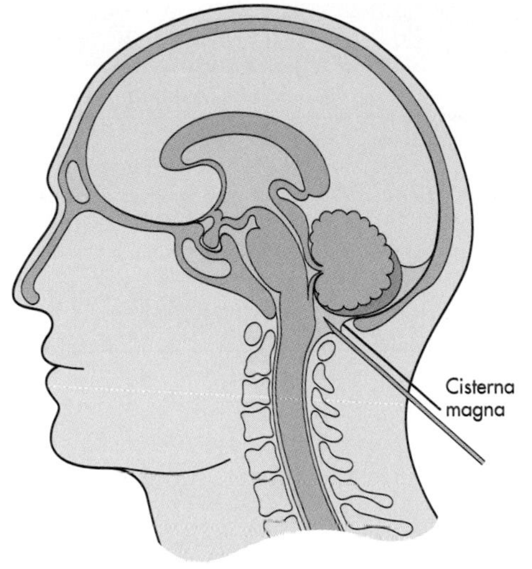

Figure 5-4 Position of the needle when a cisternal puncture is performed.

CSF fluid, which is determined by the homeostatic balance between production and resorption of CSF. Also, because the cranial venous sinuses are connected to the jugular veins, obstruction of those veins or the superior vena cava will increase intracranial pressure.

Decreased pressure is noted in hypovolemia (dehydration or shock). A chronic leakage of CSF through a previous LP site, or through a nasal sinus fracture with a dura tear, is associated with reduced pressures.

Pressures are routinely measured at the beginning and the end of an LP. If there is a significant difference in these values, one must suspect a spinal cord obstruction (tumor). In these instances, a small amount of CSF exists below the tumor. Removal of a large percentage of that fluid will drastically reduce the pressure. Large differences in opening and closing pressures are also seen in patients with hydrocephalus. If high opening pressures are noted, normal volumes of CSF should not be removed to prevent the risk of cerebellar herniation. One must be aware that children who are crying and holding their breath may have transient elevations of pressure that reduce as the child relaxes.

Color

Normal CSF is clear and colorless. Xanthochromia (usually refers to a yellow tinge) is commonly used to indicate an abnormal color of CSF. Color differences can occur with hyperbilirubinemia, hypercarotenemia, melanoma, or elevated protein levels.

A cloudy appearance may indicate an increase in the WBC count or protein level. Normally CSF contains no blood. A red tinge to the CSF indicates the presence of blood. Blood may be present because of bleeding into the subarachnoid space or because the needle used in the LP has inadvertently penetrated a blood vessel on the way into the subarachnoid space. These causes of bleeding must be differentiated because it is important to identify and document a subarachnoid bleed (Table 5-1).

With a "traumatic puncture" the blood within the CSF will clot. No clotting occurs in a patient with subarachnoid hemorrhage. Also, with a traumatic tap the fluid clears toward the end of the procedure when successive CSF samples are obtained. This clearing does not occur with a subarachnoid hemorrhage.

Table 5-1 Differential of causes of blood in the CSF

	Traumatic puncture	Subarachnoid bleeding
CSF pressure	Low	High
Duration of bleeding	Decreases when CSF is withdrawn	No change in color when CSF is withdrawn
Clotting	Present	Absent
Repeat LP	Not bloody	Bloody
Centrifugation	Clear fluid	Xanthochromia

Blood

Blood within the CSF indicates cerebral hemorrhage into the subarachnoid space or a "traumatic tap" as just described above.

Cells

The number of RBCs is merely an indication of the amount of blood present within the CSF. Except for a few lymphocytes, the presence of WBCs in the CSF is abnormal (Table 5-2). The presence of polymorphonuclear leukocytes (neutrophils) is indicative of bacterial meningitis or cerebral abscess. When mononuclear leukocytes are present, viral or tubercular meningitis or encephalitis is suspected. Leukemia or other primary or metastatic malignant tumors may cause elevated WBCs. Pleocytosis is a term used to indicate turbidity of CSF due to an increased number of cells within the fluid.

Culture and sensitivity

The organisms that cause meningitis or brain abscess can be cultured from the CSF. Organisms found also may include atypical bacteria, fungi, or *Mycobacterium tuberculosis.* A Gram stain (p. 681) of the CSF may give the clinician preliminary information about the causative infectious agent. This may allow appropriate antibiotic therapy to be initiated before the 24 to 72 hours necessary to complete the culture and sensitivity report.

The most common causes of meningitis include *Haemophilus influenzae* (in children) and *Neisseria* or *Streptococcus* in adults.

Protein

Normally very little protein is found in CSF because protein is a large molecule that does not cross the blood-brain barrier. The proportion of albumin to globulin is normally higher in CSF than in blood plasma (p. 358) because albumin is smaller than globulin and therefore can pass more easily through the blood-brain barrier. The amount of protein is usually lower in CSF obtained from the cisternal puncture and even lower still with a ventricular puncture, compared with the CSF obtained from an LP. Disease processes, however, can alter the permeability of the blood-brain barrier, allowing protein to leak into the CSF. Examples of diseases that may be associated with a more permeable blood-brain barrier include infectious or inflammatory processes such as meningitis, encephalitis, or myelitis. Furthermore, CNS tumors may produce and secrete protein into the CSF. Obstruction of CSF flow in the spinal canal caused by tumors or a disk is also associated with high protein counts because normal CSF circulation and resorption is impaired by the obstruction.

Table 5-2 Causes of leukocytes in the CSF

Cell type	Infection	Other diseases
Neutrophils	Bacterial meningitis Tubercular meningitis Cerebral abscess	Subarachnoid bleeding Tumor
Lymphocytes or plasma cells	Viral, tubercular, fungal, syphilitic meningitis	Multiple sclerosis Guillain-Barré syndrome
Eosinophils	Parasitic meningitis	Allergic reaction to radiopaque dyes
Macrophages	Tubercular, fungal meningitis	Hemorrhage, brain infarction

CSF protein electrophoresis is very important in the diagnosis of CNS diseases. Patients with multiple sclerosis, neurosyphilis, or other immunogenic degenerative central neurologic disease have elevated immunoglobulins in their CSF. Normally, less than 12% of the total protein consists of gamma globulin. An increase in the CSF level of immunoglobulin G (IgG), an increase in the ratio of IgG to other proteins (e.g., albumin), and the detection of oligoclonal gamma globulin bands are highly suggestive of inflammatory and autoimmune diseases of the CNS, especially multiple sclerosis (MS). Myelin basic protein, a component of myelin (the substance that surrounds normal nerve tissue) is elevated when demyelinating diseases (such as MS or amyotrophic lateral sclerosis) occur. This protein, detected by radioimmunoassay of the CSF, can be used to monitor the course of these deteriorating diseases.

Because albumin and prealbumin are not made in the CNS, increased levels of these specific proteins indicate increased permeability of the blood-brain barrier (as discussed previously).

Glucose

The glucose level is decreased when the bacteria or cells within the CSF increase in number and catabolize the glucose. The cells may be inflammatory cells in response to infection or inflammation or cells that are shed by tumors. A blood sample for glucose (p. 225) is usually drawn before the spinal tap is performed. A CSF glucose level less than 60% of the blood glucose level may indicate meningitis or neoplasm.

Chloride

The chloride concentration in CSF may be decreased in patients with meningeal infections, tubercular meningitis, and conditions of low blood chloride levels. An increase in the chloride level in CSF is not neurologically significant; it correlates with the blood levels of chloride (p. 141). CSF is not routinely evaluated for chloride; this test is done only if specifically requested.

Lactic dehydrogenase

Quantification of LDH (specifically, fractions 4 and 5; p. 278) is helpful in diagnosing bacterial meningitis. The source of LDH is the neutrophils that fight the invading bacteria. When the LDH level is elevated, infection or inflammation is suspected. The elevated WBC count associated with CNS leukemia is also associated with elevated LDH levels.

The nerve tissue in the CNS is also high in LDH (isoenzymes 1 and 2). Therefore, disease directly affecting the brain or spinal cord (e.g., stroke) is associated with elevated LDH levels.

Lactic acid

Elevated levels indicate anaerobic metabolism associated with decreased oxygenation of the brain. The CSF lactic acid level is increased in both bacterial and fungal meningitis but not in viral meningitis. The lactic acid level is also increased when the CSF glucose level is very low or the CSF WBC count is elevated. Because lactic acid does not readily pass through the blood-brain barrier, elevated blood lactate levels are not reflected in the CSF. Chronic cerebral hypoxemia or cerebral ischemia (hypoxic encephalopathy) is associated with elevated CSF lactic acid levels.

Cytology

Examination of cells found in the CSF can determine if they are malignant. Tumors in the CNS may shed cells from their surface. These cells can float freely in CSF. Their presence suggests neoplasm as the cause of any neurologic symptoms.

Tumor markers

Increased levels of tumor markers such as carcinoembryonic antigen, alpha-fetoprotein, or human chorionic gonadotropin may indicate metastatic tumor.

Serology for syphilis

Latent syphilis is diagnosed by performing one of many available serologic tests on CSF. These include (1) the Wassermann test, (2) the Venereal Disease Research Laboratory test (p. 403), and (3) the fluorescent treponemal antibody (FTA) test (p. 403). The FTA test is considered to be the most sensitive and specific. When test results are positive, the diagnosis of neurosyphilis is made and appropriate antibiotic therapy is initiated.

Glutamine

The CSF can be evaluated for the presence of glutamine. Elevated glutamine levels are helpful in the detection and evaluation of hepatic encephalopathy and hepatic coma. The glutamine is made by increased levels of ammonia, which are commonly associated with liver failure. (See discussion of serum ammonia on p. 49.) Levels of glutamine are also often increased in patients with Reye's syndrome.

LP is performed by a physician in approximately 20 minutes. This procedure is described as uncomfortable or painful by most patients. Some patients complain of feeling pressure from the needle. Some patients complain of a shooting pain in their legs.

Contraindications

- Patients with increased intracranial pressure
  The LP may induce cerebral or cerebellar herniation through the foramen magnum.
- Patients who have severe degenerative vertebral joint disease
  It is very difficult to pass the needle through the degenerated arthritic interspinal space.
- Patients with infection near the LP site
  Meningitis can result from contamination of CSF with infected material.

Potential Complications

- Persistent CSF leak, causing severe headache
- Introduction of bacteria into CSF, causing suppurative meningitis
- Herniation of the brain through the tentorium cerebelli or herniation of the cerebellum through the foramen magnum
  In patients with increased intracranial pressure, the quick reduction of pressure in the spinal column by release through the LP may induce herniation of the brain. This can cause compression of the brainstem, which may result in deterioration of the patient's neurologic status and death.
- Inadvertent puncture of the spinal cord, caused by inappropriately high puncture of the spinal cord
- Puncture of the aorta or vena cava, causing serious retroperitoneal hemorrhage
- Transient back pain and pain or paresthesia in the legs

CLINICAL PRIORITIES

- LP is contraindicated in patients with increased intracranial pressure because the LP may induce cerebral or cerebellar herniation.
- A basic neurologic assessment should be done prior to this test to especially evaluate the patient's legs for strength, sensation, and movement.
- If a blockage in CSF circulation is suspected in the subarachnoid space, a Queckenstedt-Stookey test may be performed.

Procedure and Patient Care

Before

- Explain the procedure to the patient. Many patients have misconceptions regarding LP. Allay the patient's fears and allow time to verbalize concerns.
- Obtain informed consent if required by the institution.
- Perform a baseline neurologic assessment of the legs by assessing the patient's strengths, sensation, and movement.
- Tell the patient that no fasting or sedation is required.
- Instruct the patient to empty the bladder and bowels before the procedure.
- Explain to the patient that he or she must lie very still throughout this procedure. Movement may cause traumatic injury. Encourage the patient to relax and take deep, slow breaths with the mouth open.

During

- Note the following procedural steps:
  1. This study is a sterile procedure that can be easily performed at the bedside. The patient is usually placed in the lateral decubitus (fetal) position (Figure 5-3, p. 580).
  2. The patient is instructed to clasp the hands on the knees to maintain this position. Someone usually helps the patient maintain this position. (A sitting position also may be used.)

3. A local anesthetic is injected into the skin and subcutaneous tissues after the site has been aseptically cleaned.
4. A spinal needle containing an inner obturator is placed through the skin and into the spinal canal.
5. The subarachnoid space is entered.
6. The insert (obturator) is removed, and CSF can be seen slowly dripping from the needle.
7. The needle is attached to a sterile manometer, and the pressure (opening pressure) is recorded.
8. Before the pressure reading is taken, the patient is asked to relax and straighten the legs to reduce the intraabdominal pressure, which causes an increase in CSF pressure.
9. Three sterile test tubes are filled with 5 to 10 ml of CSF. Usually the first tube is sent for chemical and immunologic testing because these results are not affected by any blood if a "traumatic tap" occurs. The second may be sent for culture, and the third is used for microscopic examination.
10. The pressure (closing pressure) is measured.

- Note that if blockage in CSF circulation in the spinal subarachnoid space is suspected, a *Queckenstedt-Stookey test* may be performed. For this test the jugular vein is occluded either manually by digital pressure or by a medium-sized blood pressure cuff inflated to approximately 20 mm Hg. Within 10 seconds after jugular occlusion, CSF pressure should increase 15 to 40 cm H_2O and then promptly return to normal within 10 seconds after release of the pressure. A sluggish rise or fall of CSF pressure suggests partial blockage of CSF circulation. No rise after 10 seconds suggests a complete obstruction within the spinal canal.

After

- Apply digital pressure and an adhesive dressing to the puncture site.
- Place the patient in the prone position with a pillow under the abdomen to increase the intraabdominal pressure, which will indirectly increase the pressure in the tissues surrounding the spinal cord. This retards continued CSF flow from the spinal canal.
- All testing of the CSF is ordered stat in order to diminish the false results that may occur because of cellular deterioration, etc.
- Encourage the patient to drink increased amounts of fluid with a straw to replace the CSF removed during the lumbar puncture. Drinking with a straw will enable the patient to keep the head flat.
- Usually keep the patient in a reclining position for up to 12 hours to avoid the discomfort of potential postpuncture spinal headache. Allow the patient to turn from side to side as long as the head is not raised.
- Label and number the specimen jars appropriately and deliver them to the laboratory immediately after the test. Refrigeration will alter test results. A delay between collection time and testing can invalidate results, especially cell counts.
- Assess the patient for numbness, tingling, and decreased movement of the extremities; pain at the injection site; drainage of blood or CSF at the injection site; and the ability to void. Notify the physician of any unusual findings.

Home Care Responsibilities

- The patient should be kept flat in bed for up to 12 hours to avoid a postprocedure spinal headache.
- Encourage the patient to drink increased amounts of fluid to replace CSF removed during the LP.
- Instruct the patient to report any abnormalities, such as numbness and tingling in the legs, to the physician.

Test Results and Clinical Significance

Brain neoplasm
Spinal cord neoplasm
Metastatic tumor
The CNS can be expected to be turbid, to contain malignant cells, and to have elevated protein and LDH levels.

Degenerative brain disease
Autoimmune disorder
Multiple sclerosis and other demyelinating diseases
The CSF of these patients may be turbid; it may contain increased protein levels (including myelin basic protein) and oligoclonal bands of proteins; and it may be associated with elevated LDH levels.

Neurosyphilis *Not only do these patients have elevated protein levels, increased turbidity, and increased LDH levels in their CSF, but immunologic testing is also positive.*

Subarachnoid bleeding
Cerebral hemorrhage
Traumatic lumbar puncture
The CSF in these patients has high protein levels, turbid color with xanthochromia, and RBCs.

Encephalitis
Myelitis
Hepatic encephalopathy or coma
Elevated glutamine levels are noted in these patients.

Meningitis
Encephalitis
Cerebral abscess
Elevated WBCs and proteins support the culture findings of infection.

Related Tests

- Glucose (p. 225): This test is concomitantly performed with the LP in order to assess the CSF glucose level.
- Serum protein (p. 358): Along with the LP, measurement of serum protein levels is helpful in the calculation of many formulas involved in the evaluation of CSF.

Paracentesis
(Peritoneal Fluid Analysis, Abdominal Paracentesis, Ascitic Fluid Cytology, Peritoneal Tap)

Normal Findings

Gross appearance: clear, serous, light yellow, 50 ml
RBCs: none
WBCs: <300/ml
Protein: <4.1 g/dl
Glucose: 70-100 mg/dl
Amylase: 138-404 U/L
Ammonia: <50 mg/dl
Alkaline phosphatase
  Adult male: 90-240 U/L
  Female <45 years: 76-196 U/L
  Female >45 years: 87-250 U/L
Lactic dehydrogenase (LDH): similar to serum LDH
Cytology: no malignant cells
Bacteria: none
Fungi: none
Carcinoembryonic antigen (CEA): <5.0 ng/mL

Indications

Paracentesis is performed on patients who have unexplained ascites in order to determine the cause. It is an important part of evaluating the patient with multiple trauma to rule out abdominal trauma. Paracentesis is also performed to relieve the intraabdominal pressure that accumulates with large-volume ascites.

Test Explanation

Paracentesis is an invasive procedure entailing the insertion of a needle into the peritoneal cavity (Figure 5-5) for removal of ascitic fluid. The peritoneum is defined as the space between the visceral peritoneum (thin membrane covering all the abdominal organs) and the parietal peritoneum (thin membrane covering the inside of the abdominal wall). Within the peritoneal membrane is an intricate network of capillary and lymphatic vessels. Fluid is constantly being secreted by the peritoneal membranes

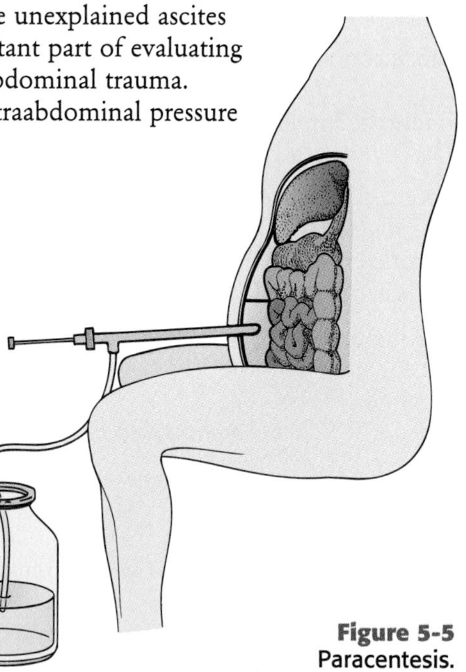

Figure 5-5
Paracentesis.

Table 5-3 Differentiation between transudate and exudate

	Transudate	Exudate
Total protein fluid/serum ratio	<0.5	>0.5
Total protein level	<3 g/dl	>3 g/dl
LDH fluid/serum ratio	<0.6	>0.6
Albumin gradient	>1.1	<1.1
Serum − Fluid = Albumin gradient		
Specific gravity	<1.015	>1.015
Clotting	None	Present
WBCs	<300/μl	>500/μl
Differential	Mononuclear	Neutrophils
Glucose	Equal to serum	<60 mg/dl
Serum − Fluid = Glucose difference	<30 mg/dl	>30 mg/dl
Appearance	Clear, thin fluid	Cloudy, viscous
Etiology	Cirrhosis, nephrosis, heart failure, low protein	Infection, inflammation, malignancy, collagen vascular diseases

and constantly being reabsorbed by those same membranes. If secretion is increased or reabsorption blocked, peritoneal fluid (ascites) will develop.

Peritoneal fluid is removed for diagnostic and therapeutic purposes. Diagnostically paracentesis is performed to obtain and analyze fluid to determine the cause of the peritoneal effusion. Peritoneal fluid is classified as transudate or exudate (Table 5-3). This is an important differentiation and is very helpful in determining the cause of the effusion. Transudates are most frequently caused by congestive heart failure, cirrhosis, nephrotic syndrome, myxedema, peritoneal dialysis, hypoproteinemia, and acute glomerulonephritis. Exudates are most often found in infectious or neoplastic conditions. However, collagen vascular disease, pulmonary infarction, gastrointestinal diseases, trauma, and drug hypersensitivity also may cause an exudative effusion.

Therapeutically this procedure is done to remove large amounts of ascitic fluid from the abdominal cavity. These patients usually experience transient relief of symptoms (shortness of breath, distention, and early satiety) due to the fluid within the abdominal cavity.

The peritoneal fluid is usually evaluated for gross appearance, RBCs, WBCs, protein, glucose, amylase, ammonia, alkaline phosphatase, LDH, cytology, bacteria, fungi, and other tests such as CEA levels. Each is discussed separately. Urea and creatinine may be measured if there is a question that the fluid may represent urine from a perforated bladder.

Gross appearance

Transudative peritoneal fluid may be clear, serous, and light yellow, especially in patients with hepatic cirrhosis. Milk-colored peritoneal fluid may result from the escape of chyle from blocked abdominal or thoracic lymphatic ducts. Conditions that may cause lymphatic blockage include lymphoma, carcinoma, and tuberculosis involving the abdominal or thoracic lymph nodes. The triglyceride value in a chylous effusion exceeds 110 mg/dl.

Cloudy or turbid fluid may result from inflammatory or infectious conditions such as peritonitis, pancreatitis, and appendicitis. Bloody fluid may be the result of a traumatic tap (the aspirating needle penetrates a blood vessel), intraabdominal bleeding, tumor, or hemorrhagic pancreatitis. Bile-stained, green fluid may result from a ruptured gallbladder, acute pancreatitis, or perforated intestines.

Cell counts

Normally no RBCs should be present. The presence of RBCs may indicate neoplasms, tuberculosis, or intraabdominal bleeding. Increased WBC counts may be seen with peritonitis, cirrhosis, and tuberculosis. Usually these counts are performed manually using a simple hemacytometer.

Protein count

Total protein levels greater than 3 g/dl are characteristic of exudates, whereas transudates usually have a protein content of less than 3 g/dl. It is now thought that the albumin gradient between serum and ascitic fluid can differentiate better between the transudate and exudate nature of ascites than can the total protein content. This gradient is obtained by subtracting the ascitic albumin value from the serum albumin value. Values of 1.1 g/dl or more suggest a transudate, which is usually caused by portal hypertension due to cirrhosis. Values less than 1.1 g/dl suggest an exudate but will not differentiate the potential cause of the exudate (malignancy from infection or inflammation).

Because there is significant overlap in protein values differentiating transudate from exudate, the total protein ratio (fluid/serum) has been considered to be a more accurate criterion. A total protein ratio of fluid to serum of greater than 0.5 is considered to indicate an exudate.

Glucose

Usually peritoneal glucose levels approximate serum glucose levels. Decreased levels may indicate tuberculous or bacterial peritonitis or peritoneal carcinomatosis.

Amylase

Increased amylase levels may be seen in patients with pancreatic trauma, pancreatic pseudocyst, acute pancreatitis, and intestinal necrosis, perforation, or strangulation. In these diseases, the amylase level is usually less than 1.5 times higher than serum levels.

Ammonia

High ammonia levels occur in ruptured or strangulated intestines and also with a ruptured appendix or ulcer.

Alkaline phosphatase

Levels of alkaline phosphatase are greatly increased in infarcted or strangulated intestines.

Lactic dehydrogenase

A peritoneal fluid/serum LDH ratio of greater than 0.6 is typical of an exudate. An exudate is identified with a higher degree of accuracy if the peritoneal fluid/serum protein ratio is greater than 0.5 and the peritoneal fluid/serum LDH ratio is greater than 0.6.

Cytology

A cytologic study is performed to detect tumors. The tumors most often seen are ovarian, pancreatic, colon, and gastric. The interpretation of cytologic changes requires that the pathologist have considerable experience in cytology. It can be difficult to differentiate malignancy from severely inflammatory mesothelial cells. In general, malignant cells tend to clump together and to have a high nucleus/cytoplasm ratio, prominent and multiple nucleoli, and unevenly distributed chromatin.

Cytologic examination of the fluid is improved by spinning down a large volume of fluid and examining the sediment. A large number of cells can be seen and compared with each other.

Bacteria

Usually the fluid is cultured and the antibiotic sensitivities are determined. Gram stains (p. 681) are often performed.

Gram stain and bacteriologic culture

The presence of bacteria may indicate a ruptured intestine, primary peritonitis, or infections such as appendicitis, pancreatitis, or tuberculosis. Culture and Gram stains identify the organisms involved in the infection and also provide information concerning antibiotic sensitivity. (See p. 681 for a more thorough discussion of Gram stain, cultures, and sensitivity.) These tests are routinely performed in order to diagnose bacterial peritonitis. If possible, these tests should be done before initiation of antibiotic therapy.

Fungi

Fungi may indicate histoplasmosis, candidiasis, or coccidioidomycosis.

Carcinoembryonic antigen

Elevated peritoneal fluid levels for CEA are associated with abdominal malignancy, usually arising from the GI tract.

Paracentesis is performed by a physician at the patient's bedside, in a procedure room, or in the physician's office in less than 30 minutes. Usually the volume removed is limited to about 4 L at any one time to avoid hypovolemia if the ascites is rapidly reaccumulated. Although local anesthetics eliminate pain at the insertion site, the patient may feel a pressurelike pain as the needle is inserted.

Contraindications

- Patients with coagulation abnormalities or bleeding tendencies
- Patients with only a small amount of fluid and extensive previous abdominal surgery

Potential Complications

- Hypovolemia if a large volume of peritoneal fluid was removed and the fluid reaccumulates, the fluid coming from the intravascular volume
- Hepatic coma in a patient with chronic liver disease
- Peritonitis
- Seeding of the needle tract with tumor when malignant ascites exists

CLINICAL PRIORITIES

- The classification of peritoneal fluid as either a transudate or an exudate helps differentiate the cause of the effusion.
- Usually the volume of peritoneal fluid removed is limited to 4 L to avoid hypovolemia if the ascites rapidly reaccumulate.
- The patient should empty the bladder before this test to avoid inadvertent puncture by the aspirating needle during the procedure.
- After this test, the patient should be carefully monitored for hemodynamic changes, especially hypotension, if a large volume of fluid was removed.

Procedure and Patient Care

Before

- Explain the procedure to the patient.
- Obtain informed consent for this procedure.
- Tell the patient that no fasting or sedation is necessary.
- Have the patient urinate or empty the bladder before the test in order to avoid inadvertent puncture of the bladder with the aspirating needle.
- Measure abdominal girth.
- Obtain the patient's weight.
- Obtain baseline vital signs.

During

- Note the following procedural steps:
  1. Position the person in a high Fowler's position in bed or in a chair with the back supported and the feet on a stool.
  2. Paracentesis is performed under strict sterile technique. A paracentesis tray usually contains all necessary supplies.
  3. The needle insertion site is aseptically cleansed and anesthetized locally.
  4. A scalpel may be used to make a stab wound into the peritoneal cavity approximately 1 to 2 inches below the umbilicus.
  5. A trocar, cannula, or needle is threaded through the incision.
  6. A plastic tubing is attached to the cannula. The other end of the tubing is placed in the collection receptacle (usually a container with a pressurized vacuum).

After

- All tests performed on peritoneal fluid should be performed immediately to avoid false results due to chemical or cellular deterioration.
- Place a small bandage over the needle site.
- Label the specimen with the patient's name, date, source of fluid, and diagnosis.
- Send the specimen promptly to the laboratory.
- Observe the puncture site for bleeding, continued drainage, or signs of inflammation.
- Measure the abdominal girth and weight of the patient; compare with baseline values.

- Monitor vital signs for evidence of hemodynamic changes. Watch for signs of hypotension if a large volume of fluid was removed.
- Write any recent antibiotic therapy on the laboratory requisition slip.
- Because of the high protein content of ascitic fluid, albumin infusions may be ordered after paracentesis to compensate for protein loss. Monitor serum protein and electrolyte (especially sodium) levels.
- Occasionally ascitic fluid continues to leak out of the needle tract after removal of the needle. A suture can stop that. If unsuccessful, a collection bag should be applied to the skin to allow for measurement of the volume of fluid loss.

Test Results and Clinical Significance

Exudate

Lymphoma *These tumors can involve the lymph nodes of the chest and abdomen. Reabsorption of fluid cannot occur, and an chylous effusion develops.*

Carcinoma *When cancer involves the peritoneal membranes, reabsorption of fluid is diminished. Furthermore, the tumors (especially ovarian) can secrete large volumes of fluid. Ascites develops.*

Tuberculosis
Peritonitis
Pancreatitis
Ruptured viscus
Infections tend to increase peritoneal capillary permeability, and fluid is secreted into the abdominal cavity.

Transudate

Hepatic cirrhosis
Portal hypertension
The capillary vessels experience an increased portal venous drainage pressure. Reabsorption is diminished and fluid accumulates.

Nephrotic syndrome
Hypoproteinemia
The nephrotic syndrome is characterized by renal albumin wasting. This and other forms of hypoproteinemia are associated with decreased intravascular oncotic pressure. The fluid tends to leak out of the intravascular space into the peritoneum.

Congestive heart failure *The venous drainage of peritoneum is diminished by the right heart failure that exists and causes increased venous pressures. Peritoneal fluid accumulates.*

Abdominal trauma
Peritoneal bleeding
Intraabdominal bleeding or ruptured viscus can be determined by identifying a bloody effusion (hemoperitoneum) or by aspirating bowel contents from the free abdominal cavity.

Related Tests

- Glucose, lactic dehydrogenase, protein, and amylase (pp. 225, 278, 357, and 51). These blood tests are performed concomitantly to assist in the evaluation of the peritoneal fluid.

Pericardiocentesis

Normal Findings

Minimal amount of clear, straw-colored fluid without evidence of any bacteria, blood, or malignant cells

Indications

Pericardiocentesis is performed to determine the cause of an unexplained pericardial effusion. It is also performed to relieve the intrapericardial pressure that accumulates with a large volume of fluid and inhibits diastolic filling.

Test Explanation

Pericardiocentesis, which involves the aspiration of fluid from the pericardial sac with a needle, may be performed for therapeutic and diagnostic purposes. Therapeutically the test is performed to relieve cardiac tamponade by removing blood or fluid to improve diastolic filling. Diagnostically pericardiocentesis is performed to remove a sample of pericardial fluid for laboratory examination to determine the cause of the fluid accumulation. This is similar to the evaluation described for pleural fluid on p. 606.

A physician usually performs this procedure in the cardiac catheterization laboratory, operating room, or emergency room in approximately 10 to 20 minutes. This procedure is associated with very little discomfort. Most patients feel pressure when the needle is inserted into the pericardial sac.

Contraindications

- Patients who are uncooperative, because of the risk of lacerations to the epicardium or coronary artery
- Patients with a bleeding disorder
  Inadvertent puncture of the myocardium may create uncontrollable bleeding into the pericardial sac, leading to tamponade.

✓ CLINICAL PRIORITIES

- Therapeutically this test can be performed to relieve cardiac tamponade by removing blood or fluid to improve diastolic filling. Diagnostically it is performed to determine the cause of a fluid accumulation.
- Atropine may be given before the procedure to prevent the vasovagal reflex of bradycardia and hypotension.
- After this test the vital signs are carefully monitored. Pericardial bleeding may be indicated by hypotension and pulsus paradoxus. Temperature elevations may indicate infection.

Potential Complications

- Laceration of the coronary artery or myocardium
- Needle-induced ventricular arrhythmias (dysrhythmias)
- Myocardial infarction
- Pneumothorax caused by inadvertent puncture of the lung
- Liver laceration caused by inadvertent puncture of that organ
- Pleural or pericardial infection caused by the aspirating needle
- Vasovagal hypotension or arrest

Procedure and Patient Care

Before

- Explain the procedure to the patient.
- Obtain informed consent for this procedure.
- Restrict fluid and food intake for at least 4 to 6 hours (if this is an elective procedure).
- Obtain IV access for infusion of fluids and cardiac medications if required.
- Administer pretest medication. Atropine is frequently given to prevent the vasovagal reflex of bradycardia and hypotension.

During

- Note the following procedural steps:
  1. The patient is placed in the supine position.
  2. An area in the fifth to sixth intercostal space at the left sternal margin (or subxyphoid) is prepared and draped. Alternatively the subxyphoid space is used for access to the pericardium.
  3. After skin anesthesia is performed, a large-bore, pericardiocentesis needle is placed on a 50-ml syringe and introduced into the pericardial sac (Figure 5-6).

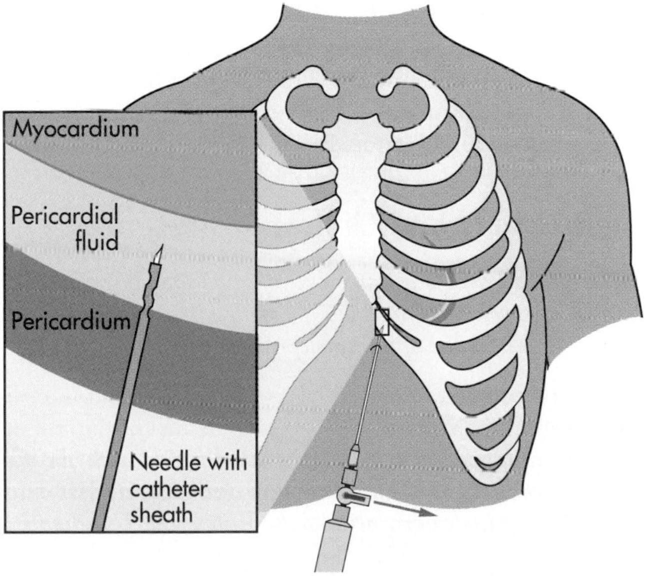

Figure 5-6 Pericardiocentesis procedure and aspiration of pericardial fluid. For recurrent cardiac tamponade and large pericardial effusion, the indwelling catheter may remain.

4. An electrocardiographic lead is often attached by a clip to the needle to identify any ST-segment elevations, which may indicate penetration into the epicardium.
5. Pericardial fluid is aspirated and placed in multiple specimen containers.
6. Some patients who have recurring cardiac tamponade may require placement of an indwelling pericardial catheter for continuous draining for 1 to 3 days. Occasionally a surgical pericardial window is necessary to prevent recurrent effusions.
7. With certain types of pericarditis, medications (e.g., antibiotics, antineoplastic drugs, corticosteroids) may be instilled during pericardiocentesis to diminish the risk of recurrent effusions.

After

- Closely monitor the patient's vital signs. An increased temperature may indicate infection. Pericardial bleeding would be marked by hypotension or pulsus paradoxus (abnormal decrease in systolic blood pressure during inspiration).
- Label and number the specimen tubes that contain the pericardial fluid and deliver them to the appropriate laboratories for examination. Note the following possibilities:
  1. Usually the fluid is taken to the chemistry laboratory, where the color, turbidity, glucose, albumin, protein, and lactic dehydrogenase levels are obtained. (See the discussion of thoracentesis on p. 606.)
  2. A tube of blood often goes to the hematology laboratory, where the quantities of red and white blood cells are recorded. (See the discussion of thoracentesis on p. 606.)
  3. The bacteriology laboratory performs routine cultures, Gram stains, fungal studies, acid-fast bacilli smears, and cultures.
  4. When malignancy is suspected, the fluid should be sent for cytologic examination.
- All tests performed on pericardial fluid should be performed immediately to avoid false results due to chemical or cellular deterioration.
- Apply a sterile dressing to the catheter if one has been left for continuing pericardial drainage.
- Establish a closed system if continued pericardial drainage is required. This is usually performed via the straight drainage method.
- Note that to minimize infection, pericardial catheters, if used, are usually removed after 2 days, although there are exceptions. After the sutures are cut and the catheter is removed, apply a sterile dressing to the puncture site.

Test Results and Clinical Significance

Pericarditis *Pericarditis can occur as a sequela to myocardial infarction; myocarditis; viral, bacterial, or tuberculous infections; or collagen vascular diseases. The fluid is usually an exudate. (See the discussion of thoracentesis on p. 606.)*

Hypoproteinemia
Nephrotic syndrome
The nephrotic syndrome is characterized by renal albumin wasting. This and other forms of hypoproteinemia are associated with decreased intravascular oncotic pressure. The fluid tends to leak out of the intravascular space into the peritoneum. This fluid is usually a transudate.

Congestive heart failure *Normally a small amount of fluid exists within the pericardial space. Fluid is constantly secreted by the pericardium and constantly reabsorbed by the pericardium. If venous pressure of the pericardium is increased as a result of passive congestion of the pericardium associated with congestive heart failure, fluid will accumulate.*

Metastatic cancer *Neoplasms affecting the pericardium primarily (mesothelioma) or secondarily (breast, lung, ovarian, lymphoma) secrete excess volume of fluid into the pleural space. This fluid is an exudate.*

Blunt or penetrating cardiac trauma

Rupture of ventricular aneurysm

These events cause sudden accumulation of blood within the closed pericardial space. As a result, diastolic filling is diminished and cardiac output diminishes. Immediate treatment is required if the patient is to survive.

Related Tests

- Glucose, lactic dehydrogenase (LDH), protein, and amylase (p. 225, 278, 357, and 51): These blood tests are performed concomitantly to assist in the evaluation of the peritoneal fluid.
- Chest radiography (p. 924): This is an important part of identifying a pericardial effusion. Furthermore a chest x-ray should be routinely performed on completion of pericardiocentesis to ensure that a pneumothorax has not iatrogenically occurred.
- Electrocardiography (p. 478): This test is simultaneously performed to indicate location of the aspirating needle.

Secretin-Pancreozymin (Pancreatic Enzymes)

Normal Findings

Volume: 2-4 ml/kg body weight

HCO_3^- (bicarbonate): 90-130 mEq/L

Amylase: 6.6-35.2 U/kg

Indications

This is a corroborative test used in the evaluation of cystic fibrosis. This test is indicated in children with recurrent respiratory tract infections, malabsorption syndromes, or failure to thrive.

Test Explanation

Cystic fibrosis is an inherited disease characterized by abnormal secretion by exocrine glands within the bronchi, small intestines, pancreatic ducts, bile ducts, and skin (sweat glands). Because of this abnormal exocrine secretion, children with cystic fibrosis develop mucus plugs that obstruct their pancreatic ducts. The pancreatic enzymes (e.g., amylase, lipase, trypsin, chymotrypsin) cannot be expelled into the duodenum and therefore are either completely absent or present only in diminished quantities within the duodenal aspirate. For the same reasons, bicarbonate and other neutralizing fluids cannot be secreted from the pancreas. In this test, secretin and pancreozymin are used to stimulate pancreatic secretion of these enzymes and bicarbonate into the duodenum. The duodenal contents are then aspirated and examined for pH, bicarbonate, and enzyme levels; amylase is the most frequently measured enzyme. Diminished values are suggestive of cystic fibrosis.

A physician performs this test in approximately 2 hours in the laboratory or at the patient's bedside. Discomfort and gagging may occur during placement of the Dreiling tube.

Procedure and Patient Care

Before

- Explain the procedure to the patient and/or parents.
- Instruct the adult patient to fast for 12 hours before testing.
- Determine pediatric fasting times according to the patient's age.

During

- Note the following procedural steps:
  1. With the use of fluoroscopy, a Dreiling tube is passed through the patient's nose and into the stomach.
  2. The distal lumen of the tube is placed within the duodenum.
  3. The proximal lumen of the tube is placed within the stomach.
  4. Both lumens are aspirated. The gastric lumen is continually aspirated to avoid contamination of the gastric contents in the duodenum aspirate.
  5. A control specimen of the duodenal juices is collected for 20 minutes.
  6. The patient is tested for sensitivity to secretin and pancreozymin by low-dose intradermal injection.
  7. If no sensitivity is present, these hormones are administered IV. Secretin can be expected to stimulate pancreatic water and bicarbonate secretion. Pancreozymin can be expected to stimulate pancreatic enzyme (lipase, amylase, trypsin, chymotrypsin) secretion.
  8. Four duodenal aspirates are collected at 20-minute intervals and placed in the specimen container.
  9. Each specimen is analyzed for pH, volume, bicarbonate, and amylase levels.

After

- Place the aspirated specimens on ice. Send them to the chemistry laboratory as soon as the test is completed.
- Remove the Dreiling tube after completion of the test. Give appropriate nose and mouth care.
- Allow the patient to resume a normal diet.

Test Results and Clinical Significance

Cystic fibrosis *These patients do not have adequate levels of exocrinic pancreatic enzymes or bicarbonates because of mucus plugging of the small pancreatic duct tributaries.*

Sprue *The pathophysiology of this observation is not definitely known. It is thought that patients with sprue have a damaged intestinal mucosa. As a result, they do not have a normal stimulatory response to secrete secretin and pancreozymin. Therefore the pancreas is chronically understimulated. When these hormones are administered, the pancreas can respond to a slight degree, but not as much as normal because of the previous prolonged periods of absence of stimulation.*

Related Tests

- Sweat electrolytes (p. 604): This is the definitive test used in the diagnosis of cystic fibrosis. Skin sweat is analyzed for sodium and chloride content.

Semen Analysis (Sperm Count, Sperm Examination, Seminal Cytology, Semen Examination)

Normal Findings

Volume: 2-5 ml
Liquification time: 20 to 30 minutes after collection
pH: 7.12-8.00
Sperm count (density): 50-200 million/ml
Sperm motility: 60% to 80% actively motile
Sperm morphology: 70% to 90% normally shaped

Indications

Semen analysis is used to evaluate the quality of sperm, to evaluate an infertile couple, and to document the adequacy of operative vasectomy.

Test Explanation

Semen production depends on the function of the testicles. Semen analysis is a measure of testicular function. Gonadotropin-releasing hormone (Gn-RH) is secreted by the hypothalamus in response to decreased levels of testosterone. Gn-RH stimulates the pituitary to produce follicle-stimulating hormone (FSH) and luteinizing hormone (LH, also called interstitial cell-stimulating hormone). The FSH stimulates the Sertoli cell growth within the seminiferous tubules (location of sperm production). LH stimulates the Leydig cells to produce testosterone, which in turn stimulates the seminiferous tubules to produce sperm. Inadequate sperm production can be the result of primary gonadal failure (due to genetic cause [Klinefelter's syndrome], infection, radiation, or surgical orchiectomy) or secondary gonadal failure (due to pituitary diseases). These forms of gonadal failure can be differentiated by measuring LH and FSH levels. In the first type, LH and FSH levels are increased. In the second, they are decreased. Stimulation tests using Gn-RH, clomiphene, or human chorionic gonadotropin are also used in the differentiation.

Semen analysis is one of the most important aspects of the fertility workup because the cause of a couple's inability to conceive often lies with the man. After 2 to 3 days of sexual abstinence, semen is collected and examined for volume, sperm count, motility, and morphology.

The freshly collected semen is first measured for volume. Men with very low or very high volumes are likely to be infertile. After liquification of the white, gelatinous ejaculate, a sperm count is done. The motility of the sperm is then evaluated; at least 60% should show progressive motility. Morphologic examination is done by staining a semen preparation and calculating the number of normal versus abnormal sperm forms. The sperm specimen is considered abnormal if greater than 70% of the sperm have abnormal forms.

A single sperm analysis, especially if it indicates infertility, is inconclusive because sperm count varies from day to day. A semen analysis should be done at least twice and possibly a third time, 3 weeks apart. Men with aspermia (no sperm) or oligospermia (20 million/ml) should be evaluated endocrinologically for pituitary, thyroid, adrenal, or testicular aberrations.

A normal semen analysis alone does not accurately assess the male factor unless the effect of the partner's cervical secretion on sperm survival is also determined. (See the discussion of the Sims-Huhner test on p. 602.) In addition to its value in infertility workups, semen analysis is also helpful in documenting adequate sterilization after a vasectomy. It is usually performed 6 weeks after the surgery. If any sperm are seen, the adequacy of the vasectomy must be suspect.

Interfering Factors

- Drugs that may cause *decreased* semen levels include antineoplastic agents (e.g., nitrogen mustard, procarbazine, vincristine, methotrexate), cimetidine, estrogens, and methyltestosterone.

CLINICAL PRIORITIES

- It is best to collect the semen for this test after 2 to 3 days of sexual abstinence.
- For best results the semen specimen should be collected in the physician's office by masturbation.
- A single sperm analysis is inconclusive because the sperm count varies from day to day. A semen analysis should be done 2 or 3 times for best results.

Procedure and Patient Care

Before

- Explain the procedure to the patient.
- Instruct the patient to abstain from sexual activity for 2 to 3 days before collecting the specimen. Prolonged abstinence before the collection should be discouraged, because the quality of the sperm cells, and especially their motility, may diminish.
- Give the patient the proper container for the semen collection.

- Instruct the patient to avoid alcoholic beverages for several days before the collection.
- For evaluation of the adequacy of vasectomy, the patient should ejaculate once or twice before the day of examination in order to clear the distal portion of the vas deferens.

During

- Note that semen is best collected by ejaculation into a clean container. For best results the specimen should be collected in the physician's office or laboratory by masturbation.
- Note that less satisfactory specimens can be obtained in the patient's home by coitus interruptus or masturbation. Note the following procedural steps:
  1. Instruct the patient to deliver these home specimens to the laboratory within 1 hour after collection.
  2. Tell the patient to avoid excessive heat and cold during transportation of the specimen.

After

- Record the date of the previous semen emission along with the collection time and date of the fresh specimen.
- Tell the patient when and how to obtain the test results. Remember that abnormal results may have a devastating effect on the patient's sexuality.

Test Results and Clinical Significance

Infertility *One of the most common causes of infertility is inadequate sperm production.*

Vasectomy (obstruction of vas deferens) *Semen analysis is necessary before vasectomy can be considered to be adequate.*

Orchitis *This is usually caused by a virus (varicella) or rarely by a bacterium.*

Testicular failure *This can be congenital (Klinefelter's syndrome) or acquired (e.g., infection). Usually, with acquired forms of testicular failure, sperm are present but in low quantities. With congenital forms of testicular failure, no sperm are seen.*

Hyperpyrexia

Varicocele

A common finding in sperm analysis is called "stress pattern." This is said to exist when greater than 20% of the sperm have abnormal appearance and sperm counts are low. The stress pattern indicates presence of a varicocele or recent febrile illness.

Pituitary pathologic condition (adenoma, infarction) *This causes hypospermia because of reduced or absent LH and FSH levels. As a result, spermatogenesis does not occur.*

Related Tests

- Antispermatozoal antibody (p. 82): These antibodies can exist in the blood of males and destroy sperm quality. Furthermore, these antibodies can be produced by women and exist in the cervical mucus, making fertility difficult.
- Sims-Huhner (p. 602): The Sims-Huhner test consists of a postcoital examination of the cervical mucus to measure the ability of the sperm to penetrate the mucus and

maintain motility. It is used in the diagnostic workup of infertility. This analysis is also helpful in documenting cases of suspected rape by testing the vaginal and cervical secretions for sperm.
- Luteinizing hormone assay and follicle-stimulating hormone (p. 296): These hormones are useful in determining the pituitary effect on gonadal function and spermatogenesis.

Sims-Huhner (Postcoital, Postcoital Cervical Mucus, Cervical Mucus Sperm Penetration)

Normal Findings

Cervical mucus adequate for sperm transmission, survival, and penetration
6 to 20 active sperm per high-power field

Indications

The Sims-Huhner test consists of a postcoital examination of the cervical mucus to measure the ability of the sperm to penetrate the mucus and maintain motility. It is invaluable in the evaluation of infertility.

Test Explanation

This study evaluates interaction between the sperm and the cervical mucus. It also measures the quality of the cervical mucus. This test can determine the effect of vaginal and cervical secretions on the activity of the sperm. This procedure is performed only after a previously performed semen analysis has been determined to be normal.

This test is performed during the middle of the ovulatory cycle because at this time the secretions should be optimal for sperm penetration and survival. During ovulation the quantity of cervical mucus is maximal, whereas the viscosity is minimal, thus facilitating sperm penetration. The endocervical mucus sample is examined for color, viscosity, and tenacity (spinnbarkeit). The fresh specimen is then spread on a clean glass slide and examined for the presence of sperm. Estimates of the total number and of the number of motile sperm per high-power field are reported. Normally 6 to 20 active sperm cells should be seen in each microscopic high-power field; if the sperm are present but not active, the cervical environment is unsuitable (e.g., abnormal pH) for their survival. After the specimen has dried on the glass slide, the mucus can be examined for ferning to demonstrate estrogen effect. (See the discussion of the cervical mucus test on p. 573.) The Sims-Huhner study is invaluable in fertility examinations; however, it is not a substitute for the semen analysis. If the results of the Sims-Huhner test are less than optimal, the test is usually repeated during the same or next ovulatory cycle.

This analysis is also helpful in documenting cases of suspected rape by testing the vaginal and cervical secretions for sperm. This procedure is performed by a physician in approximately 5 minutes. The only discomfort associated with this study is insertion of the speculum.

CLINICAL PRIORITIES

- This test is performed during the middle of the ovulation cycle, when the secretions should be optimal for sperm penetration and survival.
- Tell the female patient to remain in bed for 10 to 15 minutes after coitus to ensure cervical exposure to the semen. She should then report to the doctor within 2 hours of coitus.

Procedure and Patient Care

Before

- Explain the procedure to the patient.
- Inform the patient that basal body temperature recordings should be used to indicate ovulation.
- Tell the patient that no vaginal lubrication, douching, or bathing is permitted until after the vaginal cervical examination, because these factors will alter the cervical mucus.
- Inform the patient that this study should be performed after 3 days of male sexual abstinence.
- Instruct the patient to remain in bed for 10 to 15 minutes after coitus to ensure cervical exposure to the semen. After resting, the patient should report to her physician for examination of her cervical mucus within 2 hours after coitus.

During

- Note that the patient is in the lithotomy position; the cervix is then exposed by an unlubricated speculum. The specimen is aspirated from the endocervix and delivered to the laboratory for analysis.

After

- Tell the patient how and when she may obtain the test results.

Test Results and Clinical Significance

Infertility *This test determines the capability of the sperm to function and exist in an environment outside the male urethra. It is the final determinant of the adequacy of sperm. While semen analysis may indicate an adequate sperm count, etc., if the sperm cannot function within the vaginal or cervical environment, fertility is improbable.*

Suspected rape *The demonstration of sperm within vaginal secretions indicates that intercourse has occurred.*

Related Tests

- Semen analysis (p. 599): Semen analysis is used to evaluate the quality of sperm, to evaluate an infertile couple, and to document the adequacy of operative vasectomy.
- Antispermatozoal antibody test (p. 82): These antibodies can exist in the blood of

males and destroy sperm quality. Furthermore, these antibodies can be produced by women and exist in the cervical mucus, making fertility difficult.

- Luteinizing hormone assay and follicle-stimulating hormone (p. 296): These hormones are useful in determining the pituitary effect on gonadal function and spermatogenesis.

Sweat Electrolytes (Iontophoretic Sweat)

Normal Findings

Sodium values in children
  Normal: <70 mEq/L
  Abnormal: >90 mEq/L
  Equivocal: 70-90 mEq/L
Chloride values in children
  Normal: <50 mEq/L
  Abnormal: >60 mEq/L
  Equivocal: 50-60 mEq/L

Indications

This test is used to diagnose cystic fibrosis. The sweat electrolytes test is indicated in children with recurrent respiratory tract infections, chronic cough, early-onset asthma, malabsorption syndromes, late passage of meconium stool, or failure to thrive. This test is also used to screen children or siblings of cystic fibrosis patients for the disease.

Test Explanation

Patients with cystic fibrosis have increased sodium and chloride contents in their sweat. That forms the basis of this test, which is both sensitive and specific for cystic fibrosis. Cystic fibrosis is an inherited disease (autosomal recessive) characterized by abnormal secretion by exocrine glands within the bronchi, small intestines, pancreatic ducts, bile ducts, and skin (sweat glands). Sweat, induced by electrical current (pilocarpine iontophoresis), is collected, and its sodium and chloride contents are measured. The degree of abnormality is no indication of the severity of cystic fibrosis; it merely indicates that the patient has the disease.

Almost all patients with cystic fibrosis have sweat sodium and chloride contents 2 to 5 times greater than normal values. In patients with suspicious clinical manifestations, these levels are diagnostic of cystic fibrosis.

Abnormal sweat test results can also occur in patients with glycogen storage diseases, adrenal hypofunction, and G-6-PD deficiency.

The sweat test is not reliable during the first few weeks of life. High serum concentrations of immunoreactive trypsin may be a better test for this age group. An experienced technologist performs the sweat test in approximately 90 minutes in the laboratory or at the patient's bedside. A small electrical current is experienced during the test, but this is not painful. Generally there is no discomfort or pain associated with this test.

Interfering Factors

- In a cold room, sweating is inhibited. The room should be warmed or the child covered to maintain body heat.
- Dehydration is associated with reduced volume of sweat and increased concentration of sodium and chloride. The test results are not accurate.
- Values in pubertal adolescents may vary significantly and are not accurate.

Procedure and Patient Care

Before

- Explain the procedure to the patient and/or parents.
- Tell the patient and/or parents that no fasting is required.

During

- Note the following procedural steps:
  1. For *iontophoresis,* a low-level electrical current is applied to the test area (the thigh in infants, the forearm in older children) (Figure 5-7).
  2. The positive electrode is covered by gauze and saturated with pilocarpine hydrochloride, a stimulating drug that induces sweating.
  3. The negative electrode is covered by gauze saturated with a bicarbonate solution.
  4. The electrical current is allowed to flow for 5 to 12 minutes.
  5. The electrodes are removed, and the arm is washed with distilled water.
  6. Paper disks are placed over the test site with the use of clean, dry forceps.
  7. These disks are covered with paraffin to obtain an airtight seal, preventing evaporation of sweat.

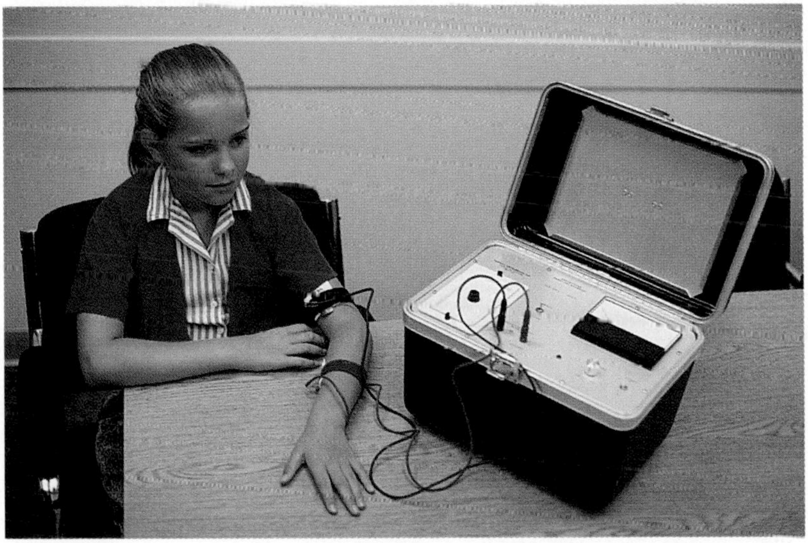

Figure 5-7 Child undergoing sweat test for cystic fibrosis.

8. After 1 hour the paraffin is removed. The paper disks are transferred immediately by forceps to a weighing jar and sent for sodium and chloride analysis.

A *screening test* may be done to detect sweat chloride levels. For screening, a test paper containing silver nitrate is pressed against the child's hand for several seconds. The test is positive when the excess chloride combines with the silver nitrate to form a white powder (silver chloride) on the paper. That is, the child with cystic fibrosis will leave a "heavy" handprint on the paper. A positive screening test is usually validated by iontophoresis.

After

- Initiate extensive education, emotional support, and counseling for the patient and/or parents if the results indicate cystic fibrosis.

Test Results and Clinical Significance

Cystic fibrosis *As indicated previously, this is the main form of testing for this inherited disease that affects children. To date, there is no cure. These children usually die of recurrent pulmonary infections.*

Related Tests

- Secretin-pancreozymin (p. 597): This is a test whereby pancreatic efflux is measured for amylase and other components. It is a corroborative test for cystic fibrosis.

Thoracentesis and Pleural Fluid Analysis
(Pleural Tap)

Normal Findings

Gross appearance: clear, serous, light yellow, 50 ml
RBCs: none
WBCs: 300/ml
Protein: <4.1 g/dl
Glucose: 70-100 mg/dl
Amylase: 138-404 U/L
Alkaline phosphatase
  Adult male: 90-240 U/L
  Female <45 years: 76-196 U/L
  Female >45 years: 87-250 U/L
Lactic dehydrogenase (LDH): similar to serum LDH
Cytology: no malignant cells
Bacteria: none
Fungi: none
Carcinoembryonic antigen (CEA): <5.0 ng/ml

Indications

Thoracentesis is performed to determine the cause of an unexplained pleural effusion. It is also performed to relieve the intrathoracic pressure that accumulates with a large volume of fluid and inhibits respiration.

Test Explanation

Thoracentesis is an invasive procedure that entails insertion of a needle into the pleural space for removal of fluid (or rarely, air) (Figure 5-8). The pleural space is defined as the space between the visceral pleura (thin membrane covering the lungs) and the parietal pleura (thin membrane covering the inside of the thoracic cavity). Within the peritoneal membrane is an intricate network of capillary and lymphatic vessels. Fluid is constantly being secreted by the pleural membranes and constantly being reabsorbed by those same membranes. If secretion is increased or reabsorption blocked, pleural fluid will develop.

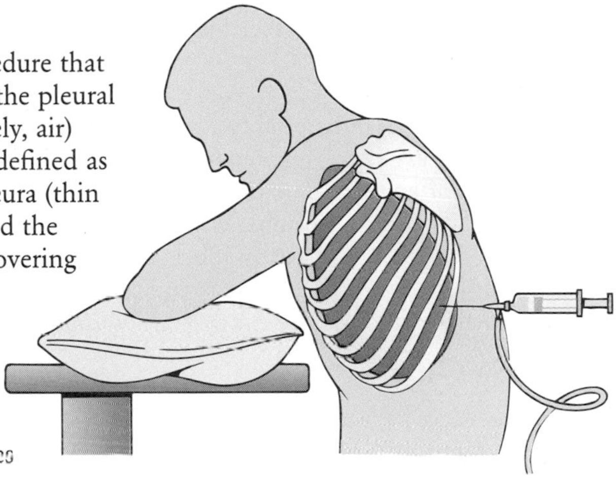

Figure 5-8 Thoracentesis.

Pleural fluid is removed for diagnostic and therapeutic purposes. *Therapeutically* it is done to relieve pain, dyspnea, and other symptoms of pleural pressure. Removal of this fluid also permits better radiographic visualization of the lung.

Diagnostically thoracentesis is performed to obtain and analyze fluid to determine the cause of the pleural effusion. Pleural fluid is classified as to transudate or exudate. This is an important distinction and is very helpful in determining the cause of the effusion. See Table 5-3 (p. 589) for differentiation between transudate and exudate. *Transudates* are most frequently caused by congestive heart failure, cirrhosis, nephrotic syndrome, and hypoproteinemia. *Exudates* are most often found in inflammatory, infectious or neoplastic conditions. However, collagen vascular disease, pulmonary infarction, trauma, and drug hypersensitivity also may cause an exudative effusion.

A decubitus chest x-ray film (p. 925) is obtained before thoracentesis to ensure that the pleural fluid is mobile and accessible to a needle placed within the pleural space.

Pleural fluid is usually evaluated for gross appearance; cell counts; protein, LDH, glucose, and amylase levels; Gram stain and bacteriologic cultures; *Mycobacterium tuberculosis* and fungus; cytology; CEA levels; and sometimes for other specific tests. Each is discussed separately.

Gross appearance

The color, optical density, and viscosity are noted as the pleural fluid appears in the aspirating syringe. Transudative pleural fluid may be clear, serous, and light yellow, especially in patients with hepatic cirrhosis. Milk-colored pleural fluid may result from the escape of chyle from blocked thoracic lymphatic ducts. An opalescent, pearly fluid is characteristic of chylothorax (chyle in the pleural cavity). Conditions that may cause lymphatic blockage include lymphoma, carcinoma, and tuberculosis involving the thoracic lymph nodes. The triglyceride value in a chylous effusion exceeds 110 mg/dl.

Cloudy or turbid fluid may result from inflammatory or infectious conditions such as empyema. Empyema is characterized by the presence of a foul odor and thick, puslike fluid. Bloody fluid may be the result of a traumatic tap (the aspirating needle penetrates a blood vessel), intrathoracic bleeding, or tumor.

Cell counts

The WBC and differential counts are determined. A WBC count exceeding 1000/ml is suggestive of an exudate. The predominance of polymorphonuclear leukocytes usually is an indication of an acute inflammatory condition (e.g., pneumonia, pulmonary infarction, early tuberculosis effusion). When over 50% of the WBCs are small lymphocytes, the effusion is usually caused by tuberculosis or tumor. Normally no RBCs should be present. The presence of RBCs may indicate neoplasms, tuberculosis, or intrathoracic bleeding. Usually these counts are performed manually using a simple hemacytometer.

Protein content

Total protein levels greater than 3 g/dl are characteristic of exudates, whereas transudates usually have a protein content of less than 3 g/dl. It is now thought that the albumin gradient between serum and pleural fluid can differentiate better between the transudate and exudate nature of pleural fluid than can the total protein content. This gradient is obtained by subtracting the pleural albumin value from the serum albumin value. Values of 1.1 g/dl or more suggest a transudate. Values of less than 1.1 g/dl suggest an exudate but will not differentiate the potential cause of the exudate (malignancy from infection or inflammation).

Because there is significant overlap in protein values differentiating transudate from exudate, the total protein ratio (fluid/serum) has been considered to be a more accurate criterion. A total protein ratio of fluid to serum of greater than 0.5 is considered to indicate an exudate.

Lactic dehydrogenase

A pleural fluid/serum LDH ratio of greater than 0.6 is typical of an exudate. An exudate is identified with a high degree of accuracy if the pleural fluid/serum protein ratio is greater than 0.5 and the pleural fluid/serum LDH ratio is greater than 0.6.

Glucose

Usually pleural glucose levels approximate serum levels. Low values appear to be a combination of glycolysis by the extra cells within an exudate and impairment of glucose diffusion because of damage to the pleural membrane. Values of less than 60 mg/dl also indicate exudate.

Amylase

In a malignant effusion, the amylase concentration is slightly elevated. Amylase levels above the normal range for serum or 2 times the serum level are seen when the effusion is caused by pancreatitis or rupture of the esophagus associated with leakage of salivary amylase into the chest cavity.

Triglyceride

Measurement of triglyceride levels is an important part of identifying chylous effusions. These effusions are usually produced by obstruction or transection of the lymphatic system caused by lymphoma, neoplasm, trauma, or recent surgery. The triglyceride value in a chylous effusion exceeds 110 mg/dl.

Gram stain and bacteriologic culture

Culture and Gram stains are routinely performed when bacterial pneumonia or empyema is a possible cause of the effusion. These tests identify the organisms involved in the infection and also provide information concerning antibiotic sensitivity. (See p. 681 for a more thorough discussion of Gram stain, cultures, and sensitivity.) If possible, these tests should be done before initiation of antibiotic therapy.

Cultures for *Mycobacterium tuberculosis* and fungus

Tuberculosis is less often a cause for pleural effusion in the United States today than it was in the past (although its incidence is now on the rise, especially among immunosuppressed patients). Fungus may be a cause of pulmonary effusion in patients with compromised immunologic defenses. (See p. 687 for more information about tuberculosis culture techniques.)

Cytology

A cytologic study is performed to detect tumors. It is positive in approximately 50% to 60% of patients with malignant effusions. Breast and lung are the two most frequent tumors; lymphoma is the third. The interpretation of cytologic changes requires that the pathologist have considerable experience in cytology. It can be difficult to differentiate malignancy from severe inflammatory mesothelial cells. In general, malignant cells tend to clump together and have a high nucleus/cytoplasm ratio, prominent and multiple nucleoli, and unevenly distributed chromatin.

Cytologic examination of the fluid is improved by spinning down a large volume of fluid and examining the sediment. A large number of cells can be seen and compared with each other. A cytologic study is performed to detect tumor cells.

Carcinoembryonic antigen

Pleural fluid CEA levels are elevated in various malignant (GI, breast) conditions.

Special tests

The pH of pleural fluid is usually 7.4 or greater. The pH is typically less than 7.2 when empyema is present. The pH may be 7.2 to 7.4 in tuberculosis or malignancy. In some instances the rheumatoid factor (p. 389) and the complement levels (p. 160) are also measured in pleural fluid. Pleural fluid antinuclear antibody (ANA) levels and the pleural fluid/serum ANA ratio are often used to evaluate pleural effusion secondary to systemic lupus erythematosus.

Thoracentesis is performed by a physician at the patient's bedside, in a procedure room, or in the physician's office in less than 30 minutes. Although local anesthetics eliminate pain at the insertion site, the patient may feel a pressurelike pain when the pleura is entered and the fluid is removed.

Contraindications

- Patients with significant thrombocytopenia, because the aspirating needle may initiate bleeding

Potential Complications

- Pneumothorax due to puncture of the lung or entry of air into the pleural space through the aspirating needle
- Intrapleural bleeding due to puncture of a blood vessel
- Hemoptysis caused by needle puncture of a pulmonary vessel
- Reflex bradycardia and hypotension
- Pulmonary edema
- Seeding of the needle tract with tumor when malignant pleural effusion exists
- Empyema caused by infection delivered by the aspirating needle

✓ CLINICAL PRIORITIES

- To prevent needle damage to the lung or pleura, the patient should remain still during this procedure. A cough suppressant may be needed if the patient has a troublesome cough.
- An x-ray film, ultrasound scan, or fluoroscopy is used to assist in localizing the pleural fluid and in determining the needle insertion site.
- Chest x-ray examinations are done after this procedure to check for pneumothorax. The lungs are carefully assessed for decreased breath sounds, which could be a sign of pneumothorax.

Procedure and Patient Care

Before

- Explain the procedure to the patient.
- Obtain informed consent for this procedure.
- Tell the patient that no fasting or sedation is necessary.
- Inform the patient that movement or coughing should be minimized to avoid inadvertent needle damage to the lung or pleura during the procedure.
- Administer a cough suppressant before the procedure if the patient has a troublesome cough.
- Note that an x-ray film or ultrasound scan is often used to assist in location of the fluid. Fluoroscopy also may be used.

During

- Note the following procedural steps:
  1. The patient is usually placed in an upright position with the arms and shoulders raised and supported on a padded overhead table. This position spreads the ribs and enlarges the intercostal space for insertion of the needle.

2. Patients who cannot sit upright are placed in a side-lying position on the unaffected side with the side to be tapped uppermost.
3. The thoracentesis is performed under strict sterile technique.
4. The needle insertion site, which is determined by percussion, auscultation, and examination of a chest x-ray film, ultrasound scan, or fluoroscopy, is aseptically cleansed and anesthetized locally.
5. The needle is positioned in the pleural space, and the fluid is withdrawn with a syringe and a three-way stopcock. Most thoracentesis kits now use a blunt-tip soft catheter over the needle. The needle is withdrawn and the soft Silastic catheter is left in place. The fluid is aspirated. The use of these soft catheters has greatly diminished the incidence of pneumothorax as a complication of this procedure.
6. Various mechanisms to stabilize the pleural needle or catheter are available to secure the needle depth during the fluid collection.
7. A short polyethylene catheter may be inserted into the pleural space for fluid aspiration; this decreases the risk of puncturing the visceral pleura and inducing a pneumothorax.
8. Also, large volumes of fluid may be collected by connecting the catheter to a gravity-drainage system.

- Monitor the patient's pulse for reflex bradycardia and evaluate the patient for diaphoresis and the feeling of faintness during the procedure.

After

- Place a small bandage over the needle site. Usually, turn the patient on the unaffected side for 1 hour to allow the pleural puncture site to heal.
- Label the specimen with the patient's name, date, source of fluid, and diagnosis. Send the specimen promptly to the laboratory.
- All tests performed on pleural fluid should be performed immediately to avoid false results due to chemical or cellular deterioration.
- Obtain a chest x-ray study as indicated to check for pneumothorax.
- Monitor the patient's vital signs.
- Observe the patient for coughing or expectoration of blood (hemoptysis), which may indicate trauma to the lung.
- Evaluate the patient for signs and symptoms of pneumothorax, tension pneumothorax, subcutaneous emphysema, and pyogenic infection (e.g., tachypnea, dyspnea, diminished breath sounds, anxiety, restlessness, fever).
- Assess the patient's lung sounds for diminished breath sounds, which could be a sign of pneumothorax.
- If the patient has no complaints of dyspnea, normal activity usually can be resumed 1 hour after the procedure.

Test Results and Clinical Significance

Exudate

Empyema
Pneumonia
Empyema is most often the result of a pneumonia. Occasionally, however, it can follow surgery, pleuritis, or trauma.

Tuberculosis effusion *This is usually a bloody effusion that is the result of the primary tuberculous infection of the lung and pleura.*

Pancreatitis *This pleural effusion is most often a "sympathetic" effusion in response to the inflammatory process below the diaphragm.*

Ruptured esophagus *The pleural fluid can occur as a result of a free communication of the ruptured esophagus with the pleural cavity. The pleura covering the mediastinum usually prevents this free communication, and the fluid is a "sympathetic" reaction to the mediastinal infection. The fluid, however, subsequently becomes infected and acts as an empyema.*

Tumors *Neoplasms affecting the pleura primarily (mesothelioma) or secondarily (breast, lung, ovarian) secrete excess volumes of fluid into the pleural space.*

Lymphoma *The tumor infiltrates the lymph nodes through which the thoracic lymphatic ducts flow. As a result, the lymph fluid is not reabsorbed and collects as a chylous effusion within the pleural space (chylothorax).*

Pulmonary infarction *This bloody effusion is also a "sympathetic" effusion in response to the necrosis of lung tissue following a pulmonary embolus.*

Collagen vascular disease: rheumatoid arthritis, systemic lupus erythematosus
Drug hypersensitivity
An immunogenic pleuritis and subsequent effusion may be the sequelae of autoimmune diseases or drug hypersensitivities as indicated previously.

Transudate

Cirrhosis
Congestive heart failure
With increased venous pressure that results from either portal vein hypertension or passive congestion from congestive heart failure, pleural fluid is not absorbed. As a result, pleural fluid accumulates.

Nephrotic syndrome
Hypoproteinemia
The nephrotic syndrome is characterized by renal albumin wasting. This and other forms of hypoproteinemia are associated with decreased intravascular oncotic pressure. The fluid tends to leak out of the intravascular space into the pleural space.

Trauma *Injury to the thorax, lungs, or great blood vessels can cause bleeding into the pleural space (hemothorax).*

Related Tests

- Glucose, lactic dehydrogenase (LDH), protein, and amylase (p. 225, 278, 357, and 51): These blood tests are performed concomitantly to assist in the evaluation of the peritoneal fluid.
- Chest radiography (p. 924): This is an important part of identifying a pleural effusion. Furthermore, a chest x-ray should be routinely performed on completion of thoracentesis to ensure that a pneumothorax has not iatrogenically occurred.

6 Manometric Studies

TESTS

Overview

Manometric studies evaluate certain areas of the body by using a manometric device to measure and record pressures. These devices can be as familiar to the patient as a blood pressure instrument or as foreign as the one used in oculoplethysmography (OPG) to record eye pressures. Commonly performed manometric studies and the areas they evaluate are shown in Table 6-1.

Procedural Care for Manometric Studies

Before

- Explain the purpose and procedure to the patient. Patient cooperation is essential in these studies.
- Fasting requirements vary according to the particular study performed. For example, no fasting is required for cystometry. The patient must be fasting for esophageal function studies.

During

- Patient positioning depends on the procedure indicated.
- A particular type of manometer is applied to the patient. For example, blood pressure cuffs are applied to the extremities for arterial and venous plethysmography. A catheter is inserted into the bladder and attached to a pressure monitor for cystometry.
- Patients must remain very still during the procedure. Movement can affect the pressure readings.

After

- Aftercare varies with each particular test. For example, some tests (e.g., venous plethysmography) require no special aftercare. OPG necessitates some specific eye precautions.

Potential Complications

There are few complications associated with these tests. The few that do occur vary markedly from test to test. For example, gastric aspiration is a potential complication of

Table 6-1 ***Manometric studies and areas of evaluation***

Test	Area evaluated
Cystometry	Bladder
Esophageal function studies	Esophagus
Oculoplethysmography	Ophthalmic artery
Plethysmography	Arterial and venous pressures
Tilt-table testing	Blood pressure
Urethral pressure profile	Urethra

esophageal function studies. Conjunctival hemorrhage is a potential complication of OPG.

Reporting of Results

Most tests are performed by a technician. The physician reviews the test results and explains them to the patient.

Cystometry (Cystometrogram [CMG])

Normal Findings

Normal sensations of fullness and temperature
Normal pressures and volumes
Maximal cystometric capacity
  Male: 350-750 ml
  Female: 250-550 ml
Intravesical pressure when bladder is empty: usually 40 cm H_2O
Detrusor pressure: <10 cm H_2O
Residual urine: <30 ml

Indications

This test is used to measure pressures within the bladder to identify patients who have bladder dysfunction. It is used in patients with bladder outlet obstruction, urinary incontinence, and questionable neurogenic bladder. It is also used to document progress in treatment of these abnormalities.

Test Explanation

The purpose of cystometry is to evaluate the motor and sensory function of the bladder when incontinence is present or neurologic bladder dysfunction is suspected. A graphic recording of pressure exerted at varying phases of the filling of the urinary bladder is produced. A pressure/volume relationship of the bladder is determined. This urodynamic study assesses the neuromuscular function of the bladder by measuring the efficiency of the detrusor muscle, intravesical pressure and capacity, and the bladder's response to thermal stimulation.

Cystometry can determine whether a bladder function abnormality is caused by neurologic, infectious, or obstructive diseases. Cystometry is indicated to elucidate the causes of frequency and urgency, especially before surgery on the urologic outflow tract. Cystometry is also part of the evaluation for the following: incontinence, persistent residual urine, vesicoureteral reflux, motor and sensory disorders affecting the bladder, and the effect of certain drugs on bladder function.

This test is performed by a urologist in approximately 45 minutes and is often performed at the same time as cystoscopy. The only discomfort is that associated with the urethral catheterization. Nocturnal examinations can be performed to evaluate nocturnal incontinence.

Contraindications

- Urinary tract infections, because of the possibility of false results and the potential for the spread of infection

CLINICAL PRIORITIES

- This is an important test for diagnosing bladder dysfunction. It can also document response to therapy.
- Certain medications can be administered during cystometry to distinguish between underactivity of the bladder due to muscle failure and underactivity due to denervation.
- This test can be done at the same time as cystoscopy.
- Patients should be carefully evaluated for infection after this test.

Procedure and Patient Care

Before

- Explain the purpose and the procedure to the patient.
- Tell the patient that no fluid or food restrictions are needed.
- Assure the patient that he or she will be draped to prevent unnecessary exposure.
- Assess the patient for signs and symptoms of urinary tract infection.
- Instruct the patient not to strain while voiding because the results can be skewed.
- If the patient has a spinal cord injury, transport him or her on a stretcher. The test will then be performed with the patient on the stretcher.

During

- Note the following procedural steps:
  1. Cystometry, usually performed in a urologist's office or a special procedure room, begins with the patient being asked to void.
  2. The amount of time required to initiate voiding and the size, force, and continuity of the urinary stream are recorded. The amount of urine, the time of voiding, and the presence of any straining, hesitancy, or terminal urine dribbling are also recorded. (See the discussion of urine flow studies, p. 631.)
  3. The patient is placed in a lithotomy or supine position.
  4. A retention catheter is inserted through the urethra and into the bladder.
  5. Residual urine volume is measured and recorded.
  6. Thermal sensation is evaluated by the instillation of approximately 30 ml of room temperature saline solution into the bladder followed by an equal amount of warm water. The patient reports any sensations.
  7. This fluid is withdrawn from the bladder.

8. The urethral catheter is connected to a cystometer (a machine used to monitor bladder pressure).
9. Sterile water, normal saline solution, or carbon dioxide gas is slowly introduced into the bladder at a controlled rate, usually with the patient in a sitting position. While the bladder is slowly filled with water, pressures are simultaneously recorded. This is called a cystometrogram.
10. Patients are asked to indicate the first urge to void and then when they have the feeling that they must void. The bladder is full at this point.
11. The pressures and volumes are plotted on a graph.
12. The patient is asked to void around the catheter, and the maximal intravesical voiding pressure is recorded.
13. The bladder is drained for any residual urine or gas.
14. If no additional studies are to be done, the urethral catheter is removed. Pressures are recorded as the catheter is slowly being removed. This allows pressure readings of the urethra. (See the discussion of the urethral pressure profile, p. 630.)

- Throughout the study, ask the patient to report any sensations, such as pain, flushing, sweating, nausea, bladder filling, and an urgency to void.
- Note that certain drugs may be administered during the cystometric examination to distinguish between underactivity of the bladder due to muscle failure and underactivity associated with denervation. Cholinergic drugs (e.g., bethanechol [Urecholine]) may be given to enhance the tone of a flaccid bladder. Anticholinergic drugs (e.g., atropine) may be given to promote relaxation of a hyperactive bladder. If these drugs are to be given, the catheter is left in place.

  After these drugs are given, the examination is repeated 20 to 30 minutes later, using the first test as a control value. The information obtained with the drugs assists in deciding whether drugs will be effective treatment.

After

- Observe the patient for any manifestations of infection (e.g., elevated temperature, chills, or dysuria).
- Examine the urine for hematuria. Notify the physician if the hematuria persists after several voidings.
- Provide a warm sitz bath or tub bath for the patient's comfort if desired.
- Note that pelvic floor sphincter electromyography (p. 506) can be performed to evaluate the urethral sphincter in cases of incontinence.

Test Results and Clinical Significance

Neurogenic bladder *With loss of motor function of the bladder, reduced filling pressures and detrusor pressures are observed. Increased residual volume of urine is also noted. Sensation of fullness and temperature is often diminished or absent. There are several different classifications of neurogenic bladder, some of which are based on the cystometry findings.*

Spina bifida, cord injury, compression, or demyelinating diseases can cause a neurogenic bladder. Diabetic neuropathy, anticholinergics, and alpha-adrenergic antagonists also diminish bladder muscle tone. Extensive pelvic surgery can interrupt the peripheral nerve fibers to the bladder, thereby creating a neurogenic bladder.

Bladder obstruction *Bladder outlet obstruction is evidenced by a reduced urine flow, increased intravesicular pressures while voiding, and residual urine volume. Although congenital causes (e.g., urethral valves, phimosis, meatal stenosis) of bladder outlet obstruction can occur, the most common cause of bladder outlet obstruction is a prostatic pathologic condition (cancer or hypertrophy). In women the most common cause of outlet obstruction is a neoplasm (usually of the cervix) or neurogenic bladder (see above).*

Bladder infection *Urgency and reduced bladder capacity are noted. Discomfort associated with bladder distention may be enhanced.*

Bladder hypertonicity *Increased pressures are noted with filling. Capacity is reduced. This occurs with some forms of spastic paralysis. This is most common with upper motor neuron disease or injury.*

Diminished bladder capacity *This may be the result of post–radiation-therapy fibrosis or an extrinsic tumor compressing the bladder. A fibrotic and inflamed bladder cannot distend adequately. Likewise, when a tumor compresses the bladder, the bladder cannot distend. Capacity is reduced.*

Related Tests

- Urine flow studies (p. 631): This is a measurement of urine flow per unit of time and is used to diagnose bladder outlet obstruction.
- Pelvic floor sphincter electromyography (p. 506): This is a measurement of the electrical activity of the periurethral sphincter function.
- Cystography (p. 948): This is an x-ray contrast study of the bladder. Outlet obstruction is evident on this study.

Esophageal Function Studies
(Esophageal Manometry, Esophageal Motility Studies)

Normal Findings

Lower esophageal sphincter pressure: 10-20 mm Hg
Swallowing pattern: normal peristaltic waves
Acid reflux: negative
Acid clearing: <10 swallows
Bernstein test: negative

Indications

This test is used to identify and document the severity of diseases affecting the swallowing function of the esophagus. It is also used to document and quantify gastroesophageal reflux. A wide variety of motor disturbances can be identified. It is commonly used on patients with heartburn, chest pain, or difficulty swallowing.

Test Explanation

Esophageal function studies include the following:

1. Determination of the lower esophageal sphincter (LES) pressure (manometry)
2. Graphic recording of esophageal swallowing waves, or swallowing pattern (manometry)
3. Detection of reflux of gastric acid back into the esophagus (acid reflux)
4. Detection of the ability of the esophagus to clear acid (acid clearing)
5. An attempt to reproduce symptoms of heartburn (Bernstein test)

Manometric studies

Two manometric studies are used in assessing esophageal function: (1) measurement of LES pressure and (2) graphic recording of swallowing waves (motility). The LES is a sphincter muscle that acts as a valve to prevent reflux of gastric acid into the esophagus. Free reflux of gastric acid occurs when the sphincter pressures are low. An example of such a disorder in adults is gastroesophageal reflux; in children, it is called chalasia (incompetent or relaxed LES).

With increased sphincter pressure, as found in patients with achalasia (failure of the LES to relax normally with swallowing) and with diffuse esophageal spasms, food cannot pass from the esophagus into the stomach. Increased LES pressures are noted on manometry. In achalasia, few if any swallowing waves are detected. In contrast, diffuse esophageal spasm is characterized by strong, frequent, asynchronous, and nonpropulsive waves.

Acid reflux with pH probe

Acid reflux is the primary component of gastroesophageal reflux. Patients with an incompetent LES will regurgitate gastric acid into the esophagus. This will then cause a drop in pH testing done by the pH probe. With the newer and smaller catheters, 24-hour pH monitoring can be performed. Episodes of acid reflux are evident. If they coincide with patient symptoms of chest pain, esophagitis can be incriminated.

Acid clearing

Patients with normal esophageal function can completely clear hydrochloric acid from the esophagus in less than 10 swallows. Patients with decreased esophageal motility (frequently caused by severe esophagitis) require a greater number of swallows to clear the acid.

Bernstein test (acid perfusion)

The Bernstein test is simply an attempt to reproduce the symptoms of gastroesophageal reflux. If the patient suffers pain with the instillation of hydrochloric acid into the esophagus, the test is positive and proves the patient's symptoms are caused by reflux esophagitis. If the patient has no discomfort, a cause other than esophageal reflux must be sought to explain the patient's discomfort.

Contraindications

- Patients who cannot cooperate
- Patients who are medically unstable

Potential Complications

- Aspiration of gastric contents

Interfering Factors

- Eating shortly before the test may affect results.
- Drugs such as sedatives can alter test results.

Procedure and Patient Care

Before

- Explain the procedure to the patient.
- Instruct the patient not to eat or drink anything for at least 8 hours before the test.
- Allay any fears and allow the patient to verbalize concerns. Be sensitive to the patient's fears about choking during the procedure.

During

- Note the following procedural steps:
  1. Esophageal studies are usually performed in the endoscopy laboratory.
  2. The fasting, unsedated patient is asked to swallow two or three very tiny tubes. The tubes are equipped so that pressure measurements can be taken at 5-cm intervals (Figure 6-1).
  3. The outer ends of the tubes are attached to a pressure transducer.
  4. All tubes are passed into the stomach; then three tubes are slowly pulled back into the esophagus. A rapid and extreme increase in the pressure readings indicates the high-pressure zone of the LES.
  5. The LES pressure is recorded.
  6. With all tubes in the esophagus, the patient is asked to swallow. Motility wave patterns are recorded.
  7. The pH indicator probe is placed in the esophagus.
  8. The patient's stomach is filled with approximately 100 ml of 0.1-N hydrochloric acid. A decrease in the pH of the esophageal pH probe indicates gastroesophageal reflux.
  9. Hydrochloric acid is instilled into the esophagus, and the patient is asked to swallow. The number of swallows is counted to determine acid clearing. More than 10 swallows to clear the acid (as determined by the pH probe) indicates decreased esophageal motility.

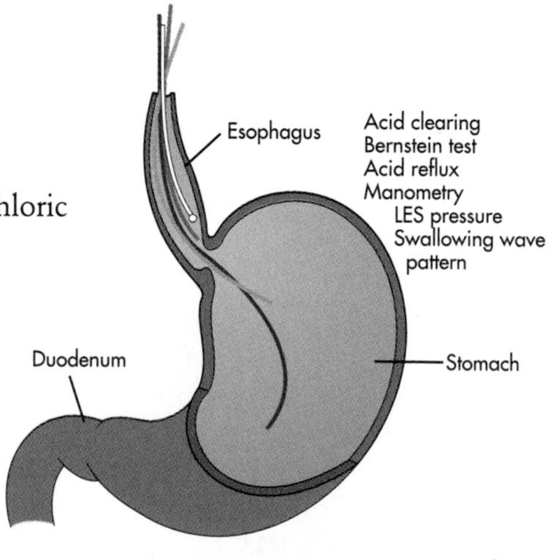

Figure 6-1 Esophageal function studies demonstrating placement of manometry tubes and a pH probe within the esophagus.

10. Finally, 0.1-N hydrochloric acid and saline solution are alternately instilled into the esophagus for the Bernstein test. The patient is not told which solution is being infused. If the patient volunteers symptoms of discomfort while the acid is running, the test is considered positive. If no discomfort is recognized, the test is negative.

- Note that these tests are performed by an esophageal technician in approximately 30 minutes.
- Inform the patient that the test results are interpreted by a physician and are available in a few hours.
- Tell the patient that except for some initial gagging when swallowing the tubes, these tests are not uncomfortable.

After

- Inform the patient that it is not unusual to have a mild sore throat after placement of the tubes.

Test Results and Clinical Significance

Presbyesophagus *This is a common motility pattern noted among the elderly. It is evident as synchronous esophageal contractions. As a result, the food is not propelled down the esophagus but, rather, becomes temporarily lodged between the two areas of contraction. This can be quite painful along with causing a functional obstruction to the passage of food.*

Diffuse esophageal spasm *Spastic synchronously occurring contractions of the esophagus do not allow the food to be propelled down the esophagus but, rather, lodge it temporarily between the two areas of contraction. This, too, can be quite painful along with causing a functional obstruction to the passage of food.*

Chalasia *Absence of tone in the lower esophageal sphincter allows for free reflux of food and gastric juices into the esophagus. This is a common cause of vomiting in newborns.*

Achalasia *This is the opposite of chalasia and most commonly occurs in young adults. The tone of the LES is significantly increased. No relaxation of the sphincter occurs. As a result, the LES acts as an obstruction to the passage of food through the esophagus.*

Gastroesophageal reflux
Reflux esophagitis
The presence of gastric contents in the esophagus causes esophagitis. The pathophysiology of gastroesophageal reflux is not completely understood. It is known that the LES tone is reduced. This allows acid to reflux into the esophagus. This is evident during pH monitoring. Esophagitis follows, and acid clearing is prolonged because the swallowing function of the inflamed esophagus is reduced.

Related Tests

- Esophagoscopy (p. 536): This is an endoscopic test of the esophagus. Reflux esophagitis, esophageal obstruction, achalasia, and other diseases, can be observed.
- Barium swallow (p. 906): This is an x-ray study of the esophagus. Diseases of the esophagus as listed for esophagoscopy can be visualized.

Oculoplethysmography
(OPG, Ocular Pressures)

Normal Findings Normal and equal blood flow in both carotid arteries

Indications

OPG is a method of indirectly determining the flow within the internal carotid artery. It is used to identify carotid arterial atherosclerotic occlusive disease. OPG is indicated in patients who have symptoms of carotid occlusive disease (e.g., transient ischemic attacks, carotid bruits, neurologic symptoms [e.g., dizziness, fainting]). This test is often performed to monitor the success of carotid endarterectomy.

Test Explanation

OPG is a noninvasive study used to indirectly measure blood flow in the ophthalmic artery. Because the ophthalmic artery is the first major branch of the internal carotid artery, its blood flow reflects the carotid blood flow and the alternative blood flow to the brain.

For this study, eye pressures are measured through suction cups placed on the eyes for the recording. If the pressures measured are reduced (compared with normal or compared with the other eye), carotid atherosclerotic occlusive disease is suspected. This procedure may be followed by cerebral angiography, if indicated. Carotid Doppler flow studies (p. 807) are more easily performed and less invasive and are therefore being used more frequently.

Contraindications

- Patients who had eye surgery within the last 2 to 6 months
- Patients who have a lens implant
- Patients who have had retinal detachment
- Patients with cataracts
- Patients who are allergic to local anesthetics

Potential Complications

- Conjunctival hemorrhage
- Corneal abrasions
  If corneal abrasions occur, the patient's eye is patched and a lubricant (e.g., Dacriose solution) is applied.
- Transient photophobia

Procedure and Patient Care

Before

- Explain the procedure to the patient.
- Instruct the patient to remove contact lenses if applicable.

- Tell patients with glaucoma to take their usual medications and eye drops.
- Tell the patient that no fasting or sedation is necessary.

During

- Note the following procedural steps:
  1. The patient is asked to lie on his or her back on a table or bed.
  2. Blood pressure in both arms is taken before the test.
  3. Electrocardiographic electrodes are applied to the patient's extremities to detect abnormal cardiac rhythms.
  4. Anesthetic eye drops are instilled in both eyes to minimize discomfort.
  5. Small detectors are attached to the earlobes to detect blood flow to the ear through the external carotid artery.
  6. Tracings for both ears are taken and compared.
  7. Suction cups resembling contact lenses are applied directly to the eyeball.
  8. Tracings of the pulsations within each eye are recorded.
  9. A vacuum source is applied to the suction cup. This increased pressure causes the pulse in both eyes to disappear temporarily because all blood flow to the eye is stopped.
  10. When the suction source is stopped, the blood flow returns to the eyes. Both pulses should return simultaneously.
  11. The time difference in the pulse rate from one eye to the other, one ear to the other, and one ear to the eye on the other side is measured in milliseconds. If internal carotid stenosis is present, blood flow to the eye, on the affected side, will be delayed.
- Note that a trained technologist performs this test in approximately 20 to 30 minutes.
- Tell the patient that eyes usually burn slightly when the ophthalmic drops are applied.
- Inform the patient that when suction is applied, he or she may feel a pulling sensation and vision may temporarily be lost.

After

- Inform the patient that the eye anesthesia usually wears off in approximately 30 minutes.
- Instruct the patient not to rub his or her eyes for at least 2 hours. If tears appear, the eye should be blotted dry.
- Inform the patient that contact lenses should not be inserted for at least 2 hours after OPG.
- Tell the patient that the eyes may appear bloodshot for several hours after the test. Artificial tears may be instilled to soothe any irritation in the eyes.
- Tell the patient to wear sunglasses if photophobia is present.

Test Results and Clinical Significance

Carotid atherosclerotic stenosis *Carotid arterial occlusive plaques can significantly reduce carotid artery blood flow as determined by OPG.*

Related Tests

- Doppler flow studies of the carotid artery (p. 785): This is an accurate and more easily performed method of identifying and monitoring carotid arterial occlusive disease.
- Cerebral angiography (p. 893): This is an x-ray examination of the carotid artery and its branches. This is an invasive method to more clearly delineate carotid anatomy and pathologic conditions.

Plethysmography, Arterial

Normal Findings

<20 mm Hg difference in systolic blood pressure of the lower extremity compared with the upper extremity

Normal pulse wave amplitude showing a steep upswing, an acute narrow peak, and a more gentle downslope containing a dicrotic notch (normal arterial pulse wave)

Indications

This is a noninvasive method of identifying and monitoring treatment of arterial occlusive disease.

Test Explanation

Plethysmography is usually performed to rule out occlusive disease of the lower extremities; however, it also can identify arteriosclerotic disease in the upper extremity. This test does require one normal extremity against which the other extremities may be compared.

Arterial plethysmography is performed by applying three blood pressure cuffs to the proximal, middle, and distal portions of the extremity. These are then attached to a pulse volume recorder (plethysmograph), and each pulse wave can be displayed. A reduction in amplitude of a pulse wave in any of the three cuffs indicates arterial occlusion immediately proximal to the area where the decreased amplitude is noted. Also, measurements of arterial pressures are performed at each cuff site. A difference in pressure greater than 20 mm Hg indicates a degree of arterial occlusion in the extremity. A positive result is reliable evidence of arteriosclerotic peripheral vascular occlusion. A negative result, however, does not definitely exclude this diagnosis because extensive vascular collateralization can compensate for even a complete arterial occlusion.

Although it is not as accurate as arteriography (p. 892), plethysmography is performed without serious complications and can be done for seriously ill patients who cannot be transported to the arteriography laboratory.

Interfering Factors

- Arterial occlusion proximal to the extremity
- Cigarette smoking, because nicotine can cause transient arterial constriction

CLINICAL PRIORITIES

- A positive result is reliable evidence of arteriosclerotic peripheral vascular occlusion.
- Patients should not smoke prior to this test because nicotine creates constriction of the peripheral arteries and alters test results.
- This test is usually performed in the noninvasive vascular laboratory or at the bedside by a technologist.

Procedure and Patient Care

Before

- Explain the procedure to the patient.
- Inform the patient that this test is painless.
- Tell the patient that he or she must lie still during the testing procedure.
- Remove all clothing from the patient's extremities.
- Instruct the patient to avoid smoking for at least 30 minutes before the test. Nicotine creates constriction of the peripheral arteries and alters the test results.
- Tell the patient that no fasting is required.

During

- Note the following procedural steps:
  1. The patient is placed in the semirecumbent position.
  2. The cuffs are applied to the extremities and then inflated to 65 mm Hg to increase their sensitivity to pulse waves.
  3. The pulse waves are recorded on the plethysmographic paper.
  4. The amplitudes and form of the pulse wave of each cuff are measured and compared. A marked reduction in wave amplitude indicates arterial occlusive disease.
- Note that this test usually is performed in the noninvasive vascular laboratory or at the patient's bedside by a noninvasive vascular technologist in approximately 30 minutes.
- Inform the patient that results are usually interpreted by a physician and are available in a few hours.
- Remind the patient that no discomfort is associated with this test.

After

- Encourage the patient to verbalize any concerns regarding the test results.

Test Results and Clinical Significance

Arterial atherosclerotic occlusive disease
Arterial trauma
Arterial embolization
Arterial occlusion is noted by a decreased pressure in the cuff immediately distal to the occlusion.

Small vessel diabetic changes *Little or no change may be noted in this disease. This type of vascular insufficiency is usually seen in diabetics.*

Vascular diseases (e.g., Raynaud's phenomenon) *Arterial occlusion that is episodic is classic for Raynaud's phenomenon. This is difficult to identify on plethysmography unless larger vessels of the wrist or hand are involved. Often this diagnosis requires that pressure-sensitive cuffs be placed on the fingers.*

Related Tests

- Arteriography (p. 892): This is an x-ray examination of the arteries of the extremities. Although more invasive and associated with greater complications, arteriography is more accurate than plethysmography.
- Doppler arterial flow studies (p. 807): This ultrasound examination determines blood flow within the artery suspected to be stenotic. This is very accurate test of arterial patency.

Plethysmography, Venous
(Cuff Pressure Test)

Normal Findings

Patent venous system without evidence of thrombosis or occlusion

Indications

This test is a noninvasive method of determining venous thrombosis and deep-vein thrombophlebitis (DVT). It is indicated on patients with a swollen extremity to diagnose DVT.

Test Explanation

Plethysmography measures changes in the volume of an extremity. Usually this test is performed on a leg to exclude DVT. During this test, blood pressure cuffs are placed on the proximal, middle, and distal portions of the extremity and attached to a pulse-volume recorder. The leg volume can then be recorded as a baseline value. The venous system is occluded by inflating the most proximal cuff (occlusion cuff); the most distal cuff (recording cuff) should record a sudden increase in venous volume. When the occlusion cuff is released, the venous volume of the leg should return to preocclusion baseline levels. In patients with venous obstruction, no initial increase in leg volume is recorded. Also, because venous outflow is obstructed, the venous volume of the leg will not dissipate quickly after release of the proximal cuff.

The results of venous plethysmography are less accurate than those of venography (p. 1002); however, no complications are associated with this noninvasive study. Plethysmography can be performed easily and quickly on any patient with suspected venous disease. Furthermore, with the use of portable plethysmography, this test can be performed at the bedside for extremely ill patients.

Doppler flow studies are now being performed to identify DVT, but Doppler flow studies are less accurate in evaluating the venous system below the knee.

Interfering Factors

- Venous occlusion more proximal to the site of the occlusion cuff

CLINICAL PRIORITIES

- This noninvasive test is usually performed on a leg to detect DVT.
- This test can be performed at the bedside for extremely ill patients.
- The results of venous plethysmography are less accurate than those of venography. However, no complications are associated with this test.

Procedure and Patient Care

Before

- Explain the procedure to the patient.
- Tell the patient that no fasting is required.
- Assure the patient that no discomfort is associated with the study.
- Instruct the patient to lie still during the testing.
- Remove all clothing from the patient's extremity to be tested.

During

- Note the following procedural steps:
  1. A large, inflatable occlusion cuff is placed on the proximal portion of the extremity, usually a leg.
  2. A second, smaller plethysmographic monitor or recording cuff is placed more distal on the leg. A third cuff may be placed in between the proximal and distal cuffs.
  3. The second cuff is inflated to 10 mm Hg to facilitate recognition of small changes in the leg's venous volume.
  4. The effects of respiration on the leg's venous volume are evaluated. If no significant changes occur with respiration, venous occlusion can be suspected.
  5. The occlusion cuff is inflated to 50 mm Hg. The monitor cuff should demonstrate a rise in venous volume, displayed on the pulse-monitor recorder.
  6. After the highest volume is recorded in the monitor cuff, the occlusion cuff is rapidly deflated. The leg should return to its preocclusion volume within 1 second. If return to preocclusion baseline values is delayed for a long period, venous thrombosis is suspected.
  7. Often this test is performed concomitantly with Doppler ultrasound of the venous system (p. 807).

- Note that this test is usually performed in the noninvasive vascular laboratory or at the patient's bedside by a noninvasive vascular technologist in approximately 30 minutes.
- Remind the patient that no discomfort is associated with this test.

After

- Note that no special aftercare is needed.

Test Results and Clinical Significance

Partial venous obstruction *This is evidenced by an appropriate rise in venous pressure with occlusion of the proximal cuff. However, the venous volume of the leg will not dissipate quickly with release of the proximal cuff. Tumor or anatomic extrinsic compression of the vein is the most common cause of partial venous occlusion.*

Total venous obstruction *This is evidenced by failure to detect any change in venous volume with proximal cuff occlusion. Thrombophlebitis is the most common cause of complete obstruction.*

Related Tests

- Venography (p. 1002): This is an x-ray study of the veins of the extremity. It is more accurate than venous plethysmography; however, it is also associated with greater risk and complications.
- Venous Doppler flow studies (p. 807): These are somewhat more accurate than plethysmography but are not able to identify DVT below the knee.

Tilt-table Testing

Normal Findings

<20 mm Hg decrease in systolic blood pressure and <10 mm increase in diastolic blood pressure

Heart rate increase <10 beats/min

Indications

The tilt-table test is a provocative test used to diagnose vasopressor syncope.

Test Explanation

Patients with this vasomotor syncope syndrome usually demonstrate symptomatic hypotension and syncope within a few to 30 minutes of being tilted upright by approximately 60° to 90°. This test is usually performed with an electrophysiologic study (p. 494). This test is often used to assess the efficacy of prophylactic pacing in some patients with vasopressor syncope. It is also used to evaluate the impact of posture on some forms of tachyarrhythmias. Normally a minimal drop in systolic blood pressure, rise in diastolic blood pressure, and increase in heart rate occur in the tilted position. Patients with vasopressor syncope demonstrate these changes in an exaggerated fashion and become lightheaded and dizzy on assuming the tilted position.

Interfering Factors

- Patients with dehydration or hypovolemia will demonstrate comparable changes in blood pressure and heart rate. This is especially true in elderly patients.
- Patients on antihypertensive medications or diuretics also may demonstrate similar changes when placed in the tilt position.

Procedure and Patient Care

Before

- Explain the procedure to the patient.
- Obtain IV access in the event emergency drugs are required.
- Note that an arterial line is often placed to accurately monitor blood pressure.
- Ask whether the patient has had excessive fluid loss (diarrhea or vomiting) in the previous 24 hours.
- Record antihypertensive or diuretic medicines that the patient may be taking.

During

- Have the patient lie supine on a horizontal tilt table.
- Obtain the patient's blood pressure and pulse as baseline values before tilting is carried out.
- Monitor these vital signs during the procedure.
- Question the patient about the presence of symptoms of dizziness and lightheadedness.
- Note that the table is progressively tilted to 60° to 80° while the patient is being monitored. Alternatively, the patient is asked to sit or stand.

After

- Monitor the arterial IV site for bleeding after removal of the vascular access.
- Firmly secure a pressure dressing to both sites (arterial and venous).

Test Results and Clinical Significance

Vasomotor syncope *Tachyarrhythmias, overmedication for hypertension or heart disease, hyperreactive vagal activity, and various forms of vasomotor instability can cause a positive tilt-test result.*

Related Tests

- Electrophysiologic study (p. 494): This is a method of studying evoked potentials within the heart. It is used to evaluate patients with syncope, palpitations, or arrhythmias.

Urethral Pressure Profile
(UPP, Urethral Pressure Measurements)

Normal Findings

Maximal urethral pressures in normal patients (cm H_2O)

Age	Male	Female
<25 years	37-126	55-103
25-44 years	35-113	31-115
45-64 years	40-123	40-100
>64 years	35-105	35-75

Indications

This test is often a part of cystometry. It is used to document reduced urethral pressures in incontinent patients (females with stress incontinence or males after prostatectomy). It is also used to indicate the degree of compression applied to the urethra from an abnormally enlarged prostate (which will increase UPP value).

Test Explanation

The UPP indicates the intraluminal pressure along the length of the urethra with the bladder at rest. Indications for this urodynamic investigation include the following:

1. Assessment of prostatic obstruction
2. Assessment of stress incontinence in females
3. Assessment of postprostatectomy sequelae of incontinence
4. Assessment of the adequacy of external sphincterotomy
5. Analysis of the effects of drugs on the urethra
6. Analysis of the effects of stimulation on urethral flow
7. Assessment of the adequacy of implanted artificial urethral sphincter devices

This test is usually performed by a urologist in less than 15 minutes. This test is only slightly more uncomfortable than urethral catheterization.

Contraindications

- Patients with urinary tract infections, because catheterization may induce bacteremia

Procedure and Patient Care

Before

- Explain the procedure to the patient.
- Because many patients are embarrassed by this procedure, assure the patient that he or she will be draped to ensure privacy.
- Tell the patient that no fasting or sedation is required.

During

- Note the following procedural steps:
  1. A catheter is placed into the bladder and attached to a pressure monitor machine.
  2. Fluids (or gas) are instilled through the catheter, which is withdrawn while the pressures along the urethral wall are measured.
  3. A constant infusion of the fluids or gas is maintained by a motorized syringe pump.
  4. The catheter is removed, and the test is completed.

After

- Give the patient a sitz bath, if requested.

Test Results and Clinical Significance

Prostatic obstruction secondary to benign prostatic hypertrophy or cancer *Increased urethral pressures are noted because of the extrinsic compression applied by the enlarged prostate.*
Urinary incontinence *Reduced urethral pressures are noted because of the reduced tone of the urethral sphincter.*

Related Tests

- Cystometry (p. 615): This test often includes UPP. This test, which can identify bladder neuromuscular pathologic conditions, is a measure of bladder pressures.

Urine Flow Studies
(Uroflowmetry, Urodynamic Studies)

Normal Findings Depend on the patient's age, gender, and volume voided

Indications

This test measures the urine flow rate during micturition. If the rate is reduced, outflow obstruction can be documented and measured. The test is used to monitor micturition for decisions concerning timing and adequacy of treatment.

Test Explanation

Uroflowmetry is the simplest of the urodynamic techniques, being noninvasive and requiring uncomplicated and relatively inexpensive equipment. This study measures the volume of urine expelled from the bladder per second. This test is indicated to investigate dysfunctional voiding or suspicious outflow tract obstruction. It is also done before and after any procedure designed to modify the function of the urologic outflow tract.

The urine flow depends greatly on the volume of urine voided. The flow rates are highest and most predictable in the urine volume range of 200 to 400 ml. When the bladder contains more than 400 ml of urine, the efficiency of the bladder muscle is greatly decreased. Nomograms of maximal flow versus voided volume may be used for accurate test result interpretation, taking into account the patient's gender and age. If the flow rates are abnormally low, the test should be repeated to check for accuracy.

Modern urine flowmeters provide a permanent graphic recording. If flowmeters are not available, the patient can time the urinary stream with a stopwatch and record the voided volume; from this the average flow is calculated.

In some cases, it is more valuable to analyze several voided volumes and flow rates rather than a single flow rate. If this is to be done, the patient is taught to use a flowmeter. A graph of flow versus volume can be plotted. Together with clinical observation, this provides very valuable information on the severity of outflow obstruction, the likelihood of urinary retention, and the state of compensation or decompensation of the detrusor muscle.

This test is often performed in conjunction with cystometry (p. 615).

Procedure and Patient Care

Before

- Explain the procedure to the patient.
- Instruct the patient how to void into the urine flowmeter.
- Determine the number of flow rates that will be needed.

During

- Note that this test should be performed when the patient has a normal desire to void and in conditions suitable for privacy. The bladder should be adequately full. Essentially all the patient must do is urinate into the flowmeter. Several different types of flowmeters are available.
- Tell the patient that no discomfort is associated with this test.
- Note that the duration of this test is several seconds.

After

- Record the position of the patient, the method of filling the bladder (it should be natural), and whether this study was part of another evaluation.

Test Results and Clinical Significance

Dysfunctional voiding *Flow rates may be normal but intermittent or delayed.*

Outflow tract obstruction *Flow rates will be diminished significantly, indicating obstruction caused by urethral stricture, prostatic cancer, or hypertrophy.*

Related Tests

- Cystometry (p. 615): This is a measurement of the pressures within the bladder during filling and micturition. Uroflowmetry may be a part of that study.

7

Microscopic Studies

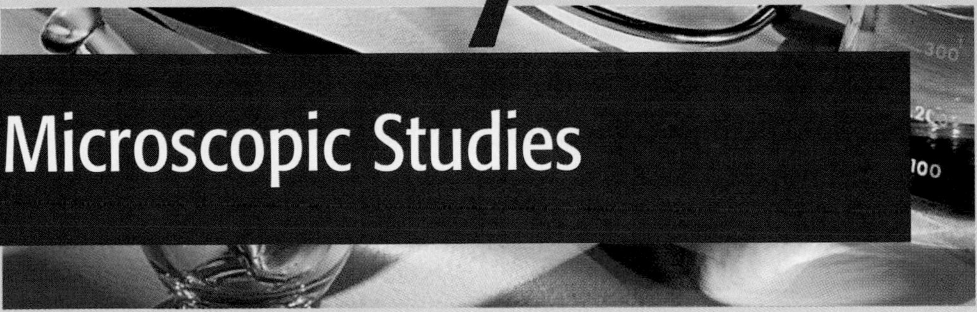

TESTS

Overview

Reasons for Obtaining Microscopic Studies

Microscopic examinations are essential for the diagnosis and treatment of numerous diseases and infectious processes. Included in this chapter are microbiologic studies and studies that require a microscopic review of tissue. Microbiologic specimens can be collected from many sources, such as tissue and organ biopsies, blood, urine, wound drainage, cervical secretions, and sputum. This testing usually takes place in the microbiology or bacteriology section of the laboratory. Microscopic examination is used in a wide variety of clinical situations, some of which include the following:

To evaluate hematologic disorders (bone marrow biopsy)
To detect sexually transmitted diseases (sexually transmitted disease culture)
To evaluate dysfunctional uterine bleeding (endometrial biopsy)
To determine liver pathologic conditions (liver biopsy)
To detect lung cancer (lung biopsy)
To screen for cancer of the vagina, cervix, and uterus (Papanicolaou smear)
To determine the sensitivity of breast cancer to hormonal therapy (estrogen and progesterone receptor assays)
To detect renal disease, such as malignancy, glomerulonephritis, and transplant rejection (renal biopsy)
To detect tuberculosis (tuberculosis culture)
To evaluate and treat infections (wound and soft tissue culture and sensitivity)

Microscopic examinations are used to evaluate histologic and cytologic specimens and to identify bacteria (and other infecting organisms). Determination of hormone receptor assay results along with chromatin identification also requires microscopic examination.

Included in microscopic studies are culture and sensitivity testing. Microscopic examination is an important part of identifying an infecting organism. A Gram stain is just one of the microscopic examinations performed with microbiology testing. A *Gram stain* is a method by which all bacteria are classified. All forms of bacteria are grossly classified as gram positive (blue staining) or gram negative (red staining). Furthermore, knowledge of the shape of the organism (e.g., spherical, rod shaped) also may be very helpful in the tentative identification of the infecting organism. For example, if the Gram stain indicates gram-negative rods, the infection may be caused by *Escherichia coli.* With knowledge of the Gram stain results, the physician can institute reasonable antibiotic treatment based on past experiences as to the organism's possible identity. The Gram stain can be reported in less than 10 minutes after smearing the specimen on a microscopic slide. Treatment can then be altered based upon the final results of culture and sensitivity testing.

The usual culture is obtained from a smear of an infected area (e.g., a wound culture). However, body fluids or tissue can be sent for culture techniques. When smeared on the appropriate culture medium, an infecting organism can be expected to grow. It is important that several different kinds of culture mediums are used in the culture process to maximize the chances of growing the infecting organism. Some bacteria or fungi grow in one medium better than another.

Most of the time the infecting organism is identified from a culture plate on which the organism is growing. In other, rarer situations the infecting organism is found by microscopic review of a tissue specimen. In still other situations the only evidence of infection is derived from serologic testing (e.g., antistreptolysin O titer). (See Chapter 2.)

While there are no *potential complications* associated with culture testing, the risks involved in obtaining tissue for microscopic examination may be considerable. They are well outlined in the discussion of each specific study.

Procedural Care for Microscopic Studies

Before

- Explain the procedure to the patient.
- Inform the patient of any special preprocedure requirements. For example, patients should not douche or tub bathe before cervical cultures for herpes. Men should not void for 1 hour before collecting urethral specimens.
- Inform the patient about the collection technique. These techniques vary from being noninvasive (throat culture) to invasive (liver biopsy).
- Invasive studies require an informed consent. Coagulation profiles are often done before invasive studies because of the risk of bleeding.
- If an invasive procedure is to be performed to obtain tissue, the patient should be prepared as if surgery were a possibility because if bleeding or organ injury occurs, the patient must be ready to go to surgery.

During

- Follow universal precautions in handling all specimens because of the risk of transmitting infection.
- Specific protocols for collection are described with each test in this chapter.
- Instruct the patient to remain still during specimen collection. The quality of the specimen depends in part on the cooperation of the patient.

After

- The specimen should be carefully labeled with the patient's name, the source, and any other pertinent information, such as antibiotic therapy.
- The specimen should be promptly transported to the laboratory or pathology department.
- Antibiotic therapy should be initiated after the specimen is collected.
- Vital signs should be carefully evaluated to detect bleeding, infection, or other potential complications of an invasive procedure.
- If the results indicate a sexually transmitted disease, sexual partners should be notified, evaluated, and treated.

Laboratory Handling of Specimens

The laboratory has protocols to minimize factors that may *interfere* with testing results. Certain specimens must be processed immediately (such as CSF cultures). Some specimens (such as urine) may be refrigerated if there will be a delay before testing. Stained smears of medically urgent specimens should be evaluated and reported immediately. Cultures should be plated immediately. This is essential to avoid bacterial deterioration. All efforts must be made to avoid the contamination of a culture to avoid incorrect results.

In addition to protocols concerning timeliness in handling of the specimen, the laboratory must also have strict guidelines for rejecting a specimen. An improperly identified specimen is the main reason for rejection. It is obvious that labeling the wrong patient with a diagnosis such as gonorrhea or some other sexually transmitted disease can have devastating consequences. Desiccated or poorly preserved specimens would be considered unsatisfactory.

Reporting of Results

Most microbiologic examinations require several days until results are available. The specimens often must go through a staining process that takes at least 24 hours. Some tissue for microscopic examination needs to be sent to reference laboratories for evaluation. Results take much longer to obtain in these cases. Preliminary culture reports and Gram stains, however, are available much sooner. The quality of microscopic study results depends on the quality of the personnel obtaining, transporting, and handling the specimens in the laboratory. The experience of the physician reporting the results is also a key component in the process. Microscopic studies are invaluable in making a diagnosis. Not only is communication among the various health care providers imperative, but also reporting must be timely, concise, and accurate.

Acid-Fast Bacilli Smear (AFB Smear)

Normal Findings No bacilli seen

Indications

This smear (usually of sputum) is used to support the diagnosis of tuberculosis (TB). The diagnosis of TB cannot be made with positive results of an AFB smear by itself. TB cultures are required. AFB smears are also used to monitor treatment of TB. The test is indicated in any patient with a persistent productive cough, night sweats, anorexia, weight loss, fever, and hemoptysis. This smear should especially be considered in high-risk patients, such as those who are immunocompromised, are alcoholic, or have had a recent exposure to TB.

Test Explanation

The most clinically significant AFB is *Mycobacterium tuberculosis.* This is the causative agent in TB. After taking up a dye such as fuchsin, *M. tuberculosis* is not decolorized by acid alcohol (i.e., it is acid-fast). It is seen under the microscope as a red, rod-shaped organism. If this bacillus is seen, the patient may have active TB. However, other species of *Mycobacterium, Nocardia,* and some fungi are acid-fast. The AFB smear is most commonly performed on sputum. At least 5,000 organisms must be present in each milliliter of specimen in order to be seen on a microscope smear. Other specimens, such as CSF, tissue, and synovial fluid, may be used. Smears may be negative as much as 50% of the time even with positive cultures. One cannot make the diagnosis of TB based only on a positive smear for AFB. Cultures (p. 687) must be positive for a definitive diagnosis. Also, cultures are the only way to obtain drug sensitivities for treatment.

AFB is also used to monitor treatment for TB. If after adequate therapy (2 months), the sputum still contains AFB (even though the culture may be negative due to anti-TB drugs), treatment failure should be considered. Cavitary disease may cause this same picture (positive smear, negative cultures).

Interfering Factors

- False negatives can occur because of faulty laboratory techniques.
- False positives can occur when water used to suspend the smear on the slide contains a non-TB organism.

CLINICAL PRIORITIES

- The AFB smear is used to support the diagnosis of TB. A definitive diagnosis requires a sputum culture and sensitivity.
- Inform the parent that sputum must be coughed up from the lungs. The first morning specimen is usually the best.
- Hold antibiotics until after the sputum has been collected.

Procedure and Patient Care

Before

- Explain the procedure for sputum collection.
- Remind the patient that the sputum must be coughed up from the lungs and that saliva is not sputum. The first morning specimen is usually best.
- Hold antibiotics until after the sputum has been collected.
- Give the patient a sterile sputum container the night before the sputum is to be collected so that the morning specimen may be obtained when the patient awakens.
- Instruct the patient to rinse out his or her mouth with water before the sputum collection to decrease contamination by particles in the oropharynx. Remind the patient not to use antiseptic mouthwash.

During

- For best results, obtain sputum collection when the patient awakens in the morning.
- Collect at least 1 teaspoon of sputum in a sterile sputum container.
- Obtain sputum by having the patient cough after taking several deep breaths.
- If the patient is unable to produce a sputum specimen, stimulate coughing by lowering the head of the patient's bed or by giving the patient an aerosol administration of a warm hypertonic solution.
- Note that other methods to collect sputum, such as endotracheal aspiration, fiberoptic bronchoscopy, and transtracheal aspiration, may be used if necessary.
- For AFB determinations, collect sputum on three separate occasions.

After

- Avoid personal contamination and wear gloves when handling all patient secretions.
- Tell the patient to notify the nurse as soon as the specimen is collected.
- Label the specimen and send it to the laboratory as soon as possible.
- Inform the patient that culture results may take 3 weeks or longer.

Test Results and Clinical Significance

Tuberculosis *Although tuberculosis is highly suspected when AFB is identified on a sputum smear, other organisms can cause positive AFB smears. They may include atypical mycobacteria and some fungi.*

Related Tests

- Tuberculosis culture (p. 687): This is the only manner in which the diagnosis of TB can be made with certainty. When TB is grown from the culture of a specimen, the diagnosis of TB can be made and treatment based on drug sensitivities can be started.
- TB skin testing (p. 1023): Purified protein derivative is administered intradermally to test for prior exposure to TB. Skin testing cannot indicate active or dormant TB. If positive, it just implies previous exposure.
- Chest radiography (p. 924): Because TB is usually infective to the lungs due to inhalation of airborne infectious material, the chest x-ray examination often demonstrates the results (Ghon complex) of the acute granulomatous infection.

Barr Body Analysis
(Sex Chromatin Body, Chromatin-Positive Body)

Normal Findings Depend on the gender of the child

Indications

This test is very easy to perform and is very inexpensive. It is used as a screening test for patients with ambiguous sex characteristics or delayed onset of puberty.

Test Explanation

Barr body (or Barr chromatin body) analysis studies may be performed when ambiguity of the newborn's genitalia makes assigning a gender to the infant difficult. This test is also done to detect sex chromosomal abnormalities, such as Turner's syndrome and Klinefelter's syndrome.

The Barr body is a chromatin mass derived from one of the X chromosomes (that is, the inactive sex chromosome). The Barr body is seen as a nucleolar satellite on histologic preparations. The number of Barr bodies is one less than the total number of X chromosomes in the cell nucleus. Therefore females (XX) normally have one Barr body and are considered to be chromatin positive; normal males (XY) have no Barr bodies and are chromatin negative. A female with Turner's syndrome (XO) would have no Barr body. These females are characterized by ovarian dysgenesis, amenorrhea, and the lack of secondary sexual maturation. A male with Klinefelter's syndrome (XXY) would have one Barr body. Klinefelter's syndrome is the most common form of male hypogonadism, which is caused by a chromosomal abnormality resulting in primary testicular failure. An XXX female would have two Barr bodies.

Scoring Barr bodies in the buccal mucosal cells is less costly than karyotype analysis (see p. 149), but the technical limitations of the test are considerable. For example, Y chromosome abnormalities cannot be identified. Because of the obvious benefit of a full cytogenic study, sex chromatin studies are less commonly performed.

Interfering Factors

- Buccal smear specimens may show false lowering of sex chromatin bodies if specimens are taken during the first week of life or during adrenocorticosteroid or estrogen therapy.
- Poor slide preparation can obscure the test results.

Procedure and Patient Care

Before

- Explain the procedure to the patient or parents.

During

- Note the following procedural steps:
  1. Sex chromatin analysis can be performed using any cell in the body. The most easily obtained cells are from the buccal mucosa. The oral mucosa is scraped, and the cells are smeared onto a glass slide.
  2. After chemical fixation and staining, the cells are studied.
  3. Assessment of the results, together with the secondary sexual characteristics and the genitalia of the patient, permits presumptive diagnosis of certain sex chromosomal abnormalities.
  4. If necessary, the results can be confirmed by chromosomal karyotyping (systematic arrangement of photographed chromosomes to demonstrate structure and number) (p. 149).
- Note that a buccal smear is performed by a technician in less than 5 minutes. A pathologist studies the slide smear.
- Tell the patient that no or minimal discomfort is associated with this test.

After

- Inform the patient how and when to obtain the test results.

Test Results and Clinical Significance

Chromosomal abnormalities (e.g., Turner's syndrome, Klinefelter's syndrome) *There are many variations in X chromosome numbers. Only one of the X chromosomes is active; the rest are inactive. Presence of a Y chromosome indicates male sex.*

Related Tests

- Chromosome karyotype (p. 149): This test is used to study an individual's chromosome makeup to determine chromosomal defects associated with disease or the risk of developing disease.

Blood Culture and Sensitivity (Blood C&S)

Normal Findings

Negative

Indications

Blood cultures are obtained to detect the presence of bacteria in the blood.

Test Explanation

Bacteremia (the presence of bacteria in the blood) can be intermittent and transient, except in endocarditis or suppurative thrombophlebitis. The episode of bacteremia is usually accompanied by chills and fever; thus the blood culture should be drawn when the patient manifests these signs to increase the chances of growing bacteria on the cultures. It is important that at least two culture specimens be obtained from two different sites. If one produces bacteria and the other does not, it is safe to assume that the bacteria in the first culture may be a contaminant and not the infecting agent. When both cultures grow the infecting agent, bacteremia exists and is due to the organism that is growing in the culture. If the patient is receiving antibiotics during the time that the cultures are drawn, the laboratory should be notified. Resin can be added to the culture medium to negate the antibiotic effect in inhibiting growth of the offending bacteria in the culture. If cultures are to be performed while the patient is on antibiotics, the blood culture specimen should be taken shortly before the next dose of the antibiotic is administered. All cultures preferably should be performed before antibiotic therapy is initiated.

Culture specimens drawn through an IV catheter are frequently contaminated, and tests using them should not be performed unless catheter sepsis is suspected. In these situations, blood culture specimens drawn through the catheter help to identify the causative agent more accurately than a culture specimen from the catheter tip.

Most organisms require approximately 24 hours to grow in the laboratory, and a preliminary report can be given at that time. Often 48 to 72 hours are required for growth and identification of the organism. Anaerobic organisms may take longer to grow. Cultures may be repeated after antibiotic therapy to assess resolution of the infection.

Interfering Factors

- Contamination of the blood specimen, especially by skin bacteria, may occur.
- Drugs that may alter test results include antibiotics.

Procedure and Patient Care

Before

- Explain the procedure to the patient.
- Tell the patient that no fasting is required.

During

- Carefully prepare the proposed venipuncture site with povidone-iodine (Betadine). Allow the skin to dry.
- Clean the tops of the Vacu-tainer tubes or culture bottles with povidone-iodine and allow them to dry. Some laboratories suggest cleaning with 70% alcohol after cleaning with Betadine and air drying.
- Collect approximately 10 to 15 ml of venous blood by venipuncture from each site in a 20-ml syringe.
- Discard the needle on the syringe and replace with a second, sterile needle before injecting the blood sample into the culture bottle.
- Inoculate the anaerobic bottle first if both anaerobic and aerobic cultures are needed.
- Mix gently after inoculation.
- Label the specimen with the patient's name, date, time, and tentative diagnosis.
- Indicate on the laboratory slip any medications that may affect test results.

After

- Transport the culture bottles immediately to the laboratory (or at least within 30 minutes).
- Notify the physician of any positive results so that appropriate antibiotic therapy can be initiated.

Test Results and Clinical Significance

Bacteremia *The bacteria growing in the blood can often be grown in the culture medium within the microbiology laboratory. When bacteremia exists, the patient must be considered gravely ill and antibiotics should be started immediately after blood cultures are obtained.*

Blood Smear (Peripheral Blood Smear, Red Blood Cell Morphology, RBC Smear)

Normal Findings

Normal quantity of RBCs, WBCs, and platelets
Normal size, shape, and color of RBCs
Normal WBC differential count

Indications

Examination of the peripheral blood smear can provide a significant amount of information concerning drugs and diseases that affect the RBCs and the WBCs. Furthermore, other congenital and acquired diseases can be diagnosed by an examination of the peripheral blood smear. When special stains are applied to the blood smear, leukemia, infection, infestation, and other diseases can be identified.

Test Explanation

When adequately prepared and examined microscopically by an experienced technologist and pathologist, a smear of peripheral blood is the most informative of all hematologic tests. All three hematologic cell lines–erythrocytes (RBCs), platelets, and leukocytes (WBCs)–can be examined. In the peripheral blood, five different types of leukocytes can routinely be identified–neutrophils, eosinophils, basophils, lymphocytes, and monocytes. The first three are also referred to as granulocytes. (See discussion of bone marrow biopsy on p. 644 for more information concerning the various elements of blood.)

Microscopic examination of the RBCs can reveal variations in RBC size (anisocytosis), shape (poikilocytosis), color, or intracellular content. Classification of RBCs according to these variables is most helpful in identifying the causes of anemia and the presence of other diseases.

RBC size abnormalities

Microcytes (small RBCs)
- Iron deficiency
- Hereditary spherocytosis
- Thalassemia

Macrocytes (larger size)
- Vitamin B_{12} or folic acid deficiency
- Reticulocytosis secondary to increased erythropoiesis (RBC production)
- Occasional liver disorder
- Postsplenectomy anemia

RBC shape abnormalities

Spherocytes (small and round)
- Hereditary spherocytosis
- Acquired immunohemolytic anemia

Elliptocytes (crescent or sickle shaped)
- Hereditary elliptocytosis
- Sickle cell anemia

Leptocytes, or "target cells" (thin cells with less hemoglobin)
- Hemoglobinopathies
- Thalassemia

Spicule cell
- Uremia
- Liver disease
- Bleeding ulcer

RBC color abnormalities

Hypochromasia (pale)
- Iron deficiency

Thalassemia
Cardiac disease
Hyperchromasia (more colored)
Concentrated hemoglobin, usually caused by dehydration

RBC intracellular structure

Nucleus–In normal RBC maturation the nucleus is lost. When increased RBC production is required (e.g., in anemia or chronic hypoxemia), the marrow floods the peripheral blood with immature nucleated forms of RBCs called normoblasts. The presence of normoblasts is considered "normal" for an infant's blood.
Physiologic response to RBC deficiency (as in hemolytic anemias, sickle cell crisis, transfusion reaction, and erythroblastosis fetalis)
Physiologic response to hypoxemia (as in congenital heart disease and congestive heart failure)
Marrow-occupying neoplasm or fibrotic tissue (as in myeloma and leukemia)
Basophilic stippling (refers to bodies enclosed or included in the cytoplasm of the RBCs)
Lead poisoning
Reticulocytosis
Howell-Jolly bodies (small, round remnants of nuclear material remaining within the RBC)
After a surgical splenectomy
Hemolytic anemia
Megaloblastic anemia
Heinz bodies (small, irregular particles of hemoglobin)
Drug-induced RBC injury
Hemoglobinopathies
Hemolytic anemia
G-6-PD deficiency

The WBCs are examined for total quantity, differential count, and degree of maturity. An increased number of immature WBCs may indicate leukemia. A decreased WBC count indicates failure of marrow to produce WBCs, resulting from drugs, chronic disease, neoplasia, or fibrosis. Finally, an experienced cell examiner also can estimate platelet number (p. 337) on a peripheral blood smear.

Procedure and Patient Care

Before

- Explain the procedure to the patient.
- Tell the patient that no fasting is required.

During

- Collect a drop of blood from a finger stick or heel stick and place it on a slide.
- If necessary, perform a venipuncture and collect the blood in a lavender-top tube.
- Note that a blood smear is first studied with an automated calculator programmed to recognize abnormal blood cell shapes and so on. A more accurate smear is performed by a technologist. Low counts may be "hand counted" to ensure accuracy. The most accurate smear requires review by a pathologist.

After

- Apply pressure or a pressure dressing to the venipuncture site.
- Assess the venipuncture site for bleeding.

Test Results and Clinical Significance

See the list in "Test Explanation."

Related Tests

- Complete blood count and differential count (p. 162): This is a battery of tests performed on the peripheral blood to measure the quantity of each blood component.
- Bone marrow biopsy (see below): This is a test on the bone marrow, which forms the components of the peripheral blood.

Bone Marrow Biopsy (Bone Marrow Examination, Bone Marrow Aspiration)

Normal Findings

Active erythroid cell line, myeloid and lymphoid cell lines, and megakaryocyte (platelet) production:

Cell Type	Range (%)
Myeloblasts	<5
Promyelocytes	1-8
Myelocytes	
Neutrophilic	5-15
Eosinophilic	0.5-3
Basophilic	<1
Metamyelocytes	
Neutrophilic	15-25
Eosinophilic	<1
Basophilic	<1
Mature myelocytes	
Neutrophilic	10-30
Eosinophilic	<5
Basophilic	<5
Mononuclear	
Monocytes	<5
Lymphocytes	3-20
Plasma cells	<1
Megakaryocytes	<5
Ratio of myeloid (WBC) to erythroid (RBC) cells (M/E ratio)	<4:1
Normoblasts	25-50
Normal iron content demonstrated by staining with Prussian blue	

Indications

Bone marrow examination is an important part of the evaluation of patients with hematologic diseases. Indications for bone marrow examination include the following:

1. To confirm the diagnosis of megaloblastic anemia
2. To diagnose leukemia or myeloma
3. To determine if the marrow is the cause of reduced blood cells in the peripheral bloodstream
4. To document deficient iron stores
5. To document bone marrow infiltrative diseases (neoplasm or fibrosis)

It is also used as staging testing for lymphomas.

Test Explanation

The bone marrow is located in the central fatty core of cancellous bone (sternum, rib, and pelvis) and the long bones (femur, tibia and humerus). There the blood-forming cells produce the blood cells and release them into the circulation (Figure 2-18, p. 457).

By examination of a bone marrow specimen the hematologist can fully evaluate hematopoiesis. Examination of the bone marrow reveals the number, size, and shape of the RBCs, WBCs, and megakaryocytes (platelet precursors) as these cells evolve through their various stages of development in the bone marrow. Samples of the bone marrow can be obtained by either aspiration or surgical removal. The latter reveals more information. Also, with aspiration a "dry tap" may occur because there is very little cellular activity or because the cells are too tightly packed to aspirate through a needle. A bone marrow biopsy is required under those circumstances to obtain marrow tissue. Microscopic examination includes estimation of cellularity, determination of the presence of fibrotic tissue or neoplasms (both primary and metastatic), and estimation of iron storage.

For the estimation of cellularity the specimen is examined and the relative quantity of each cell type determined. This is more accurately performed on a biopsy specimen than on an aspirate because the aspirate may not be truly representative of the entire marrow. Leukemias or leukemoid drug reactions are suspected when increased numbers of leukocyte precursors are present. Physiologic marrow leukemoid compensation for infection also will be recognized by finding an increased number of leukocyte precursors. Decreased numbers of marrow leukocyte precursors occur in patients with myelofibrosis, metastatic neoplasia, or agranulocytosis; in elderly patients; and following radiation therapy or chemotherapy.

Increased numbers of marrow RBC precursors occur with polycythemia vera or as physiologic compensation to hemorrhagic or hemolytic anemias. Decreased numbers of marrow RBC precursors occur with erythroid hypoplasia following chemotherapy, radiation therapy, administration of other toxic drugs, iron deficiency, or marrow replacement by fibrotic tissue or neoplasms.

Increased numbers of platelet precursors (megakaryocytes) are seen in the marrow of patients who are compensating after an episode of acute hemorrhage. They are also seen in some forms of chronic myeloid leukemia. This increase also may be compensatory in patients with secondary hypersplenism associated with portal hypertension or other conditions. In these patients the spleen prematurely extracts platelets from the circulation. Platelet counts decrease, and the marrow compensates by increasing production. Decreased numbers of megakaryocytes occur in patients who have had radiation therapy, chemotherapy, or other drug therapy and in patients with neoplastic or fibrotic marrow infiltrative diseases. Patients with aplastic anemia also have decreased numbers of megakaryocytes.

Increased numbers of lymphocyte precursors occur in chronic, viral, or mycoplasma infections (e.g., mononucleosis), lymphocytic leukemia, and lymphoma. Plasma cells (plasmocytes) are increased in number in patients with multiple myelomas, Hodgkin's disease, hypersensitivity states, rheumatic fever, and other chronic inflammatory diseases.

Estimation of cellularity also can be expressed as a ratio of myeloid (WBC) to erythroid (RBC) cells (M/E ratio). The normal M/E ratio is approximately 3:1. The M/E ratio is greater than normal in those diseases mentioned previously in which increased leukocyte precursors are present or erythroid precursors are decreased. The M/E ratio is below normal when either leukocyte precursors are decreased or erythroid precursors are increased. A more detailed list of diseases affecting the M/E ratio can be found in most hematology textbooks.

Drug-induced or idiopathic myelofibrosis can be detected by examination of the bone marrow. Using special stains, one can estimate iron stores with a marrow biopsy. Although fibrosis or neoplasia occasionally can be detected in aspiration studies, biopsy is the best method. Leukemias, multiple myelomas, and polycythemia vera can easily be detected in biopsy specimens. Similarly, lymphomas and other metastatic tumors (e.g., cancers of the breast, kidney, lung) can be seen. Bone marrow biopsy is an important part of staging for lymphomas and Hodgkin's disease.

Bone marrow aspiration is performed by a trained nurse or physician. Bone marrow biopsy-specimen removal is usually performed by a physician. The duration of these studies is approximately 20 minutes. The patient may have some apprehension when pressure is applied to puncture the outer table of the bone during biopsy-specimen removal or aspiration. The patient probably will feel pain during lidocaine infiltration and pressure when the syringe plunger is withdrawn for aspiration.

Contraindications

- Patients with acute coagulation disorders, because of the risk of excessive bleeding
- Patients who cannot cooperate and remain still during the procedure

Potential Complications

- Hemorrhage, especially if the patient has a coagulopathy
- Infection, especially if the patient is leukopenic
- Sternal fracture as a result of too aggressive application of pressure to the sternum at the time of biopsy
- Inadvertent puncture of the heart or great vessels when the test is performed on the sternum

Procedure and Patient Care

Before

- Explain the procedure to the patient.
- Obtain a written and informed consent for this procedure.

CLINICAL PRIORITIES

- Assess the results of the coagulation studies prior to bone marrow biopsy. Patients with coagulation disorders cannot have this procedure because of the risk of excessive bleeding.
- It is essential that patients remain still and cooperate during this invasive procedure.
- During bone marrow aspiration, most patients feel pain during lidocaine infiltration and pressure when the syringe plunger is withdrawn for aspiration.

- Encourage the patient to verbalize fears because many patients are anxious concerning this study.
- Assess the results of the coagulation studies. Report any evidence of coagulopathy to the physician.
- Obtain an order for sedatives if the patient appears extremely apprehensive.
- Remind the patient to remain very still throughout the procedure.

During

- Note the following procedural steps for *bone marrow aspiration,* which is performed on the sternum, iliac crest, anterior or posterior iliac spines, and proximal tibia (in children):
  1. The procedure is usually performed at the patient's bedside using local anesthesia.
  2. A preferred site is the posterior iliac crest, with the patient placed prone or on the side.
  3. The area overlying the bone is prepared and draped in a sterile manner.
  4. The overlying skin and soft tissue, along with the periosteum, is infiltrated with lidocaine.
  5. A large-bore needle containing a stylus is slowly advanced through the soft tissue and into the outer table of the bone (Figure 7-1).

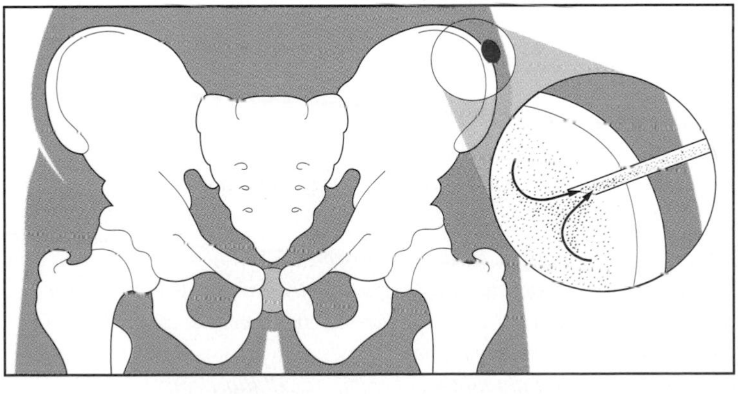

Figure 7-1 Aspiration of bone marrow.

6. Once inside the marrow the stylus is removed and a syringe is attached.
7. One-half to 2 ml of bone marrow is aspirated, smeared on slides, and allowed to dry.
8. The slides are sprayed with a preservative and taken to the pathology laboratory.

- Note the following procedural steps for *bone marrow biopsy:*

1. The skin and soft tissues overlying the bone are incised.
2. A core biopsy instrument is "screwed" into the bone.
3. The biopsy specimen is obtained and sent to the pathology laboratory for analysis.

After

- Apply pressure to the puncture site to arrest minimal bleeding.
- Apply an adhesive bandage.
- Observe the puncture site for bleeding.
- Ice packs may be used to help control bleeding.
- Assess for tenderness and erythema, which may indicate infection. Report this to the physician.
- Evaluate the patient for signs of shock (increased pulse rate, decreased blood pressure).
- Normally, place the patient on bed rest for 30 to 60 minutes after the test.
- Note that some patients complain of tenderness at the puncture site for several days after this study. Mild analgesics may be ordered.

Home Care Responsibilities

- Instruct the patient to observe the puncture site for bleeding.
- Inform the patient that tenderness and erythema may indicate infection. This should be reported to the physician.
- Mild analgesics may be needed for several days after this procedure for complaints of tenderness at the puncture site.

Test Results and Clinical Significance

Neoplasm
Myelofibrosis
Infiltrative diseases are evident histologically as to the specific cause and by demonstrating hypocellularity within the marrow.

Infection–viral, bacterial, fungal *Bacterial infection is usually associated with increased neutrophilic elements. However, in overwhelming sepsis, these elements may be depressed. Viral and some fungal infections are characterized by increases in monocytic elements.*

Agranulocytosis *The marrow has no myeloblast cells.*

Polycythemia vera *There is an abundance of erythroid cellular elements.*

Multiple myelomas
Hodgkin's disease
Lymphoma
These cancers may be associated with overwhelming presence of mononuclear elements within the marrow.

Leukemia *The myeloid precursor cells are significantly increased and crowd the marrow.*
Hypersensitivity states *This may be evident as an increase in eosinophilic and basophilic myeloblast elements.*
Acute hemorrhagic marrow hyperplasia *Following an acute hemorrhage, the erythroid (and to some extent, the myeloid) elements are greatly increased to compensate for the loss of cells in the peripheral blood system.*
Anemia *If the anemia is due to marrow failure, erythroid precursors will be deficient in number. Specifics about the appearance of the marrow cells (e.g., megaloblasts in B_{12} deficiency) may indicate the cause of the marrow failure. Special stains may reveal deficient iron storage, etc.*

Chronic inflammatory disease
Rheumatic fever
Mononuclear precursor elements may be increased.

AIDS *Decreased leukocytic elements may be noted, especially as the disease progresses.*

Related Tests

- Complete blood count (CBC) and differential count (p. 162): This is a measurement of the number and relative percentages of the myeloid, erythroid, and platelet elements in the peripheral bloodstream.

Chlamydia

Normal Findings

Negative culture
Antibodies: immunoglobulin test <1:640

Indications

Chlamydia testing is performed on patients with symptoms compatible with the wide variety of diseases this organism can cause. In the United States, its most common form is pelvic inflammatory disease. This form of sexually transmitted disease commonly presents as pelvic pain and/or vaginal discharge. Cervical cultures or smears are performed on patients who have these complaints.

Test Explanation

There are many *Chlamydia* species that cause various diseases within the human body. *Chlamydia psittaci* causes respiratory tract infections and occurs with close contact with infected birds. *C. pneumoniae,* another species, causes pneumonia. *C. trachomatis* infection is probably the most frequently occurring sexually transmitted disease in developed countries. Infections of the genitalia are most common, followed by those of the conjunctiva, pharynx, urethra, and rectum. Lymphogranuloma venereum was the first form of venereal disease recognized as a *C. trachomatis* infection; this infection is very common in central Africa. The second serotype of *C. trachomatis* causes the eye disease *trachoma,* which is the most common form of preventable blindness. A third serotype produces genital and urethral infections different from lymphogranuloma. This third type is transmitted by direct contact of the infant with the mother's cervix during vaginal delivery or by direct contact during sexual activity.

Chlamydia infection is thought to be the most widespread sexually transmitted disease in the United States. This disease is most prevalent in those younger than 20 years, in nulliparas, and in users of nonbarrier contraceptive methods. Also, in those with multiple or recent, new sexual partners, *Chlamydia* is frequently associated with gonorrhea.

Most women colonized with *Chlamydia* are asymptomatic. *Chlamydia* may be associated with pelvic inflammatory disease, particularly in adolescents.

In recognition of the rapidly increasing occurrence of *Chlamydia,* strategies to monitor prevalence, control its spread, and educate the public have been proposed. These strategies include screening all at-risk groups, particularly sexually active adolescents and those with other sexually transmitted diseases. Evaluation of those with signs and symptoms of exposure, as well as potential treatment of all females at high risk for *Chlamydia* disease, has also been proposed.

The *Chlamydia* organism can be detected in many different ways. It seems to be most accurately demonstrated by tissue culture. Although these cultures require a special cell culture line, which takes several days, they are used as the gold standard against which other methods of detection of *Chlamydia* are measured. It is now possible to detect the antigen by direct fluorescent antibody slide staining and enzyme-linked immunosorbent assay (ELISA) technique. These newer techniques are less expensive and more widely available than culture techniques; however, their sensitivity and specificity are lower.

Invasive infection with *C. trachomatis* does produce an immunogenic response. Therefore *Chlamydia* antibodies can be measured using complement fixation, microimmunofluorescence, and ELISA techniques. When a fourfold rise in IgG titer or the presence of specific IgM antibodies is documented, *Chlamydia* disease may be diagnosed.

Interfering Factors

- Women presently having their routine menses
- Patients undergoing antibiotic therapy

Procedure and Patient Care

Before

- Explain the procedure to the patient.
- Note that many different methods are used to perform chlamydial tests.

During

- Collect venous blood in a red-top tube.

CLINICAL PRIORITIES

- Due to the rapidly increasing prevalence of *Chlamydia,* screening should take place in all at-risk groups, particularly sexually active adolescents and those with other sexually transmitted diseases.
- Females are evaluated for *Chlamydia* by cervical cultures, and males are evaluated by urethral cultures.
- All affected patients should be treated with antibiotics. Sexual partners should be evaluated.

- Acute and convalescent serum should be drawn 2 to 3 weeks apart.
- A conjunctival smear is obtained by swabbing the eye lesion with a cotton-tipped applicator or scraping with a sterile ophthalmic spatula and smearing on a clean glass slide.
- Sputum cultures (p. 681) are used to check for *C. psittaci* respiratory infections.
- Note the following procedural steps:

Cervical Culture

1. The female patient should refrain from douching and bathing in a tub before the cervical culture is performed.
2. The patient is placed in the lithotomy position.
3. A nonlubricated vaginal speculum is inserted to expose the cervix.
4. The mucus is removed from the squamocolumnar junction of the cervix.
5. A sterile, cotton-tipped swab is inserted into the endocervical canal and moved from side to side for 30 seconds to obtain the culture.

Urethral Culture

1. The urethral specimen should be obtained from the man before voiding.
2. A culture is taken by gently inserting a sterile thin swab 3 to 4 cm into the urethra.

- Note that these tests are performed by a physician or nurse in several minutes.
- Tell the patient that minimal discomfort is associated with these procedures.

After

- Treat patients who have positive smears with antibiotics.
- Tell affected patients to have their sexual partners examined.

Test Results and Clinical Significance

Chlamydia infections *This organism causes many different diseases, as indicated in "Test Explanation." In the United States, this is the most significant sexually transmitted infection.*

Related Tests

- Sexually transmitted disease culture (p. 677): Discussed here are other sexually transmitted diseases and their causative agents.

Cutaneous Immunofluorescence Biopsy
(Immunofluorescence Skin Biopsy, Skin Biopsy Antibodies, Skin Immunohistopathology)

Normal Findings Normal skin histology

Indications

This test of inflamed skin is performed to evaluate and diagnose immunologically mediated dermatitis. It is indicated when an immunologic source for a skin rash is suspected.

Test Explanation

For this study a skin biopsy is obtained and evaluated by immunofluorescence methods. Deposition of human immunoglobulins and/or complement components is determined by immunofluorescent patterns. This test is useful in detecting immune complexes, complement, and immunoglobulin skin deposition in systemic and discoid lupus erythematosus, pemphigus, bullous pemphigoid, and dermatitis herpetiformis. This test is also used to confirm the histopathology of skin lesions and to monitor the results of treatment.

Procedure and Patient Care

Before

- Explain the procedure to the patient.
- Obtain an informed consent.

During

- A 4-mm punch biopsy or elliptical tissue excision is obtained.

After

- Apply a dry, sterile dressing over the biopsy site.
- Tell the patient that results may not be available for several days.
- Deliver the specimen on ice to the laboratory immediately after the biopsy is taken.

Test Results and Clinical Significance

Systemic lupus erythematosus (SLE)
Discoid lupus erythematosus
Lupus erythematosus is associated with acute, subacute, and chronic skin lesions. All are associated with deposits of immunoglobulins and complement in the epidermal basement membrane zone. The acute changes are represented by the butterfly rash of SLE. Subacute changes of SLE are represented by photosensitive ulcers. The chronic changes of discoid lupus are scalelike changes about the neck and face. Once the scale is removed, an ulcer remains until healing and scarring occur.

Pemphigus
Bullous pemphigoid
These immunologic dermatitis diseases are highlighted clinically as subepidermal blistering of skin, usually in the elderly.

Dermatitis herpetiformis *This urticarial immunologic dermatitis is often associated with gluten-sensitive enteropathy.*

Endometrial Biopsy

Normal Findings

No pathologic conditions
Presence of a "secretory-type" endometrium 3 to 5 days before normal menses

Indications

Endometrial biopsy can determine if the patient has adequate ovarian estrogen and progesterone levels. This is indicated in women who are suspected of having ovarian dysfunction (such as women who are nearing menopause, nonmenstruating, or infertile). Furthermore, it is used to evaluate women who have dysfunctional uterine bleeding.

Test Explanation

An endometrial biopsy can determine whether ovulation has occurred. A biopsy specimen taken 3 to 5 days before normal menses should demonstrate a "secretory-type" endometrium on histologic examination if ovulation and corpus luteum formation have occurred. If not, only a preovulatory "proliferative-type" endometrium will be seen.

Occasionally an endometrial biopsy is performed to indicate estrogen's effect in patients with suspected ovarian dysfunction or suspected menopause. Similarly, adequate circulating progesterone levels can be determined by identifying secretory endometrium. Another major use of endometrial biopsy is to diagnose endometrial cancer, polyps, or inflammatory conditions and to evaluate uterine bleeding.

This procedure is performed by an obstetrician/gynecologist in approximately 10 to 30 minutes. Minor discomfort (menstrual type of cramping) may be felt. It is important to recognize that an endometrial biopsy is not a substitute for a dilation and curettage (D&C). The D&C is much more extensive and tests all surfaces of the endometrium.

Contraindications

- Patients with infections (e.g., trichomonal, candidal, suspected gonococcal) of the cervix or vagina, because the infection may spread to the uterus
- Patients in whom the cervix cannot be visualized (e.g., due to abnormal position or previous surgery), because the cervix is the access to the uterus

Potential Complications

- Perforation of the uterus
- Uterine bleeding
- Interference with early pregnancy
- Infection

Procedure and Patient Care

Before

- Explain the procedure to the patient.
- Ensure that written and informed consent for this procedure is obtained from the patient.
- Tell the patient that no fasting or sedation is usually required.

During

- Note the following procedural steps:
  1. The patient is placed in the lithotomy position, and a pelvic examination is performed to determine the position of the uterus.
  2. The cervix is exposed and cleansed.
  3. A biopsy instrument is inserted into the uterus, and specimens are obtained from the anterior, posterior, and lateral walls. The biopsy can be done with a curette, suction device, or forceps. Suction endometrial biopsy is most commonly performed because it is the least painful and can be performed in the office.
  4. The specimens are placed in a solution containing 10% formalin and sent to the pathologist for histologic examination.

After

- Any temperature elevation should be reported to the physician because this procedure may activate pelvic inflammatory disease.
- Advise the patient to wear a pad because some vaginal bleeding is to be expected.
- Instruct the patient to call her physician if excessive bleeding (requiring more than one pad per hour) occurs.
- Inform the patient that douching and intercourse are not permitted for 72 hours after the biopsy.
- Instruct the patient to rest during the next 24 hours and to avoid heavy lifting to prevent increased intraabdominal pressure and uterine hemorrhage.

Home Care Responsibilities

- Instruct the patient to report any temperature elevation to her physician because this procedure may activate pelvic inflammatory disease.
- Advise the patient to wear a sanitary pad after this procedure because some vaginal bleeding is expected. Tell the patient to call her physician for excessive bleeding (more than one pad per hour).
- Tell the patient to avoid heavy lifting after this procedure to prevent increased intraabdominal pressure and possible uterine bleeding.

Test Results and Clinical Significance

Anovulation *Without ovulation the endometrium is persistently in the proliferative stage. No secretory changes are noted.*

Tumor

Polyps

Endometrial adenocarcinoma with or without squamous carcinoma components is the most common uterine cancer. Hyperplastic proliferative polyps are a common cause of dysfunctional uterine bleeding.

Inflammatory condition *Endometrial infections are rare but do occur. Ascending sexually transmitted diseases are the most common type of primary infection not associated with prior surgical instrumentation.*

Estrogen Receptor Assay
(ER Assay, ERA, Estradiol Receptor)

Normal Findings

Negative: ≤10 fmol/mg of protein
Positive: >10 fmol/mg of protein

Indications

Estrogen receptor assay is performed on breast cancer tissue to indicate tumor sensitivity to hormonal manipulative therapy and to indicate prognosis of breast cancer.

Test Explanation

The ER assay is useful in determining the prognosis and treatment of breast cancer. The assay is used to determine whether a tumor is likely to respond to endocrine medical therapy or to removal of the ovaries or adrenal gland. Tumors with a positive ER assay are more than twice as likely to respond to endocrine therapy than an ER-negative tumor. Hormone receptor assays should be done on all primary or recurrent breast carcinomas. Levels tend to be higher in postmenopausal women than in premenopausal women. In general, ER-positive tumors have a better prognosis than ER-negative tumors. ER status is now being evaluated on other gynecologic tumors, but its exact role in these patients has yet to be defined.

Slightly over 50% of patients with breast carcinoma who are ER positive respond to endocrine therapy (e.g., tamoxifen, estrogens, androgens, oophorectomy, adrenalectomy). The response is greater when the progesterone receptors (p. 672) are also positive. Patients whose breast cancers lack these hormone receptors (are ER negative) have a much lower chance of tumor response to hormone therapy and may not be candidates for this form of treatment.

Specimens are obtained by the pathologist from surgical specimens. One gram of fresh tissue used to be required. Now an ER assay can be performed by immunohistochemical methods on fixed, paraffin-embedded tissue or microscope slides. With these newer methods, much less tissue is required for assay.

Interfering Factors

- Delay in tissue fixation may cause deterioration of receptor proteins and produce lower values.
- ✗ Hormones should be discontinued before breast biopsy is performed. Antiestrogen preparations (e.g., tamoxifen [Nolvadex]) during the past 2 months may cause false-negative ER assays.
- ✗ Exogenous hormones that are taken for contraceptive purposes or menopausal hormone replacement therapy may produce lower receptor values.

Procedure and Patient Care

Before

- Explain the biopsy procedure to the patient.
- Before biopsy obtain a gynecologic history, including menopausal status and exogenous hormone use.

During

- The surgeon obtains tumor tissue.
- Place this tissue on ice, and immediately transfer it to the pathology department.
- Note that part of the tissue is used for routine histologic examination, and at least 1 g is frozen for receptor status.
- The frozen specimen is sent (in dry ice) to a central laboratory for ER analysis.
- If immunohistochemical methods of ER assay are used, the specimen is fixed as soon as it arrives at the lab. Fixed tissue is then sent for testing.

After

- Results are usually available in 2 weeks.

Test Results and Clinical Significance

Estrogen receptor positive *This cancer is more likely to be successfully treated with hormone manipulation in a therapeutic or adjuvant clinical setting.*

Related Tests

- Progesterone receptor assay (p. 672): Like estrogen receptor assay, this test predicts the likelihood of tumor response to endocrine manipulative therapy.

Herpes Simplex
(Herpesvirus Type 2, Herpes Simplex Virus Type 1 & 2 [HSV 1 & 2], Herpes Genitalis)

Normal Findings

No virus present
No HSV antigens or antibodies present

Indications

Herpes testing is performed to diagnose acute initial herpes infections. It is used on patients suspected of having an initial genital infection. It is also used in immunocompromised patients who have aggressive oral mucosal or genital eruptions compatible with the infection. Furthermore, it is used on patients (especially immunocompromised patients) who have a fever of unknown origin.

Herpes cultures are used to identify active genital herpes infection in women who are expecting to vaginally deliver a baby in the next 6 to 8 weeks.

Test Explanation

Herpes simplex virus can be classified as either type 1 or type 2. *Type 1* is primarily responsible for oral lesions (blisters on the lips–"cold sores") or even corneal lesions. About half of the patients with HSV 1 develop recurrent infections. *HSV 2* is a sexually transmitted viral infection of the urogenital tract. Vesicular lesions may occur on the penis, scrotum, vulva, perineum, perianal region, vagina, or cervix. Initial infections are often associated with generalized symptoms of fever, malaise, and so on.

Because most infants become infected if they pass through a birth canal containing HSV, determining its presence at delivery is necessary. Congenital infections may result in problems such as microcephaly, chorioretinitis, and mental retardation in the newborn. Disseminated neonatal herpesvirus infections carry a high incidence of infant mortality. A vaginal delivery is possible if no virus is present, and birth by cesarean section is needed if HSV is present. Viral testing can be performed on males or females to determine the risk of sexual transmission.

Culture is still the gold standard for HSV detection and can identify HSV in 90% of infected patients. Serologic tests are more easily and conveniently available for detection of HSV 1 and HSV 2 antigen. Unfortunately, the accuracy is not high. Only about 85% of patients who are culture positive have positive serologic results. The advantage of antigen tests is that results can be available in a day. Serologic tests for antibodies are cumbersome because they require repeated blood tests during the acute and convalescent phases of an acute viral outbreak (about 2 weeks apart). A fourfold rise in titer is expected to diagnose acute initial herpes infection. Recurrent infections are far less likely to demonstrate titer elevations. Furthermore, perhaps more than 50% of people in the United States have positive herpes antibodies. The antigen tests are done by fluorescent immunoassay or latex agglutination. The antibody tests use immunofluorescent immunoassay or enzyme-linked immunosorbent assay (ELISA) methods. Antibody testing

CLINICAL PRIORITIES

- Neonatal herpes virus infections carry a high incidence of infant mortality. A cesarean delivery may be needed if HSV is present in the pregnant mother.
- Women should refrain from douching and tub bathing 24 hours before the cervical culture.
- Men should not urinate within 1 hour of a urethral culture because voiding washes secretions out of the urethra.
- If herpes is diagnosed, it should be treated and sexual partners should be evaluated. Although acute outbreaks of herpes genitalis are treatable, this disease is not curable.

cannot diagnose whether or not there is active recurrent genital herpes. Culture testing is required to diagnose recurrent active disease.

Procedure and Patient Care

Before

- Explain the procedure to the patient.
- Tell the female patient to refrain from douching and tub bathing before the cervical culture is performed.
- Obtain the urethral specimen from the male patient before voiding.
- Note that blood study results can be diagnostic in both males and females.

During

- Obtain cultures as follows:

Urethral Culture

1. A culture is taken by inserting a sterile swab gently into the anterior urethra or genital skin lesion of the male patient.
2. It is advisable to place the male patient in the supine position to prevent falling if vasovagal syncope occurs during introduction of the cotton swab or wire loop into the urethra.
3. The patient is observed for hypotension, bradycardia, pallor, sweating, nausea, and weakness.

Cervical Culture

1. The female patient is placed in the lithotomy position, and a vaginal speculum is inserted.
2. Cervical mucus is removed with a cotton ball.
3. A sterile cotton-tipped swab is inserted into the endocervical canal and moved from side to side to obtain the culture. If a genital lesion is present, swabs from that area will be more sensitive in indicating infection.

- For *pregnant women with herpes genitalis,* note that the cervix is cultured weekly for the herpesvirus beginning 4 to 6 weeks before the due date. Vaginal delivery is possible if the following criteria are met:

1. The two most recent cultures are negative.
2. The woman is not experiencing any symptoms.
3. No lesions are visible on inspection of the vagina and vulva.
4. Throughout pregnancy the woman has not had more than one positive culture, during which she was symptom free.

Blood for Serologic Study

- Obtain 5 to 7 ml of blood in a red-top tube.

After

- Inform the patient how to obtain the test results.

Test Results and Clinical Significance

Herpes virus infection *Like other STDs, this can significantly impact patients, their children, and their sexual partners. If herpes or other STDs have been diagnosed, treatment should begin immediately and active sexual partners should be evaluated. Although acute outbreaks of herpes genitalis are treatable, the disease is not curable.*

Related Tests

- STD culture (p. 677): Discussed here are other sexually transmitted diseases and their causative agents.

Other STDs are discussed separately:

- *Chlamydia* (p. 649)
- Syphilis detection (p. 403)
- Hepatitis virus studies (p. 260)
- AIDS serology (p. 30)

Liver Biopsy

Normal Findings Normal liver histology

Indications

Liver biopsy is a safe, simple, and valuable method of diagnosing pathologic liver conditions.

Test Explanation

For this study a specially designed needle is inserted through the abdominal wall and into the liver. A piece of liver tissue is removed for microscopic examination. Percutaneous liver biopsy is used in the diagnosis of various liver disorders, such as cirrhosis, hepatitis, drug reaction, granuloma, and tumor. Biopsy is indicated for the following:

1. Patients with unexplained hepatomegaly
2. Patients with persistently elevated liver enzyme levels
3. Patients with suspected primary or metastatic tumor, as determined by other studies
4. Patients with unexplained jaundice
5. Patients with suspected hepatitis
6. Patient with suspected infiltrative diseases (e.g., sarcoidosis, amyloidosis)

The biopsy may be performed by a "blind" stick or may be directed with the use of a computed tomography (CT) or magnetic resonance imaging scan or laparoscopy. Directed biopsy is used if there is a specific focal area of the liver that is suspect and from which tissue must be obtained (e.g., a metastatic tumor). The "blind" stick is used if the liver is diffusely involved.

This test is performed by a physician in approximately 15 minutes. Minor discomfort may be experienced during injection of the local anesthetic and during needle insertion and biopsy. In the past, blind biopsies were performed with small aspiration or small tissue sampling needles. With the development of guided biopsies, larger core needles can obtain a significant amount of tissue for histologic review. This has reduced sampling errors both in placing the needle in the suspicious area and in obtaining enough tissue for histologic study.

Contraindications

- Uncooperative patients who cannot remain still and hold their breath during sustained exhalation
- Patients with impaired hemostasis
- Patients with anemia who could not tolerate major blood loss associated with inadvertent puncture of an intrahepatic blood vessel
- Patients with infections in the right pleural space or right upper quadrant, because the biopsy may spread the infection
- Patients with obstructive jaundice
  In these patients, bile within the ducts is under pressure and may subsequently leak into the abdominal cavity after needle penetration.
- Patients with a hemangioma
  This is a very vascular tumor, and bleeding after a biopsy may be severe.
- Patients with ascites, because persistent leak of fluid may occur
  Further bile leaks will not seal off.

✓ CLINICAL PRIORITIES

- Assess the coagulation profile prior to performing a liver biopsy because of the possibility of bleeding.
- After the liver biopsy, instruct the patient to remain on the right side for about 1 to 2 hours. This position decreases the risk of hemorrhage by compressing the liver capsule against the chest wall.
- Carefully evaluate the patient after this test for evidence of hemorrhage (increased pulse rate, decreased blood pressure) and peritonitis (increased temperature).

Potential Complications

- Hemorrhage caused by inadvertent puncture of a blood vessel within the liver
- Chemical peritonitis caused by inadvertent puncture of a bile duct, with subsequent leakage of bile into the abdominal cavity
- Pneumothorax (collapsed lung) caused by improper placement of the biopsy needle into the adjacent chest cavity

Procedure and Patient Care

Before

- Explain the procedure to the patient. Many patients are apprehensive about this procedure.
- Obtain an informed consent.
- Ensure that all coagulation test results are normal.
- Instruct the patient to keep on NPO status after midnight on the day of the test. Surgery may be necessary if a complication occurs. The patient must be prepared for the potential of surgery.
- Administer any sedative medications as ordered.

During

- Note the following procedural steps:
  1. The patient is placed in the supine or left lateral position.
  2. The skin area used for puncture is anesthetized locally.
  3. The patient is asked to exhale and hold the exhalation. This causes the liver to descend and reduces the possibility of a pneumothorax. Frequently the patient practices exhalation two or three times before insertion of the needle.
  4. During the patient's sustained exhalation the physician rapidly introduces the biopsy needle into the liver and obtains liver tissue.
     a. Several types of needles are available
     b. Often the biopsy needle is inserted under CT guidance. This is especially useful when tissue from a specific area of the liver is needed.
  5. The needle is withdrawn from the liver.
- If laparoscopy is used to obtain the biopsy, follow the procedure outlined for laparoscopy (p. 545).

After

- Place the tissue sample into a specimen bottle containing formalin and send it to the pathology department.
- Apply a small dressing over the needle insertion site.
- Place the patient on his or her right side for approximately 1 to 2 hours. In this position the liver capsule is compressed against the chest wall, thereby decreasing the risk of hemorrhage or bile leak.
- Assess the patient's vital signs frequently for evidence of hemorrhage (increased pulse rate, decreased blood pressure) and peritonitis (increased temperature).
- If laparoscopy was performed, provide routine postoperative care.

Test Results and Clinical Significance

Benign tumor (adenoma)
Malignant tumor
Primary (hepatoma, cholangiocarcinoma)
Metastatic (bowel, breast, lung, etc.)
Biopsies of these focal lesions can be performed and specimens obtained for histologic study. Usually these biopsies are guided by imaging studies.

Abscess
Cyst
These fluid lesions can be aspirated and catheters left for drainage.

Hepatitis
Infiltrative diseases (e.g., amyloidosis, hemochromatosis, cirrhosis, fat)
Diffuse liver abnormality is much more easily obtainable by the liver biopsy needle because more tissue contains the pathologic condition.

Related Tests

- Computed tomography scan of the abdomen (p. 933): This is an x-ray study that provides excellent visualization of the liver for guided biopsy.
- Magnetic resonance imaging (MRI) scan of the liver (p. 1009): This study uses variations in electromagnetic characteristics to provide an accurate image of the liver. Recently technology has advanced to allow the guidance of a biopsy needle to the suspect area within the liver.

Lung Biopsy

Normal Findings

No evidence of pathologic conditions

Indications

Lung biopsy is indicated to determine the nature of pulmonary parenchymal disease that has been identified on plain chest x-ray film or chest computed tomography (CT) scan. Carcinomas, granulomas, infections, and sarcoidosis can be diagnosed with this procedure. This procedure is also useful in detecting environmental exposures, infections, or familial disease, which may lead to better prevention and treatment.

Test Explanation

This invasive procedure is used to obtain a specimen of pulmonary tissue for a histologic examination by using either an open or a closed technique. The open method involves a limited thoracotomy. The closed technique includes methods such as transbronchial lung biopsy, transbronchial needle aspiration biopsy, transcatheter bronchial brushing, percutaneous needle aspiration biopsy, and video-assisted thoracostomy (VAT).

Note that this procedure is performed by a surgeon or pulmonologist in 30 to 60 minutes. Most patients describe the percutaneous biopsy procedure as painful. Postoperative incisional pain can be expected if the open technique or VAT is used.

Contraindications

- Patients with bullae or cysts of the lung, because they have a greater risk of pneumothorax with needle lung biopsy
- Patients with suspected vascular anomalies of the lung, because bleeding may occur
- Patients with bleeding abnormalities, because bleeding may occur
- Patients with pulmonary hypertension, because bleeding is more likely to occur
- Patients with respiratory insufficiency, because they are not likely to survive a pneumothorax if it occurs

Potential Complications

- Pneumothorax
- Pulmonary hemorrhage
- Empyema

✓ CLINICAL PRIORITIES

- Assess the results of the coagulation studies prior to lug biopsy because postprocedure bleeding can occur.
- The patient is usually kept on NPO status after midnight before this test.
- After this procedure carefully assess the patient for signs of bleeding (increased pulse rate, decreased blood pressure) and shortness of breath.
- A chest x-ray film is usually ordered after the procedure to check for complications (such as pneumothorax).

Procedure and Patient Care

Before

- Explain the procedure to the patient.
- Ensure that informed and signed consent is obtained.
- Instruct the patient that fasting is usually ordered. The patient may be kept on NPO status after midnight on the day of the test.
- Administer the preprocedural medications 30 to 60 minutes before the test as ordered. Atropine is usually given to decrease bronchial secretions. Meperidine (Demerol) may be used to sedate anxious patients.
- Instruct the patient to remain still during the lung biopsy. Any movement or coughing could cause laceration of the lung by the biopsy needle.

During

- Note that the patient's position depends on the method used and that the histologic lung specimen may be obtained by several different methods:

Transbronchial Lung Biopsy (See Discussion of Bronchoscopy on p. 518.)

1. This technique is performed via flexible fiberoptic bronchoscopy using cutting forceps.
2. Fluoroscopy is used to ensure proper opening and positioning of the forceps on the lesions.
3. Fluoroscopy also permits visualization of the "tug" of the lung as the specimen is removed.

Transbronchial Needle Aspiration (See Discussion of Bronchoscopy on p. 518.)

1. The specimen is obtained via a fiberoptic bronchoscope using a needle.
2. The bronchoscope is inserted, and the target site is identified by fluoroscopy.
3. The needle is inserted through the bronchoscope and into the tumor or desired area, where aspiration is performed with the attached syringe.
4. The needle is retracted within its sheath, and the entire catheter is withdrawn from the fiberoptic scope.

Transcatheter Bronchial Brushing

1. This is also performed via a fiberoptic bronchoscope. (See discussion of bronchoscopy on p. 518.)
2. During bronchoscopy a small brush is moved back and forth over the suspicious area in the bronchus or its branches.
3. The cells adhere to the brush, which is then removed and used to make microscopic slides.

Percutaneous Needle Biopsy

1. In this method for obtaining a closed specimen the biopsy is obtained after using fluoroscopic x-ray or CT scan localization of the desired site.
2. The procedure is carried out by using a cutting needle or by aspiration with a spinal type of needle to obtain a specimen.
3. The main problem with this procedure is potential damage to major blood vessels.
4. During the lung biopsy procedure, assess the patient carefully for signs of respiratory distress (e.g., shortness of breath, rapid pulse rate, cyanosis).

Open Lung Biopsy

1. The patient is taken to the operating room, and general anesthesia is provided.
2. The patient is placed in the supine or lateral position, and an incision is made into the chest wall.
3. After a piece of lung tissue is removed, the lung is sutured.
4. Chest tube drainage is used for approximately 24 hours after an open lung biopsy.
5. This procedure can be performed by thoracoscopy as described below.

Thorascopic Biopsy

1. The lung is collapsed with a double-lumen endotracheal tube placed during induction of general anesthesia.
2. With the use of a thoracoscope (similar to a laparoscope [p. 545]), the lung is grasped and a piece is cut off with the use of a cutting/stapling device. Large wedge lung resections can be obtained.
3. The scope and trocars are removed, and a small chest tube is left in place.
4. The tiny incisions are closed, and the procedure is completed.

After

- Place biopsy specimens in appropriate containers for histologic and microbiologic examination.
- Observe the patient's vital signs frequently for signs of bleeding (increased pulse rate, decreased blood pressure) and for shortness of breath.
- Assess the patient's breath sounds and report any decrease on the biopsy side.
- A chest x-ray film is ordered to check for complications (e.g., pneumothorax).
- Observe the patient for signs of pneumothorax (e.g., dyspnea, tachypnea, decrease in breath sounds, anxiety, restlessness).

Test Results and Clinical Significance

Carcinoma *Biopsies of both primary and metastatic lesions can be performed using this technique. The lesion must be peripheral enough to ensure that one of the great vessels will not be punctured.*

Granuloma *If the lesion is observed to contain calcium, it can be considered to be an old granuloma from previous granulomatous infection. If calcification is not observed, a biopsy of the lesion must be performed to rule out cancer, active fungal infection, or tuberculosis.*

Exposure lung diseases (e.g., black lung, asbestosis) *It is important to recognize and document the presence of exposure lung disease for medical (prognosis and treatment) and legal (workers' compensation or disability) reasons.*

Sarcoidosis *Sarcoidosis of the lung is an interstitial disease highlighted by chronic inflammation and fibrosis. This is obvious on lung biopsy.*

Infection *Unusual infections (such as that caused by* Pneumocystis carinii) *and unusual fungal diseases require tissue for culture and microscopic identification.*

Related Tests

- Bronchoscopy (p. 518): This endoscopic test is the access through which transbronchial biopsy and aspirations are performed.
- Computed tomography (CT) scan of the lung (p. 942): This scan utilizes the method of computerized tomography to localize a lung lesion for biopsy.

Papanicolaou Smear
(Pap Smear, Pap Test, Cytologic Test for Cancer)

Normal Findings No abnormal or atypical cells

Indications

Pap smears are the mainstay of screening for cancer of the vagina, cervix, and uterus. They are routinely performed on women over the age of 18 to 21 years or on younger women who are sexually active.

Test Explanation

A Pap smear is performed to detect neoplastic cells in cervical and vaginal secretions. This test is based on the fact that normal cells and abnormal cervical and endometrial cells are shed into the cervical and vaginal secretions. By examining these secretions microscopically, one can detect early cellular changes compatible with premalignant conditions or an existing malignant condition. The Pap smear is 95% accurate in detecting cervical carcinoma; however, its accuracy in detection of endometrial carcinoma is only approximately 40%. The cells are classified as follows:

Class 1: absence of atypical or abnormal cells (normal)
Class 2: atypical cells but no evidence of malignancy (worrisome but most frequently caused by inflammation of the cervix)
Class 3: cytologic findings suggestive of but not conclusive concerning malignancy (should be evaluated more extensively)
Class 4: cytologic findings strongly suggestive of malignancy (requires more extensive evaluation)
Class 5: cytologic findings conclusive of malignancy (requires treatment)

Abnormal smears in classes 2 to 4 do not necessarily indicate that the patient has a malignancy. Additional procedures such as cone biopsy of the cervix or colposcopy are indicated for these women.

A general movement has occurred during the last 10 years to reclassify Pap smear reporting in terms of cervical intraepithelial neoplasia (CIN). This is a simple designation of the spectrum of intraepithelial dysplasia, which usually occurs before invasive cervical cancer. In contrast to the rigid original classification, CIN reporting recognizes the continuum of cervical dysplasia and allows for some overlap. The subclasses of CIN are defined as follows:

CIN 1: mild and mild-to-moderate dysplasia
CIN 2: moderate and moderate-to-severe dysplasia
CIN 3: severe dysplasia and carcinoma in situ

In comparing CIN stratification with the previously noted classification, CIN 1 includes classes 2 and 3, CIN 2 includes class 3, and CIN 3 includes classes 4 and 5.

Most recently, the Bethesda System for reporting cervical/vaginal cytologic diagnoses was developed and revised by the National Cancer Institute. This system includes the following:

- Adequacy of specimen
  - Satisfactory for evaluation
  - Satisfactory for evaluation but limited by (specify disease)
  - Unsatisfactory for evaluation (specify reason)
- General categorization (optional)
  - Within normal limits
  - Benign cellular changes: see descriptive diagnosis
  - Epithelial cell abnormality: see descriptive diagnosis
- Descriptive diagnosis
  - Benign cellular changes
  - Infection
    - *Trichomonas*
    - Fungal organisms
    - Coccobacilli
    - Herpes simplex
    - Other
  - Reactive changes
    - Inflammation
    - Atrophy
    - Radiation
    - Intrauterine device
    - Other
- Epithelial cell abnormalities
  - Squamous cell
    - Atypical squamous cells
    - Low-grade squamous intraepithelial lesion
    - High-grade squamous intraepithelial lesion
    - Squamous cell carcinoma
  - Glandular cell
    - Endometrial cells, cytologically benign
    - Atypical glandular cell
    - Endocervical adenocarcinoma
    - Endometrial adenocarcinoma
    - Extrauterine adenocarcinoma
    - Adenocarcinoma

A Pap smear also may be performed to determine endocrine abnormalities (e.g., infertility). An abnormal maturation index is characteristic of an estrogen-progesterone imbalance. The *maturation index* (MI) is calculated by determining the ratio of parabasal cells to intermediate cells to superficial cells. The normal ovulating adult MI is 0/70/30. The MI is not a routine part of a Pap smear but can be calculated if requested. The more superficial cells present, the greater the hormone influence (ovarian estrogen, progesterone, and adrenal sex hormones). The more parabasal cells present, the less hormonal influence on vaginal mucosa. Calculation of MI cannot predict ovulation. It is used more frequently for determination of menstrual status and ovarian function.

Pap smears should be part of the routine pelvic examination, which is usually performed once a year on women over 18 years of age (or even earlier when the patient is sexually active). Opinions differ regarding the necessity for annual Pap smears. The American Cancer Society recommends that a Pap smear be taken annually for two negative examinations, then repeated once every 3 years until age 65 in asymptomatic women. More frequent testing may be indicated for patients with venereal infections, those with a family history of cervical cancer, and those whose mothers had ingested diethylstilbestrol during their pregnancies. In the past a routine cervical culture for gonorrhea was obtained during the Pap smear examination. This is no longer done. A Pap smear is obtained by a nurse or a physician in approximately 10 minutes. No discomfort, except for insertion of the speculum, is associated with this procedure.

Contraindications

- Patients presently having routine, normal menses, because this can alter test interpretation
- Patients with vaginal infections, because the infections can create cellular changes that may be misinterpreted as dysplastic

Interfering Factors

- A delay in fixing a specimen allows the cells to dry, destroys effectiveness of the stain, and makes cytologic interpretation difficult.
- Using lubricating jelly on the speculum can alter the specimen.
- Douching and tub bathing may wash away cellular deposits and interfere with the test results.
- Menstrual flow may alter test results. The best time to perform a Pap test is 2 weeks after the start of the last menses.
- Infections may interfere with hormonal cytology.
- Drugs such as digitalis and tetracycline may alter the test results by affecting the squamous epithelium.

✓ CLINICAL PRIORITIES

- Pap smears should not be collected during menstruation because results may be altered.
- A maturation index can be determined to detect endocrine abnormalities (such as estrogen-progesterone imbalance).
- Usually patients are not notified of Pap smear results unless further evaluation is needed.

Procedure and Patient Care

Before

- Explain the procedure to the patient.
- Instruct the patient not to douche or tub bathe during the 24 hours before the Pap smear. (Some physicians prefer that patients refrain from sexual intercourse for 24 to 48 hours before the test.)

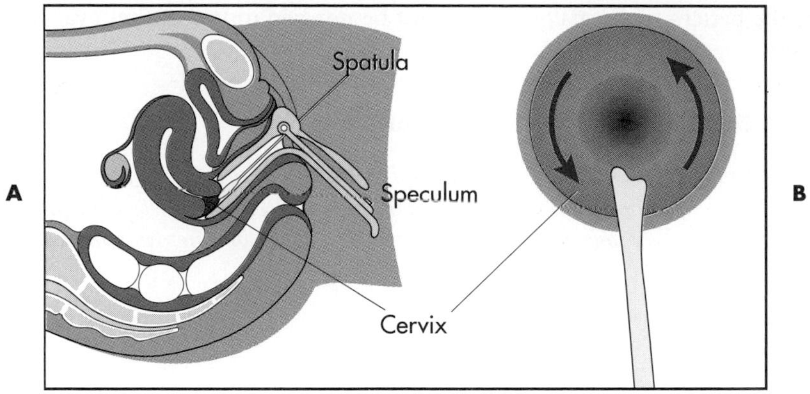

Figure 7-2 Papanicolaou (Pap) smear. **A,** Cross-sectional view of the process of obtaining a cervical specimen. **B,** Cervix is scraped with bifid end of a spatula to obtain Pap smear.

- Instruct the patient to empty her bladder before the examination. A full bladder inhibits complete palpation of pelvic structures.
- Tell the patient that no fasting or sedation is required.

During

- Note the following procedural steps:
  1. The patient is placed in the lithotomy position.
  2. A vaginal speculum is inserted to expose the cervix.
  3. Material is collected from the cervical canal by rotating a moist, saline cotton swab or spatula within the cervical canal and in the squamocolumnar junction (Figure 7-2). If a maturation index is requested for hormonal information, the smear is taken of the vaginal wall. Care is taken to exclude the cervix.
  4. The cells are immediately wiped across a clean glass slide and fixed either by immersing the slide in equal parts of 95% alcohol and ether or by using a commercial spray (e.g., Aqua Net hair spray). The secretions must be fixed before drying, because drying will distort the cells and make interpretation difficult. Furthermore, this fixing process kills any infectious organisms so that the specimen is less infectious to the personnel who handle the specimen.
  5. The slide is labeled with the patient's name, age, parity, and date of her last menstrual period.
  6. The patient's medication history (e.g., oral contraceptives) and the reason for the examination should be written on the laboratory request form.

After

- If the Pap smear has induced some bleeding, provide the patient with a perineal napkin.
- Note that once in the laboratory, the Pap smear slide is stained and reviewed microscopically by the pathologist. Several computer programs are now able to recognize abnormal cells and classify them. These programs are used to assist the pathologist in screening particularly cellular smears.

- Inform the patient that usually she will not be notified unless further evaluation is necessary.

Test Results and Clinical Significance

Cancer *This becomes evident with high class or CIN 3 cytologic results. The diagnosis of malignancy, however, can be made only on biopsy of the tumor. All suspicious or high-grade Pap smears must be more thoroughly investigated with colposcopy, cone biopsy, and/or dilation and curettage.*

Sexually transmitted diseases
Fungal infection
Parasitic infection
Herpes infection
Many of these infectious diseases cause high-grade cellular changes on Pap smears. Culture of these organisms, however, is required in order to make the diagnosis.

Infertility *Lack of estrogenic effect noted on vaginal Pap smears may indicate ovarian failure in a woman of usual menstrual age.*

Related Tests

- Colposcopy (p. 526): This is one of the follow-up tests performed for an abnormal Pap smear.

Pleural Biopsy

Normal Findings No evidence of pathologic conditions

Indications

This test is indicated when the pleural fluid obtained by thoracentesis (p. 606) is exudative fluid, which suggests infection, neoplasm, or tuberculosis. The pleural biopsy is indicated to distinguish among these disease processes. It is also performed when a plain chest x-ray film indicates a pleural-based tumor, reaction, or thickening.

Test Explanation

Pleural biopsy is the removal of pleural tissue for histologic examination. Pleural biopsy is usually performed by a percutaneous needle biopsy. It also can be performed via thoracoscopy, which is done by inserting a laparoscope into the pleural space for inspection and biopsy of the pleura. Pleural tissue also may be obtained by an open pleural biopsy, which involves a limited thoracotomy and requires general anesthesia. For this procedure a small intercostal incision is made and the biopsy of the pleura is done under direct observation. The advantage of these open procedures is that a larger piece of pleura can be obtained.

Percutaneous needle biopsies are usually performed by a physician at the patient's bedside, in a special procedure room, or in the physician's office in approximately 30 minutes. Because of the local anesthetic, little discomfort is associated with this procedure. Open biopsies are done in the operating room.

Contraindications

- Patients with prolonged bleeding or clotting times

Potential Complications

- Bleeding or injury to the lung
- Pneumothorax

Procedure and Patient Care

Before

- Explain the procedure to the patient.
- Obtain informed consent for this procedure.
- Tell the patient that no fasting or sedation is required.
- Instruct the patient to remain very still during the procedure. Any movement may cause inadvertent needle damage.

During

- Note the following procedural steps for *percutaneous needle biopsy:*
  1. This procedure is usually performed with the patient in a sitting position with his or her shoulders and arms elevated and supported by a padded overhead table.
  2. After the presence of the fluid has been determined by the thoracentesis technique, the skin overlying the biopsy site is anesthetized and pierced with a scalpel blade.
  3. A needle is inserted with a cannula until fluid is removed. (Some fluid is left in the pleural space after the thoracentesis to make the biopsy easier.)
  4. The inner needle is removed, and a blunt-tipped, hooked biopsy trocar, attached to a three-way stopcock, is inserted into the cannula.
  5. The patient is instructed to expire all air and then perform the Valsalva maneuver to prevent air from entering the pleural space.
  6. The cannula and biopsy trocar are withdrawn while the hook catches the parietal wall and takes a specimen with its cutting edge.
  7. Usually three biopsy specimens are taken from different sites at the same session.
  8. The specimens are placed in a fixative solution and sent to the laboratory immediately.
  9. After the specimens are taken, additional parietal fluid can be removed.

After

- Apply an adhesive bandage to the biopsy site.
- Note that a chest x-ray film is usually taken to detect the potential complication of pneumothorax.

- Observe the patient for signs of respiratory distress (e.g., shortness of breath, diminished breath sounds) on the side of the biopsy.
- Observe the patient's vital signs frequently for evidence of bleeding (increased pulse rate, decreased blood pressure).
- Ensure that the biopsy specimen is sent immediately to the laboratory.

Home Care Responsibilities

- Instruct the patient to report any signs of shortness of breath.
- Note any signs of bleeding, such as decreasing blood pressure or increasing pulse rate.

Test Results and Clinical Significance

Neoplasm *Pleural tumors can be primary (mesothelioma) or metastatic (breast, lung, ovarian, gastrointestinal, etc.) These tumors are often associated with a pleural effusion.*

Infection *Lung and pleural space infections can cause thickened pleura and pleural effusions (empyema). Most infections can be identified on Gram stains or cultures of the pleural fluid. However, some infections cannot be identified without tissue for culture or tissue for other forms of identification. This is especially true for the unusual infections occurring in immunocompromised patients* (Pneumocystis carinii, *an unusual fungus*).

Related Tests

- Thoracentesis and pleural fluid analysis (p. 606): This is a procedure whereby pleural fluid is aspirated from the pleural space for analysis.
- Chest radiography (p. 924): This x-ray study visualizes most surfaces of the pleura.

Progesterone Receptor Assay
(PR Assay, PRA, PgR)

Normal Findings

Negative: <10 fmol/g of tissue
Positive: >10 fmol/g of tissue

Indications

Progesterone receptor assay is performed on breast cancer tissue in order to indicate tumor sensitivity to hormonal manipulative therapy and to indicate prognosis of breast cancer.

Test Explanation

The PR assay is used in determining the prognosis and treatment of breast cancer and, to a lesser degree, other cancers. The assay helps to determine whether a tumor is likely to respond to endocrine manipulation. The test is done on breast cancer specimens when a primary or recurrent cancer is identified; it is usually done in conjunction with estrogen receptor (ER) assay (p. 655) to increase the predictability of a tumor response to hormone therapy. PR levels tend to be higher in the breast cancer of postmenopausal women than in that of premenopausal women. PR-positive tumors are suspected of being associated with a better prognosis than PR-negative tumors. Tumor response rates to medical or surgical hormonal manipulation are potentiated if the ER assay is positive. Response rates are as follows:

ER positive, PR positive: 75%
ER negative, PR positive: 60%
ER positive, PR negative: 35%
ER negative, PR negative: 25%

The test is performed in one of two ways. The standard method is to send 1 g of the breast cancer specimen to a centralized laboratory, where the PR protein is quantified in the cytoplasm or nucleus of breast cancer cells. Another method, however, is to send the actual paraffin-embedded microscope slides to that laboratory for immunohistochemical staining for PR proteins. This latter method is now considered to be more accurate.

Other tumors (such as ovarian, melanoma, uterine, or pancreatic) are occasionally studied for ER and PR assay. This is mostly done within clinical trials. To date, hormonal therapy has not been very successful with these tumors.

Interfering Factors

- Exogenous hormone use
- Use of hormones such as progesterone or estrogen may cause false-negative results.

Procedure and Patient Care

Before

- Prepare the patient for breast biopsy per routine protocol.
- Record the menstrual status of the patient.
- Record any exogenous hormone the patient may have used during the last 2 months.
- Instruct the patient to discontinue exogenous hormones before breast biopsy.

During

- Note that the surgeon obtains at least 1 g of tissue.
- Place the specimen on ice, and send it to the laboratory immediately.
- Note that in the pathology department, part of the specimen is used for routine histologic examination. The other part (at least 1 g) is frozen and sent in dry ice to a central laboratory for PR analysis.
- Note that if immunohistochemical methods of PR assay are used, the specimen is fixed as soon as it arrives at the laboratory. Fixed tissue is then sent for testing.
- Note that results are usually available in 2 weeks.

After

- Provide routine postoperative care.

Test Results and Clinical Significance

PR positive *This cancer is more likely to be successfully treated with hormone manipulation in a therapeutic or adjuvant clinical setting.*

Related Tests

- Estrogen receptor assay (p. 655): Like PR assay, this test predicts the likelihood of tumor response to endocrine manipulative therapy.

Renal Biopsy (Kidney Biopsy)

Normal Findings

No pathologic conditions

Indications

Renal biopsy is performed for the following purposes:

1. To diagnose the cause of renal disease (e.g., poststreptococcal glomerulonephritis, Goodpasture's syndrome, lupus nephritis)
2. To detect primary and metastatic malignancy of the kidney in patients who may not be candidates for surgery
3. To evaluate kidney transplantation rejection, which enables the physician to determine the appropriate dose of immunosuppressive drugs

Test Explanation

Biopsy of the kidney affords microscopic examination of renal tissue. Renal biopsy is most often obtained percutaneously (Figure 7-3). During this procedure a needle is inserted through the skin and into the kidney to obtain a sample of kidney tissue. The biopsy needle is more accurately placed when guided by ultrasonography or fluoroscopy. These localizing techniques allow more precise localization of the desired kidney tissue.

Occasionally, open renal biopsy is performed. This involves an incision through the flank and dissection to expose the kidney surgically. This procedure is performed by a physician in approximately 10 to 30 minutes. The biopsy is uncomfortable, but only minimally if enough lidocaine is used.

Contraindications

- Patients with coagulation disorders, because of the risk of excessive bleeding
- Patients with operable kidney tumors, because tumor cells may be disseminated during the procedure

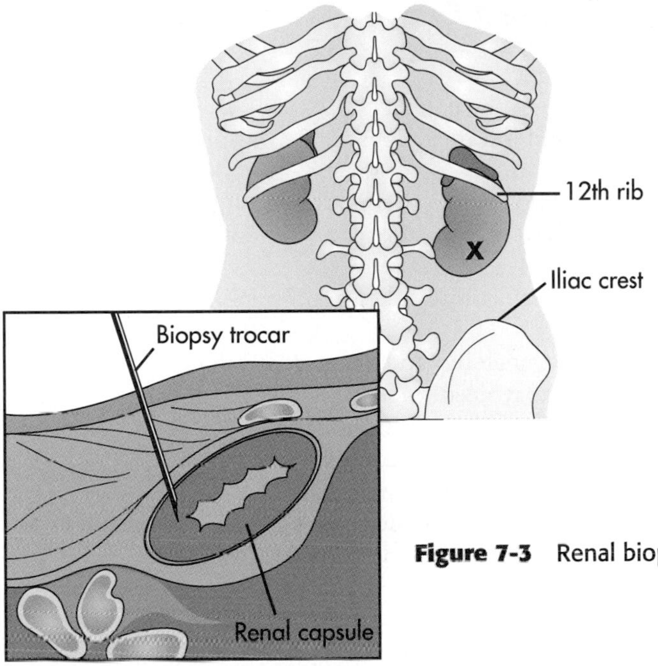

Figure 7-3 Renal biopsy.

- Patients with hydronephrosis, because the enlarged renal pelvis can be easily entered and cause a persistent urine leak requiring surgical repair
- Patients with urinary tract infections, because the needle insertion may disseminate the active infection throughout the retroperitoneum

Potential Complications

- Hemorrhage from the highly vascular renal tissue
- Inadvertent puncture of the liver, lung, bowel, aorta, and inferior vena cava
- Infection when an open biopsy is performed

✓ CLINICAL PRIORITIES

- Assess the coagulation profile before performing a kidney biopsy because of the possibility of bleeding. Often hemoglobin and hematocrit values are obtained after the procedure to check for bleeding.
- After a renal biopsy the patients usually kept in bed on his or her back for about 24 hours.
- After this test, carefully evaluate the vital signs for evidence of bleeding. Inspect the urine for gross hematuria.

Procedure and Patient Care

Before

- Explain the procedure to the patient.
- Ensure that written and informed consent for this procedure is obtained by the physician.
- Keep the patient on NPO status after midnight on the day of the test in the event that bleeding or inadvertent puncture of an abdominal organ necessitates surgical intervention.
- Assess the patient's coagulation studies (prothrombin time, partial thromboplastin time).
- Check the patient's hemoglobin and hematocrit values.
- Note that the patient may need to be typed and crossmatched for blood in the event of severe hemorrhage requiring transfusions.
- Tell the patient that no sedative is required.
- Note that the needlestick may be done at the bedside.
- If fluoroscopic or ultrasound guidance is to be used, note that the needlestick is performed in the radiology or ultrasonography department.

During

- Note the following procedural steps:
  1. The patient is placed in a prone position with a sandbag or pillow under the abdomen to straighten the spine.
  2. Under sterile conditions the skin overlying the kidneys is infiltrated with a local anesthetic (lidocaine).
  3. While the patient holds his or her breath to stop kidney motion, the physician inserts the biopsy needle into the kidney and takes a specimen.
  4. After this procedure is completed, the needle is removed and pressure is applied to the site for approximately 20 minutes.

After

- Apply a pressure dressing.
- Turn the patient on his or her back and keep in bed for approximately 24 hours.
- Check the patient's vital signs, puncture site, and hematocrit values frequently during the 24-hour period.
- Instruct the patient to avoid any activity that increases abdominal venous pressure (e.g., coughing).
- Assess the patient for signs and symptoms of hemorrhage (e.g., decrease in blood pressure, increase in pulse rate, pallor, backache, flank pain, shoulder pain, lightheadedness).
- Evaluate the patient's abdomen for signs of bowel or liver penetration (e.g., abdominal pain and tenderness, abdominal muscle guarding and rigidity, decreased bowel sounds).
- Inspect all urine specimens for gross hematuria. Usually the patient's urine will contain blood initially, but this generally will not continue after the first 24 hours. Urine samples may be placed in consecutive chronologic order to facilitate comparison for evaluation of hematuria. This is referred to as rack, or serial, urine samples.

- Encourage the patient to drink large amounts of fluid to prevent clot formation and urine retention.
- Obtain blood for hemoglobin and hematocrit level determination after the biopsy to assess for active bleeding. One purple-top tube of blood is needed.
- Instruct the patient to avoid, for at least 2 weeks, strenuous exercise (e.g., heavy lifting, contact sports, horseback riding) or any activity that could cause jolting of the kidney.
- Teach the patient the signs and symptoms of renal hemorrhage, and instruct him or her to call the physician if any of these symptoms occur.
- Instruct the patient to report burning on urination or any temperature elevations. These could indicate a urinary tract infection.

Test Results and Clinical Significance

Renal disease (e.g., poststreptococcal conditions, Goodpasture's syndrome, lupus nephritis) *These primary diseases of the kidney have classic histologic appearances. It is important to document the type of renal disease in order to ensure proper therapy. Immunofluorescent stains are often applied to the tissue to identify renal disease of immunologic origin (e.g., Goodpasture's disease).*

Primary and metastatic malignancy of the kidney *The most common cancers of the kidney are primary renal cell carcinomas. It is dangerous to perform a biopsy of this tumor because it is quite vascular. Furthermore, the biopsy could cause tumor studding along the needle tract. However, in cases of metastatic disease, or if medical conditions preclude surgery, tissue can be obtained by kidney biopsy.*

Rejection of kidney transplant *This is the definitive manner in which rejection is diagnosed. If caught early enough, the immunosuppressive medication regimen can be altered to stop the rejection process.*

Sexually Transmitted Disease Culture
(STD Culture, Culture of Cervix, Urethra, and Anus)

Normal Findings

No evidence of sexually transmitted disease (gonorrhea, *Chlamydia* [p. 649], *Trichomonas*)

Indications

These cultures and smears are performed for patients who have a vaginal discharge, pelvic pain, urethritis, or penile discharge and are at risk for sexually transmitted diseases (STDs).

Test Explanation

In the United States and other countries, some STDs have become epidemic while others have become increasingly frequent. These organisms can cause urethritis, vaginitis, endometritis, pelvic inflammatory disease, pharyngitis, proctitis, epididymitis, prostatitis, and salpingitis. Children born of infected mothers may develop conjunctivitis, pneumonia, neonatal blindness, neonatal neurologic injury, and even death.

Cultures for STD infections are performed on men and women with suggestive symptoms. If the culture is positive, sexual partners should be evaluated and treated. Cervical cultures are usually done for women; urethral cultures are done for men. Rectal and throat cultures are performed in persons who have engaged in anal and oral intercourse. Because rectal gonorrhea accompanies genital gonorrhea in a high percentage of women, rectal cultures may be recommended in all women with suspected gonorrhea. Performing a culture for gonorrhea is also part of the prenatal workup. If the STD culture is positive, treatment during pregnancy can prevent possible fetal complications (e.g., ophthalmia neonatorum) and maternal complications. Rectal and orogastric cultures should be done on the neonates of infected mothers.

Gram stains of smears or bacterial cultures should be taken before a patient begins antibiotic therapy. Bacterial cultures for gonorrhea use a special medium such as Thayer-Martin, designed for the cultivation of *Neisseria gonorrhoeae.*

Other STDs are identified by culture or smear of a genital lesion, tissue biopsy, serologic testing, and observation of classic clinical lesions. DNA probes tagged with chemoluminescent dye are also used for identification of some of these STD organisms. Each suspected organism must be specifically requested. Some laboratories do routine "genital cultures" that include gonorrhea, beta streptoccocus, and *Gardnerella* investigations.

STD cultures and smears are obtained by a physician or nurse in several minutes. Very little discomfort is associated with these procedures.

Interfering Factors

- *N. gonorrhoeae* is very sensitive to lubricants and disinfectants.
- Menses may alter test results.
- Female douching within 24 hours of a cervical culture makes fewer organisms available for culture.
- Male voiding within 1 hour of a urethral culture washes secretions out of the urethra.
- Fecal material may contaminate an anal culture.

✓ CLINICAL PRIORITIES

- If cultures for STDs are positive, sexual partners should be evaluated and treated.
- Women should not douche within 24 hours of cervical cultures because douching may decrease the number of organisms available for culture.
- Men should not urinate within 1 hour of a urethral culture because voiding washes secretions out of urethra.

Procedure and Patient Care

Before

- Explain the purpose and procedure to the patient. Use a matter-of-fact, nonjudgmental approach.
- Tell the patient that no fasting or sedation is required.

During

- Obtain cultures as follows:

Cervical Culture

1. The female patient is told to refrain from douching and tub bathing before the cervical culture.
2. The patient is placed in the lithotomy position, and a moistened nonlubricated vaginal speculum is inserted to expose the cervix (see Figure 7-2, *A*, p. 669).
3. Cervical mucus is removed with a cotton ball held in a ring forceps.
4. A sterile cotton-tipped swab is inserted into the endocervical canal and moved from side to side to obtain the culture.
5. The swab is placed in sterile saline or a transporting fluid obtained from the lab. The specimen should be plated as soon as possible. The specimen should not be refrigerated.

Anal Canal Culture

1. An anal culture of the female or male patient is taken by inserting a sterile, cotton-tipped swab approximately 1 inch into the anal canal (Figure 7-4).
2. If stool contaminates the swab, a repeat swab is taken.

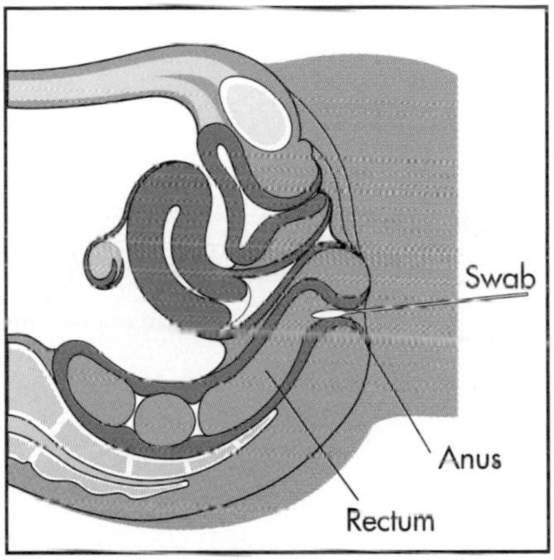

Figure 7-4 Obtaining a specimen of exudate from the rectum.

Oropharyngeal Culture

1. This culture should be obtained in male and female patients who have engaged in oral intercourse.
2. A throat culture is best obtained by depressing the patient's tongue with a wooden tongue blade and touching the posterior wall of the throat with a sterile cotton-tipped swab.

Urethral Culture

1. The urethral specimen should be obtained from the male patient before voiding. Voiding within 1 hour of collection washes secretions out of the urethra, making fewer organisms available for culture. The best time to obtain the specimen is before the first morning micturition.

2. A culture is taken by inserting a sterile swab gently into the anterior urethra (Figure 7-5).
3. It is advisable to place the male patient in the supine position to prevent falling if vasovagal syncope occurs during introduction of the cotton swab or wire loop into the urethra.
4. The patient is observed for hypotension, bradycardia, pallor, sweating, nausea, and weakness.
5. In the male, prostatic massage may increase the chances of obtaining positive cultures.

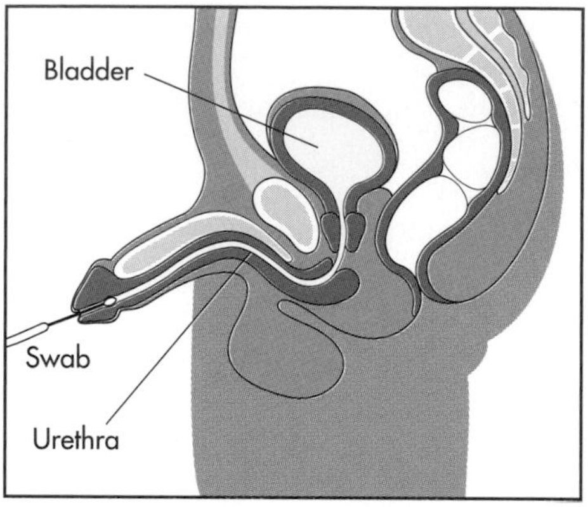

Figure 7-5 Obtaining a urethral specimen.

After

- Place the swabs for gonorrhea in a Thayer-Martin medium and roll them from side to side.
- Label and send the culture bottle to the microbiology laboratory.
- Transport the specimen to the laboratory as soon as possible.
- Handle all specimens as though they were capable of transmitting disease.
- Do not refrigerate the specimen.
- Mark the laboratory slip with the collection time, date, source of specimen, patient's age, current antibiotic therapy, and clinical diagnosis.
- Advise the patient to avoid intercourse and all sexual contact until test results are available.

Table 7-1 *Sexually Transmitted Diseases and Methods of Diagnosis*

Disease	Methods of Diagnosis
Gonorrhea	Cervical, urethral, anal, oropharyngeal cultures
Chlamydia	Cervical, urethral culture, serologic study, DNA probe testing
Lymphogranuloma venereum	
C. trachomatis	
Herpes genitalis	Culture from lesion, serologic study
Syphilis	Serologic study, fluid cultures (CNS), darkfield slide
Hepatitis	Serologic study
AIDS	Serologic study
Granuloma inguinale	Tissue biopsy
Trichomoniasis	Cervical, urethral, vaginal smear on a wet mount
Scabies	Characteristic scabies lesion, skin scraping from lesion
Molluscum contagiosum (molluscum virus)	Characteristic wartlike lesion
Condylomata acuminata (papilloma virus)	Characteristic wartlike lesion
Chancroid (*Haemophilus*)	Culture of the chancre, smear of the chancre, DNA probe
Candida (*Monilia*)	Wet mount, Gram stain, fungal culture
Pediculosis pubis (lice)	Characteristic appearance of louse
Gardnerella vaginalis	Cervical, urethral, anal cultures

- If the culture results are positive, tell the patient to receive treatment and to have sexual partners evaluated.
- Note that repeat cultures should be taken after completion of treatment to evaluate therapy.

Test Results and Clinical Significance

Gonorrhea
Chlamydia (p. 649)
Trichomonas
These and other STDs can be identified by these and other diagnostic tests (Table 7-1, p. 680).

Related Tests

Tests for the sexually transmitted diseases listed below are discussed separately:
- *Chlamydia* (p. 649)
- Herpes simplex (p. 657)
- Syphilis detection (p. 403)
- Hepatitis virus studies (p. 260)
- AIDS serology (p. 30)

Sputum Culture and Sensitivity
(Sputum C&S, Sputum Culture, and Gram stain)

Normal Findings Normal upper respiratory tract

Indications

Sputum culture is indicated in any patient with a persistent productive cough, fever, hemoptysis, or a chest x-ray picture compatible with a pulmonary infection. This test is used to diagnose pneumonia, bronchiectasis, bronchitis, or pulmonary abscess. Bacterium, fungus, or virus can be cultured.

Test Explanation

Sputum cultures are obtained to determine the presence of pathogenic bacteria in patients with respiratory infections, such as pneumonia. A *Gram stain* is the first step in the microbiologic analysis of sputum. Through sputum staining, bacteria are classified as gram positive or gram negative. This may be used to guide drug therapy until the C&S report is complete. The sputum sample is then applied to a series of bacterial culture plates. The bacteria that grow on those plates 1 to 3 days later are then identified. Determinations of bacterial sensitivity to various antibiotics (also called *drug sensitivity testing*) are done to identify the most appropriate antimicrobial drug therapy. This is done by observing a ring of growth inhibition around an antibiotic plug in the culture medium. Sputum for C&S should be collected before antimicrobial therapy is initiated, unless the test is being performed to evaluate the effectiveness of medications already being given. Pre-

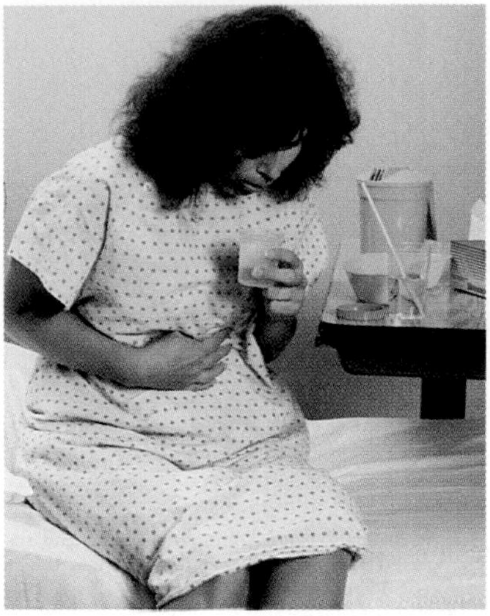

Figure 7-6 Collection of sputum specimen. The specimen should be representative of pulmonary secretions—not saliva.

liminary reports are usually available in 24 hours. Cultures require at least 48 hours for completion. Sputum cultures for fungus and *Mycobacterium tuberculosis* may take 6 to 8 weeks.

Procedure and Patient Care

Before

- Explain the procedure for sputum collection to the patient.
- Remind the patient that sputum must be coughed up from the lungs and that saliva is not sputum (Figure 7-6).
- Hold antibiotics until after the sputum has been collected.
- If an elective specimen is to be obtained, give the patient a sterile sputum container on the night before the sputum is to be collected so that the morning specimen may be obtained on arising.
- Instruct the patient to rinse out his or her mouth with water before the sputum collection to decrease contamination of the sputum by particles in the oropharynx. Antiseptic mouthwash, however, is to be avoided.

During

- Note that sputum specimens are best when the patient awakes in the morning before eating or drinking.
- Collect at least 1 teaspoon of sputum in a sterile sputum container.
- Usually obtain sputum by having the patient cough after taking several deep breaths.
- If the patient is unable to produce a sputum specimen, stimulate coughing by lowering the head of the patient's bed or giving the patient an aerosol administration of a warm, hypertonic solution.
- Note that other methods to collect sputum include endotracheal aspiration, fiberoptic bronchoscopy, and transtracheal aspiration.

After

- Tell the patient to notify the nurse as soon as the sputum is collected.
- Label the sputum, and send it to the laboratory as soon as possible.
- Note any current antibiotic therapy on the laboratory slip.

Test Results and Clinical Significance

Bacterial infection (e.g., pneumonia)
Viral infection
Atypical bacterial infection (e.g., tuberculosis)

Fungal infection

Sputum that is obtained for the above types of organisms is plated on several types of culture media in order to grow the organisms that could grow in the pulmonary tree. Some of these organisms are quite difficult to grow in the laboratory and require great attention to detail to effectively grow these pathogens and demonstrate disease.

Related Test

- Tuberculosis culture (p. 687): This is the only manner in which the diagnosis of tuberculosis (TB) can be made with certainty. When TB is grown from the culture of a specimen, the diagnosis of TB can be made and treatment based on drug sensitivities can be started.

Sputum Cytology

Normal Findings Normal epithelial cells

Indications

Sputum for cytologic examination is indicated for any patient in whom the diagnosis of cancer of the lung is considered. Bronchoscopy and percutaneous lung biopsy have supplanted the need for sputum cytology to a large degree. Now its greatest use is in patients who have abnormal chest x-ray film results, productive cough, and nothing visible on bronchoscopy. It is also used to monitor smokers who have had some atypical changes on prior examination of the lower respiratory tract.

Test Explanation

Tumors within the pulmonary system frequently slough cells into the sputum. When the sputum is gathered, the cells are examined. If the cytologic examination indicates malignant cells, a lung tumor exists within the mucosa of the trachea, bronchi, and lungs. If only normal epithelial cells are observed, either no malignancy exists or any existing tumor is not shedding cells at that time. Therefore a positive test indicates malignancy; a negative test means nothing. The test is more likely to be positive on smokers who have a chronic productive cough and/or hemoptysis. Furthermore, the more specimens obtained, the greater the accuracy of the test. This test is rarely performed, now that tissue biopsy can be easily obtained by bronchoscopic biopsy (p. 518).

Interfering Factors

- False negatives can occur as a result of poor cytologic preparation or inadequate specimen acquisition. Interpretation of cytologic changes is difficult, but most pathologists who have had experience with cytology maintain good accuracy. This is usually monitored by quality assurance studies within the pathology department.

Procedure and Patient Care

Before

- Explain the procedure for sputum collection to the patient.
- Remind the patient that sputum must be coughed up from the lungs and that saliva is not sputum.
- Give the patient a sterile sputum container the night before the sputum is to be collected so that the morning specimen may be obtained on arising.
- Instruct the patient to rinse out her or his mouth with water to decrease contamination of the sputum by particles in the oropharynx.

During

- Note that sputum specimens are best collected when the patient awakes in the morning.
- Collect at least 1 teaspoon of sputum in the sterile sputum container. The container may or may not contain alcohol as an immediate fixative–this varies according to the laboratory. Certainly if a 24-hour specimen is requested, alcohol must be within the container to diminish cellular deterioration during the collection period.
- Usually obtain sputum by having the patient cough after taking several deep breaths.
- If the patient is unable to produce a sputum specimen, stimulate coughing by lowering the head of the patient's bed or giving the patient an aerosol administration of a warm, hypertonic solution.
- Note that other methods to collect sputum include endotracheal aspiration, fiberoptic bronchoscopy, and transtracheal aspiration. Bronchial brushings can obtain excellent specimens for cytologic examination. Through the bronchoscope a brush is placed and wiped on the bronchial mucosa. It is then withdrawn back into its sheath and wiped on a dry slide, which is immediately fixed.
- Usually collect sputum for cytologic examination once daily on 3 successive days. The first morning specimen is the best.

After

- Instruct the patient to notify the nurse as soon as the sputum is collected.
- Label the specimen, and send it to the laboratory as soon as possible.

Test Results and Clinical Significance

Malignancies *Malignancies of the trachea, bronchus, and lung can be detected. Marked changes in the nuclear/cytoplasmic ratio, size of the cell, and differentiation of the cell indicate suspicious changes. It is now thought that cellular changes progress from benign, normal-looking cells to metaplastic cells, to atypical cells, to frankly cancerous cells. The cytologic report may indicate the cells are somewhere within that spectrum. The cells may be labeled benign, abnormal, suspicious, or definitely cancer. The epithelial cells of the lower respiratory system seem to make those progressive changes as the number of years the person smokes increases.*

Benign cellular changes *This is most commonly due to infection (bronchiectasis), exposure (asbestosis), or viral pneumonitis.*

Asthma *These patients often have an increased number of eosinophils within their sputum.*

Related Tests

- Bronchoscopy (p. 518): This is an endoscopic test through which pulmonary lavage can be performed and specimens for cytologic examination can be obtained.

Throat Culture and Sensitivity (Throat C&S)

Normal Findings Negative

Indications

A throat culture is obtained to diagnose bacterial, viral, gonococcal, or candidal pharyngitis. It is indicated on patients who complain of a "sore throat," have a fever of unknown cause, or may be chronic carriers of recurrent infection.

Test Explanation

Because the throat is normally colonized by many organisms, culture of this area serves only to isolate and identify a few particular pathogens (e.g., streptococci, meningococci, gonococci, *Bordetella pertussis, Corynebacterium diphtheriae*). Recognition of these organisms requires treatment. Streptococci are most often sought, because a beta-hemolytic streptococcal pharyngitis may be followed by rheumatic fever or glomerulonephritis. This type of streptococcal infection most frequently affects children between the ages of 3 and 15 years. Therefore all children with a sore throat and fever should have a throat culture done to attempt to identify streptococcal infections. In adults, however, fewer than 5% of patients with pharyngitis have a streptococcal infection. Therefore throat cultures in adults are indicated only when the patient has severe or recurrent sore throat, often associated with fever and palpable lymphadenopathy. These adults often have a history of previous streptococcal infections.

Rapid immunologic tests *(strept screen)* with antiserum against group A streptococcus antigen are now available and are very accurate for the identification of the organism without culture. With these newer kits the streptococcus organism can be identified directly from the swab specimen. With this method the streptococcus is chemically or enzymatically extracted from the swab specimen. It is then tested with the antisera containing the antibodies to group A streptococcus. Agglutination on the slide indicates group A streptococci are present. If no agglutination occurs, the specimen is still cultured for streptococcus. If that culture is negative, no streptococcus infection exists. The rapid serologic tests can be performed in about 15 minutes. The final culture report takes at least 2 days.

As a routine a throat culture uses several different type of culture media (chocolate, streptococcus-specific, and other agar) to grow various bacteria. When a specific streptococcus culture is requested or if the strept screen is negative, the specimen is plated on streptococcus-specific agar only. All cultures should be performed before antibiotic therapy is initiated. Otherwise, the antibiotic may interrupt the growth of the organism in the laboratory. More often than not, however, the physician will want to institute antibiotic therapy before the culture results are reported. In these instances, a *Gram stain* of the specimen smeared on a slide is most helpful and can be reported in less than 10 minutes. All forms of bacteria are grossly classified as gram positive (blue staining) or gram negative (red staining). Knowledge of the shape of the organism (e.g., spherical [coccus], rod shaped [bacillus]) also can be very helpful in the tentative identification of the infecting organism. With knowledge of the Gram stain results, the physician can institute a reasonable antibiotic regimen based on past experience as to the organism's possible identity and sensitivity. Most organisms take approximately 24 hours to grow in the laboratory, and a preliminary report can be given at that time. Occasionally, a period of 48 to 72 hours is required for growth and identification of the organism. Cultures may be repeated on completion of appropriate antibiotic therapy to identify resolution of the infection.

Interfering Factors

- Drugs that may affect test results include antibiotics and antiseptic mouthwashes.

Procedure and Patient Care

Before

- Explain the procedure to the patient.

During

- Obtain a throat culture by depressing the tongue with a wooden tongue blade and touching the posterior wall of the throat (Figure 7-7) and areas of inflammation, exudation, or ulceration with a sterile cotton swab. Two swabs are preferred. Growth of streptococcus from both swabs is more accurate, and the second swab can also be used in the strept screen.
- Avoid touching any other part of the mouth.
- Wear gloves and handle the specimen as if it were capable of transmitting disease.
- Place the swab in a sterile container and send it to the microbiology laboratory within 30 minutes.
- Indicate on the laboratory slip any medications that the patient may be taking that could affect test results.

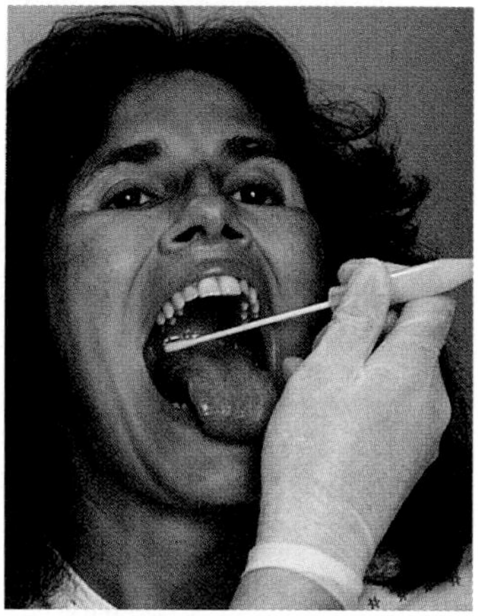

Figure 7-7 Collection of specimen from posterior pharynx.

Collections in Young Children

1. An adult should hold the child on his or her lap.
2. The person obtaining the specimen places one hand on the child's forehead to stabilize the head.
3. The collection is then obtained in a manner similar to that for adults.

After

- Notify the physician of any positive results so that appropriate antibiotic therapy can be initiated.

Test Results and Clinical Significance

Acute pharyngitis *Throat cultures are able to identify pathogenic bacteria such as streptococci,* Corynebacterium diphtheriae, *gonococci,* Bordetella pertussis, Neisseria, *corynebacteria, and staphylococci.* Candida *and* Bordetella *infections can also be identified.*

Tonsillar infections *These infections can be identified and their source determined if the swab is applied adequately to the tonsillar areas.*

Related Tests

- Antistreptolysin O titer (ASO) (p. 85): This is a serologic test that indicates a recent streptococcus infection.

Tuberculosis Culture (TB Culture, BACTEC Method, Polymerase Chain Reaction)

Normal Findings

Negative for tuberculosis

Indications

TB culture is indicated in any patient with a persistent productive cough, night sweats, anorexia, weight loss, fever, and hemoptysis. This diagnosis should be especially considered in high-risk patients, such as those who are immunocompromised, alcoholic, or have had a recent exposure to TB.

Test Explanation

The diagnosis of TB can be made only by identification and culture of *Mycobacterium tuberculosis* in the specimen. (See p. 1023 for other TB testing.) Conventional culture techniques for growth, identification, and susceptibility testing of acid-fast mycobacterium take 4 to 6 weeks. Because the patient suspected of having TB cannot be isolated from society for that duration, the disease may spread to many other people while the patient is waiting for the diagnosis. With the resurgence and increasing incidence of TB in the U.S. population (especially among immunocompromised patients with AIDS), newer, more rapid culture techniques have been identified and are now being performed.

The BACTEC method is a radiometric culture technique in which the growth medium for culturing mycobacteria is supplanted with a substrate labeled with radioactive carbon (^{14}C). This substrate is used by mycobacteria, and during metabolism, radioactive carbon dioxide ($^{14}CO_2$) is produced from the substrate. The $^{14}CO_2$ is detected quantitatively by counting the radioactivity with the Becton Dickinson Diagnostic Instrument System. The rate and amount of CO_2 produced is directly proportional to the rate and amount of growth occurring on the medium. With this technique, very small quantities of $^{14}CO_2$ can be detected. This permits quick identification of mycobacterial growth. This technique is used not only to isolate mycobacteria from clinical specimens but also to differentiate *M. tuberculosis* complex from other mycobacteria and for antimicrobial susceptibility testing.

Polymerase chain reaction culture methods also have recently been developed. With the addition of a DNA polymerase, genetic chromosomal parts can be multiplied. This allows amplification of genomes, which then can be detected by genetic DNA probes. With the newer techniques already described, *M. tuberculosis* can be identified in as little as 36 to 48 hours. With this reduction in diagnostic time, treatment can be started earlier. It is anticipated that the spread of TB therefore will be greatly reduced. The average detection time, however, is longer for extrapulmonary specimens than for sputum specimens. The time for identification is greatly reduced when numerous mycobacteria are present. Generally organisms in specimens from patients already receiving antituberculosis treatment take longer to grow.

After identification and growth of mycobacteria, antibiotic susceptibility testing is performed to identify the most effective antimycobacterial drugs. The culture can be performed on sputum, body fluids, CSF, and even biopsy tissue specimens.

Interfering Factors

- Antituberculosis drugs that have been started prior to culture could interfere with the growth of TB.

Procedure and Patient Care

Before

- Explain the procedure to the patient.
- Tell the patient that no fasting is required.

During

- For sputum, obtain an early morning specimen. It is best to induce sputum production with an ultrasonic or nebulizing device.
- Collect three to five early morning specimens. All specimens must contain mycobacteria to make the diagnosis of TB.
- For urine collection, obtain three to five single, clean-voided specimens early in the morning.
- Note that swabs, intestinal washings, and biopsy specimens should be transported to the laboratory immediately for preparation.
- Follow the institution's policy for universal specimen handling.
- Note the following procedural steps:
  1. Once the specimen is received by the laboratory, a decontamination process is applied to it to kill all nonmycobacteria. The specimen is then cultured in the appropriate medium.
  2. With the rapid growth techniques, the specimen is evaluated every 24 hours.
  3. When cultural growth is considered adequate, the organisms are stained for acid-fast bacilli and identified (p. 636).
  4. With DNA genetic probes the *Mycobacterium* species is identified.

5. At this point, if *M. tuberculosis* is present, the report will read "culture more positive for mycobacteria." If the species has been identified, this also will be reported.
6. Drug-susceptibility testing then will be carried out and subsequently reported.

After

- Instruct the patient in appropriate isolation of sputum and other body fluids to avoid potential spread of suspected TB.

Test Results and Clinical Significance

TB

Atypical mycobacterial nontuberculous disease *These organisms require special medium plates to grow. Any fluid or tissue can be used as a culture specimen. If the lungs are considered to be the sight of infection, sputum or pleural fluid is used. If the kidneys are suspected to be involved, urine should be tested. Others specimens include abdominal fluid, stomach aspirate, and bone tissue.*

Related Tests

- Acid-fast bacilli smear (p. 636): This smear is used to support the diagnosis of TB. By itself, the diagnosis of TB cannot be made. The smear (usually of sputum) is also used to monitor treatment for TB.
- Tuberculosis skin testing (p. 1023): Purified protein derivative is administered intradermally to test for prior exposure to TB. Skin testing cannot indicate active or dormant TB. If positive, it just implies previous exposure.
- Chest radiography (p. 924): Because TB is usually infective to the lungs due to inhalation of airborne infectious material, the chest x-ray examination often demonstrates the results (Ghon complex) of the acute granulomatous infection.

Wound and Soft Tissue Culture and Sensitivity (C&S)

Normal Findings Negative

Indications

A wound or soft tissue culture is indicated when a wound or soft tissue has signs of infection (redness, warmth, swelling, and pain). In a postoperative patient with a persistent fever of unknown origin, a wound may be probed and cultured even if the signs of infection are not present. Any spontaneous drainage from a wound or soft tissue should be cultured to document infection for treatment and drug sensitivities and to document the appropriateness of skin and wound isolation precautions.

Test Explanation

Wound cultures are obtained to determine the presence of pathogens in patients with suspected wound infections. Wound infections are most often caused by pus-forming organisms. All cultures should be performed before antibiotic therapy is initiated. Otherwise, the antibiotic may interrupt the growth of the organism in the laboratory. More often than not, however, the physician will want to institute antibiotic therapy after the wound is cultured but before the culture results are reported. In these instances, a *Gram stain* of the specimen smeared on a slide is most helpful and can be reported in less than 10 minutes. All forms of bacteria are grossly classified as gram positive (blue staining) or gram negative (red staining). Knowledge of the shape of the organism (e.g., spherical, rod shaped) also may be very helpful in the tentative identification of the infecting organism. With knowledge of the Gram-stain results, the physician can institute a reasonable antibiotic regimen based on past experience as to the organism's possible identity. Most organisms require approximately 24 hours to grow in the laboratory, and a preliminary report can be given at that time. Occasionally 48 to 72 hours are required for growth and identification of the organism. Cultures may be repeated after appropriate antibiotic therapy to assess for complete resolution of the infection.

It is important to recognize that many wound infections contain more than one organism. Multiple organisms may grow on culture. Deep space wounds, wounds containing necrotic debris or gas, and postoperative wounds commonly contain aerobic and anaerobic bacteria.

Interfering Factors

- Drugs that may alter test results include antibiotics.

Procedure and Patient Care

Before

- Explain the procedure to the patient.
- Assemble all equipment (Figure 7-8).

During

- Aseptically place a sterile cotton swab into the pus of the patient's wound, and then place the swab into a sterile, covered test tube. (Culturing specimens from the skin edge is much less accurate than culturing the suppurative material.)

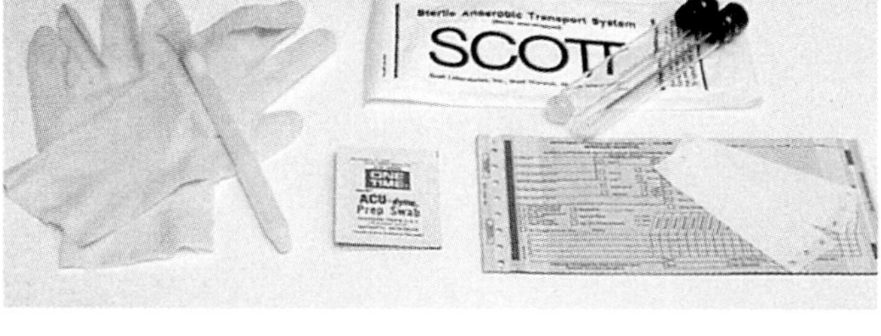

Figure 7-8 Equipment for collection of specimens from wound and decubiti.

- If an anaerobic organism is suspected, obtain an anaerobic culture tube from the microbiology laboratory. The specimen is best obtained by aspirating a closed wound and directly transferring the pus to the anaerobic culture tube.
- If wound cultures are to be obtained on a patient requiring wound irrigation, obtain the culture before the wound is irrigated.
- If any antibiotic ointment or solution has been previously applied, remove it with sterile water or saline before obtaining the culture several hours later.
- Handle all specimens carefully. These specimens are capable of transmitting disease.
- Indicate on the laboratory slip any medications the patient may be taking that could affect test results.

After

- Transport the specimen to the laboratory immediately after testing (at least within 30 minutes).
- Notify the physician of any positive results so that appropriate antibiotic therapy can be initiated.
- Note that if pus was observed in the wound or soft tissue, the patient should be immediately placed on skin and wound isolative precautions. The culture report documenting the infection does not need to be back before appropriate protective precautions are instituted.

Test Results And Clinical Significance

Wound infection *The best treatment of a wound infection is incision (widely opening the infection) and providing good drainage. Antibiotics are secondary.*

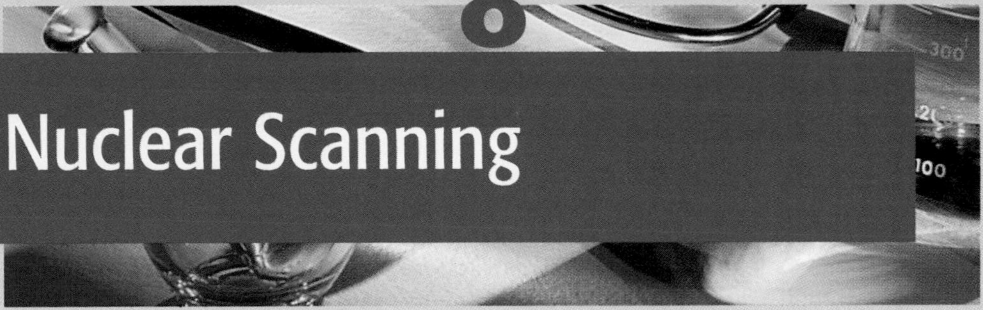

8

Nuclear Scanning

TESTS

Overview

Reasons for Performing Nuclear Medicine Studies

With the administration of a radiopharmaceutical and subsequent detection of the photons emitted from a particular organ, anatomic and functional abnormalities of various body areas can be detected. Nuclear medicine studies do not identify the specific cause (disease) of the abnormality. They provide supportive information to be used in conjunction with other diagnostic modalities. There are many indications for nuclear scanning, some of which are listed below:

1. To stage cancer by detecting metastasis to the bone (bone scan), liver (liver scan), or brain (brain scan)
2. To diagnose acute and chronic cholecystitis (gallbladder scan)
3. To identify deep vein thrombosis (fibrinogen uptake test)
4. To detect cerebral pathologic conditions (brain scan)
5. To evaluate gastric emptying (gastric emptying scan)
6. To localize sites of GI bleeding (GI bleeding scan)
7. To diagnose pulmonary embolism (lung scan)
8. To determine perfusion, structure, and function of the kidneys (renal scan) or heart (cardiac scan)
9. To evaluate thyroid nodules (thyroid scan)
10. To evaluate testicular swelling and pain (scrotal scan)

The radionuclides used in diagnostic medicine are artificially produced by either a nuclear reactor or a charged particle accelerator (cyclotron) by irradiating the nuclei and causing disruption and instability of its nucleus. Because of this instability, the nucleus of the radionuclide atom emits radioactive particles (photons in the gamma radiation range). The radionuclides used in nuclear scanning have short half-lives, which refers to the time required for 50% of the radioactive atoms to undergo decay. Technetium-99m (^{99m}Tc) is used extensively in nuclear scanning because its half-life is 6 hours and it emits low levels of gamma rays. Other commonly used radionuclides include gallium, thallium, and iodine.

To get to the desired organ, radionuclides are combined with a transport molecule. This combination of radionuclide and transport molecule is called a *radiopharmaceutical.* A radiopharmaceutical is the compound, labeled with the radionuclide, that is administered to the patient and localized in the organ to be studied. For most nuclear scans, radiopharmaceuticals are given IV. Less commonly used methods of administration include the oral and inhalation routes. Radiopharmaceuticals concentrate in target organs by various mechanisms. For example, some labeled compounds, such as iodohippurate sodium I 131 (Hippuran I 131), are cleared from the blood and excreted by the kidneys. Some phosphate compounds concentrate in the bone and infarcted tissue. Lung function can be studied by imaging the distribution of inhaled gases and aerosols.

After the radioisotope concentrates in the desired area, it emits gamma rays. The area is scanned with a gamma camera or a scintillation scanner that detects and records the emission of gamma rays. With each gamma ray detected, a light particle is emitted from the scintillation scanner. A computer translates these light readings into a two-dimensional image or scan (scintigram) that is printed in various shades of gray. Scintigrams can now be produced in color. The shades of gray or color show the distribution of the radionuclide in the organ. Hot spots are areas of increased uptake, and cold spots are areas with decreased uptake of the radionuclide. Normally the uptake of the radionuclide in an organ is diffuse and homogeneous. Hot and cold spots may mean different things on different scans. For example, a cold spot identified in the liver, spleen, or brain would indicate tumor, abscess, or some other space-occupying lesion. A cold spot detected on a thallium scan of the heart would not be suggestive of tumor but rather indicates an area of ischemia or infarction. On bone scan, hot spots may indicate areas of osteoblastic activity surrounding tumor. Arthritis or fracture may also be evident as hot spots. The scanning usually takes place in the nuclear medicine department. A large part of nuclear medicine includes blood studies and in vitro staining of microscopic slides using radioimmunoassay techniques. We have chosen to discuss these tests in Chapter 2 to avoid confusion with in vivo nuclear scanning.

Scanning can be *static*, which means that the patient and the camera are held in one position until an image is completed. Often the patient is rotated into another position for a static image of another view of the same organ. *Dynamic* scanning can also be performed and allows one to evaluate the blood flow to a certain organ, such as the brain or the liver. Single photon emission computed tomography (SPECT) is a newer technique by which a radiopharmaceutical (nearly all are single-photon emitters) is administered. The gamma camera is serially placed in multiple angles around the entire circumference of the patient. With this method, three-dimensional images can be obtained of the organ to be studied. Increased sensitivity is obtained. Still newer and less well defined is positron emission tomography (PET) scanning, which can demonstrate anatomic, functional, and biochemical abnormalities in an organ. This latter technique is still limited in its availability and is located mostly at large academic centers.

Although nuclear scanning includes a risk of radiation for the patient, the risk associated with most radionuclides is much less than that of an x-ray study. The half-lives of the radioisotopes are short, resulting in minimal radiation contamination by way of fecal and urine wastes. Nuclear scans are contraindicated in pregnant women and nursing mothers because of the risk of injury to the fetus or infant.

Procedural Care for Nuclear Scans

Before

- Explain the procedure to the patient. Assure the patient that radiation exposure is limited and minimal.
- Assess for an allergy to the radiopharmaceutical (especially when iodine is used).
- Note whether the patient has had any recent exposure to radionuclides. The previous study could interfere with the interpretation of the current study.
- Record the patient's age and current weight. This information is used to calculate the amount of radioactive substance needed.
- Many of the scanning procedures do not require any preparation. However, a few have special requirements. For example, in bone scanning the patient is encouraged to drink several glasses of water between the time of the injection of the isotope and the actual scanning.
- For some studies, blocking agents may need to be given to prevent other organs from taking up the isotope. For example, Lugol's solution may be needed to protect the thyroid gland from iodine-tagged radioisotopes. Potassium chloride may be used dur-

ing a brain scan to prevent an inordinate amount of technetium uptake by the choroid plexus, which would simulate a pathologic condition.

During

- Most radionuclides are injected IV. Often the patient is encouraged to drink water between administration of the radioisotope and the scanning. Radionuclides can also be given orally (gastric emptying scan) or by inhalation (ventilation scan).
- The area is scanned at the designated time period. The delay between administration of the radionuclide and scanning depends on the length of time required for the specific organ or tissue to take up the radionuclide and concentrate it. The patient must lie still during the scanning. Scans are usually repeated over a period that may extend from 1 hour to 3 days. The patient returns to the nuclear medicine department for each scanning.

After

- Assure the patient that only tracer doses of radioisotopes have been used and that no precautions against radioactive exposure are necessary.
- Although the amount of radionuclide excreted in the urine is very low, rubber gloves are sometimes recommended if the urine must be handled. Some doctors may advise the patient to flush the toilet several times after voiding.
- Encourage the patient to drink extra fluids to aid in excretion of the isotope from the body.
- If the isotope was injected IV, inspect the site for signs of infection, bruising, or hematoma.

Reporting of Results

Most tests are performed by a nuclear medicine technologist in the nuclear medicine department. A physician trained in diagnostic nuclear medicine interprets the test results.

Bone Scan

Normal Findings

No evidence of abnormality

Indications

The bone scan is used to identify metastatic cancer involving the bone. It is often performed on cancer patients as a routine part of staging before and after treatment. To a lesser degree, bone scanning is used to identify bone pathologic conditions that cannot be identified on plain films of the bone (e.g., osteomyelitis, old hairline fractures).

Test Explanation

The bone scan permits examination of the skeleton by a scanning camera after IV injection of a radionuclide material. Usually technetium-99m (^{99m}Tc) is the radionuclide utilized. After injection of the ^{99m}Tc, the radiopharmaceutical is taken up by the bone. Gamma rays are emitted from the ^{99m}Tc through the body and are detected by a scintillation scanner. The scintillation scanner emits light with each photon it receives from the gamma ray. When these light patterns are arranged in a spatial order, a realistic image of the bones is apparent.

The degree of radionuclide uptake is related to the metabolism of the bone. Normally a uniform concentration should be seen throughout the bones of the body. An increased uptake of isotope is abnormal and may represent tumor, arthritis, fracture, degenerative bone and joint changes, osteomyelitis, bone necrosis, osteodystrophy, or Paget's disease (Figure 8-1). These areas of concentrated radionuclide uptake are often called hot spots and are detectable months before an ordinary x-ray film can reveal the pathologic condition. Hot spots occur because new bone growth is usually stimulated around areas of abnormality. If a pathologic condition exists and there is no new bone formation around the lesion, the scan will not pick up the abnormality.

The major reason a bone scan is performed is to detect metastatic cancer to the bone. All malignancies capable of metastasis may reach the bone, especially those of the prostate, breast, lung, kidney, urinary bladder, and thyroid gland. Bone scans may be serially repeated to monitor tumor response to antineoplastic therapy.

Bone scans also provide valuable information for the evaluation of patients with trauma or unexplained pain. Bone scanning is much more sensitive than routine x-ray films in detecting small and difficult-to-find fractures, especially in the spine, ribs, face, and small bones of the extremities. Bone scans are used to determine the age of a fracture as well. If a fracture line is seen on a plain x-ray film and the uptake around that fracture is not increased on a bone scan, the injury is said to be an "old" fracture, exceeding several months in age.

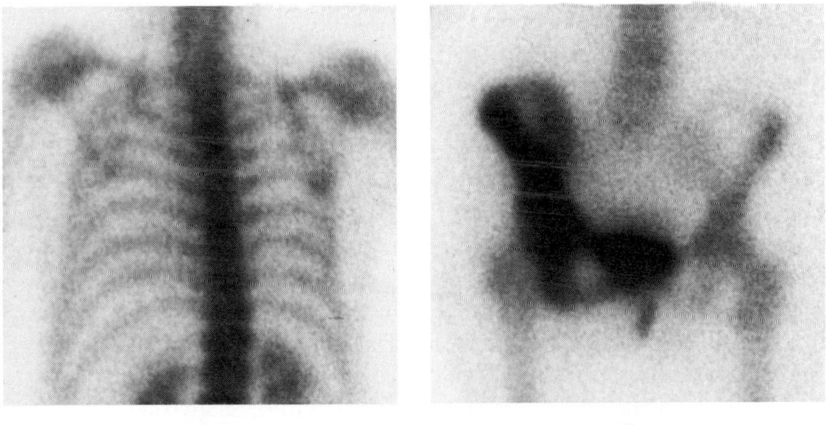

A B

Figure 8-1 Bone scan. **A,** Upper body. **B,** Lower body. There is normal uptake of radionuclide in the bones of the upper body. In the lower body view, the right iliac, ischium and pubic bones are associated with diffuse increased uptake of radionuclide, consistent with Paget's disease.

Although the bone scan is extremely sensitive, it unfortunately is not very specific. Fractures, infections, tumors, and arthritic changes all appear similar in this scan. Bone scans are helpful in identifying infection (osteomyelitis) when plain films fail to identify the classic findings of infection.

The bone scan is performed by a nuclear medicine technician in 30 to 60 minutes. It is interpreted by a physician trained in nuclear medicine imaging. The injection of the radioisotope causes slight discomfort. There may be some pain caused by lying on the hard scanning table for an hour.

Contraindications

- Patients who are pregnant, because of the risk of fetal injury
- Patients who are lactating, because of the risk of contaminating maternal milk

✓ CLINICAL PRIORITIES

- Bone scans are mainly done to detect metastatic cancer to the bone.
- Bone scans are often repeated to monitor tumor response to antineoplastic therapy.
- Bone scans should not be performed on pregnant and lactating women.

Procedure and Patient Care

Before

- Explain the procedure to the patient.
- Assure patients they will not be exposed to large amounts of radioactivity because only tracer doses of the isotope are used.
- Tell the patient that no fasting or sedation is required.

During

- Note the following procedural steps:
  1. The patient receives an IV injection of an isotope, usually sodium pertechnetate (^{99m}Tc) in a peripheral vein.
  2. The patient is encouraged to drink several glasses of water between the time of radioisotope injection and the scanning. This facilitates renal clearance of any circulating tracer not picked up by the bone. The waiting period before scanning is approximately 1 to 3 hours.
  3. The patient is instructed to urinate in order to eliminate any tracer that is in the bladder and blocking the view of the underlying pelvic bones.
  4. The patient is positioned in the supine position on the scanning table in the nuclear medicine department (Figure 8-2).
  5. A scintillation camera is placed over the patient's body and records the radiation emitted by the skeleton.

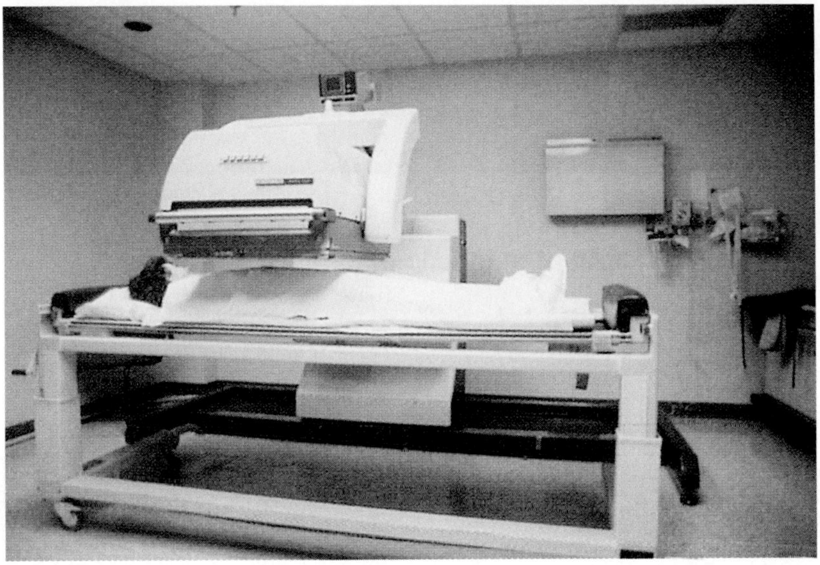

Figure 8-2 Patient prepared for bone scan. Patient's feet are tied to help maintain hips in position for maximal scanning uptake.

6. This information is translated into a two-dimensional view of the skeleton, which is then visualized on film.
7. The patient is repositioned in the prone and lateral positions during the test.

After

- Because only tracer doses of radioisotope are used, remember that no precautions need to be taken to prevent radioactive exposure to other personnel or family present.
- Assure the patient that the radioactive substance is usually excreted from the body within 6 to 24 hours.
- Encourage the patient to drink fluids to aid in the excretion of the radioactive substance.
- Observe the injection site for redness or swelling.

Test Results and Clinical Significance

Primary or metastatic tumors of the bone *These can be singular or multiple. It is difficult to specifically diagnose tumor. Serial scans may help.*

Fracture *Increased uptake in the bone of a patient with anatomic pain is very suggestive of a fracture missed on routine plain films.*

Degenerative arthritis
Rheumatoid arthritis
Increased uptake involving the joints (especially multiple joints) is classic for arthritis.

Osteomyelitis *Small islands of increased uptake within the bone of a patient with a compatible clinical history indicates infection.*
Bone necrosis *Decreased uptake (cold spot) may be present if there is not new bone growth surrounding the area of bone necrosis.*

Renal osteodystrophy
Paget's disease
These two diseases are usually evident as multiple or diffuse uptake of the tracer in the bones.

Related Tests

- Bone radiography (p. 913): The routine bone x-ray is often used to provide additional or supportive information to the bone scan.

Brain Scan (Cisternal Scan, Cerebral Blood Flow)

Normal Findings No areas of increased radionuclide uptake within the brain

Indications

In the past the brain scan was the only test available to study the brain. Since the advent of computed tomography (CT) scan of the brain (p. 939), magnetic resonance imaging (MRI) (p. 1009), and positron emission tomography (PET) (p. 737) scans, the nuclear brain scan has diminished in its usefulness. This test is used to identify pathologic conditions (tumor, infarction, infection) involving the cortex. It is used for patients with headaches, epilepsy, and other neurologic symptoms.

The nuclear cerebral blood flow brain scan is still commonly used to support the diagnosis of cerebral brain death.

Test Explanation

The brain scan permits examination of the brain by a scanning camera after IV injection of a radionuclide material (Figure 8-3). Usually technetium-99m (^{99m}Tc) is the radionuclide utilized. After injection of the ^{99m}Tc, the radiopharmaceutical is deposited anywhere in the brain where the blood-brain barrier has been disrupted by disease. Gamma rays are emitted from the ^{99m}Tc through the skull and are detected by a scintillation scanner. The scintillation scanner emits light with each photon it receives from the gamma ray. When these light patterns are arranged in a spatial order, a realistic image of the blood vessels, gray matter, and meninges of the brain and pathologic deposits are apparent. This study is performed in patients with frequent and severe headaches, stroke (cerebrovascular accident [CVA] syndrome), seizure complaints, or other neurologic complaints.

Normally the blood-brain barrier does not allow blood (containing the radionuclide) to come in direct contact with brain tissue. Frequently used isotopes (e.g., technetium-99m pertechnetate, mercury-201, radioiodinated albumin) are unable to cross this blood-brain barrier. However, in localized pathologic conditions, this normal barrier is dis-

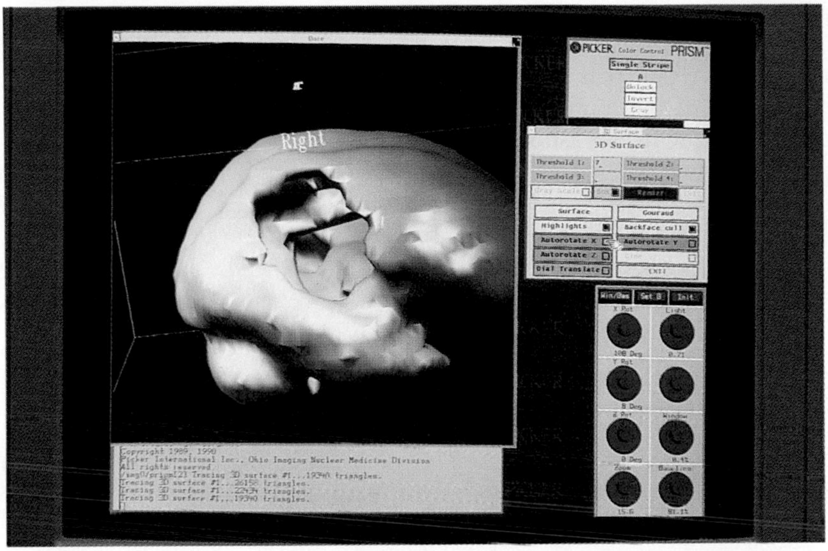

Figure 8-3 Image produced by radionuclide scan. This particular image demonstrates a deficit in cerebral blood flow caused by an arteriovenous malformation.

rupted. The isotopes are then preferentially localized or concentrated in abnormal regions of the brain.

The precise cause of the disruption of the blood-brain barrier can be any of various pathologic processes. Unfortunately, the brain scan is not a specific indicator of the exact pathologic process. Study of the location, size, and shape of the abnormality, along with the timing of the scan, may help specify the pathologic process.

The timing of brain scanning in relation to the onset of CVA-like symptoms is usually significant. For example, in cerebral infarction, scanning performed soon after the onset of symptoms may be normal and then become abnormal 2 weeks later; this combination is virtually pathognomonic of infarction. Scanning patients with cerebral thrombosis without infarction may never reveal abnormalities. Tumors and abscesses will show abnormalities on the initial scan.

The injection of isotopes followed by immediate scanning can be used to detect changes in the dynamics of cerebral blood flow by comparing one side of the brain with the other. For example, cerebrovascular occlusive disease is characterized by a decreased flow, in contrast to an arteriovenous (AV) malformation, which is associated with an increased flow rate. Technetium-99m exametazine or iodine may be used for cerebral perfusion studies. A *cerebral blood flow scan* is often used to support the findings of "brain death" by demonstrating lack of blood flow to the brain and concurrent blood flow to the scalp.

Cisternal scans may be performed by injecting radioactive material into the subarachnoid space and then taking serial scans of the head. These scans are useful in evaluating ventricular size and patency of the CSF pathways and reabsorption. Because only a small amount of CSF enters the ventricles, their uptake of radioactive material normally should be minimal. Blocks in the CSF pathways may prevent this reabsorption, however, and thus large amounts of isotopes may appear in the ventricles. Cisternal scans also may be used to evaluate CSF leakage (e.g., into the nasal sinuses) in patients with recurrent meningitis and to evaluate hydrocephalus.

The technique of single photon emission computed tomography (SPECT) has significantly improved the quality of brain scanning. With the use of radioactive carbon, nitrogen, or oxygen, anatomic and biochemical changes can be visualized within the brain. This method of brain scan approaches the usefulness of PET scans. With SPECT scanning the radionuclide is injected and the scintillation camera is placed to receive images from multiple angles (around the circumference of the head). This technique greatly increases the usefulness of nuclear brain scanning. In general, CT scans, MRI scans, and carotid duplex scans have replaced the brain scan in diagnostic neurology.

Contraindications

- Patients who are pregnant
- Patients who cannot cooperate during the testing

✓ CLINICAL PRIORITIES

- Pathologic conditions disrupt the normal blood-brain barrier and allow isotopes to concentrate in abnormal regions of the brain.
- The brain scan is not specific for indicating the cause of a pathologic process. Study of the location, shape, and size of the abnormality, along with the timing of the scan, may help delineate the problem.
- The SPECT technique has greatly improved the quality of brain scanning.

Procedure and Patient Care

Before

- Explain the procedure to the patient.
- Administer blocking agents as ordered before scanning. For example, potassium chloride prevents an inordinate amount of technetium uptake by the choroid plexus, which would simulate a pathologic cerebral condition. Similar solutions (e.g., potassium iodine, Lugol's solution) may be given orally to block thyroid uptake. Blocking agents are not necessary with the use of technetium-99m diethylenetriamine pentaacetic acid.
- Check for allergy to iodine if an iodinated solution will be used.
- Consider having a sedative ordered for agitated patients.

During

- Note the following procedural steps:
  1. After administration of the radioisotope, the patient is placed in the supine, lateral, and prone positions while a counter is placed over the head (Figure 8-4).
  2. The radioisotope counts are anatomically displayed and photographed while the patient remains very still.

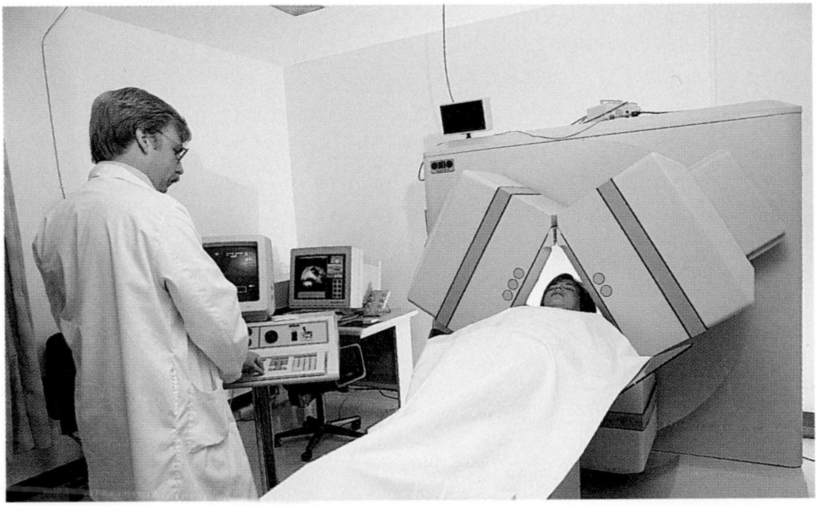

Figure 8-4 Patient positioned for a radionuclide scan of the brain. In this diagnostic study, a small amount of radioactive material crosses the blood-brain barrier to produce an image. This study is known as single photon emission computed tomography (SPECT).

3. When cerebral flow studies are performed, the counter is immediately placed over the head.
4. The counts are anatomically recorded in timed sequence to follow the isotope during its first flow through the brain.
5. Another scan is obtained 30 minutes to 2 hours later for identification of pathologic tissues.

- Note that this study is performed by a technician in the nuclear medicine department in approximately 35 to 45 minutes.
- Tell the patient that no discomfort is associated with this study other than the peripheral IV puncture required for injection of the radioisotope.

After

- Assure the patient that the radioactive material is usually excreted from the body within 6 to 24 hours.
- Because only tracer doses of radioisotopes are used, remember that no precautions need to be taken to prevent radioactive exposure to other personnel or family present.
- Encourage the patient to drink fluids to aid in the excretion of the isotope from the body.
- Observe the injection site for redness and swelling.

Test Results and Clinical Significance

Cerebral neoplasm
Brain abscess

Cerebral hemorrhage
Cancer metastasis to the brain
These pathologic conditions are associated with breakdown in the blood-brain barrier, resulting in increased uptake of radionuclide in the cerebral cortex.

Acute cerebral infarction *In the first few days to weeks following a stroke, the scan may be normal. After a few weeks, however, the blood-brain barrier is disrupted, and cortical uptake occurs. This is pathognomonic of stroke.*
Subdural hematoma *The cortex/subcortical tissue and meninges may become distorted and lateralized.*

Cerebral thrombosis
Cerebrovascular occlusive disease
Hematoma
AV malformation
Aneurysm
These vascular abnormalities are evident with cerebral flow studies.

CSF leakage *The most common site of leakage of CSF is into the nasal cavity. This can be the result of tumor or infection.*
Hydrocephalus *This is evident on cisternal scans.*

Related Tests

- Computed tomography (CT) scan of the brain (p. 939): This test is very accurate in identifying pathologic conditions of the brain. X-rays are directed to the brain from multiple circumferential angles and then gathered to produce multiple images of the brain.
- Magnetic resonance imaging scan of the brain (p. 1009): This test does not use x-rays but rather detects electromagnetic differences among the brain tissues. It visualizes the brain from similar angles as the CT scan, producing an accurate image.

Cardiac Nuclear Scanning
(Myocardial Scan, Cardiac Scan, Nuclear Cardiac Scanning, Heart Scan, Thallium Scan, MUGA Scan, Isonitrile Scan, Sestamibi Scan)

Normal Findings Normal myocardial ejection fraction and coronary perfusion

Indications

Cardiac nuclear scanning is used to detect myocardial ischemia, infarction, wall dysfunction, and decreased ejection fraction. It is commonly used as the imaging method portion of cardiac stress testing. Specific indications for cardiac nuclear scanning include the following:

1. Screening of adults for past and recent infarction
2. Evaluation of patients with chest pain and uninterpretable or equivocal electrocar-

diogram (EKG) changes caused by drugs, bundle branch block, or left ventricular hypertrophy
3. Evaluation of myocardial perfusion before and after coronary artery bypass surgery
4. Quantification and surveillance of myocardial infarction
5. Evaluation of medical and surgical therapy for coronary artery perfusion
6. Evaluation of ventricular function in patients with myocardial disease
7. Evaluation of patients receiving cardiotoxic drugs (e.g., doxorubicin [Adriamycin] chemotherapy)

Test Explanation

Cardiac radionuclear scanning is a noninvasive and safe method of recognizing alterations of left ventricular muscle function and coronary artery blood distribution. Many different radiocompound materials can be used, most often technetium-99m pertechnetate, thallium-201, or technetium-99m pyrophosphate. When these compounds are injected IV and a radiation detector is placed over the heart, an image of the heart can be recorded and photographed.

In evaluating the patency of the coronary arteries, the characteristic abnormality varies according to the type of radiocompound used. When thallium is used, all normal myocardial cells take up the substance and appear on the photoscan. Ischemic or infarcted cells do not take up the substance and appear as cold spots, devoid of nuclear material and surrounded by normal cells (Figure 8-5). Technetium-99m sestamibi (isonitrile) presents a similar picture. It is an even better cardiac imaging agent. Higher-quality images can be obtained on the first pass, providing information similar to angiocardiography. Perfusion images, ventricular function, and gated-pool ejection fractions can all be obtained with a single injection. This is often called a *myocardial perfusion scan*. Furthermore, with the use of isonitrile an ischemic area will be visible several hours after an ischemic event.

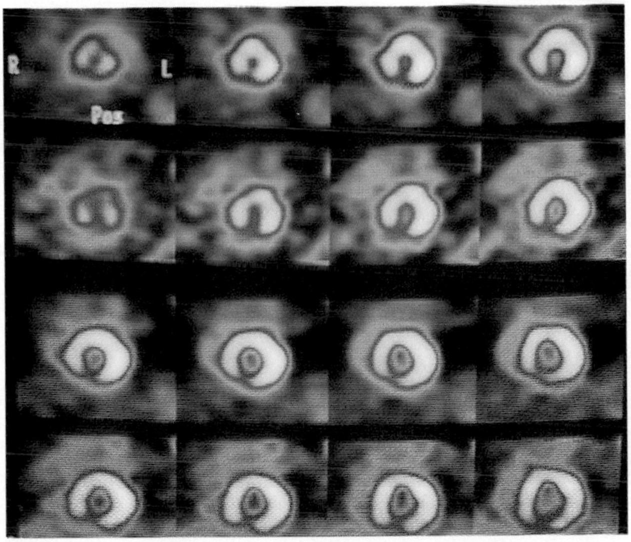

Figure 8-5 Thallium-201 scintigraphy produces a series of images of blood flow and tissue perfusion.

Technetium-99m pyrophosphate is a radionuclide that binds with calcium. When ischemia or early infarction has occurred, intracellular calcium leaks out of the cardiac muscle cells. The calcium level in the area of injury is very high. The technetium-99m pyrophosphate binds to that calcium and creates an area of increased radionuclide uptake (hot spot). This is often called a *myocardial infarction scan.* Cardiac scanning with technetium-99m pyrophosphate is particularly useful in cases where ischemia is difficult to diagnose. For example, in a patient with ventricular hypertrophy or left bundle branch block, the EKG is unreliable. If these patients have chest pain and the pyrophosphate scan is positive, muscle injury can be said to have occurred. This type of scan is also especially helpful if the patient has had chest pain 5 to 10 days prior to seeing a doctor. Because the pyrophosphate scan stays positive for that long, the delayed diagnosis of a myocardial infarction can be made.

With the radionuclides discussed cardiac nuclear scanning is used to indicate myocardial ischemia or infarction. It can be used in acute events of chest pain. Ischemia or infarction would be evident as described above. Cardiac scanning also can be used to assess myocardial ischemia during stress testing (p. 269). In some cases, no evidence of diminished blood supply to the myocardium is evident during the resting state. When stressed, however, evidence of myocardial ischemia can become quite obvious and is easily detected by nuclear stress testing. In this form of nuclear cardiac scanning the radionuclide is injected IV at the point of maximal cardiac stress. The radionuclide accumulates in the myocardium in direct proportion to the regional myocardial blood flow. The normal myocardium will have much greater radionuclide activity than the ischemic myocardium. In comparing this stress testing with a resting cardiac nuclear scan, one can see exercise-induced ischemia. This is *stress testing utilizing cardiac nuclear scanning* as the method of cardiac imaging or monitoring. This test is not only beneficial in detecting coronary occlusive disease but also successful in assessing postoperative patency of a coronary bypass graft.

For an evaluation of myocardial function, technetium-99m pertechnetate or technetium-labeled albumin is used to measure the portion of blood ejected from the ventricle during one cardiac cycle (ejection fraction). Normally, over 65% of the blood is ejected from the ventricle during systole. Values less than that indicate decreased contractility of the heart caused by ischemia, infarction, or cardiomyopathy. Computers can be synchronized with the EKG during scanning. The amount of blood ejected during sys-

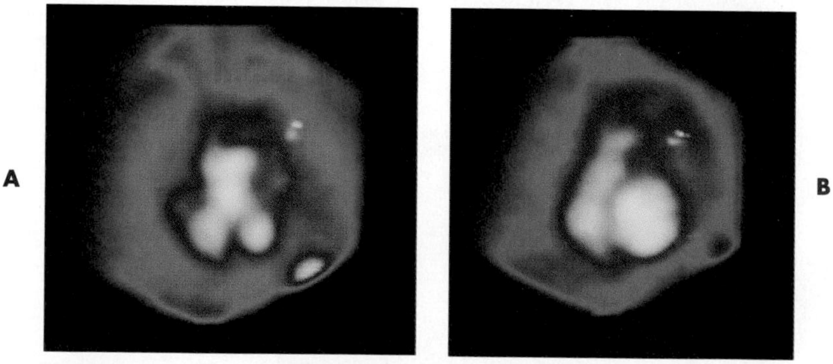

Figure 8-6 Blood pool imaging. **A,** Systolic frame. **B,** Diastolic frame.

tole also can be calculated based on the size of the heart at end-systole and end-diastole. This form of determination of ventricular function is called *gated pool imaging* or the *gated pool ejection fraction. Multigated acquisition* (MUGA) *scan* is another name for this test based on the name of the computer machinery originally required for this determination (Figure 8-6).

This computer-assisted gated (synchronized) cardiac scan can also allow the myocardial wall to be photographed while in motion. This allows visualization of the myocardium during several cardiac cycles, and contractility of the myocardium can be determined. This imaging technique is called nuclear ventriculography and can provide the same information as radiographic ventriculography, which is performed during cardiac catheterization (p. 917); however, the nuclear scans are noninvasive and much safer. Ischemic areas are seen to be hypokinetic on scans. Infarcted area are akinetic on scan. This is also evident after stress during a cardiac stress test.

In single photon emission computed tomography (SPECT) the radionuclear materials discussed emit single photons. SPECT has been used to visualize the heart from many different angles. These images are then reconstructed using techniques similar to computed tomography scanning, and three-dimensional images of the physiologic cardiac processes are obtained. Areas of myocardial ischemia can be seen with far greater resolution and can be more accurately quantified.

Contraindications

- Patients who are uncooperative
- Patients who are pregnant, because of fetal exposure to radionuclide material

Interfering Factors

- Myocardial trauma
- Recent nuclear scans (e.g., thyroid or bone scan)
- Drugs such as long-acting nitrates

✓ CLINICAL PRIORITIES

- Nuclear scanning is commonly used as the imaging portion of cardiac stress testing to assess myocardial ischemia.
- This test can be used to evaluate myocardial function by measuring the ejection fraction.
- Technetium-99m sestamibi presents a better cardiac image than thallium. It is often used to replace thallium.

Procedure and Patient Care

Before

- Explain the procedure to the patient.
- Instruct the patient that a short fasting period may be required.

During

- Take the patient to the nuclear medicine department.
- Note the following procedural steps:
  1. An IV injection of radionuclide material is performed.
  2. Depending on the radionuclide used, scanning is performed 15 minutes to 4 hours later.
  3. A gamma ray detector is placed over the precordium.
  4. The patient is placed in a supine position, then in the lateral position, and then in both the right and left oblique positions.
  5. The gamma ray scanner records the image of the heart, and a photograph is immediately developed.
  6. For a *thallium exercise stress test,* radioactive thallium is injected during exercise when the patient reaches a maximum heart rate. The patient then lies on a table, and scanning is done. A repeat scan may be done 3 to 4 hours later.
  7. If an *isonitrile stress test is* needed, the patient is injected and scanned 30 to 60 minutes later for the resting phase. Four hours later, cardiac stress testing is done. After a second injection, scanning is repeated. Milk and a muffin are usually given after each isonitrile injection to facilitate clearing of the radionuclide from the hepatobiliary system.
- Tell the patient that the only discomfort associated with this test is the venipuncture required for injection of the radioisotope.
- Note that myocardial scans are usually performed in less than 30 minutes by a nuclear medicine technician.

After

- Because only tracer doses of radioisotopes are used, note that no precautions need to be taken against radioactive exposure to personnel or family.
- Encourage the patient to drink fluids to aid in the excretion of the radioactive substance.
- Apply pressure or a pressure dressing to the venipuncture site.
- Assess the venipuncture site for bleeding.
- If stress testing was performed, evaluate the patient's vital signs at frequent intervals (as indicated).

Test Results and Clinical Significance

Coronary artery occlusive disease *This diagnosis can be made during a resting scan or during a cardiac stress nuclear scan. The manner with which this abnormality becomes evident depends on the radionuclide used.*

Decreased myocardial function associated with ischemia, myocarditis, cardiomyopathy, or congestive heart failure *These diseases affecting the myocardium are evident as hypokinesia of the cardiac wall. Infarcted areas have no wall motion.*

Decreased cardiac output *Many coronary, myocardial, and valvular diseases are associated with reduced cardiac output. A reduced ejection fraction is an indirect measurement of cardiac output. Often a reduced ejection fraction is the first sign of those diseases.*

Related Tests

- Cardiac stress testing (p. 469): This is a test whereby stress is provided to maximize the cardiac function. The heart is then often imaged with nuclear scanning to see the effect of the stress.

Fibrinogen Uptake Test with ^{125}I
(Fibrinogen Uptake Test [FUT], Radioactive Fibrinogen Scanning)

Normal Findings

No area of increased radionuclide uptake within the venous systems of the lower extremity

Indications

This nuclear study is used to identify deep venous thrombophlebitis (DVT) in patients with swollen painful legs. It is even used in asymptomatic patients who are at increased risk for DVT.

Test Explanation

The iodine-125 fibrinogen uptake test (^{125}I FUT) is a noninvasive radionuclear study used to identify thrombi in the veins of the lower extremities. When thrombi form, large amounts of fibrinogen are present at the site of clot formation. Fibrinogen is an important hemostatic factor (factor I) (see Figure 2-10, p. 156). When fibrinogen is tagged with ^{125}I and given IV, it can be detected by a gamma ray detector. At areas where clot formation is occurring (e.g., venous thromboses), the ^{125}I count will be greatly increased. The test is approximately 80% to 90% accurate in the diagnosis of DVT (even below the knee).

Although clinicians previously thought the test could recognize only clots being formed, it is now known that the ^{125}I FUT can detect established clots. This test is also useful in the early detection of subclinical DVT. Therefore immobilized patients at great risk for DVT can be identified early. However, the ^{125}I FUT has several disadvantages:

1. This test cannot detect DVT in the very proximal thigh. Normally, high quantities of fibrinogen exist in that area, and the background counts are too high to detect minimal degrees of increased uptake.
2. It is necessary to wait at least 24 hours between administering ^{125}I and detecting increased fibrinogen uptake. This is a major disadvantage when one needs to know immediately if thrombosis exists.
3. Because the fibrinogen used in this test is obtained from donated blood, the inherent risks of blood transfusion exist.

Initially this test was used to evaluate medical-surgical or obstetric patients at high risk for the formation of DVT. These patients were studied over 1 to 2 weeks to detect extremely early DVT. Patients can be studied daily for 7 to 14 days after administration of ^{125}I.

Contraindications

- Patients for whom the diagnosis of DVT is needed in less than 24 hours
- Patients with ongoing inflammation in the leg (e.g., superficial phlebitis, cellulitis, active arthritis)

Fibrinogen exists in increased levels at these areas and will give a false-positive result.

- Patients with lymphedema, because the fibrinogen level is high in the extremities
- Patients who are allergic to iodine or shellfish

A steroid-and-diphenhydramine (Benadryl) preparation may be used for these patients.

Interfering Factors

- Other areas of inflammation within the suspected extremity
- Lymphedema

✓ CLINICAL PRIORITIES

- Assess the patient for allergies to iodine.
- Lugol's solution or potassium iodide may be ordered before this test to avoid uptake of ^{125}I by the thyroid gland.
- Nursing mothers should not breast-feed their babies for 24 to 48 hours after this scan.

Procedure and Patient Care

Before

- Explain the procedure to the patient.
- Determine whether the patient is allergic to iodine or shellfish.
- Assess the patient's extremity for signs of inflammation or lymphedema.
- Tell the patient that no fasting or sedation is required.

During

- Note the following procedural steps:
  1. The patient is transferred to the nuclear medicine department, where ^{125}I fibrinogen is administered.
  2. The extremity is marked in multiple areas for subsequent examination.
  3. Countered readings are obtained 10 minutes after ^{125}I administration over the premarked sites.
  4. The patient is returned to his or her room.
  5. Twenty-four hours later, either at the patient's bedside or on return to the nuclear medicine department, the Geiger-like detector is placed over the previously marked areas for counter readings.
  6. The amount of ^{125}I identified at the premarked sites is recorded and compared with the amount present in the opposite leg or in the precordium.

7. If the amount of ^{125}I detected at any area is 15 times greater than normal extremity, heart, or baseline preinjection levels, the test is considered positive for DVT.

- To avoid uptake of ^{125}I by the thyroid gland, provide Lugol's solution or potassium iodine, if ordered, for the patient before and during the scanning procedure.
- Note that a nuclear medicine technologist performs this procedure in less than 1 hour daily.
- Tell the patient that no discomfort is associated with this test other than the fibrinogen injection.

After

- Caution all nursing mothers to refrain from breast-feeding for 24 to 48 hours after injection of ^{125}I.

Test Results and Clinical Significance

Deep-vein thrombophlebitis *Increased uptake in the lower extremity, especially, indicates active DVT.*

Related Tests

- Venography (p. 1002): This is an accurate test to identify DVT. It uses iodinated contrast with its inherent risks.
- Doppler venous duplex scan (p. 807): This uses ultrasound to identify DVT. However, it is not accurate for DVT below the knee (a common location of clotting).
- Plethysmography, venous (p. 626): This is an accurate test to detect venous thrombosis by manometric testing.

Gallbladder Nuclear Scanning

(Hepatobiliary Scintigraphy, Hepatobiliary Imaging, Biliary Tract Radionuclide Scan, Cholescintigraphy, DISIDA Scanning, HIDA Scanning, IDA Gallbladder Scanning)

Normal Findings

Gallbladder, common bile duct, and duodenum visualize within 60 minutes after radionuclide injection. (This confirms patency of the cystic and common bile ducts.)

Indications

Cholescintigraphy is valuable in evaluating patients for suspected gallbladder disease. The primary use of this study is to diagnose acute cholecystitis in patients who have acute right upper quadrant abdominal pain. When gallbladder ejection fraction is calculated, chronic cholecystitis can be diagnosed. This study is also used to assist in the diagnosis of extrahepatic biliary obstruction.

Test Explanation

Through the use of iminodiacetic acid analogues (IDAs) labeled with technetium-99m (^{99m}Tc), the biliary tract can be evaluated in a safe, accurate, and noninvasive manner. These radionuclide compounds are extracted by the liver and excreted into the bile. Gamma rays are emitted from the ^{99m}Tc in the bile through the body and are detected by a scintillation camera. The scintillation camera emits light with each photon it receives from the gamma ray. When these light patterns are arranged in a spatial order, a realistic image of the biliary tree is apparent.

Failure to visualize the gallbladder 60 to 120 minutes after injection of the radionuclide dye is virtually diagnostic of an obstruction of the cystic duct, which instigates the pathophysiology of acute cholecystitis. Delayed filling of the gallbladder is associated with chronic or acalculus cholecystitis. This procedure is also helpful in diagnosing biliary duct obstructions. The identification of the radionuclide in the biliary tree but not in the bowel is diagnostic of common bile duct obstruction.

This procedure is superior to oral cholecystography, IV cholangiography, ultrasonography, and computed tomography (CT) of the gallbladder in the detection of cholecysti-

Table 8-1 Comparison of methods of visualizing the gallbladder and biliary system

Test	Advantages	Disadvantages
Cholecystography	Easily performed, inexpensive	Will not visualize if other inflammatory processes are in the abdomen Will not visualize if bilirubin >2.0 Will not visualize if patient vomits or has diarrhea
IV cholangiography	Easily performed, inexpensive	Will not visualize if bilirubin >2.0
Endoscopic retrograde cholangiopancreatography (ERCP)	Good visualization of the bile duct Stones can be extracted Stents can be placed to drain bile	Technically difficult May not visualize the gallbladder Invasive procedure
Percutaneous transhepatic cholangiography (PTC)	Good visualization of the biliary tree Stents can be placed to drain bile	Invasive procedure May not visualize the gallbladder.
Ultrasound	Easily performed, accurate, inexpensive	May not be accurate for common bile duct pathologic conditions Cannot diagnose acute cholecystitis with certainty
Scintigraphy (nuclear scanning)	Indicates acute cholecystitis Can visualize the biliary tree even if bilirubin is >2.0	Not accurate for chronic cholecystitis More complicated to perform Takes several hours to identify pathologic condition May give false-positive results if other inflammatory processes are occurring within the abdomen

tis (Table 8-1). Also, with cholescintigraphy, gallbladder function can be numerically determined by calculating the capability of the gallbladder to eject its contents. It is believed that an ejection fraction below 35% indicates primary gallbladder disease.

Occasionally morphine sulfate is given IV during nuclear scanning. The morphine causes increased ampullary contraction. Not only can this reproduce the patient's symptoms of biliary colic, but it also serves to force the bile containing the radionuclide into the gallbladder. If no radionuclide is seen in the gallbladder with the use of morphine within 15 to 60 minutes, the diagnosis of acute cholecystitis is nearly certain. This greatly decreases the scanning time because without morphine it requires 4 hours to obtain a definitive diagnosis of acute cholecystitis.

A nuclear medicine technologist performs this study in 1 to 4 hours in the nuclear medicine department. A physician trained in interpretation of diagnostic nuclear medicine interprets the test in a few minutes. The only discomfort associated with this procedure is the IV injection of radionuclide.

Contraindications

- Pregnancy, because of the risk of fetal injury

Interfering Factors

- If the patient has not eaten for more than 24 hours, the radionuclide may not fill the gallbladder. This would produce a false-positive result.

CLINICAL PRIORITIES

- Gallbladder scanning is primarily used to diagnose acute cholecystitis in patients who have acute right upper quadrant pain.
- This procedure is superior to oral cholecystography, IV cholangiography, ultrasonography, and CT of the gallbladder in the diagnosis of cholecystitis.
- This procedure can also determine the ejection fraction of the gallbladder.
- Morphine sulfate can be administered IV during scanning to markedly reduce the scanning time from 4 hours to less than 1 hour.

Procedure and Patient Care

Before

- Explain the procedure to the patient.
- Assure the patient that he or she will not be exposed to large amounts of radioactivity.
- Instruct the patient to fast for at least 2 hours before the test. This fasting is preferable but not mandatory.

During

- Note the following procedural steps:
  1. After IV administration of a ^{99m}Tc-labeled IDA (e.g., DISIDA, PIPIDA, HIDA), the right upper quadrant of the abdomen is scanned.

2. Serial images are obtained over 1 hour.
3. Subsequent images can be obtained at 15- to 30-minute intervals.
4. If the gallbladder, common bile duct, or duodenum is not visualized within 60 minutes after injection, delayed images are obtained up to 4 hours later.
5. Images are recorded on film.
6. When an *ejection fraction* is to be determined, the patient is given a fatty meal or cholecystokinin is administered to evaluate emptying of the gallbladder. The gallbladder is continually scanned to measure the percentage of isotope ejected.

After

- Obtain a meal for the patient, if indicated.

Test Results and Clinical Significance

Acute cholecystitis *No visualization of the gallbladder will be seen because a gallstone is stuck in the cystic duct, causing acute cholecystitis. The rest of the biliary tree is visualized.*

Chronic cholecystitis
Acalculus cholecystitis
Cystic duct syndrome
Delayed visualization of the gallbladder is seen after several hours. The gallbladder ejection fraction is below 35%. The pathophysiology of cystic duct syndrome is not well known.

Common bile duct obstruction secondary to gallstones, tumor, or stricture *This is evident when the radionuclide is seen in a large bile duct but not in the bowel. Obstruction of the bile duct must be present.*

Related Tests (Table 8-1, p. 712)

- Ultrasonography of the gallbladder (p. 778): With the use of ultrasound, gallstones can be identified to be within the gallbladder. The diagnosis of acute cholecystitis cannot be made with the same degree of certainty as it can using biliary scintigraphy.
- Oral cholecystography (p. 930): This is an x-ray study of the gallbladder using orally administered dye. The diagnosis of acute cholecystitis cannot be made with the same degree of certainty as it can using biliary scintigraphy.

Gallium Scan

Normal Findings

Diffuse, low level of gallium uptake, especially in the liver and spleen
No increased gallium uptake within the body

Indications

Gallium becomes concentrated in areas of the body where WBCs tend to congregate (areas of tumor, infection, and inflammation). It is used to stage gallium-avid tumors (e.g., lymphomas, lung cancer). It is used to locate infection or inflammation in patients with fever of unknown origin. Finally, it is used to monitor response to treatment of infection, inflammation, or tumor.

Test Explanation

A gallium scan of the total body is usually performed 24, 48, and 72 hours after an IV injection of radioactive gallium. Gallium is a radionuclide that is concentrated by areas of inflammation and infection, by abscesses, and by benign and malignant tumors. Not all types of tumors, however, will concentrate gallium (gallium avid). Lymphomas are particularly gallium avid. Other tumors that can be detected by a gallium scan include sarcomas, hepatomas, and carcinomas of the GI tract, kidney, uterus, stomach, and testicle.

This test is useful in detecting metastatic tumor, especially lymphoma, even when other diagnostic imaging tests are normal. The gallium scan also is useful in demonstrating a source of infection in patients with a fever of unknown origin. Gallium can be used to identify noninfectious inflammation within the body in patients who have an elevated sedimentation rate. Unfortunately, this test is not specific enough to differentiate among tumor, infection, inflammation, and abscess.

Some organs (liver, spleen, bone, colon) normally retain gallium. Therefore a normal total-body gallium scan study would demonstrate some uptake in these organs, but this uptake is much less concentrated than in pathologic areas (e.g., tumor, inflammation).

A nuclear medicine technologist performs each scan in approximately 30 to 60 minutes. Repeated scanning, however, is required. Repeated injections are not necessary. The test results are interpreted by a physician trained in nuclear medicine and are usually available 72 hours after the injection. No pain or discomfort is associated with this procedure other than the IV injection. However, it occasionally can be uncomfortable to lie still on a hard table for the duration required.

Contraindications

- Pregnancy, because of the risk of fetal injury

✓ CLINICAL PRIORITIES

- Gallium scanning is useful in detecting metastatic tumor, even when other diagnostic imaging tests are normal.
- Gallium is normally retained in the liver, colon, spleen, and bone. Therefore it is normal to demonstrate small amounts of uptake in these organs during scanning.
- Scanning can be repeated without additional injections of the radionuclide.

Procedure and Patient Care

Before

- Explain the procedure to the patient.
- Usually administer a cathartic or enema to the patient to minimize increased gallium uptake within the bowel.

During

- Note the following procedural steps:
  1. The unsedated patient is injected with gallium.
  2. A total-body scan may be performed 4 to 6 hours later by slowly passing a scintillation camera over the body.
  3. The images provided by the scintillation camera are recorded on film.
  4. Additional scans are usually taken 24, 48, and 72 hours later.
  5. During the scanning process the patient is positioned in the supine, prone, and lateral positions.

After

- Assure the patient that only tracer doses of radioisotopes have been used and that no precautions against radioactive exposure to others are necessary.

Test Results and Clinical Significance

Tumor
Noninfectious inflammation (sarcoidosis, rheumatoid arthritis)
Infection
Abscess
These processes can concentrate gallium, but not with 100% accuracy. These pathologic conditions may exist in patients in whom results of the gallium scan are normal.

Gastric Emptying Scan

Normal Findings

No delay in gastric emptying
Gastric emptying complete in 90-120 minutes for *solids*, 15-75 minutes for *liquids*

Indications

This scan is used to determine the rate of gastric emptying. It is performed on patients who have postcibal nausea, vomiting, bloating, early satiety, or belching.

Test Explanation

In this study the patient ingests a solid or liquid "test meal" containing a radionuclide such as technetium (Tc). The stomach is then scanned until gastric emptying is complete. This study is used to assess the stomach's ability to empty solids or liquids and to evaluate disorders that may cause a delay in gastric emptying, such as obstruction (caused by peptic ulcers or gastric malignancies) and gastroparesis. This scan is also useful in determining the patency of a GI anastomosis.

This procedure lasts approximately 90 to 120 minutes, depending on the gastric emptying time. The test is interpreted by a nuclear medicine physician. Results are available the same day. There is no discomfort associated with the test.

Contraindications

- Patients who are pregnant or lactating, because the radionuclide may cause fetal or newborn injury

Procedure and Patient Care

Before

- Explain the procedure to the patient.
- Assure the patient that no pain is associated with this study.
- Inform the patient that only a small dose of nuclear material is ingested. Reassure the patient that this is a safe dose.
- Instruct the patient to keep an NPO status after midnight on the day of the test.

During

- Note the following procedural steps:
    1. In the nuclear medicine department the patient is asked to ingest a test meal. In the solid-emptying study the patient eats a cooked egg white containing Tc. In the liquid-emptying study the patient drinks orange juice or water containing technetium-99m diethylenetriamine pentaacetic acid (DTPA) or indium-111 DTPA.
    2. After ingestion of the test meal the patient lies supine under a gamma camera that records gastric images. This scan is repeated at short intervals (about 15 minutes) until gastric emptying has been complete. This may take several hours, although each particular timed scan takes only a few minutes.

With the use of computer calculations of timed images, the rate of gastric emptying can be determined.

After

- Assure the patient that he or she has ingested only a small amount of nuclear material. No radiation precautions need to be taken against the patient or his or her bodily secretions.

Test Results and Clinical Significance

Gastric obstruction caused by gastric ulcer or cancer *Tumors located at the gastric outlet can obstruct or delay gastric emptying. Ulcers, particularly in the duodenum, can cause edema and scarring, which also can cause delay in gastric emptying. The scan, while not specific as to the cause of the obstruction, will demonstrate prolonged gastric emptying.*

Nonfunctioning GI anastomosis *Postoperative edema is suspected to be the cause of delayed gastric emptying after gastric surgery. Gastroparesis also may play a role.*

Gastroparesis *The muscle function required for gastric emptying can be affected by nerve damage caused by diabetes or other neuropathies. There may be endocrine factors (gastrin related) affecting gastric emptying. This process is not uncommon after prolonged periods of gastric obstruction. Here, again, the gastric emptying scan will be prolonged.*

Related Tests

- Gastroesophageal reflux scan (see below): This is very similarly performed but evaluates the patient for reflux of the gastric contents into the esophagus.

Gastroesophageal Reflux Scan
(GE Reflux Scan, Aspiration Scan)

Normal Findings No evidence of gastroesophageal reflux

Indications

This scan is performed on patients who complain of heartburn, reflux of food, water brash (sour taste in the mouth), aspiration, or paroxysmal nocturnal dyspnea (from nocturnal aspiration). It can detect gastroesophageal reflux and/or aspiration.

Test Explanation

GE reflux scans are used to evaluate patients with symptoms of heartburn, regurgitation, vomiting, and dysphagia. Also, these scans are used to evaluate the medical or surgical treatment of patients with GE reflux. Finally, aspiration scans may be used to detect aspiration of gastric contents into the lungs and evaluate swallowing function.

This procedure is performed in the nuclear medicine department in approximately 30 minutes. There is no discomfort associated with this test.

Contraindications

- Patients who cannot tolerate abdominal compression
- Patients who are pregnant or lactating, because the radionuclide could cause injury to the fetus or newborn

Age-related concerns

- Aspiration scans can be used to evaluate *infants* for chalasia.
- The tracer is added to the formula or feeding. Films are taken over the next hour with delayed films taken as needed.

Procedure and Patient Care

Before

- Explain the procedure to the patient.
- Assure the patient that no pain is associated with this test.
- Instruct the patient to eat a full meal just before the study.

During

- Note the following procedural steps:

GE Reflux Scan

1. The patient is placed in the supine position and asked to swallow about 100 to 150 ml of a tracer cocktail (e.g., orange juice, diluted hydrochloric acid, and technetium-99m–labeled colloid).
2. Images are immediately taken of the patient over the esophageal area.
3. The patient is asked to assume other positions to determine whether GE reflux occurs and, if so, in what position.
4. A large abdominal binder that contains an air-inflatable cuff is placed on the patient's abdomen. This is insufflated to increase abdominal pressure.
5. Images are again taken over the esophageal area to determine if any GE reflux occurs.

Aspiration Scans

1. These scans may be performed by adding a radionuclide to the patient's evening meal and keeping the patient in the supine position until the next morning.
2. Images are made over the lung fields to detect esophagotracheal aspiration of the tracer.
3. In infants being evaluated for chalasia, the tracer is added to the feeding or formula. Nuclear tracer films are then taken over the next hour, with delayed films as needed.

After

- With the use of computer calculations based on the images of the scans, the severity and percentage of reflux can be calculated.
- Assure the patient that he or she has ingested only a small dose of nuclear material. No radiation precautions need to be taken against the patient or his or her bodily secretions.

Test Results and Clinical Significance

Gastroesophageal reflux *The radionuclide can be seen to reflux from the stomach into the esophagus. This should diminish or disappear with successful medical or surgical treatment.*

Pulmonary aspiration *This can be the result of severe gastroesophageal reflux or the result of faulty swallowing function.*

Related Tests

- Gastric emptying scan (p. 716): This is a similarly performed scan designed to identify delayed gastric emptying, which can contribute to gastroesophageal reflux.

Gastrointestinal Bleeding Scan
(Abdominal Scintigraphy, GI Scintigraphy)

Normal Findings No collection of radionuclide in GI tract

Indications This study is mainly used to localize sites of GI bleeding.

Test Explanation

The GI bleeding scan is a test used to localize the site of bleeding in patients who are having active GI hemorrhage. The scan also can be used in patients who have suspected intraabdominal (nongastrointestinal) hemorrhage from an unknown source. Localization of the source of GI or other bleeding can be quite difficult. When surgery is required under these circumstances, it is difficult, cumbersome, and prolonged. The surgeon may have extreme difficulty finding the source of bleeding. The bleeding scan helps localize the bleeding for the surgeon.

Box 8-1 provides an overview of the diagnostic procedures used in evaluating GI bleeding. Many of these studies have limitations that warrant the need for the GI bleeding scan. For example, endoscopy has proved to be extremely useful in determining the source of intestinal bleeding; however, endoscopy is not helpful if the source is within the small intestine or the colon. Although colonoscopy allows excellent visualization of the colon when it is cleared out, it is extremely difficult to see when acute, active intestinal bleeding is occurring. Arteriography has three limitations in its evaluation of GI bleeding. First, arteriography can determine the site of bleeding, but the rate of bleeding must exceed 0.5 ml/min for detection. Second, if GI bleeding is intermittent, the results of the arteriogram can be falsely negative. Third, arteriography visualizes only the blood vessels to the small bowel, right colon, and transverse colon through a superior mesenteric angiogram. If the left colon and sigmoid vessels are to be visualized (most bleeding comes from these areas), an inferior mesenteric angiogram must be requested. This is more difficult to perform.

Box 8-1 Diagnostic procedures for gastrointestinal bleeding

UPPER GI BLEEDING (hematemesis or blood in the nasogastric [NG] tube)
Esophagogastroduodenoscopy
Celiac angiography
Aortography (to rule out aortoduodenal fistula)

LOWER GI BLEEDING (hematochezia or melena)
Pass NG tube to eliminate upper GI bleeding
Proctoscopy to eliminate hemorrhoids
Colonoscopy if patient is stable and bowel is relatively free of stool
Arteriography if bleeding is fast enough
GI scintigraphy if bleeding is slow but persistent
Barium enema if other tests cannot localize bleeding and bleeding is persistent

The GI bleeding scan has several advantages over arteriography. The GI bleeding scan can detect bleeding if the rate is in excess of 0.05ml/min. Also, with the use of technetium-labeled RBCs, delayed films (as long as 24 hours) can be obtained indicating the site of an intermittent or extremely slow intestinal bleed.

A GI scintigram is much more sensitive in locating the site of GI bleeding; however, it is not very specific in pinpointing the site or the cause of bleeding. Usually, when positive, the exact source of bleeding cannot be localized any more accurately than indicating the affected quadrant of the abdomen (e.g., right upper, left lower). This test is usually performed by injecting sulfur colloid labeled with technetium-99m (^{99m}Tc) or ^{99m}Tc-labeled RBCs into the patient. If the patient is bleeding at a rate in excess of 0.05 ml/min, pooling of the radionuclide will ultimately be detected in the abnormal segment of the intestine. Few false-positive results occur. Again, it is important to recognize that the test will only localize the bleeding; it will not indicate the exact pathologic condition causing the bleeding. With this test result, if surgery is required, the surgeon is directed to the abnormal area and hopefully can detect and resect the pathologic bleeding source.

It is important to realize that this test can take at least 1 to 4 hours to obtain useful information. Unstable patients should not leave the intensive care environment for that long. Furthermore, the unstable patient may need to go to surgery in minutes and the surgeon may not have the luxury of taking several hours to determine the region of active bleeding.

Contraindications

- Patients who are pregnant or lactating
- Medically unstable patients whose stay in the nuclear medicine department may be risky

Interfering Factors

- Barium within the GI tract may mask a small source of bleeding.

CLINICAL PRIORITIES

- GI bleeding scans can localize the bleeding. They cannot indicate the cause of the bleeding.
- Because this test requires several hours, unstable patients may not be candidates for it. They may be unable to leave the intensive care unit for that long.
- Delayed films may be taken up to 24 hours later to detect slow, intermittent, or chronic bleeding.

Procedure and Patient Care

Before

- Explain the procedure to the patient.
- Assess the patient's vital signs to ensure that they are stable for the patient's transfer to and from the nuclear medicine department.
- Accompany the patient to the nuclear medicine department if vital signs are questionably stable.

- Assure the patient that only a small amount of nuclear material will be administered.
- Instruct the patient to notify the nuclear medicine technologist if he or she has a bowel movement during the test. Blood in the GI tract can act as a cathartic.
- Inform the patient that no pretest preparation is required.
- Instruct the nuclear medicine technologist to notify the nurse of all bloody bowel movements that occur while the patient is in the nuclear medicine department.

During

- Note the following procedural steps:
  1. Ten millicuries of freshly prepared ^{99m}Tc-labeled sulfur colloid is administered IV to the patient. If ^{99m}Tc-labeled RBCs are to be used, 3 to 5 ml of the patient's own blood is combined with the ^{99m}Tc and reinjected into the patient.
  2. Immediately after administration of the radionuclide, the patient is placed under a scintillation camera.
  3. Multiple images of the abdomen are obtained at short intervals (5 to 15 minutes). Delayed films may be performed as late as 6 to 24 hours later in order to detect slow, intermittent, or chronic bleeding. The scintigrams are recorded on film.
  4. Detection of radionuclide in the abdomen indicates the site of bleeding. If no bleeding sites are noted in the first hour, the scan is repeated at hourly intervals for as long as 24 hours.
- Note that areas of the bowel hidden by the liver or spleen may not be adequately evaluated by this procedure. Also, the rectum cannot be easily evaluated because other pelvic structures (e.g., the bladder) obstruct the view. If the initial study is negative and subsequent films give evidence of active bleeding, a repeat scan may be performed.
- Note that this test is usually performed in approximately 20 to 30 minutes by a technologist in the nuclear medicine department.
- Tell the patient that the only discomfort associated with this study is the injection of the radioisotope.

After

- Reevaluate the patient's vital signs on return to the nursing unit.
- Assure the patient that only tracer doses of radioisotopes have been used and that no precautions against radioactive exposure to others are necessary.

Test Results and Clinical Significance

Ulcers
Tumors
Angiodysplasia and other vascular malformations
Polyps
Diverticulosis
Inflammatory bowel disease
The mucosa and submucosa in the areas of these diseases are quite friable and can bleed profusely.

Aortoduodenal fistulas *These usually present as rapid exsanguinating and recurrent upper GI bleeding episodes in a patient who has had prior aortic aneurysm surgery or prior radiation therapy to the area of the midabdomen to upper abdomen.*

Related Tests

- Arteriography (p. 892): This is a radiographic study used to evaluate the patient with GI bleeding at a rate greater than 1 ml/min.

Liver/Spleen Scanning (Liver Scanning)

Normal Findings

Normal size, shape, and position of the liver and spleen with no filling defects

Indications

This test allows for visualization of the liver and spleen. It is indicated in patients with cancer to rule out metastatic tumor to the liver. It is a routine part of tumor staging. It is also indicated in patients with primary tumors (hepatomas) or in patients with cirrhosis who are at high risk for the development of primary hepatomas. Patients with abnormal liver enzymes will also have their liver visualized. Liver scanning is used to monitor liver diseases and response to therapy.

Test Explanation

This radionuclide procedure is used to outline and detect structural changes of the liver and spleen. A radionuclide, usually technetium-99m–labeled sulfur colloid, is administered IV. Later, a scintillation camera is placed over the right upper and left upper quadrants of the patient's abdomen. This records the distribution of the radioactive particles emitted from the liver and spleen. Images are obtained that are comparable to the gamma ray emission and are recorded on film.

Because the scan can demonstrate only filling defects greater than 2 cm in diameter, false-negative results may occur in patients with space-occupying lesions (e.g., tumors, cysts, granulomas, abscesses) smaller than 2 cm. The scan may be incorrectly interpreted as positive for filling defects in patients with cirrhosis because of the distortion of the patient's liver parenchyma. The liver scan can detect tumors, cysts, granulomas, abscesses, and diffuse infiltrative processes affecting the liver (e.g., amyloidosis, sarcoidosis).

When a liver filling defect is observed, the most common cause is a benign hemangioma. This can be differentiated from tumor with the use of technetium-labeled RBCs. The patient's own RBCs are labeled with technetium (Tc) and reinjected into the patient. Immediate uptake of the radionuclide by the filling defect is suggestive of a hemangioma, for which no therapy is usually required.

In general, computed tomography (CT) scans and magnetic resonance imaging scans have replaced the liver scan in diagnostics. Single photon emission computed tomography (SPECT) has significantly improved the quality and accuracy of liver scanning. With SPECT scanning the radionuclide is injected and the scintillation camera is placed to receive images from multiple angles (around the circumference of the liver). This greatly increases the usefulness of nuclear liver scanning. With the use of radioactive carbon, nitrogen, or oxygen, anatomic and biochemical changes can be visualized within the liver. This method of liver scanning is called positron emission tomography (PET) scanning (p. 737).

The liver scan can be used to identify subpulmonic or subdiaphragmatic abscesses, or a combination lung/liver scan can be performed. Both organs are visualized by the synchronous performance of a liver and a lung scan. Usually, the liver is immediately subadjacent to the lung. If this liver/lung space is widened, a collection exists between the organs, indicating either a subpulmonic or subdiaphragmatic abscess. With the increased availability and accuracy of CT body scans, the use of a combination lung/liver scan to diagnose abscesses in these spaces has been reduced significantly.

The liver scan can also identify portal hypertension. Normally, most of the radionuclide administered during a liver scan is taken up by the liver. If the liver-to-spleen ratio is reversed (that is, the spleen takes up more of the radionuclide), reversal of hepatic blood flow exists as a result of portal hypertension.

Splenic hematoma, abscess, cyst, tumor, infarction, and infiltrate processes such as granulomas also can be detected. SPECT scanning can also be used to improve visualization of the spleen.

Contraindications

- Patients who are pregnant or lactating, because of risk of damage to the fetus or infant

Interfering Factors

- Barium in the GI tract overlying the liver or spleen will produce defects on the scan that may be mistaken for masses.

✓ CLINICAL PRIORITIES

- This test is a routine part of tumor staging. It is used to rule out metastasis to the liver in cancer patients.
- False negatives can occur in patients with lesions smaller than 2 cm.
- A combination lung-liver scan can be performed to identify subpulmonic or subdiaphragmatic abscesses.

Procedure and Patient Care

Before

- Explain the procedure to the patient.
- Tell the patient that no fasting or premedication is required.
- Assure the patient that he or she will not be exposed to large amounts of radiation because only tracer doses of isotopes are used.

During

- Note the following procedural steps:

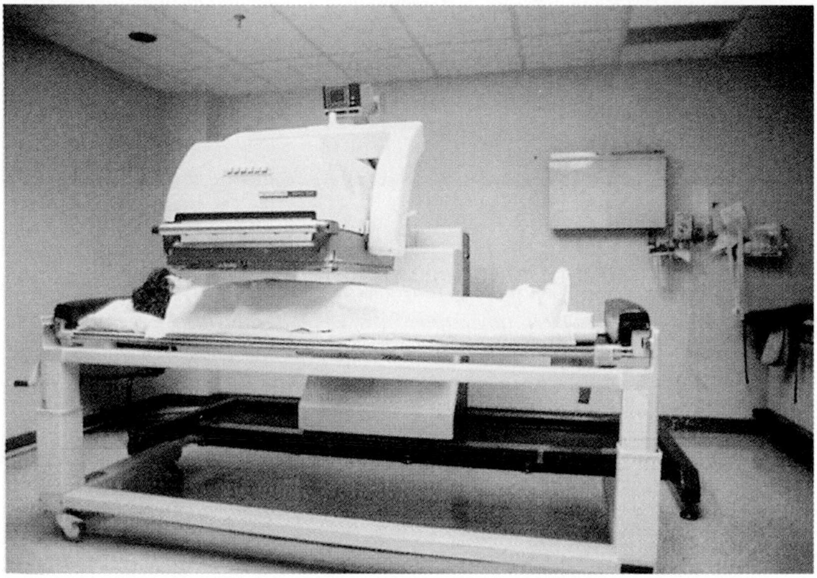

Figure 8-7 Patient prepared for liver scan.

1. The patient is taken to the nuclear medicine department, where the radionuclide is administered IV. (For inpatients a nuclear medicine technologist may administer the radionuclide at the bedside.)
2. Thirty minutes after injection, a gamma ray detector is placed over the right upper quadrant of the patient's abdomen.
3. The patient is placed in supine, lateral, and prone positions so that all surfaces of the liver can be visualized (Figure 8-7).
4. The radionuclide image is recorded on Polaroid or x-ray film.

- Note that this procedure is performed by a trained technologist in approximately 1 hour. A physician trained in nuclear medicine interprets the results.
- Tell the patient that the only discomfort associated with this procedure is the IV injection of the radionuclide.

After

- Because only tracer doses of radioisotopes are used, inform the patient that no precautions need to be taken by others against radiation exposure.

Test Results and Clinical Significance

Primary or metastatic tumor of the liver or spleen
Abscess of the liver or spleen
Hematoma of the liver or spleen
Hepatic or splenic cyst
Hemangioma
These diseases are evident as localized filling defects within the liver-spleen parenchyma.

Lacerations of the liver or spleen *The organ can be seen to be fractured, with a hematoma within the laceration.*

Infiltrative processes (e.g., sarcoidosis, amyloidosis, tuberculosis, or granuloma of the liver or spleen)
Cirrhosis
These diseases are apparent as diffuse irregularity in the uptake of the radionuclide within the liver or spleen.

Portal hypertension *There is reversal of the normal liver/spleen ratio of uptake of the radionuclide. Usually the liver takes up most of the radionuclide. In portal hypertension, with reversal of hepatic portal blood flow, the spleen takes up more of the radionuclide.*
Accessory spleen *The radionuclide aggregates in extrasplenic sites. This is very helpful to the surgeon who is planning a splenectomy and removal of all spleen tissue for patients with autoimmune thrombocytopenia or hemolytic anemia.*
Splenic infarction *This is evident as a localized space-filling defect within the spleen in a patient with sudden onset of left upper quadrant pain.*

Related Tests

- Computed tomography (CT) scan of the liver and spleen (p. 933): This is probably a more accurate test for the evaluation of these organs. However, to make the diagnosis of hemangioma, liver scanning with autologous RBCs labeled with Tc is superior in accuracy to a CT scan.
- Magnetic resonance imaging (MRI) scan of the liver and spleen (p. 1009): This is considered to be more accurate than the nuclear scans; however, it is more difficult to obtain and more expensive.

Lung Scan (Ventilation/Perfusion Scanning [VPS], Pulmonary Scintiphotography, V/Q Scan)

Normal Findings

Diffuse and homogeneous uptake of nuclear material by the lungs

Indications

The lung scan is very helpful in making the diagnosis of pulmonary embolism. It is easily and rapidly performed on patients who have sudden onset of noncardiac chest pain or shortness of breath. It is often performed on patients who have unexplained tachycardia or hypoxemia (Box 8-2).

Test Explanation

This nuclear medicine procedure is used to identify defects in blood perfusion of the lung in patients with suspected pulmonary embolism. Blood flow to the lungs is evaluated us-

Box 8-2 Diagnosis of pulmonary embolism

SYMPTOMS
Chest pain
Shortness of breath
Feelings of impending doom
Pleurodynia (pain with deep inspiration)

SIGNS
Tachycardia
Hypoxemia
S_4 gallop

TESTS	RESULTS
Chest x-ray	Normal, although if the pulmonary embolism (PE) progresses to pulmonary infarction, a wedge-shaped abnormality can be identified.
Electrocardiography	Normal, although if the PE is large enough, right heart strain may be evident (i.e., S wave in lead I, Q wave in lead III, and inverted T wave in lead III).
Arterial blood gases	Po_2 is reduced. O_2 saturation is reduced. Pco_2 may be slightly increased.
Lung scan	Poor perfusion to an isolated segment of lung is observed.
V/Q scan	Mismatch of ventilation and perfusion is evident.
Pulmonary angiography	Cutoff of blood flow to one or more segments of the lung and filling defects in the pulmonary arteries or arterioles is observed.

ing a macroaggregated albumin (MAA) tagged with technetium (Tc), which is injected into the patient's peripheral vein. Because the diameter of the radionuclide aggregates is larger than that of the pulmonary capillaries, the aggregates become temporarily lodged in the pulmonary vasculature. A scintillation camera detects the gamma rays from within the lung microvasculature. With the use of light conversion a realistic image of the lung is obtained on film.

A homogeneous uptake of particles that fills the entire pulmonary vasculature conclusively rules out pulmonary embolism. If a defect in an otherwise smooth and diffusely homogeneous pattern is seen, a perfusion abnormality exists (Figure 8-8). This can indicate pulmonary embolism. Unfortunately, many other serious pulmonary parenchymal lesions (e.g., pneumonia, pleural fluid, emphysematous bullae) also cause a defect in pulmonary blood perfusion. Therefore, although the scan may be sensitive, it is not specific because many different pathologic conditions can cause the same abnormal results.

The chest x-ray film aids in the interpretation of the perfusion scan because a defect on the perfusion scan seen in the same area as a pulmonary parenchymal abnormality on the chest x-ray film does not indicate pulmonary embolism. Rather, the defect may represent pneumonia, atelectasis, effusion, and so on. When a perfusion defect occurs in an area of the lung that is normal on a chest x-ray study, however, pulmonary embolism is very likely.

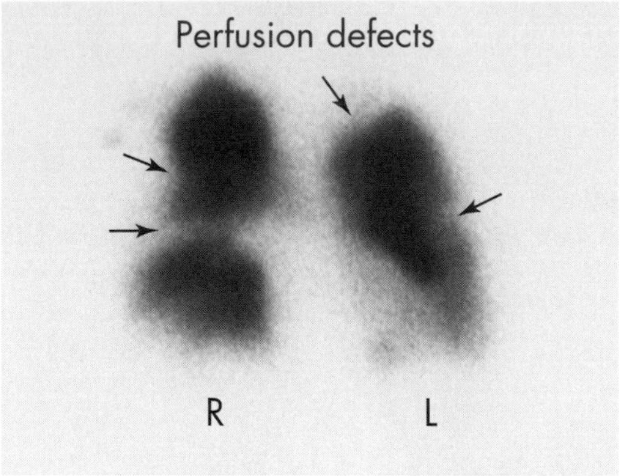

A

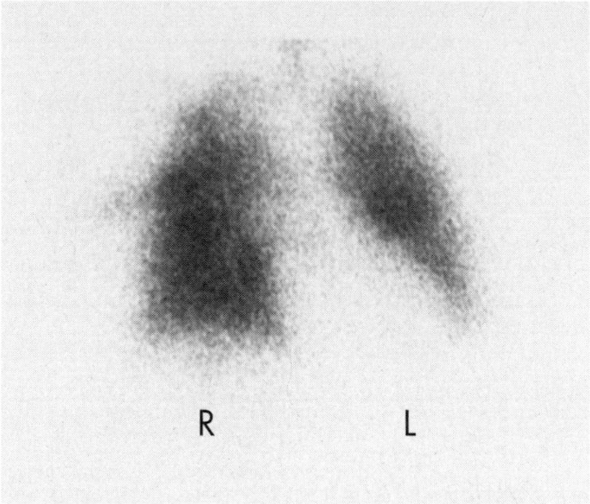

B

Figure 8-8 Lung scan. **A**, Perfusion. **B**, Ventilation. There are multiple perfusion defects noted on the perfusion lung scan. However, the uptake of radionuclide on the ventilation scan is normal. This combination of findings is due to pulmonary emboli.

Specificity of a perfusion scan also can be enhanced by the concomitant performance of a *ventilation lung scan,* which detects parenchymal abnormalities in ventilation (e.g., pneumonia, pleural fluid, emphysematous bullae). The ventilation scan reflects the patency of the pulmonary airways using krypton gas or Tc diethylenetriamine pentaacetic acid (DTPA) as an aerosol. When vascular obstruction (embolism) is present on a perfusion scan, ventilation scans will demonstrate a normal wash-in and a normal wash-out of radioactivity from the embolized lung area. If parenchymal disease (e.g., pneumonia) is responsible for the perfusion abnormality, however, wash-in or wash-out will be abnormal. Therefore the "mismatch" of perfusion and ventilation is characteristic of embolic disorders, whereas the "match" is indicative of parenchymal disease. When ventilation and perfusion scans are performed synchronously, this is called a *ventilation/perfusion (V/Q) scan.*

It is important to obtain a chest x-ray study around the same time as a perfusion lung scan to identify any parenchymal abnormalities that may affect perfusion. If the lung scan results are suspicious or equivocal, a pulmonary angiogram should be performed. Likewise, if anticoagulation is risky to the patient, an angiogram is required to make the diagnosis of pulmonary embolism with certainty. Most nuclear physicians place the lung scan results in one of several categories: negative for pulmonary embolism, low probability of pulmonary embolism, high probability of pulmonary embolism, or positive for pulmonary embolism.

Contraindications

- Patients who are pregnant

Interfering Factors

- Patients with known pulmonary parenchymal or pleural problems (e.g., pneumonia, emphysema, pleural effusion, tumors)
  These problems will give the picture of a perfusion defect and simulate pulmonary embolism.

✓ CLINICAL PRIORITIES

- This nuclear medicine procedure is mainly used to detect pulmonary embolism.
- Because lung scans are sensitive but not specific, several types of pulmonary problems (other than pulmonary embolism) can cause a defect in pulmonary blood perfusion.
- The specificity of a perfusion scan can be improved by the performance of a ventilation scan. When they are performed together, this is called a ventilation/perfusion (V/Q) scan.
- The chest x-ray study aids in the interpretation of the lung scan.

Procedure and Patient Care

Before

- Explain the procedure to the patient.
- Obtain informed consent if required by the institution.
- Assure the patient that he or she will not be exposed to large amounts of radioactivity because only tracer doses of isotopes are used.
- Although rarely done, if iodine-131 will be administered, give the patient 10 drops of Lugol's solution several hours before the test as a blocking agent for the thyroid gland. This will prevent iodine uptake by the thyroid gland.
- Tell the patient that no fasting is required.
- Note that a recent (within the last 24-48 hours) chest x-ray film should be obtained.
- Instruct the patient to remove jewelry around the chest area.

During

- Note the following procedural steps:
  The unsedated, nonfasting patient suspected of having a pulmonary embolism is taken to the nuclear medicine department (Figure 8-9).

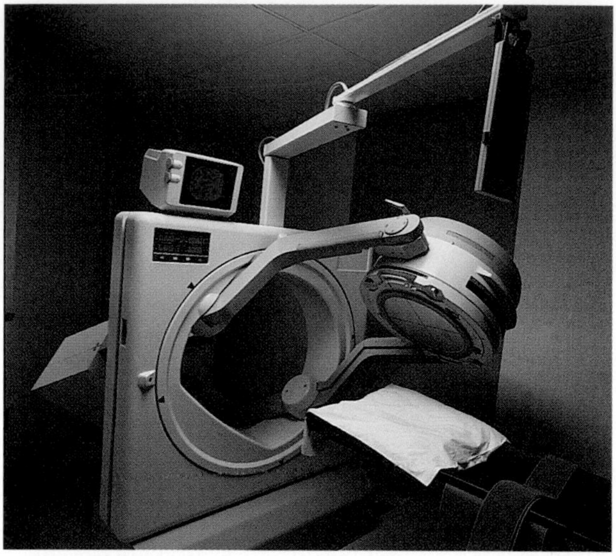

Figure 8-9 Clinical setting for lung scanning.

Perfusion Scan

1. The patient is given a peripheral IV injection of radionuclide-tagged MAA.
2. While the patient lies in the appropriate position, a gamma ray detector is passed over the patient and records radionuclide uptake on Polaroid or x-ray film.
3. The patient is placed in the supine, prone, and various lateral positions, which allows for anterior, posterior, and lateral and oblique views, respectively.
4. The results are interpreted by a physician trained in diagnostic nuclear medicine.

Ventilation Scan

1. The patient breathes through a closed-system face mask with a mouthpiece. The radionuclide tracer is then administered into the system.
2. Less patient cooperation is needed with a krypton tracer. Ventilation scans can even be performed on comatose patients using krypton. Krypton images can be obtained before, during, or after perfusion images.
3. In contrast, Tc DTPA images are usually done before perfusion images and require patient cooperation with deep breathing and appropriate use of breathing equipment to prevent contamination.

- Note that this test is usually performed by a physician in approximately 30 minutes.
- Tell the patient that no discomfort is associated with this test other than the peripheral venipuncture.

After

- Inform the patient that no radiation precautions are necessary.

Test Results and Clinical Significance

Pulmonary embolism *This is evident as a perfusion defect on a perfusion lung scan. It is also apparent as a "mismatch" of ventilation and perfusion on a V/Q scan. Positive results are definitive, but negative results can be false.*

Pneumonia
Tuberculosis
Asthma
Chronic obstructive pulmonary disease
Tumor
Atelectasis
Bronchitis

These parenchymal abnormalities can cause perfusion defects. When a defect is apparent on the plain chest x-ray film or a ventilation lung scan, a ventilation/perfusion "match" is identified. Matched defects are not due to pulmonary emboli, but rather to the above-noted parenchymal disease.

Related Tests

- Pulmonary angiography (p. 979): This is the definitive test for determining the diagnosis of pulmonary embolism.
- Arterial blood gases (p. 97): Hypoxemia is the hallmark of pulmonary embolism.
- Electrocardiography (p. 278): While the EKG is usually normal with pulmonary embolism, right heart strain can be identified with large acute pulmonary emboli.
- Chest radiography (p. 925): Although pulmonary embolisms are not evident on the plain chest x-ray film, parenchymal abnormalities are important to identify to accurately interpret the perfusion lung scan.

Meckel's Diverticulum Nuclear Scan

Normal Findings

No increased uptake of radionuclide in the right lower quadrant of the abdomen

Indications

This scan is designed to identify a Meckel's diverticulum that contains ectopic gastric mucosa. It is indicated in patients who have recurrent lower abdominal pain or in pediatric or young adult patients who have occult GI bleeding.

Test Explanation

Meckel's diverticulum is the most common congenital abnormality of the intestinal tract. It is a persistent remnant of the omphalomesenteric tract. The diverticulum usually occurs in the ileum, approximately 2 feet proximal to the ileocecal valve. Approximately 20% to 25% of Meckel's diverticula are lined internally by ectopic gastric mucosa. This gastric mucosa can secrete acid and cause ulceration of the intestinal mucosa nearby. Bleeding, inflammation, and intussusception are other potential complications of this congenital abnormality. The majority of these complications occur by 2 years of age.

Both normal gastric mucosa within the stomach and ectopic gastric mucosa in

Meckel's diverticulum concentrate technetium-99m pertechnetate. When this radionuclide is injected IV, it is concentrated in the ectopic gastric mucosa of Meckel's diverticulum. One can then expect to see a hot spot in the right lower quadrant of the abdomen at about the same time as the normal stomach mucosa is visualized. This is a very sensitive and specific test for this congenital abnormality.

It is possible that Meckel's diverticulum is present but contains no ectopic gastric mucosa within. Usually this is not symptomatic. No concentration of radionuclide will occur within the diverticulum. This test is not helpful in these cases.

Other conditions can simulate a hot spot compatible with Meckel's diverticulum containing ectopic gastric mucosa. Usually these are associated with inflammatory processes within the abdomen (e.g., appendicitis, Crohn's disease, or ectopic pregnancy).

Procedure and Patient Care

Before

- Explain the procedure to the patient.
- Advise the patient to refrain from eating or drinking anything for 6 to 12 hours before the examination.
- A histamine H_2-receptor antagonist is usually given for 1 to 2 days before the scan. This blocks secretion of the radionuclide from the ectopic gastric mucosa and improves visualization of Meckel's diverticulum.

During

- The patient lies in a supine position, and a large-view nuclear detector camera is placed over the patient's abdomen to identify concentration of nuclear material after IV injection.
- Images are taken at 5-minute intervals for 1 hour.
- Patients may be asked to lie on their left side to minimize the excretion of the radionuclide from the normal stomach, flooding the intestine with radionuclide and precluding visualization of Meckel's diverticulum.
- Occasionally glucagon is provided to prolong intestinal transit time and avoid downstream contamination with the radionuclide.
- Occasionally gastrin is given to increase the uptake of the radionuclide by the ectopic gastric mucosa.
- There is no pain associated with this test.

After

- The patient is asked to void, and a repeat image is obtained. This is to ensure that Meckel's diverticulum has not been hidden by a distended bladder.
- Inform the patient that no precautions need to be taken by others against radiation because only tracer doses of radioisotopes are used.

Test Results and Clinical Significance

Increased uptake in the right lower quadrant is compatible with Meckel's diverticula containing ectopic gastric mucosa. *As indicated above, if the diverticulum does not contain ectopic gastric mucosa, the test will not be positive. Furthermore, one must be aware that other inflammatory diseases can cause false-positive results.*

Octreotide Scan (Carcinoid Nuclear Scan, Neuroendocrine Nuclear Scan)

Normal Findings No evidence of increased uptake throughout the body

Indications

Octreotide scans are used to identify and localize neuroendocrine primary and metastatic tumors. This scan is indicated in patients with known neuroendocrine tumors (e.g., carcinoid tumors and gastrinomas). It is used preoperatively to direct the surgeon to primary and metastatic tumors. This scan is also used to monitor therapy of these tumors.

Test Explanation

Most neuroendocrine cells have a somatostatin receptor on the cellular membrane. Neuroendocrine tumors retain these receptors. Octreotide is an analogue of somatostatin. When combined with a radiopharmaceutical (such as iodine-123 or indium-111 DTPA), the radiolabeled octreotide will attach to the somatostatin receptors of the neuroendocrine tumor cells. With the use of a scintillation camera the uptake can be observed and localized.

In patients with known neuroendocrine tumors, this test is used to direct the surgeon to the primary and metastatic sites within the body (especially the abdomen). This test is also used in the surveillance of patients who have been or are being treated for these neuroendocrine tumors. When this test is used as a monitor of disease, recurrence or progression can be identified quite easily and accurately. The liver, however, is more difficult to evaluate with octreotide scanning. The use of single photon emission computed tomography (SPECT) imaging improves the sensitivity of this test. Many different types of hormone-producing tumors can be detected by this scan. Most notable include carcinoid, gastrinoma, insulinoma, glucagonoma, pheochromocytoma, and small cell lung cancer. Other abnormalities can pick up octreotide, including granulomatous infections (such as sarcoidosis or tuberculosis), rheumatoid arthritis, and nonhormonal cancers (breast, lymphoma, and non–small cell lung cancers).

The imaging procedure is performed by a trained technologist in approximately 30 minutes. A physician trained in nuclear medicine interprets the results. The only discomfort associated with this procedure is the IV injection of the radionuclide.

Contraindications

Patients who are pregnant or lactating, because of risk of damage to the fetus or infant

Interfering Factors

- Barium in the GI tract overlying the liver or spleen will produce defects on the scan that may be mistaken for masses.

Procedure and Patient Care

Before

- Explain the procedure to the patient.
- Tell the patient that no fasting or premedication is required.
- Assure the patient that he or she will not be exposed to large amounts of radiation because only tracer doses of isotopes are used.
- If an iodinated radionuclide is to be used, ensure that the patient does not have an allergy to iodine.
- If an iodinated dye is to be used, administer 5 drops of Lugol's solution (iodine) daily for 3 days. This will avoid uptake of the radionuclide by the thyroid gland.
- If the patient has been receiving octreotide as a form of antineoplastic treatment, this must be discontinued for 2 weeks prior to scanning.

During

- Note the following procedural steps:
  1. The patient is taken to the nuclear medicine department, where the radionuclide is administered IV. (For inpatients a nuclear medicine technologist may administer the radionuclide at the bedside.)
  2. One hour after injection, a gamma camera is successively placed over the entire body.
  3. The patient is placed in supine, lateral, and prone positions so that all surfaces can be visualized.
  4. The radionuclide image is recorded on film. SPECT images may also be performed.
  5. Usually the patient is given a fatty meal 2 hours after octreotide injection to clear the radiopharmaceutical from the gallbladder.
  6. After 4 hours the patient is given a strong laxative to clear the octreotide from the bowel.
  7. Repeat scanning is again performed at 2, 4, 24, and 48 hours after administration of the octreotide.

After

- Inform the patient that no precautions need to be taken by others against radiation exposure because only tracer doses of radioisotopes are used.

Test Results and Clinical Significance

Carcinoid tumors *This tumor consists of neuroendocrine argentaffin cells that have somatostatin receptors. They usually arise from the appendix, small bowel, or colon. However, any organ can be the primary site of a carcinoid tumor.*

Neuroendocrine tumors *Neuroendocrine tumors and other tumors as listed above can take up octreotide.*

Granulomatous infections such as sarcoidosis and tuberculosis *The pathophysiology of this observation is not well understood.*

Oncoscint Scan (Immunoscintigraphy)

Normal Findings

No increased uptake of radionuclide in the body

Indications

This scan is used to identify recurrent ovarian or colorectal cancer. It is indicated in patients who are suspected to have recurrence on the basis of elevated blood tumor markers (CA-125 and carcinoembryonic antigen [CEA], respectively).

Test Explanation

Immunoscintigraphy is a new procedure. At present it is used to detect recurrent metastatic colorectal or ovarian cancer. The radionuclide indium chloride-111 or indium-111 satumomab pendetide is attached to a monoclonal antibody that is commonly on the cell surface of colorectal and ovarian cancer cells. When injected, this radionuclide-antibody conjugate attaches to the cancer cells. With the use of a scintillation camera, whole-body images are obtained. Areas of increased uptake may represent tumor.

This scan is not 100% accurate and can be incorrectly negative up to 30% of the time. When positive, however, its accuracy meets or exceeds the accuracy of a computed tomography (CT) scan. This new diagnostic procedure can assist in the decision making of patients with metastatic or recurrent colorectal or ovarian adenocarcinoma. It is very helpful in determining the source of a rising tumor marker (carcinoembryonic antigen, p. 137, or CA-125, p. 125) in patients with an otherwise normal diagnostic evaluation. It is particularly helpful in determining extrahepatic abdominal and pelvic recurrent tumors. Also, it is very helpful in differentiating postsurgical or postradiation changes from recurrent cancer. The former do not take up tracer; the latter does. One must be aware that uptake of the radionuclide normally occurs in the liver, spleen, and bowel.

With knowledge of the suspected recurrent tumor, the surgeon can more easily locate recurrent tumor for resection. This scan is therefore helpful preoperatively.

This scan is the first of many of its kind that have and will find their way to clinical medicine. It makes use of monoclonal antibody technology. A radionuclide is tagged to a monoclonal antibody that is specific for the target to be identified. This will lead to much more specific test results. More sensitive and specific monoclonal antibodies are expected in the near future. These monoclonal antibodies do have an effect on subsequent immunoassays. For example, the mouse antibody used in the oncoscint scan distorts subsequent CEA testing, which is performed by radioimmunoassay.

Contraindications

- Nursing mothers, because the radionuclide may be harmful to the newborn.

Procedure and Patient Care

Before

- Explain the procedure to the patient.
- Explain that no fasting is required before the test.

CLINICAL PRIORITIES

- This new diagnostic procedure can assist in diagnosing metastatic or recurrent colorectal or ovarian adenocarcinoma.
- This test is helpful in determining the source of rising CEA or CA-125 levels.
- This test is one of the first of many tests that make use of monoclonal antibodies. For this test, a radionuclide attached to a monoclonal antibody is injected into the body and attaches to cancer cells.

- Because the radionuclide can be concentrated in areas of degenerative joint disease, abdominal aortic aneurysms, abdominal inflammatory processes, or inflammatory bowel disease, a careful history should be obtained before scanning. Usually a CT scan of the abdomen (p. 933) is performed prior to this test. The above-noted diseases would have been identified by the CT scan.

During

- The patient is injected with the radiolabeled monoclonal antibody.
- Initial images are obtained 48 to 72 hours after IV infusion.
- The patient is asked to lie on a padded table.
- A scintigraphy camera is placed over the anterior or posterior surface of the chest, abdomen, and pelvis. Approximately 10 minutes is required for each view.
- The patient may be asked to return the following day or the day after that for repeated images.
- Little or no discomfort is associated with this procedure.
- The procedure takes approximately 1 hour each day for at least 1 to 4 days.
- This procedure is performed in the nuclear medicine department.
- If a significant amount of radionuclide occurs in the bowel so as to obscure the vision of the rest of the abdomen, a cathartic or enema may be administered.

After

- Inform the patient that no precautions need to be taken by others against radiation exposure because only tracer doses of radioisotopes are used.

Test Results and Clinical Significance

Recurrent colorectal cancer
Ovarian cancer
These cancers are often obvious (by CT, bone, and magnetic resonance imaging [MRI] scans) when bulky recurrent tumors exist. However, it is important to identify these tumors at the earliest point of recurrence in the hopes that surgical excision will affect survival. Therefore CEA and CA-125 blood studies are routinely performed. When elevated, these blood tests results may be the earliest evidence of tumor. The tumor burden may be too small to identify with CT, bone, and MRI scans. Oconscint is very useful at this stage in supporting the diagnosis of recurrence and in locating the recurrent tumor.

Positron Emission Tomography (PET)

Normal Findings

Normal patterns of tissue metabolism

Indications

This new generation of imaging scans is not routinely used outside large medical institutions. Positron emission techniques have been used to identify pathophysiologic conditions of the brain, heart, lungs, and other tissues and organs.

Test Explanation

PET is a unique technique that combines the early biochemical assessment of pathologic conditions achieved by nuclear medicine with the precise localization achieved by computed tomography (CT). PET is able to penetrate the body's metabolism by recording tracers of nuclear annihilations in body tissue. The dose of radioactive material given to the patient, either a gas or injection, produces a radiation exposure comparable to that of other nuclear medicine studies. The selected tracers are chemically designed to measure body processes (e.g., blood flow and volume, protein metabolism). Table 8-2 lists radionuclides used in PET scanning.

A chemical compound with the desired biologic activity is labeled with a radioactive isotope that decays by emitting a positron (or positive electron). The positron combines with an electron, and the two are mutually annihilated with emission of two gamma rays. The gamma rays penetrate the surrounding tissue and are recorded outside the body by a circular array of detectors. Because the gamma rays travel in almost exactly opposite directions, their source can be established with a high degree of accuracy. A computer reconstructs the spatial distribution of the radioactivity for a selected plane within the patient and displays the resulting image on a cathode ray screen. PET provides noninvasive regional assessment of many biochemical processes essential to the functioning of the organ being studied (Figure 8-10, *A-B*).

Table 8-2 ***Radionuclides used in PET scanning***

Radionuclide	Application
Carbon-11	Cerebral, cardiac, pulmonary perfusion Detection of myocardial infarction Cerebral function
Nitrogen-13	Cerebral and cardiac perfusion Pulmonary inhalation Liver function
Oxygen-15	Cerebral perfusion and oxygen utilization
Fluorine-18	Cerebral function and glucose metabolism
Gallium-68	Cerebral perfusion Lymphoreticular function

A

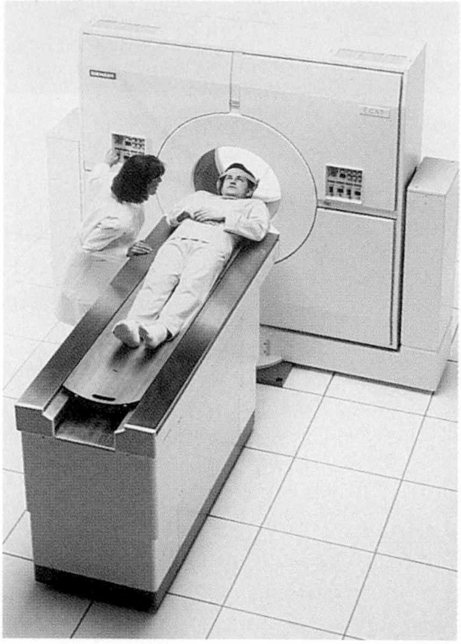

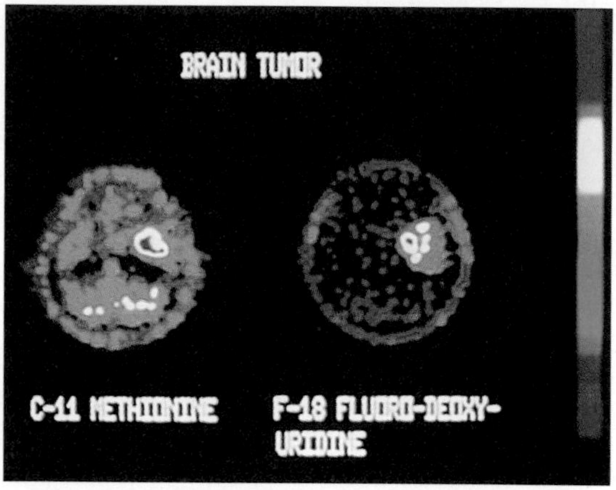

B

Figure 8-10 Positron emission tomography (PET). **A,** Clinical setting for PET. Shown are the Siemens ECAT Scanner gantry and patient bed. **B,** Images received from PET scan with different radioisotopes such as carbon-11 and fluorine-18. This study positively identified a brain tumor.

The technology of PET is now well developed, and both its capabilities and limitations are being increasingly understood. Many PET studies are being carried out with results that cannot be obtained by other techniques. These include the following:

1. Determination of regional metabolism in the heart and brain (e.g., radioactive glucose used to map biochemical activity in the brain)
2. Studies of tissue permeability
3. Measurement of the size of infarcts in the heart from a coronary occlusion
4. Investigation into the physiology of psychosis
5. Assessment of the effects of drugs on diseased or malfunctioning tissues
6. Possibility of measuring the effects of cancer treatment by changes in malignant tissues and by biochemical reactions in surrounding normal tissues

The cost of PET technology is high; it requires a cyclotron, appropriate chemical or radiation facilities, computer equipment, and effective group work by physicians, chemists, mathematicians, physiologists, and physicists. This procedure, once regarded as exotic, may now be on the threshold of becoming a fundamental tool in diagnostic medicine.

Interfering Factors

- Recent use (within 24 hours) of caffeine, alcohol, or tobacco may affect test results.
- Excessive anxiety may affect brain function evaluation.
- Drugs that may influence results include tranquilizers and sedatives.

CLINICAL PRIORITIES

- Test results can be affected by recent use of caffeine, alcohol, or tobacco.
- Tell patients that no sedatives or tranquilizers should be taken because they may need to perform mental activities during the test.
- After the test, patients should be encouraged to drink fluids and urinate frequently to aid in removal of the radioisotope from the bladder.

Procedure and Patient Care

Before

- Explain the procedure to the patient. Because most patients have not heard of this study, they are often anxious and require emotional support.
- Obtain informed consent if required by the institution.
- Inform the patient that he or she may have two IV lines inserted, one for infusion of the radioisotope and the other for serial blood samples.
- Inform the patient that he or she does not need to restrict food or fluids on the day of the test; however, the patient should refrain from alcohol, caffeine, and tobacco for 24 hours.
- Instruct diabetic patients to take their pretest dose of insulin at a meal 3 to 4 hours before the test.
- Tell the patient that no sedatives or tranquilizers should be taken, because he or she may need to perform certain mental activities during the test.
- Tell the patient to empty the bladder before the test for comfort.

During

- Note the following procedural steps:
  1. The patient is positioned in a comfortable, reclining chair.
  2. Two IV lines are inserted.
  3. The radioactive material can be infused through an IV line or be inhaled as a radioactive gas.
  4. The gamma rays that penetrate the tissues are recorded outside the body by a circular array of detectors and are displayed by a computer.
  5. If the brain is being scanned, the patient may be asked to perform different cognitive activities (e.g., reciting the Pledge of Allegiance) to measure changes in brain activity during reasoning or remembering.
  6. Extraneous auditory and visual stimuli are minimized by a blindfold and ear plugs.
- Note that this procedure is performed by a physician or trained technologist in approximately 60 to 90 minutes.
- Tell the patient that the only discomfort associated with this study is insertion of the two IV lines.

After

- Instruct the patient to change position slowly from lying to standing to avoid postural hypotension.
- Encourage the patient to drink fluids and urinate frequently to aid in removal of the radioisotope from the bladder.

Test Results and Clinical Significance

Myocardial infarction
Coronary artery disease
Areas of ischemia or infarction are associated with decreased flow and viability (with decreased metabolism).

Cerebrovascular accident (stroke) *These areas are evident as decreased blood flow, decreased oxygen utilization, and anaerobic metabolism.*

Epilepsy *Focal areas of increased metabolism are evident during seizure activity. Decreased metabolism and blood flow are noted between seizures.*

Parkinson's disease *Changes of increased metabolism deep in the brain may be evident.*

Dementia
Alzheimer's disease
PET scans are said to be able to differentiate Alzheimer's disease from other forms of dementia.

Schizophrenia
Huntington's disease
These diseases have variable findings. The physiologic changes indicate reduced metabolic activity.

Brain tumor *Differing tumor histologic characteristics and grades cause differing PET characteristics.*

Neoplasia *New growth becomes quite evident by increased metabolism.*

Related Tests

- Computed tomography (CT) scanning (p. 933): This uses a technique that recognizes differences in density coefficients to visualize different organs and tissues. Unlike PET, a CT scan cannot provide information concerning metabolism or function.

Radioactive Iodine Uptake
(RAIU, Iodine Uptake Test, ^{131}I Uptake)

Normal Findings

2 hours: 4% to 12% absorbed
6 hours: 6% to 15% absorbed
24 hours: 8% to 30% absorbed
Actual values may vary according to the laboratory.

Indications

This test is a measure of thyroid function and was once a necessary part of the evaluation of thyroid function. However, it is rarely performed now that direct assays are available for both thyroxine and triiodothyronine. It is still used to evaluate defects in thyroid hormone production.

Test Explanation

The RAIU is a useful guide to thyroid function. This test is based on the ability of the thyroid gland to trap and retain iodine. In this procedure a known quantity of radioactive iodine is given orally to the patient. A gamma ray detector placed over the thyroid gland determines the quantity or percentage of radioactive iodine taken up by the gland over a specific time.

Performing the measurement at different times after the iodine is given allows several aspects of thyroid function to be evaluated. Uptake determination at 30 minutes reflects the ability of the thyroid gland to trap iodine. When uptake is measured at 6 hours, the ability of the thyroid gland to bind iodine organically is evaluated. Maximal iodine uptake is observed within 24 hours. Determinations of iodine uptake after this time measure the ability of the gland to release iodine in the form of thyroid hormone.

Increased thyroid uptake of radioactive iodine is seen in patients with hyperthyroid states. Decreased uptake occurs in patients with hypothyroid conditions. The RAIU tends to be more accurate for diagnosing hyperthyroidism than hypothyroidism.

Contraindications

- Patients who are allergic to iodine or shellfish
- Patients who are pregnant

Potential Complications

- Radioactive exposure to the thyroid gland, which is minimized when ^{123}I or ^{125}I is used instead of ^{131}I

Interfering Factors

- In patients taking exogenous iodine preparations the iodine will increase the body's iodine pool and decrease uptake by the thyroid gland.
- Iodine deficient patients will trap increased amounts of iodine, resulting in increased uptake.
- Rebound thyroid stimulation after discontinuation of suppressive doses of thyroid medications results in falsely elevated RAIU levels.
- Recent x-ray studies using iodinated contrast material will decrease uptake for the same reasons as described above.
- Diarrhea will result in decreased absorption of tracer from the GI tract and result in decreased RAIU levels.

- Drugs that may cause *increased* levels include barbiturates, estrogen, lithium, phenothiazines, and thyroid-stimulating hormone.
- Drugs that may cause *decreased* levels include adrenocorticotropic hormone, antihistamines, corticosteroids, Lugol's solution, nitrates, saturated solution of potassium iodine, thyroid and antithyroid drugs, and tolbutamide.

Procedure and Patient Care

Before

- Explain the procedure to the patient.
- Assess the patient for allergies to iodine.
- Note that some laboratories prefer to keep the patient on NPO status after midnight on the day of the test.
- Restrict iodine and thyroid preparations 1 week before testing if indicated by the institution.
- Evaluate the patient's drug history for interfering factors.

During

- Note the following procedural steps:
  1. A tasteless dose of radioactive iodine, usually ^{123}I, is given by mouth to the patient. If RAIU is to be determined at 2 hours, the iodine is administered IV.
  2. The patient is given written instructions regarding the times to return to the radiology department for scanning.
  3. The patient is informed that he or she may usually eat 45 minutes to 1 hour after the dose of iodine has been given.
  4. For the scanning the patient is asked to lie in a supine position.
  5. A gamma ray detector is placed over the patient's thyroid gland to determine RAIU.
- List on the laboratory slip the x-ray studies and drugs the patient has received that could affect test results.
- Note that this test is performed in approximately 30 minutes by a radiologic technologist.
- Inform the patient that this test is not uncomfortable.

After

- Inform the patient that the dose of radioactive iodine used in this test is minute and harmless. Tell him or her that no isolation or special urine precautions are necessary.

Test Results and Clinical Significance

Increased levels

Hyperthyroidism *There are many causes and classifications of hyperthyroidism. All are associated with increased RAIU. However, if the cause of the hyperthyroidism is excess iodine ingestion, the RAIU will be diminished.*

Decreased levels

Hypothyroidism *Diminished thyroid function is associated with reduced uptake and metabolism of iodine by the thyroid, along with reduced production of thyroid hormone. RAIU is therefore decreased.*

Related Tests

- Triiodothyronine (T_3), thyroxine (T_4), thyroid-stimulating hormone (TSH) (pp. 435, 417, and 413): These tests are the most common manner in which thyroid function is measured. They are more accurate than RAIU, and no radioactive material needs to be administered to the patient.
- Thyroid scanning (p. 754): This is a commonly performed test when evaluating thyroid enlargement or mass.

Red Blood Cell Survival Study
(RBC Survival Study, Splenic Sequestration Study)

Normal Findings

Half-life of RBC: 26-30 days
Spleen/liver ratio: 1:1
Spleen/pericardium ratio: <2:1

Indications

This nuclear test is used to identify reduced RBC survival as a result of hemolysis. It is used in the evaluation of hemolytic anemia. It is also helpful in the determination of RBC survival in patients with splenomegaly and anemia.

Test Explanation

In patients with hemolytic anemia, the RBCs are destroyed and normally sequestered in the spleen. As a result of this ongoing RBC destruction, the RBC life span will be significantly reduced. This reduction in RBC survival indicates that active hemolysis is occurring and is the cause of the patient's anemia.

Although hemolysis can be identified by determination of the catabolic products of hemoglobin (which are increased), by measuring the level of circulating haptoglobin (which is decreased, p. 247), or by measuring the transport globulin that binds heme (which is decreased), the determination of the RBC life span by nuclear studies can provide a semiquantitative measurement of the degree of hemolysis. This quantitation can be best performed by determining the half-life of the RBC within the circulation. This portion of the test is performed by extracting some of the patient's RBCs, labeling them with chromium-51 (^{51}Cr), and reinjecting them into the patient. Subsequent blood levels of ^{51}Cr indicate the half-life of the labeled RBCs. As RBC survival decreases, more labeled RBCs are sequestered by the spleen. As a result, the amount of ^{51}Cr activity in the blood decreases.

The second portion of the test is the imaging of the spleen, liver, and pericardium. In patients with hemolytic anemia associated with abnormal splenic sequestration, the spleen/liver ratio is in excess of 1:1. However, this same abnormally high ratio can also occur without hemolysis in patients who have splenomegaly caused by a disease other than hemolytic anemia. To eliminate that confusion, the spleen/pericardium ratio is determined; a ratio greater than 2:1 indicates abnormal splenic sequestration of hemolyzed RBCs. A normal spleen/pericardium ratio with an increased spleen/liver ratio indicates splenomegaly due to portal hypertension, for example.

This second portion of the splenic sequestration study is also helpful in determining which patients with hemolytic anemia will benefit from splenectomy. Patients with increased splenic sequestration can be expected to improve after splenectomy.

This test requires 2 to 3 weeks for completion. The study is performed by a nuclear medicine technologist or physician. No pain or discomfort is associated with this procedure. The patient must lie still during the nuclear imaging portion of the test.

Contraindications

- Patients who are pregnant, because of the risk of fetal damage caused by the radiation exposure

Interfering Factors

- Factors that can *decrease* RBC survival include recent RBC transfusion, increased RBC production, active bleeding, high WBC counts in excess of 25,000, and high platelet counts greater than 500,000.
- Splenomegaly can *increase* spleen/pericardium ratios.
- Splenic infarctions can *decrease* spleen/pericardium ratios.

Procedure and Patient Care

Before

- Explain the procedure to the patient.
- Assure the patient that he or she will not be exposed to large amounts of radioactivity because only tracer doses of the isotope are used.
- Tell the patient that no preparation or sedation is required.
- Notify the nuclear medicine technologist or physician if blood transfusion or hemorrhage has occurred shortly before or during the study.
- Note that usually a hematocrit, WBC count, platelet count, and reticulocyte count are performed before testing.

During

- Note the following procedural steps:
  1. Approximately 20 ml of blood is withdrawn from the patient, and the RBCs are labeled with ^{51}Cr.
  2. The tagged RBCs are reinjected into the patient.
  3. On the first day of testing, 10 ml of blood is withdrawn by a peripheral venipuncture into a red-top tube.
  4. The RBCs are quantified for ^{51}Cr counts per minute.
  5. Nuclear imaging of the spleen, liver, and pericardium is carried out.
  6. This process is repeated 3 times a week for 2 to 3 weeks.
  7. The peripheral venous blood ^{51}Cr counts are plotted on a graph, and the half-life is determined.
  8. The spleen/liver and spleen/pericardium ratios and nuclear counts are determined.

After

- Inform the patient that because only tracer doses of radioisotopes are used, no precautions need to be taken against radioactive exposure.

Test Results and Clinical Significance

Increased splenic sequestration

Hemolysis (immunogenic, hemoglobinopathies, nutritional deficiencies, uremia, etc.) *Hemolysis will result in increased splenic sequestration because it is the spleen that predominantly extracts old or injured RBCs from the circulation. Therefore, ^{51}Cr "light-up" of the spleen is expected.*

Splenomegaly *This usually is evident as an increase in the spleen/liver ratio of 1:1. However, the spleen/pericardium ratio is still less than 2:1. This pattern is due to splenomegaly caused by diseases such as portal hypertension, infiltrative diseases, or neoplastic disease.*

Decreased RBC survival

Hemolysis (immunogenic, hemoglobinopathies, nutritional deficiencies, uremia, etc.) *Hemolysis will be associated with a reduced RBC survival curve as the ^{51}Cr levels are plotted over time.*

Hemorrhage *If ongoing acute or chronic (e.g., chronic GI loss) hemorrhage is present, ^{51}Cr curves will indicate reduced RBC survival. In reality, the ^{51}Cr is lost to the circulation by virtue of the bleeding.*

Abnormally increased erythropoiesis *If the RBC is malformed or contains abnormal hemoglobin, the RBC survival could be reduced, yet active hemolysis is not occurring.*

Recent transfusion *The RBC survival of transfused RBCs is significantly less than native RBC. After transfusions, one can expect a ^{51}Cr curve and scan to be compatible with reduced RBC survival.*

8 NUCLEAR SCANNING

Related Tests

- Haptoglobin (p. 247): This is a blood glycoprotein that acts as a transport for free hemoglobin. In the presence of hemolysis, haptoglobin levels diminish.
- Protein, blood (p. 357): Globulin levels are reduced in the presence of hemolytic anemia.

Renal Scanning (Kidney Scan, Radiorenography, Renography, Radionuclide Renal Imaging, Nuclear Imaging of the Kidney, DMSA Renal Scan, DTPA Renal Scan, Captopril Renal Scan)

Normal Findings Normal size, shape, and function of the kidney

Indications

Renal scans are used to indicate the perfusion, function, and structure of the kidneys. They are also used to indicate the presence of obstruction or renovascular hypertension.

Because this study uses no iodinated dyes (except when iodohippurate is used), it is safe to use on patients who have iodine allergies or compromised renal function. Renal scans are used to monitor renal function in patients with known renal disease. This scan also plays a large part of the diagnosis of renal transplant rejection.

Test Explanation

This nuclear medicine procedure provides visualization of the urinary tract after IV administration of a radioisotope. The radioactive material is detected by a scintillation camera, which can detect the gamma rays emitted by the radionuclide in the kidney. The scintillation camera information can be translated into light and thereby create a realistic image of the renal structure. That information can also be collated by a computer, and the amount of gamma ray emission per unit of time can be calculated to determine renal function, vascular insufficiency, or renal obstruction. Scans do not interfere with the normal physiologic process of the kidney. The resultant image (scan) indicates distribution of the radionuclide within the kidney and ureters.

There are several different kinds of renal scans, depending on what information is needed. Different isotopes may be more suitable for different scans, based on the manner in which the kidney handles the radioisotope.

Renal blood flow (perfusion) scan

This type of renal scan is used to evaluate the blood flow to each kidney. It is used to identify renal artery stenosis, renovascular hypertension, and rejection of renal transplant. Also, it is used to demonstrate hypervascular lesions (renal cell carcinoma) in the kidney.

The basic test is performed by rapid IV injection of the radionuclide (usually technetium-99m diethylenetriamine pentaacetic acid [^{99m}Tc DTPA], ^{99m}Tc disodium monomethane arsonate [DMSA], or iodohippurate sodium ^{131}I) while the patient is under the scintigraphy camera. Computers collate the data obtained by the camera and create a curve of gamma activity per unit of time. Each kidney is compared to the opposite and to the aorta. Decreased gamma activity is noted in the kidney with arterial stenosis or renovascular hypertension. Decreased activity relative to the aorta is noted in a transplanted kidney that is experiencing rejection. Increased gamma activity is noted in the kidney that contains a hypervascular tumor (cancer).

Renal structural scan

This type of renal scan is performed to outline the structure of the kidney to identify a pathologic condition that may alter normal anatomic structure (e.g., tumor, cyst, abscess). Congenital disorders (e.g., hypoplasia or aplasia of the kidney, malposition of the kidney) can also be detected. Also, information following renal transplants can be obtained with this scan. A filling defect in the renal parenchyma may indicate a tumor, cyst, abscess, or infarction. Horseshoe-shaped kidney, pelvic kidney, or absence of a kidney may be evident. Anatomic alterations in the parenchymal distribution of tracer may indicate transplant rejection.

^{99m}Tc DTPA or ^{99m}Tc DSMA can be used for this scan. DSMA is particularly good because it is rapidly taken up by the kidney but excreted very slowly, allowing good visualization of the renal structure.

Renal function scan (renogram)

Renal function can be determined by documenting the capability of the kidney to take up a particular radioisotope and excrete it. A well-functioning kidney can be expected to rapidly assimilate the isotope and then excrete the same isotope. A poorly functioning kidney will not be able to take up the isotope rapidly or excrete it in a timely manner. Each radioactive tracer is handled by the kidney in a different manner. Different renal functions can be tested according to which isotope is used:

^{99m}Tc DTPA measures glomerular filtration.

^{99m}Tc DMSA measures tubular cell secretion.

Iodohippurate sodium ^{131}I or iodohippurate sodium ^{133}I measures both glomerular filtration and tubular cell secretion.

In this study the dose of radionuclide is determined by calculation of the body weight or surface area. The patient is placed under the scintigraphy camera. The radioisotope is injected, and a computer analyzes the data obtained from the camera. Activity per unit of time equals the function of the kidney, which is plotted on graph paper. This is called a renogram curve (isotope renography). The function tested depends on the radioisotope being used. Disappearance of the isotope is also plotted as part of that same curve and is a measurement of excretory function of the kidney. The curves are plotted, and their shapes can be compared to expected normals and to the opposite kidney. Furthermore, renal function can be monitored by serially repeating this test and comparing results. Renal function can be noted to be improved or deteriorating, depending on serial comparisons of the curves.

The kidney with diminished renal function (e.g., glomerulonephritis) or decreased blood supply can be expected to not have rapid uptake of activity and rapid disappearance (excretion) of the radionuclide. The curve will be much flatter. This can also be seen in rejection after transplantation. Impending renal failure can be identified with this scan.

Renal hypertension scan

This scan is used to determine the presence and the source of renovascular hypertension. This scan usually uses an angiotensin-converting enzyme (ACE) inhibitor (such as captopril). The captopril scan (captopril renography/scintigraphy) determines the functional significance of a renal artery or arteriole stenosis. After the administration of captopril, the glomerular filtration rate (GFR) in a kidney with a partial vascular obstruction is reduced despite the preservation of renal plasma flow. The GFR in the contralateral kidney is maintained. This would be demonstrated as delayed radioactivity in the affected kidney after injection of a radionuclide. These scans may predict the response of the blood pressure to medical treatment, angioplasty, or surgery.

Renal obstruction scan

This scan is performed to identify obstruction of the outflow tract of the kidney due to obstruction of the renal pelvis, ureter, or bladder outlet. In this study the radionuclide is rapidly injected while the patient is under the scintigraphy camera. Activity is measured and plotted per unit of time. After about 10 minutes, a diuretic (Lasix) is administered. The radionuclide in the unobstructed kidney can be seen to rapidly wash out (be excreted) from the kidney. A slow excretion without a wash-out is seen in an obstructed but still functioning kidney. Furthermore, when the collecting system does become visible, it is observed to be dilated.

Often several of these scans are combined to obtain the maximum amount of information about the renal system. A *triple renal study* may use all of these techniques to evaluate renal blood perfusion, structure, and excretion.

Renal scans are superior to other testing in determining renal function, identifying renal infarction, monitoring renovascular hypertension, and identifying primary renal diseases and transplant rejection. This radionuclear scan is also helpful in the evaluation of the following:

- Arterial atherosclerosis or trauma; the renal uptake of the radionucleated material will be delayed or absent on the affected side or sides
- Pathologic renal or ureteral conditions in patients who cannot have IV pyelography (IVP) (p. 953) because of dye allergies or poor renal function
- Renal tumors, abscesses, or cysts in patients who may have an allergy to iodine; these appear as cold spots because of the nonfunctioning tissue
- Renal or ureteral disease in patients whose renal function is already poor and who would be at risk for further reduction in function if iodinated dye were to be administered

Contraindications

- Patients who are pregnant, because of the risk of fetal injury

✓ CLINICAL PRIORITIES

- There are several different types of renal scans (such as blood flow, structure, function, obstruction, hypertension) that can be done, depending on what information is needed. Various isotopes are used, depending on how the kidney handles the radioisotopes.
- A renal scan should not be scheduled within 24 hours after an IVP because the iodinated dye may diminish renal function.
- Renal scans can be used to evaluate rejection of a transplant.

Procedure and Patient Care

Before

- Explain the procedure to the patient.
- Do not schedule a renal scan within 24 hours after an IVP. The iodinated dye may temporarily diminish renal function.
- Assure the patient that he or she will not be exposed to large amounts of radioactivity because only tracer doses of isotopes are used.
- Note that Lugol's solution (10 drops) may be ordered if iodohippurate sodium ^{131}I will be used. This minimizes thyroid uptake of the radioisotope.
- Remind the patient to void before the scan.
- Tell the patient that no sedation or fasting is required but that good hydration is essential.
- Instruct the patient to drink two to three glasses of water before the scan.

During

- Note the following procedural steps:
  1. The unsedated, nonfasting patient is taken to the nuclear medicine department.
  2. A peripheral IV injection of radionuclide is given. It takes only minutes for the radioisotopes to be concentrated in the kidneys.
  3. While the patient assumes a prone or sitting position, a gamma ray scintigraphy camera is passed over the kidney area and records the radioactive uptake on film.
  4. For a *Lasix renal scan* or a *diuretic renal scan,* the patient is imaged with DTPA. Images are obtained for 10 to 20 minutes, then 40 mg of Lasix is administered IV, and another 20 minutes of images are obtained.
  5. For the *captopril renal scan,* the patient is scanned after the administration of an ACE inhibitor, such as captopril.
  6. Scans may be repeated at different intervals after the initial isotope injection. For the *renal blood flow* and the *renal function scans,* scanning is started immediately after the injection.
  7. For *structural renal scans,* the patient is asked to lie still for the entire time of the scan (30 minutes).
- Note that the duration of this test varies from 1 to 4 hours, depending on the specific information required. Perfusion scans are done in approximately 20 minutes and functional scans in less than 1 hour. Static structure scans require 20 minutes to 4 hours for completion.
- Note that this study is performed by a nuclear medicine technologist or physician.
- Tell the patient that no pain or discomfort is associated with this procedure.
- Inform the patient that he or she must lie still during this study.

After

- Inform the patient that because only tracer doses of radioisotopes are used, no precautions need to be taken against radioactive exposure.
- Tell the patient that the radioactive substance is usually excreted from the body within 6 to 24 hours. Encourage the patient to drink fluids.

Test Results and Clinical Significance

Urinary obstruction *This is obvious on a renal obstruction scan. After diuresis the obstructed kidney fails to demonstrate excretion (wash-out) of the radionuclide. Prolonged obstruction ultimately leads to total loss of function of the obstructed kidney. That kidney will not light up after injection of a radionuclide.*

Renovascular hypertension *The renal hypertension scan is performed after administration of captopril. The time for the affected kidney to light up is significantly prolonged.*

Renal infarction *This can be seen as a wedge-shaped defect on the structural scan and perhaps as decreased blood flow on the perfusion scan.*

Renal arterial atherosclerosis *This is evident as delayed light-up on the perfusion scan. The plotted curve is flatter than normal.*

Glomerulonephritis
Pyelonephritis
Acute tubular necrosis
Absence of kidney function

If significant enough to affect renal function, these diseases are evident on the renal function scans. The affected kidney does not light up as quickly as normal. The plotted curves of function per unit of time are flatter than normal. No uptake is seen with absence of renal function.

Renal tumor
Renal abscess
Renal cyst
These abnormalities are apparent as filling defects on the renal structural scan.

Congenital abnormalities such as renal aplasia, hypoplasia, and malposition *These abnormalities are evident on the renal structural scan.*

Renal trauma *With arterial injury, the renal blood flow scan will demonstrate prolonged or no visualization of the affected kidney. The renal structural scan may demonstrate a laceration of the kidney with extravasation of radionuclide out of the renal capsule.*

Transplant rejection *This is apparent with many of the scans described in this section. With rejection of a transplanted kidney, one may see reduced blood flow to the transplanted kidney, reduced function of the transplanted kidney, and/or alterations in renal structure of the transplanted kidney.*

Related Tests

- Intravenous pyelography (p. 953): This is an x-ray examination of the kidneys and lower urologic tract. With the use of iodinated IV contrast, this test can also provide information about renal function, blood flow, and structure. Also renal obstruction can be demonstrated.
- Computed tomography (CT) (p. 933): This scan is an x-ray study utilizing the technology of computed tomography. This test can provide information about renal function, blood flow, and structure. Also, renal obstruction can be demonstrated.

Schilling Test (Vitamin B_{12} Absorption Test)

Normal Findings

Excretion of 8% to 40% of radioactive vitamin B_{12} within 24 hours

Indications

This test is performed on patients who have been found to have vitamin B_{12} deficiency (pernicious anemia). It is useful to determine the cause of that deficiency. Abnormal Schilling test results indicate a defect in absorption of vitamin B_{12}.

Test Explanation

The Schilling test is performed to detect vitamin B_{12} absorption. Normally, ingested vitamin B_{12} combines with intrinsic factor, which is produced by gastric mucosa, and is absorbed in the distal part of the ileum. Pernicious anemia results when absorption of vitamin B_{12} is inadequate. This may be caused by a primary malabsorption problem of the intestinal tract or by lack of intrinsic factor.

The two-stage Schilling test can detect a defect in vitamin B_{12} absorption. With normal absorption the ileum absorbs more vitamin B_{12} than the body needs and excretes the excess into the urine. With impaired absorption, however, little or no vitamin B_{12} is excreted into the urine.

In the Schilling test, urinary B_{12} levels are measured after the ingestion of radioactive vitamin B_{12}. The test can be performed in one stage (without intrinsic factor) or two stages (with intrinsic factor). Patients with pernicious anemia from lack of intrinsic factor will have abnormal results for the first stage and normal results for the second stage of the Schilling test. Patients with malabsorption from an intestinal source will have abnormal results for the first- and second-stage Schilling test. A combined one-stage and two-stage test is now commonly used.

All bone marrow and hematologic studies along with determination of serum vitamin B_{12} levels must be done before the Schilling test. The vitamin B_{12} that is administered during this test can significantly alter those test results.

Contraindications

- Patients who are pregnant
- Patients who are lactating

Interfering Factors

- Radioactive nuclear material received 10 days before testing may affect results.
- Renal insufficiency may cause reduced excretion of radioactive vitamin B_{12}.
- Patients who are elderly, diabetic, or hypothyroid may have reduced excretion of vitamin B_{12}.
- Inadequate collection of urine can falsely reduce the vitamin B_{12} in the urine.
- Stool in the urine specimen will alter test results.
- Drugs that may affect test results include laxatives because they could decrease the rate of vitamin B_{12} absorption.

CLINICAL PRIORITIES

- This test is used to detect pernicious anemia, which is due to inadequate absorption of vitamin B_{12}.
- Pernicious anemia may be caused by a malabsorption problem in the bowel or by a lack of intrinsic factor.
- A combined one-step and two-step test is now commonly used for this test.

Procedure and Patient Care

Before

- Explain the procedure to the patient.
- Instruct the patient to remain on NPO status except for water 8 to 12 hours before the test. Food should not be given until after the patient receives the injections.
- Instruct the patient not to take laxatives during the test period.

During

- Note the following procedural steps:

First-Stage Schilling Test (Without Intrinsic Factor)

1. Radioactive vitamin B_{12} is administered orally to the patient.
2. Shortly thereafter, nonradioactive vitamin B_{12} is administered to the patient IM to saturate tissue-binding sites and to permit some excretion of radioactive vitamin B_{12} in the urine if it is absorbed.
3. A 24- to 48-hour urine collection for vitamin B_{12} is obtained.
4. The patient is encouraged to drink fluids.

Second-Stage Schilling Test (With Intrinsic Factor)

1. If indicated, the second stage is performed approximately 1 week after the first stage.
2. The fasting patient is provided radioactive vitamin B_{12} combined with human intrinsic factor.
3. As before, an IM injection of nonradioactive vitamin B_{12} is administered.
4. Again, 24- to 48-hour collections are begun.

Combined One-Stage and Two-Stage Schilling Test

1. The fasting patient receives a capsule of vitamin B_{12} labeled with cobalt-57 plus intrinsic factor.
2. A second capsule of vitamin B_{12} labeled with cobalt-58 is also given.
3. One hour later, an IM injection of nonradioactive vitamin B_{12} is administered.
4. Again, the urine is collected for 24 to 48 hours.
5. Percentages of ^{57}Co and ^{58}Co are calculated. ^{57}Co-labeled vitamin B_{12} will be present only in patients with pernicious anemia secondary to lack of intrinsic factor. No vitamin B_{12} will be present in the urine of patients whose pernicious anemia is caused by primary bowel malabsorption.

After

- Ensure that the urine specimens are promptly transported to the laboratory.

Test Results and Clinical Significance

Decreased levels

Pernicious anemia *Pernicious anemia is a megaloblastic anemia that results from vitamin B_{12} deficiency. This may occur as a result of lack of intestinal absorption of vitamin B_{12} due to deficiency of intrinsic factor.*

Intestinal malabsorption *With poor absorption of nutrients from the gut, vitamin B_{12} levels diminish despite the presence of normal amounts of intrinsic factor.*

Hypothyroidism
Liver disease
These diseases are also associated with abnormal vitamin B_{12} absorption and metabolism.

Related Tests

- Vitamin B_{12} (p. 750): This is a direct measurement of B_{12} levels in the blood.

Scrotal Nuclear Imaging
(Scrotal Scan, Testicular Imaging)

Normal Findings Symmetric and prompt blood flow to both testicles

Indications

Scrotal imaging is helpful in the diagnosis of patients with a sudden onset of unilateral testicular swelling and pain. Scrotal imaging can differentiate unilateral testicular torsion from other causes of testicular pain (e.g., acute epididymitis, torsion of the testicular appendage, orchitis, strangulated hernia, testicular hemorrhage).

Test Explanation

Testicular torsion is a surgical emergency requiring prompt surgical exploration to salvage the involved testicle. To provide immediate surgical care the surgeon must differentiate it from other causes of painful testicular swelling, which do not require surgery. Use of radionuclide scrotal imaging enables the surgeon to diagnose testicular torsion. This study is usually performed on an emergency basis and in the nuclear medicine department.

The patient is positioned under the gamma camera with the scrotum supported between the abducted thighs. Technetium-99m pertechnetate is administered, and a dynamic radionuclide nuclear angiogram is obtained. Static images are obtained immediately afterward. An area of decreased perfusion corresponding to the involved testes indicates a high probability of torsion of the testicle. If the clinically involved testes is normally perfused or hypervascular, a disease other than torsion of the testicle (as described earlier) exists. In 95% of all cases of testicular torsion, the scrotal image will make the diagnosis. This information can be obtained in 30 to 45 minutes after injection of the nuclear material.

Procedure and Patient Care

Before

- Explain the procedure to the patient.
- Tell the patient that no fasting or premedication is required.
- Assure the patient that he will not be exposed to large amounts of radiation because only tracer doses of isotope are used.
- If the patient is a child, encourage the parent(s) to be present.

During

- The patient is placed on a padded table in the supine position.
- The patient's legs are abducted, and the testicles are supported with tape or a lead shield. The penis is taped to the lower abdomen.
- A small IV injection of technetium-99m pertechnetate is administered.
- Radionuclide imaging is then immediately performed over both testicles. Both dynamic and static images are obtained.

After

- Inform the patient that because only tracer doses of radioisotopes are used, no precautions need to be taken by others against radiation exposure.
- If the patient is identified as having torsion of the testicle, prepare the patient for surgery.

Test Results and Clinical Significance

Increased testicular blood flow

Epididymitis
Torsion of the testicular appendage
Orchitis
Trauma
These abnormalities may be associated with increased blood flow to the testicle.

Decreased testicular blood flow

Testicular torsion of the spermatic cord *Torsion of the testicle inhibits blood flow to the testicle. This will ultimately lead to infarction of the testicle if not treated immediately.*

Related Tests

- Scrotal ultrasonography (p. 801): Although this test is usually used to identify neoplasm of the testicle, one may expect to see some swelling and edema with an ischemic testicle.

Thyroid Scanning (Thyroid Scintiscan)

Normal Findings

Normal size, shape, position, and function of the thyroid gland
No areas of decreased or increased uptake

Indications

This test is used to visualize the thyroid gland when disease of the thyroid is suspected. It is particularly useful in the evaluation of patients with a suspected thyroid nodule. With thyroid nuclear scanning the nodule can be classified and more appropriately treated.

Test Explanation

Thyroid scanning allows the size, shape, position, and physiologic function of the thyroid gland to be determined with the use of radionuclear scanning. A radioactive substance such as technetium-99m is given to the patient to visualize the thyroid gland. A scintigraphy camera is passed over the neck area, and an image is recorded on film.

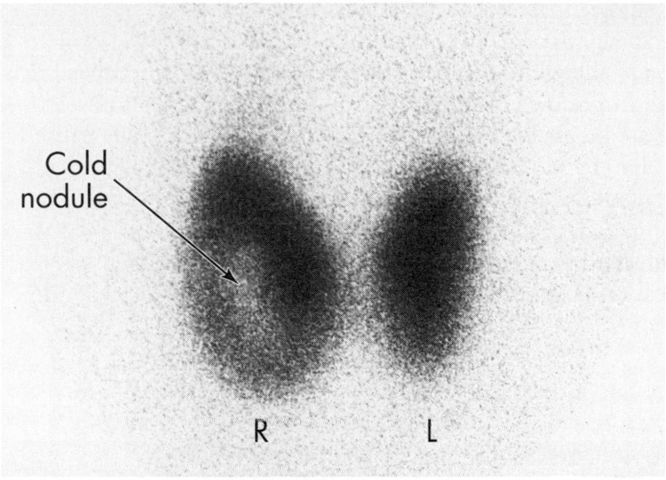

Figure 8-11 Thyroid scan. Note the cold nodule in the right (larger) lobe of the thyroid gland. This finding is consistent with tumor, cyst, or goiter.

Thyroid nodules are easily detected by this technique. Nodules are classified as functioning *(warm/hot)* or nonfunctioning *(cold)* depending on the amount of radionuclide taken up by the nodule (Figure 8-11). A functioning nodule could represent a benign adenoma or a localized toxic goiter. A nonfunctioning nodule may represent a cyst, carcinoma, nonfunctioning adenoma or goiter, lymphoma, or localized area of thyroiditis.

Scanning is useful in the following clinical situations:

1. Patients with a neck or substernal mass.
2. Patients with a thyroid nodule. Thyroid cancers are usually nonfunctioning (cold) nodules.
3. Patients with hyperthyroidism. Scanning will assist in differentiating Graves' disease (diffusely enlarged hyperfunctioning thyroid gland) from Plummer's disease (nodular hyperfunctioning gland).
4. Patients with metastatic tumors without a known primary site. A normal scan excludes the thyroid gland as a possible primary site.
5. Patients with a well-differentiated form of thyroid cancer.

Another form of thyroid scan is called the *whole-body thyroid scan.* This scan is performed on patients who have previously had a thyroid cancer treated. Iodine-125 (^{125}I) is injected IV, and the entire body is scanned to look for metastatic thyroid tissue. A hot spot would indicate recurrent tumor. Before this test can be performed, all of the thyroid tissue in the neck must be either surgically excised or ablated with radioactive ^{131}I. If the patient is on thyroid replacement therapy, the thyroid medicine must be discontinued at least 6 weeks prior to testing. This makes any metastatic thyroid tissue particularly iodine avid. A high thyroid-stimulating hormone blood level assures that any thyroid cancer tissue will take up the administered radioactive iodine. This test is routinely (every 1 to 2 years) performed on patients who have had a thyroid cancer larger than 1 cm. Smaller cancers are unlikely to metastasize. Much of the procedure is similar to thyroid scanning.

Contraindications

- Patients who are allergic to iodine or shellfish, because sometimes ^{125}I is used as the radionuclide
- Patients who are pregnant, because the radionuclear tracer may cause fetal injury

Potential Complications

- Radiation-induced oncogenesis
  This complication is eliminated if technetium or low-radioactive iodine isomers are used instead of ^{131}I.

CLINICAL PRIORITIES

- Thyroid nodules are classified as hot or cold, depending on the amount of radionuclide taken up by the nodule.
- The entire body can be scanned to detect metastatic thyroid tissue by the *whole-body thyroid scan.*
- Iodine in foods or x-ray contrast agents should be avoided prior to thyroid scanning.

Interfering Factors

- Iodine-containing foods affect results because the iodine may saturate all the iodine binding sites and very little iodine tracer will be taken up by the thyroid. Also, if large quantities of iodine are ingested, the thyroid may shut down and even technetium tracer will not be taken up by the thyroid.
- Recent administration of x-ray contrast agents affects results because these agents contain large quantities of iodine. For the reasons described above, contrast agents should be avoided prior to thyroid scanning.
- Drugs that may affect test results include cough medicines, multiple vitamins, some oral contraceptives, and thyroid drugs.

Procedure and Patient Care

Before

- Explain the procedure to the patient.
- Check the patient for allergies to iodine.
- Instruct the patient about medications that need to be restricted for 6 weeks before the test (e.g., thyroid drugs, medications containing iodine).
- Obtain a history concerning previous contrast x-ray studies, nuclear scanning, or intake of any thyroid-suppressive or antithyroid drugs.
- Tell the patient that fasting is usually not required. Check with the laboratory.

During

- Note the following procedural steps:
  1. A standard dose of radioactive technetium is usually given to the patient by mouth. The capsule is tasteless.
  2. Scanning is usually performed 24 hours later. If technetium is used, scanning may be performed 2 hours later.
  3. At the designated time, the patient is placed in a supine position and a scintigraphy camera is placed over the thyroid area.
  4. The radioactive counts are recorded and displayed.
- Note that this study is performed by a radiologic technologist in less than 30 minutes.
- Tell the patient that no discomfort is associated with this study.

After

- Assure the patient that the dose of radioactive technetium used in this test is minute and therefore harmless. No isolation and no special urine precautions are needed.

Test Results and Clinical Significance

Adenoma *This may be evident as a hot nodule if it is functioning or a cold nodule if it is not functioning.*

Toxic and nontoxic goiter *The toxic goiter will be apparent as a hot nodule. The nontoxic goiter will be a cold nodule.*

Cyst
Carcinoma
Lymphoma
Thyroiditis
Metastasis
These diseases are usually evident as cold nodules or filling defects in the normal thyroid tissue.

Graves' disease *This disease is evident on thyroid scan as diffuse increased uptake of radionuclide involving the entire thyroid gland.*

Plummer's disease *This disease produces a single or multiple nodular areas of increased uptake.*

Hyperthyroidism
Hypothyroidism
In general, hyperthyroid patients have increased uptake of radionuclide, and hypothyroid patients have reduced uptake.

Hashimoto's disease *This often is apparent as mottled uptake of radionuclide.*

Related Tests

- Thyroid ultrasonography (p. 803): This is an important part of evaluation of the thyroid gland. In general, all solid nodules on ultrasound that are cold on thyroid scan should be considered suggestive of cancer.
- Triiodothyronine (T_3), thyroxine (T_4), thyroid-stimulating hormone (TSH) (pp. 435, 417, and 410): These tests are the most common methods by which thyroid function is

measured. They are more accurate than radioactive iodine uptake and thyroid scanning. No radioactive material needs to be administered to the patient. These tests should be a part of every thyroid evaluation.

WBC Scan (Inflammatory Scan)

Normal Findings No signs of WBC localization outside the liver or spleen

Indications

This scan is used to identify and localize occult inflammation or infection. It is used for patients who have a fever of unknown origin, suspected osteomyelitis, or inflammatory bowel disease. It is used to indicate whether or not an abnormal mass (e.g., a pancreatic pseudocyst) is infected.

Test Explanation

This test is based on the fact that WBCs are attracted to areas of infection or inflammation. When the patient is suspected of having an infection or inflammation, yet the site cannot be localized, the injection of radiolabeled WBCs may identify and localize that area of inflammation or infection. Appropriate treatment can then be performed. This is especially helpful in patients who have a fever of unknown origin, suspected occult intraabdominal infection, or suspected (yet radiographically unapparent) osteomyelitis. The scan can differentiate infectious from noninfectious processes. Areas of noninfectious inflammation (e.g., inflammatory bowel disease) also take up the radiolabeled WBCs.

This scan requires drawing about 40 to 50 ml of blood from the patient, separating out the WBCs, labeling the WBCs with technetium or indium, and reinjecting them into the patient. Four to 24 hours later, imaging of the whole body may show an area of increased radioactivity suggestive of accumulation of the radiolabeled WBCs in an area of infection or inflammation.

The imaging procedure is performed by a trained technologist in approximately 30 minutes. A physician trained in nuclear medicine interprets the results. The only discomfort associated with this procedure is the IV injection of the radionuclide.

Interfering Factors

- The reticuloendothelial system (liver, spleen, and bone marrow) tends to accumulate these radiolabeled cells normally.

Procedure and Patient Care

Before

- Explain the procedure to the patient.
- Assure the patient that he or she will not be exposed to large amounts of radioactivity because only tracer doses of the isotope are used.

- Tell the patient that no preparation or sedation is required.

During

- Note the following procedural steps:
  1. Approximately 40 to 50 ml of blood is withdrawn from the patient, and the WBCs are extracted from the rest of the blood cells. This is usually done by centrifugation. With leukopenia, the WBC count is so low that separating them out from the other blood cellular components would be very difficult. In these instances, donor WBCs are used instead of autologous WBCs. Donor WBCs are also used for HIV-positive patients to minimize the risk to laboratory workers.
  2. The WBCs are suspended in saline and tagged with technetium-99m (^{99m}Tc) or indium-111 (^{111}In) lipid-soluble product. ^{99m}Tc is preferable to ^{111}In because its half-life is longer. Therefore it is cheaper and more readily available for the infrequent times this scan is requested.
  3. The tagged WBCs are reinjected into the patient.
  4. In 4, 24, and 48 hours after injection, a gamma camera is placed over the body.
  5. The patient is placed in supine, lateral, and prone positions so that all surfaces of the body can be visualized.
  6. The radionuclide image is recorded on film.

After

- Inform the patient that because only tracer doses of radioisotopes are used, no precautions need to be taken against radioactive exposure.

Test Results and Clinical Significance

Infection (abscess, osteomyelitis, or poststernotomy infections) *The WBCs are localized to the area of infection and show up as increased radionuclear uptake (hot spot).*

Inflammation (e.g., inflammatory bowel disease, arthritis) *Like infection, areas of noninfectious inflammation attract the radiolabeled WBCs.*

9

Stool Tests

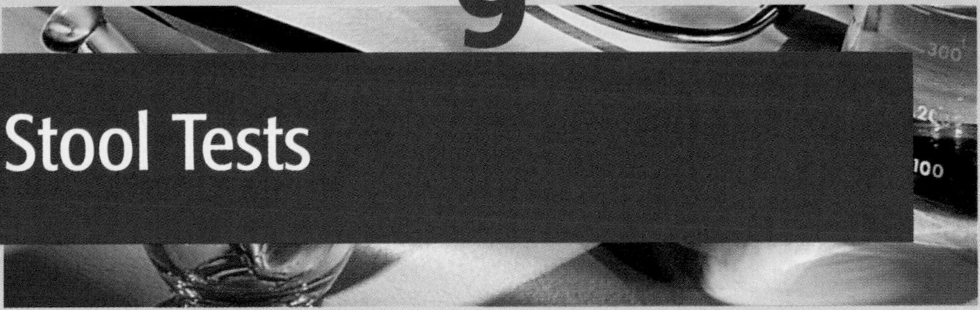

TESTS

Overview

Reasons for Performing Stool Studies

Stool represents the waste products of digested food. It also includes bile, mucus, shed epithelial cells, bacteria, and other inorganic salts. Normally food is passed through the stomach, into the duodenum, and into the small bowel. There, most of the nutrient and electrolyte absorption occurs. The liquid stool is then passed into the colon, where most of the water is reabsorbed.

Stool studies are used to evaluate the function and integrity of the bowel. These studies are performed to evaluate patients with intestinal bleeding, infections, infestations, inflammation, malabsorption, and diarrhea.

In this chapter, we have listed some stool studies that are commonly performed. Other testing can be done on the stool but is more often performed on other specimens. In those situations, the study is listed in the appropriate chapter for the specimen that is more commonly used.

Although it may be unpleasant to obtain, handle, and examine a stool specimen, the information obtained from these studies is invaluable to proper care of the patient with GI diseases.

Procedural Care for Stool Studies

Before

- Explain the method of stool collection to the patient. Be matter-of-fact to avoid any embarrassment to the patient.
- Instruct the patient not to mix urine or toilet paper with the stool specimen.
- Instruct the patient to use an appropriate collection container.
- Observe universal precautions when handling stool specimens.

During

- Ask the patient to defecate into a clean bedpan.
- Place a small amount of stool in a sterile collection container.
- If a rectal swab is to be used, wear gloves and insert the cotton-tipped swab at least 1 inch into the anal canal. Then rotate the swab for 30 seconds and place it in the clean container.

After

- Handle the stool specimen carefully, as though it were capable of causing infection. Wear gloves when obtaining and handling the specimen.
- Promptly send the stool specimen to the laboratory. Delays in transfer of the specimen may affect test results. If there will be a delay in laboratory handling of the stool specimen, follow laboratory procedures or guidelines concerning storage. Stools for ova and parasites should be kept warm. Stools for enteric pathogens and *Clostridium difficile* should be refrigerated. Another option is to add a preservative to the stool. For example, for stool culture, a buffered glycerol-saline solution may be combined with the stool as a preservative.

Reporting of Results

It may take several days or even weeks to obtain results of some stool specimens. However, most stool study results are available within 24 hours.

Clostridial Toxin Assay (*Clostridium difficile*, Antibiotic-associated Colitis Assay; Pseudomembranous Colitis Toxic Assay, *C. diff.*)

Normal Findings Negative (no *Clostridium* toxin identified)

Indications

This test is indicated in patients with diarrhea who have been on antibiotics for more than 5 days. It is also performed on immunosuppressed patients with diarrhea even though they are not on antibiotics. Occasionally a patient will present with abdominal bloating and fever without diarrhea.

Test Explanation

Clostridium difficile bacterial infection of the intestine may occur in patients who are immunocompromised or taking broad-spectrum antibiotics (e.g., clindamycin, ampicillin, and cephalosporins). The infection results from depression of the normal flora of the bowel through the administration of antibiotics. This increases the number of *C. difficile* bacteria within the intestines. The overgrowth of *C. difficile* causes diarrhea that is usually watery and voluminous. Abdominal cramps, fever, and leukocytosis are noted in most patients. Symptoms usually begin 4 to 10 days after the initiation of antibiotic therapy.

The clostridial bacterium releases a toxin that causes necrosis of the colonic epithelium. The detection of this toxin in the stool is therefore diagnostic of clostridial enterocolitis (pseudomembranous colitis). This toxin is identified by stool immunoassay techniques. *C. difficile* can also be diagnosed by obtaining colonic-rectal tissue for this toxin. Finally, stool cultures (p. 767) for *C. difficile* can be performed. Stool culture takes longer for results to be available.

Management of this antibiotic-associated colitis includes immediate cessation of the broad-spectrum antibiotics (if possible), IV replacement of fluid and electrolytes, and institution of metronidazole (Flagyl) or vancomycin (Vancocin) antibiotic therapy.

Procedure and Patient Care

Before

- Explain the method of stool collection to the patient. Be matter-of-fact to avoid embarrassment to the patient.
- Instruct the patient not to mix urine and toilet paper with the stool specimen.
- Handle the specimen carefully, as though it were capable of causing infection. If the nurse is assisting with the specimen collection, gloves should be worn.

During

- Ask the patient to defecate into a clean container. A rectal swab cannot be used, because it collects inadequate amounts of stool. The stool cannot be retrieved from the toilet.
- Note that a stool specimen also can be collected by proctoscopy.
- Place the specimen in a closed container and then transport it to the laboratory to prevent deterioration of the toxin.
- If the specimen cannot be processed immediately, refrigerate it.

After

- Maintain enteric isolation precautions on all patients until appropriate therapy is completed.

Test Results and Clinical Significance

Antibiotic-related pseudomembranous colitis
Clostridium difficile colitis
Multiple names exist for the same clinical entity. This infection can progress to toxic megacolon and even death. In the extreme cases of this disease, medical therapy may not be adequate, and a total colectomy may be required.

Related Tests

- Sigmoidoscopy (p. 550): This endoscopic test is used to support the diagnosis of pseudomembranous colitis. Also, through this test, good specimens can be obtained for clostridial toxin testing.
- Stool culture (p. 767): This study is performed to identify pathogenic bacteria growing within the bowel.

Fecal Fat (Fat Absorption, Quantitative Stool Fat Determination)

Normal Findings

Fat: 5 g/24 hr
Retention coefficient: ≥95%

Indications

This test is performed to confirm the diagnosis of steatorrhea. Steatorrhea is suspected when the patient has large, greasy, and foul-smelling stools. Determining an abnormally high fecal fat content confirms the diagnosis.

Test Explanation

The fecal fat test measures the fat content in the stool. The total output of fecal fat per 24 hours in a 3-day stool collection provides the most reliable measurement.

Children with cystic fibrosis have mucous plugs that obstruct the pancreatic ducts. The pancreatic enzymes (amylase, lipase, trypsin, and chymotrypsin) cannot be expelled into the duodenum and are therefore either completely absent or present only in diminished quantities within the G.I. tract. Lipase and bicarbonate are lipolytic, and without them fat is not digested for absorption. This results in impaired fat absorption (malabsorption). These patients have large, greasy, and foul-smelling stools; this is known as steatorrhea.

Although reliable, analysis of fecal fat is not specific to cystic fibrosis. Any condition that may cause malabsorption (e.g., sprue, Crohn's disease, Whipple's disease) or maldigestion (e.g., bile duct obstruction, pancreatic duct obstruction secondary to tumor or gallstones) is also associated with increased fecal fat. Short-gut syndrome is also associated with high fecal fat output.

Interfering Factors

- Drugs that may *increase* levels of fecal fat include enemas and laxatives, especially mineral oil.
- Drugs that may *decrease* levels of fecal fat include Metamucil and barium.

Age-related concerns

- Children with cystic fibrosis have mucous plugs that obstruct the pancreatic ducts. This prevents fat absorption (malabsorption).
- A fat retention coefficient is used in infants and children to determine the difference between ingested fat and fecal fat.
- The fat retention coefficient should be at least 95%. A low value indicates steatorrhea.

Procedure and Patient Care

Before

- Explain the procedure to the patient.
- Give the patient instructions regarding the appropriate diet (a diet diary may be requested by the laboratory):
  1. For adults, usually 100 g of fat per day is suggested for 3 days before and throughout the collection period.
  2. Children, and especially infants, cannot ingest 100 g of fat. Therefore, a *fat retention coefficient* is determined by measuring the difference between ingested fat and fecal fat and then expressing that difference (the amount of fat retained) as a percentage of the ingested fat:

$$\frac{\text{Ingested fat} - \text{Fecal fat}}{\text{Ingested fat}} \times 100\% = \text{Fat coefficient}$$

- Note that the fat retention coefficient in normal children and adults is 95% or greater. A low value indicates steatorrhea.

- Instruct the patient to defecate into a dry, clean container. Occasionally a tongue blade is required to transfer the stool to the specimen container.
- Tell the patient not to urinate into the stool container.
- Inform the patient that even diarrheal stools should be collected.
- Instruct the patient that toilet paper should not be placed in the stool container.
- Tell the patient not to take any laxatives or enemas during this test because they will interfere with intestinal motility and alter test results.

During

- Collect each stool specimen and send immediately to the laboratory during the 24- to 72-hour testing period.
- Label each specimen and include the time and date of collection.
- If the specimen is collected at home, give the patient a large stool container to keep in the freezer.

After

- Inform the patient that a normal diet can be resumed.

Test Results and Clinical Significance

Increased levels

Cystic fibrosis *These patients experience maldigestion of fat because their pancreatic function is poor. They cannot absorb fat from the gut. As a result, they have steatorrhea.*

Malabsorption secondary to sprue, celiac disease, Whipple's disease, Crohn's disease (regional enteritis), or radiation enteritis *The absorptive capability of the stool is markedly reduced. Transit time is markedly decreased. As a result of these changes, fat is not absorbed. Steatorrhea is the result.*

Maldigestion secondary to obstruction of the pancreatobiliary tree (e.g., cancer, stricture, gallstones) *Exocrine secretion of the pancreatobiliary tree is necessary for digestion of dietary fat. When disease affects these organs, steatorrhea results.*

Short-gut syndrome secondary to surgical resection, surgical bypass, or congenital anomaly *The transit time in these patients is markedly diminished. The time available for digestion and absorption of fat is inadequate. Steatorrhea results.*

Related Tests

- D-Xylose absorption (p. 461): This test is used to evaluate the absorptive capability of the intestines. It is used in the evaluation of patients suspected of having malabsorption.

Stool Culture (Stool for Culture and Sensitivity [Stool C&S], Stool for Ova and Parasites [O&P])

Normal Findings Normal intestinal flora

Indications

Stool cultures are indicated in patients who have unrelenting diarrhea, fever, and abdominal bloating. One is especially suspicious if the patient has been drinking well water, has been on prolonged antibiotics, or has traveled out of the United States.

Test Explanation

Normally stool contains many bacteria and fungi. The more common bacteria include *Enterococcus, Escherichia coli, Proteus, Pseudomonas, Staphylococcus aureus, Candida albicans, Bacteroides,* and *Clostridium*. Bacteria are indigenous to the bowel; however, several bacteria act as pathogens within the bowel. These include *Salmonella, Shigella, Campylobacter, Yersinia,* pathogenic *Escherichia coli, Clostridium,* and *Staphylococcus*. Parasites also may affect the stool. Common parasites are *Ascaris* (hookworm), *Strongyloides* (tapeworm), and *Giardia* (protozoans), and *Cryptosporidium* (especially in AIDS patients). Identification of any of these pathogens in the stool incriminates that organism as the cause of the infectious enteritis.

Sometimes the normal stool flora can become pathogenic if overgrowth of the bacteria occurs as a result of antibiotics, immunosuppression, or overaggressive catharsis (e.g., *Clostridium difficile*). *Helicobacter pylori* can be found in the stool but indicates an increased risk of peptic ulcer disease and gastritis. Usually, however, this is better cultured from the stomach or determined by a serologic test on the blood.

Infections of the bowel from bacteria, virus, or parasites usually present as acute diarrhea, excessive flatus, abdominal discomfort, and fever. This may progress to toxic megacolon.

Interfering Factors

- Urine may inhibit the growth of bacteria. Therefore urine should not be mixed with the feces during collection of a stool sample.

✓ CLINICAL PRIORITIES

- Stool cultures are usually done on patients with unrelenting diarrhea, fever, and abdominal bloating.
- The normal stool flora can become pathogenic if bacterial overgrowth occurs as a result of antibiotics, immunosuppression, or excessive catharsis.
- Wear gloves when obtaining and handling a stool specimen. Handle the specimen as though it were capable of causing infection.

- Recent barium studies may obscure the detection of parasites.
- Drugs that may affect test results include antibiotics, bismuth, and mineral oil.

Procedure and Patient Care

Before

- Explain the method of stool collection to the patient. Be matter-of-fact to avoid any embarrassment to the patient.
- Instruct the patient not to mix urine or toilet paper with the stool specimen.
- Instruct the patient to use an appropriate collection container.

During

- Ask the patient to defecate into a clean bedpan.
- Place a small amount of stool in a sterile collection container.
- Send mucus and blood streaks with the specimen.
- If a rectal swab is to be used, wear gloves and insert the cotton-tipped swab at least 1 inch into the anal canal. Then rotate the swab for 30 seconds and place it in the clean container.

Tape Test

- Use this test when pinworms (*Enterobius*) are suspected.
- Place a clear tape in the patient's perianal region. (This is especially helpful in children.)
- Because the female worm lays her eggs at night around the perianal area, apply the tape before bedtime and remove it in the morning before the patient gets out of bed.
- Press the sticky surface of the tape directly to a glass slide and examine microscopically for pinworm ova.

After

- Handle the stool specimen carefully, as though it were capable of causing infection. Wear gloves when obtaining and handling the specimen.
- Indicate on the laboratory slip any antibiotics that the patient may be taking.
- Promptly send the stool specimen to the laboratory. Delays in transfer of the specimen may affect viability of the organism. If long delays are necessary, obtain a buffered glycerol-saline solution to be combined with the stool and used as a preservative.
- Note that some enteric pathogens occasionally take as long as 6 weeks to isolate.
- When pathogens are detected, maintain isolation of the patient's stool until therapy is completed. Other people who have had close contact with the patient should be tested to prevent spread of the infection.

Test Results and Clinical Significance

Bacterial enterocolitis
Protozoan enterocolitis
Parasitic enterocolitis

These infections can be grown on special culture plates. The parasites can also be detected on smear of the stool. Treatment of these infections must be prompt, especially in children, who can dehydrate rapidly and become septic.

Related Tests

- Clostridial toxin assay (p. 763): This test allows one to make the diagnosis of pseudomembranous colitis due to the bacterium *Clostridium difficile.*

Stool for Occult Blood (Stool for OB)

Normal Findings No occult blood within stool

Indications

This test is a part of every routine physical examination. Furthermore, it is a part of every evaluation for abdominal pain. It is also a part of routine screening of asymptomatic individuals over the age of 50 years.

Test Explanation

Normally only minimal quantities of blood are passed into the GI tract. Usually this bleeding is not significant enough to cause a positive result in stool for OB testing. This test can detect OB when as little as 5 ml of blood are lost per day.

Tumors of the intestine grow into the lumen and are subjected to repeated trauma by the fecal stream. Eventually the friable tumor ulcerates and bleeding occurs. Most often, bleeding is so slight that gross blood is not seen in the stool. The blood can be detected only by chemical assay through the OB testing of the stool.

Benign and malignant GI tumors, ulcers, inflammatory bowel disease, arteriovenous malformations, diverticulosis, and hematobilia (hemobilia) can all cause OB within the stool. Other more common abnormalities (e.g., hemorrhoids, swallowed blood from oral or nasal pharyngeal bleeding) may also cause OB within the stool.

It has been well documented that vigorous exercise can create OB within the stool. It is important to note that many drugs and the ingestion of red meats (such as beef and pork) may cause a false-positive OB stool test (red meats contain animal hemoglobin). The more sensitive the test, the more false positives will be obtained.

When OB testing is properly performed, a positive result obtained on multiple specimens performed on successive days warrants a thorough GI evaluation. There is no consensus, however, about how many specimens need to be positive before a thorough evaluation is indicated. Most would agree that four positive results out of six specimens constitute criteria for a more thorough evaluation. Patients with chronic and prolonged OB loss in the stool may have iron deficiency anemia.

Interfering Factors

- Bleeding gums following a dental procedure may affect results.
- Ingestion of red meat within the 3 days before testing may affect results.
- Ingestion of fish, turnips, and horseradish may affect results.
- Drugs that may cause GI bleeding include anticoagulants, aspirin, colchicine, iron preparations (large doses), nonsteroidal antiarthritics, and steroids.
- Drugs that may cause false-positive results include colchicine, iron, oxidizing drugs (e.g., iodine, bromides, boric acid), and rauwolfia derivatives.
- Drugs that may cause false-negative results include vitamin C.

✓ CLINICAL PRIORITIES

- This test is part of the routine screening done on people over the age of 50 years.
- Red meats need to be avoided for 3 days before the test. Otherwise, false positives could be obtained because red meats contain animal hemoglobin.
- Positive test results for OB indicate the need for a thorough GI evaluation.

Procedure and Patient Care

Before

- Explain the procedure to the patient.
- Instruct the patient to refrain from eating any red meat for at least 3 days before the test.
- Instruct the patient to refrain from drugs known to interfere with OB testing.
- Instruct the patient in the method of obtaining appropriate stool specimens. Many procedures are available (e.g., specimen cards, tissue wipes, test paper). Tests may be done at home with specimen cards (Hemoccult) and mailed to a local testing laboratory or doctor's office when collected.
- Instruct the patient not to mix urine with the stool specimen.
- Inform the patient about the need for multiple specimens obtained on separate days to increase the test's accuracy.
- Note that in some centers a high-residue diet is recommended to increase the abrasive effect of the stool.
- Note on the laboratory slip any anticoagulant medications that the patient may be taking.
- Be gentle in obtaining stool by digital rectal examination. Traumatic digital examination can cause a false-positive stool, especially in patients with prior anorectal disease such as hemorrhoids.

During

Hemoccult Slide Test

1. Place a stool sample on one side of guaiac paper.
2. Place 2 drops of developer on the other side.
3. Note that a bluish discoloration indicates OB in the stool.

Tablet Test

1. Place a stool sample on the developed paper.
2. Place a tablet on top of the stool specimen.
3. Put 2 or 3 drops of tap water on the tablet and allow to flow onto the paper.
4. Note that a bluish discoloration indicates OB in the stool.

After

- Inform the patient as to the results.
- If the tests are positive, inquire whether the patient violated any of the preparation recommendations.

Test Results and Clinical Significance

GI tumor (cancers and polyps) *The mucosa overlying neoplasm is friable. Bleeding occurs when stool passes by.*

Peptic diseases (esophagitis, gastritis, and ulceration) *In peptic disease, the mucosa becomes inflamed, thickened, and friable. Bleeding easily occurs. Ulcers can erode into blood vessels within the wall of the gut.*

Varices *Caused by portal hypertension, these large venous complexes are covered by a thin lining of mucosa. With increased intraabdominal pressure, these can rupture and bleed.*

Inflammatory bowel disease (ulcerative colitis, Crohn's disease) *The inflammatory reaction causes a thickened and friable mucosa, which causes bleeding.*

Ischemic bowel disease *The mucosa of the bowel is the first layer to be affected by diminished blood supply. This mucosa easily sloughs, and minor bleeding can occur.*

GI trauma *Penetrating or blunt trauma can cause bleeding into the gut.*

Recent GI surgery *Small amounts of bleeding occur at the new GI anastomosis.*

Hemorrhoids and other anorectal problems *An anorectal pathologic condition is the most common nonneoplastic cause of blood in the stool.*

Related Tests

- Colonoscopy (p. 522): This test allows endoscopic evaluation of the entire colon.
- Esophagogastroduodenoscopy (p. 536): This endoscopic procedure visualizes the esophagus, stomach, and duodenum.
- Barium enema (p. 900): This test uses barium to provide x-ray visualization of the colon.
- Upper GI series (p. 999): This test uses barium to provide x-ray visualization of the upper GI tract.
- Small bowel series (p. 991): This test uses barium to provide x-ray visualization of the small intestines.

These tests are performed successively if a patient has OB identified on multiple specimens.

10

Ultrasound Studies

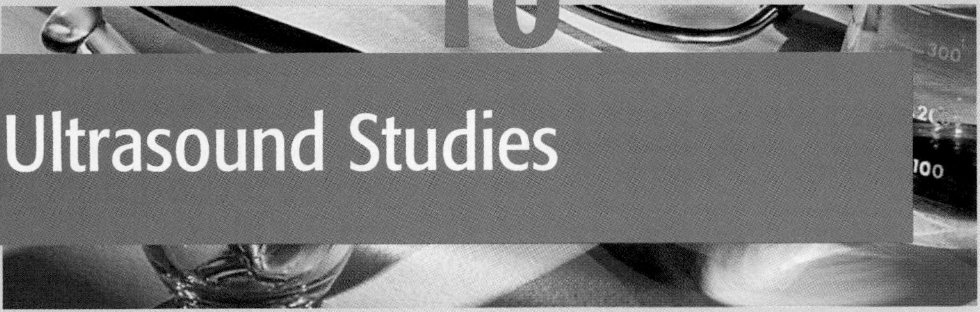

TESTS

Overview

Ultrasonography is a diagnostic technique in which high-frequency sound waves (ultrasonic waves) are directed at internal body structures, and a record is made of the wave pulses as they are reflected back (echoed) through the tissues. Different acoustic densities differentiate between solid and cystic structures and thereby form an "image" of the organ being studied.

Reasons for Performing Ultrasound Procedures

Ultrasonography is performed for any of the following reasons:

1. To determine whether a lump or other abnormality is a fluid-filled cyst or a solid tumor (e.g., kidney, thyroid, breast lesions).
2. To monitor therapy (e.g., to determine whether thyroid suppression therapy of a thyroid nodule is successful).
3. To guide needle-directed biopsy of a suspected tumor site to establish a diagnosis (e.g., prostate cancer).
4. To stage a tumor (e.g., esophageal cancer, rectal cancer).
5. To evaluate pregnancy and placental status.
6. To detect ectopic pregnancy.
7. To determine fetal status, size, and growth.
8. To evaluate disorders of arteries (e.g., aneurysm) and veins (e.g., deep vein thrombosis).

Principles of Ultrasonography

Tissues of different composition reflect sound waves differently, which permits differentiation of normal and diseased tissue. Sound waves are transmitted well through fluid, but not through air, bone, or contrast medium (e.g., barium).

The advantages of ultrasonography are that it is noninvasive and requires no ionizing radiation. Therefore, repeated studies can be performed and multiple images obtained with no risk. Because no radiation exposure occurs, ultrasonography can be performed in an office or laboratory or at the bedside. Ultrasonography is less expensive than either computed tomography (CT) or magnetic resonance imaging (MRI).

Ultrasonography is painless. The skin overlying the body area to be evaluated (e.g., heart, gallbladder) is covered with a lubricating gel to provide an air-free barrier between the skin and the ultrasonographic probe, which contains a transducer. The probe is passed over the specific body area, and ultrasonic waves, with frequencies in a range above human hearing, are transmitted through the tissues. The transducer converts the echoes to electric impulses and transforms them into visual images, or sonograms, which can be viewed singly (like a photograph), or in rapid sequence (like a movie), to evaluate the data obtained. Light (lucent) or dark (dense) areas seen on an ultrasonogram are a result of the manner in which various tissues reflect ultrasonic waves.

In some types of ultrasonography, the probe (transducer) is placed within the body. For example, in transesophageal echocardiography (TEE), the transducer is incorporated in the tip of a fiberoptic endoscope, which is placed in the esophagus, behind the heart;

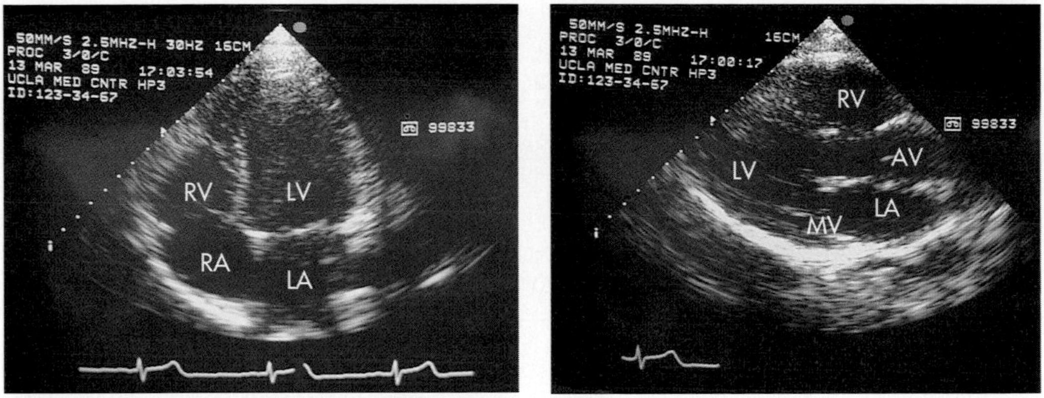

Figure 10-1 Two-dimensional echocardiogram. *RA,* right atrium; *RV,* right ventricle; *LA,* left atrium; *LV,* left ventricle; *MV,* mitral valve.

in rectal or prostate ultrasonography, the transducer is introduced through the anus into the rectum; and during surgery, the transducer can be held directly on the organ to be evaluated (e.g., the liver).

Various scans and techniques can be used to display the ultrasonic echoes. Some of these are as follows:

1. *B-scan:* A B-scan image is made up of a series of dots, each indicating a single ultrasonic echo. The position of a dot corresponds to the time elapsed, and the brightness of a dot corresponds to the strength of the echo. Movement of the transducer over the skin yields a two-dimensional cross-sectional image (Figure 10-1).
2. *M-mode scan:* Image obtained with M-mode echocardiography shows the motion (M) of the heart over time.
3. *Real-time imaging:* Multiple transducers are used to display a rapid sequence of images (like a movie) instantaneously while an object is being examined. Over the past several years, real-time ultrasound scanners have replaced static B-mode scanners as the main type in clinical use. Real-time imaging allows visualization of fetal movement or motion of the heart, for example.
4. *Doppler ultrasound:* As opposed to static ultrasound where the sound wave returning to the transducer is the same frequency as that which was emitted, Doppler ultrasound uses a different technique. In Doppler ultrasound of blood vessels, the RBCs within the vessel distort the frequency of the ultrasound waves. The change in frequency of the ultrasound wave is proportional to the velocity of the RBC. The better the blood flow, the faster the RBCs move by the stationary ultrasound beam, the greater the frequency distortion (or Doppler shift).

   With this technique sound waves are transformed into audible sounds or linear graphic recordings. This is important for assessing blood flow through arteries and veins. It is also used with pregnant women to assess the fetal heart rate and with increasing frequency to determine blood flow to organs (e.g., kidney, testicles).

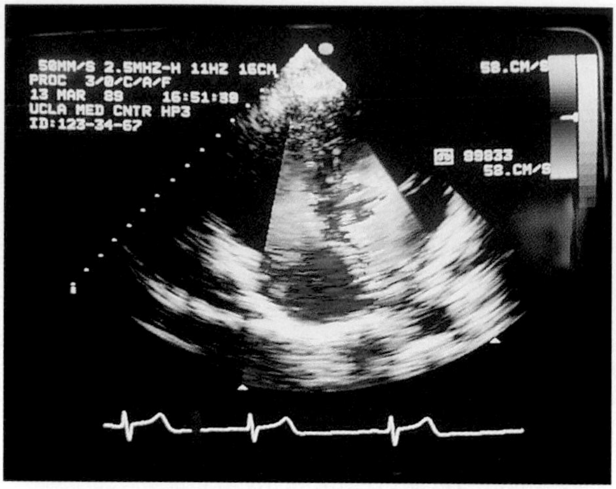

Figure 10-2 Color flow Doppler echocardiography. Flow, or signals, moving toward the transducer are recorded in shades of yellow and red, and those moving away from the transducer are recorded as blue.

5. *Color flow Doppler imaging:* This imaging technique is used to determine direction (recorded as colors) and velocity (shades) of blood flow in the chambers of the heart (Fig. 10-2). This technique is important in evaluating heart valve regurgitation and blood shunting in patients with heart defects.
6. *Duplex scanning:* Real-time imaging and color flow Doppler imaging combine to demonstrate how the arteries and veins are functioning and velocity and turbulence within the vessels. Duplex scanning is useful to detect plaque within arteries, demonstrate aneurysms, and assess renal or liver transplants for rejection.

Ultrasonography is often used in conjunction with other diagnostic testing. For example, if a CT scan of the kidney demonstrates a filling defect, an ultrasound scan can indicate whether that defect is a benign fluid-filled cyst or a malignant solid tumor.

Procedural Care for Ultrasonography

Before

- Most ultrasound procedures require little or no preparation. However, patients undergoing pelvic scanning must have a full bladder, which may become uncomfortable. Patients undergoing ultrasound examination of the gallbladder cannot be given anything orally, to overt gallbladder contraction that usually follows ingestion of a meal. A contracted gallbladder is difficult to identify with ultrasonography.
- Consent is needed if the transducer will be inserted into a body cavity.

During

- Ultrasound examinations are usually performed in an ultrasonography room (Figure 10-3), but can be performed on the patient unit or in a physician's office.
- A greasy paste, or "coupling agent," is applied to the tissue overlying the organ to be studied. Air impedes transmission of sound waves, and this lubricant ensures good contact between the skin and the transducer. Thus sound transmission and reception are enhanced.

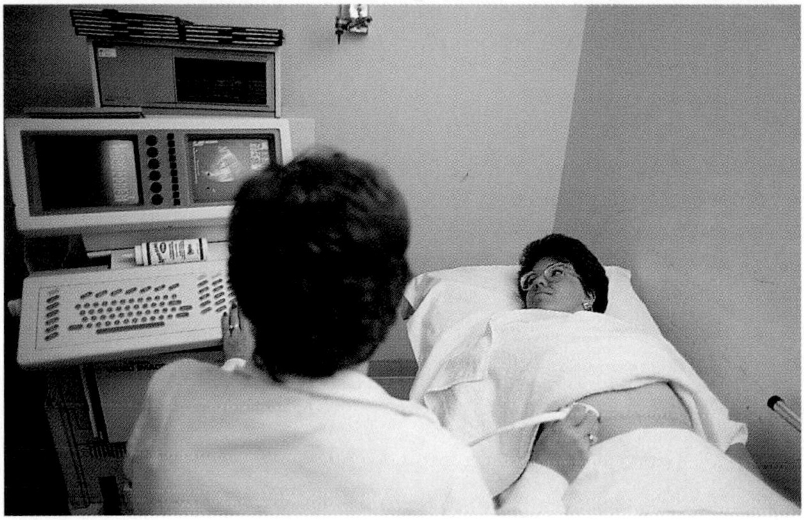

Figure 10-3 Ultrasonography room.

After

- Because ultrasonography is noninvasive, no special nursing measures are needed after the study except to help the patient remove the ultrasound paste.
- Ultrasound examinations can be repeated as often as necessary without harm to the patient. No cumulative effects have been noted.

Interfering Factors

- Air impedes transmission of ultrasonic waves into the body. The use of a lubricant is essential to ensure good transmission of sound waves to and from the body.
- Barium blocks transmission of ultrasonic waves. For this reason, ultrasonography of the abdomen should be performed before any barium contrast studies.
- Large amounts of gas in the bowel will distort visualization of abdominal organs, because bowel gas reflects sound. Likewise, ultrasonic evaluation of the lungs yields poor results.
- Obesity may affect the results of the study, because sound waves are altered by fatty tissue. For this reason, it may be difficult to obtain an accurate scan in an obese patient.
- Movement causes artifacts. Some patients may need to be sedated to remain still. Uncooperative patients (especially children) may not be candidates for ultrasonography.
- Because ultrasonography requires direct contact of the transducer and the skin, it may not be possible to perform this study in postoperative patients with dressings.

Potential Complications

No potential complications have been directly related to ultrasonography at the intensities used for medical diagnosis. However, in some procedures (e.g., TEE), complications may occur as a result of the invasive method used to place the ultrasound probe inside the body. These complications are described for individual tests.

Reporting of Results

The patient can usually observe the scan on a monitor in the room. The technician may point out some findings at that time. Later, the physician will review the scan and explain the results to the patient.

Abdominal Ultrasonography (Abdominal Sonography; Echography; Ultrasonography of the Kidney, Liver, Pancreatobiliary System, Gallbladder, Pancreas, Biliary Tree)

Normal Findings

Normal abdominal aorta, liver, gallbladder, bile ducts, pancreas, kidney, ureters, and bladder

Indications

This technique is used to visualize the abdomen and the organs within it. Its uses are many, as described.

Test Explanation

Through use of reflected sound waves, ultrasonography provides accurate visualization of the abdominal aorta, liver, gallbladder, pancreas, bile ducts, spleen, kidneys, ureters, and bladder. The technique of ultrasonography requires the emission of high-frequency sound waves from the transducer to penetrate the organ being studied. The sound waves are bounced back to the transducer and electronically converted to a pictorial image that is recorded on film. Real-time ultrasound provides an accurate picture of the organ being studied. Doppler ultrasound provides information about blood flow to those organs.

The *kidney* is evaluated ultrasonographically to (1) diagnose and locate renal cysts, (2) differentiate renal cysts from solid renal tumors, (3) demonstrate renal and pelvic calculi, (4) document hydronephrosis, and (5) guide a percutaneously inserted needle for cyst aspiration or biopsy (Figure 10-4). Ultrasound of the urologic tract is used to detect malformed or ectopic kidneys and perinephric abscesses. Renal transplantation surveillance is possible with ultrasonography. One advantage of kidney sonography over intravenous pyelography (p. 953) is that it can be performed in patients with impaired renal function, because no intravenous contrast medium is required.

The *testes* (p. 801) can be evaluated for neoplasm, abscess, infection, inflammation, or torsion. The *prostate gland* (p. 799) can be examined for neoplasm, hypertrophy, or infection. Ultrasonography is used to guide biopsy of the prostate gland.

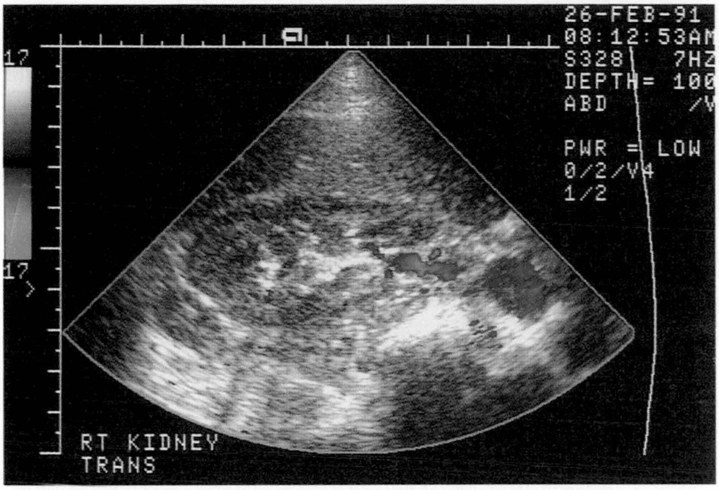

Figure 10-4 Ultrasonogram of the kidney.

The *abdominal aorta* can be assessed for aneurysmal dilation. Sonographic evidence of an aortic aneurysm >5 cm in greatest dimension, or any aneurysm that is documented to be significantly enlarging is an indication for abdominal aortic aneurysm resection. Ultrasonography is also an ideal way to monitor aneurysms before and after surgery.

Ultrasonography is used to detect cystic structures of the *liver* (e.g., benign cysts, hepatic abscesses, dilated hepatic ducts) and solid intrahepatic tumors (primary and metastatic). Hepatic ultrasonography can also be performed intraoperatively with a sterile probe. This technique allows accurate location of small, nonpalpable hepatic tumors or abscesses. The *gallbladder* and *extrahepatic ducts* can be visualized for evidence of gallstones (Figure 10-5), polyps, or dilation secondary to obstructive strictures or tumors. The

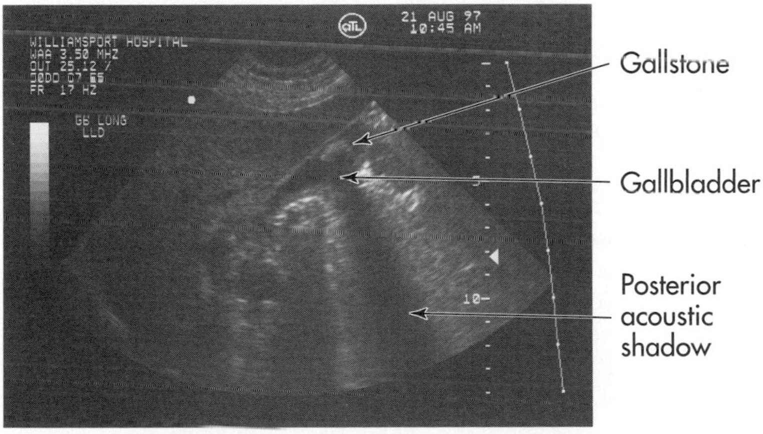

Figure 10-5 Ultrasonogram of the gallbladder. Long axis view of the gallbladder containing a gallstone. Note the posterior acoustic shadowing, typical for gallstones.

pancreas is examined for evidence of tumor, pseudocysts, acute or chronic inflammation, or pancreatic abscess. Repeated ultrasound scans of the pancreas are frequently obtained to document resolution of acute pancreatic inflammatory processes. Often the pancreas is better visualized if the stomach and duodenum are filled with water.

Because ultrasonography requires no contrast material or radiation, it is especially useful in patients who are allergic to contrast media or are pregnant. Fasting is desirable but not mandatory. (See discussion of pelvic ultrasonography [p. 796] for evaluation of pelvic organs.)

Interfering Factors

- Barium and gas distort the sound waves and alter test results. This test should be performed before any x-ray testing with barium contrast.
- Ultrasound is only as good as the skills of the sonographer.

✓ CLINICAL PRIORITIES

- Because this study requires no contrast material and no associaed radiation, it is especially useful in patients allergic to dyes and in pregnant patients.
- The need for preprocedure fasting depends on the organ to be examined.
- Ultrasound of the kidney can be used to evaluate rejection of a kidney transplant.

Procedure and Patient Care

Before

- Explain the procedure to the patient.
- Tell the patient that no discomfort is associated with the procedure.
- Tell the patient that fasting may or may not be required, depending on the organ to be examined. No fasting is required for ultrasonography of the abdominal aorta, kidney, liver, spleen, or pancreas, but is preferred before ultrasonography of the gallbladder and biliary tree.

During

- Procedure:
  1. The patient is placed on the ultrasonography table in the prone or supine position, depending on the organ to be examined.
  2. A greasy conductive paste is applied to the patient's skin, to enhance sound wave transmission and reception.
  3. A transducer is placed over the skin (Figure 10-6).
  4. Images are made of the reflections from the organ being studied.
- For water distention of the stomach, the patient is asked to drink 8 to 10 oz of water while standing.
- The test is completed in approximately 20 minutes, usually by an ultrasound technologist, and later is interpreted by a radiologist.

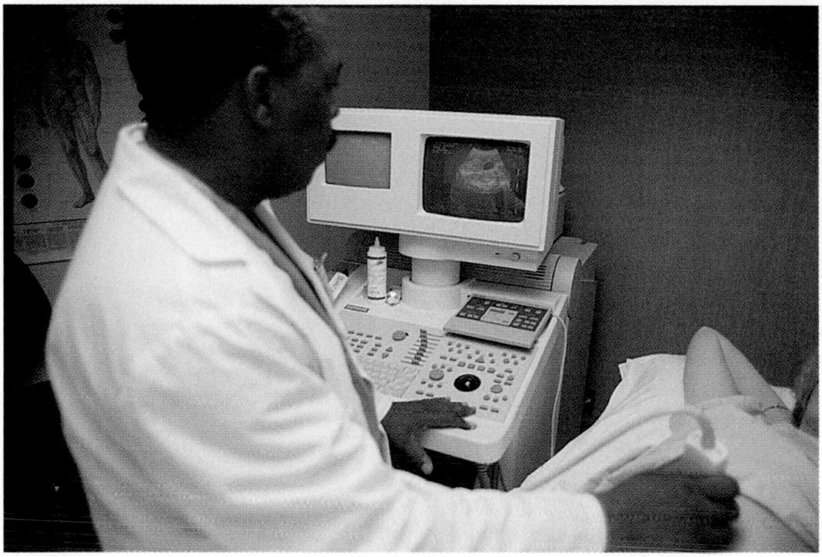

Figure 10-6 Abdominal ultrasonography.

After

- Remove the coupling agent (grease) from the patient's skin.
- If a biopsy was performed, refer to the specific organ (e.g., liver biopsy, kidney biopsy).

Test Results and Clinical Significance

Kidney

Renal cysts and polycystic kidney *Renal cysts appear as dark (echo free, or hypoechoic) areas with smooth, well-defined walls. In polycystic kidney, these cysts are of various sizes.*

Renal tumor *Renal tumors appear as white (hyperechoic) areas.*

Renal calculi
Hydronephrosis
Ureteral obstruction
Obstruction is inferred by identification of dilation of the collecting system.

Perinephric collection (e.g., perirenal abscess, perirenal hematoma) *Perirenal collections of pus or blood appear as a hypoechoic (dark) halo surrounding the kidney.*

Primary renal disease (e.g., glomerulonephritis, pyelonephritis) *Primary renal disease is evidenced by small, isoechoic kidneys, especially at the end stage.*

Pancreas

Tumor *Pancreatic tumor is evident as an echogenic (solid) mass, usually in the head of the pancreas.*

Cysts or pseudocysts *These appear as dark (hypoechoic) masses. Neoplastic cysts are difficult to differentiate from pseudocysts. Malignant cystic tumors cannot be differentiated from benign cysts.*
Abscess *Hypoechoic (dark) areas in an inflamed pancreas could be cysts or abscesses, which cannot be differentiated.*
Inflammation *Acute inflammation of the pancreas is seen as an enlarged edematous pancreas. Chronic inflammation is apparent as a small, contracted echogenic (dense) pancreas.*

Gallbladder

Polyps
Tumor
Neoplasms appear as echogenic (solid) masses in the gallbladder that do not move with change in position.

Gallstone *Ultrasound is accurate for detection of gallstones. An echogenic mass with "shadowing" behind it is the classic appearance of a gallstone.*

Liver

Tumor: primary or metastatic *The ultrasound appearance of liver metastasis is variable. In general, liver neoplasms are echogenic.*

Abscess
Cysts
Liver abscesses and cysts cannot be differentiated with certainty with ultrasonography.

Bile ducts

Gallstone
Tumor
Tumors and gallstones appear as echogenic masses with posterior acoustic "shadowing" within the bile duct.

Dilation due to stricture, stones, or tumor
Intrahepatic dilated bile ducts
The entire biliary tree is seen as a hypoechoic tube in the portal area or liver.

Abdominal aorta

Aneurysm *The aorta appears as a hypoechoic tubular structure in the retroperitoneum. Aortic aneurysm is evident as a saccular dilation.*

Abdominal cavity

Ascites *Ultrasound is sensitive for detection of fluid within the abdomen. As little as 10 ml of fluid can be detected.*
Abscess *Abscesses secondary to appendicitis or diverticulitis are easily demonstrated. Phlegmon (inflammatory involvement of tissue) may surround an abscess.*

Related Tests

- Ultrasonography of the prostate gland, testes, uterus, and ovaries is discussed separately (pp. 799, 801, and 796, respectively).

Breast Ultrasonography (Ultrasound Mammography)

Normal Findings No evidence of cyst or tumor

Indications

Ultrasound examination of the breast is most commonly performed to determine if a mammographic abnormality or a palpable lump is a cyst (fluid filled) or solid tumor (benign or malignant).

Test Explanation

In diagnostic real-time ultrasonography, harmless high-frequency sound waves are emitted and penetrate the breast. The sound waves are reflected back to the sensor and arranged in a pictorial image by electronic conversion. Ultrasonography of the breast is useful to (1) differentiate cystic from solid breast lesions, (2) identify masses in women with breast tissue too dense for accurate mammography, and (3) monitor a cyst to determine whether it enlarges or disappears. Ultrasonography is also useful for examination of symptomatic breasts in women in whom the radiation of mammography is potentially harmful. These include:

1. Pregnant women. Radiation may be harmful to the fetus.
2. Women younger than age 25, who may be at greater oncologic risk from the radiation of mammography.
3. Women with silicone augmented breasts. The prosthesis can be penetrated by the ultrasound beam. Ordinarily, these prostheses would obscure residual tissue on physical examination and mammography.
4. Women who refuse mammography because of unreasonable fear of diagnostic radiation.

Ultrasound is especially useful in patients with an abnormal mass identified on a mammogram, because the nature (cystic or solid) of the mass can be determined. Most cysts are benign.

Diagnostic accuracy is improved when breast ultrasonography is combined with mammography (see p. 963). Ultrasound can be used to locate a nonpalpable breast abnormality for biopsy or aspiration.

Procedure and Patient Care

Before

- Explain the procedure to the patient and assure the patient that no discomfort is associated with the examination.
- Inform the patient that no fasting or sedation is required. Instruct the patient not to apply any lotions or powders to the breasts on the examination day.

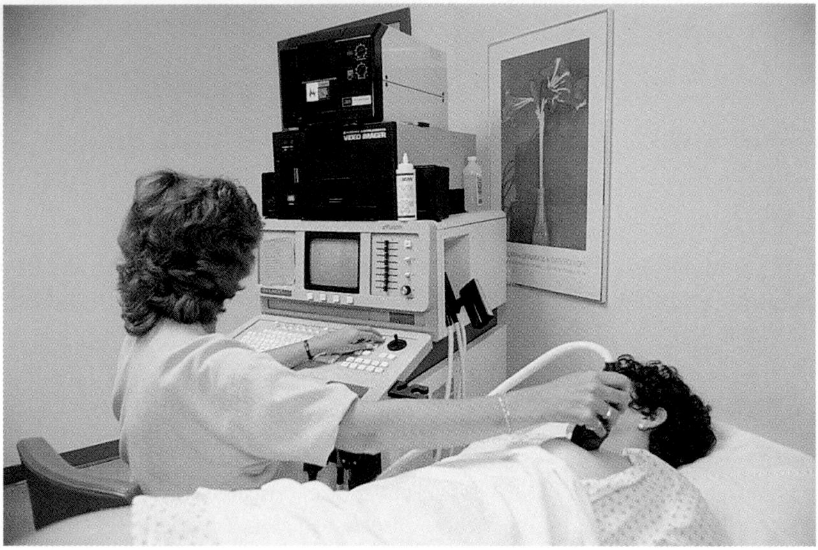

Figure 10-7 Ultrasonography of the breast.

During

- Note the following procedural steps:
  1. The patient lies prone on the examining table, which contains a tank that holds heated and chlorinated water.
  2. One breast at a time is immersed in the water.
  3. The transducer that produces the ultrasound waves and detects their echoes is positioned at the bottom of the water tank.
  4. Alternatively, the patient is placed supine, a conductive paste is applied, and a hand-held transducer is placed directly on the skin overlying the breast.
- The test is performed by an ultrasound technician in approximately 15 minutes.
- Although no discomfort is associated with the procedure, women with back problems or limited flexibility may have difficulty maintaining the necessary position.

After

- After the test is completed, the breasts are dried or the conductive paste is removed.

Test Results and Clinical Significance

Cyst
Hematoma
Abscess
These appear as a hypoechoic (dark) well-circumscribed mass with acoustic "shadowing" behind the back wall.

Cancer
Fibroadenoma
These appear as an echogenic (white) lesion within the breast. Benign and malignant lesions cannot be differentiated as well with ultrasonography as with mammography.

Fibrocystic disease *This is evident as diffuse echogenic localized tissue within the breast.*

Related Tests

- Mammography (p. 963): This x-ray study of the breast can detect breast abnormalities but cannot differentiate between cystic and solid masses, as ultrasonography can.

Carotid Artery Duplex Scanning
(Carotid Doppler Ultrasound)

Normal Findings Carotid artery free of plaques and stenosis

Indications

This Doppler ultrasound test is performed to identify occlusive disease in the carotid artery or its branches. It is recommended in patients with headaches and with neurologic symptoms such as transient ischemic attacks (TIA), hemiparesis, paresthesia, or acute speech or visual deficits.

Test Explanation

Carotid duplex scanning is a noninvasive, ultrasound test used to directly detect occlusive disease of the extracranial carotid artery. A pulsed Doppler probe is used to evaluate flow velocity and direction in the artery, and to measure the amplitude and waveform of the carotid arterial pulse. A two-dimensional image of the carotid artery enables direct visualization of possibly stenotic or occluded arteries and arterial flow disruption.

This test is performed by an ultrasound technologist in the ultrasound or radiology department in approximately 15 to 30 minutes. Results are interpreted by a radiologist, usually the same day. No discomfort is associated with the test.

Procedure and Patient Care

Before

- Explain the procedure to the patient.
- Tell the patient that no special preparation is required.
- Assure the patient that the study is painless.

During

- Place the patient supine with the head supported to prevent lateral motion.
- Note the following procedural steps:
  1. A water-soluble gel is used to couple the sound from the transducer to the skin surface.
  2. Images of the carotid artery and pulse waveform are obtained.

After

- Remove the water-soluble gel from the patient's skin.

Test Results and Clinical Significance

Carotid artery occlusive disease *Narrowing of the lumen of the carotid artery or any of its branches can be accurately determined as a percentage of the vessel occluded (e.g., 90% occlusion). Most often occlusion is a result of atherosclerotic disease.*

Related Tests

- Angiography, Carotid (p. 892): This is a more accurate test of the carotid system, and is performed if surgery is contemplated. The angiogram demonstrates where and how extensive occlusive plaques are.

Contraceptive Device Localization
(Intrauterine Device [IUD] Localization)

Normal Findings

An IUD contraceptive device is located in the endometrial cavity

Indications

This ultrasound test is performed to locate an IUD when its string cannot be palpated.

Test Explanation

When a woman is unable to visualize or palpate the string of an IUD, ultrasonography is indicated to determine whether the IUD has perforated the uterus, been evacuated, or been incorporated with an intrauterine pregnancy. IUDs have a particular type-specific structure and can be easily recognized on a sonogram. If an IUD can be seen on an abdominal x-ray film but cannot be demonstrated in the endometrial cavity on a sonogram, the IUD most likely has perforated the uterus.

IUD localization is performed in approximately 20 minutes. No discomfort is associated with this study other than having a full bladder and the urge to urinate.

Interfering Factors

- Recent gastrointestinal contrast studies, because barium severely distorts reflective sound waves
- Air-filled bowel loops, because gas does not transmit sound waves well
- Failure to fill the bladder, which is often used as a reference point for pelvic sonography

Procedure and Patient Care

Before

- Explain the procedure to the patient.
- Give the patient three to four glasses (200 to 300 ml) of water or other liquid 1 hr be-

fore the examination, and instruct her not to void until after the procedure is completed. This will allow the bladder to fill and to be used as a reference point.
- Tell the patient that no fasting or sedation is required.

During

- Note the following procedural steps:
  1. The patient is taken to the ultrasound room and placed supine on the examination table.
  2. The ultrasonographer, usually a radiologist, applies a greasy, conductive paste to the abdomen to enhance sound transmission and reception.
  3. A transducer is passed vertically and horizontally over the skin.
  4. Pictures are taken of the sound waves, and a real-time image is produced.

After

- Remove the lubricant from the patient's skin.
- Provide an opportunity for the patient to void.

Test Results and Clinical Significance

Perforation of the uterus *If an IUD is seen on a plain film of the abdomen but cannot be found in the uterus at ultrasonography, it can be suspected that the IUD has perforated the uterus and is outside it.*

Expulsion of the IUD *The IUD cannot be located in the uterus or on a plain film of the abdomen.*

Incorporation of the IUD in an intrauterine pregnancy *The IUD was in place when pregnancy occurred and has become incorporated in the pregnancy.*

Echocardiography (Cardiac Echography, Heart Sonography, Transthoracic Echocardiography [TTE])

Normal Findings

Normal position, size, and movement of the cardiac valves and heart muscle wall
Normal directional flow of blood within the heart chambers

Indications

Echocardiography is performed most commonly to evaluate heart wall motion (a measure of heart wall function) and to detect valvular disease, evaluate the heart during stress testing, and identify and quantify pericardial fluid.

Test Explanation

Echocardiography is a noninvasive ultrasound procedure used to evaluate the structure and function of the heart. In diagnostic ultrasonography, harmless, high-frequency sound waves emitted from a transducer penetrate the heart and are reflected back to the transducer as a series of echoes (Figure 10-8). These echoes are amplified and displayed on a cathode ray tube. Tracings also can be recorded on moving graph paper or videotape. The

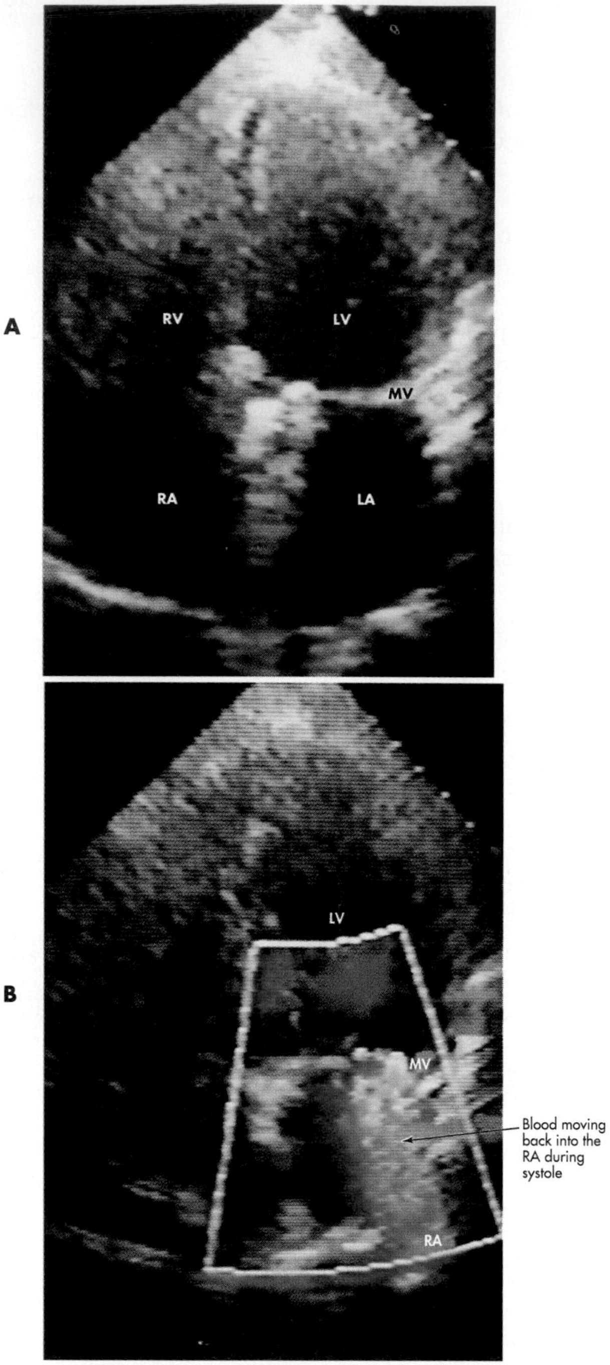

Figure 10-8 Echocardiogram, **A,** Two-dimensional (2D) echocardiography (black and white) **B,** Color Doppler echocardiography. The heart is oriented with the ventricles on the upper portion of the picture and the atria on the lower portion. The four chambers of the heart are easily identified. The right side of the heart is seen on the left side of the figure. *RV,* right ventricle; *LV,* left ventricle; *RA,* right atrium; *LA,* left atrium; *MV,* mitral valve leaflets (white line) closed during systole. On the Color Doppler echocardiogram, the blue indicates abnormal reversal of blood flowing from the left ventricle and into the left atrium during systole due to mitral valve regurgitation.

study usually includes M-mode recordings, two-dimensional recordings, and a Doppler study.

M-mode echocardiography produces a one-dimensional recording of the amplitude and rate of motion (M) of the heart structures in real time. This allows the various cardiac structures to be located and studied regarding their movement during a cardiac cycle.

In *two-dimensional echocardiography,* the ultrasonic beam is moved within one sector of the heart. Computer reconstruction produces a two-dimensional image of the spatial relationships within the heart.

Color flow Doppler imaging demonstrates the direction and velocity of blood flow within the heart and great vessels. These variations in blood flow and velocity alter the ultrasound frequency. By assigning computerized weighted numbers to these altered frequencies, origins of velocity change and blood turbulence can be mapped. Altered direction and velocity of blood flow are coded as colors and shades, respectively (e.g., blue and red represent the direction of blood flow; various hues from dull to bright represent blood velocity). The most useful application of the color flow Doppler imaging is to determine the direction and turbulence of blood flow across regurgitant or narrowed valves. Color flow Doppler imaging also may be helpful in assessing proper functioning of prosthetic valves.

Echocardiography is used to diagnose pericardial effusion, valvular heart disease (e.g., mitral valve prolapse, stenosis, regurgitation), subaortic stenosis, myocardial wall abnormalities (e.g., cardiomyopathy), infarction, aneurysm, and cardiac tumors (e.g., myxomas). Atrial and ventricular septal defects and other congenital heart diseases, and post-infarction mural thrombi are also recognized with this testing.

Echocardiography is fast becoming the method of choice for cardiac stress testing. During an exercise or chemical cardiac stress test, ischemic muscle areas are evident as hypokinetic areas within the myocardium. Echocardiography is being used increasingly in emergent evaluation of chest pain. If the myocardium is normal and without areas of hypokinesia, no coronary artery occlusive disease is suspected. A hypokinetic or akinetic area, however, indicates ischemia or infarction and that the chest pain is cardiac in origin.

It is now possible to perform echocardiography through the esophagus using a transducer mounted on an endoscope. This procedure is referred to as transesophageal echocardiography (TEE) (p. 804). Fetal echocardiograms enable identification of significant congenital heart disease before birth.

Echocardiography usually takes approximately 45 minutes, and is performed by an ultrasound technician in a darkened room in the cardiac laboratory or radiology department. No discomfort is associated with this study other than that the transmission gel is usually cooler than body temperature.

Contraindications

- Patients who are uncooperative

Interfering Factors

- Patients with chronic obstructive pulmonary disease (COPD) have a substantial amount of air between the heart and the chest cavity. Air space does not conduct ultrasound waves well.

CLINICAL PRIORITIES

- Echocardiography is rapidly becoming the method of choice of heart imaging for stress testing.
- This test is frequently used in the emergency evaluation of chest pain.
- Because of the large amount of air between the heart and the chest cavity, it is difficult to evaluate patients with COPD with echocardiography. Transesophageal echocardiography is a better test in these patients.

- In obese patients, the space between the heart and the transducer is greatly enlarged; therefore, accuracy of the test is decreased.

Procedure and Patient Care

Before

- Assure the patient that the study is painless.
- Include pertinent patient history on the echocardiogram request form.

During

- Note the following procedural steps:
  1. The patient is placed supine.
  2. Electrocardiographic (EKG) leads are placed (p. 478).
  3. A gel, which allows better transmission of sound waves, is placed on the chest wall, over which the transducer is passed.
  4. Ultrasonic waves are directed at the heart, and appropriate tracings are obtained (Figures 10-9 and 10-10).

After

- Remove gel from the patient's chest wall.
- Inform the patient that the physician must interpret the study and that the results will be available in a few hours.

Test Results and Clinical Significance

Valvular heart disease (e.g., stenosis, regurgitation, mitral valve prolapse) *This is readily evident on echocardiograms. All valves can be easily seen with the linear mode. The circulatory effects of valvular disease are apparent on Doppler studies.*

Pericardial effusion *Fluid around the heart is easily evident. Echocardiography can be used to guide a needle into the pericardial space for aspiration of fluid for analysis and treatment.*

Ventricular or atrial mural thrombi *When these are evident, anticoagulation therapy is required. These thrombi may be the result of previous myocardial infarction, ventricular aneurysm, congestive heart failure, or cardiomyopathy.*

Myxomas *These tumors are often evident as a mass partially attached to the endocardium.*

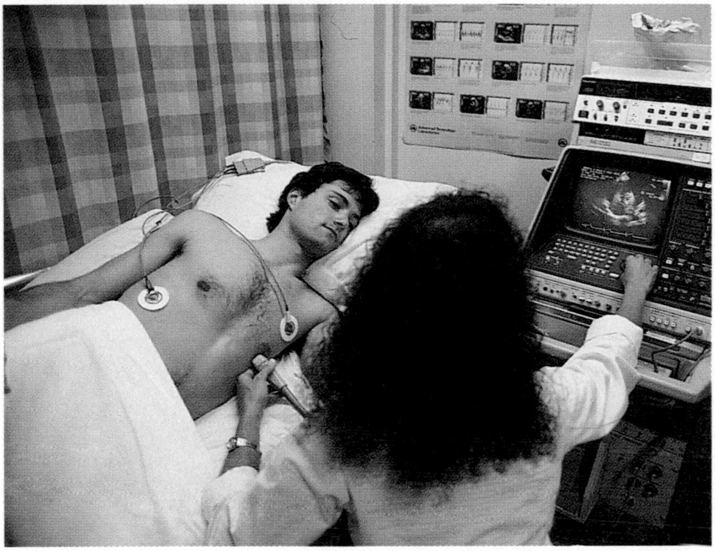

Figure 10-9 Echocardiography laboratory.

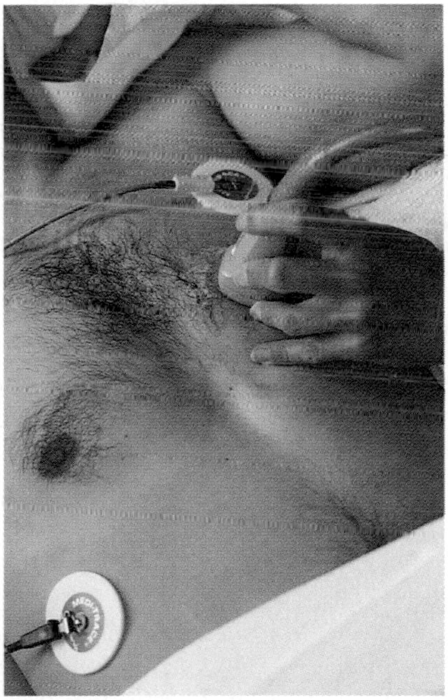

Figure 10-10 Placement of chest leads and transducer on precordium.

Poor ventricular muscle motion *Hypokinesia is evident in a portion of or in the entire myocardial wall in patients with myocardial ischemia, cardiomyopathy, and congestive heart failure.*

Ventricular hypertrophy *This chronic disease is evident as an unusually thickened myocardium.*

Endocarditis *Vegetations are readily evident on the valves. Aggressive antibiotic or anticoagulation therapy, or both, is needed.*

Septal defects *Left-to-right shunting is readily evident with color flow Doppler imaging.*

Related Tests

- Transesophageal echocardiography (TEE) (p. 804) provides information similar to that obtained with transthoracic echocardiography, but TEE allows better visualization of the posterior portion of the heart and thoracic vessels.

Fetal Biophysical Profile (BPP)

Normal Findings Score of 8 to 10 points (if amniotic fluid volume is adequate)

Critical Values Score of less than 4 may necessitate immediate delivery.

Indications

The premise behind the BPP is that assessment of variable factors of fetal biophysical activity are more reliable than examination of a single parameter (e.g., fetal heart rate). Indications for BPP include postdate pregnancy, maternal hypertension, diabetes mellitus, vaginal bleeding, maternal Rh factor sensitization, maternal history of stillbirth, and premature rupture of membranes. The BPP is probably more useful in identifying a fetus that is in jeopardy than in predicting future fetal well-being. Testing usually begins at about 32 weeks, but can be done earlier if maternal complications exist.

Test Explanation

The BPP is a method of evaluating antepartal fetal status on the basis of five variables: fetal heart rate, fetal breathing movement, gross fetal movement, fetal muscle tone, and amniotic fluid volume. Fetal heart rate reactivity is measured with the nonstress test (p. 504); the other four parameters are measured with ultrasonography. Each variable is scored as either 2 or 0. Therefore, 10 is a perfect score, and 0 is the lowest score.

1. *Fetal heart rate reactivity.* Fetal heart rate reactivity is measured and interpreted in the same way as with the nonstress test (p. 504). Fetal heart rate is considered reactive when there are movement-associated fetal heart rate accelerations of at least 15 beats/min above baseline and 15 seconds in duration, over a 20 minute time period. A score of 2 indicates reactivity; a score of 0 indicates that fetal heart rate is nonreactive.

2. *Fetal breathing movements.* This variable is assessed on the assumption that fetal breathing movements indicate fetal well-being, and their absence may indicate hypoxemia. Rate and uniformity of fetal breathing become increasingly regular after week 36 of gestation. At least one episode of fetal breathing lasting a minimum of 60 seconds within a 30-minute observation period is scored as 2; absence of this breathing pattern is scored as 0. Several factors can alter fetal breathing movements. For example, fetal breathing movements increase during the second and third hours after maternal meals and also at night. Fetal breathing movements may decrease in conditions such as hypoxemia, hypoglycemia, nicotine use, and alcohol ingestion.

3. *Fetal body movements.* Fetal activity is a reflection of neurologic integrity and function. The presence of at least three discrete episodes of fetal movement within a 30-minute observation period is scored as 2; two or fewer fetal movements in 30 minutes is scored as 0. Fetal activity is greatest 1 to 3 hours after the mother has consumed a meal. For this reason, it is often suggested that this test be scheduled in relation to mealtime.

4. *Fetal muscle tone.* In the uterus, the fetus is normally in a position of flexion, but also stretches, rolls, and moves. The arms, legs, trunk, and head may be flexed and extended. If there is at least one episode of active extension with return to flexion (e.g.,

opening and closing of a hand), it is scored as 2; slow extension with return to only partial flexion, fetal movement not followed by return to flexion, limbs or spine in extension, and an open fetal hand are scored as 0.

5. Amniotic fluid volume. Measurement of amniotic fluid volume is an effective method of predicting fetal distress. Oligohydramnios (too little amniotic fluid) has been associated with fetal anomalies, intrauterine growth retardation, and postterm pregnancy. Immediate delivery is recommended in postterm pregnancy with oligohydramnios because of the high risk of associated problems such as umbilical cord compromise. If there is at least one pocket of amniotic fluid that measures 1 cm in two perpendicular planes, the score is 2; if either fluid is absent in most areas of the uterine cavity or the largest pocket measures 1 cm or less in the vertical axis, the score is 0.

A score of 8 or 10 with an acceptable amount of amniotic fluid is normal. A score of 8 with oligohydramnios or a score of 4 to 6 is equivocal and is interpreted as possibly abnormal. Some clinicians recommend repeating the test within 24 hours; others advocate extending testing after any equivocal test result. A score of 0 or 2 is abnormal and indicates the need for assessment of immediate delivery.

Although the BPP is fairly new, it has already been modified. Some physicians omit the nonstress test if the ultrasound parameters are normal; some include placental grading as a sixth parameter. Information about fetal size, position, and location of the placenta can also be obtained.

Additional information about fetal well-being can be gained from Doppler ultrasound evaluation of the placenta and the *umbilical artery flow velocity.* Changes in umbilical artery flow or direction may indicate fetal stress or illness.

Interfering Factors

- Maternal hyperglycemia may increase fetal biophysical activity.
- Hypoxemia and trauma may decrease fetal biophysical activity.
- Maternal or fetal infection will affect fetal biophysical activity.
- Occasionally no movement will be noted. If no eye movement or respiratory movement is noted, the fetus may be sleeping.
- Central nervous system stimulants, such as catecholamines, can increase fetal biophysical activity.
- Magnesium sulfate, analgesics, anesthetics, sedatives, and nicotine can depress fetal biophysical activity.

CLINICAL PRIORITIES

- The BPP is more useful in identifying a fetus in jeopardy than in predicting future fetal well-being.
- The BPP is usually indicated in women with high-risk pregnancies. Testing usually begins around week 32 of gestation, but can be done earlier if there are maternal complications.
- Several BPP variables are affected by the maternal blood glucose level. For this reason, it is often recommended that this test be performed 1 to 3 hours after the mother has eaten.

Procedure and Patient Care

Before

- Explain the procedure to the patient.
- Inform the patient that no fasting is required.

During

- Fetal heart rate reactivity is measured and interpreted from a nonstress test (p. 504).
- Fetal breathing movements, fetal body movements, fetal muscle tone, and amniotic fluid volume are determined by ultrasound imaging (see obstetric ultrasonography, p. 796).

After

- If test results are abnormal or equivocal, support the patient in the next phase of the fetal evaluation process.

Test Results and Clinical Significance

Fetal asphyxia
Congenital anomalies
Oligohydramnios
Intrauterine growth retardation
Postterm pregnancy
Fetal distress or death

Related Tests

- Contraction (p. 474) and nonstress testing (p. 504): These tests are performed to monitor fetal heart rate and movement.
- Pelvic ultrasonography (p. 796): This test is used in the obstetric patient to identify a tubal or molar pregnancy, indicate the number of fetuses, and determine fetal age, rate of growth, position, and size.

Ocular and Orbit Ultrasonography

Normal Findings Normal pattern of orbital and posterior orbital structures

Indications

Ocular ultrasound is used to examine the eye when the extraocular and intraocular spaces cannot be adequately evaluated by other methods because of disease, scarring, or surgery, and to evaluate the posterior bulbar area for tumors and cysts.

Test Explanation

Ultrasound of the eye is used to detect intraocular disease such as vitreous hemorrhage, retinal or choroidal detachment, and intraocular foreign bodies. It is also used to identify retro-ocular abnormalities such as tumor (e.g., glioma, meningioma), benign cysts (e.g., dermoid, mucocele), and cavernous hemangioma. Changes in corneal and ocular shape as a result of disease, surgery, or trauma can be identified. CT and MRI are also excellent methods to evaluate the ocular and retrobulbar spaces. The orbital fossae and eyes can be evaluated in the fetus by ultrasound if cranial or ocular abnormalities are suspected.

Procedure and Patient Care

Before

- Explain the procedure to the patient.
- Topical anesthetic drops are administered to the eyes 5 to 10 minutes before the study.

During

- The ultrasound probe is applied directly to the eye.
- Ultrasound images are obtained.
- Alternatively, ultrasound immersion technique can be performed (i.e., the probe is immersed in a water bath).

After

- Inform the patient that the cornea is still anesthetized and that because no discomfort can be appreciated, it is important to refrain from rubbing or otherwise contacting the eye.

Test Results and Clinical Significance

Retinal or choroidal detachment *This can result from senile deterioration, trauma, or posterior ocular bleeding.*

Thickened orbit *The most common cause is hyperthyroidism (Graves' disease).*

Vitreous opacities *These "floaters" or dark spots in vision can be caused by foreign bodies, desquamated cells, or hemorrhage.*

Neoplasm *These include posterior ocular tumors such as melanoma, hemangioma, or metastatic tumors, retrobulbar tumors such as glioma, meningioma, neurofibroma, or metastatic tumor.*

Pelvic Ultrasonography (Obstetric Echography, Pregnant Uterus Ultrasonography, Pelvic Ultrasonography in Pregnancy, Obstetric Ultrasonography, Vaginal Ultrasonography)

Normal Findings Normal fetal and placental size and position

Indications

Pelvic ultrasonography is used in obstetric patients to evaluate the pregnancy and the fetus. It is especially important in high-risk pregnancies. In nonpregnant women, it is used to evaluate the genital tract for disease and to monitor known pelvic disease (e.g., benign ovarian cysts).

See rectal sonography (p. 799) for discussion of pelvic ultrasound examination in male patients.

Test Explanation

Ultrasound examination is a harmless, noninvasive method of evaluating the female genital tract and the fetus. In real-time diagnostic ultrasound, high-frequency sound waves are emitted from the transducer and penetrate the structure to be studied (e.g., uterus, ovaries, parametria, placenta, fetus). These sound waves are reflected back to a sensor within the transducer, and by electronic conversion are arranged into a pictorial image of the studied structure.

Pelvic ultrasonography can be performed with the transducer placed on the anterior abdomen, or in the vagina with a specially designed vaginal probe, which provides the best view of the pelvic organs in a nonpregnant woman. The images obtained with both transducers are complementary. Vaginal ultrasound provides significant accuracy in identifying paracervical, endometrial, and ovarian disease that may not be detected with the anterior abdominal probe. Occasionally, abdominal organs fall into the pelvis and preclude good pelvic visualization with the anterior abdominal probe. Vaginal ultrasound provides better visualization under these circumstances. In the obese patient, the thick abdominal wall inhibits good transmission of ultrasonic waves, and vaginal ultrasound is preferred. The anterior abdominal probe, however, provides better visualization of the upper pelvis than does the vaginal probe, especially in pregnant women.

Pelvic ultrasonography may be useful in the obstetric patient in the following circumstances:

1. To make an early diagnosis of normal pregnancy or abnormal pregnancy (e.g., tubal pregnancy).
2. To identify multiple pregnancies.
3. To differentiate a tumor (e.g., hydatidiform mole) from a normal pregnancy.
4. To determine the age of the fetus from the diameter of the head.
5. To measure fetal growth rate.
6. To identify placental abnormalities such as abruptio placentae and placenta previa.

7. To determine the position of the placenta (ultrasound localization of the placenta is done before amniocentesis).
8. To make differential diagnoses of various uterine and ovarian enlargements (e.g., polyhydramnios, neoplasms, cysts, abscesses).
9. To determine fetal position.
10. To diagnose ectopic pregnancy.

Pelvic ultrasonography is useful in nonpregnant women to monitor the endometrium in patients who take tamoxifen and to aid in the diagnosis of:

1. Ovarian cyst.
2. Ovarian tumor.
3. Tubo-ovarian abscess.
4. Uterine fibroids.
5. Uterine cancer.
6. Pelvic inflammatory disease (PID).
7. Uterine stripe (endometrium).

The procedure is performed in approximately 20 minutes. No discomfort is associated with the study, other than having a full bladder and the urge to void. Some patients may be uncomfortable lying on a hard table.

Contraindications

- Patients with latex allergy, because vaginal ultrasound requires placement of the probe in a latex condomlike sac

Interfering Factors

- Patients who have recently undergone barium contrast studies, because barium creates severe distortion of reflective sound waves
- Patients with air-filled bowels, because gas does not transmit sound waves well
- Obesity or failure to fill the bladder, because the image may be uninterpretable

Procedure and Patient Care

Before

- Explain the procedure to the patient.

CLINICAL PRIORITIES

- Pelvic ultrasound can be performed with the transducer placed on the anterior abdomen or in the vagina.
- Vaginal ultrasound is preferred in the obese patient because a thick abdominal wall inhibits transmission of sound waves.
- A full bladder is essential in patients undergoing transabdominal ultrasonography, to provide a reference point for interpreting pelvic ultrasonograms.
- No discomfort is associated with the study other than having a full bladder and the urge to void.

- Assure the patient that the study has no known deleterious effect on maternal or fetal tissues, even if repeated several times.
- Give the patient three to four glasses (200 to 350 ml) of water or other liquid 1 hr before the examination, and instruct her not to void until after the procedure is completed. This will permit visualization of the bladder, which is used as a reference point in pelvic anatomy. The full bladder also displaces the bowel from the pelvis and pushes the uterus and ovaries away from the pubis. The fluid in the bladder acts as a window to the pelvis for transmission of sound waves.
- No water is required if ultrasonography is to be done vaginally only.
- If a transabdominal ultrasound is required urgently and there is no time to fill the bladder by ingestion or administration of fluids, the bladder can be filled by means of a bladder catheter.
- Tell the patient that no fasting or sedation is required.

During

- Note the following precedural steps:
  1. The patient is taken to the ultrasound room and placed supine on the examining table.
  2. The ultrasonographer, usually a radiologist, applies a greasy, conductive paste to the abdomen to enhance sound wave transmission and reception.
  3. A transducer is passed vertically and horizontally over the skin.
  4. If a vaginal probe is used, it is inserted in the vagina and angled to identify the various parts of the pelvis.
  5. The sound waves are reflected back by the transducer, and an image appears on the cathode ray tube.
  6. During the examination, fetal structures are pointed out to the mother.

After

- Remove the lubricant from the patient's skin.
- Provide an opportunity for the patient to void.

Test Results and Clinical Significance

Abdominal or tubal pregnancy *Extrauterine pregnancy is evident when the placental complex is external to the uterus.*

Hydatidiform mole *Molar pregnancy can be diagnosed and monitored by ultrasound.*

Intrauterine growth retardation
Fetal hydrocephalus
Multiple fetuses
Fetal death
Abnormal fetal position (e.g., breech, transverse)
Polyhydramnios
Fetal characteristics are easily evaluated with ultrasound. (see fetal biophysical profile [p. 792]).

Abnormal position of the placenta (e.g., placenta previa, abruptio placentae) *Placenta position and quality can be evaluated with ultrasonography. Doppler ultrasound can be used to evaluate placental blood flow.*

Neoplasm of the ovaries, uterus, or fallopian tubes *Ultrasound is sensitive in detection of tumors of the female genital tract. The uterine stripe (endometrial lining of the uterus) is monitored in patients taking medications associated with hyperplasia or cancer (e.g., tamoxifen).*
Cysts *Ultrasound is the most accurate method to differentiate an ovarian cyst from a solid ovarian tumor. Pure cysts (well-defined hypoechoic mass with clean walls) are more likely to be benign than are complex cysts (containing echogenic material).*
Pelvic inflammatory disease and abscesses *Abscesses (tubo-ovarian) appear similar to ovarian cysts but can be differentiated by means of their clinical features.*
IUD localization (p. 786).

Related Tests

- Contraceptive device localization (p. 786): An IUD can be located with ultrasound when its string cannot be palpated.
- Sonography of the rectum (see below): This is used in the staging of rectal tumors in men and women.

Prostate and Rectal Sonography

Normal Findings Normal size, contour, and consistency of the prostate gland

Indications

Prostate or rectal sonography is helpful in the detection of prostate cancer in patients with an elevated prostate-specific antigen (PSA) titer. This study can also be used to stage and monitor rectal cancer and to detect other perirectal diseases.

Test Explanation

Rectal ultrasound of the prostate is a valuable tool in the early diagnosis of prostate cancer. When combined with rectal digital examination and PSA testing (p. 356), very small prostate cancers can be identified. Rectal prostate sonography is also helpful in evaluating the seminal vessels and other perirectal tissue. Ultrasound is helpful in guiding prostate biopsy, and can be helpful in quantifying the volume of prostate cancer. When radiation therapy implantation is required for treatment, ultrasound is used to map the exact location of the prostate cancer. Rectal ultrasound is helpful in staging rectal cancers as well. The depth of transmural involvement and presence of extrarectal extension can be accurately assessed.

Real-time ultrasonography requires the emission of high-frequency sound waves from a special transducer placed in the rectum. The sound waves are reflected back to the transducer and electronically converted into a pictorial image. This test can be performed in the ultrasound section of the radiology department, and is now being routinely performed in most urologists' offices. Results are available almost immediately.

Contraindications

- Patients with latex allergy, because rectal ultrasound requires placement of the probe in a latex condomlike sac

Interfering Factors

- Stool in the rectum

CLINICAL PRIORITIES

- By combining rectal or prostate sonography with a digital rectal examination and PSA test, small prostate cancers can be identified.
- This test can be easily performed in the office of most urologists.
- This test cannot be performed in patients with latex allergy.

Procedure and Patient Care

Before

- Explain the procedure to the patient.
- Tell the patient that a small-volume enema is required approximately 1 hr before the ultrasound examination.

During

- The patient is placed in the left lateral decubitus position.
- A digital rectal examination may be performed to assess the prostate gland or rectal tumor.
- A draped and lubricated ultrasound probe is placed within the rectum.
- Scans are obtained in various spatial planes.

After

- Provide the patient with tissue material to cleanse the perianal area.

Test Results and Clinical Significance

Prostate cancer
Benign prostatic hypertrophy
An enlarged solid prostate mass anterior to the rectum is suggestive of prostate disease.

Prostatitis *An enlarged bulgy echogenic gland indicates inflammation.*
Seminal vesicle tumor *An echogenic mass in the region of the seminal vesicle may indicate tumor.*

Prostate abscess
Perirectal abscess
A hypoechoic fluid-filled mass that is well circumscribed indicates abscess, especially if surrounded by a phlegmonous reaction.

Intrarectal or perirectal tumor *Extent of tumor can be accurately assessed with ultrasound. Lymph node metastasis, if present, is evident.*

Related Tests

- Pelvic ultrasonography (p. 796): Discussion of this test describes pelvic ultrasound of the female genital tract and the pregnant uterus.

Scrotal Ultrasonography (Ultrasound of Testes)

Normal Findings Normal size, shape, and configuration of the testicles

Indications

Ultrasonography of the scrotum allows thorough evaluation of the testes and other scrotal structures for evidence of suspected disease.

Test Explanation

Scrotal ultrasound is a noninvasive, nonionizing, rapid method for scrotal examination. Through the use of reflected sound waves, ultrasonography provides accurate visualization of the scrotum and its contents. Ultrasonography requires the emission of high-frequency sound waves from the transducer to penetrate the organ being studied. The sound waves are reflected back to the transducer and electronically converted into a pictorial image.

Present uses for scrotal ultrasound include:

1. Evaluation of scrotal masses.
2. Measurement of testicular size.
3. Evaluation of scrotal trauma.
4. Evaluation of scrotal pain.
5. Evaluation of occult testicular neoplasm.
6. Surveillance in patients with previous primary or metastatic contralateral testicular neoplasms.
7. Follow-up of testicular infections.
8. Localization of undescended testes.
9. Ultrasound guided needle biopsy of a suspected testicle tumor.

The scrotum is examined with real-time ultrasound. The testes and extratesticular intrascrotal tissues are examined. The accuracy of scrotal ultrasound is 90% to 95%. Both benign and malignant tumors (primary and metastatic) can be identified with ultrasound. Benign abnormalities (e.g., testicular abscess, orchitis, testicular infarction, testicular torsion) can be identified. Extratesticular lesions such as hydrocele (fluid in the scrotum), hematocele (blood in the scrotum), and pyocele (pus in the scrotum) can be identified. Scrotal and groin ultrasound has been helpful in locating cryptorchid (undescended) testes.

Very little discomfort is associated with testicular ultrasound. The study is usually performed by an ultrasound technologist, and the results are interpreted by an ultrasound physician.

Procedure and Patient Care

Before

- Explain the procedure to the patient.
- Tell the patient that no fasting is required.

During

- Note the following precedural steps:
  1. Careful examination of the scrotum is performed by the physician. Usually, a short history is obtained.
  2. The scrotum is supported by a towel or cradled by the examiner's gloved hand.
  3. A greasy, conductive paste is applied to the scrotum before scanning. This paste enhances sound wave transmission and reception.
  4. Thorough scanning in the sagittal, transverse, and oblique projections is performed.
- The test takes approximately 20 to 30 minutes.

After

- Remove the coupling agent (grease) from the patient's scrotum.

Test Results and Clinical Significance

Benign testicular tumor
Malignant testicular tumor
Seminoma of the testicle is evident as a hypoechoic mass in the testicle. Other cancers may appear as hyperechoic dense masses in the testicle.

Occult testicular tumor
Testicular infection (e.g., orchitis)
Hydrocele: fluid around the testicle
Hematocele: blood around the testicle
Pyocele: pus around the testicle
Varicocele: venous varicosities in the cord, usually on the left side
Spermatocele: cystic collection surrounding the cord or epididymis
These abnormalities appear as hypoechoic (dark) areas surrounding the testicle or cord.

Epididymitis *This is apparent as an enlarged epididymis. It is a painful infection involving the epididymis.*

Scrotal hernia *Bowel contents can be seen in the scrotum and indicate hernia.*

Cryptorchidism *Cryptorchid (undescended) testes can be located anywhere from the retroperitoneum to the inlet of the scrotum. It is important to locate these organs and evaluate their consistency, because undescended testes are at high risk of becoming malignant.*

Hematoma *A testicular hematoma from trauma is seen as a hypoechoic mass in the parenchyma of the testicle.*

Testicular torsion *Inadequate suspension of the testicle in the scrotum results in the testicle twisting around on its blood supply. The testicle appears to have an irregular texture, with echogenic areas that correspond to areas of intratesticular hemorrhage. Doppler ultrasound can indicate reduced blood flow to the testicle.*

Related Tests

- Scrotal nuclear imaging (p. 753): This nuclear scan of the testicle is the preferred method to diagnose testicular torsion. It can also be used to identify space-occupying lesions (e.g., tumors or hematoma).

Thyroid Ultrasonography
(Thyroid Echography, Thyroid Sonography)

Normal Findings Normal size, shape, and position of the thyroid gland

Indications

The primary purpose of thyroid ultrasound is to indicate whether a thyroid nodule is a fluid-filled cyst (likely benign) or a solid tumor (possibly malignant). Ultrasound is also used to monitor the medical treatment or observation of a thyroid nodule, and to monitor the contralateral thyroid lobe when one side was surgically removed because of cancer.

Test Explanation

Ultrasound examination of the thyroid gland is valuable to distinguish cystic from solid thyroid nodules. If the nodule is found to be purely cystic (fluid filled), the fluid can simply be aspirated (cysts are not cancerous), and surgery is avoided. If the nodule has a mixed or solid appearance, however, a tumor may be present, and surgery may be required for diagnosis and treatment.

This study may be repeated at intervals to determine the response of a thyroid mass to medical therapy. This test is the procedure of choice for studying the thyroid gland in pregnant women, because no radioactive material is used.

An ultrasound technologist usually performs this study in approximately 15 minutes; a radiologist interprets the results. No discomfort is associated with this study.

Procedure and Patient Care

Before

- Explain the procedure to the patient.
- Tell the patient that breathing or swallowing will not be affected by the placement of a transducer on the neck.
- Inform the patient that a liberal amount of lubricant will be applied to the neck to ensure effective transmission and reception of sound waves.
- Tell the patient that no fasting or sedation is required.

During

- Note the following precedural steps:
  1. The patient is taken to the ultrasonography department (usually in the radiology department) and placed supine with the neck hyperextended.
  2. Gel is applied to the patient's neck.
  3. A transducer is passed over the nodule.
  4. Photographs are taken of the image displayed.

After

- Assist the patient in removing the lubricant from the neck.

Test Results and Clinical Significance

Cyst *A thyroid cyst is evident as a hypoechoic, well-circumscribed mass in the thyroid gland.*

Thyroid adenoma
Thyroid carcinoma
Goiter
These are evident as a solid echogenic mass within the thryroid gland.

Related Tests

- Thyroid scanning (p. 754): This nuclear medicine study allows visualization of the thyroid gland after intravenous administration of a radionuclide. Cysts, tumors, and goiters appear as space-occupying filling defects (cold nodule) within the thyroid gland. This study is often performed with ultrasonography of the thyroid. A cold nodule that is solid at ultrasonography is the type of lesion with the greatest chance of being a cancer.

Transesophageal Echocardiography (TEE)

Normal Findings

Normal position, size, and movement of the heart muscle, valves, and chambers

Indications

An ultrasonography probe, placed endoscopically in the distal esophagus or proximal stomach, provides accurate information about the heart muscle, heart valves, and heart function. It is also capable of providing accurate information about the thoracic aorta.

Test Explanation

TEE provides ultrasonic imaging of the heart from a retrocardiac vantage point, avoiding interference by the interposed subcutaneous tissue, bony thorax, and lungs. A high-frequency ultrasound transducer placed in the esophagus at endoscopy provides better resolution than that of images obtained with routine transthoracic echocardiography (p. 787). For TEE, the distal end of the endoscope is advanced into the esophagus. The transducer is positioned behind the heart (Figure 10-11). Controls on the handle of the endoscope permit the transducer to be rotated and flexed in the anteroposterior, and right and left lateral planes. TEE images have better resolution than those obtained by routine transthoracic echocardiography because of the higher frequency sound waves and closer proximity of the transducer to the cardiac structures.

TEE is helpful in evaluation of structures that are inaccessible or poorly visualized by the transthoracic probe approach, especially in patients who are obese or have large lung-air spaces (e.g., chronic obstructive pulmonary disease).

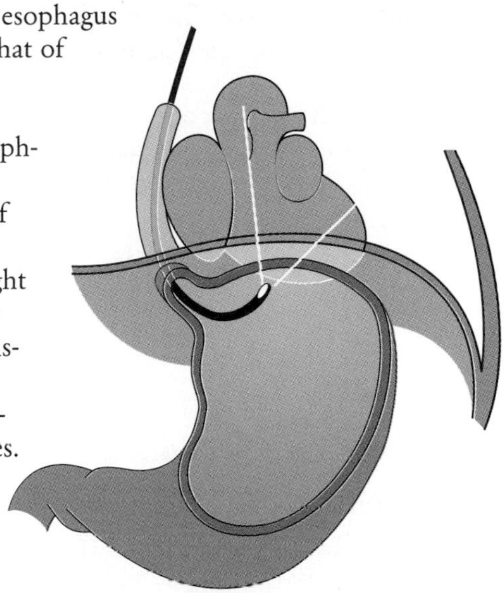

Figure 10-11 Transesophageal echocardiography. Diagram illustrates location of the transesophageal endoscope in the esophagus.

TEE is performed for the following reasons:

1. To better visualize the mitral valve.
2. To differentiate intracardiac from extracardiac masses and tumors.
3. To better visualize the atrial septum (for atrial septal defects).
4. To diagnose thoracic aortic dissection.
5. To better detect valvular vegetation indicative of endocarditis.
6. To determine cardiac sources of arterial embolism.
7. To detect coronary artery disease by identifying areas of muscle wall hypokinesia.

Also, TEE can be used intraoperatively to monitor high-risk patients for ischemia. Ischemic muscle movement is much different from normal muscle movement. Because TEE is a sensitive indicator of myocardial ischemia it can be used to monitor patients undergoing major abdominal, peripheral vascular, and carotid artery procedures who are at high risk for intraoperative ischemia because of coronary artery disease.

Transesophageal echocardiography is more sensitive than electrocardiography (EKG) for detecting ischemia. TEE is also used intraoperatively to evaluate surgical results of valvular or congenital heart disease and to detect air emboli, a serious complication of neurosurgery performed with the patient in the upright position (e.g., cervical laminectomy).

TEE is performed by a cardiologist or a gastrointestinal endoscopist in approximately 20 minutes in the endoscopy suite or at the bedside. Little discomfort is associated with this test, and light sedation is administered.

Contraindications

- Patients with known upper esophageal disease
- Patients with known esophageal varices

- Patients with Zenker's diverticulum
- Patients with esophageal abnormalities (e.g., stricture diverticula, scleroderma, esophagitis)
- Patients with bleeding disorders
- Patients who have recently undergone esophageal surgery
- Patients who cannot cooperate with the procedure

Potential Complications

- Esophageal perforation or bleeding
- Cardiac arrhythmias

✓ CLINICAL PRIORITIES

- TEE is especially useful in patients who are obese or have chronic obstructive pulmonary disease.
- TEE can be used intraoperatively to monitor patients at high risk for ischemia.
- TEE is the most sensitive technique for detecting air emboli, a serious complication of neurosurgery performed with the patient in the upright position (e.g., cervical laminectomy).

Procedure and Patient Care

Before

- Explain the procedure to the patient.
- Instruct the patient to fast for 4 to 6 hours before the test.
- Remove all oral prostheses.
- Obtain intravenous access.

During

- Intravenous sedation is commonly provided with a short-acting benzodiazepine. Other sedation may be provided.
- Apply EKG leads and continually monitor heart rhythm.
- Apply a blood pressure cuff and monitor blood pressure periodically.
- Occasionally pulse oximetry is monitored to determine oxygen saturation in heavily sedated patients.
- Note the following procedural steps:
  1. The pharynx is anesthetized with a locally applied topical agent to depress the gag reflex.
  2. The patient is placed in the left lateral decubitus position.
  3. The endoscope is inserted through the mouth and into the upper esophagus.
  4. The patient is asked to swallow, and the transducer is positioned behind the heart by manipulation through the endoscope.
  5. The room is darkened, and the ultrasound images are displayed on a monitor. Printouts of the ultrasound image can be obtained if desired.

After

- Naloxone or flumazenil may be administered to reverse the sedative effects of the narcotics.
- Observe the patient closely for approximately 1 hr after the procedure, until the effects of sedation have worn off.

Test Results and Clinical Significance

Myocardial ischemia
Myocardial infarction
These are suspected by presence of abnormal (hypokinetic) wall motion.

Valvular heart disease *Motion of heart valves is evaluated.*
Intracardiac thrombi *These can be a cause of arterial emboli. Thrombi usually form in the area of akinetic muscle due to myocardial infarction or myocardial aneurysm.*
Cardiac valvular vegetation *This is a result of endocarditis and is a cause of arterial emboli.*
Cardiomyopathy *Heart muscle is hypokinetic, may or may not be thickened, and may or may not be dilated.*
Marked cardiac chamber dilatation *This is usually due to chronic congestive heart failure.*
Cardiac tumors *The most common (although, rare) cardiac tumor is a myxoma.*
Thoracic aortic aneurysm *TEE is considered the standard for diagnosis of dissecting thoracic aortic aneurysm.*

Related Tests

- Echocardiography (p. 787): While providing the same information as TEE, the posterior portion of the heart is not so well seen as with TEE.

Vascular Doppler Studies
(Venous Doppler Studies and Arterial Doppler Studies)

Normal Findings

Venous

Normal Doppler venous signal with spontaneous respiration
Normal venous system without evidence of occlusion

Arterial

Normal arterial Doppler signal with systolic and diastolic components
No reduction in blood pressure in excess of 20 mm Hg compared with the normal extremity
Normal ankle-to-brachial artery blood pressure index of 0.85 or greater
No evidence of arterial occlusion

Indications

This ultrasound study provides information about arterial and venous patency without the use of invasive techniques. Arterial Doppler studies are used in patients with suspected arterial insufficiency (e.g., claudication, poorly healing skin ulcer, cold and pale leg, pulseless extremity, resting pain). Venous ultrasound is used to evaluate the patency of the venous system in patients with a swollen painful leg, venous varicosities of the upper or lower extremities, or edematous extremities.

Test Explanation

Doppler studies are used to identify occlusion of the veins or arteries of an extremity. Venous patency is demonstrated with Doppler ultrasound by detecting moving red blood cells (RBCs) within the vein. The Doppler transducer directs an ultrasound beam at the vein. Moving RBCs scatter the frequency of the beam. The change in frequency of the sound wave reflected back to the transducer is proportional to the velocity of the blood flow. Venous Doppler studies are not accurate for detection of venous occlusive disease of the lower calf.

With the use of duplex scanning, an accurate representation of the vessel anatomy and patency can be obtained. With a single-mode transducer, the blood flow can be heard audibly and is augmented by an audio speaker as a swishing noise. If the vein is occluded, no swishing sounds are detected.

With single-mode arterial Doppler studies, peripheral arteriosclerotic occlusive disease of the extremities can be identified and located. By slowly deflating blood pressure cuffs placed on the calf and ankle, systolic pressure in the arteries of the extremities can be accurately measured by detecting the first evidence of blood flow with the Doppler transducer. The extremely sensitive Doppler ultrasound detector can recognize the swishing sound of even the most minimal blood flow. Normally, systolic blood pressure is slightly higher in the arteries of the arms than in the legs. If the difference in blood pressure exceeds 20 mm Hg, occlusive disease is believed to exist immediately proximal to the area tested.

Arterial studies can also be performed with duplex Doppler scanning. The duplex concept is based on the ability to define the arterial walls within a two-dimensional image, and a pulsed Doppler probe is used to evaluate flow velocity and direction. This technique can measure the amplitude and the waveform of the vascular pulse. Furthermore,

CLINICAL PRIORITIES

- Venous patency is demonstrated with Doppler ultrasound, which detects moving RBCs within a vein.
- Flow velocity and direction within an artery can be evaluated with duplex Doppler scanning.
- Because nicotine can cause vasoconstriction, cigarette smoking is prohibited before and during this test.
- An ankle-to-brachial artery index less than 0.85 indicates significant arterial occlusive disease in the extremity.

a two-dimensional image of the artery can be produced. As a result, possibly stenotic or occluded arteries and arterial flow disruption can be directly visualized. Lower extremity arterial bypass graft patency can also be assessed with Doppler ultrasound.

Interfering Factors

- Venous or arterial occlusive disease proximal to the site of testing
- Cigarette smoking, because nicotine can cause constriction of the peripheral arteries and alter the results

Procedure and Patient Care

Before

- Explain the procedure to the patient.
- Inform the patient that the procedure is painless.
- Remove all clothing from the extremity to be examined.
- Instruct the patient to abstain from cigarette smoking for at least 30 min before the test.

During

- Note the following precedural steps:

Venous Doppler Studies

1. A conductive gel is applied in multiple areas to the skin overlying the venous system of the extremity
2. In the lower extremity, the deep venous system is usually identified in the ankle, calf, thigh, and groin.
3. The characteristic "swishing" sound indicates a patent venous system. Failure to detect this signal indicates venous occlusion.
4. Usually, both the superficial and venous systems are evaluated.

Arterial Doppler Studies

1. Blood pressure cuffs are placed around the thigh, calf, and ankle.
2. A conductive paste is applied to the skin overlying the artery distal to the cuffs.
3. The proximal cuff is inflated to a level above systolic blood pressure in the normal extremity.
4. The Doppler ultrasound transducer is placed immediately distal to the inflated cuff.
5. The pressure in the cuff is slowly released.
6. The highest pressure at which blood flow is detected by the characteristic swishing Doppler signal is recorded as the blood pressure of that artery.
7. The test is repeated at each successive level.
8. An ankle-to-brachial artery index less than 0.85 indicates significant arterial occlusive disease in the extremity.

- These studies are usually performed in the vascular laboratory or radiology department, and take approximately 30 minutes.

After

- Encourage the patient to verbalize fears in terms of test results.
- Remove the transducer gel from the extremity.
- Inform the patient that the radiologist must interpret the studies and that results will be available in a few hours.

Test Results and Clinical Significance

Venous occlusion, secondary to thrombosis or thrombophlebitis *Complete or partial occlusion is apparent at any level above the upper calf. Results are not accurate below the upper calf.*

Venous varicosities *Doppler ultrasound can recognize flow reversal as a result of incompetent valves of varicose veins.*

Small or large vessel arterial occlusive disease
Spastic arterial disease (e.g., Raynaud's phenomenon)
Small vessel arterial occlusive disease (as in diabetes)
Embolic arterial occlusion
Arterial aneurysm
These vascular diseases are most evident with duplex Doppler scanning. Color flow Doppler imaging can be done, in which designated colors demonstrate flow velocity and direction. Partial or complete occlusion is readily visualized. Turbulence, as with an aneurysm, is obvious. Reversal of flow that may occur distal to an occluded artery will be evident.

Related Tests

- Venography (p. 1002): This is a radiographic study of the veins of an extremity. It is more accurate for detection of deep venous thrombosis in the lower calf, but no more accurate than Doppler studies in the more proximal extremity. Intravenous iodinated contrast medium used for this test may precipitate an allergic reaction or renal failure.

11

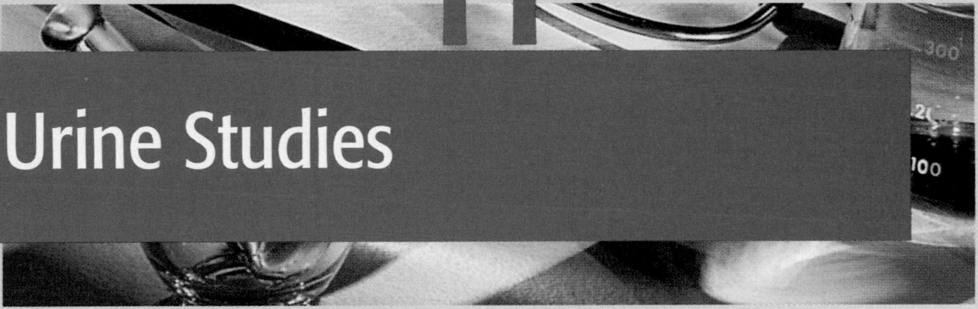

Urine Studies

TESTS

Overview

Urine is derived from filtration of the blood by the nephrons in the kidney. Blood enters the kidney through the renal artery and passes into small capillaries in the glomerulus. There, solute and water are filtered through the capillary and into Bowman's capsule. This fluid progressively passes through the capsule and into the renal tubule. More capillaries surround the tubule, and water and other solutes can pass through the tubule into and out of the capillaries according to the body's needs. Within the renal medulla, the collecting system collects all the urine from each nephron and transports it to the renal pelvis. The urine then passes through the ureters and into the bladder. At micturition (voiding), the urine passes through the urethra and out of the body.

Urine is nearly all water, with a small percentage of solutes. All end products of metabolism and all potentially harmful materials are excreted in the urine to maintain normal acid/base, fluid and electrolyte balance, and homeostasis.

In general, the urine reflects the blood level for any analyte. If the blood level is elevated and the kidneys are working well, the urine level for that same product can be expected to be high. If the urine level is not high, the kidneys may be diseased, resulting in high levels in the blood. In some instances, certain blood solute products are not filtered from the blood unless "threshold" levels of the solute are exceeded. For example, glucose is not excreted by the kidney unless blood levels exceed around 180 mg/dl.

Reasons for Obtaining Urine Specimens

The urine specimen has been referred to as a "fluid biopsy" of the urinary tract. It is usually painlessly obtained, and provides a great deal of information quickly and economically. Like other specimen tests, urine tests must be carefully performed and properly controlled. Most urine tests are performed for one of the following reasons:

1. To diagnose renal or urinary tract disease (e.g., proteinuria may indicate glomerulonephritis).
2. To monitor renal or urinary tract disease (e.g., urine cultures may be used to monitor the effectiveness of antibiotic therapy for urinary tract infections).
3. To detect metabolic or systemic diseases not directly related to the kidneys (e.g., glucose in the urine may be indicative of diabetes mellitus or Cushing's syndrome).

Although blood tests provide valuable information about the body, urinalysis is preferred for several reasons:

1. Identification of urinary tract infection (UTI) requires a urine specimen.
2. A 24-hour urine collection will reflect homeostasis and disease better than a blood specimen obtained at a random moment of the day.
3. Some products to be tested for are rapidly cleared by the kidneys and may not be apparent in the blood (e.g., Bence Jones protein). Results of a blood test may be normal while urinalysis indicates the presence of these products.
4. The serum product being tested may be affected by renal clearance (e.g., sodium). Therefore, a urine specimen to measure the sodium concentration will add significant additional information to a serum sodium level.
5. Urine testing is easily performed and does not require an invasive skin puncture.
6. Many urine tests are cheaper than blood tests. The urine test may be less accurate or only qualitative, but may be all that is needed.

Types of Urine Specimens

The type of urine specimen collected and the collection procedure depend on the test needed. There are five basic types of urine specimens. In addition, other body fluids can be evaluated to determine whether they contain urine.

First morning specimen. To collect a first morning specimen, the patient voids before going to bed. Immediately on rising, the patient collects a urine specimen. The benefits of a first morning specimen are multiple. First, the urine in the bladder overnight represents all of the urine for the previous 6 to 8 hours. Unlike a random spot urine sample, it is a more accurate reflection of the patient's 24-hour urine. Second, postural changes that may affect the urine can be avoided by obtaining the urine specimen immediately on arising. Third, diurnal variations may affect test results. Collecting the first morning specimen allows one to factor in the timing of the testing. Finally, because the urine has been retained in the bladder during a relative overnight fast, it is concentrated, and testing is more likely to detect positive findings. This specimen is ideal for detecting substances such as proteins and nitrates, and is often used to confirm a diagnosis of orthostatic proteinuria.

Although the first morning specimen is frequently the specimen of choice, it is not the most convenient to obtain. It requires that the patient be given instructions and the collection container at least 1 day before the specimen is needed. In addition, the specimen must be preserved if it is not going to be delivered to the laboratory within 2 hours of collection.

Random urine specimen. Random urine specimens are usually obtained during daytime hours and without any prior patient preparation. For ease and convenience, routine screening is most often performed on a random specimen. Random testing is usually performed when the substance to be tested does not have significant diurnal variation and its normal concentration is adequate to be detected in a small volume of urine. Random urine is also the specimen of choice for illegal drug screening. This is to avoid patient tampering with results or changing behavior in anticipation of testing.

Timed urine collection. Because substances such as hormones, proteins, and electrolytes are variably excreted over 24 hours, and because of the effects of exercise, posture, hydration, and body metabolism on excretion rates, quantitative urine tests often require a timed collection. These time periods may range anywhere from 2 to 24 hours. Timed collections are of two types. One type includes urine specimens collected at a predetermined time. For example, glucose is often measured 2 hours after a meal (postprandial), because that is when the urine is expected to contain the maximum glucose level. A 2-hour postprandial specimen can be collected after any meal. The second type includes specimens collected at a specific time of day. For example, a specimen for urobilinogen testing is best collected between 2:00 and 4:00 PM, when bilinogen is maximally excreted. Depending on the substance being measured and the type of collection, a preservative may be needed to ensure stability throughout the collection period. In addition, certain foods and drugs may need to be avoided during the collection period. Box 11-1 lists some of the more common errors in collecting timed urine specimens.

To collect a timed specimen, the patient is instructed to void and discard the first specimen. This is noted as the start time of the test. All subsequent urine is saved in a special container for the designated period of time. At the end of the specified time period, the patient voids and adds this urine to the specimen container, completing the collection process.

Box 11-1 Sources of error in timed urine specimens

Loss of specimen
Inadequate preservative used
Inclusion of two first morning specimens
Inaccurate total volume measurement
Transcription error

Double-voided specimen. This collection method is performed to obtain and evaluate fresh urine, and is often used to monitor urine glucose and ketone concentrations. To obtain this specimen, the patient first empties the bladder. Shortly thereafter, the patient voids again. The second specimen in the double-voided specimen is the freshest urine and is used for testing. It accurately reflects blood concentrations at that particular time.

Urine specimen for culture and sensitivity. This specimen is collected for examination of bacteria. The specimen must be collected in a sterile container as aseptically as possible. This requires meticulous cleansing of the urinary meatus with an iodine preparation to reduce contamination of the specimen by external organisms. A midstream collection technique will cleanse the urethral canal of contaminant bacteria. The specimen should be cultured within 1 hour of collection.

Other body fluids. Body fluids can be tested for blood urea nitrogen (BUN) and creatinine to determine whether the fluid is urine. This is done commonly after pelvic surgery. Abdominal fluid serous drainage can look like urine. If the BUN and creatinine concentrations in that fluid are the same as in serum, the fluid is considered to be serous drainage or ascites. If, however, the concentration of BUN and creatinine in the fluid is more than three times that in serum, the fluid is urine. This testing is also helpful in obstetrics to differentiate amniotic fluid from urine.

Collection Methods

Collection methods vary from those requiring no patient preparation to invasive-type procedures. The reason for the test and the clinical situation determine the appropriate collection method.

Common collection methods

Routine Void Specimen

A routine void specimen requires no preparation and is collected by having the patient urinate into an appropriate nonsterile container. Random and first morning specimens are collected in this manner.

Midstream and Clean-Catch Specimens

If a culture and sensitivity study is required or if the specimen is likely to be contaminated by vaginal discharge or bleeding, a clean-catch or midstream specimen is collected. For a clean-catch specimen, meticulous cleansing of the urinary meatus with an iodine preparation is necessary to reduce contamination of the specimen by external organisms. In male patients, the foreskin is retracted and the meatus cleansed. Then the cleansing agent must be carefully removed, because it may inhibit growth of any bacteria in the specimen, which would affect the culture and sensitivity determination. For a midstream collection, the patient begins to urinate into a bedpan, urinal, or toilet, then stops. This washes the urine out of the distal urethra. The patient voids 3 to 4 oz of urine into a sterile container, which is then capped, and the patient is allowed to finish voiding.

Twenty-four-Hour Urine Collection

The patient is instructed to void and discard the first specimen (for example, at 8:00 AM on day 1). This is noted as the start time of the 24-hour collection. The patient collects all urine voided up to and including that at 8:00 AM the following morning (day 2). In the laboratory, the total volume of the sample is recorded. After the specimen is thoroughly mixed, a measured sample is withdrawn for analysis.

If any urine is removed or discarded during a timed collection, the entire timed collection is invalid. Twenty-four hour urine collections are more accurate than specimens collected over a shorter time. Some analytes are excreted at different rates throughout the day or night, and random specimens may miss the time of maximal excretion. Also, because greater concentrations of an analyte are present in a 24-hour collection, the chance of a false-negative result is reduced.

Special collection methods

Special collection methods are indicated when a specimen cannot be obtained by the more common techniques.

Urethral Catheterization

A catheterized specimen is obtained by inserting a sterile catheter through the urethra into the bladder. Although catheterization may cause infection, this collection method is used when patients are unable to void or cannot void when the specimen is required (e.g., during trauma).

In patients with an indwelling urinary catheter in place, a specimen is obtained by attaching a small-gauge needle to a syringe and aseptically inserting the needle into the catheter at a point distal to the sleeve leading to the balloon. Many kinds of tubes have a rubber access area for this type of collection technique. Urine is aspirated and placed in a sterile urine container. (Usually the catheter tubing distal to the puncture site needs to be clamped for 15 to 30 minutes before the aspiration of urine to allow urine to fill the tubing. After the specimen is withdrawn, the clamp is removed.) The urine that accumulates in a plastic reservoir bag should never be used for a urine test.

Suprapubic Aspiration

In suprapubic aspiration, urine is collected directly from the bladder by inserting a needle through the abdominal wall and into the bladder. The urine is aspirated into a syringe and sent for analysis. This method is mainly used to obtain urine for anaerobic culture, when specimen contamination is unavoidable, and in infants and young children. Complications are rare.

Pediatric Collections

Urine specimens from infants and young children are often collected using a pediatric collection bag. This clear, pliable, polyethylene bag has a hypoallergenic skin-adhesive backing around the opening. The perineal skin is cleansed and dried before the specimen bag is applied to the skin. The bag is placed over the penis in male children and around the vagina (excluding the rectum) in female children. Once the bag is in place, the patient is checked every 15 minutes until the urine is collected. The specimen bag should be removed as soon as the urine is collected. Bags may be folded and self-sealed for transportation. If a 24-hour specimen is needed, a tube is attached to the bag and connected to a storage container. This avoids repeated skin preparation and reapplication of adhesive to the child's sensitive skin.

Transport, Storage, and Preservation

Disposable plastic containers (100-200 ml capacity) with lids are sufficient for most routine urine tests. Screw-top containers are preferred because they are less likely to leak during transportation. Wax-coated cardboard containers should not be used, because of the possibility of contaminating the specimen with fatty material. Sterile kits are available for bacterial cultures. Kits usually contain a disposable plastic urine container and cleansing pads.

Rigid, brown, light-resistant plastic containers (approximately 3000 ml capacity) are suitable for most 12- and 24-hour urine collections. These containers have a wide mouth and a leak-proof screwcap. Preservatives may be added to these containers. One-gallon glass jugs may also be used.

Specimen containers must be correctly labeled. Labels should not be placed on the lid, because when the lid is removed the specimen is unlabeled. The patient identification label should be placed directly on the container.

Specimens should be promptly transported to the laboratory. If this is not possible and specimen transportation will be delayed 2 hours or longer, precautions need to be taken to preserve the integrity of the specimen. A variety of changes can occur in an unpreserved specimen. Physical, chemical, and microscopic examinations can all be affected by oxidation, precipitation, and overgrowth of bacteria. Therefore, appropriate handling and storage are necessary to ensure that changes do not occur and that accurate results are obtained. Laboratories have written criteria describing when to reject a urine specimen as unsuitable for testing. Box 11-2 lists common criteria for rejecting a urine specimen.

Many analytes require preservatives to maintain viability during the collection period. The proper preservative depends on the type of collection, the delay before testing, and the tests to be performed. No single urine preservative suits all testing requirements.

Box 11-2 Criteria for rejection of a urine sample

Improper sample identification
Incorrect urine preservation
Insufficient urine quantity
Improper specimen collection
Missing or incomplete request form
Visible contamination (e.g., stool)

Some analytes require an acidic pH for stability; others are stable in an alkaline pH. For example, acetic acid can be used as a preservative to maintain acidity. Sodium carbonate is used to maintain alkalinity. Boric acid is commonly used to inhibit bacterial multiplication. Some analytes are best preserved by refrigeration, which is the easiest means of preserving many urine specimens. If possible, all timed urine specimens should be refrigerated throughout the collection period. Timed specimens may also require the addition of a chemical preservative. For example, sodium fluoride is used to preserve glucose in a 24-hour urine collection. Some analytes need to be protected from light by using a dark collection container or by wrapping the container with foil. Urine for the evaluation of tumor cells is usually collected into an equal amount of 50% alcohol. Fixatives (e.g., Saccomanno's) also can be used to preserve cytologic specimens.

Collection preservatives may differ among laboratories, depending on (1) testing methods, (2) units of measurement, (3) how often the test is performed, (4) time delays, or (5) transportation to reference laboratories.

Urine Reagent Strips

The urine reagent strip has replaced many complicated individual chemical analyses for determination of various components in the urine. For example, estimation of glucose, albumin, hemoglobin, and bile concentrations, as well as urinary pH, specific gravity, protein, ketone bodies, nitrates, and leukocyte esterase, can be easily determined using a dipstick. Dipsticks are small strips of paper impregnated with a chemical that reacts to products in the urine by changing color. The color correlates with concentrations of the analyte in the urine. Many tests can be performed with one dipstick.

This method of testing involves dipping a "fresh" (not outdated) reagent strip or dipstick into urine and observing the color change on the strip. The color is compared with the color chart on the bottle of reagent strips at the *exact* time indicated. Dipstick testing is accurate and somewhat quantitative. However, a large number of products in a urine specimen can cause false-positive or false-negative results. Dipstick testing is considered preliminary or for screening. Often more definitive and quantitative studies are necessary to confirm the results.

Reporting of Results

Accurate results depend on appropriate collection, transport, storage, and preservation of the urine specimen. To be clinically useful, test results must be promptly reported, because delays can make the data useless. The report must also be delivered to the appropriate medical record keeper and must be presented in a manner that is clear and easily interpreted.

The report should include the test results, reporting units, and reference ranges. Reference ranges vary from institution to institution. Comments may be included to help interpret results. For example, the technologist may note that the urine specific gravity is too low for proper interpretation of results. Proper reporting of "critical" or "panic" values (well outside the usual range of normal) is essential because such results generally require immediate intervention. If these results are called in to a physician or nurse, verification of notification must be properly documented.

Amylase

Normal Findings

3-35 IU/hr, 6-30 Wohlgemuth units/ml, up to 5000 Somogyi units/24 hr, or 6.5-48.1 U/hr. (Amylase clearance: <2)

Indications

The urine amylase concentration is used to assist in making the diagnosis of pancreatitis, although other nonpancreatic diseases can cause elevated urine amylase levels. Urine amylase levels rise later than blood amylase levels. Several days after onset of the disease process, serum amylase levels may be normal while urine levels are significantly elevated. Urine amylase concentration is particularly useful in detecting pancreatitis late in the disease course.

Test Explanation

Amylase is normally secreted from the pancreatic acinar cells into the pancreatic duct and then into the duodenum. Once in the intestine, it aids catabolism of carbohydrates to their component simple sugars. Destruction of acinar cells (as in pancreatitis) or obstruction to the pancreatic duct flow (as in pancreatitic carcinoma) causes outpouring of this enzyme into the bloodstream.

Because the kidneys rapidly clear amylase, disorders that affect the pancreas cause elevated amylase levels in the urine. Serum levels of amylase rise transiently, but usually return to normal 1 to 2 days after resolution of the acute phase of disease. Levels of amylase in the urine, however, remain elevated 5 to 7 days after onset of disease. This is an important indicator of pancreatitis in patients who have had symptoms for 3 days or longer.

As with serum amylase (p. 51), urine amylase is sensitive but not specific for pancreatitic disorders. Other diseases, such as parotiditis (mumps), cholecystitis, perforated bowel, penetrating peptic ulcer, ectopic pregnancy, and renal infarction, can cause elevated urine levels; however, urine levels are usually highest with pancreatitis. A comparison of the renal clearance ratio of amylase to creatinine provides more specific diagnostic information than either the urine amylase level or the serum amylase level alone. When the amylase/creatinine clearance ratio is 5% or more, the diagnosis of pancreatitis can be made with certainty. A ratio less than 5% in a patient with elevated serum and urine amylase levels is indicative of nonpancreatic pathologic conditions (e.g., perforated bowel, macroamylasemia).

Interfering Factors

- Intravenous dextrose solutions can cause a false-negative result.
- Drugs that may cause *elevated* amylase levels include aminosalicylic acid, aspirin, azathioprine, corticosteroids, dexamethasone, ethyl alcohol, glucocorticoids, iodine-

CLINICAL PRIORITIES

- Urinary levels of amylase remain elevated for 5 to 7 days after disease onset. This is helpful in diagnosing pancreatitis after serum levels have returned to normal.
- When the amylase/creatinine clearance ratio is 5% or higher, the diagnosis of pancreatitis can be made with certainty.

containing contrast media, loop diuretics (e.g., furosemide), methyldopa, narcotic analgesics, oral contraceptives, and prednisone.
- Drugs that may cause *decreased* levels include citrates, glucose, and oxalates.

Procedure and Patient Care

Before

- Explain the procedure to the patient.
- Tell the patient that no fasting is required.
- Record the exact times of urine collection.

During

- Begin the 24-hour urine collection. Discard the initial specimen, and collect all urine voided during the next 24 hours.
- A 2-hour spot urine specimen can be sent instead of the 24-hour urine collection.
- Show the patient where to store the urine specimen.
- Keep the specimen on ice or refrigerated during the collection period. No preservative is needed.
- Post the hours for urine collection in a prominent place to prevent accidentally discarding the specimen.
- Instruct the patient to void before defecating so that urine is not contaminated by stool.
- Remind the patient not to put toilet paper in the urine collection container.
- Collect the last specimen as close as possible to the end of the collection period. Add this urine to the container.
- List on the laboratory slip any medications that may affect test results.

After

- Send the urine specimen to the laboratory promptly.

Test Results and Clinical Significance

Increased levels

Acute pancreatitis
Chronic relapsing pancreatitis
Damage to pancreatic acinar cells (as in pancreatitis) causes outpouring of amylase into the intrapancreatic lymph system and the free peritoneum. Blood vessels draining the free peritoneum and ab-

sorbing the lymph pick up the excess amylase. The amylase is then cleared by the kidneys, and urine levels rise. Amylase clearance can be expected to be >5.

Penetrating peptic ulcer into the pancreas
Gastrointestinal disease
In patients with perforated peptic ulcer, necrotic bowel, perforated bowel, or duodenal obstruction, amylase leaks out of the gut and into the free peritoneal cavity. The amylase is picked up by the blood and lymphatic vessels of the peritoneum. The amylase is cleared by the kidneys, and urine levels rise. Amylase clearance is between 2 and 5.

Acute cholecystitis
Parotiditis (mumps)
Ruptured ectopic pregnancy
Amylase is present in the salivary glands, gallbladder, and fallopian tubes. Diseases that affect these organs are associated with elevated urine and blood levels of amylase. Amylase clearance will be between 2 and 5.

Diabetic ketoacidosis
Pulmonary infarction
Post-endoscopic retrograde pancreatography
These clinical situations are sometimes associated with high urine amylase levels.

Related Tests

- Serum amylase (p. 51): Amylase can be detected in the serum earlier than in the urine. This test is more easily performed and therefore used more frequently to monitor the course of disease.
- Lipase (p. 287): Lipase is similar to amylase but is more specific for the pancreas.

Bence Jones Protein

Normal Findings

No Bence Jones protein present

Indications

Bence Jones protein in the urine (especially high levels) most commonly indicates multiple myeloma. The test is used to detect and monitor the treatment and clinical course of multiple myeloma and similar diseases.

Test Explanation

Bence Jones protein consists of immunoglobulin light chains, and is found in 75% of patients with multiple myeloma. This protein is most notably made by the plasma cells in these patients. It may also be associated with tumor metastases to bone, chronic lymphocytic leukemia, lymphoma, macroglobulinemia, and amyloidosis.

Normally, there is no protein in the urine because the glomerular spaces do not allow filtration of large molecules such as proteins. Bence Jones protein, however, is very small and easily filtrated by the kidneys and excreted into the urine. Because Bence Jones protein is rapidly cleared from the blood by the kidneys, it is difficult to detect in the blood; therefore only urine is used for this study. Normally, urine should contain no Bence Jones protein.

Routine urine testing for proteins using reagent strips often does not reflect the type or amount of proteins in the urine. In fact, the strip may even show a negative result despite large amounts of Bence Jones protein. Classically, Bence Jones protein was detected by heating the specimen to 60° F. Protein precipitated out, only to disappear when the specimen was boiled. The protein reappeared with cooling. Sulfosalicylic or acetic acid can also be used to precipitate out proteins in the urine. When compared with known standards, the protein can be semiquantitated. Urine electrophoresis and immunoelectrophoresis have become the procedures of choice, especially when the amount of proteins needs to be quantitated.

Interfering Factors

- Dilute urine may yield a false-negative result.

Procedure and Patient Care

Before

- Explain the procedure to the patient.
- Instruct the patient not to contaminate the urine specimen with toilet paper or stool.

During

- Instruct the patient to collect an early morning specimen of at least 50 ml of uncontaminated urine in a container. If it would be helpful to know the amount of Bence Jones protein excreted over 24 hours, a 24-hour collection is ordered.

After

- Immediately transport the specimen to the laboratory. If it cannot be taken to the laboratory immediately, refrigerate the specimen, because heat-coagulable proteins can decompose, causing false-positive test results.

Test Results and Clinical Significance

Increased levels

Multiple myeloma (plasmacytoma) *Only about 2% of patients with myeloma do not produce Bence Jones protein. Detection of Bence Jones protein at high levels (>60 mg/L) is most common with this malignant disease.*

Chronic lymphocytic leukemia
Lymphoma
Metastatic colon, breast, lung, or prostate cancer
Several neoplastic disorders are associated with monoclonal gammaglobinopathies. Some can produce Bence Jones protein.

Amyloidosis *Primary amyloidosis can produce immunoglobulin light chains similar to those of Bence Jones protein.*

Waldenstrom's macroglobulinemia *This malignant lymphoproliferative disease is highlighted by lymphadenopathy, hepatosplenomegaly, anemia, hyperviscosity, and Bence Jones proteinuria (about 20% of the patients).*

Related Tests

- Urinalysis (p. 859): Urinalysis includes determination of protein in the urine. If positive, urine electrophoresis (similar to serum protein electrophoresis) can be performed (p. 361).

Bilirubin

Normal Findings

No bilirubin in urine

Indications

Bilirubin identification and semiquantitation is included in routine urinalysis.

Test Explanation

Bile, which is formed in the liver, has many constituents, including bile salts, phospholipids, cholesterol, bicarbonate, water, and bilirubin. Bilirubin metabolism begins with the breakdown of red blood cells (RBCs) in the reticuloendothelial system (see Fig. 2-7, p. 110). Hemoglobin is released from lysed RBCs and broken down to heme and globin molecules. Heme is catabolized to form biliverdin, which is transformed to *unconjugated* (indirect) bilirubin. In the liver, indirect bilirubin is conjugated with a glucuronide, resulting in *conjugated* (direct) bilirubin. Conjugated bilirubin is excreted from the liver cells and into the intrahepatic canaliculi, then to the hepatic ducts, the common bile duct, and the bowel, where it is excreted.

If bilirubin excretion is inhibited, conjugated (direct) hyperbilirubinemia will result. Obstruction of the bile duct by a gallstone is the classic example of obstructed bilirubin excretion causing conjugated hyperbilirubinemia. Unlike the unconjugated form, conjugated bilirubin is water soluble and can be excreted into the urine. Therefore, bilirubin in urine suggests disease affecting bilirubin metabolism after conjugation or defects in excretion (e.g., gallstones).

Determination of bilirubin concentration is included in routine urinalysis. This test is no longer very useful as a monitor of liver disease or as an indicator of severity of liver disease. Serum bilirubin is more appropriate for those purposes. For screening, however, elevated urine bilirubin concentration can indicate previously unsuspected liver injury due to disease, gallstones, or drug toxicity. Bilirubin in the urine will color the urine dark yellow or orange.

Interfering Factors

- Bilirubin is not stable in urine, especially when exposed to light.
- Phenazopyridine (Pyridium) colors the urine orange. This may give the false impression that the patient has jaundice.
- Drugs that may cause *increased* bilirubin levels include allopurinol, antibiotics, barbiturates, chlorpromazine, diuretics, ethoxazene (Serenium), oral contraceptives, phenazopyridine, steroids, and sulfonamides.
- Drugs that can cause false-negative results include indomethacin (Indocin) and ascorbic acid (vitamin C).

Procedure and Patient Care

Before

- Explain the procedure to the patient.
- Tell the patient that no food or drink restrictions are necessary.

During

- Note that this is a spot urine test.
- Collect at least 10 ml of urine for quick, simple testing.
- Use reagent strips (e.g., Multistix) or tablets (e.g., Icotest) for quick, simple testing.

Multistix

- This is a firm, plastic strip with seven separate areas for testing pH, protein, glucose, ketones, bilirubin, blood, and urobilinogen.
- For testing bilirubin, obtain a fresh urine specimen and examine it as soon as possible.
- Immerse the dipstick in the well-mixed urine, then remove it immediately to avoid dissolving other reagents.
- Tap the dipstick against the rim of the urine container to remove excess urine.
- Hold the strip horizontally and compare it with the color chart on the label of the bottle after 20 to 30 seconds, according to directions. Results are given in the range of 0 to 3.

Icotest tablets

- Place 5 drops of urine on the special test mat. Add 2 drops of water.
- Results are positive if the mat turns blue or purple within 30 seconds.
- This test is more sensitive than reagent strips for detecting bilirubin.

After

- Do not reuse reagent strips or tablets.
- Whether using strips or tablets or if sending the urine to the laboratory, list any medications that may affect test results.

Test Results and Clinical Significance

Increased levels of bilirubin in the urine
Gallstones

Extrahepatic duct obstruction (e.g., tumor, inflammation, gallstone, scarring, or surgical trauma)
Extensive liver metastasis
Direct physical obstruction of flow of bile from the biliary tree causes elevated serum levels of conjugated (direct) bilirubin, which leads to elevated urine levels of bilirubin.

Cholestasis from drugs *Some drugs affect bilirubin metabolism and excretion after glucuronide conjugation. Elevated serum levels of conjugated (direct) bilirubin lead to elevated urine levels of bilirubin.*

Dubin-Johnson syndrome
Rotor's syndrome
These congenital defects in bilirubin metabolism occur after glucuronide conjugation. This causes elevated serum levels of conjugated (direct) bilirubin, which leads to elevated urine levels of bilirubin.

Related Tests

- Serum bilirubin (p. 109): This is a measurement of bilirubin in serum.
- Urinalysis (p. 859): Urine bilirubin is included in routine urinalysis.
- Urobilinogen (p. 875): This urine test detects urobilinogen, a metabolite of bilirubin made in the bowel. It is elevated in the urine of patients with jaundice if excretion of bilirubin is not inhibited.

Calcium
(Urine Calcium, Quantitative Calcium)

Normal Findings

Vary with diet
Normal diet: 100-400 mg/day or 2.50-7.50 mmol/day (SI units)
Low-calcium diet: 50-150 mg/day or 1.25-3.75 mmol/day (SI units)

Indications

This test measures the calcium concentrate in the urine. It is used most commonly to identify and support a diagnosis of hypercalcemia. It is not commonly used because more direct blood measurements can more accurately and rapidly provide the same information.

Test Explanation

Nearly all the calcium excreted from the body is done so in the stool. Much smaller quantities are excreted in the urine. This quantitative test measures the amount of calcium excreted in the urine in 24 hours. (This test differs from the older, less accurate, qualitative Sulkowitch reagent test, rarely performed today, in which results are measured from 0, +1 [normal] to +4).

Excretion of calcium in the urine is increased in all patients with hypercalcemia. A thorough discussion of calcium metabolism is found on p. 130. Primary hyperparathyroidism is one of the most common causes of hypercalcemia and is the most common reason for measurement of urinary calcium. With the development of assays for parathyroid hormone, the need for determination of urine calcium concentration has decreased. The test is still helpful in determining the cause of recurrent nephrolithiasis. Urinary calcium levels far in excess of dietary intake are abnormal and lead to mobilization of calcium stores (bone and teeth). When calcium is excreted in the urine at high levels, nephrolithiasis and nephrocalcinosis are possible.

Urinary calcium levels are decreased in patients with hypocalcemia (p. 130). A common cause of hypocalcemia is hypoparathyroidism.

Disagreement exists as to whether the specimen should be collected from patients who ingest a normal diet, a normal diet except for milk products, or a controlled diet limited to 100 to 200 mg of calcium. Reference values vary according to the type of diet.

Interfering Factors

- Alkaline urine decreases urine calcium.
- Urine obtained in patients ingesting a high- or low-calcium diet can factitiously elevate or lower urine calcium measurements.
- Prolonged immobilization can be associated with mobilization of calcium from the bones and therefore be associated with high urine calcium levels.
- Drugs that may *increase* urine calcium levels include antacids, anticonvulsant agents, carbonic anhydrase inhibitors, diuretics, calcitonin, calcium salts, steroids, mithramycin, and phosphates.
- Drugs that may *decrease* urine calcium levels include estrogen, lithium bicarbonate, and oral contraceptives.

Procedure and Patient Care

Before

- Explain the procedure to the patient.
- Determine the diet regimen recommended by the specific laboratory.
- Give the patient written and oral instructions regarding dietary restrictions.

During

- Begin the 24-hour urine collection. Discard the initial specimen, and collect all urine voided by the patient during the next 24 hours.
- Post the hours for urine collection in a prominent location.
- Remind the patient to void before defecating so that the urine is not contaminated by feces.
- Instruct the patient not to place toilet paper in the collection container.
- Encourage the patient to drink fluids during the 24 hours, unless contraindicated for medical purposes.
- Collect the last specimen as close as possible to the end of the 24 hours.
- Indicate the time the last specimen was collected on the laboratory slip or urine container.

- Store the 24-hour collection in a plastic urine container or an acid-washed glass bottle.
- Keep the collected urine on ice or refrigerated during the collection period.
- Note that some laboratories add a preservative to the container to prevent precipitation. Check with the laboratory.
- List on the laboratory slip any medications that may affect test results.

After

- Send the 24-hour specimen to the laboratory as soon as it is complete.

Test Results and Clinical Significance

For more detail on pathophysiology, see p. 130.

Increased levels (hypercalciuria)

Primary hyperparathyroidism
Hyperparathyroidism
Nonparathyroid PTH–producing tumor (e.g., lung or renal carcinoma)
In patients with hypercalcemia, urine calcium excretion is increased.

Milk-alkali syndrome *Increased calcium intake is associated with increased urine calcium excretion.*

Cushing's syndrome
Granulomatous infections (e.g., sarcoidosis, tuberculosis)
By enhancing vitamin D activity, serum and urine calcium levels increase.

Osteoporosis
Metastatic tumor to the bone
Paget's disease of bone
Prolonged immobilization
Destruction of the bone is followed by hypercalcemia, with increased urinary calcium.

Renal tubular acidosis
Acidic environment
Idiopathic hypercalciuria

Decreased levels (hypocalciuria)

Hypoparathyroidism
Vitamin D deficiency
Malabsorption disorder
Renal failure
As serum calcium decreases, so does urinary calcium.

Related Tests

- Calcium, blood (p. 130) This is a direct measurement of calcium levels in the blood.

Chloride (Cl)

Normal Findings

Adult/elderly: 110-250 mEq/day or 110-250 mmol/day (SI units)
Child: 15-40 mmol/day
Infant: 2-10 mmol/day

Indications

This test is used with other urinary electrolytes to indicate the state of electrolyte or acid/base imbalance.

Test Explanation

Chloride is the major extracellular anion. Its main purpose is to maintain electrical neutrality, mostly as a salt with sodium. It follows sodium (cation) losses and accompanies sodium excesses to maintain electrical neutrality. For example, when aldosterone encourages sodium reabsorption, chloride follows to maintain electrical neutrality. Because water moves with sodium and chloride, chloride also affects water balance. Finally, chloride serves as a buffer to assist in acid-base balance. As carbon dioxide (and H cation) increases, bicarbonate must move from the intracellular space to the extracellular space. To maintain electrical neutrality, chloride shifts back into the cell.

A 24-hour urine collection for chloride is useful to evaluate the electrolyte composition of urine to evaluate electrolyte and acid-base imbalances. It is also useful to evaluate the effectiveness of diets with restricted salt (sodium chloride). If sodium and chloride levels are high, the patient is not complying with the diet.

Interfering Factors

- Urine volume and perspiration can affect chloride levels.
- Dietary salt intake or saline infusion affects urinary levels.
- Drugs that may cause *increased* levels include bromides, diuretics, and steroids.

Procedure and Patient Care

Before

- Explain the procedure to the patient.
- Tell the patient that no special diet is required.

During

- Begin the 24-hour urine collection. Discard the initial specimen, and collect all urine voided by the patient during the next 24 hours.
- Show the patient where to store the urine container.
- Keep the specimen on ice or refrigerated during the 24-hour period.
- Indicate the starting time on the urine container and laboratory slip.

- Post the hours for the urine collection in a prominent location to prevent accidental discarding of the specimen.
- Instruct the patient to void before defecating so that the urine is not contaminated by feces.
- Remind the patient not to put toilet paper in the collection container.
- Encourage the patient to drink fluids during the 24 hours.
- Instruct the patient to collect the last specimen as close as possible to the end of the 24 hours.

After

- Transport the urine specimen to the laboratory promptly.

Test Results and Clinical Significance

Increased levels

Dehydration
Starvation
Diuretic therapy
Addison's disease
Sodium (followed by chloride) reabsorption is decreased.

Increased salt intake
Intravenous saline infusion
Output must equal input to maintain homeostasis. Therefore, urinary chloride increases with increased intake.

Decreased levels

Cushing's syndrome
Conn's syndrome
Steroid therapy
Congestive heart failure
Sodium (followed by chloride) reabsorption is increased.

Malabsorption syndrome
Prolonged gastric suction or vomiting
Diarrhea
Pyloric obstruction
Diaphoresis
Reduced salt intake
Serum chloride levels are decreased. Therefore, urinary chloride is decreased.

Related Tests

- Urinary electrolytes (pp. 847, 851): These are measurements of sodium and potassium electrolytes.
- Chloride, blood (p. 141): This is a measurement of serum chloride level.

Cortisol (Hydrocortisone, Urine Cortisol)

Normal Findings

Adult/elderly: 10-100 mg/24 hr or 27-276 nmol/day (SI units)
Adolescent: 5-55 mg/24 hr
Child: 2-27 mg/24 hr

Indications

This test, a measure of urinary cortisol, is performed in patients with suspected hyperfunction or hypofunction of the adrenal gland.

Test Explanation

An elaborate feedback mechanism for cortisol exists to coordinate the function of the hypothalamus, pituitary gland, and adrenal glands. Corticotropin-releasing hormone (CRH) is made in the hypothalamus. This stimulates adrenocorticotropic hormone (ACTH) production in the anterior pituitary gland. ACTH, in turn, stimulates the adrenal cortex to produce cortisol. The rising levels of cortisol act as a negative feedback and curtail further production of CRH and ACTH. The cortisol is excreted in the urine. Elevated urine levels reflect elevated serum cortisol levels.

Cortisol is a potent glucocorticoid released from the adrenal cortex. This hormone affects the metabolism of carbohydrates, proteins, and fats. It has an especially profound effect on glucose serum levels. Cortisol tends to increase glucose by stimulating gluconeogenesis from glucose stores. It also inhibits the effect of insulin and thereby inhibits glucose transport into the cells.

Interfering Factors

- Pregnancy causes increased cortisol levels.
- Physical and emotional stress can elevate cortisol levels.
  Stress is stimulatory to the pituitary-cortical mechanism, which thereby stimulates cortisol production.
- Drugs that may cause *increased* levels include oral contraceptives, danazol, hydrocortisone, and spironolactone (Aldactone).
- Drugs that may cause *decreased* levels include dexamethasone, ethacrynic acid, ketoconazole, and thiazides.

Procedure and Patient Care

Before

- Explain the procedure to the patient.
- Assess the patient for signs of physical stress (e.g., infection, acute illness) or emotional stress, and report these to the physician.

During

- Begin the 24-hour urine collection. Discard the initial specimen, and collect all urine passed by the patient during the next 24 hours.
- Post the hours for urine collection in a prominent spot.
- Note that it is not necessary to measure each urine specimen.
- Remind the patient to void before defecating so that the urine is not contaminated by feces.
- Tell the patient not to put toilet paper in the collection container.
- Encourage the patient to drink fluids during the 24 hours unless contraindicated for medical reasons.
- Collect the last specimen as close as possible to the end of the 24 hours. Add this to the collection.
- Place the 24-hour urine collection in a plastic container and keep on ice or refrigerated. Use a preservative.
- Note on the laboratory slip the date and time that the specimen collection began and ended.
- Indicate on the laboratory slip any medications that may affect test results.

After

- Send the specimen to the laboratory promptly.

Test Results and Clinical Significance

Increased levels

Cushing's disease
Ectopic ACTH-producing tumors
Stress
ACTH is overproduced as a result of neoplastic overproduction of ACTH in the pituitary gland or elsewhere in the body by an ACTH-producing cancer. Stress is a potent stimulus to ACTH production. Cortisol levels rise as a result.

Cushing's syndrome (adrenal adenoma or carcinoma) *Neoplasm produces cortisol without regard to the normal feedback mechanism.*

Hyperthyroidism *Metabolic rate is increased and cortisol levels rise accordingly to maintain elevated glucose needs.*

Obesity *All sterols are increased in the obese, perhaps because fatty tissue may act as a depository or location of synthesis.*

Decreased levels

Adrenal hyperplasia *Congenital absence of important enzymes in the synthesis of cortisol prevents adequate serum levels.*

Addison's disease *As a result of hypofunctioning of the adrenal gland, cortisol levels drop.*

Hypopituitarism *ACTH is not produced by the pituitary gland destroyed by disease, neoplasm, or ischemia. The adrenal gland is not stimulated to produce cortisol.*

Hypothyroidism *Normal cortisol levels are not required to maintain the reduced metabolic rate in patients with hypothyroidism.*

Related Tests

- ACTH stimulation test (p. 26): This test is used to evaluate the differential diagnosis of Cushing's syndrome or Addison's disease.
- ACTH hormone (p. 23): The serum ACTH study is a test of anterior pituitary gland function that affords the greatest insight into the causes of Cushing's syndrome (overproduction of cortisol) and Addison's disease (underproduction of cortisol).
- Blood cortisol (p. 167): This is direct measurement of cortisol blood level.

δ-Aminolevulinic Acid
(Aminolevulinic Acid [ALA], δ-ALA)

Normal Findings 1-7 mg/24 hr or 11.1-57.2 mmol/24 hr (SI units)

Critical Values >20 mg/24 hr

Indications

This test is used to diagnose porphyria, and in the evaluation of subclinical forms of lead poisoning in children.

Test Explanation

The basic precursor for the porphyrins (p. 844), δ-ALA is needed for the normal production of porphobilinogen, which ultimately leads to heme synthesis in erythroid cells. Heme is used in the synthesis of hemoglobin. Genetic disorders (e.g., porphyria) are associated with lack of a particular enzyme vital to heme metabolism. These disorders are characterized by accumulation of porphyrin products in the liver or RBCs. The liver porphyrias are much more common. Symptoms of liver porphyrias include abdominal pain, neuromuscular signs and symptoms, constipation, and, occasionally, psychotic behavior. This group of disorders results from enzymatic deficiency in synthesis of heme (a portion of hemoglobin). Acute intermittent porphyria is the most common form of liver porphyria and is caused by a deficiency in uroporphyrinogen-I synthase (also called porphobilinogen deaminase).

Most patients with acute intermittent porphyria have no symptoms (latent phase) until the acute phase is precipitated by medication or some other factor (see Box 2-8, p. 449). The acute phase is characterized by abdominal and muscular pain, nausea, vomiting, hypertension, mental symptoms (e.g., anxiety, insomnia, hallucinations, paranoia), sensory loss, and urinary retention. Hemolytic anemia also may develop during the acute phase. These acute symptoms are associated with increased serum and urine levels of porphyrin precursors (aminoleuvulinic acid, porphyrins, and porphobilinogens).

In lead intoxication, heme synthesis is similarly diminished by the inhibition of ALA dehydrase. This enzyme assists in the conversion of ALA to porphobilinogen. As a result of lead poisoning, ALA accumulates in the blood and urine.

Interfering Factors

- Drugs that may cause *increased* ALA levels include penicillin, barbiturates, and griseofulvin (see also Box 2-8, p. 449).

Procedure and Patient Care

Before

- Explain the procedure to the patient.

During

- Begin the 24-hour urine collection. Discard the initial specimen, and collect all urine passed by the patient during the next 24 hours.
- Show the patient where to store the urine container.
- Keep the specimen on ice or refrigerated during the collection period.
- Keep the urine in a light-resistant container with a preservative.
- Indicate the starting time on the urine container and on the laboratory slip.
- Post the hours for the urine collection in a noticeable place to prevent accidental discarding of the specimen.
- Instruct the patient to void before defecating so that urine is not contaminated by feces.
- Remind the patient not to put toilet paper in the collection container.
- Encourage the patient to drink fluids during the 24 hours unless contraindicated for medical reasons.
- Collect the last specimen as close as possible to the end of the 24 hours. Add this to the urine collection.
- If the patient has a Foley catheter in place, cover the drainage bag to prevent exposure to light.
- Indicate on the laboratory slip any drugs that may affect test results.

After

- Transport the urine specimen promptly to the laboratory.

Test Results and Clinical Significance

Increased levels

Porphyria (acute intermittent, variegate, and coproporphyria) *During the acute phase, porphyrin precursors (including ALA) accumulate in the blood and urine.*

Lead intoxication *Chonic lead intoxication may be associated with increased ALA, which accumulates in the blood and urine.*

Chronic alcoholic liver disorders

Diabetic ketoacidosis

These disease are associated with increased ALA. The pathophysiology of these observations is complex and not well defined.

Related Tests

- Uroporphyrinogen-I-synthase (p. 449): This test is used to identify persons at risk for development of porphyria, and to diagnose porphyria in the acute and latent stages.
- Porphyrin and porphobilinogen, urine (p. 844): This is a quantitative measurement of porphyrins and porphobilinogen in the urine. Helps to define a porphyrin pattern that can classify the type of porphyria.

Glucose (Urine Sugar, Urine Glucose)

Normal Findings

Random specimen: Negative
24-hour specimen: <0.5 g/day or <2.78 mmol/day (SI units)

Indications

Testing for glucose in the urine is part of routine urinalysis. If present, it reflects the degree of glucose elevation in the blood. Urine glucose tests are also used to monitor the effectiveness of therapy for diabetes mellitus.

Test Explanation

A qualitative glucose test is part of routine urinalysis. This screening test for the presence of glucose within the urine may indicate the likelihood of diabetes mellitus or other causes of glucose intolerance (see glucose, p. 225). This diagnosis must be confirmed by other tests (e.g., fasting glucose, glucose tolerance, glycosylated hemoglobin). Urine glucose tests are also used to monitor the effectiveness of diabetes therapy; however, this is largely supplanted today by finger stick determinations of blood glucose levels.

In patients with diabetes that is not well controlled with hypoglycemic agents, blood glucose levels can become very high. Normally, glucose is filtered from the blood by the glomeruli of the kidney. In the glomerular filtrate, the glucose concentration is the same as in the blood. Normally, all of the glucose is reabsorbed in the proximal renal tubules. When the blood glucose level exceeds the capability of the renal threshold to reabsorb the glucose (about 180 mg/dl), it begins to spill over into the urine (glycosuria). As the blood glucose level increases, the amount of glucose spilling into the urine also increases.

Glucosuria is not always abnormal. It may occur immediately after eating a high-carbohydrate meal, and in patients with otherwise normal glucose levels or prediabetic patients receiving dextrose-containing IV fluids. Further, glucosuria does not always indicate diabetes, but can occur normally or in diseases that affect the renal tubule or in genetic defects in metabolism and excretion of glucose. In these diseases, the renal threshold for glucose is abnormally low. Despite a normal blood glucose concentration, the kidney cannot reabsorb the normal glucose load. As a result, surplus glucose is spilled into the urine. In these patients, results of glucose tolerance tests are normal.

Interfering Factors

- Drugs that may cause false-positive results with reagent tablets (e.g., Clinitest) but not with enzyme-impregnated strips (Clinistix, Tes-Tape) include acetylsalicylic acid, aminosalicylic acid, ascorbic acid, cephalothin, chloral hydrate, nitrofurantoin, ascorbic acid, streptomycin, and sulfonamides.
- Any substance that can reduce copper in the Clinitest can produce positive results. This may include other sugars (e.g., galactose, fructose, lactose).
- Drugs that may cause false-negative tests include ascorbic acid (Clinistix, Tes-Tape), levodopa (Clinistix), and phenazopyridine (Clinistix, Tes-Tape).
- Drugs that may cause *increased* urine glucose levels include aminosalicylic acid, cephalosporins, chloral hydrate, chloramphenicol, dextrothyroxine, diazoxide, loop and thiazide diuretics, estrogen, glucose infusions, isoniazid, levodopa, lithium, nafcillin, nalidixic acid, and nicotinic acid (large doses).

Procedure and Patient Care

Before

- Explain the procedure to the patient.
- Read the directions on the bottle or container of reagent strips.
- Check the expiration date on the bottle before use.
- Inform the patient that urine tests for glucose may be performed at specified times during the day, generally before meals and at bedtime, and that test results may be used to determine insulin requirements.

During

- Because accuracy is necessary, collect a "fresh" urine specimen. Stagnant urine that has been in the bladder for several hours will not accurately reflect the serum glucose level at testing.
- Preferably, obtain a double-voided specimen by the following method:
  1. Collect a urine specimen 30 to 40 minutes before the time the urine specimen is actually needed.
  2. Discard this first specimen.
  3. Give the patient a glass of water to drink.
  4. At the required time, obtain a second specimen, to be tested for glucose.
- Inform the patient that testing for glucose can be easily performed using enzyme tests such as Clinistix, Diastix, or Tes-Tape.
- Remember that urine glucose also can be determined using the Clinitest (a copper-reducing method).
- If a 24-hour specimen is required, refrigerate the urine during the collection period.

After

- Record the urine glucose level on the patient's glucose chart.

Test Results and Clinical Significance

Increased levels

Diabetes mellitus and other causes of hyperglycemia

Pregnancy *Glycosuria is common in pregnant women. Persistent and significantly high levels may indicate gestational diabetes or other obstetric illness. Also, lactosuria is common in nursing women. Lactose is a reducing substance that may cause false-positive results for glucose, depending on the method of testing.*

Renal glycosuria *It can occur normally or in patients with diseases that affect the renal tubule. It can also result from genetic defects in the metabolism and excretion of glucose. In these diseases, the renal threshold for glucose is abnormally low. Despite a normal blood glucose level, the kidney cannot reabsorb the glucose it should. As a result, the surplus glucose is spilled into the urine.*

Fanconi's syndrome *Associated with transport defects in the proximal renal tubules, causing glycosuria, this genetic defect can also affect the metabolism and excretion of amino acids and electrolytes.*

Hereditary defects in metabolism of other reducing substances (e.g., galactose, fructose, pentose) *These reducing substances may cause false-positive tests for glucose, depending on the method of testing.*

Increased intracranial pressure (e.g., from tumors, hemorrhage) *The pathophysiology for this observation is not well defined, although many theories exist.*

Nephrotoxic chemicals (e.g., carbon monoxide, mercury, lead) *These chemicals injure the kidney and lower the renal threshold.*

Related Tests

- Glucose (p. 225): This is the main screening test for diagnosis of diabetes.
- Glycosylated hemoglobin (p. 238): This is an accurate method for indicating glucose tolerance in the recent past.
- Glucose tolerance (p. 233): This is a test of a patient's capability to handle a glucose load.
- Timed postprandial glucose (p. 229): This is a timed glucose measurement after a carbohydrate meal.
- Glucagon (p. 223): This is a direct measurement of glucagon, which acts to increase glucose in the blood.
- Insulin (p. 272): This is a direct measurement of insulin, which acts to decrease glucose in the blood.

17-Hydroxycorticosteroids (17-OCHS)

Normal Findings

Male
- <8 years: <1.5 mg/24 hr
- <12 years: <4.5 mg/24 hr
- Adult: 4.5-10.0 mg/24 hr
- Elderly: Values lower than for adult

Female
- <8 years: <1.5 mg/24 hr
- <12 years: <4.5 mg/24 hr
- Adult: 2.5-10.0 mg/24 hr
- Elderly: Values lower than for adult

Indications

This urine study is used to assess adrenocortical function by measuring the cortisol metabolites (17-OCHS) in a 24-hour urine collection.

Test Explanation

Elevated levels of 17-OCHS are noted in patients with adrenal hyperfunction (Cushing's syndrome), whether the condition is caused by a pituitary or adrenal tumor, bilateral adrenal hyperplasia, or ectopic tumors producing adrenocorticotropic hormone (ACTH). Low levels of 17-OCHS are seen in patients with adrenal hypofunction (Addison's disease) as a result of destruction of the adrenal glands (by hemorrhage, infarction, metastatic tumor, or autoimmunity), surgical removal of an adrenal gland without appropriate steroid replacement, congenital enzyme deficiency, hypopituitarism, or adrenal suppression after prolonged exogenous steroid ingestion.

Testing the urine for this hormone metabolite is an indirect measure of adrenal function. Urine and plasma levels of cortisol (see p. 829 and p. 167) provide a much more accurate measurement of adrenal function. Because excretion of cortisol metabolites follows a diurnal variation, 24-hour urine collection is necessary.

Interfering Factors

- Emotional and physical stress (e.g., infection) and licorice ingestion may cause increased adrenal activity.
- Drugs that may cause *increased* 17-OCHS levels include acetazolamide, chloral hydrate, chlorpromazine, colchicine, erythromycin, meprobamate, paraldehyde, quinidine, quinine, and spironolactone.
- Drugs that may cause *decreased* levels include estrogen, oral contraceptives, phenothiazines, and reserpine.

Procedure and Patient Care

Before

- Explain the procedure to the patient.
- Note that drugs are usually withheld several days before urine collection. Check with the physician and laboratory for specific guidelines.
- Assess the patient for signs of stress, and report these to the physician.

During

- Do not administer any drugs that may interfere with test results.
- Begin the 24-hour urine collection. Discard the initial specimen, and collect all urine voided by the patient during the next 24 hours.
- Post the hours for the urine collection in a prominent spot.
- Note that it is not necessary to measure each urine specimen.
- Tell the patient to void before defecating so that the urine is not contaminated by feces.
- Inform the patient that toilet paper should not be placed in the collection container.

- Encourage the patient to drink fluids during the 24 hours, unless contraindicated for medical reasons.
- Collect the last specimen as close as possible to the end of the 24 hours. Add this to the container.
- Keep the urine specimen refrigerated or on ice during the collection period.

After

- Send the urine to the chemistry laboratory as soon as the test is completed.
- List on the laboratory slip any medications the patient may be taking that can affect test results.

Test Results and Clinical Significance

Increased levels

Cushing's disease
Ectopic ACTH-producing tumors
Overproduction of ACTH results from ACTH-producing cancers in the pituitary gland or elsewhere in the body.

Stress
Stress is a potent stimulus to ACTH production. Cortisol and 17-OCHS levels rise as a result.

Cushing's syndrome (Adrenal adenoma or carcinoma) *The neoplasm produces cortisol without regard to the normal feedback mechanism, and 17-OCHS levels rise.*

Hyperthyroidism *Metabolic rate is increased, and cortisol and 17-OCHS levels rise accordingly to maintain the elevated glucose needs.*

Obesity *All sterols are increased in obese patients, perhaps because fatty tissue acts as a depository or location of synthesis.*

Decreased levels

Adrenal hyperplasia (Adrenogenital syndrome) *Congenital absence of important enzymes in the cortisol synthesis process prevents adequate serum and urine levels.*

Addison's disease due to adrenal infarction, adrenal hemorrhage, surgical removal of the adrenal glands, congenital enzyme deficiency, or adrenal suppression from steroid therapy *As a result of hypofunctioning of the adrenal gland, cortisol and 17-OCHS levels are decreased.*

Hypopituitarism *ACTH is not produced by the pituitary gland destroyed by disease, neoplasm, or ischemia. The adrenal glands are not stimulated to produce cortisol and 17-OCHS.*

Hypothyroidism *Normal cortisol levels are not required to maintain the reduced metabolic rate in patients with hypothyroidism. Cortisol and 17-OCHS levels are decreased.*

Related Tests

Serum cortisol (p. 167): This test is a measure of serum cortisol, and is performed in patients with suspected adrenal gland hyperfunction or hypofunction.

5-Hydroxyindoleacetic Acid (5-HIAA)

Normal Findings

2-6 mg/24 hr or 10.4-31.2 mmol/day (SI units).
Concentrations in female patients are lower than in male patients.

Indications

This test is used to identify patients with carcinoid tumor and to monitor their therapy.

Test Explanation

Quantitative analysis of urine 5-HIAA is performed to detect and monitor the clinical course of carcinoid tumors. Carcinoid tumors are serotonin-secreting tumors that may grow in the appendix, intestine, lung, or any tissue derived from the neuroectoderm. These tumors contain argentaffin-staining (enteroendocrine) cells, which produce serotonin and other powerful neurohormones that are metabolized by the liver to 5-HIAA and excreted in the urine. These powerful neurohormones are responsible for the clinical symptoms (e.g., bronchospasm, flushing, diarrhea) of carcinoid syndrome. This test is used not only to identify carcinoid tumors but also to reevaluate known tumors by means of serial levels of urinary 5-HIAA. Increasing levels of 5-HIAA indicate progression of tumor; decreasing levels indicate a therapeutic response to antineoplastic therapy. To some extent, larger tumors are associated with higher blood levels than smaller tumors are.

Interfering Factors

- Bananas, plantain, pineapple, kiwi, walnuts, plums, pecans, and avocados can factitiously elevate 5-HIAA levels.
- Drugs that may cause *increased* 5-HIAA levels include acetanilid, acetophenetidin (phenacetin), glyceryl guaiacolate (guaifenesin [Robitussin]), methocarbamol, acetaminophen, and reserpine.
- Drugs that may cause *decreased* levels include chlorpromazine, ethyl alcohol, heparin, imipramine (Tofranil), isoniazid (INH), levodopa, monoamine oxidase (MAO) inhibitors, methenamine, methyldopa (Aldomet), phenothiazines, promethazine (Phenergan), aspirin, and tricyclic antidepressants.

Procedure and Patient Care

Before

- Explain the procedure to the patient.
- Instruct the patient to refrain from eating foods containing serotonin (e.g., plums, pineapples, bananas, eggplant, tomatoes, avocados, walnuts) for several days (usually 3) before and during testing.

During

- Begin the 24-hour urine collection. Discard the initial specimen, and collect all urine voided by the patient during the next 24 hours.
- Show the patient where to store the urine specimen.
- Keep the specimen on ice or in a refrigerator during the collection period. A preservative is needed to maintain an appropriate pH.
- Post the hours for urine collection in a noticeable place to prevent accidental discarding of the specimen.
- Instruct the patient to void before defecating so that urine is not contaminated by stool.
- Tell the patient not to put toilet paper in the urine container.
- Collect the last specimen as close as possible to the end of the 24-hour collection period. Add this urine to the container.

After

- Send the urine specimen to the laboratory promptly.
- List on the laboratory slip any medications that may affect the test results.

Test Results and Clinical Significance

Increased levels

Carcinoid tumor of the appendix, bowel, lung, breast, or ovary *Serotonin is produced by the argentaffin-staining (enteroendocrine) cells within the tumor. The serotonin is metabolized by the liver to 5-HIAA, which is then excreted into the urine.*

Noncarcinoid illness
Cystic fibrosis
Intestinal malabsorption
These conditions may be associated with elevated 5-HIAA levels. The pathophysiology of these observations is not clear.

Decreased levels

Depression
Migraine
Serotonin deficit has been noted in these illnesses. The cause is unknown.

17-Ketosteroids (17-KS)

Normal Findings

Male: 7-25 mg/24 hr or 24-88 mmol/day (SI units)
Female: 4-15 mg/24 hr or 14-52 mmol/day (SI units)
Elderly: Values decrease with age
Child:
 <12 yr: <5 mg/24 hr
 12-15 yr: 5-12 mg/24 hr

Indications

This urine test is performed to assist in evaluation of adrenal cortex function, especially as it relates to androgenic function. It is especially useful for evaluation and monitoring of adrenal hyperplasia (adrenogenital syndrome) and adrenal tumors.

Test Explanation

This urine test is used to measure adrenocortical function by measuring 17-KS in the urine. 17-KS are metabolites of testosterone and other androgenic sex hormones. The principal 17-KS is dehydroepiandrosterone (DHEA). In men, approximately one third of the hormone metabolites come from testosterone, produced in the testes, and two thirds come from other androgenic hormones, produced in the adrenal cortex; in women and children, almost all 17-KS are nontestosterone androgenic hormones, produced in the adrenal cortex. Therefore this test is useful in diagnosing adrenocortical dysfunction. It is important to note that 17-KS are not metabolites of cortisol and do not reflect levels of cortisol production. Elevated 17-KS levels are frequently noted in congenital adrenal hyperplasia and androgenic tumors of the adrenal glands. In these diseases, excess steroid synthesis is of the "noncortisol" androgenic sterols. These diseases frequently cause virilization syndromes. Testicular tumors rarely cause elevated 17-KS levels.

Low levels of 17-ketosteroids have little clinical significance, because of the inaccuracy of determining low levels. The most common cause of low 17-ketosteroid levels is stress. During stress, the adrenal glands produce less androgen and more cortisol. In this regard, low 17-KS levels may reflect states of good health.

Interfering Factors

- Stress may decrease adrenal androgenic activity.
- Drugs that may cause *increased* 17-KS levels include antibiotics, chloramphenicol, chlorpromazine, dexamethasone, meprobamate, phenothiazines, quinidine, secobarbital, and spironolactone (Aldactone).
- Drugs that may cause *decreased* levels include estrogen, oral contraceptives, probenecid, promazine, reserpine, salicylates (prolonged use), and thiazide diuretics.

Procedure and Patient Care

Before

- Explain the procedure to the patient.
- Withhold all drugs (with physician approval) for several days before the test.
- Assess the patient for signs of stress, and report these to the physician.

During

- Begin the 24-hour urine collection. Discard the initial specimen, and collect all urine voided by the patient during the next 24 hours.
- Post the hours for urine collection in a prominent spot.
- Remember that it is not necessary to measure each urine specimen.

- Tell the patient to void before defecating so the urine is not contaminated by lose.
- Inform the patient that toilet paper should not be placed in the collection container.
- Encourage the patient to drink fluids during the 24 hours, unless contraindicated for medical reasons.
- Remember that the urine collection needs a preservative.
- Keep the collected urine on ice or refrigerated.
- Collect the last specimen as close as possible to the end of the 24 hours. Add this to the urine collection.

After

- Indicate on the laboratory slip the start and end times of the specimen collection.
- List on the laboratory slip any medications that may affect test results.
- Send the specimen to the laboratory as soon as the test is completed.

Test Results and Clinical Significance

Increased levels

Congenital adrenal hyperplasia *In congenital hyperplasia, an enzyme defect results in underproduction of cortisol. By the normal feedback mechanism, ACTH is maximally produced. The result is maximum noncortisol adrenal (androgenic) sterol production. Levels of 17-KS are therefore elevated. This often causes masculinizing syndrome in female patients and precocious puberty in male patients. Congenital adrenal hyperplasia is the most common cause of elevated 17-KS levels in children.*

Pregnancy *Pregnancy is associated with slightly higher levels of androgens. 17-KS levels are therefore elevated.*

ACTH administration
ACTH-secreting ectopic tumors
Hyperpituitarism
ACTH stimulates adrenal cortisol and to a lesser degree androgenic sterol production. 17-KS levels are therefore elevated in these three clinical situations.

Testosterone- or androgenic-secreting tumors of the adrenal glands, ovaries, or testes *These tumors are most often associated with elevated 17-KS levels in adults, and can produce very high androgen levels. 17-KS levels also can be very high. Adrenal androgenic (mostly DHEA)–producing cancers or adenomas also can produce very high levels of 17-KS.*

Cushing's syndrome *17-KS production varies depending on the cause of adrenal overproduction.*

Stein-Leventhal syndrome *This masculinizing syndrome is not well understood. Elevated 17-KS levels have been noted.*

Decreased levels

Severe debilitating disease
Severe stress or infection
Chronic disease
In serious illness, the adrenal glands produce more cortisol and less androgenic hormone. 17-KS levels are therefore low.

Addison's disease *With diminished adrenal function, production of androgenic hormones is reduced. 17-KS levels are therefore low.*

Hypogonadism (Klinefelter's syndrome)
Castration
With reduced testosterone production, 17-KS levels are low.

Hypopituitarism *Reduced production of ACTH reduces the activity of the adrenal cortex. 17-KS levels are therefore low.*

Related Tests

17-Hydroxycorticosteroids (p. 835): This urine test measures the metabolites of cortisol and function of the adrenal cortex.

Osmolality (Urine Osmolality)

Normal Findings

12- to 14-hour fluid restriction: >850 mOsm/kg H_2O (SI units)
Random specimen: 50-1200 mOsm/kg H_2O (SI units), depending on fluid intake

Critical Values

<100 mOsm/kg H_2O in overhydration
>800 mOsm/kg H_2O in dehydration

Indications

This test is used to evaluate fluid and electrolyte abnormalities. It is an accurate determination of the kidney's concentrating capabilities. It is also used to investigate antidiuretic hormone (ADH) abnormalities (e.g., diabetes insipidus) and inappropriate ADH secretion.

Test Explanation

Urine osmolality is the measurement of the number of dissolved particles in the urine. It is a more exact measurement of urine concentration than specific gravity is, because specific gravity depends on the weight and density of the particles in the urine. Specific gravity also requires correction for the presence of glucose or protein, as well as for temperature; in contrast, osmolality depends only on the number of particles of solute in a unit of solution. Osmolality can be measured over a wider range than specific gravity, and with greater accuracy.

Osmolality is used in precise evaluation of the concentrating ability of the kidney. This test is also used to monitor fluid and electrolyte balance. Osmolality is valuable in the workup of patients with renal disease, inappropriate ADH secretion, and diabetes insipidus. Osmolality may be measured during urinalysis if the patient has glycosuria or proteinuria or has undergone tests that require use of contrast medicine. In these situations, the urine osmolar gap is increased as a result of other organic osmolar particles. The osmolar gap is the sum of all the particles expected to be in the urine (e.g., electrolytes, urea, glucose) compared with the actual osmolality. Normally, the osmolar gap is 80-100 mOsm/kg H_2O.

Urine osmolality is more easily interpreted when the serum osmolality is simultaneously measured. Urine osmolality is measured by determining the freezing point or by measuring vapor pressure of the specimen. The freezing point is more commonly determined, and is very accurate.

CLINICAL PRIORITIES

- This test provides valuable information about fluid and electrolyte abnormalities.
- Urine osmolality is a more exact measure of urine concentration than is specific gravity.
- Urine osmolality is more easily interpreted when the serum osmolality is also measured.

Procedure and Patient Care

Before

- Explain the procedure to the patient.
- Tell the patient that no special preparation is necessary for a random urine specimen.
- Inform the patient that preparation for a fasting urine specimen may require ingestion of a high-protein diet for 3 days before the test.
- Instruct the patient to eat a dry supper the evening before the test and to drink no fluids until the test is completed the next morning.

During

- Collect a first-voided urine specimen for a random sample.
- For a fasting specimen, instruct the patient to empty the bladder at approximately 6:00 AM and to discard the urine. Collect the test urine at 8:00 AM.
- Indicate on the laboratory slip the patient's fasting status.

After

- Send the specimen to the laboratory.
- Provide food and fluids for the patient.

Test Results and Clinical Significance

Increased levels

Syndrome of inappropriate ADH (SIADH) secretion *Several illnesses can produce SIADH secretion. ADH is inappropriately secreted despite factors that normally would inhibit its secretion. As a result, large quantities of water are reabsorbed by the kidney. Less free water is excreted and the urine osmolality rises.*

Paraneoplastic syndromes associated with carcinoma (e.g., lung, breast, colon) *These cancers act as an autonomous ectopic source for secretion of ADH. The pathophysiology is the same as is described for SIADH.*

Shock *The normal physiologic response to shock is to minimize the loss of free body water. The kidneys therefore absorb all the free water possible. Urine osmolality rises.*

Hepatic cirrhosis
Congestive heart failure
These illnesses are associated with water retention due to reduced perfusion of the kidneys. Less free body water is excreted, and urine osmolality rises.

Decreased levels

Diabetes insipidus *Insufficient secretion of ADH despite physiologic stimulation by increased serum osmolality diminishes the kidneys' capability to concentrate urine. Urine osmolality decreases.*

Excess fluid intake *Free water overload is excreted into the urine. Urine osmolality decreases.*

Renal tubular necrosis
Severe pyelonephritis
The concentrating capability of the kidneys is reduced. Excess free water is excreted. Urine osmolality decreases.

Related Tests

- Serum osmolality (p. 314): This is a measurement of osmolality of the serum. When combined with urine osmolality, more accurate interpretation of either test is possible.
- ADH (p. 62): This provides a direct measurement of ADH in the blood.
- ADH suppression test (p. 65): This test is helpful in evaluation of ADH abnormalities.

Porphyrins and Porphobilinogens

Normal Findings

Total porphyrins (μg/24 hr):
  Male: 8-149
  Female: 3-78
Uroporphyrin (μg/24 hr):
  Male: 4-46
  Female: 3-22
Coproporphyrin (μg/24 hr):
  Male: <96
  Female: <60
Porphobilinogens (0--2 mg/24/hr or 0-8.8 mmol/day (SI units)

Indications

This test is a quantitative measurement of porphyrins and porphobilinogen. It is used along with aminolevulinic acid (ALA) to identify the various forms of porphyria.

Test Explanation

Porphyria is a group of genetic disorders associated with enzyme deficiencies involved with porphyrin synthesis. Porphyrins (e.g., uroporphyrin, coproporphyrin) and porphobilinogens are important building blocks in the synthesis of heme. Heme is incorporated into hemoglobin within the erythroid cells. Porphyrias are classified according to location of the accumulation of the porphyrin precursors. In most forms of porphyria, increased levels of porphyrins and porphobilinogen are found in the urine.

Variable symptoms are associated with different types of porphyrias. Erythropoietic porphyria is associated with photosensitivity of the eyes and skin. Intermittent porphyria and less often variegate and hereditary coproporphyria are associated with abdominal pain and neurologic symptoms. Heavy metal (e.g., lead) intoxication is associated with increased porphyrins in the urine. Certain drugs can induce porphyria and cause elevated porphyrin levels in the urine (see Box 2-18, p. 449). This test is a quantitative analysis of urinary porphyrins and porphobilinogens. If porphyrins are present, the urine may be colored amber red or burgundy, or even darker after standing in the light.

Urine tests for porphyrins are not as accurate as plasma measurements and pattern identification for the various forms of porphyria, but are accurate in screening for porphyria, especially the intermittent variety. Although the test can also be done on a fresh stool specimen, random and 24-hour urine collections are more accurate. Colorimetric methods (or spectrophotometry) are used most often. Fractionation of the various types of porphyrins within the urine allows identification of patterns commonly associated with the various porphyrias. High-performance liquid chromatography is used for that. The diagnosis of porphyria and interpretation of test results are difficult. The American Porphyria Foundation can provide assistance to health care providers in this area.

Interfering Factors

- Drugs that may alter test results include aminosalicylic acid (PAS), barbiturates, chloral hydrate, chlorpropamide (Diabinese), ethyl alcohol, griseofulvin, morphine, oral contraceptives, phenazopyridine (Pyridium), procaine, and sulfonamides (see also Box 2-18, p. 449).

Procedure and Patient Care

Before

- Explain the procedure to the patient.
- Tell the patient that no fasting is required.

During

Porphobilinogens

- Collect a freshly voided urine specimen.
- Protect the specimen from light.
- For both porphobilinogens and porphyrins, indicate on the laboratory slip any drugs that may affect test results.

Porphyrins

- Begin the 24-hour urine collection. Discard the initial specimen, and collect all urine voided by the patient during the next 24 hours.
- Instruct the patient to avoid alcohol use during the collection period.
- Show the patient where to store the urine container.
- Keep the specimen on ice or refrigerated during the 24 hours.
- Keep the urine in a light-resistant specimen bottle with a preservative to prevent degradation of the light-sensitive porphyrin.
- Indicate the starting time on the urine container and the laboratory slip.
- Post the times for urine collection in a prominent place to prevent accidental discarding of the specimen.
- Instruct the patient to void before defecating so that urine is not contaminated by feces.
- Remind the patient not to put toilet paper in the collection container.
- Encourage the patient to drink fluids during the 24 hours unless contraindicated for medical reasons.
- Collect the last specimen as close as possible to the end of the 24 hours. Add this urine to the collection.

After

- Transport the urine specimen promptly to the laboratory.

Test Results and Clinical Significance

Increased levels

PORPHYRIAS

Acute intermittent porphyria *Porphobilinogen and to a lesser degree porphyrin levels are elevated during the acute phase. No real increase is noted during the latent phases.*
Congenital erythropoietic porphyria *Porphobilinogen level is elevated.*
Hereditary coproporphyria *Coproporphyrin and porphobilinogen levels are elevated.*
Variegate porphyria *In acute episodes, porphobilinogen and ALA (p. 831) levels are elevated.*
Lead poisoning *ALA level is most significantly elevated, although porphyrin levels are slightly elevated.*

Related Tests

- Uroporphyrinogen-I-synthase (p. 449): Used to identify persons at risk for development of porphyria, and to diagnose porphyria in the acute and latent stages.
- Urine for ALA (p. 831): Used to diagnose porphyria and in evaluation of children with subclinical forms of lead poisoning.

Potassium (K)

Normal Findings

25-120 mEq/L/day or 25-120 mmol/day (SI units). Values vary greatly with diet.

Indications

This test measures the amount of K in a spot or 24-hour urine collection to aid in determining electrolyte balance.

Test Explanation

Potassium is the major cation within the cell. The electrolyte balance of K can be measured in a spot or a 24-hour urine collection. A 24-hour collection is especially important to evaluate electrolyte (especially hypokalemia) balance, acid-base balance, and renal and adrenal diseases.

The serum K concentration depends on many factors. Aldosterone, and to a lesser extent glucocorticosteroids, tends to increase renal losses of potassium. If sodium blood levels are diminished, the renal tubules can reabsorb sodium in exchange for K, which is then excreted at increased rates. Acid-base balance depends to a small degree on K excretion. In alkalotic states, H^+ can be reabsorbed in exchange for K^+. The kidneys cannot reabsorb K. Therefore, K intake is balanced by kidney excretion through the urine.

Interfering Factors

- Dietary intake affects K levels.
- Excessive intake of licorice may cause increased levels of K in the urine because licorice acts like aldosterone and increases K excretion.
- Drugs that may cause *increased* levels include diuretics, glucocorticoids, and salicylates.

Procedure and Patient Care

Before

- Explain the procedure to the patient.
- Tell the patient that no special diet is required.

During

- Begin the 24-hour urine collection. Discard the initial specimen, and collect all urine voided by the patient during the next 24 hours.
- Show the patient where to store the urine container.
- Keep the specimen on ice or refrigerated during the entire 24 hours.
- Indicate the starting time on the urine container and the laboratory slip.
- Post the hours for urine collection in a noticeable place to prevent accidental discarding of the specimen.

- Instruct the patient to void before defecating so that the urine is not contaminated by feces.
- Remind the patient not to put toilet paper in the collection container.
- Encourage the patient to drink fluids during the 24 hours.
- Instruct the patient to collect the last specimen as close as possible to the end of the 24 hours. Add this urine to the container.

After

- Transport the urine specimen promptly to the laboratory.

Test Results and Clinical Significance

Increased levels

Chronic renal failure *Sodium loss is increased in some forms of renal failure due to loss of reabsorptive capabilities of the kidneys. Potassium follows sodium loss.*

Renal tubular acidosis *Reduced excretion of H^+ increases excretion of K^+.*

Starvation *To provide energy, protein- and fat-containing tissues are broken down. The cells in those tissues expel K into the bloodstream. The K is then excreted, at increased levels, into the urine.*

Cushing's syndrome
Hyperaldosteronism
Aldosterone increases K urinary excretion. Because glucocorticosteroids have an aldosterone-like effect, K excretion is also increased in Cushing's syndrome.

Excessive intake of licorice *Licorice has an aldosterone-like effect, as described on p. 847.*

Alkalosis *H^+ is reabsorbed in the renal tubules in exchange for K excretion.*

Diuretic therapy *Most diuretics are K wasting and increase K urinary excretion.*

Decreased levels

Dehydration *Decreased renal blood flow associated with dehydration diminishes urinary excretion of K.*

Addison's disease *This disease is associated with diminished aldosterone effect on the kidneys. Because aldosterone increases urinary excretion of K, reduced levels of aldosterone are associated with reduced urinary K levels.*

Malnutrition
Vomiting
Diarrhea
Malabsorption
Diminished intake of K is matched by diminishing urinary excretion of K.

Acute renal failure *Urinary excretion of K is diminished. This is the most common cause of hyperkalemia.*

Related Tests

- Urine for sodium (p. 851): These electrolytes are often measured with K. Metabolically, they are intermingled.
- Potassium, (p. 342): Direct measurement of K in serum.

Pregnanediol

Normal Findings

Variable	Pregnanediol (mg/day)
Age (yr)	
<9	<0.1
10-15	0.1-1.2
Adult male	0-1.9
Adult female	
Follicular phase	<2.6
Luteal phase	2.6-10.6
Pregnancy (trimester)	
1st	10-35
2nd	35-70
3rd	70-100

Indications

This test measures pregnanediol, a metabolite of progesterone. It is used in the evaluation and decision making in women who are having difficulty becoming pregnant or maintaining a pregnancy. It is also used to monitor "high risk" pregnancies.

Test Explanation

Urinary pregnanediol is measured to evaluate progesterone production by the ovaries and placenta. The main effect of progesterone is on the endometrium. It initiates the secretory phase of the endometrium in anticipation of implantation of a fertilized ovum. Normally, progesterone is secreted by the ovarian corpus luteum after ovulation. Both serum progesterone levels and urine concentration of progesterone metabolites (pregnanediol and others) are significantly increased during the second half of an ovulatory cycle. Pregnanediol is the most easily measured metabolite of progesterone.

Because pregnanediol levels rise rapidly after ovulation, this study is useful in documenting whether ovulation has occurred and, if so, exactly when. This is useful information for a woman who has difficulty becoming pregnant. During pregnancy, pregnanediol levels normally rise because of placental production of progesterone. Repeated assays can be used to monitor the status of the placenta in high-risk pregnancy.

Hormone assays for urinary pregnanediol are primarily used to monitor progesterone supplementation in patients with an inadequate luteal phase to maintain an early pregnancy. Urinary assays may be supplemented by plasma assays (progesterone assay, p. 351), which are quicker and more accurate.

Interfering Factors

- Drugs that may cause *increased* levels include adrenocorticotropic hormone (ACTH).
- Drugs that may cause *decreased* levels include oral contraceptives and progesterone.

Procedure and Patient Care

Before

- Explain the procedure to the patient.
- Tell the patient that usually no special diet is required.
- Inform the patient that no sedation or fasting is necessary.

During

- Begin the 24-hour urine collection. Discard the initial specimen, and collect all urine voided by the patient during the next 24 hours.
- Show the patient where to store the urine collection.
- Keep the specimen on ice or refrigerated during the 24 hours.
- Check with the laboratory to see if a preservative is needed.
- Indicate the starting time on the urine container and the laboratory slip.
- Post the hours for urine collection in a noticeable place to prevent accidental discarding of the specimen.
- Instruct the patient to void before defecating so that the urine is not contaminated by feces.
- Remind the patient not to put toilet paper in the collection container.
- Encourage the patient to drink fluids during the 24 hours.
- Instruct the patient to collect the last specimen as close as possible to the end of the 24 hours. Add this urine to the container.

After

- Record on the laboratory slip the date of the last menstrual period or the week of gestation during pregnancy.

Test Results and Clinical Significance

Increased levels

Ovulation *Ovulation occurs with development of a corpus luteum, which makes progesterone. Pregnanediol is a metabolite of progesterone.*

Pregnancy *A healthy placenta produces progesterone. Pregnanediol is a metabolite of progesterone.*

Molar pregnancy *Hydatidiform mole can produce progesterone, although at lower levels than during pregnancy.*

Luteal cysts of ovary *The corpus luteum produces progesterone in the nonpregnant woman and in the early stages of pregnancy. Cysts can also produce progesterone for prolonged periods of time. Pregnanediol is a metabolite of progesterone.*

Arrhenoblastoma of ovary *This tumor can secrete sex hormones or their metabolites (usually testosterone). 17-hydroxyprogesterone is a precursor of sex hormones. Pregnanediol is a metabolite of progesterone.*

Hyperadrenocorticism
Adrenocortical hyperplasia
Adrenal cortical hormones are secreted at increased rates. 17-Hydroxyprogesterone is a precursor of these cortical hormones. Pregnanediol is a metabolite of progesterone.

Choriocarcinoma of ovary *This tumor produces progesterone.*

Decreased levels

Preeclampsia
Toxemia of pregnancy
Threatened abortion
Placental failure
Fetal death
These obstetrical emergencies are associated with decreased placental viability. Progesterone is made by the placenta during pregnancy. Pregnanediol is a metabolite of progesterone, which is decreased when placental viability is threatened.

Ovarian neoplasm *Ovarian epithelial cancers can destroy functional ovarian tissue. Progesterone levels may decrease.*

Amenorrhea
Ovarian hypofunction
Without ovulation, a corpus luteum will not develop. Progesterone will not be secreted, and progesterone and pregnanediol levels will be lower than expected.

Related Tests

- Progesterone assay (p. 351): Direct measurements of progesterone in serum.

Sodium (Na⁺)

Normal Findings

24-hour collection: 40-220 mEq/L/day or 40-220 mmol/day (SI units)
Spot urine collection: >20 mEq/L

Indications

This test is used to evaluate fluid and electrolyte abnormalities, especially Na. It can also be used to monitor therapy for these abnormalities.

Test Explanation

This test is used to evaluate Na balance in the body by determining the amount of Na excreted in urine over 24 hours. Na is the major cation in the extracellular space. Measuring the amount of Na in the urine is useful for evaluating patients with volume depletion, acute renal failure, adrenal disease, and acid-base imbalance. This test is important, especially when the serum Na concentration is low. For example, in patients with hyponatremia caused by inadequate Na intake, the urine Na level will be low. In patients with hyponatremia caused by chronic renal failure or Addison's disease, however, the urine Na concentration will be high.

Many factors regulate Na balance. Aldosterone causes conservation of Na by stimulating the kidneys to reabsorb Na and decreasing renal losses. Natriuretic hormone, or third factor, is stimulated by increased Na levels. This hormone decreases renal absorption and increases renal losses of Na. Antidiuretic hormone (ADH), which controls the reabsorption of water at the distal tubules of the kidney, affects Na urine levels by dilution or concentration.

Interfering Factors

- Dietary salt intake may increase Na levels.
- Drugs that may cause *increased* urine levels include antibiotics, cough medicines, caffeine, laxatives, and diuretics (e.g., spironolactone)
- Drugs that may cause *decreased* urine levels includes steroids.

Procedure and Patient Care

Before

- Explain the procedure to the patient.
- Tell the patient that no fasting is required.

During

- Begin the 24-hour urine collection. Discard the initial specimen, and collect all urine voided by the patient during the next 24 hours.
- Show the patient where to store the urine specimen.
- Keep the specimen on ice or refrigerated during the 24 hours.
- Indicate the starting time on the urine container and on the laboratory slip.
- Post the hours for urine collection in a noticeable place to prevent accidental discarding of the specimen.
- Instruct the patient to void before defecating so that urine is not contaminated by feces.
- Remind the patient not to put toilet paper in the collection container.
- Encourage the patient to drink fluids during the 24 hours.
- Instruct the patient to collect the last specimen as close as possible to the end of the 24 hours. Add this urine to the container.
- A spot urine specimen can be obtained and sent to the laboratory if information about urine Na is needed sooner than 24 hours. In this situation, ask the patient to void in a nonsterile container, and transport the entire volume to the laboratory. The more urine available, the more accurately the spot urine specimen will reflect the 24-hour urine results.

After

- Transport the urine specimen promptly to the laboratory.

Test Results and Clinical Significance

Increased urine levels

Dehydration *Free water is maximally reabsorbed by the kidney, and urine Na is more concentrated.*

Adrenocortical insufficiency *Aldosterone and corticosteroids stimulate Na reabsorption in the distal renal tubules. With inadequate levels of these hormones, Na will not be reabsorbed, and large amounts are wasted into the urine.*

Diuretic therapy *Most diuretics work by diminishing Na reabsorption and increasing Na loss in the kidney.*

Syndrome of inappropriate ADH secretion (SIADH) *ADH stimulates free water reabsorption in the kidney. With inappropriately high secretion of ADH, free water in the urine is diminished and Na is more concentrated.*

Diabetic ketoacidosis *The osmotic diuresis due to hyperglycemia tends to diminish Na reabsorption in the kidney. Further, Na salts combine with some ketotic products to further increase Na losses into the urine.*

Chronic renal failure *Renal reabsorption of Na and many other products is diminished in a diseased, nonfunctioning kidney. Urine Na levels increase.*

Decreased urine levels

Congestive heart failure *Renal blood flow is diminished with reduced cardiac output. The renin-angiotensin system is stimulated (see p. 381), and aldosterone production is stimulated. Aldosterone stimulates renal reabsorption of Na, and urine levels diminish.*

Malabsorption
Diarrhea
Intestinal absorption of Na is reduced. The physiologic response is to reduce Na excretion in the urine.

Cushing's disease *Corticosteroids have an aldosterone-like effect on the kidney, which tends to stimulate renal reabsorption of Na, and urine levels diminish.*

Aldosteronism *Aldosterone stimulates renal reabsorption of Na, and urine levels diminish.*

Inadequate Na intake *Intestinal absorption of Na is very efficient. Therefore it is rare for a nutritional deficiency to occur as Na insufficiency severe enough to significantly diminish renal excretion. However, with Na deficit or ongoing Na loses treated with inadequate Na replacement, serum Na levels significantly diminish and the kidneys are maximally stimulated to reabsorb Na. Urine Na levels diminish.*

Related Tests

- Serum Na (p. 396): This is a direct measurement of Na levels in blood.
- Aldosterone (p. 37): More than any other hormone, aldosterone has a significant effect on blood Na levels.
- ADH (p. 62): By affecting free body water excretion, Na levels are affected by virtue of dilution or concentration.

Toxicology

Normal Findings

See Tables 11-1 and 11-2 for blood toxicology and urine toxicology, respectively.

Indications

Toxicology is used to evaluate for drug abuse, overdose, or poisoning.

Test Explanation

Detection of the most commonly abused nonprescription mood-altering drugs is discussed. These drugs are most commonly used in suicide attempts and chemical poisonings.

Testing for drug overdose and poisoning is best performed on blood. Results indicate immediate drug levels, which can indicate or alter therapy. Screening for use or abuse of nonprescription drugs is usually done on urine. Urine specimens are easily obtained without any invasive procedure. Often the specimen is obtained several hours or days after the drug administration. Blood levels are low, but urine levels are high. Further, drug

Table 11-1 ***Blood toxicology screening***

Drug	Type	Therapeutic level*	Toxic level*
Acetaminophen	Analgesic, antipyretic	Depends on use	>250 μg/ml
Alcohol	–	None	80-200 mg/dl (mild to moderate intoxication) 250-400 mg/dl (marked intoxication) >400 mg/dl (severe intoxication)
Amobarbital	Sedative, hypnotic	0.5-3.0 μg/ml	>10 μg/ml
Butabarbital	Sedative, hypnotic	0.5-3.0 μg/ml	>10 μg/ml
Carboxyhemoglobin (COHb, carbon monoxide)	Gas	None	>30% COHb (beginning of coma)
Glutethimide	Sedative	0.5-3.0 μg/ml	>10 μg/ml
Lead	–	None	>40 μg/dl
Lithium	Manic episodes of manic-depression psychosis	0.8-1.2 mEq/l	>2.0 mEq/l
Meprobamate	Antianxiolytic	0.5-3.0 μg/ml	>10 μg/ml
Methyprylon	Hypnotic	0.5-3.0 μg/ml	>10 μg/ml
Phenobarbital	Anticonvulsant	15-30 μg/ml	>40 μg/ml
Phenytoin (Dilantin)	Anticonvulsant	10-20 μg/ml	>20 μg/ml
Salicylate	Antipyretic, anti-inflammatory, analgesic	100-250 μg/ml	>300 μg/ml

*Varies according to institution performing the test.

Table 11-2 Urine toxicology screening for amphetamines

Drug	Therapeutic level*	Toxic level*
Amphetamine	2-3 μg/ml	>3 μg/ml
Dextroamphetamine	0.1-1.5 μg/ml	>15 μg/ml
Methamphetamine	3-5 μg/ml	>40 μg/ml
Phenmetrazine	5-30 μg/ml	>50 μg/ml

*Varies according to institution performing the test.

metabolic products exist in the urine for longer periods, allowing detection of drug use in the past few hours or days. The disadvantages of urine drug tests are that they cannot indicate with any degree of accuracy when the drug was used and if the drug had any effect on the person's actions at any time. Also, the urine can be altered easily by changing the concentration (by drinking large volume of water or adding water to the specimen), changing the pH, or adding foreign substances. Urine temperature, specific gravity, and creatinine concentration are often determined in urine specimens to ensure the specimen has not been altered. It is important to define the appropriate chain of transfer of the specimen from the moment it is obtained to the point of testing to prevent tampering.

Because of the impact on a person's life (socially, financially, and legally), positive results must be substantiated by another equally accurate test method. A popular combination is to screen with thin-layer or gas chromatography to separate out the constituents in the specimen, followed by mass spectrometry to identify those constituents.

Toxicology studies are used to incriminate drugs as a cause of or factor in a death. They are also used to assess patients when drug abuse or poisoning is contributing to an illness. Drug abuse is important to recognize in the workplace because of safety issues and in prisons because of disciplinary concerns.

Commonly Abused Drugs

Marijuana (cannabis). Marijuana is usually detected by identifying one of its metabolites (tetrahydrocannabinol [THC]) in the urine. Most laboratories detect carboxy-THC, and use 100 ng/ml as a cutoff. Lower levels from passive inhalation of marijuana may be detected, but are not prosecutable in court. These metabolites can exist in the urine 1 hour after use, and for 1 to 3 days afterward.

Cocaine (including crack). Benzoylecgonine is a metabolite of cocaine. It is easily detectable in urine 1 to 4 hours after use, and for 2 or 3 days. To indicate the timing of cocaine use, serum levels of cocaine must be determined.

Phencyclidine (PCP). PCP or one of its metabolites is detectable in urine about 6 to 18 hours after use and for as long as 3 days.

Amphetamines (especially methamphetamine). Amphetamines are identifiable in urine about 3 hours after use and for about 1 or 2 days. One must be careful in assuming abuse with detection of amphetamines, because many over-the-counter cold medicines and weight loss medicines contain amphetamine analogs.

Morphine and other narcotic alkaloids. Heroin, morphine, and codeine can be identified in the urine glucuronide conjugated forms 2 hours after use and for 2 to 3 days. Like amphetamines, one must be careful in assuming abuse with detection of codeine, because many over-the-counter pain relievers and cough-suppressive medicines contain codeine.

Barbiturates. Barbiturates can be detected in the blood, urine, or gastric contents by direct immunoassay.

Common Toxins

Lead. Lead diminishes the activity of ALA dehydrase, which converts δ-ALA to porphobilinogen in the synthesis of heme for hemoglobin within erythroid cells. As a result, δ-ALA accumulates in the blood and urine.

Other heavy metals. Heavy metals such as mercury, arsenic, bismuth, and antimony can be identified in the urine.

Interfering Factors

- Detergents, bicarbonates, salt tablets, or blood can all foil accurate drug testing in the urine.

Procedure and Patient Care

Before

- Explain the procedure to the patient or significant others.
- If the specimen is obtained for medicolegal testing, ensure that the patient or family member has signed a consent form.
- Obtain as much information as possible about the drug type, amount, and ingestion time.
- Carefully assess the patient for respiratory distress, a common adverse reaction to drug overdose.

During

- Collect blood or urine specimens as indicated. Urine specimens are collected in the presence of a trained health care professional.
- Collect gastric contents for analysis if indicated.
- Note that hair and nail samples may be used to detect or document exposure to arsenic and mercury.
- Immediately identify the sample and mark the patient's name on the specimen.

After

- Apply pressure or a pressure dressing to the venipuncture site.
- Assess the venipuncture site for bleeding.
- Assess the patient for respiratory distress, a common adverse reaction to drug overdose.
- Refer the patient for appropriate drug and psychiatric counseling.
- Follow the predetermined chain of transfer of the specimen to the laboratory for testing. Each person involved in handling the specimen must document his or her place in its handling.
- Remind the patient that all positive screening results must be confirmed.

Test Results and Clinical Significance

Abuse or use of nonprescription drugs *Urine is most often used for this testing.*
Heavy metal and lead poisoning *Blood, urine, CSF, and tissue specimens may all be used to identify these poisons.*
Suicide attempts *Determination of toxic levels of drugs is much more accurately determined with blood tests, although urine may also be used.*

Related Tests

- Ethanol (p. 206): This is a direct measurement of alcohol level in the blood.
- Carboxyhemoglobin (p. 135): This test is used to detect carbon monoxide poisoning.
- Aminolevulinic acid (p. 831): This test is used to identify lead poisoning.
- Drug monitoring (p. 194): These tests are used to help identify toxic levels of therapeutic drugs such as aspirin and acetaminophen, commonly involved in suicide attempts.

Uric Acid

Normal Findings 250-750 mg/24 hr or 1.48-4.43 mmol/day (SI units)

Indications

Uric acid levels can be measured in both blood and urine. Urine levels of uric acid are helpful in evaluating uric acid metabolism in gout and for assessing hyperuricosuria in renal calculus formation. This test also helps to identify persons at risk for stone formation.

Test Explanation

Uric acid is a nitrogenous compound that is the final breakdown product of purine (a deoxyribonucleic acid [DNA] building block) catabolism. (See p. 466 for blood uric acid level.) Seventy-five percent of uric acid is excreted via the kidneys, and 25% by way of the intestinal tract. Elevated uric acid levels (hyperuricemia) may be indicative of gout, a form of arthritis due to deposition of uric acid crystals in periarticular tissue. Elevated uric acid in the urine is called uricosuria. Uric acid can become supersaturated in the urine and crystalize to form kidney stones, which can block the renal system.

Uric acid is produced primarily in the liver. Urinary excretion of uric acid depends on uric acid levels in the blood, along with glomerular filtration and tubular secretion of uric acid into the urine. Elevated uric acid levels can cause nephrolithiasis and ureterolithiasis. Uric acid is less well saturated in acidic urine. As the urine pH rises, more uric acid can exist without crystallization and stone formation. Therefore, urine known to have a high uric acid level can be alkalinized by ingestion of a strong base to prevent stone formation.

Interfering Factors

- Recent use of radiographic contrast agents may increase uric acid levels in the urine.
- Drugs that may interfere with test results include alcohol, anti-inflammatory preparations, salicylates, thiazide diuretics, vitamin C, and warfarin.

CLINICAL PRIORITIES

- This test is helpful in evaluating uric acid metabolism and gout.
- In persons with high uric acid levels, the urine should be kept alkaline to prevent precipitation of kidney stones.

Procedure and Patient Care

Before

- Explain the procedure to the patient.
- Tell the patient that no special diet is usually required.

During

- Begin the 24-hour urine collection. Discard the initial specimen, and collect all urine voided by the patient during the next 24 hours. A preservative may be used.
- Show the patient where to store the urine container.
- Keep the specimen on ice or refrigerated during the entire 24 hours. (Note that some laboratories do not require that the specimen be kept cool.)
- Indicate the starting time on the urine container and laboratory slip.
- Post the hours for the urine collection in a noticeable place to prevent accidental discarding of the specimen.
- Instruct the patient to void before defecating so the urine is not contaminated by feces.
- Remind the patient not to put toilet paper in the collection container.
- Encourage the patient to drink fluids during the 24 hours.
- Instruct the patient to collect the last specimen as close as possible to the end of the 24 hours. Add this urine to the container.

After

- Transport the urine specimen to the laboratory promptly.

Test Results and Clinical Significance

Increased levels (uricosuria)

Gout *Uric acid levels are high in blood. With normal glomerular filtration, levels are high in urine.*

Metastatic cancer
Multiple myeloma

Leukemias
Cancer chemotherapy
Rapid cell destruction associated with rapidly growing cancers (with high cell turnover), and especially after chemotherapy for those rapidly growing tumors, causes the cells to lyse and spill their nucleic acids into the blood stream. In the liver, these free nucleic acids are converted to uric acid. Blood and urine levels of uric acid increase.

High purine diet *With increased uric acid production caused by a diet high in purines, uric acid levels in the urine will be increased.*
Uricosuric drugs (e.g., ascorbic acid, calcitonin, citrate, dicumarol, estrogens, steroids, iodinated dyes, glyceryl guaiacolate, phenolsulfonphthalein, probenecid, salicylates, and outdated tetracyline) *These drugs increase uric acid excretion into the urine.*
Lead toxicity *Heavy-metal poisoning is associated with increased uric acid tubular secretion.*

Decreased levels

Kidney disease *With decreased glomerular filtration rate and decreased tubular secretion of uric acid, urine levels fall.*
Eclampsia *The pathophysiology of this observation is not well known.*
Chronic alcohol ingestion *Chronic acidosis from excessive alcohol ingestion decreases renal tubular secretion of uric acid into the urine.*
Acidosis (ketotic [diabetic or starvation], lactic) *Renal tubular secretion of uric acid into the urine is decreased. Ketoacids, as occur in diabetic or alcoholic ketoacidosis, may compete with uric acid for tubular excretion, which is another cause of decreased uric acid excretion.*

Related Tests

- Uric acid in blood (p. 446): Used to diagnose gout.

Urinalysis (UA)

Normal Findings

Appearance: clear
Color: amber yellow
Odor: aromatic
pH: 4.6-8.0 (average, 6.0)
Protein
  0-8 mg/dl
  50-80 mg/24 hr (at rest)
  <250 mg/24 hr (during exercise)
Specific gravity
  Adult: 1.005-1.030 (usually, 1.010-1.025)
  Elderly: values decrease with age
  Newborn: 1.001-1.020

Leukocyte esterase: negative
Nitrites: none
Ketones: none
Crystals: none
Casts: none present
Glucose (see urine glucose, p. 833)
Fresh specimen: none present
24-hour specimen: <0.5 g/day or <2.78 mmol/day (SI units)
White blood cells (WBCs): 0-4 per low-power field
WBC casts: none
Red blood cells (RBCs): ≤2
RBC casts: none

Indications

Urinalysis is part of routine diagnostic and screening evaluations. It can reveal a significant amount of preliminary information about the kidneys and other metabolic processes. Urinalysis is routinely done in all patients admitted to the hospital, pregnant women, and presurgical patients. It is done diagnostically in patients with abdominal or back pain, dysuria, hematuria, or urinary frequency. It is part of routine monitoring in patients with chronic renal disease and some metabolic diseases. It is the most frequently ordered urine test.

Test Explanation

Total urinalysis involves multiple routine tests on a urine specimen. This specimen is not necessarily a clean-catch specimen. However, if urinary tract infection is suspected, often a midstream, clean-catch specimen is obtained. This urine is then split into two portions. One is sent for urinalysis, and the other is held in the laboratory refrigerator for culture (see p. 873) if results of urinalysis indicate infection. Routinely, urinalysis includes remarks as to the color, appearance, and odor; pH; and presence of proteins, glucose, ketones, blood, and leukocyte esterase. In addition, the urine is examined microscopically for RBCs, WBCs, casts, crystals, and bacteria. Because this is a spot urine test, volume is not measured. Volume of urine may be important in many clinical situations, and a full 24-hour specimen is required.

Laboratory examination

Appearance and Color

Urine appearance and color are noted as part of routine urinalysis. A normal urine specimen should be clear. Cloudy urine may be caused by the presence of pus (necrotic WBCs), RBCs, or bacteria; however, normal urine also may be cloudy because of ingestion of certain foods (e.g., large amounts of fat, ureates, phosphates). Urine ranges from pale yellow to amber because of the pigment urochrome (product of bilirubin metabolism). The color indicates the concentration of the urine and varies with specific gravity. Dilute urine is straw colored, and concentrated urine is deep amber.

Abnormally colored urine may result from a pathologic condition or the ingestion of certain foods or medicines. For example, bleeding from the kidney produces dark red

Table 11-3 Frequently used drugs that may affect urine color

Generic and brand names	Drug class	Urine color
Anisindione (Miradon)	Oral anticoagulant	Red-orange in alkaline urine
Cascara sagrada	Stimulant laxative	Red in alkaline urine; yellow-brown in acid urine
Chloroquine (Aralen)	Antimalarial	Rusty yellow or brown
Chlorzoxazone (Paraflex)	Skeletal muscle relaxant	Orange or purple-red
Docusate calcium (Doxidan, Surfak)	Laxative	Pink to red to red-brown
Furazolidone (Furoxone)	Anti-infective, antiprotozoal	Brown
Iron preparations (Ferotran, Imferon)	Hematinic	Dark brown or black on standing
Levodopa	Antiparkinsonian agent	Dark brown on standing
Methylene blue (Urolene Blue)	Antimethemoglobinemic	Blue-green
Nitrofurantoin (Macrodantin, Nitrodan)	Antibacterial	Brown
Phenazopyridine (Pyridium)	Urinary tract analgesic	Orange to red
Phenindione (Eridione)	Anticoagulant	Red-orange in alkaline urine
Phenolphthalein (Ex Lax)	Contact laxative	Red or purplish pink in alkaline urine
Phenothiazines (e.g., prochlorperazine [Compazine])	Antipsychotic, neuroleptic, antiemetic	Red-brown
Phenytoin (Dilantin)	Anticonvulsant	Pink, red, red-brown
Riboflavin (vitamin B)	Vitamin	Intense yellow
Rifampin	Antibiotic	Red-orange
Sulfasalazine (Azulfidine)	Antibacterial	Orange-yellow in alkaline urine
Triamterene (Dyrenium)	Diuretic	Pale blue fluorescence

urine, whereas bleeding from the lower urinary tract produces bright red urine. Dark yellow urine may indicate the presence of urobilinogen or bilirubin. *Pseudomonas* organisms may produce green urine. Beets may cause red urine, and rhubarb can color the urine brown. Many frequently used drugs also may affect urine color (Table 11-3).

Odor

Determination of urine odor is part of routine urinalysis. The aromatic odor of fresh, normal urine is caused by the presence of volatile acids. Urine of patients with diabetic ketoacidosis has the strong, sweet smell of acetone. In patients with a urinary tract infection, the urine may have a foul odor. Urine with a fecal odor may indicate an enterovesicle fistula.

pH

Analysis of the pH of a freshly voided urine specimen indicates the acid-base balance. The urine reflects the work of the kidneys to maintain normal pH homeostasis. Just as the lungs (respiratory component) help compensate for acid-base imbalance, so do the kidneys (metabolic component). The kidneys assist in acid-base balance by reabsorption of sodium and excretion of hydrogen.

An alkaline pH is obtained in a patient with alkalemia. Bacteria, urinary tract infection, or a diet high in citrus fruits or vegetables may cause increased urine pH. Certain medications (e.g., streptomycin, neomycin, kanamycin) are effective in treating urinary tract infections when the urine is alkaline. Acidic urine is generally obtained in patients with acidemia, which can result from metabolic or respiratory acidosis, starvation, dehydration, or a diet high in meat products or cranberries.

The urine pH is useful in identifying crystals in the urine and determining the predisposition to form a given type of stone. Acidic urine is associated with xanthine, cystine, uric acid, and calcium oxalate stones. To treat or prevent these urinary calculi, urine should be kept alkaline. Alkaline urine is associated with calcium carbonate, calcium phosphate, and magnesium phosphate stones. To treat or prevent these urinary calculi, urine should be kept acidic.

Protein

Evaluation of protein is a sensitive indicator of kidney function. Normally, protein is not present in the urine because the spaces in the normal glomerular filtrate membrane are too small to allow its passage. If the glomerular membrane is injured, as in glomerulonephritis, the spaces become much larger, and protein (usually albumin, because it is a smaller molecule than the globulins) seeps into the filtrate and then into the urine. If this persists at a significant rate, hypoproteinemia can develop as a result of severe protein loss through the kidneys. This decreases the normal capillary oncotic pressure that holds fluid within the vasculature, and causes severe interstitial edema. The combination of proteinuria and edema is known as nephrotic syndrome.

Proteinuria is probably the most important indicator of renal disease. The urine of all pregnant women is routinely checked for proteinuria, which can be an indicator of preeclampsia. Urinary protein is used to screen for nephrotic syndrome and for complications of diabetes mellitus, glomerulonephritis, amyloidosis, and multiple melanoma (see test for Bence Jones protein, p. 820).

If significant protein is noted at urinalysis, a *24-hour urine* specimen should be collected so that the quantity of protein can be measured. This test can be repeated as a method of monitoring renal disease and its treatment. Usually, protein loss of >3000 mg/24 hr leads to the signs and symptoms of nephrotic syndrome.

Glucose

See discussion on page 833.

Specific Gravity

Specific gravity is a measure of the concentration of particles (including wastes and electrolytes) in the urine. High specific gravity indicates concentrated urine; low specific gravity indicates dilute urine. Specific gravity refers to the weight of the urine compared with that of distilled water (which has a specific gravity of 1.000). Particles in the urine give it weight, or specific gravity.

Specific gravity is used to evaluate the concentrating and excretory power of the kidneys. Renal disease tends to diminish concentrating capability. As a result, chronic renal diseases are associated with low specific gravity. Specific gravity must be interpreted in light of the presence or absence of glycosuria and proteinuria. Specific gravity is also a measurement of hydration status. With overhydration, the urine will be more dilute, with lower specific gravity, whereas with dehydration, specific gravity can be expected to be abnormally high. Measurement of urine specific gravity is easier and more convenient than measurement of osmolality (see p. 842). Specific gravity correlates roughly with osmolality. Knowledge of specific gravity is needed to interpret the results of most parts of the urinalysis. Specific gravity is usually evaluated with a refractometer (which measures the amount of light that can pass through a drop of urine) or a dipstick.

Leukocyte Esterase (WBC Esterase)

Leukocyte (WBC) esterase is a screening test used to detect leukocytes in the urine. Positive results indicate urinary tract infection. Some patients have no symptoms of urinary tract infection (e.g., pain or burning on urination). For this examination, chemical testing is performed with a leukocyte esterase dipstick; a shade of purple is considered a positive result. Some laboratories have established screening protocols in which a microscopic examination (see below) is performed only if results of a leukocyte esterase test are positive. Leukocyte esterase is nearly 90% accurate in detecting WBCs in urine.

Nitrites

Like the leukocyte esterase screen, the nitrite test is a screening test for identification of urinary tract infections. Some patients have no symptoms of urinary tract infection (e.g., pain or burning on urination). This test is based on the principle that many bacteria produce an enzyme called reductase, which can reduce urinary nitrates to nitrites. Chemical testing is done with a dipstick containing a reagent that reacts with nitrites to produce a pink color, thus indirectly suggesting the presence of bacteria. A positive test result indicates the need for a urine culture. Nitrite screening enhances the sensitivity of the leukocyte esterase test to detect urinary tract infections. Nitrite testing is only about 50% accurate in detecting WBCs in the urine.

Ketones

Normally, no ketones are present in the urine; however, a patient with poorly controlled diabetes and hyperglycemia may have massive fatty acid catabolism. The purpose of this catabolism is to provide an energy source when glucose cannot be transferred into the cell because of insulin insufficiency. Ketones (β-hydroxybutyric acid, acetoacidic acid, and acetone) are the end products of this fatty acid breakdown. As with glucose, ketones spill over into the urine when blood levels in diabetic patients are elevated. Ketonuria is usually associated with poorly controlled diabetes. This test for ketonuria is also important in evaluating ketoacidosis associated with alcoholism, fasting, starvation, high-protein diets, and isopropanol ingestion. Ketonuria may occur with acute febrile illnesses, especially in infants and children.

Bilirubin and Urobilinogen

See discussion on p. 822.

Microscopic examination of urine sediment

Microscopic examination of the sediment from a centrifuged urine specimen provides substantial information about the urinary system. Because many different methods can be used to prepare the sediment for microscopic review, normal values may vary significantly among laboratories. Reference ranges are provided here to recognize marked abnormalities.

Crystals

Crystals found in the urinary sediment on microscopic examination indicate that renal stone formation is imminent, if not already present. By themselves, crystals cause no symptoms until they form stones. Even then, stones produce symptoms only when they obstruct the urinary tract. Uric acid crystals occur in patients with high serum uric acid levels (e.g., gout). Phosphate and calcium oxalate crystals occur in the urine of patients with parathyroid abnormalities or malabsorption states. The type of crystal found varies with the disease and the pH of the urine (see above discussion on urinary pH).

Casts

Casts are clumps of materials or cells that form in the renal distal and collecting tubules, where the material is maximally concentrated. These amorphous clumps of material and cells are shaped like tubules, thus the term cast. For casts to form, the pH must be acidic and the urine concentrated. Casts are usually associated with some degree of proteinuria and stasis within the renal tubules. There are two kinds of casts: hyaline and cellular. Casts are best seen on low power of the light microscope. Some casts are nearly clear (hyaline), and the condenser lamp must be dimmed to see them well.

Hyaline casts

Hyaline casts are conglomerations of protein and are indicative of proteinuria. A few hyaline casts are normally present, especially after strenuous exercise.

Cellular casts

Granular casts. Granular casts result from the disintegration of cellular material into granular particles within a WBC or epithelial cell cast. Granular casts are found after exercise and in various renal diseases. Their basic component is the same as the cellular material.

Fatty casts. In some diseases, the epithelial cells desquamate into the renal tubule. As the cell degenerates, fatty deposits within the cell coalesce and become incorporated with protein into casts. If casts are not formed, these fatty droplets coalesce to bigger droplets called free oval fat bodies. These are all associated with nephrotic syndrome or nephrosis. Free oval fat bodies may also be associated with fatty emboli, which occur in patients with bone fractures.

Waxy casts. Waxy casts may be cell casts, hyaline casts, or renal failure casts. Waxy casts probably represent further degeneration of granular casts. They occur when urine flow through the renal tubule is diminished, giving time for granular casts to degenerate. Waxy casts are associated with chronic renal diseases and chronic renal failure. They also occur in diabetic nephropathy, malignant hypertension, and glomerulonephritis.

Epithelial cells and casts (renal tubular casts). Epithelial cells can enter the urine anywhere during the process of urinary excretion. These cells can be shed from the bladder as a result of tumor, infection, or polyps. They can result from cellular contamination of the urine by vaginal or urethral secretions. They can also result from desquamation of renal tubule cells into the lumen of the tubules and collecting system. These cells can form epithelial casts. The material in these cells can disintegrate first into coarse granules and then into fine granules, making granular casts. The presence of occasional epithelial cells is not remarkable; large numbers, however, are abnormal. Tubular (epithelial) casts are most suggestive of glomerulonephritis.

White blood cells and casts. Normally, few WBCs are found in the urine sediment on microscopic examination. The presence of five or more WBCs in the urine indicates a urinary tract infection involving the bladder or kidneys, or both. A clean-catch urine culture should be done for further evaluation. WBC casts are most frequently found in infections of the kidney (e.g., acute pyelonephritis), and are also seen in poststreptococcal glomerulonephritis or inflammatory nephritis (e.g., lupus nephritis).

Red blood cells and casts. Any disruption in the blood-urine barrier, whether at the glomerular, tubular, or bladder level, will cause RBCs to enter the urine. Hematuria can be microscopic or gross. Bladder, ureteral, and urethral diseases are the most common causes of RBCs in the urine. Pathologic conditions (e.g., tumors, trauma, stones, infection) that involve the mucous membrane in the collecting system can also cause hematuria. Hematuria is detected easily with routine urinalysis. RBC casts suggest glomerulonephritis (which may be present in patients with acute bacterial endocarditis, renal infarct, Goodpasture's syndrome, vasculitis, sickle cell disease, or malignant hypertension), interstitial nephritis, acute necrosis, pyelonephritis, renal trauma, or renal tumor.

Interfering Factors

Appearance and color

- Sperm remaining in the urethra after recent or retrograde ejaculation can cause the urine to appear cloudy.
- Urine that has been refrigerated for longer than 1 hour can become cloudy.
- Certain foods affect urine color. Carrots may cause dark yellow urine; beets may cause red urine; rhubarb may cause reddish or brownish urine.
- Urine darkens with prolonged standing, due to oxidation of bilirubin metabolites.
- Many drugs, given the right environment, can alter the color of urine. See Table 11-3.

Odor

- Some foods (e.g., asparagus) produce characteristic urine odor.
- When urine stands for a long time and begins to decompose, it has an ammonia-like smell.

pH

- Urine pH becomes alkaline on standing, because of the action of urea-splitting bacteria, which produce ammonia.
- The urine pH of an uncovered specimen will become alkaline because carbon dioxide vaporizes from the urine.
- Dietary factors affect urine pH. Ingestion of large quantities of citrus fruits, dairy products, and vegetables produces alkaline urine, whereas a diet high in meat and certain foods (e.g., cranberries) produces acidic urine.
- Drugs that *increase* urine pH include bicarbonate antacids, carbonic anhydrase inhibitors, and acetazolamide.
- Drugs that *decrease* urine pH include ammonium chloride, mandelic acid, and chlorothiazide.

Protein

- Transient proteinuria may be associated with severe emotional stress, excessive exercise, and cold baths.

- Radiopaque contrast media administered within 3 days may cause false-positive results for proteinuria when turbidity is used as a measure of protein in the urine.
- Urine contaminated with prostate or vaginal secretions may cause proteinuria.
- Diets high in protein can cause proteinuria.
- Highly concentrated urine may have a higher concentration of protein than more dilute urine.
- Hemoglobin may cause a positive result with the dipstick method.
- Bence Jones protein may not appear with the dipstick method.
- Drugs that may cause *increased* protein levels include acetazolamide, aminoglycosides, amphotericin B, cephalosporins, colistin, griseofulvin, lithium, methicillin, nafcillin, nephrotoxic drugs (e.g., arsenicals, gold salts), oxacillin, penicillamine, penicillin G, phenazopyridine, polymyxin B, salicylates, sulfonamides, tolbutamide, and vancomycin.

Specific gravity

- Recent use of radiographic dyes increases urinary specific gravity.
- Cold causes falsely high specific gravity.
- Drugs that may cause *increased* specific gravity include dextran and sucrose.

Leukocyte esterase

- False-positive results may occur in specimens contaminated by vaginal secretions (e.g., heavy menstrual discharge, *Trichomonas* infection, parasites) that contain WBCs.
- False-negative results may occur in specimens containing high levels of protein or ascorbic acid.

Ketones

- Special diets (carbohydrate-free, high protein, high fat) may cause ketonuria.
- Drugs that may cause false-positive results include bromosulfophthalein, isoniazid, isopropanol, levodopa, paraldehyde, phenazopyridine, and phenolsulfonphthalein (phenol red).

Crystals

- Radiographic contrast media may cause precipation of urinary crystals.

WBCs

- Vaginal discharge may contaminate the urine specimen and factitiously cause WBCs in the urine.

RBCs

- Strenuous physical exercise may cause RBC casts.
- Traumatic urethral catheterization may cause RBCs in the urine.
- Overaggressive anticoagulant therapy or bleeding disorders tend to cause RBCs in the urine without concomitant disease.

Procedure and Patient Care

Before

- Explain the procedure to the patient.

✓ CLINICAL PRIORITIES

- The most common cause of RBCs in the urine is from contamination due to menses. Before a more thorough evaluation is begun, determine whether the patient was having a period when the urine specimen was obtained.
- Leukocyte esterase and nitrate tests are screening tests used to detect urinary tract infections. Positive test results indicate the need for urine culture.
- If a urinary tract infection is suspected, a midstream, clean-catch specimen is needed.
- If a 24-hour urine collection is needed, it should be refrigerated during the collection period. A preservative may also be necessary.

During

- Collect a fresh urine specimen in a urine container.
- If the urine specimen contains vaginal discharge or bleeding, a clean-catch or midstream specimen will be needed. This requires meticulous cleaning of the urinary meatus with an iodine preparation to reduce contamination of the specimen by external organisms. The cleansing agent must then be completely removed so as not to contaminate the specimen. The midstream collection is obtained as follows:
  1. Have the patient begin to urinate into a bedpan, urinal, or toilet, then stop urinating. This washes urine out of the distal part of the urethra.
  2. Correctly position a sterile urine container and have the patient void 3 to 4 oz of urine.
  3. Cap the container.
  4. Allow the patient to finish voiding.
- Testing for ketones can be performed immediately after urine collection by placing a drop of urine on a reagent tablet (acetest). If acetone is present, shades of lavender will appear. Or dip a reagent stick (Ketostix) into the urine specimen. Read the strip in 15 seconds by comparing it with the color chart.
- For testing urine specific gravity, a first-voided specimen is best.
- Specific gravity can be measured with a refractometer. Light passes through the specimen, and the refractive index (difference between the velocity of light passing through air and the specimen) is determined.
- An easier method of measuring specific gravity is the dipstick method. A dipstick is placed in the specimen, and the resulting color is compared with a color chart.
- To test for protein, a first-voided specimen is best. Occasionally, however, a 24-hour urine collection is preferred.
- Most laboratories use the dipstick method to determine protein in the urine.
- The dipstick method is not as accurate as sulfosalicylic acid turbidimetric methods.
- Nitrite, leukocyte esterase, pH, and ketones are measured with the dipstick method and the results determined by comparison with a color chart.
- Urine sediment is obtained by centrifuging a small volume (10 ml) of urine and discarding the supernatant. The remaining urine is a concentrated sediment that can be microscopically examined.

After

- Transport the urine specimen to the laboratory promptly.
- If the specimen cannot be processed immediately, refrigerate it.
- If a 24-hour urine collection is requested, the specimen should be refrigerated or preserved with formalin during the collection time.
- Casts will break up as urine is allowed to sit. Urine examinations for casts should be performed with fresh specimens.

Test Results and Clinical Significance

Appearance and color

Infection *Infection may cause turbid, foul-smelling urine.* Pseudomonas *infection can give a green tint to urine.*

Gross hematuria *RBCs in the urine cause the urine to be red. This is always a pathologic sign unless the blood is found to be from a source other than the urinary tract. Tumors, trauma, stones, and infection anywhere in the urinary tract can cause RBCs in the urine. Glomerulonephritis, interstitial nephritis, acute necrosis, and polynephritis are also associated with hematuria.*

Drug therapy (see Table 11-3)

Overhydration, diabetes insipidus, diuretic therapy, glycosuria *These states produce nearly colorless urine.*

Fever, excessive sweating, dehydration, jaundice *These states cause dark yellow or orange urine.*

Hemoglobinuria, myoglobinuria, porphyria *These illnesses cause wine-colored or even dark brown urine.*

Odor

Ketonuria *Associated with poor glucose tolerance, ketones in the urine cause a fruity smell.*

Urinary tract infection *Most infections cause foul smelling urine.*

Enterovesicle fistula *This condition causes urine to smell like stool.*

Maple sugar urine *This congenital defect in protein metabolism causes the urine to smell like burnt sugar.*

Phenylketonuria *This disease causes the urine to smell musty.*

pH

Increased levels

Alkalemia *The renal component of pH homeostasis is to excrete excess base to try to correct acid-base imbalance.*

Urinary tract infections *Urea-splitting bacteria cause the urine to be alkaline as urea is converted to ammonia.*

Gastric suction
Vomiting
Renal tubular acidosis
These are all associated with reduced hydrogen ion excretion. Urine pH is increased.

Decreased levels

Acidemia *To maintain homeostasis, the kidneys attempt to excrete hydrogen ions, causing the urine pH to be reduced.*

Diabetes mellitus
Starvation
Ketone acids associated with starvation or poor glucose metabolism cause acid urine.

Respiratory acidosis
Chronic obstructive pulmonary disease (COPD)
CO_2 retention is compensated for by renal excretion of hydrogen ions. The urine becomes acidotic.

Protein

Increased levels

Nephrotic syndrome, glomerulonephritis, malignant hypertension, diabetic glomerulosclerosis, polycystic disease, lupus erythematosus, Goodpasture's syndrome, heavy-metal poisoning, bacterial pyelonephritis, nephrotoxic drug therapy *Renal disease involving the glomeruli is associated with proteinuria.*

Trauma *Protein can spill into the urine as a result of traumatic destruction of the blood-urine barrier.*

Macroglobulinemia *With increased globulin within the blood, albumin is excreted in an attempt to maintain oncotic homeostasis.*

Multiple myelomas *Classically, multiple myelomas produce large amounts of proteins (e.g., Bence Jones protein) in the urine.*

Preeclampsia
Congestive heart failure
The pathophysiology of these observations are many. Suffice it to say that albumin leaks from the glomeruli, which are temporarily damaged by these illnesses.

Orthostatic proteinuria *As many as 20% of normal male patients have small amounts of protein in the urine when specimens are obtained from patients in the upright position. The pathophysiology is not known with certainty. It may be associated with passive congestion of the kidney in the upright position. This phenomenon can be diagnosed by obtaining a urine specimen before arising, and another after the patient has been up for 2 hours. The first has no protein, the latter does.*

Severe muscle exertion *Prolonged muscular exertion can be associated with small amounts of protein in the urine.*

Renal vein thrombosis *Congestion of the kidney is associated with proteinuria.*

Bladder tumor *Tumors of the bladder secrete protein into the lumen of the bladder.*

Urethritis or prostatitis *Inflammation in the periurethral glands or urethra can cause proteinuria.*

Amyloidosis *Often associated with proteinuria, it may be so severe as to cause nephrotic syndrome. Usually, amyloidosis of the kidney is due to other severe, ongoing disease.*

Specific Gravity

Increased levels

Dehydration *The kidneys reabsorb all available free water; thus excreted urine is concentrated.*

Pituitary tumor or trauma *SIADH syndrome results in excessive water reabsorption and concentrated urine.*
Decreased renal blood flow (as in heart failure, renal artery stenosis, or hypotension) *Urine is concentrated through secretion of ADH and the renin-angiotensin system.*
Glycosuria and proteinuria *These particles of glucose and protein increase specific gravity.*

Water restriction
Fever
Excessive sweating
Vomiting
Diarrhea
The above five clinical situations are associated with diminished blood volume. They cause concentrated urine mediated through secretion of ADH and the renin-angiotensin system.

Decreased levels

Overhydration *Excess water is excreted, causing dilute urine with low specific gravity.*
Diabetes insipidus *Inadequate ADH secretion causes decreased water reabsorption. Excess water is excreted, causing dilute urine with low specific gravity.*
Renal failure *In chronic renal failure the kidney loses its ability to concentrate urine through water reabsorption. Excess water is excreted, causing dilute urine with low specific gravity.*
Diuresis *Diuretics tend to cause dilute, voluminous urine flow.*

Leukocyte esterase

Possible urinary tract infection *Detection of leukocyte esterase indicates the presence of WBCs in the urine (pyuria), indicative of urinary tract infection.*

Nitrites

Possible urinary tract infection *Reductase produced by bacteria reduces nitrates to nitrites. The presence of nitrites indicates bacterial infection somewhere in the urinary tract.*

Ketones

Poorly controlled diabetes mellitus
Starvation
Alcoholism
Weight-reduction diets
Prolonged vomiting
Anorexia
Fasting
High-protein diets
Glycogen storage diseases
Impaired glucose metabolism causes catabolism of fat for production of energy. Ketones (β-hydroxybutyric acid, acetoacetic acid, and acetone) are formed and spill into the urine.

Febrile illnesses in infants and children
Hyperthyroidism
Severe stress or illness
Hypermetabolic states cause excessive utilization of glucose. Fats are then broken down. Ketones form and spill over into the urine.

Excessive aspirin ingestion *Aspirin toxicity is associated with reduced glucose production. Ketones form and spill over into the urine.*
Anesthesia *The pathophysiology of this observation is probably multiple. Drug effect, starvation, and severe illness can all affect ketone formation.*

Crystals

Renal stone formation *Stones form with crystals as a nidus for production. Crystals in small quantities are not pathologic. Crystals do give some insight into metabolic diseases, (e.g., gout, hyperparathyroidism) and other congenital defects of protein metabolism.*
Urinary tract infection Proteus *infection, in particular, is associated with crystal formation, especially if chronic.*

Granular casts and waxy casts

Acute tubular necrosis
Urinary tract infection
Glomerulonephritis
Pyelonephritis
Nephrosclerosis
Chronic lead poisoning
Exercise
Stress
Renal transplant rejection
Coarse and fine granular casts represent further degeneration of cellular casts. They appear when urine flow through the collecting system is diminished, allowing time for further degeneration. As a result, nearly any renal disease or toxicity can be associated with granular cast formation. Waxy casts represent further deterioration of granular casts over time.

Fatty casts

Nephrotic syndrome
Diabetic nephropathy (Kimmelstiel-Wilson syndrome)
Glomerulonephritis associated with streptococcal infection
Chronic renal disease (glomerulonephritis)
Mercury poisoning
Classically, fatty casts are associated with nephrotic syndrome. Any disease or poison that affects the tubular cells causes them to degenerate and desquamate into the lumen. The fatty deposits within those cells coalesce to mix with protein, to make fatty casts or oval fat bodies.

Fat embolism *About 50% of fat embolisms are associated with urinary fat.*

Epithelial casts

Glomerulonephritis
Eclampsia
Heavy-metal poisoning
Diseases that affect the renal tubule cells and diminish urine flow are associated with epithelial cast formation.

Epithelial cells

Acute renal allograft rejection
Acute tubular necrosis

Acute glomerulonephritis due to streptococcal infection
Acute tubule cell injuries cause those cells to be destroyed and desquamate into the lumen of the tubule, to be excreted in the urine.

Hyaline casts

Orthostatic proteinuria
Fever
Strenuous exercise
Stress
These clinical states are often associated with short-term proteinuria and decreased urine flow through the renal collecting system. Proteinaceous (or hyaline) casts develop.

Glomerulonephritis
Pyelonephritis
Congestive heart failure
Chronic renal failure
These diseases are associated with chronic proteinuria and hyaline cast formation.

RBCs and casts

Increased RBC levels

Primary renal diseases (e.g., glomerulonephritis, interstitial nephritis, acute tubular necrosis, pyelonephritis) *These diseases are associated with the deterioration of the blood-urine barrier.*
Renal tumor *Renal neoplasms are friable and hypervascular. RBCs are common with cancers of the kidney.*
Renal trauma *Lacerations, contusions, and hematomas ultimately lead to blood in the urine.*

Renal stones
Cystitis
Prostatitis
Tumors of the ureters and bladder
Traumatic bladder catheterization
Bladder trauma
Any mucosal injury or disease will cause bleeding directly into the urine. Hematuria is usually gross (visible to the naked eye).

Increased RBC cast levels

Glomerulonephritis
Subacute bacterial endocarditis
Renal infarct
Goodpasture's syndrome
Vasculitis
Sickling
Malignant hypertension
Systemic lupus erythematosus
Bleeding from the kidney when associated with reduced urine flow through the kidney can be associated with RBC casts. RBC casts exclude the lower urinary tract as a source of bleeding.

WBCs and casts

Increased WBC levels

Bacterial infection in the urinary tract *WBCs in response to bacterial infections anywhere in the urinary tract can cause leukouria. It may be difficult to differentiate cystitis from urethritis, but it can be done with the two-specimen technique. Ask the patient to void about 20 ml of urine into one container and the rest into another container. More WBCs in the first container indicates urethritis; more in the second container indicates cystitis.*

Increased WBC cast levels

Acute pyelonephritis
Glomerulonephritis
Lupus nephritis
Infectious or inflammatory diseases affecting the kidney can be associated with WBC cast formation. The presence of casts excludes the lower urinary tract as a source of the infection or inflammation.

Related Tests

- Blood glucose (p. 225): This test is included in routine urinalysis. It warrants separate discussion, however, because of its importance.
- Urine culture and sensitivity (see below): If urinalysis indicates the possibility of infection, a culture and sensitivity test should be performed.

Urine Culture and Sensitivity (Urine C&S)

Normal Findings

Negative: <10,000 bacteria/ml urine
Positive: >10,000 bacteria/ml urine

Indications

This test is used to diagnose urinary tract infection (UTI) in patients with dysuria, frequency, or urgency. It is also indicated when patients have fever of unknown origin or when urinalysis suggests infection.

Test Explanation

Urine culture and sensitivity tests are performed to determine the presence of pathogenic bacteria in patients with suspected urinary tract infections. Most often, urinary tract infections are limited to the bladder, although the kidneys, ureters, bladder, or urethra can be the source of infection. All cultures should be performed before antibiotic therapy is initiated, because the antibiotic may interrupt the growth of the organism in the laboratory. Most organisms require approximately 24 hours to grow in the laboratory, and a preliminary report can be given at that time. Occasionally, 48 to 72 hours are required for growth and identification of an organism. Cultures may be repeated after appropriate antibiotic therapy to assess for complete resolution of the infection, especially urinary tract infections.

To save money in some institutions, urine is collected and split. Half is sent for urinalysis, and the other half is held in the laboratory refrigerator and evaluated only if results of urinalysis indicate a possible infection (e.g., increased number of WBCs, bacteria, high pH, leukocyte esterase).

An important part of any routine culture is assessment of the sensitivity to various antibiotics of any bacteria that are growing in the urine. The physician can then prescribe the safest, least expensive, and most effective antibiotic therapy for the specific bacteria.

Interfering Factors

- Contamination of the urine with stool, vaginal secretions, hands, or clothing will cause false positive results.
- Drugs that may affect test results include other antibiotics.

Procedure and Patient Care

Before

- Explain to the patient the procedure for collecting a clean-catch (midstream) urine specimen.
- Withhold antibiotics until after the urine specimen has been collected.
- Provide the patient with the necessary supplies for the collection.

During

- Note that a *clean-catch* or *midstream* urine collection is required for culture and sensitivity testing. This requires meticulous cleansing of the urinary meatus with an iodine preparation to reduce contamination of the specimen by external organisms. The foreskin must be retracted in male patients. The cleansing agent must be completely removed so it will not contaminate the urine specimen. The midstream collection is obtained as follows:
  1. Have the patient begin to urinate into a bedpan, urinal, or toilet, and then stop urinating. This washes urine from the distal portion of the urethra.
  2. Correctly position a sterile urine container so the patient can void 3 to 4 oz of urine.
  3. Cap the container.
  4. Allow the patient to finish voiding.
- Note that *urinary catheterization* may be needed for patients unable to void. This procedure is not usually performed, however, because of the risk of introducing organisms into the bladder and because of patient discomfort.
- For inpatients with an *indwelling urinary catheter,* obtain a specimen by attaching a small-diameter (e.g., 25 gauge) needle to a syringe and aseptically inserting the needle into the catheter at a point distal to the sleeve leading to the balloon. Aspirate the urine, and place it in a sterile urine container. Usually the catheter tubing distal to the puncture site needs to be clamped for 15 to 30 minutes before aspiration of urine to allow urine to fill the tubing. After the specimen is withdrawn, remove the clamp.

Most modern catheter-bag systems have a rubber port through which urine can be aspirated.
- Collect specimens from infants and young children in a disposable pouch called a U bag. This bag has adhesive backing around the opening to attach to the child' pubic skin. Clean the urinary meatus before applying the bag.
- Note that *suprapubic aspiration* of urine is a safe method of obtaining urine in neonates and infants. The abdomen is prepared with an antiseptic, and a 25-gauge needle is inserted into the suprapubic area 1 inch above the symphysis pubis. Urine is aspirated into the syringe, then transferred to a sterile urine container.
- Note that in patients with a *urinary diversion* (e.g., ileal conduit), catheterization should be performed through the stoma. Urine should not be collected from the ostomy pouch.
- Indicate on the laboratory slip any medications that may affect test results.
- Urine for culture and sensitivity testing should not be taken from a bedpan or brought from home, because it will be contaminated.

After

- Transport the specimen to the laboratory immediately (within 30 minutes). If this is not possible, the specimen may be refrigerated up to 2 hours. Urine for cytomegalovirus culture, however, will be destroyed by refrigeration.
- Notify the physician of any positive results so that appropriate antibiotic therapy can be initiated.

Test Results and Clinical Significance

Urinary tract infection *Urine is a good culture medium for bacteria. In case of urinary stasis, obstruction, or incomplete emptying, bacteria infect the urine. Urinary tract infections can occur as a result of ascending infections from the urethra, especially in female patients.*

Related Tests

- Urinalysis (p. 859): Often performed before culture and sensitivity testing. The presence of WBCs, leukocyte esterase, nitrites, or bacteria indicates a urinary tract infection.

Urobilinogen

Normal Findings

Spot urine: 0.01-1.0 Ehrlich units/ml

Indications

This test is used to support the diagnosis of hemolysis. The test is not commonly performed, however, because there are better tests for that diagnosis. It is included in routine urinalysis.

Test Explanation

When RBCs are lysed within the reticuloendothelial system (spleen or liver), hemoglobin is broken down to heme and globin. The heme is catabolized to bilirubin (see p. 109 for discussion of bilirubin metabolism). The bilirubin is excreted by way of the bile ducts into the bowel. There some of the bilirubin is transformed into urobilinogen by the action of bacteria in the bowel. Most of the urobilinogen is excreted in stool; some is reabsorbed by the bowel through the enterohepatic circulation. Most of the urobilinogen is excreted from the liver back into the bowel, but some is excreted by the kidneys. If bilirubin levels are high due to overproduction, which may result from increased RBC lysis, urobilinogen levels will be elevated. If bilirubin is high due to defects in bilirubin metabolism or obstruction of excretion, urobilinogen levels will not be elevated, because excretion of bilirubin to the bowel is needed for formation of urobilinogen. It is easier to determine the cause of elevated bilirubin levels by fractionating the bilirubin into its direct and indirect components.

Interfering Factors

- pH can affect urobilinogen levels. Alkaline urine indicates higher levels; acidic urine may show lower levels.
- Cholestatic drugs may reduce urobilinogen levels.
- Antibiotics reduce intestinal flora, which in turn reduces urobilinogen levels.

Procedure and Patient Care

Before

- Explain the procedure to the patient.
- Tell the patient that no food or drink restrictions are necessary.

During

- Note that this is a spot urine test.
- Collect at least 10 ml of urine for quick, simple testing.
- Transport the specimen to the laboratory immediately to avoid oxidation of the urobilinogen.

After

- If urine cannot be evaluated soon, refrigerate the specimen.

Test Results and Clinical Significance

Increased levels

Hemolytic anemia
Pernicious anemia
Hemolysis due to drugs
Hemolysis results in increased RBC destruction. This causes more heme to be catabolized into bilirubin. Increased bilirubin is excreted into the bowel. More urobilinogen is made in the bowel. More urobilinogen is reabsorbed from the gut. More urobilinogen is excreted by the kidneys into the urine.

Hematoma
Excessive ecchymosis
RBCs in these areas break down, causing large amounts of heme to be catabolized into bilirubin. Increased bilirubin is excreted into the bowel. More urobilinogen is produced in the bowel. More urobilinogen is reabsorbed from the gut. More urobilinogen is excreted by the kidneys into the urine.

Decreased levels

Biliary obstruction
Cholestasis
No bilirubin reaches the bowel for conversion into urobilinogen. Therefore, urine levels of urobilinogen are reduced.

Related Tests

- Bilirubin (p. 822): This test should be performed with urobilinogen testing to assist in interpretation of the results.
- Urinalysis (p. 859): Urobilinogen testing is routine.

Vanillylmandelic Acid (VMA) and Catecholamines (Epinephrine, Norepinephrine, Metanephrine, Normetanephrine, Dopamine)

Normal Findings

VMA

Adult/elderly: 2-7 mg/24 hr or 10-35 μmol/24 hr (SI units)
Adolescent: 1-5 mg/24 hr
Child: 1-3 mg/24 hr
Infant: <2 mg/24 hr
Neonate: <1 mg/24 hr

Catecholamines

Epinephrine
Adult/elderly: 0.5-20.0 μg/24 hr or <275 nmol/24 hr (SI units)
Child:
0-1 yr: 0-2.5 μg/24 hr
1-2 yr: 0-3.5 μg/24 hr
2-4 yr: 0-6.0 μg/24 hr
4-7 yr: 0.2-10.0 μg/24 hr
7-10 yr: 0.5-14.0 μg/24 hr

Metanephrine
24-96 mg/24 hr

Catecholamines, cont'd

Norepinephrine
Adult/elderly: 15-80 μg/24 hr
Child:
0-1 yr: 0-10 μg/24 hr
1-2 yr: 0-17 μg/24 hr
2-4 yr: 4-29 μg/24 hr
4-7 yr: 8-45 μg/24 hr
7-10 yr: 13-65 μg/24 hr

Dopamine
Adult/elderly: 65-400 μg/24 hr
Child:
0-1 yr: 0-85 μg/24 hr
1-2 yr: 10-140 μg/24 hr
2-4 yr: 40-260 μg/24 hr
>4 yr: 65-400 μg/24 hr

Normetanephrine
75-375 μg/24 hr

Indications

This 24-hour urine test for VMA and catecholamines is primarily performed to diagnose hypertension secondary to pheochromocytoma. It is also used to detect the presence of neuroblastomas and other rare adrenal tumors.

Test Explanation

A pheochromocytoma is a tumor of the chromaffin cells within the adrenal medulla that frequently secretes abnormally high levels of epinephrine and norepinephrine. These hormones cause episodic or persistent severe hypertension by producing peripheral arterial vasoconstriction. Dopamine is the precursor of epinephrine and norepinephrine. Metanephrine and normetanephrine are catabolic products of epinephrine and norepinephrine, respectively. VMA (3-methoxy-4-hydroxymandelic acid) is the product of catabolism of both metanephrine and normetanephrine. In pheochromocytoma one or all of these substances is present in excessive quantities in a 24-hour urine collection. These hormones may be measured singularly in the urine, but the collective metabolic end product, VMA, is more easily detected because VMA concentration is much higher than any one catecholamine component.

A 24-hour urine test is preferable to a blood test, because catecholamine secretion from the tumor may be episodic and potentially could be missed at any time during the day. The urine provides the laboratory with a specimen that reflects catecholamine production over an entire day. It is best to perform testing when symptoms (hypertension) of the potential adrenal tumor are significant. At that time, catecholamine production is greatest and can be more assuredly identified.

Interfering Factors

- Increased levels of VMA may be caused by certain foods (e.g., tea, coffee, cocoa, vanilla, chocolate, cider vinegar, soda, licorice).
- Vigorous exercise, stress, and starvation may cause increased VMA levels.
- Falsely decreased levels of VMA may be caused by uremia, alkaline urine, and radiographic iodine contrast agents.
- Drugs that may cause *increased* VMA levels include caffeine, epinephrine, levodopa, lithium, and nitroglycerin.
- Drugs that may cause *decreased* VMA levels include clonidine, disulfiram (Antabuse), guanethidine, imipramine, monoamine oxidase (MAO) inhibitors, phenothiazines, and reserpine.
- Drugs that may cause *increased* catecholamine levels include alcohol (ethyl), aminophylline, caffeine, chloral hydrate, clonidine (prolonged therapy), contrast media (iodine containing), disulfiram, epinephrine, erythromycin, insulin, methenamine, methyldopa, nicotinic acid (large doses), nitroglycerin, quinidine, riboflavin, and tetracyclines.
- Drugs that may cause *decreased* catecholamine levels include guanethidine, reserpine, and salicylates.

CLINICAL PRIORITIES

- This test is primarily used to evaluate the hypertensive patient for pheochromocytoma.
- A VMA-restricted diet is essential for 2 to 3 days before and throughout the 24-hour urine collection period.
- This 24-hour urine collection requires a preservative and should be placed on ice or refrigerated.

Procedure and Patient Care

Before

- Explain the dietary restrictions and the 24-hour urine collection procedure to the patient.
- For 2 or 3 days before and throughout the 24-hour collection for VMA, place the patient on a VMA-restricted diet. Instruct the patient to avoid coffee, tea, bananas, chocolate, cocoa, licorice, citrus fruit, all foods and fluids containing vanilla, and aspirin. Obtain specific restrictions from the laboratory.
- Restrict the patient from taking antihypertensive medications, and sometimes all medications, during this period and possibly longer.

During

- Collect the 24 hour urine specimen. Use a preservative.
- Begin the 24-hour urine collection. Discard the initial specimen, and collect all urine voided by the patient during the next 24 hours. Refrigerate the specimen or keep it on ice during the collection period.
- Post the hours for the urine collection in a prominent place to avoid accidental discarding of the specimen.
- Remind the patient to void before defecating so that the urine is not contaminated by feces.
- Instruct the patient not to put toilet paper in the collection container.
- Encourage the patient to drink fluids during the 24 hours unless contraindicated for medical purposes.
- Collect the last specimen as close as possible to the end of the 24 hours. Add this urine to the container.
- Indicate the time the last specimen was collected on the laboratory slip or urine container.
- Identify and minimize factors contributing to patient stress and anxiety. Excessive physical exercise and emotion may alter catecholamine test results by causing increased secretion of epinephrine and norepinephrine.

After

- Send the specimen to the laboratory as soon as the test is completed.
- Allow the patient to have foods and drugs that were restricted in preparation for the test.

Test Results and Clinical Significance

Increased levels

Pheochromocytomas
Neuroblastomas
Ganglioneuromas
Ganglioblastomas
These tumors can produce catecholamines. VMA levels will be elevated.

Severe stress
Strenuous exercise
Acute anxiety
Catecholamines are elevated during physical (serious illness) or emotional stress or after heavy exercise. VMA levels will be elevated.

12

Radiographic Studies

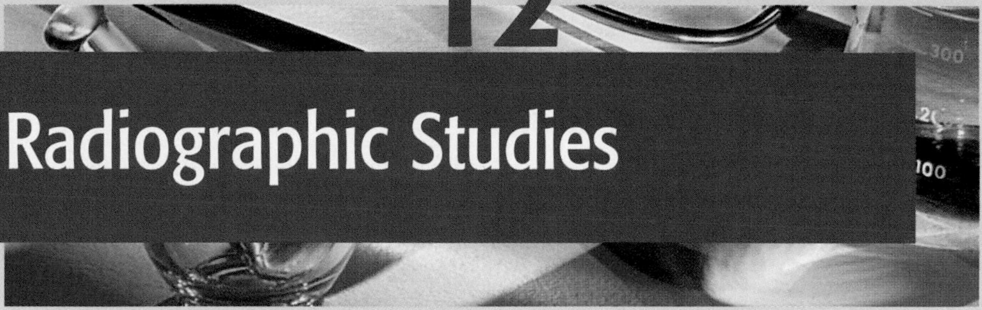

TESTS

Overview

Reason to Perform X-ray Studies

Because x-rays can penetrate human tissue, radiographic studies provide a valuable picture of body structures. These studies can be as simple as routine chest radiography or as complex as dye-enhanced cardiac catheterization. With the increasing concern about radiation exposure, the patient may want to know if the proposed benefit outweighs the risk involved.

X-ray studies are used in a wide variety of clinical conditions, such as the following:

1. To evaluate dye excretion in the urinary system (e.g., intravenous pyelography [IVP], antegrade pyelography, retrograde pyelography).
2. To evaluate arterial occlusive disease (e.g., arteriography of the kidney, adrenal glands, or cerebrum).
3. To evaluate a joint after injection of a radiopaque substance (arthrography).
4. To evaluate the gastrointestinal tract with barium contrast medium (e.g., barium enema, upper gastrointestinal series).
5. To evaluate bone disorders such as fractures, infections, and arthritis (long bone x-ray films).
6. To evaluate the tracheobronchial tree (bronchography).
7. To visualize the heart chambers, arteries, and great vessels (cardiac catheterization).
8. To evaluate the pulmonary and cardiac systems (chest radiography).
9. To guide needles for biopsy of tumors and aspiration of fluid.
10. To evaluate abdominal organs (computed tomography [CT] of the abdomen).
11. To provide an accurate clinical picture of the liver (CT portogram).
12. To determine patency of the fallopian tubes (hysterosalpingography).
13. To evaluate abdominal pain or trauma (kidneys, ureter, and bladder [KUB] or obstruction series).
14. To detect breast cancer (mammography).
15. To diagnose a pulmonary embolus (pulmonary angiography).

Principles of Radiology

X-ray films are radiographs of body structures and look like negatives of photographs. Radiography is based on the ability of x-rays to penetrate tissues and organs differently according to tissue density. X-rays are generated by a machine that passes a high-voltage electrical current through a tungsten filter in a vacuum tube (x-ray tube). As the x-ray passes through body tissues, images are formed on photographic film positioned on the other side of the body. Images are produced in varying degrees of dark and light, according to the amount of x-rays that penetrate the tissues. The greater the amount of energy absorbed, the less x-rays reach the film and the whiter the image appears on the film. For example, bones appear white (radiopaque) because the x-rays cannot penetrate bone to reach the film. When bones are fractured, the break is visible as a black (radiolucent) line. Because patients with osteoporosis have less calcium in their bones, the bones appear gray and porous on x-ray films. Because x-rays can easily penetrate air, areas filled with air or gas (e.g., lungs, bowel) appear black or very dark on x-ray films. Muscles, blood, organs, and other tissues in the body appear as various shades of gray because they are denser than air but not so dense as bone.

By orienting the radiographic machine at different angles in relation to the body or a body part, different views (projections) can be obtained. The two basic views are anteroposterior (AP), in which the x-rays pass through the front of the body (anterior) to the back (posterior), and lateral, in which the x-rays pass through the body from the side. For posteroanterior (PA) views, the x-rays pass through the back of the body to the front. Oblique views are obtained when the x-rays pass through the body at different angles according to how the patient is positioned.

Some of the many types of x-ray procedures include the following.

Plain Radiography

Plain radiography is performed without contrast material or other augmentation techniques. This procedure is used for routine examination of areas such as the chest, skull, abdomen, and bones.

Fluoroscopy

In this radiologic procedure, x-rays pass through the body to a fluorescent viewing screen that is coated with calcium tungstate. The radiologist can not only view the body organs but can also observe their motion. For example, while a patient swallows barium, its flow through the upper gastrointestinal tract can be followed, or after administration of a barium enema, the flow of barium through the colon can be observed. Fluoroscopy is used in angiography procedures to guide the catheter to its desired position (e.g., through the heart during cardiac catheterization). Single films (spot films) can be obtained for a permanent record of findings. Videotapes of fluoroscopic procedures (cineradiography) can provide a record of movement for study at a later time. Tapes can be viewed in slow motion to aid in determining abnormal function. The major disadvantage of fluoroscopy is that it exposes the patient to more radiation than standard x-ray procedures do.

Tomography

In tomography, a sequence of x-ray films is obtained, each representing a section ("slice") of tissue at a different level. Usually the slices are 0.5 to 1.0 cm apart throughout the organ being studied. Tomography permits examination of a single layer of tissue that would otherwise be obscured from surrounding tissue on an ordinary film.

For tomography, the x-ray tube and film cassette are rapidly moved in opposite directions while the x-ray film is obtained. This technique effectively blurs all the tissues except in the plane or slice being studied. Indications for tomography have greatly decreased since the advent of CT. In CT, computers re-create a three-dimensional, cross-sectional view of body structures after obtaining x-ray information from the entire circumference of the body.

The CT scan results from passing x-rays through the body organs at many angles through 360°. The variation in density of each tissue allows for variable penetration of the x-rays. Each degree of density is given a numeric value called a *density coefficient,* which is digitally computed into a shade of gray. An image is then displayed on a cathode ray tube as thousands of dots in various shades of gray. The image can be enhanced by repeating the CT procedure after intravenous administration of iodine-containing contrast dye. The images can be recorded on film.

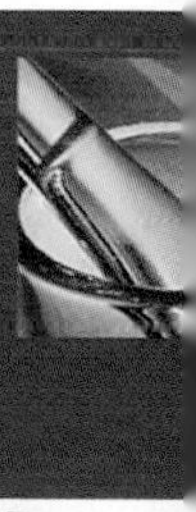
12 RADIOGRAPHIC STUDIES

Box 12-1 Clinical priorities associated with use of barium sulfate

- Barium may interfere with subsequent x-ray studies (e.g., IVP, CT). Tests requiring the use of barium should be performed after other x-ray studies.
- Cathartics are required before tests that require barium, to prevent the possibility of false-positive findings due to food in the bowel.
- Cathartics should always be administered after tests that require barium, to diminish the possibility of barium or fecal impaction.
- The patient should observe the color of stool to ensure that all barium (white) has been eliminated from the intestinal tract.
- Barium should not be administered in patients with acute colitis, especially ulcerative colitis, because it can precipitate development of toxic megacolon.
- Barium should not be administered if gastrointestinal perforation is suspected. Extravasation of barium from the GI tract may be associated with multiple and recurrent abdominal abscesses.

Contrast Studies

In some areas of the body, a contrast agent is necessary to provide better visualization of organs being studied. Contrast material can be administered orally, rectally, intravenously, percutaneously, by inhalation, or through urinary catheterization. For angiography, contrast agent is injected into a blood vessel.

The most commonly used contrast media are barium sulfate, for gastrointestinal studies (Box 12-1); organic iodine, for vascular and renal studies; and iodized oils, for myelography. These substances are radiopaque (i.e., they block the passage of x-rays) and thus provide excellent contrast to bodily structures. Air can also be used as a contrast medium, although is much less commonly used lately.

In addition to radiation risks associated with all radiology procedures, contrast studies pose additional potential complications. For example, iodinated dyes may cause a severe allergic reaction, and barium sulfate may cause constipation and bowel impaction.

Xeroradiography

Xeroradiography uses a photoelectric developing process other than the photochemical process of conventional x-ray studies. The images are printed on paper much like that of an office copier. This procedure provides a "positive" picture rather than the "negative" x-ray film. This procedure is used primarily for soft tissue evaluation, such as radiography of the breast.

Digital Subtraction Angiography

Digital subtraction angiography is a type of computerized fluoroscopy in which venous or arterial catheterization is performed to visualize the arteries, especially the carotid and cerebral arteries. The procedure enables small differences in x-ray absorption between an artery and the surrounding tissues to be converted to digital information and stored. It is especially useful when bone blocks visualization of the blood vessel being studied. This study is valuable for preoperative and postoperative evaluation of patients undergoing vascular and tumor surgery.

An image "mask" is made of the area of clinical interest and stored in a computer. After intravenous injection of contrast material, subsequent images are made. The computer then subtracts the preinjection mask image from the postinjection image. This removes all undesired tissue images (e.g., bone) and leaves an arterial image of high contrast. Venous injection of the dye, rather than arterial injection, averts the complications and risks associated with conventional arteriography. However, arterial injection of contrast material is more often used.

Risks of Radiation Exposure

All x-ray procedures carry the risk of exposure to radiation. In general, there are three possible types of damage to the body from radiologic procedures.

1. *Somatic effects* ultimately occur in patients exposed to the harmful agent. These may include short-term effects such as blood cell problems or long-term effects such as cancer.
2. *Genetic effects* include damage to future generations as a result of exposure of parent germ cells to a harmful agent. Depending on the type of damage to the germ cell, genetic effects can range from mild to severe (e.g., mental retardation).
3. *Fetal effects* occur as a result of exposure to a harmful agent during the embryonal or fetal stage of development. This type of damage is highly dependent on timing of the exposure with respect to gestational age. Damage can range from mild birth defects to childhood malignancies. The fetus is at greatest risk during early pregnancy, when organs are developing. Radiation exposure during later pregnancy, after development is complete and only growth is occurring, is far less risky to the fetus.

Because of the risks of radiation exposure, x-ray studies should not be performed more often than necessary. For this reason, patients should be adequately prepared for each test, to reduce the need for repeated studies. Patients should be shielded from unnecessary exposure with lead aprons and gloves. During or within 10 to 12 days after normal menses, women can safely undergo diagnostic x-ray studies. Otherwise, no women in the childbearing years should undergo x-ray examination unless a pregnancy test is performed and the results are negative. These restrictions exist to avoid exposure and subsequent injury to a fetus when a woman is unknowingly pregnant.

Contraindications

Pregnancy is a contraindication for all x-ray studies. However, sometimes the benefits of diagnostic x-ray examination outweigh the risks. In those cases, every attempt should be made to minimize exposure of the fetus to x-rays (e.g., use of a lead apron). The contraindications listed below relate to specific types of x-ray studies. Specific details relative to each type of radiographic procedure are discussed later in this chapter.

1. Iodinated dye (e.g., IVP cardiac catheterization)
   - Patients allergic to shellfish or iodinated dye (Table 12-1)
   - Patients with renal disorders, because iodinated contrast is nephrotoxic.
   - Patients who are dehydrated, because they are especially susceptible to dye-induced renal failure.
   - Patients with pheochromocytoma, because a hypertensive crisis may be precipitated by the use of iodine.
2. Arterial or venous puncture *(e.g., cardiac catheterization, angiography)*
   - Patients with a bleeding disorder, because the arterial or venous puncture site may not stop bleeding.

Table 12-1 Signs, symptoms, and treatment of iodine contrast allergy

	Minor reaction	Intermediate reaction	Severe or life-threatening reaction
Incidence	1 of 25	1 of 150	1 of 5000
Signs and symptoms	Nausea, vomiting, mild urticaria	Facial, tongue, or laryngeal edema; bronchospasm; chest pain; chills and fever	Laryngeal and pulmonary edema, hypotension, myocardial depression, cardiac arrhythmias, seizure, ventilatory failure
Treatment	Antihistamines	Antihistamines, possibly steroids, IV fluids, observation, bronchodilators	Antihistamines, steroids, IV fluids, bronchodilators, intubation and ventilation, pressors, antiseizure medications

3. *Barium (e.g., upper gastrointestinal series, barium enema)*
   - Patients with suspected perforation of the colon or upper GI tract. In these patients, meglumine diatrizoate (Gastrografin), a water-soluble contrast medium, should be used.

Interfering Factors

Factors that can obscure x-ray visualization include:

- Presence of metallic objects (e.g., hemostasis clips, jewelry).
- Barium retained from previous studies.
- Large amounts of fecal material or gas in the bowel.
- Improper positioning.
- Excessive movement.

Procedure and Patient Care

Specific procedures are presented with the discussion of each test.

Before

- Explain the procedure to the patient. Cooperation is necessary, because the patient must lie still during the procedure.
- Obtain informed consent if required by the institution.
- Assess the patient for allergy to iodine or shellfish if iodinated dye will be used.
- Instruct the patient to remove all jewelry from the area to be imaged.
- Inform the patient of any fasting requirements.
- Depending on the type of test, the patient may be given nothing orally for 2 to 8 hours before testing.
- Mark the site of the patient's peripheral pulses with a pen before arterial catheterization, to permit assessment of the peripheral pulses after the procedure.
- Ensure that the appropriate coagulation studies have been performed and that the results are normal.
- For cerebral angiography, perform a baseline neurologic assessment for comparison with subsequent assessments.

- Administer sedation if indicated.
- Assist the patient with bowel preparation if indicated. For example, a barium contrast study necessitates bowel preparation and, possibly, cleansing enemas.

During

- Instruct the patient to remain motionless throughout the testing. Sometimes patients are asked to hold their breath for certain periods of time while images are being taken.

After

- If an iodine contrast dye has been used, assist the patient to drink fluids to avoid dye-induced renal failure and to promote dye excretion.
- If barium contrast was used, laxatives may be indicated to prevent constipation and bowel obstruction.
- Monitor the patient's vital signs. Changes may be noted due to medications used during the tests or from complications such as bleeding.
- Evaluate the patient for delayed reaction to dyes. These may occur within 2 to 6 hours after the test.

Potential Complications

- Allergic reaction to iodinated dye. Allergic reactions can include flushing, itching, urticaria, and even severe life-threatening anaphylaxis (evidenced by respiratory distress, decreased blood pressure, or shock). In the unusual event of anaphylaxis, diphenhydramine (Benadryl), steroids, and epinephrine are included in resuscitative efforts. Oxygen and endotracheal equipment should be on hand for immediate use.
- Catheter-induced embolic stroke (cerebral vascular accident, myocardial infarction).
- Complications associated with the catheter insertion, such as arterial thrombosis, embolism, or pseudoaneurysm.
- Infection at the catheter insertion site.
- Renal failure, especially in elderly patients with chronic dehydration or mild renal failure. Adequate hydration may reduce the likelihood of this complication.

Reporting of Results

Radiographs are carefully reviewed and the findings reported by the radiologist. Results may be discussed with the patient at the time of testing or within a few days.

Adrenal Venography

Normal Findings

Normal adrenal veins and normal adrenal vein hormone assay

Indications

With adrenal venography, adrenal disease can be localized in preparation of proposed surgical extirpation.

Test Explanation

Adrenal venography is performed to obtain blood samples from the adrenal veins and to detect adrenal disease. Once the veins are identified, a catheter can be placed in them and blood selectively obtained from each adrenal vein.

In patients with Cushing's syndrome, the blood is analyzed for plasma cortisol. If the plasma cortisol level in the blood obtained from one side is much higher than that of the other, a unilateral adrenal tumor is causing the Cushing's syndrome. If plasma cortisol levels are bilaterally elevated, it can be concluded that the Cushing's syndrome is caused by bilateral adrenal hyperplasia.

In patients with a pheochromocytoma, adrenal venous blood is analyzed for catecholamines. If the catecholamine level on one side is much higher than that on the other, a unilateral pheochromocytoma exists on the side with the elevated levels. If the blood catecholamine levels on both sides are equally elevated, bilateral adrenal pheochromocytoma probably exists. If the adrenal venous blood levels are not elevated on either side in a patient with elevated peripheral blood catecholamine levels, the pheochromocytoma exists outside the adrenal gland (i.e., extra-adrenal pheochromocytoma).

The venous blood also can be evaluated for aldosterone, androgens, and other substances. This procedure is usually performed by an angiographer (radiologist) in approximately 1 hour. The only discomfort is the groin puncture necessary for venous access.

Contraindications

- Allergy to shellfish or iodinated dye
- Bleeding disorders, because bleeding at the venous puncture site (usually in the groin) may be difficult to stop

Potential Complications

- Allergic reaction to iodinated dye
  Allergic reactions may vary from mild flushing, itching, and urticaria to severe, life-threatening anaphylaxis, (evidenced by respiratory distress, decreased blood pressure, or shock). In the unusual event of anaphylaxis, the patient is given diphenhydramine (Benadryl), steroids, and epinephrine. Oxygen and endotracheal equipment should be on hand for immediate use.
- Adrenal hemorrhage or necrosis caused by the pressure of dye injection, which may cause Addison's disease (adrenal insufficiency)
- Cellulitis
- Thrombophlebitis
- Bacteremia

Procedure and Patient Care

Before

- Explain the procedure to the patient.
- Ensure that written, informed consent has been obtained.
- Assess the patient for allergy to iodinated dye. Inform the radiologist if an allergy to

iodinated contrast is suspected. The radiologist may prescribe a diphenhydramine-steroid preparation, to be administered before testing. Usually, hypoallergenic non-ionic contrast material is used for the test.

- Administer propranolol (Inderal), a β-adrenergic blocker, and phenoxybenzamine (Dibenzyline), an α-adrenergic blocker, in patients with suspected pheochromocytoma, to prevent a potentially fatal catecholamine-induced hypertensive episode.

During

- Bring the fasting patient to the angiography laboratory (usually in the radiology department).
- Place the patient in the supine position on the x-ray table.
- Note the following procedural steps:
  1. The patient's groin is prepared and draped in a sterile manner.
  2. After the venipuncture site is locally anesthetized, the femoral vein is catheterized.
  3. The catheter is passed into the adrenal vein.
  4. Dye is injected to visualize the adrenal veins and to ensure that the catheter is in the adrenal vein.
  5. Blood is obtained and sent to the chemistry laboratory for assays.

After

- Evaluate the patient's vital signs frequently for signs of bleeding or hemorrhage.
- Assess the patient with a suspected pheochromocytoma for signs and symptoms of a hypertensive episode. If such an episode occurs, notify the physician immediately to obtain an order for appropriate α- and β-adrenergic blocking agents.
- Assess the groin site for redness, pain, swelling, and bleeding with each vital sign check.
- Apply cold compresses to the puncture site if needed to reduce discomfort or swelling.

Home Care Responsibilities

- After the test, assess the patient for signs of bleeding (e.g., increased pulse, decreased blood pressure).
- If there is a possibility of pheochromocytoma, carefully monitor the blood pressure for a hypertensive episode.
- Assess the groin for redness, swelling, pain, or bleeding.

Test Results and Clinical Significance

Unilateral adrenal tumor *Disease is limited to one side, indicating a tumor.*
Bilateral adrenal hyperplasia *Disease exists on both sides.*

Unilateral pheochromocytoma
Bilateral pheochromocytoma
Extra-adrenal pheochromocytoma

If the catecholamine level is elevated on one side and not the other, unilateral pheochromocytoma is present. If elevated on both sides, bilateral pheochromocytomas are present. If catecholamine levels are not elevated on either side, yet elevated catecholamine levels are noted in the peripheral blood, the site of the pheochromocytoma is outside the adrenal glands. This is important information for the endocrine surgeon to be aware of preoperatively.

Related Tests

- Urine for catecholamines (p. 877): This test is used to identify pheochromocytoma in patients with aggressive hypertension.

Antegrade Pyelography

Normal Findings Normal outline, size, and position of the ureters and bladder

Indications

This procedure provides visualization of the ureters when they cannot be demonstrated with contrast-enhanced radiography (e.g., IVP, retrograde pyelography).

Test Explanation

Occasionally a kidney with poor dye uptake at IVP cannot be adequately examined by means of retrograde pyelography either, because the ureter is impassable from below (e.g., obstructed) or a cystoscopic procedure is clinically contraindicated. In such cases, the upper collecting system may be visualized at antegrade pyelography, with injection of contrast material through percutaneous needle puncture of the renal pelvis or calyx. This test is usually performed when attempts at retrograde catheterization (retrograde pyelography) have been unsuccessful. Antegrade pyelography is specifically indicated in the following conditions:

1. Localization of ureteral obstruction caused by a stricture, nonopaque ureteral stone, or tumor.
2. Evaluation of ureteral obstruction after a urinary diversion procedure.
3. Hydronephrosis in a child with poor IVP dye uptake, to identify ureteropelvic and ureterovesical obstruction.

This test is performed by a radiologist or urologist in less than 1 hour. The only discomfort is local anesthesia, used to numb the skin overlying the pelvis.

Potential Complications

- Hemorrhage at the needle puncture site, because the kidney is highly vascular.
- Allergic reaction to iodinated dye, which rarely occurs because the dye is not administered intravenously.

Procedure and Patient Care

Before

- Explain the procedure to the patient. Allay the patient's fears, and allow time for the patient to verbalize concerns.
- Obtain informed consent.
- Check for allergy to iodine or shellfish, and inform the physician.

During

- Place the patient in a prone position.
- Note the following procedural steps:
  1. The renal pelvis is localized by means of ultrasound or fluoroscopy. A dilated collecting system is more easily identified than is a normal collecting system.
  2. Skin overlying the desired site is marked and antiseptically prepared.
  3. With the patient under local anesthesia, the skin is incised and a needle with a stylet is inserted toward the renal pelvis.
  4. While the patient suspends respiration, a smaller, thin-walled needle with a stylet is advanced through the needle into the lumen of the renal pelvis. Flexible tubing connects the syringe to the needle to aspirate urine.
  5. Contrast material is injected to outline the upper collection system to the point of obstruction below.
  6. X ray films in PA, oblique, and AP views are obtained.

After

- Apply a small pressure dressing to the incision site.
- Assess the incision site for bleeding.
- Because the kidney is highly vascular, check vital signs as ordered to detect any evidence of bleeding.
- Note that antibiotic drugs are often recommended for several days to avoid infection, which may be caused by instrumentation at a level above the ureteral obstruction.
- Evaluate for signs of allergic reaction to dye (e.g., dyspnea, rash, tachycardia, hives).

Home Care Responsibilities

- Check the incision site for bleeding.
- Evaluate vital signs for evidence of bleeding (e.g., increased pulse, decreased blood pressure).
- Antibiotics may be ordered prophylactically after the procedure to avoid infection.

Test Results and Clinical Significance

Ureteral stone
Ureteral obstruction from tumor or adhesions
Ureteropelvic or ureterovesical obstruction from a stone, tumor, or scarring
Congenital or acquired hydronephrosis
These conditions are evident as complete obstruction of contrast medium in the ureter.

Related Tests

- Retrograde pyelography (p. 981): The ureters are visualized by filling them with contrast medium from below (during cystoscopy [p. 528]).
- Intravenous pyelography (p. 953): The ureters are visualized with contrast medium injected intravenously and concentrated in the kidney. This test also allows visualization of the kidneys.

Arteriography (Angiography; Renal, Adrenal, Cerebral, and Lower Extremity Arteriography)

Normal Findings Normal arterial vasculature

Indications

Arteriography of the adrenal glands, kidneys, brain, and lower extremity is used to evaluate arterial occlusive disease of these organs, and is helpful in evaluation of suspected neoplasms arising from these organs. Arteriography provides the vascular surgeon with an accurate picture of the vascular anatomy of these structures. This is especially important in artero-occlusive disease involving the arteries to these organs.

Test Explanation

With the injection of radiopaque contrast material into arteries, blood vessels can be visualized to determine arterial anatomy, vascular disease, or neoplasms. With a catheter usually placed through the femoral and into the desired artery, radiopaque contrast material is rapidly injected while x-ray films are obtained. Blood flow dynamics, abnormal blood vessels, vascular anomalies, normal and abnormal vascular anatomy, and tumors can be seen.

Digital subtraction angiography (DSA) allows bony structures to be obliterated from the picture. DSA is a sophisticated type of computerized fluoroscopy that, when used with arterial angiography, enables better visualization of the arteries, especially the carotid and cerebral arteries. DSA enables small differences in x-ray absorption between an artery and the surrounding tissues to be converted to digital information and stored. It is especially useful when adjacent bone inhibits visualization of the blood vessel to be evaluated. For DSA, an image (mask) is made of the area of clinical interest and stored in the computer program. After intra-arterial injection of contrast material, subsequent images are made. The computer then subtracts the preinjection mask image from the postinjection image. This removes all the undesired images (e.g., bone) and leaves the arterial image of high contrast and quality.

While nearly all major blood vessels can be visualized through the technique of arteriography, the kidneys, adrenal glands, brain, and abdominal aorta (with lower extremities) are most usually visualized. Coronary arteriography is described under cardiac catheterization (p. 917).

Renal angiography permits evaluation of blood flow dynamics, demonstration of ab-

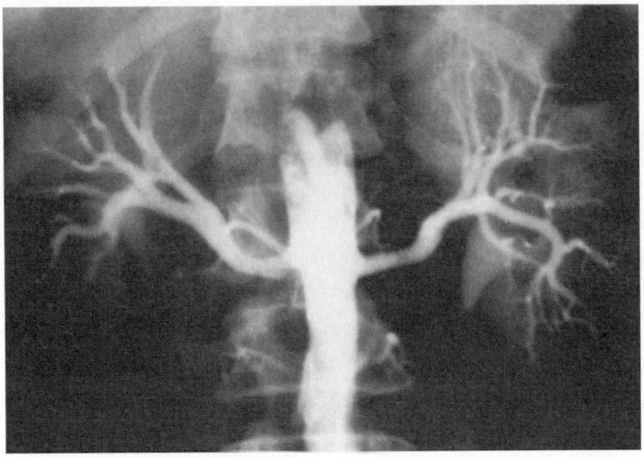

Figure 12-1 Renal arteriogram.

normal blood vessels, and differentiation of a vascular renal cyst from hypervascular renal cancers (Figure 12-1). Arteriosclerotic narrowing (stenosis) of the renal artery is best demonstrated with this study. The angiographic location of the stenotic area is helpful for the vascular surgeon considering repair. Complete transection of the renal artery by blunt or penetrating trauma can also be seen as total vascular obstruction. Highly vascular renal cancers can produce a "blush" of contrast material during angiography.

The adrenal gland and its arterial system can also be visualized by *adrenal arteriography*. Both benign and malignant tumors of the adrenal gland, as well as bilateral adrenal hyperplasia, can be detected easily with this technique.

Cerebral angiography provides radiographic visualization of the cerebral vascular system with the injection of radiopaque dye into the carotid or vertebral arteries (Figure 12-2). With this procedure, abnormalities of the cerebral circulation (e.g., aneurysms, occlusions, stenosis, arteriovenous malformations) can be identified. A vascular tumor is seen as a mass containing small, abnormal blood vessels. A nonvascular tumor, abscess, or hematoma appears as a mass that distorts the normal vascular contour.

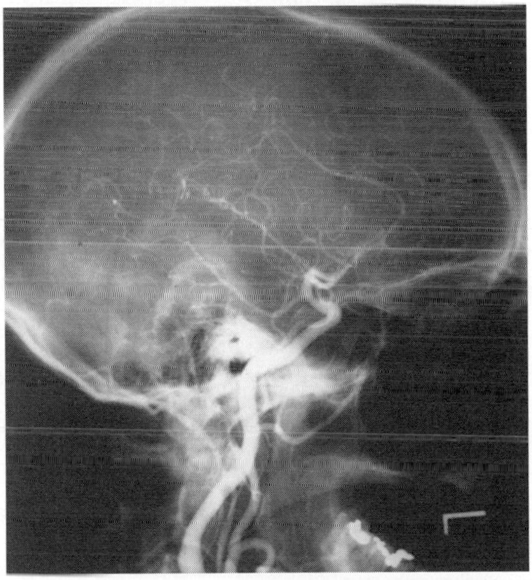

Figure 12-2 Carotid angiogram.

Lower extremity arteriography enables accurate identification and location of occlusions within the abdominal aorta and lower extremity arteries. After the catheter is placed in the aorta or more selectively into the femoral artery, radiopaque dye is injected. X-ray films are obtained in timed sequence to allow radiographic visualization of the arterial system of the lower extremities. Total or near-total occlusion of the flow of dye is seen in arteriosclerotic vascular occlusive disease. Emboli are seen as total occlusions of the artery. Arterial traumas such as lacerations or intimal tears (laceration of the arterial inner lining) likewise appear as total or near-total obstruction of the flow of dye. Aneurysmal dilatation of the aorta or its branches also can be seen. Unusual arterial disorders (e.g., thromboangiitis obliterans [Buerger's disease], fibromuscular dysplasia) demonstrate classic arterial "beading," which is pathognomonic.

Lower extremity arteriography is usually performed electively in patients with symptoms and signs of peripheral vascular disease. Emergency arteriography, however, is needed when the blood flow to an extremity has ceased suddenly. Immediate surgical therapy is needed and is most effective when the surgeon has knowledge of the cause and location of sudden occlusion. This knowledge can be obtained only with arteriography.

Arterial vascular balloon dilation can be performed if a short-segment arterial stenosis is identified. In these instances, the wire is left in place and a balloon catheter is inserted over it. The dilating balloon is inflated, and the arteriosclerotic plaque is gently and persistently dislodged.

This procedure is usually performed by an angiographer (radiologist) in approximately 1 to 2 hours. During the dye injection, remind the patient that an intense, burning flush may be felt throughout the body, but lasts only a few seconds. The only discomfort is in the area of the groin puncture necessary for arterial access, and discomfort from lying on a hard x-ray table for a long time.

Age-related concerns

- The elderly patient with chronic dehydration or who has mildly decreased renal function is at high risk for dye-induced renal failure.
- The post-procedure urinary output in the elderly patient needs to be carefully monitored. Fluids should be encouraged.

Contraindications

- Patients allergic to shellfish or iodinated dye
- Patients who are uncooperative or agitated
- Patients who are pregnant
- Patients with renal disorders, because iodinated contrast is nephrotoxic
- Patients with a propensity for bleeding, because the arterial puncture site may not stop bleeding
- Patients with unstable cardiac disorders
- Patients with dehydration, because they are especially susceptible to dye-induced renal failure

Potential Complications

- Allergic reaction to iodinated dye

  Allergic reactions may vary from mild flushing, itching, and urticaria to severe, life-threatening anaphylaxis, evidenced by respiratory distress, drop in blood pressure, and shock. In the unusual event of anaphylaxis, diphenhydramine (Benadryl), steroids, and epinephrine are added to routine resuscitative efforts. Oxygen and endotracheal equipment should be on hand for immediate use.

- Hemorrhage from the arterial puncture site used for arterial access
- Arterial embolism from dislodgement of arteriosclerotic plaque
- Soft tissue infection around the puncture site
- Renal failure, especially in elderly patients with chronic dehydration or mild renal failure
- Dissection of the intimal lining of the artery causing complete or partial arterial occlusion
- Development of pseudoaneurysm as a result of failure of the puncture site to seal
- Hypertensive crisis
  With adrenal angiography, fatal hypertensive crisis may occur in patients with pheochromocytoma. Propranolol (Inderal), a β-adrenergic blocker, and phenoxybenzamine (Dibenzyline), an α-adrenergic blocker, are given for several days before the study to avert precipitation of a malignant hypertensive episode.
- In adrenal angiography, hemorrhage of the adrenal gland, which may lead to adrenal insufficiency

✓ CLINICAL PRIORITIES

- Assess for allergies to iodinated dye.
- Perform a baseline assessment of the patient's peripheral pulses before arterial catheterization.
- Be certain that coagulation studies (PT, PTT, bleeding time) are normal before the test, because of the risk of bleeding.
- After the test, the patient is kept on bed rest for approximately 8 hours to allow complete sealing of the arterial puncture.

Procedure and Patient Care

Before

- Explain the procedure to the patient. Allay any fears, and allow the patient to verbalize concerns.
- Ensure that written, informed consent for this procedure is in the patient's chart.
- Inform the patient that a warm flush may be felt when the dye is injected.
- Assess the possibility of allergy to iodinated dye. Inform the radiologist if an allergy to iodinated contrast is suspected. The radiologist may prescribe diphenhydramine (Benadryl) and steroid preparation to be administered before the test. Usually, hypoallergenic nonionic contrast agent is used during the test.
- Determine whether the patient has been taking anticoagulants.
- The patient is given nothing orally for 2 to 8 hours before testing.
- Mark the site of the patient's peripheral pulses with a pen before arterial catheterization, to permit assessment of the peripheral pulses after the procedure.
- If the patient does not have peripheral pulses before arteriography, document that fact so that arterial occlusion will not be suspected at the postangiographic assessment.
- Administer preprocedural medications as ordered.
- If a pheochromocytoma is suspected, administer propranolol and phenoxybenzamine as ordered, to prevent a potentially fatal hypertensive episode.

- Ensure that the appropriate coagulation studies have been performed and that the results are normal.
- For cerebral angiography, perform a baseline neurologic assessment for comparison with subsequent assessment, potentially to diagnose stroke that may be precipitated by the study.
- Remove all valuables and dental prostheses.
- Instruct the patient to void before the study, because iodinated dye can act as an osmotic diuretic.
- Inform the patient that bladder distention may cause some discomfort during the study.

During

- Note the following procedural steps:
  1. The patient may be sedated before being taken to the angiography room, which is usually within the radiology department.
  2. The patient is placed on the x-ray table in supine position (see Figure 12-3).
  3. If the femoral artery is to be used, the groin is shaved, prepared, and draped in a sterile manner.
  4. The femoral artery is cannulated, and a wire is threaded up the artery and into or near the opening of the artery to be examined (Figure 12-4).
  5. A catheter is placed over that wire. The wire and catheter are both placed under fluoroscopic visualization. Because the catheter and wire have curled tips, both can be manipulated directly into the artery to be studied. The wire is removed.
  6. Iodinated contrast material is injected through the catheter with an automated injector at a preset, controlled rate, over several seconds.
  7. Serial x-ray films are obtained in timed sequence to show the arterial injection, and subsequent x-ray films are taken to show the venous phase of the injection.

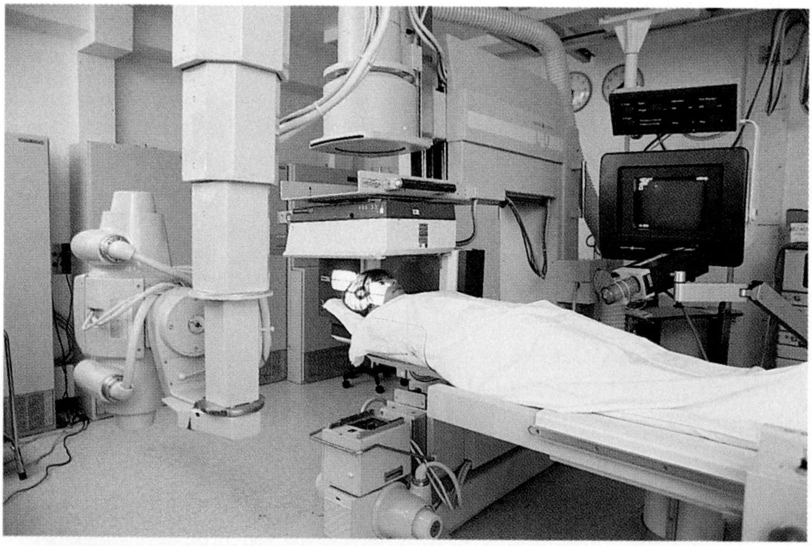

Figure 12-3 Positioning of patient for cerebral angiography.

- During adrenal angiography, monitor blood pressure for evidence of malignant hypertensive storm.

After

- X-ray studies are completed, the catheter is removed, and a pressure dressing is applied to the puncture site.
- Monitor the patient's vital signs for indications of hemorrhage.
- Assess the peripheral arterial pulse in the extremity used for vascular access and compare it with the preprocedural baseline values.
- If cerebral arteriography was performed, perform a neurologic assessment for any signs of catheter-induced embolic stroke syndrome.
- Observe the arterial puncture site frequently for signs of bleeding or hematoma.
- Maintain pressure at the puncture site with a 1- to 2-pound sand bag or IV bag.
- Keep the patient on bed rest for about 8 hours after the procedure to allow complete sealing of the arterial puncture site.
- Assess the patient's extremities for signs of loss of blood supply (e.g., loss of pulses, numbness, pallor, tingling, pain, loss of sensory or motor function).
- Note and compare the color and temperature of the extremity with that of the uninvolved extremity.
- Administer mild analgesics for minor discomfort at the arterial puncture site.
- Notify the physician if the patient has severe, continuous pain.
- Have the patient drink fluids to prevent dehydration caused by the diuretic action of the dye.
- Evaluate the patient for delayed allergic reaction to the dye (dyspnea, rash, tachycardia, hives). This usually occurs within 2 to 6 hours after the test.

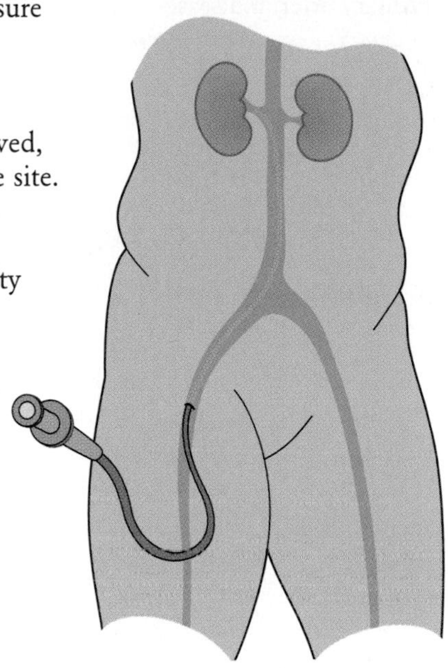

Figure 12-4 Catheter insertion for renal angiography.

Test Results and Clinical Significance

Adrenal angiography

Pheochromocytoma
Adrenal adenoma
Adrenal carcinoma
These are evident as avascular filling defects within the gland. Pheochromocytomas are epinephrine- or norepinephrine-producing tumors that can precipitate a hypertensive crisis during angiography.

Bilateral adrenal hyperplasia *Adrenal glands are usually larger and more vascular.*

Arteriography of lower extremity

Arteriosclerotic occlusion *This is evident as a segment of narrowing in an otherwise normal vessel.*

Embolus occlusion *An embolus may come from the heart or an abdominal aortic aneurysm. Complete interruption in the flow of dye within the blood vessel is seen.*

Primary arterial diseases (e.g., fibromuscular dysplasia, Buerger's disease) *Often arteriograms demonstrate findings that are classic for the particular disease.*

Aneurysm *This is a saccular dilation of a blood vessel. It can rupture or throw off emboli.*

Aberrant arterial anatomy *Variations in arterial anatomy are well known and usually well delineated by arteriography.*

Tumor neovascularity *Vascular tumors often have classic findings of arteriovenous shunting, which causes blood to pool in these areas.*

Neoplastic arterial compression *Nonvascular tumors compress or distort the normal vasculature.*

Brain arteriography

Vascular aneurysm
Vascular occlusion or stenosis
Vascular arteriovenous malformations
Cerebral vascular thrombosis
Arteriographic findings are similar to those described for the lower extremities.

Tumor
Abscess
Hematoma
These abnormalities distort the normal arterial anatomy.

Kidney arteriography

Anatomic aberrant blood vessels *Anatomic abnormalities involving the kidneys are common.*

Renal cyst *This is an avascular mass in a kidney.*

Renal solid tumor *Most renal cell carcinomas are very vascular.*

Atherosclerotic narrowing of the renal arteries *Stenosis or total occlusion of the renal arteries causes decreased blood flow to the kidneys. Vasopressin is stimulated through the angiotensin system (p. 381). Hypertension results.*

Arthrography (Arthrogram)

Normal Findings

Normal bursae, menisci, ligaments, and articular cartilage of the joint

Indications

Arthrography affords radiographic visualization of a joint after injection of a radiopaque substance, air, or both into the joint cavity to outline the soft tissue structures not normally seen on routine x-ray films.

Test Explanation

Arthrography is usually performed on the knee and shoulder joints, but can also be performed on other joints, such as the ankles, hips, wrists, or temporomandibular joint.

Bones, menisci, cartilage, and ligaments are clearly visualized with this procedure. Joint derangement and synovial cysts are diagnosed with arthrography. This procedure is usually performed in patients with persistent, unexplained joint pain, swelling, or dysfunction.

The physician performs this procedure in approximately 30 minutes. Pressure or a tingling sensation may be felt as the contrast medium is injected, along with some discomfort in the joint.

Contraindications

- Pregnancy
- Active arthritis, because the injection may worsen the arthritis
- Joint infection, because the injection may worsen or spread the infection

Potential Complications

- Infection at the puncture site
- Allergic reaction to iodinated dye; rare, because the dye is not administered intravenously

Procedure and Patient Care

Before

- Explain the procedure to the patient.
- Obtain informed consent if required by the institution.
- Tell the patient that no fasting or sedation is required.

During

- Place the patient supine on the examining table.
- Note the following procedural steps:
  1. The skin overlying the joint is aseptically cleansed and anesthetized.
  2. A needle is inserted into the joint space.
  3. Joint effusion fluid is aspirated to minimize dilution of the contrast material, which could diminish the quality of the x-ray films.
  4. With the needle still in place the aspirating syringe is removed, and a syringe containing dye is inserted.
  5. The contrast agent is injected.
  6. The needle is removed, the joint is manipulated to help distribute the contrast material.
  7. The patient may be asked to walk several steps or to perform range-of-motion exercise pertinent to the joint.
  8. X-ray films are obtained with the joint held in various positions. Traction may be applied to separate the bones of the joint to allow better visualization of the space and structures within.

After

- Assess the joint for swelling. Apply ice if necessary.
- Administer a mild analgesic (e.g., aspirin, acetaminophen) if the patient has mild discomfort.

- Report any increase in pain or swelling to the physician.
- Inform the patient that crepitant noises (like crackling tissue paper) in the joint may be heard after the test. They are caused by the air injected into the joint during the procedure, and usually disappear in 1 to 2 days.

Test Results and Clinical Significance

Joint derangement *Many significant joint injuries (e.g., dislocations, subluxations, cartilaginous tears) are recognized by means of arthrography.*
Baker's cyst *This is seen as a collection of dye posterior to the knee and represents herniation of the joint capsule.*
Arthritis *Characteristic findings of degenerative and rheumatoid arthritis are visualized with arthrography.*
Fractured knee meniscus *This is seen as a radiopaque line in the meniscus.*
Synovial tumor *This is evident as a mass protruding into or extending out of the joint space.*
Synovitis
Muscle or tendon tears (rotator cuff injuries)
Cartilaginous diseases (e.g., chondromalacia)
Ligamentous injury
These common injuries have characteristic arthrographic findings, depending on the joint being studied.

Related Tests

- MRI of the joint space (p. 1009): Allows better visualization of the joint space and other joint structures.

Barium Enema (BE, Lower GI Series)

Normal Findings

Normal filling, contour, and patency of the colon
Normal filling of the appendix and terminal ileum

Indications

Lower GI barium contrast study (BE) enables visualization of the colon, distal small bowel, and occasionally the appendix. It is indicated in patients with the following conditions:

Abdominal pain (but contraindicated in patients with acute abdominal pain)
Obvious or occult blood in the stools
Inflammatory bowel disease
Suspected cancer (bowel or abdominal)
Abnormal results of an obstruction series of radiographs (see p. 972), indicating volvulus or colon obstruction

Test Explanation

The BE study consists of a series of x-ray films that visualize the colon. It is used to demonstrate the presence and location of polyps, tumors, and diverticula. Anatomic abnormalities (e.g., malrotation) also can be detected. Therapeutically, the BE may be used to reduce nonstrangulated ileocolic intussusception in children. Bleeding from diverticula can cease after a BE.

The BE is occasionally used to assess filling of the appendix. When clinical findings suggest possible appendicitis, failure of the appendix to fill with barium may support the diagnosis. Although the colon is the main organ evaluated with a BE, reflux of barium into the terminal ileum also allows adequate visualization of the distal portion of the small intestine. Diseases that affect the terminal ileum, especially Crohn's disease (regional enteritis), can be identified. Inflammatory bowel disease and fistulas involving the colon can be demonstrated with BE.

In many cases, air is insufflated into the colon after instillation of barium. This provides air contrast to the barium. With air contrast, the colonic mucosa can be much more accurately visualized. This is called an *air contrast barium enema (ACBE) or double-contrast barium enema,* and is used especially when small polyps are suspected. The accuracy of the BE to detect small colonic tumors is approximately 60%, whereas the accuracy of the ACBE to detect small colonic tumors exceeds 85% (Figure 12-5).

This test is usually performed in the radiology department by a radiologist in approximately 45 minutes. Abdominal bloating and rectal pressure occur during instillation of barium.

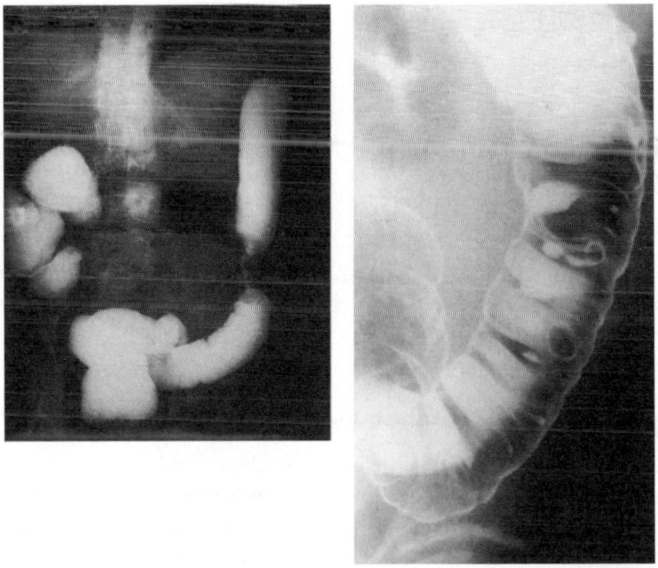

Figure 12-5 **A,** Single-contrast barium study illustrates obstructing circumferential carcinoma of the sigmoid colon. **B,** Double-contrast barium study shows multiple colonic diverticula. Diverticula on dependent surfaces are barium-filled; diverticula on nondependent surfaces are seen as ring shadows.

Contraindications

- Suspected perforation of the colon
  In these patients, diatrizoate (Gastrografin), a water-soluble contrast medium, is used. No bowel preparation is performed.
- Patients who are unable to cooperate
  This test requires the patient to hold the barium in the rectum and colon, which is especially difficult for elderly patients.
- Megacolon
  Barium may worsen this condition.

Potential Complications

- Colonic perforation, especially when the colon is weakened by inflammation, tumor, or infection
- Barium fecal impaction

Interfering Factors

- Barium in the abdomen from previous barium contrast tests
  Barium in the abdomen may interfere with visualization of portions of the colon.
- Significant residual stool in the colon
  Stool precludes adequate visualization of the entire bowel wall. Stool may be confused as polyps.
- Spasm of the colon
  Spasm can mimic the radiographic signs of a cancer. The use of IV glucagon minimizes spasm.

Procedure and Patient Care

Before

- Explain the procedure to the patient. Encourage the patient to verbalize questions and fears.
- Assist the patient with bowel preparation, which varies among institutions. In elderly patients, this preparation can be exhaustive and can cause severe dehydration. Bowel preparation usually includes diet restriction, hydration, orally ingested cathartic, and cleansing enemas. Typical preparation in most adults includes the following:
  Day before examination:
    Give the patient clear liquids (no dairy products) for lunch and supper.
    Have the patient drink one glass of water or clear fluid every hour for 8 to 10 hours.
    2:00 PM: Administer one full bottle (10 z) of magnesium citrate or X-Prep (extract of senna fruit).
    7:00 PM: Administer three 5-mg bisacodyl (Dulcolax) tablets.
    Keep the patient NPO after midnight.
  Day of examination:
    Keep the patient NPO.
    6:00 AM: Administer a bisacodyl suppository or a cleansing enema, or both.

Age-related concerns: Pediatrics

- Typical preparation in a child may include the following:

Age ≤ 2 years:
  Clear-liquid diet for 24 hours before the test
  NPO for 4 hours before testing
  Pediatric Fleet enema the night before testing, repeated 3 hours before testing

Age >2 years:
  Low-residue diet for 2 days before testing
  Clear-liquid diet (excluding milk) for 24 hours before testing
  NPO for 3 hours before testing
  Castor oil the day before testing:
    Age 2-4 years: 1 oz
    Age 5-9 years: 1.5 oz
    Age 10-16 years: 2 oz
  Saline solution enemas the night before testing only if good results were not obtained with castor oil
  Pediatric Fleet enemas until clear, 3 hours before testing

- Be aware of dehydration and electrolyte abnormalities. Instruct the parent to hydrate the child well with electrolyte-containing fluids after the BE.
- The colon in the young child will not tolerate the volume and pressure of instillation of barium that the adult colon can. Both should be reduced.
- A child cannot retain the barium long enough for complete filling of the colon. Thus a rectal tube with a balloon on the end is used. The small balloon is inflated minimally, and the buttocks are taped tightly to prevent premature defecation of the barium.

Age-related concerns: Elderly

- Bowel preparation may be difficult for the elderly. Often these patients live alone and cannot administer an enema. Their social support system should be evaluated before the day of the BE.
- The elderly become dehydrated easily. Hypovolemia and orthostasis can lead to falling. Further, electrolyte abnormalities may develop, which can alter cardiac rhythm. Bowel preparation may have to be decreased or prolonged over several days to avert these complications. Hydration with electrolyte-containing fluids is vital.
- The elderly have reduced muscle tone, and often cannot retain barium long enough for adequate visualization of the colon. A rectal tube with a balloon at the end is inserted into the rectum, and the balloon is inflated to diminish premature defecation of barium.
- Elimination of residual barium is especially important in chronically constipated elderly patients. Be sure to instruct patients to use a mild cathartic after testing and to continue the cathartic daily until the stool is no longer white.

- Determine whether the bowel is adequately cleansed. When the fecal return is clear, preparation is adequate. If large, solid fecal waste is still being evacuated, preparation is inadequate. Notify the radiologist, who may want to extend the bowel preparation.
- In patients with suspected bowel obstruction, no oral cathartic should be administered. If catharsis is ineffective and enemas are not evacuated, colon obstruction may be present, and the physician should be notified immediately.
- Suggest that the patient take reading material to the x-ray department to occupy the time while expelling the barium.

During

- Note the following procedural steps:
  1. A balloon rectal catheter is placed.
  2. The balloon on the catheter is inflated tightly against the anal sphincter to hold the barium in the colon.
  3. The patient is asked to roll in the lateral, supine, and prone positions.
  4. Barium is dripped into the rectum by gravity.
  5. Barium flow is monitored fluoroscopically.
  6. The colon is thoroughly examined as the barium progresses through the large colon and into the terminal ileum.
  7. The barium is drained out.
  8. If an ACBE has been ordered, air is insufflated into the large bowel.
  9. The patient is asked to expel the barium, and a postevacuation x-ray film is obtained.
  10. The standard procedure for administering barium through a colostomy is to instill the contrast medium through an irrigation cone placed in the stoma. When the x-ray series is completed, the barium is allowed to be expelled from the stoma. A gentle stream of clean water for irrigation is helpful in expelling residual barium. See Box 12-2 for special care of the patient with a colostomy.

After

- Ensure that the patient defecates as much barium as possible. Laxatives may be ordered.

Box 12-2 Special care for the patient with a colostomy

- Bowel preparation is the same, except enemas are not administered.
- The patient may be asked to irrigate the colostomy with saline solution about 4 hours before the test.
- If a loop colostomy is present (usually in the right upper quadrant of the abdomen), ask the physician which area of the colon is to be studied. If only the distal colon is to be evaluated, oral cathartics will not contribute to the cleansing process. Irrigation and enemas alone are used. If the proximal colon is to be studied, cathartics and proximal irrigation are used.
- Because barium cannot be retained, a balloon catheter is used.
- Elimination of barium is important. Cathartics and irrigation should be administered until the stool is no longer white.

- Inform the patient that bowel movements will be white. When all the barium has been expelled, the stool will return to normal color.
- Suggest the use of soothing ointments on the anal area to minimize anorectal pain that may result from the aggressive test preparation.
- Encourage ingestion of fluids containing electrolytes to avoid dehydration or electrolyte abnormalities caused by the cathartic agents.
- Encourage rest after the procedure. The cleansing regimen and BE procedure may be exhausting.

Test Results and Clinical Significance

Malignant tumor *This is evident as an "apple core"–looking filling defect in the barium column.*

Polyps *These are evident as round filling defects in the barium column. Stool can create this same picture. Persistence in location throughout the study suggests polyps.*

Diverticula *These are evident as outpouchings of the colon. Diverticulosis refers only to the presence of diverticula. Diverticulitis indicates an infectious inflammation surrounding the colon, and is evident as narrowing of the barium column.*

Inflammatory bowel disease (e.g., ulcerative colitis, Crohn's disease) *This is evident as narrowing of the barium column as a result of inflammation surrounding the colon. A cobblestone-like pattern is classic for ulcerative colitis. Areas devoid of barium are classic for Crohn's disease. The rectum is usually involved in ulcerative colitis, but spared in Crohn's disease. Fistulas may be evident in Crohn's disease.*

Colonic stenosis secondary to ischemia, infection, or previous surgery *This is evident as a "non–apple core"–like narrowing of the barium column.*

Perforated colon *Leakage of contrast is seen with perforation. The most common cause of perforation is cancer or diverticulitis. If perforation is suspected, a water-soluble iodine-containing contrast agent should be used, because it can be absorbed by the body. Barium cannot be absorbed, and can cause persistence of infection.*

Colonic fistula *This is evident as leakage of contrast agent from the colon to another organ (e.g., urinary bladder) or area of the bowel.*

Appendicitis *Although a diagnosis of appendicitis cannot be made with certainty, it can be supported by lack of barium filling during a BE. The appendix does not fill in 30% to 60% of normal appendixes.*

Extrinsic compression of the colon from extracolonic tumors (e.g., ovarian) or abscess *This is evident as a convex, rounded distortion of the barium column.*

Malrotation of the gut *In this congenital abnormality, the cecum, normally in the right lower quadrant of the abdomen, is in the left upper quadrant.*

Colon volvulus *The cecum or sigmoid portion of the colon can turn on its mesentery and cut off flow of barium to that area of bowel. Sometimes, instillation of barium is therapeutic and can reduce the volvulus.*

Intussusception *When proximal bowel is invaginated into the distal bowel (intussusception) the flow of barium stops at the tip of the intussusceptum. Sometimes, instillation of barium is therapeutic and can reduce the intussusception. In children the intussusception is usually caused by enlarged lymph nodes in the ileal colic area. In adults, a polypoid tumor usually is the leading pathology of the intussusceptum.*

Hernia *Large groin (usually sliding hernias) or ventral hernias can contain the colon, which is seen outside the abdomen in the hernia sac.*

Related Tests

- Colonoscopy (p. 552): Provides direct visualization of the colon mucosa. It is more accurate than BE, and enables endoscopic surgery (e.g., biopsy, polypectomy).
- Small bowel series (p. 991): Provides visualization of the small intestine.

Barium Swallow (Esophagogram)

Normal Findings

Normal size, contour, filling, patency, and position of the esophagus

Indications

The barium swallow provides visualization of the lumen of the esophagus. It is indicated in patients with the following symptoms:

Dysphagia
Noncardiac chest pain
Painful swallowing
Swallowing abnormalities (see swallowing examination [videoflurosocopy], p. 995)
Gastroesophageal reflux

Test Explanation

This barium contrast study is a more thorough examination of the esophagus than that provided by most upper GI series (p. 999). As in most barium contrast studies, defects in normal filling and narrowing of the barium column indicate tumor, strictures, or extrinsic compression from extraesophageal masses, or an abnormally enlarged heart and great vessels. Varices also can be seen as serpiginous linear-filling defects. Anatomic abnormalities such as hiatal hernia, Schatzski's rings, and diverticula (Zenker or epiphrenic) can be seen as well.

In patients with esophageal reflux, the radiologist may identify reflux of the barium from the stomach into the esophagus. Muscular abnormalities such as achalasia, as well as diffuse esophageal spasm, can be easily detected. If perforations or rupture of the esophagus is suspected, it is best not to use barium, but a water-soluble contrast medium. Anatomic abnormalities such as sliding or paraesophageal hiatal hernias can also be detected.

This procedure is usually performed in the radiology department by a radiologist in approximately 15 to 20 minutes. No discomfort is associated with this test.

Contraindications

- Evidence of bowel obstruction or severe constipation
  Barium may create a stonelike impaction.

- Perforated viscus
  If barium were to leak, the degree and duration of infection would be much worse. Usually when perforation is suspected, diatrizoate (Gastrografin), a water-soluble iodine-containing contrast medium, is used.
- Unstable vital signs
- Patients who are unable to cooperate during the test

Potential Complications

- Barium-induced fecal impaction

Interfering Factors

- Food in the esophagus, which prevents adequate visualization

CLINICAL PRIORITIES

- This study provides a more thorough examination of the esophagus than is provided by most upper gastrointestinal x-ray studies.
- Barium is not used if perforation or rupture of the esophagus is suspected. In these cases, a water-soluble contrast agent is used.
- After the test, cathartics are recommended to aid in evacuating the barium.

Procedure and Patient Care

Before

- Explain the procedure to the patient.
- Instruct the patient to remain NPO for at least 8 hours before the test. Usually the patient is kept NPO after midnight on the day of the test.
- Assess the patient's ability to swallow. If the patient tends to aspirate, inform the radiologist.

During

- Note the following procedural steps:
  1. The fasted patient is asked to swallow the contrast medium. Usually this is barium sulfate in milkshake-like form; however, if a perforated viscus is possible, diatrizoate (Gastrografin) is used.
  2. As the patient drinks the contrast agent through a straw, the x-ray table is tilted to the near-erect position.
  3. The patient is asked to roll into various positions so that the entire esophagus can be adequately visualized.
  4. With fluoroscopy or videofluoroscopy, the radiologist observes the flow of contrast medium through the entire esophagus.

After

- Inform the patient of the need to evacuate all the barium. Cathartics are recommended. Initially, stool will be white, but should return to normal color with complete evacuation.

Test Results and Clinical Significance

Total or partial esophageal obstruction *Usually this is caused by a cancer. However, achalasia or stricture can be so severe as to cause obstruction. Patients complain of dysphagia.*
Cancer *This is most evident as narrowing in the esophagus or diminished gastroesophageal function.*
Peptic or corrosive (e.g., lye) esophagitis or ulceration *This can cause bleeding, perforation, scarring and stricture.*
Scarred strictures *These are usually a sequela of untreated peptic or corrosive esophagitis.*
Lower esophageal rings *May be congenital or acquired as a result of long-term reflux.*
Varices *Submucosal venous varices can result from prolonged portal hypertension.*
Chalasia or achalasia *Chalasia occurs in infants who have no lower esophageal sphincter function. These children have gastroesophageal reflux. Achalasia is usually acquired, but may be congenital. These patients cannot relax the lower esophageal sphincter, and esophageal obstruction (dysphagia) develops.*
Esophageal motility disorders (e.g., presbyesophagus, scleroderma, diffuse esophageal spasm) *Elderly patients may have asynchronous motility, which prevents swallowed food from progressing through the esophagus.*
Diverticula *These can be in the upper esophagus (Zenker's) and be due to spasm of the cricopharyngeus muscle (upper esophageal sphincter), or in the lower esophagus (epiphrenic) and be due to paraesophageal infection.*
Extrinsic compression from extraesophageal tumors, cardiomegaly, or aortic aneurysm *Distorts the normal esophageal anatomy.*

Related Tests

- Endoscopic esophagogastroscopy (p. 536): Enables direct visualization of the esophageal lumen.

Bone Densitometry
(Bone Mineral Content [BMC], Bone Absorptiometry, Bone Mineral Density [BMD])

Normal Findings

Normal: <1.0 SD below normal (>-1.0)
Osteopenia: 1.0-2.5 SD below normal (-1.0 to -2.5)
Osteoporosis >2.5 SD below normal (<-2.5)

Indications

Bone densitometry systems determine bone mineral content and density to diagnose osteoporosis. Indications include:

- Early premenopausal oophorectomy or estrogen deficiency syndromes (e.g., amenorrhea)
- Plain films indicating osteopenia
- Endocrinopathies known to be associated with osteopenia (e.g., hyperparathyroidism, prolactinoma, Cushing's syndrome, male hypogonadism, hyperthyroidism)
- Unexplained or multiple fractures
- Anorexia
- Multiple myeloma
- Prolonged immobility
- GI malabsorption (proteins and calcium)
- Chronic renal diseases (secondary and tertiary hyperparathyroidism)
- Treatment-related osteopenia (e.g., long-term heparin, anticonvulsant, or steroid therapy)
- Monitoring of treatment of osteoporosis (e.g., hormone replacement therapy, exercise, calcitonin analog, vitamin D, calcium supplements)
- Onset of menopause, to make a better informed decision regarding the risk and benefits of hormone replacement therapy

Test Explanation

Osteoporosis and osteopenia, or decreased bone mass, most commonly develop in postmenopausal women. Bones become weak and fracture easily. Diseases associated with osteoporosis include renal failure, hyperparathyroidism, GI malabsorption syndrome, prolonged steroid therapy, and prolonged immobility. The consequences of osteoporosis are vertebral crush fractures and hip fractures. Nationally, these fractures cost billions of health care dollars for medical treatment and long-term custodial care. More important, however, about 20% of patients older than 45 years will die within 1 year as a consequence of hip fracture.

Methods to identify the early stages of osteoporosis are available. The earlier osteoporosis is recognized, the more effective the treatment and the milder the clinical course. If the diagnosis of osteoporosis is delayed until fractures occur or plain film x-rays demonstrate "thin" bones, the success of treatment is less likely.

The diagnosis of osteoporosis should lead to aggressive medical therapy, which can be expensive and not without risks. Therefore the diagnosis of osteoporosis must be based on accurate data. Bone densitometry was developed to provide accurate and precise measurement of bone strength based on bone density. Several groups of bones are routinely evaluated because they accurately represent the entire skeleton. The lumbar spine is the best representative of cancellous bone. The radius is the most easily studied cortical bone. The proximal hip (neck of the femur) is the best representative of cancellous and cortical mixed bone. Specific bone sites can be evaluated if they are symptomatic.

There are two methods of determining bone density.

1. *Single-photon densitometry (absorptiometry).* With this technique, a radioactive radionuclide (photon emitter) is placed in a tube and passed over the bony area to be studied (usually the distal radius). A scintillator photon detector is placed on the opposite side of the bone. The greater the density of the bone in the scanning path, the greater the number of photons absorbed by the bone and the fewer the number of photons that reach the detector in the scintillator. The relative absorption is calibrated to express bone mineral and mass per unit length of bone

(grams per centimeter). This technique is used primarily to evaluate the radius or other bones not surrounded by soft tissue.

2. *Dual-energy densitometry (absorptiometry).* This method uses a dual-photon source to measure the density of the bone. There are two different sources of dual-photon energy, and therefore two methods of performing dual-energy densitometry. *Dual-photon absorptiometry (DPA)* typically uses gadolinium 153 as a gamma source for 44- and 100-keV gamma ray photons. With *dual-energy x-ray absorptiometry (DEXA),* x-rays are used in place of the radionuclide to provide two different x-ray energies to produce dual photons in the x-ray spectrum. Because DPA and DEXA use two photons, more energy is produced so that bones (spine and hip [femoral neck]) surrounded by more soft tissue can be more easily penetrated. The radius can be measured with either of these dual-energy techniques.

The diagnosis of osteoporosis can be made when vertebral bone density is more than 10% below what is expected for sex, age, height, weight, and race. Patients with values between 0.8 and 0.99 g/cm^2 have a 20% or less chance of spontaneous fractures, whereas patients with values $<0.62\ g/cm^2$ have a nearly 100% chance of spontaneous fractures. Usually, bone density is reported in terms of standard deviation from mean values. *T* scores compare the patient's results with those of a group of young healthy adults. *Z* scores compare the patient's results with those of a group of age-matched controls. *T* scores are probably more accurate in predictive value of risk for fracture. The World Health Organization has defined osteopenia as bone density value >1 SD below peak bone mass levels in young women, and osteoporosis as a value of >2.5 SD below that same measurement scale. Most clinicians believe therapeutic intervention should be begun in patients with osteopenia, to prevent progression to osteoporosis.

The data are interpreted by a radiologist or a physician trained in nuclear medicine. Bone density studies take about 30 to 45 minutes to perform and are free of any discomfort. Only minimal radiation is used (the total dose of radiation exposure is less than for a chest x-ray study). In the future, advances in bone densitometry will be directed toward reducing the time to perform the study. Advances in DPA and DEXA are presently being studied. Furthermore, quantitative computed tomography (QCT) is being studied as a means to measure bone density. With this technique, the CT scanner is modified to provide low-dose single- or dual-photon energy.

Interfering Factors

- Barium may falsely increase the density of the lumbar spine. Bone density measurements should not be performed within about 10 days after barium studies.
- Posterior vertebral calcific arthritic sclerosis can falsely increase bone density of the spine.
- Calcified abdominal aortic aneurysm may falsely increase bone density of the spine.
- Internal fixation devices of the hip or radius will falsely increase bone density of those bones.
- Overlying metal jewelry or other objects may falsely increase bone density.
- Previous fractures of the bone to be studied can falsely increase its bone density.
- Metallic clips placed in the plane of the vertebra in patients who have had previous abdominal surgery can falsely increase bone density.
- Previous bone scans can falsely decrease bone density because the photons generated

✓ CLINICAL PRIORITIES

- Bone densitometry was developed to provide accurate and precise measurement of bone strength based on bone density.
- According to the WHO, *osteopenia* is present if the bone density value is >1 SD below peak bone mass levels in young women, and *osteoporosis* is present if the value is >2.5 SD below the same level.
- This test should not be performed within 10 days after barium studies, because barium may falsely increase the bone density of the lumbar spine.

from the bone as a result of the previously administered radionuclide will be detected by the scintillator counter.

Procedure And Patient Care

Before

- The densitometer is usually calibrated by the x-ray or nuclear medicine technician before the patient's arrival.
- Tell the patient that no fasting or sedation is required.
- Explain the procedure to the patient.
- Ask the patient to remove all metallic objects (e.g., belt buckles, zippers, coins, keys, jewelry) that might be in the scanning path.

During

- The patient lies on an imaging table (Figure 12-6) with the legs supported on a padded box to flatten the pelvis and lumbar spine.
- Under the table, a photon generator is slowly passed under the lumbar spine.
- Above the table, a scintillation (gamma or x ray) detector camera is passed over the patient parallel to the generator. Images of the lumbar and hip bones are projected on a computer monitor.
- Next, the foot is applied to a brace that internally rotates the nondominant hip, and the procedure is repeated over the hip. A similar procedure is performed to evaluate the radius. When the radius is examined, the nondominant arm is preferred unless there is a history of fracture to that bone.

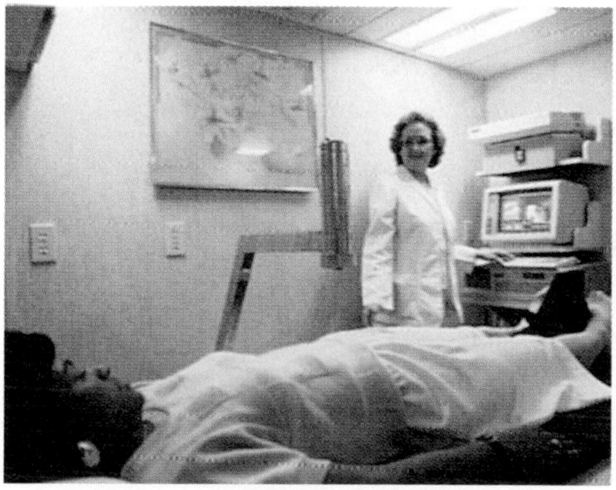

Figure 12-6 Bone densitometry.

After

- On the computer screen, a small window of the lumbar spine, femoral neck, or distal radius is drawn. The computer calculates the amount of photons not absorbed by the bone, or bone mineral content (BMC). Bone mineral density (BMD) is computed as follows:

$$\text{BMD} = \frac{\text{BMC (g/cm}^2\text{)}}{\text{Surface area of the bone}}$$

- Findings are compared with data from healthy 25- to 35-year-old women, and the SD above or below the curve is determined. This is the *T* score. Positive *T* scores indicate bone stronger than normal; negative *T* scores indicate bone weaker than normal. *Z* scores are calculated in the same way, but the comparisons are made to those in patients matched for age, sex, race, height, and weight.

Test Results And Clinical Significance

Osteopenia
Osteoporosis
Osteopenia precedes osteoporosis. The most common cause of osteoporosis is lack of sexual hormones (estrogen in the female, testosterone in the male). Osteopenia may result from primary ovarian failure secondary to menopause or oophorectomy, or pituitary disease. In male patients, osteopenia usually occurs in children with congenital hormone deficiencies.

Hyperparathyroidism *Excess parathyroid hormone mobilizes calcium from the bone, causing demineralization and bone weakening.*

Chronic renal insufficiency *Excess phosphates that accumulate as a result of reduced glomerular filtration reduce the calcium in the blood. Parahormone is stimulated to increase calcium levels. Excess parathyroid hormone mobilizes calcium from the bone, causing demineralization and weakening of the bones (secondary hyperparathyroidism). If after persistent parathyroid stimulation the parathyroid glands become autonomous and secrete elevated parahormone despite normal calcium levels, tertiary hyperparathyroidism develops. The bone changes are the same as described above.*

GI malabsorption *Calcium and protein cannot be absorbed. The bones are depleted of their minerals, and bone density is reduced.*

Cushing's syndrome
Chronic steroid therapy
Glucocorticosterols inhibit bone mineralization and decrease bone density.

Chronic heparin therapy *Heparin binds calcium and other minerals. These minerals are therefore not available for bone growth. Further, these minerals are mobilized from their bone stores. Bone density diminishes.*

Chronic immobility *The pathophysiology of bone demineralization in the immobilized patient is not clearly understood.*

Related Tests

- Long bone radiography studies (p. 913): Plain films can identify advanced bone demineralization and indicate severe osteoporosis.

Bones (Long), Radiography

Normal Findings

No evidence of fracture, tumor, infection, or congenital abnormalities

Indications

This x-ray study is performed to evaluate any bone for fracture, infection, arthritis, tendinitis, or bone spurs. Bone age can be determined in children to evaluate growth and development. Primary and metastatic tumors can be identified.

Test Explanation

X-ray films of the long bones are usually obtained when the patient has complaints about a pertinent body area. Fractures or tumors are readily detected by x-ray studies. Severe or chronic infection involving a bone (osteomyelitis) may be detected. X-ray studies of the long bones also can detect joint destruction and bone spurring as a result of persistent arthritis. Growth patterns can be followed by serial x-ray studies of long bones, usually the wrists and hands. Healing of a fracture can be documented and monitored. X-ray films of the joints reveal the presence of joint effusions and soft tissue swelling. Calcifications in the soft tissue indicate chronic inflammatory changes of the nearby bursa or tendons. Soft tissue swelling can also be seen on these similar x-ray films. Because the cartilage and tendons are not directly visualized, cartilage fractures or sprains, and ligamentous injuries cannot be seen.

At least two films obtained at a 90-degree angle are required so that the bone region being studied can be visualized from two different angles (usually anteroposterior and lateral). Some bone studies (e.g., skull, spine, hip) require oblique views to visualize all the parts that need to be seen.

Interfering Factors

- Jewelry or clothing can obstruct radiographic visualization of part of the bone to be evaluated.
- Previous barium studies can diminish full radiographic visualization of some of the bones surrounding the abdomen (e.g., spine, pelvis).

✓ CLINICAL PRIORITIES

- This test can determine bone age to evaluate growth and development. Usually the bones of the wrists and hands are used for this determination.
- When obtaining x ray films, shield the patient's testes or ovaries, and abdomen, if pregnant, to prevent radiation exposure.

Procedure and Patient Care

Before

- Explain the procedure to the patient.
- Carefully handle any injured parts of the patient's body.
- Instruct the patient to keep the extremity still while the x-ray film is being obtained. This can sometimes be difficult, especially when the patient has severe pain associated with a recent injury.
- Shield the patient's testes, ovaries, or pregnant abdomen to prevent exposure from scattered radiation.
- Tell the patient that no fasting or sedation is required.

During

- In the radiology department, the patient is asked to place the involved extremity in several positions. An x-ray film is obtained of each position.
- Note that this test is routinely performed by a radiologic technologist within several minutes.
- Tell the patient that no discomfort is associated with this test except perhaps from moving the extremity.

After

- Administer an analgesic for relief of pain, if indicated.

Test Results and Clinical Significance

Fractures

Congenital bone disorders (e.g., achondroplasia, dysplasia, dysostosis)
Multiple disorders associated with bone, absence of a bone, or growth and development of bone or bone groups are detected.

Tumors (osteogenic sarcoma, Paget's disease, myeloma, metastases) *These can be evident as osteoblastic destruction (radiolucent defects in bone) or osteoclastic reaction (radiopaque areas of bone) to the tumor.*

Infection or osteomyelitis *These are evident as soft tissue swelling around the bone infection. Further signs may include periosteal reaction and bony destruction of the affected bone.*

Osteoporosis or osteopenia *Bone demineralization and thinning indicate osteoporosis. Patients are at increased risk for traumatic and atraumatic fractures.*

Joint destruction (arthritis) *Degenerative and rheumatoid arthritic degenerative changes are seen as narrowing of the joint space due to cartilaginous destruction. Bone spurs and other changes can be noted.*

Bone spurs *Exophytic growths of bone at pressure points (heels and feet) can cause significant pain.*

Abnormal growth pattern *Bony development can be evaluated with x-ray films of the wrists, arms, pelvis, and skull. Comparison of findings with those normal for chronological age provides insight and perspective into possible abnormalities in growth and development.*

Joint effusion *Swelling and some increased radiodensity of the joint indicate effusion. This may be the result of bleeding, trauma, inflammation, or infection.*

Foreign bodies *X-ray films of the extremities can demonstrate foreign bodies (usually in the hands and feet).*

Bronchography (Bronchogram, Laryngography)

Normal Findings

Normal tracheobronchial tree

Indications

Bronchography enables visualization of the tracheobronchial tree. It is used to identify bronchiectasis.

Test Explanation

A bronchogram is an x-ray examination of the tracheobronchial tree produced after the instillation of an iodinated dye into the bronchi via a catheter or bronchoscope. Positioning of the patient and the catheter allows the radiopaque material to coat all portions of the tracheobronchial tree so that their outlines can be recorded on a chest x-ray film. X-ray films demonstrate the outline and structure of the trachea, bronchi, and entire tracheobronchial tree.

Bronchography is indicated to diagnose bronchiectasis, to identify obstruction in the distal bronchi, and to detect congenital or acquired forms of tracheobronchial malformation and tracheoesophageal fistula. Bronchography may be used in the evaluation of patients for possible surgery, and those with recurring, localized pneumonia, or severe hemoptysis. Bronchography should not be performed in patients with exacerbation of cough or sputum production. The test should be performed after the symptoms are treated and when mucous secretions are minimal. Because of the alterations in pulmonary function, as well as occasional inflammatory reactions induced by this procedure, studying one lung at a time is safer than studying both. The indications for bronchography have diminished since the development of flexible fiberoptic bronchoscopy, which provides direct visualization of the tracheobronchial tree.

Bronchography is performed by a radiologist in approximately 45 minutes. Usually the only discomfort associated with this test is the urge to cough.

Contraindications

- Pregnancy
- Acute pulmonary infections, because of the distortion of the bronchial tree that may already exist
- Respiratory insufficiency, because the study may temporarily reduce pulmonary function

Potential Complications

- Bronchospasm or laryngospasm
- Allergic reaction to iodinated dye
  Allergic reaction is rare because the dye is not administered intravenously.

CLINICAL PRIORITIES

- Bronchography should not be performed if the patient has an exacerbation of cough. Coughing will prevent adequate bronchiolar filling and expel the contrast agent before the test is completed.
- Because of alterations in pulmonary function induced by this procedure, it is safer to study one lung at a time.
- After the procedure, the patient should not eat or drink until the tracheobronchial anesthesia has worm off and the gag reflex has returned.

Interfering Factors

- Excessive coughing or sputum production can inhibit bronchiolar filling and cause premature expulsion of the contrast material.

Procedure and Patient Care

Before

- Explain the procedure to the patient. Allay any concerns and allow the patient to express any fears.
- Obtain informed consent if required by the institution.
- Check for allergies to iodine dye and shellfish.
- Keep the patient NPO after midnight the day of the test.
- Instruct the patient to perform thorough mouth care the night before and the morning of the test to minimize the risk of introducing bacteria into the lungs during the procedure.
- Consider postural drainage to promote expulsion of mucus or exudate from the lungs.
- Remove and safely store the patient's dentures and glasses or contact lenses.
- Administer preprocedural medications as ordered. Medications may include atropine to decrease secretions and to minimize vagally induced bradycardia, and diazepam (Valium) for its sedative effect.
- Instruct the patient not to swallow the local anesthetic sprayed into the throat. Provide an emesis basin for expectoration.
- Ask the patient to make every effort to suppress coughing during the procedure. Coughing will prevent adequate bronchiolar filling and expel the contrast substance before the test is completed. Rapid, shallow breathing will help to suppress the cough reflex. If the patient has a productive cough, an expectorant is administered and postural drainage is performed for 1 to 3 days before the procedure.

During

- Place the patient in a sitting position.
- Note the following procedural steps:
  1. After spraying a local anesthetic into the patient's nose or mouth to suppress the gag reflex, a catheter or bronchoscope is passed into the trachea.

2. The pharynx, larynx, and major bronchi are anesthetized before introduction of the radiopaque dye.
3. The position of the patient and the placing of the catheter allow the radiologist to selectively fill regions of interest with radiopaque material.
4. The positions assumed by the patient are usually the reverse of those used in postural drainage.
5. Multiple x-ray views are obtained.

After

- If indicated, perform postural drainage to help remove the radiopaque dye from the tracheobronchial tree.
- Instruct the patient not to eat or drink anything until the tracheobronchial anesthesia has worn off and the gag reflex returns, usually in approximately 2 hours.
- Observe the patient closely for evidence of impaired respiration or laryngospasm. Vocal chords may become spasmodic after intubation. Emergency resuscitation equipment should be readily available.
- Encourage the patient to cough, which will help clear the tracheobronchial tree.
- Inform the patient that slight temperature elevation often occurs for 2 to 3 days after the test.
- Inform the patient that sore throat often develops. This can be relieved by gargling or using throat lozenges.
- Note that follow-up x-ray films may be obtained to ascertain if any dye remains in the tracheobronchial tree.
- Tell the patient that normal activities may usually be resumed 24 hours after the test.

Test Results and Clinical Significance

Bronchiectasis *This is associated with bronchial destruction and pockets of infection in the bronchioles.*
Bronchial obstruction *This is usually caused by a cancer, mucus plug, or foreign body.*
Tracheobronchoesophageal fistula *This is evidenced by seeing some of the contrast material in the esophagus.*

Related Tests

- Bronchoscopy (p. 518): With the advent of bronchoscopy, which allows direct visualization of the proximal tracheobronchial tree, the use of bronchography has considerably diminished.

Cardiac Catheterization
(Coronary Angiography, Angiocardiography, Ventriculography)

Normal Findings

Normal heart-muscle motion, normal and patent coronary arteries, normal great vessels, and normal intracardiac pressure and volume

Indications

Cardiac catheterization is used to visualize the heart chambers, arteries, and great vessels. It is used most often to evaluate chest pain. The study is used to locate the region of coronary occlusion in patients with positive stress test results and to determine the effects of valvular heart disease. Right heart catheterization is the most accurate method to determine cardiac output, and is also used to identify pulmonary emboli (see pulmonary angiography, p. 979).

Test Explanation

Cardiac catheterization enables examination of the heart, great blood vessels (aorta, inferior vena cava, pulmonary artery, and pulmonary vein), and coronary arteries. A catheter is passed into the heart through a peripheral vein (for right heart catheterization) or artery (for left heart catheterization). Through the catheter, pressures are recorded and radiographic dyes are injected. With the assistance of computer calculations, cardiac output

Tables 12-2 *Pressures and volumes used in cardiac monitoring*

	Description	Normal value
PRESSURES		
Routine blood pressure	Routine brachial artery pressure	90-140/60–90 mm Hg
Systolic left ventricular pressure	Peak pressure in the left ventricle during systole	90-140 mm Hg
End-diastolic left ventricular pressure	Pressure in the left ventricle at the end of diastole	4-12 mm Hg
Central venous pressure	Pressure in the superior vena cava	2-14 cm H_2O
Pulmonary wedge pressure	Pressure in the pulmonary venules, an indirect measurement of left atrial pressure and left ventricular end-diastolic pressure	Left atrial: 6-15 mm Hg
Pulmonary artery pressure	Pressure in the pulmonary artery	15–28/5-16 mm Hg
Aortic artery pressure	Same as routine blood pressure	
VOLUMES		
End-diastolic volume (EDV)	Amount of blood present in the left ventricle at the end of diastole	50-90 ml/m^2
End-systolic volume (ESV)	Amount of blood present in the left ventricle at the end of systole	25 ml/m^2
Stroke volume (SV)	Amount of blood ejected from the heart in one contraction (SV = EDV − ESV)	45 ± 12 ml/m^2
Ejection fraction (EF)	Proportion (fraction) of EDV ejected from the left ventricle during systole (EF = SV/EDV)	0.67 ± 0.07
Cardiac output (CO)	Amount of blood ejected by the heart in 1 min	3-6 L/min
Cardiac index (CI)	Amount of blood ejected by the heart in 1 min per square meter of body surface area (CI = CO/body surface area)	2.8-4.2 L/min/m^2 in a patient with 1.5 m^2 of body surface area

and other measures of cardiac function can be determined. Cardiac catheterization is indicated for the following reasons:

1. To identify, locate, and quantify the severity of atherosclerotic, occlusive coronary artery disease
2. To evaluate the severity of acquired and congenital cardiac valvular or septal defects
3. To determine the presence and degree of congenital cardiac abnormalities, such as transposition of the great vessels, patent ductus arteriosus, and anomalous venous return to the heart
4. To evaluate the success of previous cardiac surgery or balloon angioplasty
5. To evaluate cardiac muscle function
6. To identify and quantify ventricular aneurysms
7. To identify and locate acquired disease of the great vessels, such as atherosclerotic occlusion or aneurysms within the aortic arch
8. To evaluate acute myocardial infarction and to facilitate infusion of thrombolytic agents into occluded coronary arteries
9. To insert a catheter to monitor right-sided heart pressures, such as pulmonary artery and pulmonary wedge pressures, and to measure cardiac output. Cardiac output can be measured only during right heart catheterization. (Table 12-2 provides pressures and volumes used in cardiac monitoring.)
10. To dilate stenotic coronary arteries (angioplasty), to place coronary artery stents, or to perform laser atherectomy.

Cardiac catheterization is performed under sterile conditions. In right heart catheterization, usually the subclavian, brachial, or femoral vein is used for vascular access (Figure 12-7). In left heart catheterization, usually the right femoral artery is cannulated, or alter-

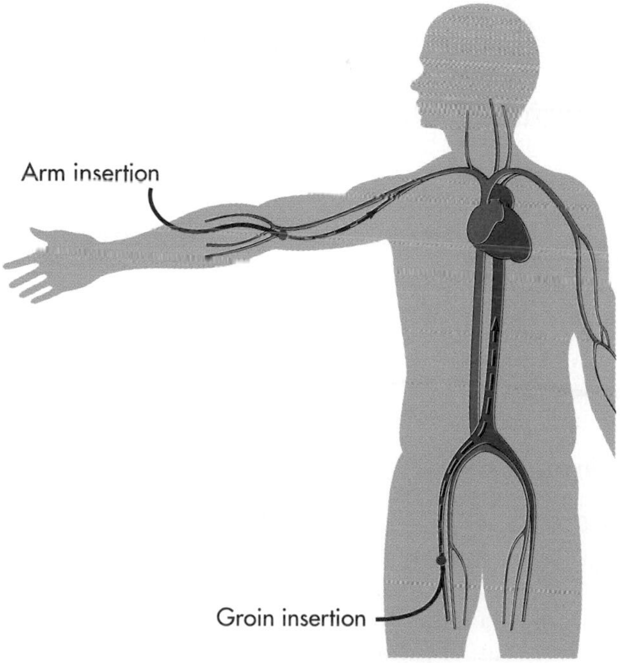

Figure 12-7 Insertion sites for cardiac catheterization.

natively, the brachial or radial artery. As the catheter is placed into the great vessels of the heart chamber, pressures are monitored and recorded. Blood samples for analysis of oxygen content are also obtained. The catheter is advanced with appropriate guidance into the desired position. After pressures are obtained, angiographic visualization of the heart chambers, valves, and coronary arteries is achieved with the injection of radiographic dye.

Transluminal coronary angioplasty is a therapeutic procedure that can be performed during coronary angiography in medical centers where open heart surgery is available. During this procedure, a specially designed balloon catheter is introduced into the coronary arteries and placed across the stenotic area of the coronary artery. This area can then be dilated by controlled inflation of the balloon. The coronary arteriogram is then repeated to document the effects of the forceful dilation of the stenotic area. Coronary arterial stents can be placed at the site of previous stenosis after angioplasty, and maintain patency for longer periods of time. Likewise, *laser atherectomy* can be performed to more permanently open coronary arteries with hard, atheromatous plaque deposits.

Cardiac catheterization is usually performed by a cardiologist in approximately 1 hour. During the dye injection the patient may experience a severe hot flush, which may be uncomfortable but lasts only 10 to 15 seconds. Some patients have a tendency to cough as the catheter is placed in the pulmonary artery. Verbally support the patient as the x-ray films are obtained, because the possibly loud noises may frighten the patient.

Age-related concerns

- Elderly patients with chronic dehydration or mild renal failure are at high risk for dye-induced renal failure.
- Urinary output must be carefully monitored after the procedure. Fluid intake needs to be encouraged, because dehydration may be induced by the diuretic action of the dye.

Contraindications

- Patients who are unable to cooperate during the test
- Patients who would refuse intervention if an amenable lesion were found
- Patients with an iodine dye allergy who have not received preventive medication for allergy
- Patients who are pregnant, because of radiation exposure to the fetus
- Patients with renal disorders, because iodinated contrast material is nephrotoxic
- Patients with a bleeding propensity, because the arterial or venous puncture site may not seal

Potential Complications

- Cardiac arrhythmias (dysrhythmias)
- Perforation of the heart myocardium
- Catheter-induced embolic cerebrovascular accident (stroke) or myocardial infarction
- Complications associated with the catheter insertion site, such as arterial thrombosis, embolism, or pseudoaneurysm

- Allergic reaction to iodinated dye
  Allergic reaction varies from flushing, itching, and urticaria to severe, life-threatening anaphylaxis (evidenced by respiratory distress, decreased blood pressure, or shock). In the event of anaphylaxis, the patient is given diphenhydramine (Benadryl), steroids, and epinephrine. Oxygen and endotracheal equipment should be on hand for immediate use.
- Infection at the catheter insertion site
- Pneumothorax after subclavian vein catheterization of the right side of the heart

CLINICAL PRIORITIES

- Assess for allergy to iodinated dye.
- Perform a baseline assessment of the patient's peripheral pulses before catheterization.
- After the test, keep the patient on bed rest for 4 to 8 hours to allow complete sealing of the arterial puncture.
- Assess the puncture site for bleeding, hematoma, and absence of pulse.

Procedure and Patient Care

Before

- Explain the procedure to the patient.
- Obtain written, informed consent.
- Allay the patient's fears and anxieties about the test. Although this test creates tremendous fear in a patient, it is performed often, and complications are rare.
- Instruct the patient to abstain from oral intake for at least 4 to 8 hours before the test.
- Prepare the catheter insertion site by shaving and scrubbing the skin.
- Determine whether the patient is allergic to iodine dye. If so diphenhydramine (Benadryl) and steroids should be provided several days before the test if possible. Nonionic iodine contrast dye should be used during the test.
- Mark the patient's peripheral pulses with a pen before catheterization. This will facilitate postcatheterization assessment of the pulses in the affected and nonaffected extremities.
- Provide appropriate precatheterization sedation as ordered by the physician.
- Instruct the patient to void before going to the catheterization laboratory.
- Remove all valuables and dental prostheses before transporting the patient to the catheterization laboratory.
- Obtain IV access for delivery of fluids and cardiac drugs if necessary.

During

- Take the patient to the cardiac catheterization laboratory (Figure 12-8).
- Note the following procedural steps:
  1. The chosen catheter insertion site is prepared and draped in a sterile manner.
  2. The desired vessel is punctured with a needle.
  3. A wire is placed through the needle and into the catheter.

A

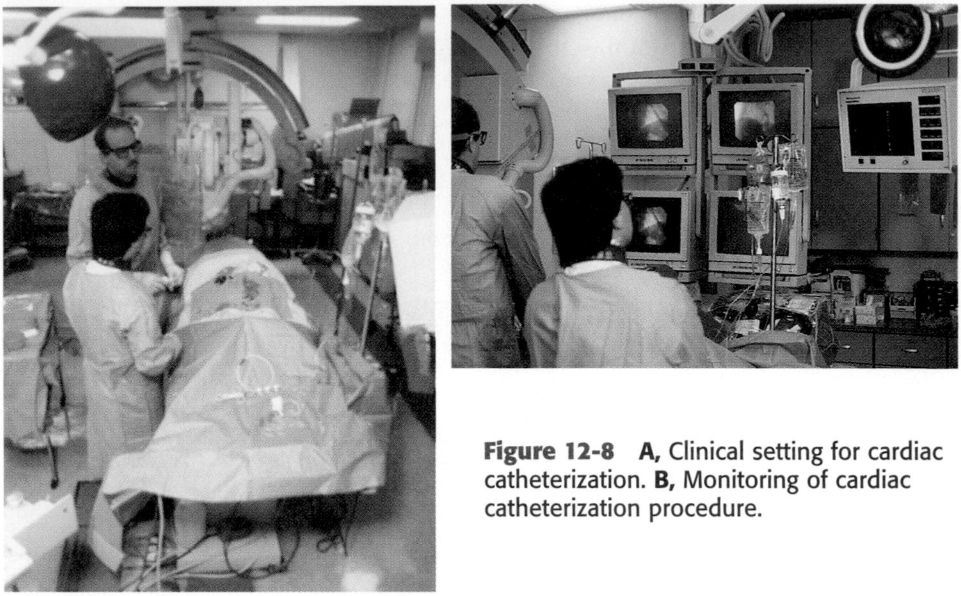

B

Figure 12-8 **A,** Clinical setting for cardiac catheterization. **B,** Monitoring of cardiac catheterization procedure.

4. The angiographic catheter is threaded on top of the wire.
5. Once the catheter is in the desired location, the appropriate cardiac pressures and volumes are measured.
6. Cardiac ventriculography is performed with controlled injection of contrast material.
7. Each coronary artery is catheterized. Cardiac angiography is then carried out with controlled injection of contrast material.
8. During the injection, x-ray films are rapidly obtained.
9. The patient's vital signs must be monitored constantly during the procedure.
10. If *angioplasty* is performed, the following procedural steps are carried out:
    a. The cardiologist appropriately places the catheter and balloon at the stenotic area.
    b. As the EKG tracing is observed, the balloon is inflated and the stenotic areas are forcefully dilated.
    c. If signs of myocardial ischemia develop, the balloon is immediately deflated.
    d. Usually, the balloon is inflated for only a few seconds.
11. After obtaining all required information, the catheter is removed.

After

- Monitor the patient's vital signs.
- Apply pressure to the site of vascular access.
- Keep the patient on bed rest for 4 to 8 hours to allow complete sealing of the arterial puncture.
- Keep the affected extremity extended and immobilized with sandbags to decrease bleeding.
- Assess the puncture site for signs of bleeding, hematoma, or absence of pulse.

- Assess the patient's pulses in both legs. Compare with preprocedural baseline values.
- Encourage the patient to drink fluids to maintain adequate hydration. Dehydration may be caused by the diuretic action of the dye.
- Evaluate the patient for delayed reaction to the dye (dyspnea, tachycardia, rashs, hives). This usually occurs within the first 2 to 6 hours after the test. Treat with antihistamines or steroids.
- Inform the patient that the angiograms will be reviewed by the cardiologist and that the results will be available in 1 or 2 days.

Test Results and Clinical Significance

Coronary artery occlusive disease *Stenosis in one or more of the coronary arteries (or branches) can be easily identified and located for revascularization with angioplasty or coronary artery bypass grafting.*

Anatomic variation of the cardiac chambers and great vessels *Ventricular and atrial septal defects, patent ductus arteriosus, and transposition of the great vessels are among many abnormalities that can be identified*

Ventricular aneurysm *Aneurysmal dilatation of part of the wall muscle due to infarction and weakness is evident at ventriculography.*

Ventricular mural thrombi
Intracardiac tumor
Altered blood flow dynamics
Ventricular wall motion deficits
Acquired or congenital septal defects and valvular abnormalities
Ventricular abnormalities are most evident during the ventriculography portion of the study. Some of these abnormalities also cause hemodynamic effects, which are recognized by pressure readings performed during cardiac catheterization.

Aortic root arteriosclerotic or aneurysmal disease
Anomalies in pulmonary venous return
Pulmonary emboli
Anomalies and diseases of the great vessels are evident following the outflow of dye after ventriculography.

Pulmonary hypertension *This condition is recognized by pressure readings performed during cardiac catheterization.*

Reduced cardiac output *Cardiac output is most accurately assessed by right heart catheterization. The right side is catheterized if cardiac output readings are required or valvular diseases of the right side are suspected.*

Arterial oxygen desaturation *Arterial oxygen saturation may be decreased when mixing of venous and arterial blood occurs. This may be seen with septal defects, transposition of the great vessels, or congenital shunting.*

Related Tests

- Cardiac nuclear scanning (p. 704): Can provide similar information concerning ventricular wall function and motion. Ejection fraction (a measure of cardiac output) and blood flow dynamics can also be determined. With newer radioisotopes, sites of coronary artery occlusion can be seen.

Chest Radiography (Chest X-ray, CXR)

Normal Findings Normal lungs and surrounding structures

Indications

This is the most commonly obtained x-ray study because it can indicate so much information about the heart, lungs, bony thorax, mediastinum, and great vessels.

Test Explanation

Chest radiography is important in the complete evaluation of the pulmonary and cardiac systems. This procedure is often part of the general admission screening workup in adult patients. Much information can be provided by the chest x-ray study (Figure 12-9). Repeated studies enable identification and monitoring of the following conditions:

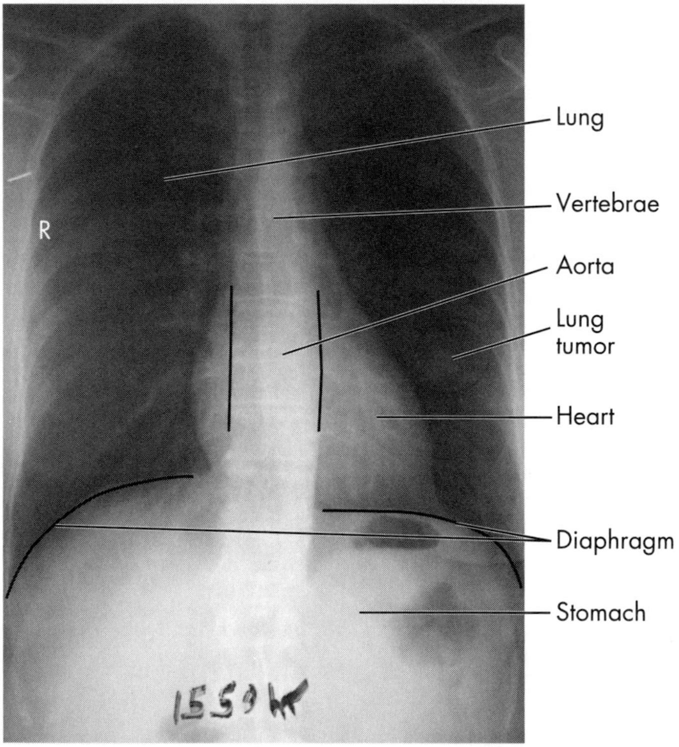

Figure 12-9 Chest x-ray. The diaphragm *(D)* separates the abdominal contents (including the stomach *[S]*) from the chest. The heart *(H)* is situated in the middle of the chest. The air-filled lungs *(L)* are represented as dark spaces on either side of the chest. The tubular opaque structure running vertically along the vertebrae *(V)* represents the aorta *(A)*. The ribs, clavicle, and other bony structures can also be seen as part of the thoracic cage.

1. Tumors of the lung (primary and metastatic), heart (myxoma), chest wall (soft-tissue sarcomas), and bony thorax (osteogenic sarcoma)
2. Inflammation of the lung (pneumonia), pleura (pleuritis), and pericardium (pericarditis)
3. Fluid accumulation in the pleura (pleural effusion), pericardium (pericardial effusion), and lung (pulmonary edema)
4. Air accumulation in the lung (chronic obstructive pulmonary disease) and pleura (pneumothorax)
5. Fractures of the bones of the thorax or vertebrae
6. Diaphragmatic hernia
7. Heart size, which may vary depending on cardiac function
8. Calcification, which may indicate large-vessel deterioration or old lung granulomas
9. Location of centrally placed intravenous access devices

Most chest x-ray films are obtained at a distance of 6 feet, with the patient standing (Figure 12-10). The sitting or supine position also can be used, but x-ray films obtained with the patient supine will not demonstrate fluid levels or pneumothorax. For a *posteroanterior (PA)* view (projection) the x-rays pass through the back of the body (posterior) to the front (anterior). For an anteroposterior view, the x-rays pass through the body from front to back. For a *lateral* view, the x-rays enter from the side. For *oblique* views, x-rays pass through the body at various angles. *Lordotic* views, obtained with the patient recumbent, provide visualization of the apices (rounded upper portions) of the lungs and are usually used to detect tuberculosis. *Decubitus* films are obtained with the patient in the recum-

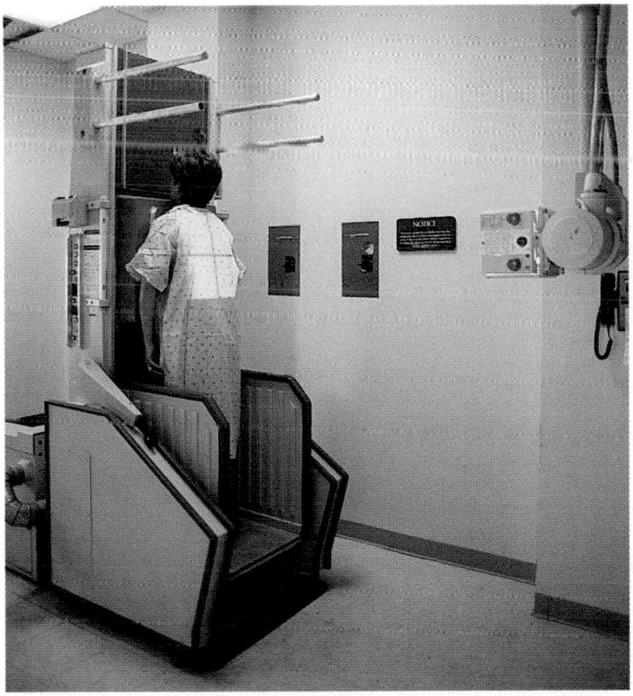

Figure 12-10 Patient positioned for chest x-ray study.

Table 12-3 Patient position required to identify suspected problems

Suspected problem	Position required
Pneumothorax	Erect
Effusion	Lateral decubitus
Widened mediastinum	Erect
Cardiac enlargement	Erect
Fractured rib	Oblique
Tuberculosis	Lordotic

bent lateral position, to demonstrate and localize fluid, which becomes dependent in the pleural space (pleural effusion). Table 12-3 shows the view required for detection of various problems.

Chest x-ray studies are best performed in the radiology department. Studies using a portable x-ray machine may be done at the bedside and are often performed in critically ill patients who cannot leave the nursing unit.

Contraindications

- Pregnancy

Interfering Factors

- Conditions (e.g., severe pain) that prevent the patient from taking and holding a deep breath
- Scarring from previous lung surgery (makes interpretation difficult)
- Obesity (requires more x-rays to penetrate the body to provide a readable x-ray film)

✓ CLINICAL PRIORITIES

- Chest x-ray studies are best performed in the radiology department, but can be performed at the bedside if the patient cannot leave the nursing unit.
- Patient positioning during the test depends on the suspected condition (see Table 12-3).
- To prevent radiation-induced abnormalities, a lead shield is used to cover the testicles in men and the ovaries in women.

Procedure and Patient Care

Before

- Explain the procedure to the patient.
- Tell the patient that no fasting is required.

- Instruct the patient to remove clothing to the waist and to put on an x-ray gown.
- Instruct the patient to remove all metal objects (e.g., necklaces, pins) so they do not block visualization of part of the chest.
- Tell the patient that he or she will be asked to take a deep breath and hold it while the x-ray films are obtained.
- Ensure that the testicles in men and the ovaries in women are covered with a lead shield to prevent radiation-induced abnormalities.

During

- After the patient is correctly positioned, tell him or her to take a deep breath and hold it until the x-ray films are obtained.
- Note that x-ray films are obtained by a radiologic technologist in several minutes.
- Inform the patient that no discomfort is associated with chest radiography.

After

- No special care is required after chest radiography.

Test Results and Clinical Significance

Lung

Lung tumors (primary or metastatic) *These are evident as soft tissue masses in the lung fields.*

Pneumonia *Increased opacity (lightness) in the lung field indicates pneumonia or atelectatic lung tissue.*

Pulmonary edema *Increased opacity of the lung is indicative of pulmonary edema, most commonly from congestive heart failure.*

Pleural effusion *Fluid in the chest wall is evident as increased opacity outside the lung fields, in particular, in the costophrenic margins. A lateral decubitus film will show layering out of free pleural fluid. Entrapped fluid, however, will not layer out.*

Chronic obstructive pulmonary disease *Increased lung space is classic for COPD.*

Pneumothorax *Air outside the lung space (pneumothorax) is always abnormal. If large enough, chest tube insertion is required.*

Atelectasis *Collapse of pulmonary alveoli is evident as white patches or lines in the lung fields.*

Tuberculosis *Usually in the upper lobes, chronic TB is usually associated with calcification.*

Lung abscess *Lung abscess is evident as a lung mass with a hollow (radiolucent) center. Sometimes, fungus can grow inside an abscess.*

Congenital lung diseases (hypoplasia) *Congenital aplasia or hypoplasia of the lung tissue is evident by reduced lung tissue on the affected side.*

Pleuritis *A thickened pleura indicates pleuritis, due to a viral, bacterial, neoplastic, or other cause.*

Foreign body in the chest, bronchus, or esophagus *Swallowed, aspirated, or penetrating (bullets) foreign bodies can be easily seen.*

Heart

Cardiac enlargement *When the heart is more that 50% to 60% of the horizontal width of the chest, cardiac enlargement due to congestive heart failure or cardiomyopathy is present.*

Pericarditis
Pericardial effusion
These conditions are evident as an enlarged heart shadow.

Chest wall

Soft tissue sarcoma
Osteogenic sarcoma
These primary tumor masses of the bony thorax and chest wall soft tissue are evident as masses arising from those areas.

Fracture of ribs or thoracic spine *Best seen on lateral or oblique x-ray films, fractures may be displaced or well aligned. They are usually associated with other chest trauma.*
Thoracic scoliosis *Alterations in thoracic spinal alignment are obvious on chest x-ray films.*
Metastatic tumor to bony thorax *Osteolytic (dark) or osteoblastic (white) nodules can be seen in the bony thorax. Breast, prostate, kidney, and lung are among the most common cancers to metastasize to the bones in this region.*

Diaphragm

Diaphragmatic or hiatal hernia *This condition is evident as increased opacity in the posteroinferior mediastinum.*

Mediastinum

Aortic calcinosis *This is evident as white lines indicating the walls of the calcified aorta.*
Enlarged lymph nodes *Central masses in the mediastinum indicate enlarged lymph nodes, usually of neoplastic origin.*
Dilated aorta *This may indicate aneurysm.*

Thymoma
Lymphoma
Substernal thyroid
These abnormalities often are evident as large soft tissue masses in the anterosuperior mediastinum.

Widened mediastinum *Cardiac enlargement, aneurysm, lymph node enlargement, or hematoma may be the cause.*

Related Tests

- Computed tomography, chest (p. 942): Allows more detailed information concerning pathologic conditions of the chest and its structures.

Chest Tomography
(Tomogram, Tomography of the Lung)

Normal Findings

Normal lungs and surrounding structures

Indications

This plain film chest x-ray allows visualization of a section ("slice") of lung at any vertical plane. It is useful in demonstrating the characteristics (border, central area, and presence of calcification) of a lung nodule. Chest CT scanning, however, is more easily performed and the results more accurate.

Test Explanations

Tomography is a radiographic examination in which a sequence of x-ray films is obtained, each representing a section of the organ being studied. Usually, the sections are demonstrated at 0.5 to 1.0 cm intervals. Tomography permits examination of a single layer or plane of tissue that would otherwise be obscured by surrounding tissue on an ordinary film.

For tomography, the x-ray tube and film cassette are rapidly moved in opposite directions while the x-ray film is obtained. This technique effectively blurs all the tissue planes except that being studied. Tomography is often a helpful adjunct to routine chest x-ray examination for several reasons:

1. It may reveal properties of a lung lesion (e.g., cavitation, tumor margins) that are normally not seen on chest x-ray films.
2. It provides better visualization of many structures (e.g., the hilus, trachea, mediastinum) that are not clearly seen on a routine chest x-ray film.
3. It may demonstrate many small lesions (e.g., metastases) that are normally seen on a routine chest x-ray film.

Indications for chest tomography have greatly decreased since the advent of computed tomography (CT) of the chest (see p. 942).

Contraindications

- Pregnancy

Interfering Factors

- Conditions (e.g., severe pain) that prevent the patient from taking and holding a deep breath

Procedure and Patient Care

Before

- Explain the procedure to the patient.
- Tell the patient that no fasting is required.
- Instruct the patient to put on an x-ray gown.
- Instruct the patient to remove all metal objects (e.g., necklaces, pins) so that they do not block visualization of part of the chest.
- Tell the patient that he or she will be asked to take a deep breath and hold it while x-ray films are obtained.
- Ensure that the testicles in men and the ovaries in women are covered with a lead shield to prevent radiation-induced abnormalities.

During

- Take the nonfasting patient to the radiology department.
- Note the following procedural steps:
  1. With the patient remaining completely still, an x-ray tube is rapidly moved back and forth while the film cassette is rapidly moved in the opposite direction. Excursion of this movement regulates the plane of tissues photographed.

2. Prone and supine positions may be required.
- Tell the patient that he or she will be unable to detect the fine, synchronized movements of the x-ray tube and film.
- A radiologist performs this test in approximately 15 minutes.
- Tell the patient that no discomfort is associated with chest tomography.

After

- No special care is required after the test.

Test Results and Clinical Significance

Lung tumor *Tomography aids in defining the borders of tumors. Poorly defined borders indicate cancer.*

Tuberculosis *Tomography is helpful in identifying calcification in lung lesions. The presence of calcification indicates a granulomatous infection (e.g., tuberculosis, sarcoidosis).*

Lung abscess *The central portion of a fluid-filled lung lesion is more likely an abscess than a neoplasm.*

Bronchiectasis *Small bronchiolar pockets of infection in the midlung are classic for bronchiectasis.*

Related Tests

- Chest CT scan (p. 942): Similar to chest tomography, but more accurate and easily performed.

Cholecystography
(Oral Cholecystogram, Gallbladder Series, GB Series)

Normal Findings

Good visualization of gallbladder
No filling defects
No stones

Indications

This test is used to evaluate the gallbladder in patients with chronic right upper quadrant abdominal pain, dyspepsia, heartburn, or fatty food intolerance.

Test Explanation

Oral cholecystography provides x-ray visualization of the gallbladder after oral ingestion of a radiopaque, iodinated dye in pill form. Adequate visualization of the gallbladder requires concentration of this dye within the gallbladder. The following factors are necessary for adequate dye concentration within the gallbladder:

1. Ingestion of all the dye tablets.

2. Adequate absorption of the dye from the gastrointestinal tract. Vomiting or diarrhea may preclude this absorption.
3. Abstinence from a meal on the morning of the test. A fatty meal eaten before x-ray films are obtained induces gallbladder emptying of the concentrated dye, and the gallbladder cannot be visualized.
4. Excretion of the dye into the bile. This excretion is inhibited by inadequate hepatocellular function or bilirubin level >2 mg/dl.
5. Patency of the cystic duct. The dye is secreted by the liver through the hepatic duct and enters the gallbladder through the cystic duct. Obstruction of the cystic duct (as in acute cholecystitis) will prevent the dye from entering the gallbladder.
6. Concentration of the dye within the gallbladder. The mucosa of a chronically inflamed gallbladder is unable to absorb the bile waters and concentrate the dye adequately for visualization.

On x-ray film, the biliary calculi (gallstones) are visualized as radiolucent shadows within a dye-filled gallbladder (Figure 12-11). Gallbladder polyps and tumors occasionally also can be seen as filling defects.

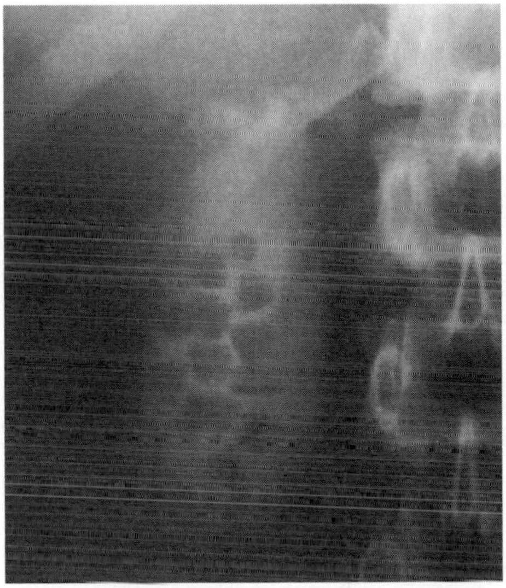

Figure 12-11 Oral cholecystogram. Gallstones are visualized as negative filling defects.

Occasionally the gallbladder is not visualized after a single dose of dye tablets is ingested. The test should then be repeated with a double dose. Nonvisualization after a double dose is reliable evidence of chronic cholecystitis if none of the listed factors necessary for adequate dye concentration have been violated.

Oral cholecystography is less accurate than gallbladder ultrasound. It is also more cumbersome to perform. It may take several days to obtain an accurate result. Fasting is required. Gallbladder ultrasonography, however, can be performed on an emergency basis. Fasting is preferred but not necessary for ultrasonography. When positive, the accuracy of gallbladder ultrasound is unparalleled (see p. 778). Ultrasound has now replaced cholecystography as the method of choice in the diagnosis of gallstones.

The x-rays take only a few minutes to obtain. They are interpreted by a radiologist, and the results are available the same day. No discomfort is associated with the test.

Contraindications

- Allergy to iodine dye
  This is a relative contraindication. Most patients who are allergic to iodine dye react only when the dye is administered intravenously.

- Pregnancy
- Bilirubin level >2 mg/dl
  Excretion of the dye into the bile is inhibited.
- Another inflammatory process within the abdomen
  Absorption of the orally ingested dye is not adequate for visualization.
- Diarrhea or vomiting
  Precludes absorption of the dye.

Potential Complications

- Adverse reaction or allergy to dye
  Rare, because the dye is not administered intravenously.

Interfering Factors

- Barium within the abdomen (usually as a result of an upper GI series or barium enema) precludes visualization of the gallbladder.
- Vomiting or diarrhea affects absorption of the radiopaque dye.

✓ CLINICAL PRIORITIES

- This test provides visualization of the gallbladder after the oral ingestion of radiopaque, iodinated dye in pill form.
- Vomiting or diarrhea may preclude absoption of the dye from the GI tract. This prevents adequate dye concentration in the gallbladder.
- The gallbladder cannot be visualized with this test if the bilirubin level is >2 mg/dl.

Procedure and Patient Care

Before

- Explain the procedure to the patient.
- Instruct the patient about the importance of ingesting the appropriate dose of radiopaque dye.
- Be sure the serum bilirubin level is <1.8 mg/dl.
- Instruct the patient to ingest a low-fat or fat-free meal the evening before testing.
- Assess for iodine dye allergy before administering radiopaque dye. The dye tablets are usually taken 2 hours after dinner. Usually, six 0.5 g iopanoic acid tablets are administered. These are best taken one tablet at a time at 5-minute intervals.
- Inform the radiologist if vomiting or diarrhea occurs after ingestion of the radiopaque dye tablets.
- Instruct the patient to remain NPO except for water after taking the contrast tablets.

During

- Note the following procedural steps:
  1. In the radiology department, several plain x-ray films of the patient's right upper quadrant are obtained.

2. If the patient is to receive a fatty meal, a palatable liquid is ingested.
3. Repeated x-ray films of the right upper quadrant are performed.

After

- If the gallbladder is not visualized, note that the patient may be instructed to repeat the procedure with a double dose of radiopaque dye tablets.
- Inform the patient that the radiopaque dye is eventually excreted in the urine. Some patients may report slight dysuria following cholecystography.

Test Results and Clinical Significance

Gallstones *Stones may be seen in the gallbladder.*
Gallbladder polyps *A single filling defect is seen in the gallbladder.*

Chronic cholecystitis
Cholesterolosis
Gallbladder cancer
Cystic duct obstruction
These abnormalities produce "nonvisualization" of the gallbladder after a double dose of dye tablets.

Related Tests

- Ultrasound, gallbladder (p. 778): Provides similar information as does the cholecystography. It is more easily performed, and probably more accurate when results are positive.

Computed Tomography, Abdomen
(CAT Scan, Abdomen; CT Scan, Abdomen)

Normal Findings No evidence of abnormality

Indications

CT is used in evaluating abdominal organs. CT can be used to guide needles during biopsy of tumor and aspiration of fluid, in staging known neoplasms, and to monitor abdominal disease when serially and repeatedly performed.

Test Explanation

CT of the abdomen is a noninvasive, yet accurate radiographic procedure used to diagnose pathologic conditions (e.g., tumors, cysts, abscesses, inflammation, perforation of the bowel, intra-abdominal bleeding, intestinal or ureteral obstruction, vascular aneurysms, and calculi) in the abdominal and retroperitoneal organs. The CT image results from passing x-rays through the abdominal organs at many angles. The variation in density of each tissue allows variable penetration of the x-rays. Each density is given a numeric value called a density coefficient, which is digitally computed into shades of gray. This is then displayed on a television screen as thousands of dots in various shades of

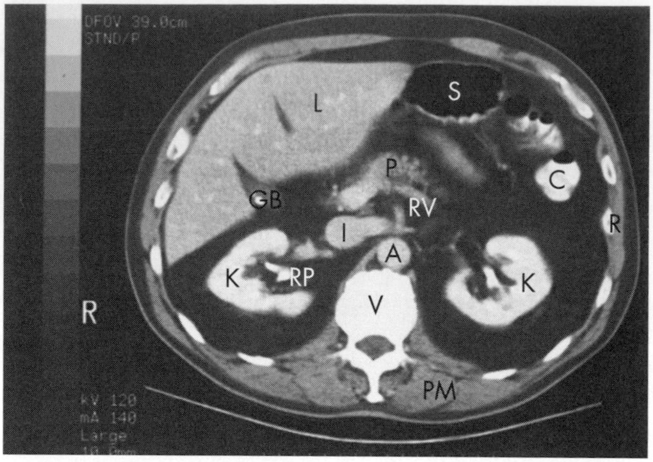

Figure 12-12 CT of the abdomen. Normally many abdominal structures can be seen on a CT scan. *L,* Liver; *GB,* gallbladder (containing a gallstone-radiolucent area); *K,* kidney; *RV,* left renal vein; *RP,* pelvis of the right renal collecting system; *V,* vertebra; *I,* inferior vena cava; *A,* aorta; *C,* the splenic flexure of the colon (contrast filled); *S,* air/contrast filled stomach; *P,* pancreas; *R,* bony ribs of the lower chest; *PM,* paraspinal muscles of the back.

gray. The final display appears as a photograph of the anatomic area sectioned by x-rays (Figure 12-12). The image can be enhanced by repeating the CT scan after IV administration of iodine-containing contrast material. These images can be recorded on x-ray film.

Liver tumors, abscesses, trauma, cysts, and anatomic abnormalities can be seen, as well as pancreatic tumors, pseudocysts, inflammation, calcification, bleeding, and trauma. The kidneys and urinary outflow tract are well visualized.

Renal tumors and cysts, ureteral obstruction, calculi, and congenital renal and ureteral abnormalities are easily seen with the use of IV contrast material. Extravasation of urine secondary to trauma or obstruction can also be easily demonstrated. Adrenal tumors and hyperplasia are best diagnosed with CT. Some radiology literature indicates that the histology of the tumor can be suggested based on the density coefficients shown on the scan.

Although the bowel can be better visualized by an upper GI series, small bowel follow-through, or barium enema, large tumors and perforations of the bowel can be identified with CT, especially when oral contrast material is ingested. The spleen can be well visualized for hematoma, laceration, fracture, tumor infiltration, and splenic vein thrombosis with CT. The retroperitoneal lymph nodes can be evaluated. These are usually present, but all nodes with a diameter >2 cm are considered abnormal. The abdominal aorta and its major branches can be evaluated for aneurysmal dilatation and intramural thrombi, and the pelvic structures (including the uterus, ovaries, fallopian tubes, prostate gland, and rectum) and musculature can be evaluated for tumors, abscesses, infection, or hypertrophy. Ascites and hemoperitoneum can easily be demonstrated on a CT scan.

With the development of new and faster scanners, *dynamic CT scanning* (see CT portography, p. 945) can be performed during arterial injection of dye to the organ being studied. Dynamic scanning can indicate blood flow and degree of vascularity of an organ or part of an organ in the abdomen.

CT is usually performed by a radiologist in less than 30 minutes. If dye is used, the procedure time may be doubled, because the abdomen is scanned both before and after administration of the dye. The only discomfort associated with this study is lying still on a hard table and the peripheral venipuncture. Mild nausea is common when contrast dye is used; thus an emesis basin should be readily available. Some patients may experience a salty taste, flushing, and warmth during the dye injection.

CT can be used to aspirate fluid from the abdomen or an abdominal organ, for cultures and other studies; to guide biopsy needles into areas of abdominal tumors to obtain tissue for study; and to guide catheter placement for drainage of intra-abdominal abscesses.

CT is an important part of staging and monitoring of many tumors before and after therapy. Treatment of tumors of the colon, rectum, hepatic system, breast, lungs, prostate gland, ovaries, uterus, kidneys, lymph glands, and adrenal gland commonly fails, and this can be detected early with CT.

Contraindications

- Allergy to iodinated dye or shellfish
- Pregnancy
- Unstable vital signs
- Profound obesity (usually >300 lb), because the CT table cannot support that much weight
- Claustrophobia

Potential Complications

- Allergic reaction to iodinated dye
  Allergic reactions vary from flushing, itching, and urticaria to severe, life-threatening anaphylaxis (evidenced by respiratory distress, decreased blood pressure, or shock). In the unusual event of anaphylaxis, diphenhydramine (Benadryl), steroids, and epinephrine are included in routine resuscitative efforts. Oxygen and endotracheal equipment should be available for immediate use.
- Acute renal failure from dye infusion
  Adequate hydration before the procedure may reduce the likelihood of this complication.

Interfering Factors

- Presence of metallic objects (e.g., hemostasis clips)
- Retained barium from previous studies
- Large amounts of fecal material or gas in the bowel

✓ CLINICAL PRIORITIES

- Check the patient for allergy to iodinated dyes.
- Mild nausea is common when the contrast dye is injected. For this reason, patients are usually kept NPO for 4 hours before the test.
- Most patients who are mildly claustrophobic can tolerate this study after appropriate medication with antianxiety drugs.
- Adequate hydration before the test may decrease the possibility of acute renal failure from dye infusion.
- CT can be used to guide needles into abdominal tumors for biopsy or to guide catheters into intra-abdominal abscesses for drainage.

Procedure and Patient Care

Before

- Explain the procedure to the patient. Cooperation is necessary, because the patient must lie still during the procedure.
- Obtain informed consent if required by the institution.
- Assess the patient for allergies to iodinated dye or shellfish.
- Inform the radiologist if an allergy to iodinated contrast material is suspected. The radiologist may prescribe a diphenhydramine and steroid preparation to be administered before testing. Usually a hypoallergenic, nonionic contrast agent is used.
- Show the patient a picture of the CT machine. Encourage the patient to verbalize concerns, because some patients may have claustrophobia. Most patients who are mildly claustrophobic can be scanned after appropriate premedication with antianxiety drugs.
- Keep the patient NPO for at least 4 hours before the test if oral contrast agent is to be administered; however, this test can be performed on an emergency basis in patients who have recently eaten.

During

- Note the following procedural steps:
  1. The patient is taken to the radiology department and placed on the CT table (Figure 12-13).
  2. The patient then is placed in an encircling body scanner (gantry). The x-ray tube travels around the gantry, and images (scans) of the various levels of the abdomen and pelvis are obtained. Any motion will cause blurring and streaking of the final scan. Therefore, the patient is asked to remain motionless during x-ray exposure. Television monitoring equipment allows immediate display of the CT image, which is then recorded on Polaroid or x-ray film. In a separate room, the technicians manipulate the CT table, and determine the level of the abdomen to be scanned (see Figure 12-14). Through audio communication, the patient is instructed to hold his or her breath during x-ray exposure.
  3. Better results are obtained with oral or IV iodinated contrast dye. The GI organs can be accurately differentiated from other abdominal organs, and the vessels and ureters are contrasted with the surrounding structures. Contrast agent can sometimes be administered rectally to enable visualization of the pelvic organs.

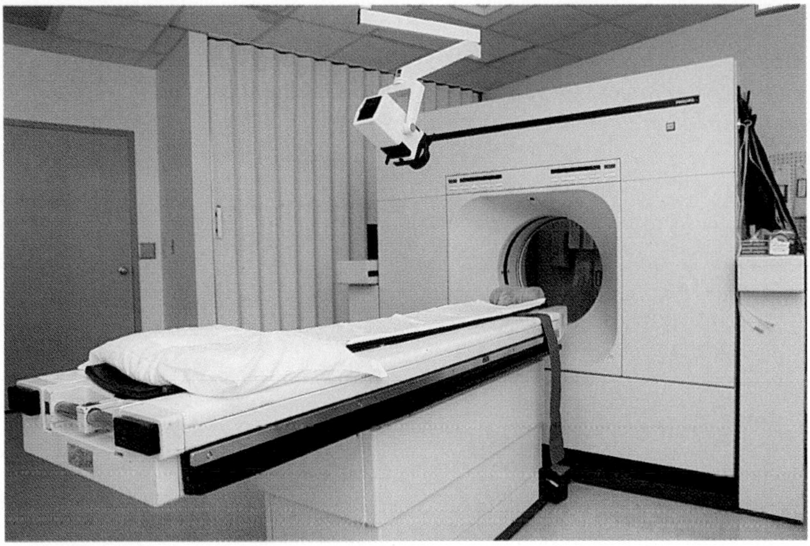

Figure 12-13 CT equipment.

After

- Encourage the patient to drink fluids to avoid dye-induced renal failure and to promote dye excretion.
- Inform the patient that diarrhea may occur after ingestion of the oral contrast agent.
- Evaluate the patient for delayed reaction to dye (e.g., dyspnea, rash, tachycardia, hives). This may occur 2 to 6 hours after the test. Treat with antihistamines or steroids.

Test Results and Clinical Significance

Liver

Tumor, abscess, bile duct dilation *These are evident as radiolucent (dark) filling defects in the liver parenchyma.*

Pancreas

Tumor, pseudocyst, inflammation, bleeding *These are evident as solid or cystic masses of the pancreas.*

Spleen

Hematoma, fracture, laceration, tumor, venous thrombosis *CT of the spleen is the most accurate method of accurately indicating splenic trauma. Tumors, hematomas, and cysts are well demonstrated.*

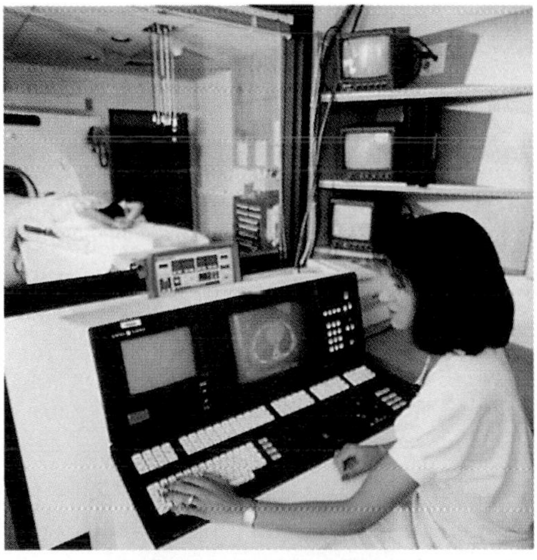

Figure 12-14 X-ray technician performs CT.

Gallbladder/biliary system

Gallstones, tumor, bile duct dilation *Gallstone are sometimes difficult to see. However, an inflammatory response around the gallbladder is evident. Bile duct dilatation is usually evident by demonstration of dilated ducts in the liver parenchyma.*

Kidneys

Tumor, cyst, ureteral obstruction, calculi, congenital abnormalities *Hydronephrosis is easily evident on a CT scan. Likewise, tumors and cysts can be seen. The density of the renal mass can be computed. If the mass is the same density as water, it can safely be assumed the mass is due to a cyst. The CT scan is not as good as IVP in identifying ureteral calculi or ureteral anatomic abnormalities.*

Adrenal gland

Adenoma, cancer, pheochromocytoma, hemorrhage, myelolipoma, hyperplasia *CT is the most accurate method of evaluating the adrenal glands. It is not only used to diagnose tumors, but also to monitor neoplastic diseases that affect the adrenal glands.*

GI tract

Perforation, tumor, inflammatory bowel disease, diverticulitis, appendicitis *Although CT findings are nonspecific as to the cause of an inflammatory mass, CT is sensitive in identification of such a mass. The location and surrounding structures aid in diagnosis of the underlying pathologic process.*

Uterus, fallopian tubes, ovaries

Tumor, abscess, infection, hydrosalpinx, cyst, fibroid *CT is accurate in evaluation of the pelvis for neoplasms of the ovaries, uterus, or cervix. Likewise, infections and abscess can be identified and drained with CT guidance.*

Prostate

Hypertrophy, tumor *An enlarged prostate is easily seen on a CT scan. However, benign and malignant disease cannot be differentiated.*

Retroperitoneum

Tumor, lymphadenopathy *Sarcomas, lymphomas, and inflammation may be evident as masses of increased density in the retroperitoneum.*

Abdominal aneurysm *The presence of an aortic aneurysm can be determined by CT scanning. Repeated scanning can be performed to see if the aneurysm is expanding. A leak or rupture in the aneurysm can also be identified.*

Peritoneum

Ascites, hemoperitoneum

Abscess

Free and localized fluid can be seen on CT scans especially if GI contrast agent has been used. Sometimes loops of bowel can look like abscess.

Related Tests

- MRI (p. 1009): This test is less accurate than CT for identification of abdominal disease. However, in certain abdominal areas (e.g., liver and pelvis) it may be better.

Computed Tomography, Brain (CT Scan, Brain; Computerized Axial Transverse Tomography [CATT])

Normal Findings

No evidence of disease

Indications

The first use of CT scanning was in the evaluation of the brain. The brain is well imaged with CT. This test is indicated when CNS disease is suspected. Specifically, CT is useful in the diagnosis of brain tumors, infarction, bleeding, and hematomas. Information about the ventricular system can also be obtained by CT scanning. Multiple sclerosis and other degenerative abnormalities can be identified.

Test Explanation

Computed tomography of the brain consists of a computerized analysis of multiple tomographic x-ray films taken of the brain tissue at successive layers, providing a three-dimensional view of the cranial contents. The CT image provides a view of the head as if one were looking down through its top. The variation in density of each tissue allows for variable penetration of the x-ray beam. An attached computer calculates the amount of x-ray penetration of each tissue and displays this as shades of gray. The image is placed on a television screen and photographed. The final result is a series of anatomic pictures of coronal and sagittal sections of the brain.

The CT scan is used in the differential diagnosis of intracranial neoplasms, cerebral infarction, ventricular displacement or enlargement, cortical atrophy, cerebral aneurysms, intracranial hemorrhage and hematoma, and arteriovenous (AV) malformation.

Visualization of a neoplasm, previous infarction, or any pathologic process that destroys the blood-brain barrier may be enhanced by IV injection of an iodinated contrast dye. CT may be repeated serially to monitor the progress of any disease or to monitor the healing process. In many cases, CT scanning has eliminated the need for more invasive procedures such as cerebral arteriography and pneumoencephalography. In many institutions, MRI of the brain has replaced the use of CATT.

CT of the brain is performed by a radiology technician in less than 1 hr, and the scans are interpreted by a radiologist. If dye is administered, the procedure time is doubled, because CT scans are obtained before and after administration of the contrast dye. The only discomfort associated with CT is lying still on a hard table and peripheral venipuncture. Mild nausea is common when contrast dye is used, and an emesis basin should be readily available. Some patients may experience a salty taste, flushing, and warmth during the dye injection.

Contraindications

- Allergy to iodinated dye or shellfish
- Claustrophobia
- Pregnancy
- Unstable vital signs
- Profound obesity (usually >300 lb), because the CT table cannot support the weight

Potential Complications

- Allergic reaction to iodinated dye
  Allergic reactions vary from mild flushing, itching, and urticaria to severe, life-threatening anaphylaxis (evidenced by respiratory distress, decreased blood pressure, or shock). In the unusual event of anaphylaxis, diphenhydramine (Benadryl), steroids, and epinephrine are included in routine resuscitation. Oxygen and endotracheal equipment should be available for immediate use.
- Acute renal failure from dye infusion
  Adequate hydration before the procedure may reduce the likelihood of this complication.

CLINICAL PRIORITIES

- Check the patient for allergy to iodinated dyes.
- Mild nausea is common when the contrast dye is injected. For this reason, patients are usually kept NPO for 4 hours before the test.
- Most patients who are mildly claustrophobic can tolerate this study after appropriate medication with antianxiety drugs.
- Adequate hydration before the test may decrease the possibility of acute renal failure from dye infusion.

Procedure and Patient Care

Before

- Explain the procedure to the patient. Cooperation is necessary, because the patient must lie still during the procedure.
- Obtain informed consent if required by the institution. Show the patient a picture of the CT machine and encourage verbalization of concerns, because some patients may have claustrophobia. Most patients who are mildly claustrophobic can be scanned after appropriate premedication with antianxiety drugs.
- Keep the patient NPO for 4 hours before the study, because contrast dye may cause nausea. It is not usually known before the test if enhanced visualization with dye injection will be indicated. If a contrast agent will not be used, food and fluids may be taken. In emergency situations, no fasting is required.
- Instruct the patient that wigs, hairpins, clips, or partial dentures cannot be worn during the procedure, because they hamper visualization of the brain.

- Assess the patient for allergy to iodinated dye or shellfish.
- Inform the radiologist if allergy to iodinated contrast agent is suspected. The radiologist may prescribe a diphenhydramine-steroid preparation to be administered before testing. Usually, a hypoallergenic, nonionic contrast agent is used during the test.
- Tell the patient that he or she may hear a clicking noise as the scanner moves around the head.

During

- Note the following precedural steps:
  1. The patient lies supine on an examining table with the head resting on a snug-fitting rubber cap within a water-filled box or with the head stabilized in a locked head brace. The patient's head is enclosed only to the hairline (as under a hair dryer). The face is not covered, and the patient can see out of the machine at all times. Sponges are placed along the side of the head to ensure it does not move during the study.
  2. The scanner passes an x-ray beam through the brain from one side to the other. The machine then rotates, and the procedure is repeated at each degree through a 180-degree arc. The machine is then moved, and the entire procedure is repeated at 0.5 to 1.0 cm planes.
  3. Remember that iodinated dye usually is used. A peripheral IV line is started, and the iodine dye is administered through it. The entire scanning process is repeated.

After

- Encourage the patient to drink fluids, because dye is excreted by the kidneys and causes diuresis.
- Evaluate the patient for delayed reaction to dye (e.g., dyspnea, rash, tachycardia, hives). This usually occurs 2 to 6 hours after the test. Treat with antihistamines or steroids.

Test Results and Clinical Significance

Intracranial neoplasm (benign and malignant) *These tumors usually are evident as soft tissue masses of increased radiolucency (darkness). Adjacent structures are distorted by the tumor's presence. Some benign tumors have calcification within.*

Cerebral infarction *An infarction can be seen and its age determined with fair accuracy.*

Ventricular displacement
Ventricular enlargement
Hydrocephalus
The fluid-filled ventricles are obvious on CT scans as the least dark areas of the brain. Enlargement may indicate hydrocephalus, with or without increased intracranial pressure. Distortion of the ventricles may be due to tumor or hemorrhage.

Cortical atrophy *Brain tissue lucency may change, and the cortical tissue appears thinner.*

Cerebral aneurysm
AV malformation
Aneurysms and AV malformations are seen when intravenous contrast agent is used.

Intracranial hemorrhage
Hematoma
Abscess
These space-occupying lesions are difficult to differentiate. Serial CT scans may be helpful. In time, hemorrhage will become more diffuse. Hematoma will liquify and become less radiolucent, and even calcify later. Abscess is often surrounded by edema and will slowly enlarge. Epidural and subdural hematomas are evident as isodense areas of swelling that distort the nearby brain tissue.

Multiple sclerosis *Classic CT findings with contrast agent can indicate multiple sclerosis with a moderate degree of accuracy. White matter atrophy, periventricular plaques, and spontaneous hypolucent areas in the periventricular area are usually present.*

Related Tests

- MRI of the brain (p. 1009): This test provides an image of the brain that is superior to CT scans. In many institutions, MRI has replaced CT in evaluation of the CNS.

Computed Tomography, Chest (Chest CT Scan)

Normal Findings

No evidence of disease

Indications

This test is used to more thoroughly evaluate suspected disease in the chest. Questionable or vague abnormalities on the routine chest x-ray can be more thoroughly evaluated with CT scanning of the chest.

Test Explanation

CT of the chest is a noninvasive, yet accurate radiographic procedure for diagnosing and evaluating pathologic conditions such as tumors, nodules, hematomas, parenchymal coin lesions, cysts, abscesses, pleural effusion, and enlarged lymph nodes affecting the lungs and mediastinum. Tumors and cysts of the pleura and fractures of the ribs can also be seen. When an IV contrast material is given, vascular structures can be identified, and a diagnosis of aortic or other vascular abnormality can be made. With oral contrast material, the esophagus and upper GI structures can be evaluated for tumor and other conditions. CT provides a cross-sectional view of the chest and is especially useful in detecting small differences in tissue density, demonstrating lesions that cannot be seen with conventional radiography and tomography. The mediastinal structures can be visualized in a manner that cannot be equaled with conventional x-ray films and tomographic scans.

The x-ray image results from using a body scanner (x-ray tube in a circular gantry) to deliver x-rays through the patient's chest at many different angles. The variation in density of each tissue allows for variable penetration of the x-rays. Each density is given a numeric value called a coefficient, which is digitally computed into shades of gray. This is then displayed on a television screen as thousands of dots in various shades of gray. The final display appears as a photograph of the anatomic area sectioned by the x-rays.

This procedure is performed by a radiologist in 30 to 45 minutes. If dye is administered, the procedure time may be doubled, because CT scanning is done before and after administration of the contrast dye. The only discomfort associated with this study is lying still on a hard table, and the peripheral venipuncture. Mild nausea is common when contrast dye is used, and an emesis basin should be readily available. Some patients may experience a salty taste, flushing, and warmth during the dye injection.

Contraindications

- Pregnancy
- Allergy to iodinated dye or shellfish
- Claustrophobia
- Profound obesity (usually >300 lb)
- Unstable vital signs

Potential Complications

- Allergic reaction to iodinated dye
  May vary from mild flushing, itching, and urticaria to severe, life-threatening anaphylaxis (evidenced by respiratory distress, decreased blood pressure, or shock). In the unusual event of anaphylaxis, diphenhydramine (Benadryl), steroids, and epinephrine are included in routine resuscitation. Oxygen and endotracheal equipment should be available for immediate use.
- Acute renal failure from dye infusion
  Adequate hydration beforehand may reduce the likelihood of this complication.

CLINICAL PRIORITIES

- Check the patient for allergy to iodinated dyes.
- Mild nausea is common when the contrast dye is injected. For this reason, patients are usually kept NPO for 4 hours before the test.
- Most patients who are mildly claustrophobic can tolerate this study after appropriate medication with antianxiety drugs.
- Adequate hydration before the test may decrease the possibility of acute renal failure from dye infusion.

Procedure and Patient Care

Before

- Explain the procedure to the patient. Cooperation is necessary, because the patient must lie still during the procedure.
- Obtain informed consent if required by the institution.
- Assess the patient for allergies to iodinated dye or shellfish.
- Inform the radiologist if an allergy to iodinated contrast is suspected. The radiologist may prescribe a diphenhydramine-steroid preparation to be administered before testing. Usually, a hypoallergenic, nonionic contrast dye is used for the test.

- Show the patient a picture of the CT machine and encourage verbalization of concerns about claustrophobia. Most patients who are mildly claustrophobic can tolerate this study after appropriate premedication with antianxiety drugs.
- Keep the patient NPO for 4 hours before the test in the event that contrast dye is administered.

During

- Note the following procedural steps:
  1. The patient is taken to the radiology department and asked to remain motionless in a supine position. Any motion will cause blurring and streaking of the final scan.
  2. An encircling x-ray camera (body scanner) takes pictures at varying intervals and levels over the chest area. Monitor equipment allows immediate display, and the image is recorded on x-ray film.
  3. Occasionally, IV dye is administered to enhance the chest image, and the x-ray studies are repeated.

After

- Encourage patients who received dye injection to increase their fluid intake, because the dye is excreted by the kidneys and causes diuresis.
- Evaluate the patient for delayed reaction to the dye (e.g., dyspnea, rashes, tachycardia, hives). This usually occurs 2 to 6 hours after the test. Treat with antihistamines or steroids.

Test Results and Clinical Significance

Lung

Lung tumor (primary or metastatic) *This is evident as soft tissue masses in the lung fields.*
Pneumonia *Increased lucency in the lung field indicates pneumonia or atelectatic lung.*
Pleural effusion *Fluid in the chest wall is evident as increased lucency outside the lung fields, particularly in the costophrenic margins.*
Chronic obstructive pulmonary disease *Increased lung space is classic for COPD.*
Atelectasis *Collapse of pulmonary alveoli is evident as white patches or lines in the lung fields.*
Tuberculosis *Usually in the upper lobes, chronic TB and other granulomatous diseases are usually associated with calcification.*
Lung abscess *Lung abscess is evident as a lung mass with a hollow (radiolucent) center. Sometimes fungus grows inside the abscess.*
Pleuritis *A thickened pleura indicates pleuritis, from a viral, bacterial, neoplastic, or other cause.*

Heart

Pericarditis
Pericardial effusion
Evident as thickened pericardium with or without fluid around the heart.

Chest wall

Soft tissue sarcoma
Osteogenic sarcoma

Primary tumor masses of the bony thorax and chest wall soft tissue, they are evident as masses arising from those areas of the chest.

Fracture (ribs or thoracic spine) *This is usually associated with other chest trauma.*

Metastatic tumor to bony thorax *Osteolytic (dark) or osteoblastic (white) nodules can be seen in the bony thorax. Breast, prostate, kidneys, and lungs are among the most common cancers to metastasize to the bones in this region.*

Diaphragm

Diaphragmatic or hiatal hernia *This is evident as increased lucency in the posteroinferior mediastinum.*

Mediastinum

Aortic calcinosis *Evident as white lines indicating the walls of the calcified aorta.*

Enlarged lymph nodes *Central-occurring masses in the mediastinum indicate enlarged lymph nodes, usually of a neoplastic etiology.*

Dilated aorta *This is indicative of aneurysm. Dissection, if present, is obvious on CT scans of the chest.*

Thymoma
Lymphoma
Substernal thyroid
These are often evident as large soft tissue masses in the anterosuperior mediastinum.

Metastatic tumor to mediastinum *Esophageal and upper stomach cancers may metastasize to the mediastinal lymph nodes.*

Perforation of esophagus (spontaneous [Boerhaave's syndrome] or iatrogenic [following esophageal dilation]). *Meglumine diatrizoate (Gastrografin) that was previously ingested will be seen free in mediastinum.*

Related Tests

- Chest radiography (p. 924): Routine part of every thorough evaluation of the cardiopulmonary system. While not so accurate as CT, it provides a tremendous amount of information easily.

Computed Tomography Portogram
(CT Portogram)

Normal Findings

No evidence of liver abnormalities

Indications

The CT portogram provides an accurate picture of the liver. It is used when small tumors (usually metastases) are suspected, and is particularly helpful to the surgeon contemplating liver resection.

Test Explanation

A CT scan of the liver (see p. 933) is inaccurate in identifying liver tumors <2 cm in greatest dimension. A CT portogram can accurately identify liver abnormalities as small as 5 mm. The difference between CT of the liver and CT portography is the manner in which the contrast dye is injected. In routine CT, dye is injected through a peripheral vein. In CT portography, dye is injected through a catheter placed in the splenic artery. The dye passes through the spleen and into the splenic vein, and subsequently into the portal vein and its tributaries. Hepatic tumors and cysts, however, do not take up dye. On the portogram, these lesions appear as filling defects (dark spots) in the liver. Tumors take up the dye, and appear as white spots in the liver. Use of this test is limited to identification of suspected smaller neoplasms in the liver. It is used in cancer patients with suspected metastatic lesions in the liver. The number and location of these metastatic lesions are best visualized with CT portography. Conventional CT scanning of the liver may miss the smaller tumors.

Placement of the arterial catheter by a radiologist takes about 30 minutes and is minimally uncomfortable. CT scanning by a technician takes about 15 minutes and is not uncomfortable. The CT scans are interpreted by a radiologist.

Contraindications

- Allergy to shellfish or iodinated dye
- Uncooperative or agitated patients
- Pregnancy
- Renal disorders, because iodinated contrast is nephrotoxic
- Bleeding propensity, because it may be difficult to stop the bleeding at the femoral arterial puncture site
- Unstable cardiac disorders
- Dehydration, because of the risk for dye-induced renal failure

Potential Complications

- Allergic reactions to iodinated dye
  These reactions may vary from mild flushing, itching, and urticaria to severe, life-threatening anaphylaxis (evidenced by respiratory distress, decreased blood pressure,

✓ CLINICAL PRIORITIES

- Check the patient for allergies to iodinated dyes.
- Dehydrated patients are susceptible to dye-induced renal failure. The elderly are at high risk for this complication.
- Mark the site of the patient's peripheral pulses before arterial catheterization. This will enable easier assessment of the peripheral pulses after the procedure.
- Monitor vital signs carefully for indications of hemorrhage after the procedure. Usually a 1- to 2-lb sandbag or IV bag is placed over the puncture site for several hours.

and shock). In the unusual event of anaphylaxis, diphenhydramine (Benadryl), steroids, and epinephrine are included in routine resuscitative efforts. Oxygen and endotracheal equipment should be available for immediate use.

- Hemorrhage from the arterial puncture site used for arterial access
- Arterial embolism from dislodgement of arteriosclerotic plaque
- Soft tissue infection around the puncture site
- Renal failure, especially in elderly patients with chronic dehydration or mild renal failure
- Pseudoaneurysm development as a result of failure of the puncture site to seal

Procedure and Patient Care

Before

- Explain the procedure to the patient. Allay any fears, and allow the patient to verbalize concerns.
- Ensure that written, informed consent for this procedure is in the patient's chart.
- Assess the possibility of allergy to iodinated dye. Inform the radiologist if an allergy to iodinated contrast is suspected. The radiologist may prescribe diphenhydramine and a steroid preparation to be administered before the test. Usually, hypoallergenic, nonionic contrast material is used during the test.
- Determine if the patient has been taking anticoagulants.
- Keep the patient NPO for at least 2 to 4 hours before testing.
- Mark the site of the patient's peripheral pulses with permanent ink before arterial catheterization. This will enable assessment of the peripheral pulses after the procedure.

During

- Note the following precedural steps:
  1. The patient may be sedated before being taken to the angiography room, which is usually in the radiology department.
  2. The patient is placed supine on the x-ray table.
  3. If the femoral artery is to be used, the groin is shaved, prepared, and sterile draped.
  4. The femoral artery is cannulated, and a wire is threaded up the artery and into or near the opening of the splenic artery.
  5. A catheter is placed over the wire and into the splenic artery.
  6. The patient is transferred to the CT unit, also usually in the radiology department.
  7. Through the catheter, iodinated contrast material is injected into the splenic artery.
  8. The patient is positioned in the CT scanner (see CT scanning of the body, p. 937).
  9. CT scans are obtained immediately subsequent to injection of dye into the indwelling catheter.

After

- After scanning is completed, the catheter is removed and a pressure dressing applied to the puncture site.
- Monitor the patient's vital signs for indications of hemorrhage.
- Assess the peripheral pulse in the extremity used for vascular access and compare it with the preprocedural baseline values.

- Maintain pressure at the puncture site with a 1- to 2-lb sandbag or an IV bag for several hours.
- Keep the patient on bed rest for about 4 to 8 hours after the procedure to permit complete sealing of the arterial puncture site.
- Evaluate the patient for delayed allergic reaction to the dye (e.g., dyspnea, rash, tachycardia, hives). Reactions usually occur within 2 to 6 hours after the test. Treat with antihistamines or steroids.

Test Results and Clinical Significance

Hepatic tumor *Tumors as small as 3-5 mm are apparent as radiopaque (white) areas in the liver parenchyma.*

Hepatic cyst *This is evident as radiolucent (dark) areas in the liver parenchyma.*

Hepatic hemangioma *This is evident as bright radiopaque areas in the liver parenchyma.*

Related Tests

- CT scan of the body (p. 933): Similar to CT portography except the dye is injected intravenously. Liver imaging is not as sensitive or accurate.

Cystography (Cystourethrography, Voiding Cystography, Voiding Cystourethrography)

Normal Findings

Normal bladder structure and function

Indications

Cystography enables radiographic visualization of the bladder. It is useful in patients with hematuria, recurrent urinary tract infections, and suspected bladder trauma.

Test Explanation

Filling the bladder with contrast material provides visualization of the bladder for radiographic study. Either fluoroscopic or x-ray films demonstrate bladder filling and collapse after emptying. Filling defects or shadows in the bladder indicate primary bladder tumors. Extrinsic compression or distortion of the bladder is seen with pelvic tumor (e.g., rectal, cervical) or hematoma (secondary to pelvic bone fractures). Extravasation of the dye is seen with traumatic rupture, perforation, and fistula of the bladder. Vesicoureteral reflux (abnormal backflow of urine from bladder to ureters), which can cause persistent or recurrent pyelonephritis, also may be demonstrated during cystography. Although the bladder is visualized during IVP (p. 953), primary pathologic bladder conditions are best studied by means of cystography.

A radiologist performs the study in approximately 15 to 30 minutes. This test is moderately uncomfortable if bladder catheterization is required.

Contraindications

- Urethral or bladder infection or injury
  Gram-negative sepsis can occur as a result of catheterization. Existing bladder injury may be made worse by instillation of dye into the bladder.

Potential Complications

- Urinary tract infection
  May result from catheter placement or instillation of contaminated contrast material.
- Allergic reaction to iodinated dye
  Rare, because the dye is not administered intravenously.

✓ CLINICAL PRIORITIES

- Assess for allergy to iodinated dyes.
- After the test, assess the patient for urinary tract infection, which may result from catheter placement or instillation of contaminated contrast material.
- Encourage the patient to drink fluids to eliminate the dye and to prevent accumulation of bacteria.

Procedure and Patient Care

Before

- Explain the procedure to the patient.
- Obtain informed consent if required by the institution.
- Give clear liquids for breakfast on the morning of the test.
- Assure the patient that he or she will be draped to prevent unnecessary exposure.
- Insert a Foley catheter if ordered.

During

- Note the following procedural steps:
  1. The patient is taken to the radiology department and placed in a supine or lithotomy position.
  2. Unless a catheter is already present, one is placed.
  3. Approximately 300 ml (much less for children) of air or radiopaque dye is injected through the catheter into the bladder, and the catheter is clamped.
  4. X-ray films are taken.
  5. If the patient is able to void, the catheter is removed and the patient is asked to urinate while films are taken of the bladder and urethra *(voiding cystourethrogram)* (Figure 12-15).
  - Ensure that in male patients a lead shield is placed over the testes to prevent irradiation of the gonads.
  - The ovaries in female patients cannot be shielded without blocking bladder visualization. Ensure that female patients are not pregnant.

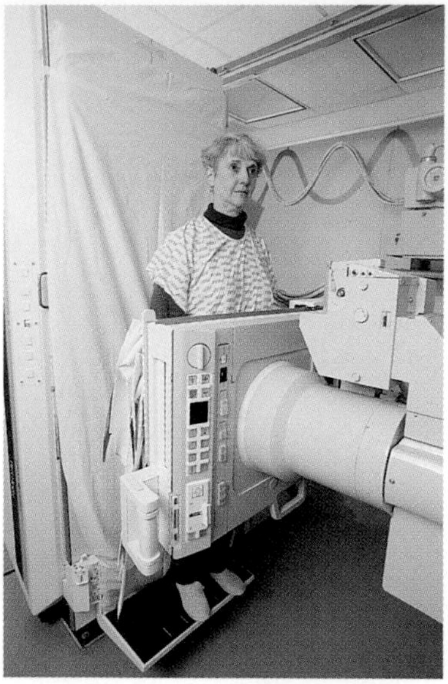

Figure 12-15 Position for voiding cystourethrography.

After

- Assess the patient for signs of urinary tract infection.
- Encourage the patient to drink fluids to eliminate the dye and to prevent accumulation of bacteria.

Test Results and Clinical Significance

Bladder tumor *Primary cancers of the bladder are evident as filling defects (radiolucent shadow) in the bladder.*

Pelvic tumor or hematoma *Any mass that distorts the pelvic anatomy is seen as external compression of the dye-filled bladder.*

Bladder trauma *Laceration or perforation of the bladder is evident by the finding of dye outside the bladder. This is usually best demonstrated on the postvoid film.*

Vesicoureteral reflux *Reflux of urine or dye from the bladder into the ureter is obvious with distention of the bladder with dye.*

Hysterosalpingography (Uterotubography, Uterosalpingography, Hysterogram)

Normal Findings

Patent fallopian tubes
No defects in uterine cavity

Indications

This test is part of a workup for infertility. The result can indicate patency or obstruction of the fallopian tubes.

Test Explanation

In hysterosalpingography, the uterine cavity and fallopian tubes are visualized radiographically after the injection of contrast material through the cervix. Uterine tumors, intrauterine adhesions, and developmental anomalies can be seen. Tubal obstruction of the fallopian tubes caused by internal scarring, tumor, infection, or kinking also can be detected. A possible therapeutic effect of this test is that passage of dye through the tubes may clear mucous plugs, straighten kinked tubes, or break up adhesions. This test also may be used to document adequacy of surgical tubal ligation. Its main purpose is in the evaluation of infertility to see if there is any obstruction of the fallopian tubes.

This procedure is performed by a physician in approximately 15 to 30 minutes. The patient may feel occasional, transient menstrual-type cramping and may have shoulder pain caused by subphrenic irritation from the dye as it leaks into the peritoneal cavity.

Contraindications

- Infections of the vagina, cervix, or fallopian tubes, because of risk of extending the infection
- Uterine bleeding, because contrast material may enter the open blood vessels. Further, clots may be pushed out of the uterus and into the fallopian tubes, causing obstruction
- Pregnancy, because contrast material may induce abortion

Potential Complications

- Infection of the endometrium (endometritis)
- Infection of the fallopian tubes (salpingitis)
- Uterine perforation
- Allergic reaction to iodinated dye or shellfish (rare because the dye is not administered intravenously)

Interfering Factors

- Fecal material or gas in the bowel, which may obscure visualization
- Tubal spasm or excessive traction, which may cause the appearance of a stricture in a normal fallopian tube
- Excessive traction, which may displace adhesions, thereby making tubes appear normal

✓ CLINICAL PRIORITIES

- Check the patient for allergy to iodinated dyes.
- This test is not performed if pregnancy is suspected, because the contrast material might induce abortion.
- After the test, evaluate the patient for signs and symptoms of infection (e.g., fever, increased pulse rate, pain).

Procedure and Patient Care

Before

- Explain the procedure to the patient. Ask the patient when she had her last menstrual period. If pregnancy is suspected, the test is not performed.
- Obtain informed consent if required by the institution.
- Assess the patient for allergy to iodine dye or shellfish. Report positive findings to the radiologist. Allergic reactions in this study are rare, because the dye is not administered intravenously.

- Instruct the patient to take laxatives the night before the test, if ordered.
- Administer enemas or suppositories on the morning of the test, if ordered.
- Administer sedatives (e.g., diazepam [Valium]) or antispasmodics, if ordered, before the test.
- Tell the patient that no food or fluid restrictions are needed.

During

- Note the following procedural steps:
  1. A plain x-ray film of the abdomen is often obtained before the test to ensure that preparation adequately eliminated gastrointestinal gas and feces.
  2. After voiding, the patient is placed on the fluoroscopy table in the lithotomy position.
  3. A speculum is inserted into the vagina, and the cervix is visualized and cleansed.
  4. Contrast material is injected during fluoroscopy, and x-ray films are obtained.
  5. More dye is injected so that the entire upper genital tract (uterus and fallopian tubes) can be filled.
  6. This test can be considered satisfactorily performed only if the uterus and the tubes are distended to their maximal capacity or fluid flows through the fallopian tubes.

After

- Inform the patient that a vaginal discharge (sometimes bloody) may be present for 1 or 2 days after the test. A perineal pad should be worn.
- Evaluate the patient for delayed reaction to dye (e.g., dyspnea, rash, tachycardia, hives). Treat symptoms with antihistamines or steroids.
- Inform the patient that cramping and dizziness may occur after the study.
- Evaluate the patient for signs and symptoms of infection (e.g., fever, increased pulse rate, pain). Instruct the patient to call her physician and report these symptoms if they occur.

Test Results and Clinical Significance

Uterine tumor (e.g., leiomyoma, cancer) *Filling defects in the uterus may indicate tumor.*

Developmental anomaly of the uterus (e.g., uterus bicornis) *The anatomy of the uterus can be well visualized and evaluated.*

Intrauterine adhesions *Usually from previous infection, these adhesions within the uterus can cause infertility.*

Uterine fistula *Usually traumatic (iatrogenic [e.g., during dilatation and curettage]), a fisutla is evident as extravasation of dye from the uterus.*

Obstruction, kinking, or twisting of the fallopian tubes secondary to adhesions *This is indicated by stenosis or complete obstruction. Fertility is unlikely unless tubal patency is reestablished.*

Extrauterine pregnancy *Early tubal pregnancy can be demonstrated with this study, but there are better and easier ways to determine tubal pregnancy (e.g., CT of the pelvis [p. 933]).*

Tumor of the fallopian tubes *Tumors are evident as tubal filling defects.*

Intravenous Pyelography (IVP, Excretory Urography [EUG], Intravenous Urography [IUG, IVU])

Normal Findings

Normal size, shape, and position of the kidneys, renal pelvis, ureters, and bladder
Normal kidney excretory function as evidenced by the length of time for passage of contrast material through the kidneys

Indications

The IVP is the most commonly used radiologic test for evaluation of the urinary system, because much information about the kidneys, ureters, bladder, and prostate can be obtained. It is indicated in patients with:

Pain compatible with urinary stones
Blood in the urine
Proposed pelvic surgery, to locate the ureters
Trauma to the urinary system
Urinary outlet obstruction
Suspected kidney tumor

Age-related concerns

- In pediatric patients, fluid restrictions should be modified based on age and clinical symptoms.
- Elderly patients are particularly vulnerable to compromised renal function. Fluid restrictions are modified for the elderly and for patients with chronic dehydration (e.g., from chronic diarrhea).
- Because of the combination of fasting and catharsis necessary for test preparation, elderly and debilitated patients are at high risk for weakness and injury. These patients should ambulate only with assistance.

Test Explanation

IVP is a radiologic study in which radiopaque contrast material is used to visualize the kidneys, renal pelvis, ureters, and bladder. The dye is injected intravenously, filtered in the kidney by the glomeruli, and passes through the renal tubules. X-ray films obtained at set intervals over the next 30 minutes will show passage of the dye through the kidneys and ureters and into the bladder (Figure 12-16).

If the artery leading to one of the kidneys is blocked, the dye cannot enter that part of the renal system and it will not be visualized. If the artery is partially blocked, it will take longer before the contrast material is visualized.

With primary glomerular disease (e.g., glomerulonephritis), the glomerular filtrate is reduced, which causes a reduction in the quantity of dye filtered. Therefore, more time is required for enough dye to enter the kidney to enable renal opacification. As a result, kidney visualization is delayed. This indicates an estimate of renal function.

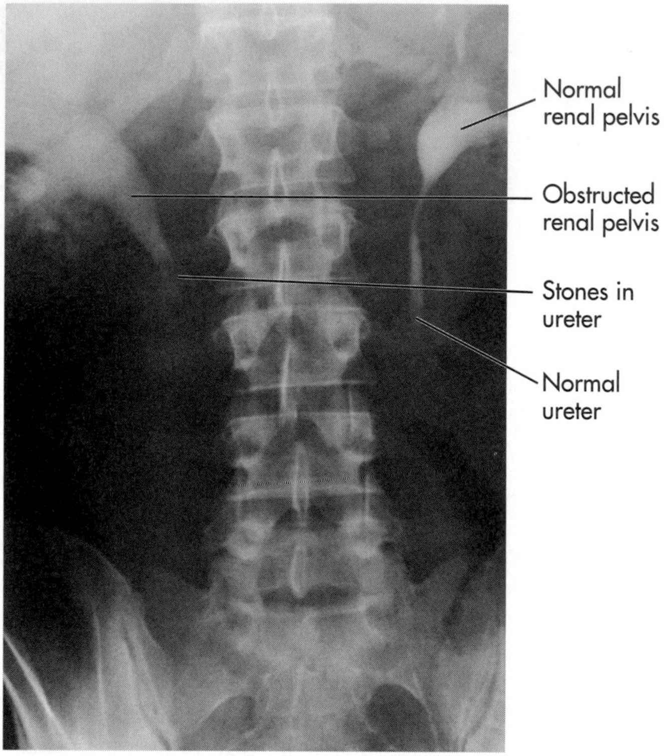

Figure 12-16 IVP. Note the distended obstructed urinary collecting system obstructed by a stone in the right ureter (left side of figure). The left collecting system is normal sized and unobstructed.

Defects in dye filling of the kidney can indicate renal tumors or cysts. Often, intrinsic and extrinsic tumors, stones, and scarring can partially or completely obstruct the flow of dye through the collecting system (pelvis, ureters, bladder). If the obstruction has been of sufficient duration, the collecting system proximal to the obstruction will be dilated (hydronephrosis). Retroperitoneal and pelvic tumors, aneurysms, and enlarged lymph nodes also can produce extrinsic compression and distortions of the opacified collecting system.

IVP is used to assess the effect of trauma on the urinary system. Renal hematomas distort the renal contour. Renal artery laceration is suggested by nonopacification of one kidney. Laceration of the kidneys, pelvis, ureters, or bladder often causes urine leaks, which are identified by dye extravasation from the urinary system.

IVP is used to assess for congenital absence or malposition of the kidneys. Horseshoe kidneys (connection of the two kidneys), double ureters, and pelvic kidneys are typical congenital abnormalities.

Nephrotomography provides radiographic visualization of the kidney using tomographic technique after IV injection of radiopaque dye. Tomography is a radiologic technique by which a sequence of x-ray films, each representing a visual section ("slice") through the

Table 12-4 Tests for visualization of the urinary system

Portion of the urinary system	Test
Kidney	CT
Renal pelvis and ureters	IVP or retrograde pyelography
Bladder	Cystography or cystoscopy
Urethra	Urethrography or cystoscopy

organ, is obtained. Tomography permits examination of a single layer or plane of the organ that would otherwise be obscured by the surrounding structures. Nephrotomography permits visualization of different planes of the kidney to differentiate solid renal and adrenal tumors from benign renal cysts.

Table 12-4 describes diagnostic tests used to evaluate the urinary system.

Contraindications

- Allergy to shellfish or iodinated dyes
  Premedication with prednisone and diphenhydramine (Benadryl) may be ordered.
- Severe dehydration, which can cause renal shutdown and failure
  Geriatric patients are particularly vulnerable.
- Renal insufficiency, as evidenced by a blood urea nitrogen (BUN) value > 40 mg/dl, because the iodinated nephrotoxic dye can worsen kidney function
- Multiple myeloma, because the iodinated nephrotoxic dye can worsen renal function

Potential Complications

- Allergic reaction to iodinated dye
  Allergic reactions vary from mild flushing, itching, and urticaria to severe, life-threatening anaphylaxis (evidenced by respiratory distress, decreased blood pressure, or shock). In the unusual event of anaphylaxis, the patient may be given diphenhydramine (Benadryl), steroids, and epinephrine. Oxygen and endotracheal equipment should be available for immediate use.
- Infiltration of contrast dye
  Avoided by ensuring patency of the IV line. In the event of infiltration, a local injection of hyaluronidase may be given to hasten absorption of iodine and resolution of the reaction.
- Renal failure
  Most often occurs in elderly patients with chronic dehydration before the dye injection.

Interfering Factors

- Fecal material, gas, or barium in the bowel may obscure visualization of the renal system.

CLINICAL PRIORITIES

- Check the patient for allergy to iodinated dyes.
- Evaluate for adequacy of renal function (BUN/creatinine) before IVP.
- Barium studies should be scheduled after IVP.

- Abnormal renal function studies may prevent adequate visualization of the urinary tract.
- Retained barium from previous studies may obscure visualization. Studies with barium (e.g., barium enema) should be scheduled after IVP.

Procedure and Patient Care

Before

- Explain the procedure to the patient. Inform the patient that several x-ray films will be obtained over 30 minutes.
- Obtain informed consent if required by the institution.
- Check the patient for allergy to iodinated dye or shellfish.
- Inform the radiologist if an allergy to iodine is suspected. The radiologist may prescribe a diphenhydramine-steroid preparation to be administered before the test. Usually, hypoallergenic, nonionic contrast material is used during the test.
- Give the patient a laxative (e.g., castor oil) or a cathartic, as ordered, the evening before the test.
- Inform the patient of the required food and fluid restrictions. Some institutions prefer abstinence from solid foods for 8 hours before testing; some allow a clear-liquid breakfast on the test day. For pediatric, elderly, and debilitated patients, fasting times will be ordered on an individual basis.
- Ensure adequate hydration (IV or oral) before and after the test to prevent dye-induced renal failure.
- In patients receiving high rates of IV fluids, infusion rates may be decreased for several hours before the study to increase the concentration of the dye within the urinary system.
- Assess BUN and creatinine levels. Abnormal renal function could deteriorate as a result of the dye injection.
- Give the patient an enema or suppository on the morning of the study, if ordered.
- Schedule any barium studies after completion of IVP.

During

- Note the following procedural steps:
  1. The patient is taken to the radiology department and placed in the supine position.
  2. A plain film of the abdomen (KUB) is taken to ensure that no residual stool obscures visualization of the renal system. This also screens for calculi in the renal collecting system.

3. Skin testing for iodine allergy is often done.
4. A peripheral IV line is started (if not in place), and a contrast dye (e.g., Hypaque, Renografin) is given.
5. X-ray films are obtained at specific times (usually at 1, 5, 10, 15, 20, and 30 minutes, and sometimes longer after dye administration) to follow the course of the dye from the cortex of the kidney to the bladder.
6. Tomography may be performed to identify a mass.
7. The patient is taken to the bathroom and asked to void.
8. A post-voiding film is obtained to visualize the empty bladder.

- Occasionally it is necessary to partially occlude the ureters temporarily to obtain a better film of the collecting system in the upper part of the ureters. This is done by compressing the abdomen with an inflatable rubber tube wrapped tightly around the abdomen slightly below the umbilicus.
- For nephrotomography, the x-ray tube and cassette are rapidly moved in opposite directions while the film is obtained. This technique effectively blurs all tissue planes (slices) except that being studied.
- The test is performed by a radiologist in approximately 45 minutes.
- Inform the patient that the dye injection often causes transitory flushing of the face, a feeling of warmth, a salty taste in the mouth, or even transient nausea. Initial IV needle placement and lying on a hard x-ray table are the only other discomforts associated with IVP.

After

- Assess urinary output. Decreased output may be an indication of renal failure.
- Evaluate the patient for delayed reaction to dye (e.g., dyspnea, rash, tachycardia, hives). Reactions usually occur within the first 2 to 6 hours after the test. Treat with antihistamines or steroids.
- Encourage the patient to drink fluids to counteract fluid depletion caused by the test preparation procedures.
- Evaluate elderly and debilitated patients for weakness, because of the combination of fasting and catharsis necessary for test preparation. Instruct these patients to ambulate only with assistance.
- Maintain adequate oral or IV hydration for several hours after IVP.

Home Care Responsibilities

- After the test, patients must be encouraged to drink a lot of fluids to reestablish their normal state of hydration.
- Instructions to patients regarding urinary output are crucial. Decreased urine output may be an indication of impending renal failure.

Test Results and Clinical Significance

Pyelonephritis or glomerulonephritis *Primary renal disease usually is evident as reduced opacification of the kidney with dye. This is because it takes longer for enough dye to be filtered to the renal system to opacify the kidney.*

Kidney tumor (benign or malignant)
Renal hematoma, laceration
Cyst or polycystic disease of the kidney
These are usually evident as a radiolucent (dark) filling defect in the kidney parenchyma. Ultrasound of the kidney (p. 778) is diagnostic for cysts.

Congenital abnormality of the urologic tract *Congenital anomalies may include absence of a kidney or altered shape, size, or location of a kidney. The collecting system can be duplicated, with more than one ureter per kidney. The bladder can be divided by a congenital septum into two small bladders.*
Renal or ureteral calculi *Calculi (stones) are evident as radiolucent filling defects that can obstruct the ureters.*
Trauma to the kidneys, ureters, or bladder *Injury may be evident as leakage of dye from the injured organ. Hematomas are seen as filling defects or radiolucent shadows.*
Tumor of the collecting system *This can partially or completely obstruct the collecting system.*
Hydronephrosis *This condition is due to prolonged obstruction of the collecting system distal to the hydronephrotic area.*
Extrinsic compression of the collecting system (e.g., caused by tumor, aneurysm) *Nonurologic tumors or masses can distort or obstruct the ureters or bladder.*
Bladder tumor *This is seen as a radiolucent (dark shadow) filling defect in the bladder.*
Prostate enlargement *This is evident as an extrinsic protrusion into the base of the bladder and inadequate emptying of the bladder due to outlet obstruction.*

Related Tests

- CT of the abdomen (p. 933): Allows better visualization of the kidneys. The ureters are better studied with IVP.
- Cystography (p. 948): Study of the bladder after placement of dye directly into the bladder. With this study, the dye is more concentrated, and more information concerning the bladder can be obtained.

Kidney, Ureter, and Bladder Radiography
(KUB) (Flat Plate of the Abdomen, Plain Film of the Abdomen, Scout Film)

Normal Findings

No evidence of calculi
Normal gastrointestinal (GI) gas pattern

Indications

This screening x-ray strategy is used to rapidly evaluate the abdomen in patients with abdominal pain or trauma. It can demonstrate pathologic conditions of the urinary or gastrointestinal system.

Test Explanation

The KUB is a flat plate, or simple x-ray film, of the abdomen. It is often referred to as a *plain film,* or *scout film.* The KUB is similar to the supine view on an obstruction series (see p. 972), and can be performed to demonstrate the size, shape, location, and any malformations of the kidneys and bladder. The KUB can also be used to identify calculi in these organs and in the ureters. This is often one of the first studies done to diagnose other intra-abdominal diseases, such as intestinal obstruction, soft tissue masses, and a ruptured viscus (Figure 12-17). The KUB is useful in detecting abnormal accumulations of gas within the GI tract and identifying ascites. No contrast medium is used for this study.

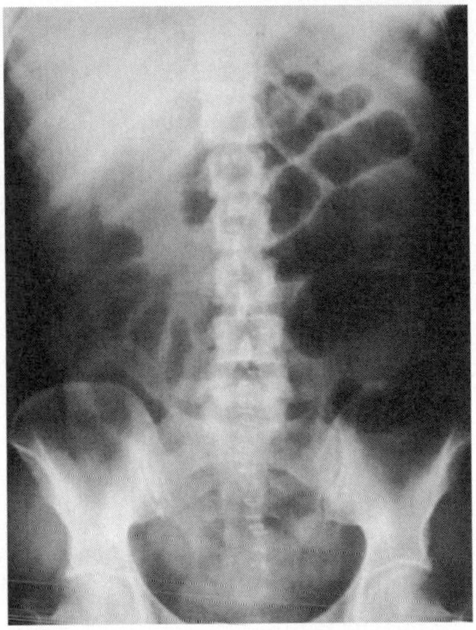

Figure 12-17 Flat plate of abdomen depicts multiple, somewhat dilated loops of small bowel consistent with postoperative ileus.

Contraindications

- Pregnancy

Interfering Factors

- Barium retained from previous studies can obscure visualization.

✓ CLINICAL PRIORITIES

- This test is also called a *plain film* or *scout film* of the abdomen.
- This test involves no contrast dye.
- This is often one of the first tests used in the evaluation of abdominal problems.
- This test should be scheduled before any barium studies.

Procedure and Patient Care

Before

- Explain the procedure to the patient.
- Tell the patient that no fasting or sedation is required.
- Schedule this study before any barium studies.
- In male patient the testicles should be shielded with a lead apron to prevent their irradiation.
- In female patients, the ovaries cannot be shielded because of their proximity to the kidneys, ureters, and bladder.

During

- In the radiology department, the patient is placed in the supine position. X-ray films are obtained of the patient's abdomen (Figure 12-18).
- Note that the KUB is performed by a radiologic technologist in a few minutes, and is interpreted by a radiologist.
- Inform the patient that results are available in approximately 1 hour.
- Tell the patient that no discomfort is associated with this study.

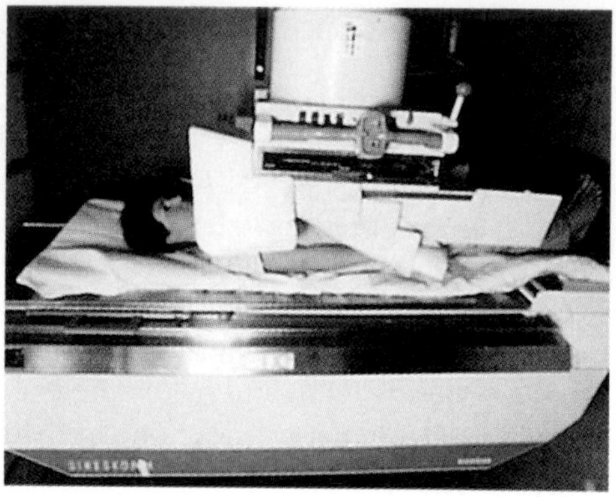

Figure 12-18 KUB equipment.

After

- If indicated, schedule intravenous pyelography or GI studies after completion of the KUB.

Test Results And Clinical Significance

Calculi *A calcified stone in the area of the KUB where the ureters would be is indicative of a ureteral calculi. This requires supportive evidence, as obtained with IVP (p. 953).*

Abnormal accumulation of bowel gas *Abnormal accumulation of bowel gas can indicate intestinal obstruction or paralytic ileus.*

Ascites *The classic "ground glass" appearance of the entire abdomen on the KUB films indicates peritoneal effusion.*

Soft tissue masses *Large soft tissue masses can be seen surprisingly well on this plain film without use of any contrast material.*

Ruptured viscus *Free air (i.e., air outside the bowel but inside the abdomen) is indicative of a perforated viscus.*

Congenital anomalies (e.g., location, size, and number of kidneys) *Because the kidneys can be well visualized with KUB, anomalies are fairly easily detected.*

Organomegaly or bladder distention *An enlarged liver or spleen is seen as a large soft tissue mass in the right or left upper quadrant, respectively. A large soft tissue mass in the midline or pelvis is usually a distended bladder.*

Related Tests

- Obstruction series (p. 972): This study includes a KUB as part of the series of plain film x-rays obtained to evaluate abdominal pain.

Lymphangiography
(Lymphangiogram, Lymphography)

Normal Findings Normal-sized lymph nodes containing no filling defects

Indications

Lymphangiography provides an x-ray examination of the thoracoabdominal lymphatic system after injection of contrast medium into a lymphatic vessel in the foot or hand.

Test Explanation

The lymphatic system consists of lymph vessels and lymph nodes. Assessment of this system is important because cancer (lymphomas and Hodgkin's disease) often spreads via the lymphatic system. With the help of lymphangiography, pathologic lymph nodes can be localized for surgical removal or inclusion in radiation therapy ports.

Lymphangiography is especially useful in patients with suspected lymphatic cancer (e.g., lymphoma, metastatic tumor). The test enables demonstration of the extent and level of lymphatic metastasis. Lymphangiography is also useful in staging lymphomas and evaluating the results of chemotherapy or radiation therapy. Because the contrast medium remains in the lymph nodes for 6 months to 1 year, repeated plain x-ray films may be obtained for continued follow-up of disease progression or response to treatment.

This test is also useful in the evaluation of chronic leg swelling. Lack of flow of the dye into the pelvic lymphatic vessels indicates lymphatic vessel obstruction as the cause of leg edema.

Contraindications

- Allergy to iodine dye or shellfish
- Severe chronic lung diseases, cardiac disease, or advanced kidney or liver disease
  Lipid-containing radiopaque dye may further injure these organs.

✓ CLINICAL PRIORITIES

- Lymphangiography can demonstrate the extent and level of lymphatic metastasis. It is helpful in staging lymphomas and evaluating chemotherapy or radiation therapy.
- Check the patient for allergy to iodinated dyes.
- Excessive infiltration or IV administration of the dye may create a transient bluish tint to the skin.

Potential Complications

- Lipoid (lipid) pneumonia
  Develops if the contrast medium flows into the thoracic duct and causes micropulmonary emboli. These small emboli usually disappear after several weeks or months.

- Allergic reaction or allergy to iodine dye
  Allergic reactions vary from flushing, itching, and urticaria to severe, life-threatening anaphylaxis (evidenced by respiratory distress, decreased blood pressure, or shock). In the event of anaphylaxis, the patient may be given diphenhydramine (Benadryl), steroids, and epinephrine. Oxygen and endotracheal equipment should be available for immediate use.

Procedure and Patient Care

Before

- Explain the procedure to the patient.
- Obtain informed consent if required by the institution.
- Tell the patient that no fasting or sedation is required.
- Inform the radiologist if an allergy to iodinated contrast is suspected. The radiologist may prescribe a diphenhydramine-steroid preparation to be administered before testing. Usually, a hypoallergenic, nonionic contrast is used during the test.
- Inform the patient that if a blue-colored dye is used, a bluish tinge may be noted in the urine. Excessive infiltration or IV administration of the lymphatic stain may create a transient bluish tint to a portion of or the entire skin surface.

During

- Note the following procedural steps:
  1. In the radiology department, the patient is placed supine on an x-ray table.
  2. A lymphatic stain is injected into the subcutaneous tissue between each of the first three toes in each foot to outline the lymphatic vessels (Figure 12-19). (The stain can also be injected into the web of the skin between the fingers.)
  3. After the stain is taken up by the lymphatic vessels, they can be easily seen.
  4. A local anesthetic is injected.
  5. A small incision is made on the top of the foot (or hand).
  6. The lymphatic vessel is identified and cannulated to infuse the iodine contrast agent.
  7. The dye is slowly infused into the vessel, usually with a low-rate infusion pump. The patient must lie very still during the injection.
  8. The flow of iodine dye is observed with fluoroscopy.
  9. When the dye reaches the upper lumbar level, the flow of dye is discontinued.
  10. X-ray films are taken of the chest, abdomen, and pelvis to demonstrate filling of the lymph nodes. Often, the patient is asked to return in 24 hours for additional x-ray studies.
  11. On completion of the injection, the cannula is removed and the incision is sutured.
- Note that this procedure is performed by a radiologist in approximately 3 hours. Additional x-ray films are usually obtained after 24 to 48 hours.

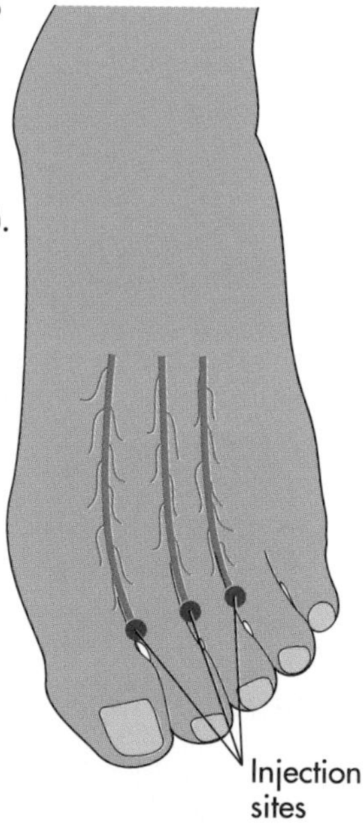

Figure 12-19 Lymphangiogram. Sites for dye injection.

- Inform the patient that discomfort may be felt when the stain is injected subcutaneously and the feet are locally anesthetized.

After

- Observe the injection and incision sites for evidence of cellulitis. Instruct patients who are returning to home to evaluate the site for redness, pain, and swelling.
- Inform the patient that the sutures should be removed 7 to 10 days after the test.

Test Results and Clinical Significance

Metastatic tumor involving the lymph glands
Lymphoma or Hodgkin's disease
Tumor in lymph nodes causes a radiolucent filling defect and enlargement of the involved lymph node.

Lymphedema of an extremity *The more proximal lymph vessels and lymph nodes do not contain any dye after injection, because of obstruction in the lymph vessels in a more distal location.*

Mammography (Mammogram)

Normal Findings

No tumor noted

Indications

Mammography enables detection of breast cancers, benign tumors, and cysts before they are even palpable. Mammography can be performed for screening or diagnostic purposes.

Screening mammography

- Women aged 50 to 80 years should undergo two-view mammography annually.
- Women of any age with a history of breast cancer should undergo mammography annually.
- Women aged 40 to 50 years:
  American Cancer Society recommendation: annual mammography.
  NIH Consensus Panel recommendation:
  Average risk of breast cancer: mammography every 1-2 years.
  Increased risk: mammography annually. This includes women with (1) a personal history of breast cancer, (2) lumpy or dense breasts, (3) genetic susceptibility to breast cancer, (4) more than four first- or second-degree relatives with breast cancer, especially breast cancer or ovarian cancer in each generation, (5) a close relative with breast cancer, or (6) first pregnancy after age 30 years.

Diagnostic mammography

- Women older than 25 years should undergo two-view diagnostic mammography if they have breast symptoms such as a palpable nodule or lump, breast skin thickening or indentation, nipple discharge or retraction, erosive sore of the nipple, or breast pain.

Test Explanation

Mammography is an x-ray examination of the breast. Careful interpretation of these x-ray films can identify cancers. In many cases, breast cancers can be detected before they become palpable. It is believed that early detection of breast cancer may improve patient survival. Radiographic signs of breast cancer include fine, stippled, clustered calcifications (white specks on the breast x-ray films); a poorly defined spiculated mass; asymmetric density; and skin thickening.

Although mammography is not a substitute for breast biopsy, results are reliable and accurate when interpreted by a skilled radiologist. The accuracy of detection of breast cancer with mammography has been approximately 85%. This means that 15% of breast cancers are missed at mammography, despite the fact that in most institutions mammograms are interpreted by more than one radiologist. Usually cancers that are not detected by mammography are in areas of the breast not well imaged by x-ray films (e.g., the high axillary tail of the breast). Almost 35% of breast cancers are not palpable and are detected only with mammography. Therefore the combination of mammography and close physical examination provides the best approach to detect breast cancer at its earliest stage.

Some controversy surrounds the role of mammography in screening asymptomatic patients. Several large U.S. studies have encouraged mammography yearly after age 40 years. Women older than 50 years should have a mammogram yearly. Women who are at great risk for breast cancer (e.g., those who have had a cancer in the contralateral breast) should have mammograms yearly, regardless of age.

Mammography also can detect other diseases of the breast, such as acute suppurative mastitis, abscess, fibrocystic changes, cysts, benign tumors (e.g., fibroadenoma), and intraglandular lymph nodes.

In the past, radiation exposure was significant with mammography. Today, however, because of fast-speed film, little radiation is required to expose mammographic film. Therefore, the patient receives minimal radiation exposure during this test (about 0.5 rads per view). The risk for breast cancer may begin to increase after the direct exposure of about 1800 rads. Therefore, a woman can safely undergo mammography annually for 900 years before there is a significant increase in breast cancer risk. Women younger than 25 years, however, are most susceptible to the neoplastic effects of ionizing radiation. Mammography is rarely performed in women in this age group.

Xeromammography provides the same information as routine mammography and has the same risks. Unlike regular x-ray films, which are negative films, xeromammograms are positive prints. The form of mammography used depends on the preference of the radiologist who must interpret the mammogram; however, the use of xeroradiography is decreasing. Newer, "dedicated" mammography units provide more accurate and easily interpretable x-ray films.

The American College of Radiology (ACR) has recommended standardization of mammography reports, as follows:

Class I: Negative
Class II: Benign
Class III: Benign; short-term follow-up suggested
Class IV: Suspicious for cancer; further evaluation suggested
Class V: Cancer highly suspected

Results of mammography can only suggest a diagnosis of breast cancer. The diagnosis of cancer must be confirmed with microscopic histologic review of a biopsy specimen.

Mammography is performed by a certified radiologic technologist in approximately 10 minutes. The ACR also accredits the mammography machine for quality of picture and accuracy of x-ray dose. The x-ray films are interpreted by an accredited radiologist. Moderate discomfort is associated with mammography. This is caused by the pressure required to compress the breast tissue while the x-ray films are obtained. In patients with tender breasts, this may be especially painful.

Mammography can also be used to locate a mammographically identified lesion (i.e., not palpable) for biopsy. The most common method is *preoperative mammogram localization* of the abnormality, followed by open biopsy. For this procedure, patient is taken to the mammography room after having received preoperative preparation and instruction. A grid is applied to the breast containing the abnormality. Craniocaudal and direct lateral views are obtained. With the grid still in place, the radiologist numbs the skin and places a needle into the abnormal area. A wire is then disengaged into the breast. Repeated mammograms are obtained. The patient is then taken to the operating room. After appropriate anesthesia, an incision is made along the wire, to the abnormal area, which is then removed for biopsy.

Nonoperative *stereotactic biopsy* with needle or *mammotomy* probes is the newest and least invasive manner of obtaining tissue from a nonpalpable mammographic abnormality. For this procedure the patient is placed prone on a special table. Through a hole in the table, the breast is placed in a mammography machine under the table (Figure 12-20). The mammogram is connected to a computer that can identify the exact location of the mammographic abnormality (Figure 12-21). The machine sets up a core biopsy needle or mammotome probe in alignment. When fired, the biopsy equipment is in the center of the lesion, and specimens are obtained for biopsy. No surgery or sutures are required. Further, only minimal pain is experienced, because a breast in compression has little skin pain sensation.

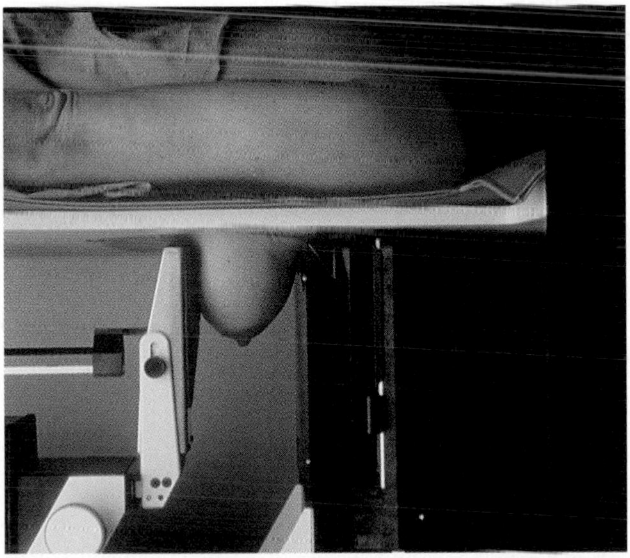

Figure 12-20 Stereotaxic breast biopsy. The patient is positioned on the table with the breast pendulus through the aperture. The breast is compressed with the target lesion centered in the biopsy window.

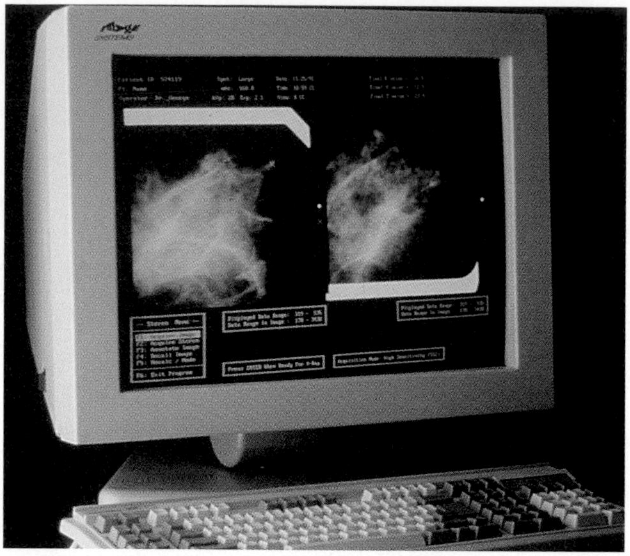

Figure 12-21 The mammography film is placed on the digitizer, and coordinates of the breast lesion are determined and displayed. These coordinates guide the needle to the precise location of the lesion, and the aspirate is drawn for biopsy.

Contraindications

- Pregnancy, because the risk of fetal damage
- Women younger than 25 years

Interfering Factors

- Talcum powder can give the impression of calcifications within the breast.
- Jewelry worn around the neck can preclude total visualization of the breast.
- Breast augmentation implants prevent total visualization of the breast.
- Previous breast surgery can distort mammographic findings.

CLINICAL PRIORITIES

- The combination of mammography and close physical examination provides the best approach for detecting breast cancer at its earlier stage.
- During mammography, radiation exposure is minimal.
- Some discomfort may be experienced during breast compression. Compression is necessary for visualization of the breast.

Procedure and Patient Care

Before

- Explain the procedure to the patient.
- Inform the patient that some discomfort may be experienced during breast compression. Compression allows better visualization of the breast tissue. Assure the patient that the breast will not be harmed by compression.

- Tell the patient that no fasting is required.
- Explain to the patient that a minimal radiation dose will be used during the test.
- Instruct the patient to disrobe above the waist and put on an x-ray gown.
- Instruct the patient to report the location of any symptom or lump she may have noted.

During

- Note the following procedural steps:
  1. The patient is taken to the radiology department and stands in front of a mammogram machine.
  2. One breast is placed on the x-ray plate.
  3. The x-ray cone is brought down on top of the breast to compress it gently between the broadened cone and the x-ray plate (see Figure 12-22).
  4. The x-ray film is exposed, for a *craniocaudal view.*
  5. The x-ray plate is turned about 45 degrees medially and placed on the inner aspect of the breast.
  6. The broadened cone is brought in medially and again gently compresses the breast. A *mediolateral view* is obtained.
  7. Occasionally *direct lateral* (90-degree) or *magnified spot views* are obtained to more clearly visualize an area of suspicion. Elongated or small cones are applied to the x-ray tube to enhance visualization of a specific area of the breast.

After

- Take the opportunity to instruct the patient in breast self-examination.
- Support the patient in her concerns if additional views are required. It is always frightening if further views are required. Usually these additional views include spot magnified views, which allow the radiologist to better visualize an area of the breast.

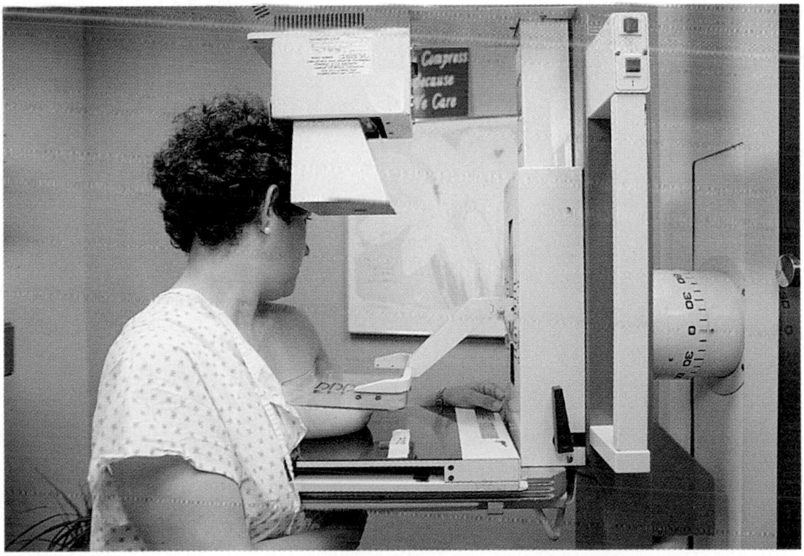

Figure 12-22 Mammography procedure.

Test Results and Clinical Significance

Breast cancer *This can be evident as a radiodense (white) stellate or spiculated mass, a cluster of calcifications, or vague asymmetric radiodensity. When cancer invades the skin, the skin will appear thickened. Also, the nipple can appear inverted if a subareolar cancer exists.*

Benign tumor (e.g., fibroadenoma) *Benign tumors are usually well-rounded masses with discrete borders. Sometimes fibroadenomas can degenerate, and calcifications can develop within. Colloid or medullary cancers can appear similarly well rounded.*

Breast cyst *Cysts are seen as well-rounded masses with discrete borders. Ultrasound of the breast demonstrates the cysts to be fluid filled.*

Fibrocystic disease *This is the most common breast finding. Nearly every women has some degree of fibrocystic disease. On mammograms, this is seen as a vague asymmetric radiodensity (white). It can also be evident as calcifications.*

Breast abscess
Suppurative mastitis
The mammographic findings of infection are increased thickness of the skin, with increased radiodensity of the breast tissue.

Related Tests

- Ultrasound of the breast (p. 783): An important adjunct to mammography, ultrasound can differentiate between cystic and solid lesions.

Myelography (Myelogram)

Normal Findings Normal spinal canal

Indications

Myelography provides radiographic visualization of the subarachnoid space of the spinal canal. The cord, nerve roots, and surrounding meninges can be seen. This test is indicated in patients with severe back pain or localized neurologic signs that suggest the canal is the location of disease (e.g., herniated lumbar disk).

Test Explanation

By placing radiopaque dye or air into the subarachnoid space of the spinal canal, the contents of the canal can be fluoroscopically outlined. Cord tumors, meningeal tumors, metastatic spinal tumors, herniated intervertebral disks, and arthritic bone spurs can be readily detected with this study. These lesions appear as spinal canal narrowing or as varying degrees of obstruction to the flow of the dye column within the canal. The entire canal (from lumbar to cervical areas) can be examined. Because this test is usually performed with lumbar puncture (LP; see p. 579), all the potential complications of that procedure exist.

Various types of contrast material can be used for myelography. Iophendylate (Pantopaque) is most often used as the *oil-based* medium. Because oil-based dye persists indefinitely, as much as possible must be aspirated after the procedure before the spinal needle is removed. The patient's head is then kept elevated above the level of the spine to prevent upward dispersion of the dye, which can cause meningeal irritation. Oil-based dye is heavier than CSF, and stays in the lower canal. After the dye is removed, the patient may be kept supine for up to 12 hours.

A *water-soluble* contrast material, metrizamide (Amipaque), is now frequently used for myelography. This dye is absorbed by the blood and excreted by the kidneys. Metrizamide has two advantages over oil-based medium. First, metrizamide need not be removed at the end of the procedure, because it is water soluble and will be completely absorbed. This feature reduces the duration of the procedure and minimizes the discomfort associated with dye removal. Second, metrizamide is less viscous than iodine, oil-based dye and therefore enables better visualization of small areas (e.g., nerves, nerve roots, nerve sheaths). Also, metrizamide can flow freely through narrow canals, and affords better differentiation of complete and incomplete spinal blockages. The disadvantage associated with metrizamide is that it may precipitate seizure activity after the procedure. To prevent this, the patient should be well hydrated and given no medications that could decrease the seizure threshold (e.g., phenothiazines, tricyclic antidepressants, CNS stimulants, amphetamines). Another water-soluble contrast agent, iohexol (Omnipaque), is associated with a significantly lower risk of CNS toxicity than is metrizamide and is now more routinely used.

After the procedure, the patient's head and thorax should be elevated 30 to 50 degrees for approximately 6 to 8 hours to reduce upward dispersion of the dye and to prevent contact of the water-soluble agent with the cerebral meninges, which could precipitate a seizure. Bed rest may be ordered for up to 24 hours.

To avert some of the side effects associated with radiopaque substances, some neurosurgeons prefer to use *air-contrast* myelography. After air myelography, the patient is positioned with the head lower than the trunk to prevent air from gravitating to the cerebral space and causing headache. This position is usually maintained for approximately 48 hours. Most of the air will be absorbed by this time, and the head can then be elevated.

Myelography is performed by a radiologist in approximately 45 minutes. Patient response varies from mild discomfort to severe pain.

Contraindications

- Multiple sclerosis, because exacerbation may be precipitated by myelography
- Increased intracranial pressure, because LP may cause herniation of the brain
- Infection near the LP site, because this may precipitate bacterial meningitis
- Allergy to shellfish or iodinated dye

Potential Complications

- Headache
- Meningitis
- Herniation of the brain
- Seizures

- Allergic reaction to iodinated dye
  Allergic reactions vary from mild flushing, itching, and urticaria to severe, life-threatening anaphylaxis (evidenced by respiratory distress, decreased blood pressure, or shock). In the unusual event of anaphylaxis, the patient may be given diphenhydramine (Benadryl), steroids, and epinephrine. Oxygen and endotracheal equipment should be available for immediate use.

CLINICAL PRIORITIES

- Myelography can be performed with different types of contrast materials. Pantopaque is an oil-based medium; Amipaque and Omnipaque are water-soluble contrast media. Air-contrast myelography can also be performed.
- To avoid herniation of the brain, this test is contraindicated in patients with increased intracranial pressure.

Procedure and Patient Care

Before

- Explain the procedure to the patient.
- Ensure that the physician has obtained written, informed consent for this procedure.
- Assess the patient for allergy to iodinated contrast dye or shellfish.
- Inform the radiologist if an allergy to iodinated contrast is suspected. The radiologist may prescribe a diphenhydramine (Benadryl)-steroid preparation to be administered before testing. Usually, hypoallergenic, nonionic contrast material is used during the test.
- If a water-soluble contrast agent (e.g., metrizamide) will be used, ascertain whether the patient has recently taken phenothiazines, tricyclic antidepressants, CNS stimulants, or amphetamines. These medications can decrease the seizure threshold.
- Have the patient empty the bladder and bowel before myelography, if possible.
- Explain to the patient that he or she must lie very still during the procedure.
- Food and fluid restrictions vary according to the type of dye used. Check with the radiology department for specific restrictions.
- Inform the patient that he or she will be tilted into an up-and-down position on the table so that the dye can properly fill the spinal canal and provide adequate visualization of the desired area.

During

- Note the following procedural steps:
  1. Lumbar puncture or cisternal puncture (see p. 579) is performed.
  2. Fifteen milliliters of CSF is withdrawn, and 15 ml or more of radiopaque dye or air is injected into the spinal canal. Because the specific gravity of the dye is greater than that of CSF, the direction of dye flow will depend on the tilt of the table and the patient's position.
  3. With the needle in place, the patient is placed prone on the tilt table, with the

head tilted down. A foot support and shoulder brace or harness will keep the patient from sliding.
4. The lights are turned off, and the column of dye is followed in a cephalad direction with fluoroscopy.
5. Representative x-ray films are obtained.
6. Obstruction to the flow of the dye is evident, and the level of a lesion is easily detected.
7. After myelography is performed, the needle is removed and a dressing is applied.
8. The patient is returned to the unit on a gurney and kept on bed rest.

After

- Note that nursing interventions after the procedure depend on the type of contrast agent used.
- The patient usually is placed on bed rest for several hours, as indicated. Position the patient as specifically ordered by the physician in consultation with the radiologist.
- The head position varies according to the dye used. For example, the head is usually elevated if an oil-based or water-soluble contrast agent was used. After an air-contrast study, the head is positioned lower than the trunk.
- Observe the patient for signs and symptoms of meningeal irritation (e.g., fever, stiff neck, occipital headache, photophobia).
- If metrizamide was used, observe the patient for seizure activity. Do not administer medications that may precipitate seizure activity (e.g., phenothiazines).
- Monitor the patient's vital signs and ability to void.
- Encourage the patient to drink fluids to enhance excretion of the dye and to hasten replacement of CSF.
- Evaluate the patient for delayed reaction to dye (e.g., dyspnea, rash, tachycardia, hives). This usually occurs within the first 2 to 6 hours after the test. Treat symptoms with antihistamines or steroids.

Home Care Responsibilities

- After myelography, safe positioning of the patient's head is determined by the type of dye used in the procedure.
- Encourage the patient to drink fluids to enhance excretion of the dye and to replace CSF.
- Tell the patient to report any signs of meningeal irritation (e.g., fever, stiff neck, occipital headache, photophobia).

Test Results and Clinical Significance

Spinal cord tumors (e.g., astrocytoma, neurofibroma, meningioma) *These are seen as radiolucent filling defects in the column of radiopaque dye in the canal.*

Metastatic spinal tumor *Extrinsic spinal tumors (usually metastatic) are evident as extrinsic radiolucent filling defects in the column of radiopaque dye in the canal.*

Cervical ankylosing spondylosis
Arthritic lumbar stenosis from arthritic bone spurs
These bony changes can compress the spinal canal, and are evident as distortion of the cord or nerve roots.

Herniated intravertebral disk *A herniated disk acts as external compression on the spinal cord or the nerve root. The most common areas of disk herniation are L4-L5 and L5-S1.*
Avulsion of nerve roots *Traumatic avulsion of the nerve root can cause profound neurologic changes.*
Cysts *Cysts of the cord or meninges surrounding the cord are evident as extrinsic radiolucent filling defects in the column of radiopaque dye in the canal.*

Related Tests

- MRI (p. 1009): This test is more accurate than myelography for viewing the spinal cord and its surrounding structures. However, some patients are too claustrophobic to undergo MRI.

Obstruction Series

Normal Findings

No evidence of bowel obstruction
No abnormal calcifications
No free air

Indications

This x-ray series is used for the evaluation of abdominal pain or suspected obstruction of the intestinal tract.

Test Explanation

The obstruction series is a group of x-ray films of the abdomen in patients with suspected bowel obstruction, paralytic ileus, perforated viscus, abdominal abscess, kidney stones, appendicitis, or foreign body ingestion. The series of films usually consists of at least two x-ray studies. The first is an *erect abdominal* film, which should include visualization of both diaphragms. The film is examined for evidence of free air under either diaphragm, which is pathognomonic for perforated viscus. This view is also used to detect air-fluid levels within the intestine; the presence of an air-fluid level is compatible with bowel obstruction or paralytic ileus. Occasionally, patients are too ill to stand erect. In this case, an x-ray film can be taken with the patient in the left lateral decubitus position. If free air is present, it will be seen between the liver and the right side of the abdominal wall. Air-fluid levels also can be detected.

The second view in the obstruction series is usually a *supine abdominal* x-ray study, similar to the KUB study (p. 958). An abdominal abscess may be seen as a cluster of tiny bubbles within a localized area. A calcification within the ureter could indicate a kidney ureteral stone. A small calcification in the right lower quadrant in a patient with pain in this quadrant may be an appendicolith. A gas-filled, distended bowel is compatible with bowel obstruction or paralytic ileus.

The obstruction series can also be used to monitor the clinical course of GI disease. For example, repeated obstruction series in patients with partial small bowel obstruction or paralytic ileus can indicate clinical worsening or improvement.

Frequently, a *cross-table lateral* view of the abdomen is included in an obstruction series, to detect abdominal aorta calcification, which often occurs in older patients. The calcification represents the anterior wall of the aorta. If an aortic aneurysm exists, this calcification will be seen to protrude from the spine.

Finally, the *supine abdominal* x-ray study can be used as a scout film before performing GI or abdominal contrast material–enhanced x-ray studies (e.g., barium enema [p. 900] or IVP [p. 953]), to ensure nothing is obstructing adequate visualization of what needs to be studied.

The obstruction series is performed in minutes in the radiology department by a radiologic technologist; however, it can be performed at the bedside with a portable x-ray machine. A radiologist interprets the films. No discomfort is associated with the study.

Contraindications

- Pregnancy

Interfering Factors

- Previous GI barium contrast study
  Although barium within the GI tract can preclude identification of other important calcifications (e.g., kidney stones), it can be helpful in outlining the GI anatomy.

Procedure and Patient Care

Before

- Explain the procedure to the patient.
- Ensure that all radiopaque clothing has been removed.
- Remind the patient that no contrast agent will be used.

During

- Although the procedure varies among facilities, usually a supine abdominal x-ray film, erect abdominal film, and perhaps a lower erect chest film are obtained. Often a cross table lateral x-ray film is also included.

After

- No special care is needed.

Test Results and Clinical Significance

Abdominal aortic calcification or abdominal aortic aneurysm *Abdominal aortic aneurysm is evident by calcification in the anterior wall of the aorta, displaced significantly anterior from the vertebrae.*

Calculi *A calcified stone in the area where the ureters would be is indicative of ureteral calculi. This finding requires further supportive evidence by means of IVP (p. 953). Appendicolithiasis (stone in the appendix) is suspected when a patient with right lower quadrant abdominal pain is seen to have a stone in that quadrant.*

Abdominal accumulation of bowel gas *Abnormal accumulations of bowel gas can indicate intestinal obstruction or paralytic ileus.*

Ascites *The classic ground-glass appearance of the entire abdomen on the KUB study indicates peritoneal effusion.*

Soft tissue masses *Large soft tissue masses or abscesses can be seen surprisingly well on this plain film x-ray, without contrast material enhancement.*

Ruptured viscus *Free air (i.e., air outside the bowel but inside the abdomen) is indicative of a perforated viscus.*

Congenital anomalies in the location, size, and number of kidneys *Because the kidneys are well seen, abnormalities of these features are easily detected.*

Organomegaly or bladder distention *An enlarged liver or spleen is seen as a large soft tissue mass in the right or left upper quadrant, respectively. A large soft tissue mass in the midline or pelvis is usually a distended bladder.*

Foreign body *A bullet or other projectile is obvious on x-ray films. A surgical sponge or instrument left during surgery is also visible.*

Related Tests

- KUB (p. 958): This is only one component of the obstruction series and therefore does not contribute as much information as does an obstruction series.

Pelvimetry (Radiographic Pelvimetry)

Normal Findings

Transverse diameter of the midpelvis 10.5 cm

Indications

Although this test is rarely indicated, measurement of the maternal pelvic diameter compared with the fetus head circumference is performed if cephalopelvic disproportion is suspected. This test is also used if the fetus is malpositioned and there is a question as to whether the mother's pelvis is adequate for vaginal delivery.

Test Explanation

Although most abnormalities of the pelvis can be suspected with clinical measurements, x-ray pelvimetry is the most accurate means of determining adequacy of the pelvic bony structures for a normal vaginal delivery. With pelvimetry, the capacity of the pelvis can be compared with the size of the head of the infant, and any cephalopelvic disproportion can be discovered.

Radiographic pelvimetry is not used often in modern obstetrics because of the risks associated with radiation; however, this study may be indicated in the following situations:

1. Suspected abnormal fetal position when vaginal delivery is anticipated
2. Injury or disease of the bony pelvis or hips that may have caused pelvic distortion
3. Clinically abnormal pelvic measurements
4. Debilitating disease and a clinically small or unfavorable pelvis
5. History of difficult vaginal delivery
6. Early labor with the fetus's head unengaged
7. Admission for trial labor to rule out contracted pelvis
8. Dysfunctional labor, especially when the physician is considering oxytocin administration

Although measuring the pelvis clinically is less accurate than x-ray determination, it is adequate in most patients. Radiographic pelvimetry is important only late in pregnancy or during labor. If pelvimetry indicates a difficult or dangerous vaginal delivery, cesarean section is recommended. Cesarean section is now more frequently performed when vaginal delivery is clinically suspected to be difficult. As a result, x-ray pelvimetry rarely affects the physician's decision concerning the type of delivery. In those rare situations in which vaginal delivery is attempted despite an anticipated difficult delivery, radiographic pelvimetry is performed more for legal purposes than for medical benefits. Ultrasound measurements of fetal size in comparison with pelvic measurements is another method of determining cephalopelvic disproportion.

Contraindications

- Early pregnancy, because x-ray exposure at this time may injure the fetus

Procedure and Patient Care

Before

- Explain the procedure to the patient.
- Tell the patient that no fasting or sedation is required.
- Instruct the patient to remove all clothing and don a long x-ray gown.

During

- Note the following procedural steps:
  1. In the radiology department, a lateral x-ray film is obtained with the patient standing, to detect the effect of gravity on engagement and to indicate the position of the fetal head when it reaches the lower birth canal.
  2. The patient may then be placed in the supine, lateral, or semirecumbent position.
  3. During film exposure, the patient is asked to stop breathing.
  4. Generally the patient is instructed to hyperventilate and then stop breathing while the film is obtained.
  5. After the x-ray films are obtained, multiple measurements are made at various pelvic angles and diameters to measure the pelvic inlet, true pelvis, and birth canal.
- Note that a radiologic technologist performs this study in approximately 15 minutes.
- Tell the patient that no discomfort is associated with this study.

After

- Provide emotional support for the patient at this difficult time. Most patients are concerned that some problem exists.

Test Results and Clinical Significance

Cephalopelvic disproportion
Abnormal fetal position
If maternal pelvis diameter is inadequate for vaginal delivery, cesarean section is recommended.

Percutaneous Transhepatic Cholangiography (PTC, PTHC)

Normal Findings

Normal gallbladder and biliary ducts

Indications

This procedure allows visualization of the bile ducts and sometimes the pancreatic duct. Patients with jaundice can be evaluated for tumors, gallstones, and other diseases.

Test Explanation

By passing a needle through the liver and into an intrahepatic bile duct, iodinated dye can be directly injected into the biliary system. The intrahepatic and extrahepatic biliary ducts, and occasionally the gallbladder can be visualized and studied for partial or total obstruction from gallstones, benign strictures, malignant tumors, congenital cysts, and anatomic variations. This is especially helpful in patients with jaundice. If the jaundice is a result of extrahepatic obstruction, a catheter can be left in the bile duct and used for external drainage of bile. Furthermore, a stent can be placed across a stricture to decompress the biliary system internally.

PTC and endoscopic retrograde cholangiopancreatography (ERCP, p. 532) are the only methods available to visualize the biliary tree in patients with jaundice. ERCP is used more frequently because of its lower complication rate. PTC, however, is the only way to visualize the biliary tree after most gastric surgery. Occasionally (if the pancreatic duct and the common bile duct are from a common channel), part or all of the pancreatic duct can be filled with dye from the same injection. See Table 12-5 for a list of diagnostic tests to visu-

Table 12-5 ***Diagnostic tests to visualize the pancreatobiliary system***

Test	Advantages	Disadvantages
Intravenous cholangiography	Easy to perform	Poor visualization of ducts
Oral cholecystography	Easy to perform	Visualizes only the gallbladder
ERCP	Good visualization of the pancreas and bile ducts; able to decompress the biliary system	Difficult to perform; complications possible
PTC	Good visualization of the ducts; able to decompress the biliary system	Difficult to perform; complications possible
Nuclear radioscintigraphy	Easy to perform	Poor visualization of the biliary system; not specific as to disease

alize the pancreatobiliary system, along with their advantages and disadvantages.

PTC is performed by a radiologist in approximately 1 hour, during which time the patient must lie still. Abdominal pain may be felt for several hours after the test. Occasionally the patient also may have right shouldertop pain because of diaphragmatic irritation of leaking bile or blood.

Contraindications

- Allergy to iodine or shellfish
- Evidence of mild cholangitis
  Dye injections increase biliary pressure and cause bacteremia, which may lead to septicemia and shock.
- Inability of the patient to cooperate and remain still
- Prolonged clotting time

Potential Complications

- Allergic reaction to iodinated dye
  Allergic reactions may vary from mild flushing, itching, and urticaria to severe, life-threatening anaphylaxis (evidenced by respiratory distress, decreased blood pressure, or shock). In the unusual event of anaphylaxis, the patient may be given diphenhydramine (Benadryl), steroids, and epinephrine. Oxygen and endotracheal equipment should be available for immediate use.
- Peritonitis caused by bile extravasation from the liver after the needle has been removed
- Bleeding caused by inadvertent puncture of a large hepatic blood vessel
- Sepsis and cholangitis from injection of the dye into an already infected and obstructed bile duct
  The pressure of injection pushes the bacteria into the blood stream, causing bacteremia.

Interfering Factors

- The presence of barium from a previous upper GI series or barium contrast study may preclude visualization of the biliary tree.

✓ CLINICAL PRIORITIES

- Check the patient for allergy to iodinated dyes.
- Verify that results of coagulation studies are within the normal range before this test, because bleeding is a potential complication.
- Abdominal pain after the test may be an indication of bleeding or bile extravasation.

Procedure and Patient Care

Before

- Explain the procedure to the patient.

- Obtain informed consent.
- Assess the patient for allergy to iodinated dye or shellfish.
- Inform the radiologist if an allergy to iodinated contrast material is suspected. The radiologist may prescribe a diphenhydramine steroid preparation to be administered before the test. Usually a hypoallergenic, nonionic contrast agent is used during the test.
- Type and cross match the patient's blood. The patient may bleed and require a transfusion or surgery.
- Verify that results of coagulation studies are within the normal range.
- Keep the patient NPO after midnight on the day of the test. A laxative may be ordered.
- Premedicate the patient as indicated, usually with atropine and meperidine.

During

- Note the following procedural steps:
  1. The patient is placed supine on an x-ray table in the radiology department.
  2. The abdominal wall or lower chest wall (over the liver) is anesthetized with lidocaine (Xylocaine).
  3. With the use of televised fluoroscopic monitoring, the needle is advanced through the skin and into the liver (Figure 12-23).
  4. When bile flows freely through the needle, radiographic dye is injected.
  5. X-ray films are obtained immediately.
  6. If an obstruction is found, a catheter or stent is placed over a guide wire and left temporarily in the biliary tract to establish drainage and decompression of the biliary tract.

After

- Keep the patient on bed rest for several hours.
- If indicated, place a sandbag over the needle insertion site.
- Observe the patient for hemorrhage or bile leakage. A small amount of bleeding is normal.
- Keep the patient NPO for a few hours after the test in the event intra-abdominal bleeding or bile extravasation develops that requires surgery.

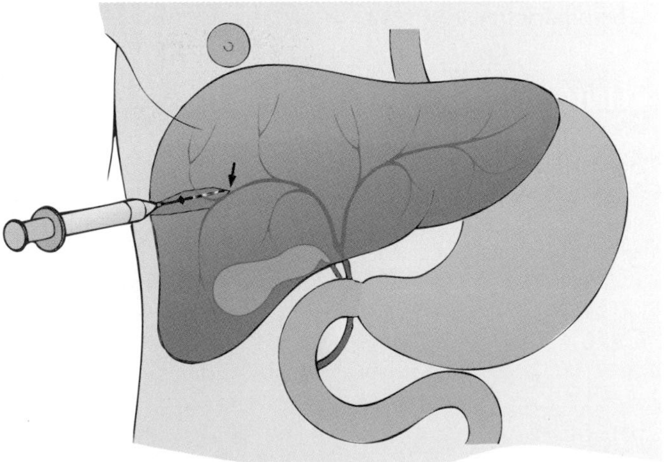

Figure 12-23 Percutaneous transhepatic cholangiography (PTHC).

- Repeatedly assess the patient's vital signs for evidence of hemorrhage.
- Assess the patient for signs of bacteremia or sepsis.
- If a catheter is left in the biliary tract, establish a sterile, closed drainage system.
- Withhold high doses of pain medications that may blunt the abdominal signs associated with hemorrhage or bile extravasation.

Test Results and Clinical Significance

Tumors, strictures, or gallstones of the hepatic or common bile duct *These diseases cause partial or complete obstruction of the biliary tree. Tumors usually cause long strictures. Benign strictures are more likely to cause short segment narrowings. Gallstones usually are evident as rounded radiolucent (dark) filling defects in the bile duct. When they obstruct the bile duct, the obstruction is seen as a soft convex cutoff of the bile duct.*

Sclerosing cholangitis
Biliary sclerosis
These conditions are due to inflammatory or fibrotic changes around the bile ducts; this leads to a long stricture in most of the biliary tree and its radicals.

Cysts of the common bile duct *These congenital outpouchings of the bile duct may vary in size from tiny and barely noticeable to large and voluminous. The pressure surrounding these cysts can obstruct the normal portion of the bile duct in the closed space of the right upper quadrant of the abdomen.*

Tumors, strictures, inflammation, or true or pseudocysts of the pancreatic duct *If the pancreatic duct is visualized, these abnormalities can be identified. Pancreatic tumors are evident as long strictures. Postinflammatory strictures are usually short segment narrowings. Neoplastic cysts may be connected to the main pancreatic duct and fill with dye. Pseudocysts, due to pancreatic duct disruption that follows severe pancreatitis, nearly always connect with the main pancreatic duct and therefore fill with dye.*

Anatomic biliary or pancreatic duct variations *Duplications, aberrant entry of the pancreatobiliary ducts into the intestine, and other anomalies can be identified.*

Related Tests

- ERCP (p. 532): This is the preferred method of visualizing the pancreatobiliary tree in the patient with jaundice.

Pulmonary Angiography (Pulmonary Arteriography, Bronchial Angiography)

Normal Findings

Normal pulmonary vasculature

Indications

Pulmonary angiography is indicated most commonly in patients with suspected pulmonary embolism and the lung scan yields inconclusive results, and in whom anticoagulation represents a moderate risk.

Box 12-3 Diagnosis of pulmonary embolism

SYMPTOMS
Shortness of breath
Feeling of imminent death
Pleuritic chest pain

SIGNS
Hypoxemia
Tachycardia
Pleural rub
Cardia gallop
Concomitant phlebitis
Diagnostic tests
EKG: right heart strain
Chest x-rays: may be normal
Pulmonary infarct may be evident as radiodensity in affected parenchyma
Arterial blood gases: hypoxemia, hypocapnia
Lung scan: blood perfusion defect
Pulmonary angiography: clot in pulmonary artery

Test Explanation

With injection of a radiographic contrast material into the pulmonary arteries, pulmonary angiography permits visualization of the pulmonary vasculature. Angiography is used to detect pulmonary embolism and a variety of congenital and acquired lesions of the pulmonary vessels. See Box 12-3 for an overview of the diagnosis of pulmonary embolism.

When pulmonary embolism is suspected, lung scanning should be performed first. If the lung scan is normal, pulmonary embolism is ruled out. If the scan is equivocal, however, the diagnosis of pulmonary embolism is questionable, because pathologic parenchymal processes (e.g., emphysema, pneumonia) also may cause abnormalities on the lung scan. Definitive diagnosis of pulmonary embolism may require pulmonary angiography. This may be especially important in patients with peptic ulcers or bleeding disorders, in whom anticoagulant treatment of pulmonary embolism may be associated with significant risk. Also, in rare instances pulmonary embolectomy rather than anticoagulation is considered critical for patient survival. In these cases, angiographic localization of the clot is important.

Bronchial angiography is being performed in some facilities to identify bleeding sites in the lungs. Catheters are placed transarterially into the orifice of the bronchial arteries. Radiopaque material is injected, and the arteries are visualized. If a bleeding site is identified, a sclerosing agent can be injected to prevent further bleeding.

This test is performed by a physician in approximately 1 hour. During injection of dye, the patient may feel a burning sensation and warm flush throughout the body.

Contraindications

- Allergy to shellfish or iodinated dye
- Pregnancy
- Bleeding disorders

Potential Complications

- Allergic reaction to iodinated dye
  Allergic reactions may vary from mild flushing, itching, and urticaria to severe, life-threatening anaphylaxis (evidenced by respiratory distress, decrease in blood pressure, or shock). In the unusual event of anaphylaxis, the patient may be given diphenhydramine (Benadryl), steroids, and epinephrine. Oxygen and endotracheal equipment should be immediately available.
- Cardiac arrhythmia (dysrhythmia)
  Premature ventricular contractions during right-sided heart catheterization may lead to ventricular tachycardia and ventricular fibrillation.

✓ CLINICAL PRIORITIES

- Check the patient for allergies to iodinated dyes.
- Because of the invasiveness of this test, it should not be performed in patients with bleeding disorders.
- After this test, evaluate the patient for a delayed reaction to the dye. This usually occurs within 2 to 6 hours after the test, and is treated with antihistamines or steroids.

Procedure and Patient Care

Before

- Explain the procedure to the patient.
- Ensure that written, informed consent is obtained.
- Inform the patient that a warm flush will be felt when the dye is injected.
- Check the patient for allergies to iodinated dyes and shellfish.
- Inform the radiologist if an allergy to iodine is suspected. The radiologist may prescribe a diphenhydramine-steroid preparation to be administered before the test. Usually, a hypoallergenic, nonionic contrast is used during the test.
- Determine if the patient has ventricular arrhythmias (dysrhythmias).
- Keep the patient NPO after midnight on the day of the test.
- Administer preprocedural medications as ordered. Atropine is given to decrease secretions. Meperidine may be used for sedation and relaxation.

During

- Note the following procedural steps:
  1. The patient is placed supine on an x-ray table.
  2. Electrocardiographic electrodes are attached for cardiac monitoring.

3. The catheter is placed into the femoral vein and passed into the inferior vena cava.
4. With fluoroscopic visualization, the catheter is advanced to the right atrium and the right ventricle.
5. The catheter is manipulated into the main pulmonary artery, where the dye is injected.
6. X-ray films of the chest are obtained immediately in timed sequence. This allows all vessels visualized by the injection to be photographed. If filling defects are seen in the contrast-filled vessels, pulmonary emboli are present.
7. If *bronchial angiography* is performed, the femoral artery is cannulated instead of the vein. The remainder of the procedure is similar to that for pulmonary angiography.

After

- Observe the catheter insertion site for inflammation, hemorrhage, and hematoma.
- Assess the patient's vital signs for evidence of bleeding (decreased blood pressure, increased pulse).
- Apply cold compresses to the puncture site if needed to reduce swelling or discomfort.
- Inform the patient that coughing may occur after this study.
- Educate the patient regarding the need for bed rest for 12 to 24 hours after the test.
- Evaluate the patient for delayed reaction to the dye (e.g., dyspnea, rash, tachycardia, hives). This usually occurs within 2 to 6 hours after the test. Treat with antihistamines or steroids.

Test Results and Clinical Significance

Pulmonary embolism *This is evident if one or more venous tributaries contain a clot. There may be an abrupt cutoff of the vessels as a result of complete obstruction secondary to the embolic clot.*

Congenital and acquired lesions of the pulmonary vessels (e.g., pulmonary hypertension) *Congenital anomalies in pulmonary arterial anatomy are not rare. This technique is also used for right heart cardiac catheterization (p. 917). Bronchial arterial evaluation is usually used for pulmonary symptoms (e.g., hemoptysis).*

Tumor *Bronchial tumors may bleed, and bronchial angiography may indicate the location.*

Related Tests

- Lung nuclear scan (p. 726): When clearly positive, this is a very accurate method of indicating the presence of a pulmonary embolism. A negative scan is also accurate in indicating the absence of an embolism. However, all too commonly, an unclear nuclear scan is obtained. Pulmonary angiography is helpful in these situations.

Retrograde Pyelography

Normal Findings

Normal outline and size of the ureters and bladder
No evidence of ureteral obstruction

Indications

Retrograde pyelography provides x-ray visualization of the ureter distal to an obstruction. It is performed in patients with known obstruction of unknown cause.

Text Explanation

Retrograde pyelography enables radiographic visualization of the urinary tract through ureteral catheterization and injection of contrast material. The ureters are catheterized during cystoscopy. Radiopaque material is injected into the ureters, and x-ray films are obtained (Figure 12-24). This test can be performed even if the patient is allergic to IV contrast dye, because none of the dye injected into the ureters is absorbed.

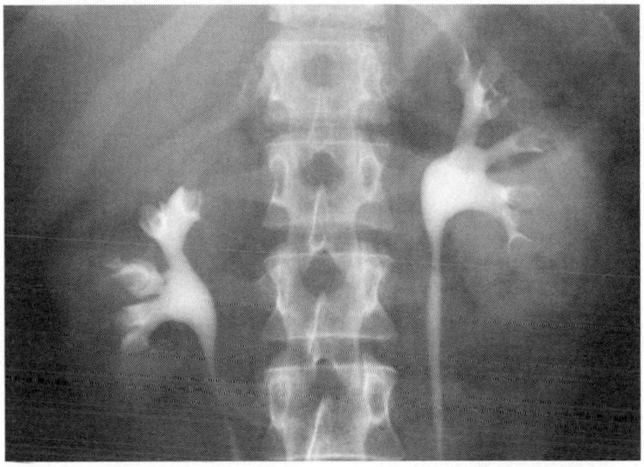

Figure 12-24 Retrograde pyelography with patient in lithotomy position.

Retrograde pyelography aids in radiographically examining the ureters when visualization with IVP (p. 953) is inadequate or contraindicated. When a ureter is obstructed, IVP enables visualization of only the ureter proximal to the obstruction, if anything. To visualize the distal portion of the ureter, retrograde pyelography is necessary. Also, in patients with unilateral renal disease, the involved kidney and collecting system are not visualized, because renal function is so poor. As a result, no dye is filtered into the collecting system by the nonfunctioning kidney. To rule out ureteral obstruction as a cause of unilateral kidney disease, retrograde pyelography must be performed. Tumors, benign strictures, tortuous ureters, stones, scarring, and extrinsic compression may cause ureteral obstruction. Retrograde pyelography provides complete visualization of the ureters.

Retrograde pyelography is performed by a urologist in approximately 1 hour in a cystoscopy room or operating room. The study is uncomfortable. If awake, the patient will feel pressure and an urge to void. If general anesthesia is used, no postoperative pain is noted.

Potential Complications

- Urinary tract infection
  Infections may result because of the invasive nature of this procedure.
- Sepsis by seeding the blood stream with bacteria from infected urine
- Perforation of the bladder or ureter
- Hematuria as a result of urologic instrumentation
- Temporary obstruction to ureteral urine flow
  Manipulation of the ureters may cause edema, which can result in temporary, partial obstruction to urine flow.

- Allergic reaction to iodinated dye
  Rare, because the dye is not administered IV.

Interfering Factors

- Retained barium from previous x-ray studies can obscure visualization.

Procedure and Patient Care

Before

- Explain the procedure to the patient.
- Ensure that informed consent is obtained.
- If enemas are ordered to clear the bowel, assist the patient as needed, and record the results.
- If the procedure will be performed with the patient under local anesthesia, allow the patient to have a liquid breakfast.
- If the procedure will be performed with the patient under general anesthesia, follow routine general anesthesia precautions. Keep the patient NPO after midnight on the day of the test.
- Fluids may be given IV.
- Administer preprocedural medications as ordered 1 hour before the study. Sedatives decrease spasm of the bladder sphincter, thus decreasing patient discomfort.
- Check the patient for allergy to iodinated dye.

During

- Note the following procedural steps:
  1. The ureteral catheters are passed into the ureters by means of cystoscopy (see p. 529, Figure 4-6).
  2. Radiopaque contrast material (Hypaque or Renografin) is injected into the ureteral catheters, and x-ray films are obtained.
  3. The entire ureter and pelvis are demonstrated.
  4. As the catheters are withdrawn, more dye is injected and more x-ray films are taken to visualize the complete outline of the ureters.
  5. A delayed film is often obtained to assess the emptying capabilities of the ureter. This is usually done in about 5 minutes after the last injection.
  6. If obstruction is noted, a stent may be left in the ureter so that the ureter can drain.

After

- Check and record the patient's vital signs as ordered. Watch for decreased blood pressure and increased pulse as indications of bleeding.
- Observe the patient for signs and symptoms of sepsis (e.g., elevated temperature, flush, chills, decreased blood pressure, increased pulse).
- Assess the patient's ability to void for at least 24 hours. Urinary retention may be secondary to edema caused by instrumentation.
- Note the color of the urine; a pink tinge is typically present. Report bright red blood or clots to the physician.

- Encourage the patient to increase intake of fluids. Dilute urine decreases dysuria. Fluids also maintain a constant flow of urine to prevent stasis and accumulation of bacteria in the bladder.
- Monitor the patient for bladder spasm. Often, belladonna-opium suppositories are given to relieve bladder spasm.
- Administer analgesics as needed.

Home Care Responsibilities

- Observe vital signs for indications of bleeding (e.g., decreased blood pressure, increased pulse) and sepsis (e.g., temperature, flush, chills).
- Monitor urine output over the first 24 hours to detect urinary retention.
- Encourage the patient to drink lots of fluids to prevent stasis and accumulation of bacteria in the bladder.

Test Results and Clinical Significance

Tumor or strictures *Primary tumors of the ureter, but most often extrinsic contiguous tumors, involve the ureters and cause partial or complete obstruction. Strictures from radiation fibrosis or primary retroperitoneal fibrosis can also cause strictures of varying degree.*

Stones *Stones, the most common cause of ureteral obstruction, are evident on retrograde pyelography, and can be removed by cystoscopy.*

Congenital anomaly *Congenital duplications, ureteral cysts, bands, or ureteral kinking are evident with this study.*

Related Tests

- Intravenous pyelography (IVP) (p. 953): This is an x-ray study of the kidneys, ureter, and bladder using an IV contrast agent. Visualization of obstructed ureters is limited.

Sella Turcica Radiography

Normal Findings

No abnormalities

Indications

This plain film of the sella turcica is used to screen for pituitary adenomas.

Test Explanation

X-ray films are obtained of the sella turcica, an area of the bony cranium at the base of the skull that contains the pituitary gland. Pituitary adenomas can be easily detected by

Table 12-6 Functioning pituitary adenomas

Syndrome	Hormone	Pituitary adenoma
Acromegaly	Growth hormone	Acidophilic
Galactorrhea	Prolactin	Chromophobe
Cushing's syndrome	ACTH	Basophilic
Hypogonadism	Insufficient FSH or LH	Chromophobe
Double vision	None	Chromophobe compression of chiasm

ACTH = adrenocroticotropic hormone, FSH = follicle-stimulating hormone, LH = luteinizing hormone.

identifying erosion and destruction of the normal sella turcica. Pituitary tumors may produce biologically active hormones (Table 12-6). CT (p. 939) or MRI (p. 1009) of the brain is usually performed if a pituitary tumor is suspected.

Procedure and Patient Care

Before

- Explain the procedure to the patient.
- Tell the patient that all objects above the neck must be removed.
- If a glass eye is present, note this on the x-ray examination request, because it will produce a confusing shadow on the film.

During

- Axial (submentovertical), half-axial (Towne), posteroanterior, and lateral views of the skull are usually taken.
- Tell the patient that this test is painless.
- A radiologic technologist performs this test in a few minutes.

After

- No special aftercare is needed.

Test Results and Clinical Significance

Pituitary tumor *Tumors cause enlargement of the sella turcica, which is evident on skull x-ray films.*

Destruction of the sella turcica *Caused by tumor, aneurysm, or other disease, the bony surrounding of the pituitary is destroyed.*

Related Tests

- CT (p. 939) or MRI (p. 1009) of the brain: These are more accurate methods of identifying pituitary tumors.

Sialography

Normal Findings

No evidence of disease in the salivary ducts and related structures

Indications This test is used to identify calculi in the salivary ducts.

Test Explanation

Sialography is an x-ray procedure used to examine the salivary ducts (parotid, submaxillary, submandibular, sublingual) and related glandular structures after injection of a contrast medium into the desired duct. The procedure is used to detect calculi, strictures, tumors, or inflammatory disease in patients with pain, tenderness, or swelling in these areas. CT of the salivary ducts is more reliable for detection of salivary parenchymal tumors or inflammation. Sialography is effective for ductule calculi or strictures.

A radiologist performs this procedure in the radiology department in less than 30 minutes. The patient may feel a little pressure as the contrast medium is injected into the ducts.

Contraindications

- Mouth infections (e.g., yeast infection), because they may be spread to the salivary glands

Potential Complications

- Allergic reaction to iodinated dye
  This is rarely, because the dye is not administered IV.

Procedure and Patient Care

Before

- Explain the procedure to the patient. The thought of dye injection in the mouth is frightening to many patients. Provide emotional support.
- Obtain informed consent if required by the institution.
- Instruct the patient to remove jewelry, hairpins, and dentures, which could obscure x-ray visualization.
- Instruct the patient to rinse the mouth with an antiseptic solution to reduce the possibility of introducing bacteria into the ductal structures.

During

- Note the following procedural steps:
  1. X-ray studies are taken before the dye injection to ensure that radiopaque stones are not present, which could prevent the contrast material from entering the ducts.
  2. The patient is placed supine on an x-ray table.

3. The contrast medium is injected directly into the desired orifice through a cannula or special tiny catheter.
4. X-ray films are obtained with the patient in various positions.
5. The patient is given a sour substance (e.g., lemon juice) orally to stimulate salivary excretion of the dye.
6. Another set of x-ray studies is obtained to evaluate ductal drainage.

After

- Encourage the patient to drink fluids to eliminate the dye.

Test Results and Clinical Significance

Calculi
Strictures
These cause obstruction of the duct draining the salivary gland.

Tumor *Most tumors of the salivary glands are benign, and in the parotid gland. These tumors are demonstrated as radiolucent filling defects or distortion of the glandular ductules within the gland.*

Inflammatory disease *Sialitis (especially parotitis) can result from viral illnesses (e.g., mumps) or bacterial infections.*

Skull Radiography

Normal Findings

Normal skull and surrounding structures

Indications

This x-ray is used to evaluate the skull and paranasal sinuses for trauma or disease.

Test Explanation

An x-ray film of the skull provides visualization of the bones making up the skull, the nasal sinuses, and any CNS calcification. This study is indicated when a pathologic condition is suspected in any of these structures.

Skull fractures are easily seen as abnormal radiolucent lines in an otherwise radiopaque skull bone (Figure 12-25). Metastatic tumors of the skull can easily be seen as radiolucent spots on an otherwise normal film. Opacification of the nasal sinuses may indicate sinusitis, hemorrhage, or tumor.

Located in the middle of the brain, the pineal gland is thought to regulate biorhythms in mammals. This gland may become calcified after puberty. When calcified, the pineal gland is a useful marker, and allows the midline of the brain to be easily identified on skull x-ray films. Conditions such as unilateral hematoma or tumor will cause a shift of the midline structures (and the calcified pineal gland) to the side opposite the site of the pathologic condition. Simple skull x-ray films therefore allow easy detection of these unilateral, space-occupying lesions.

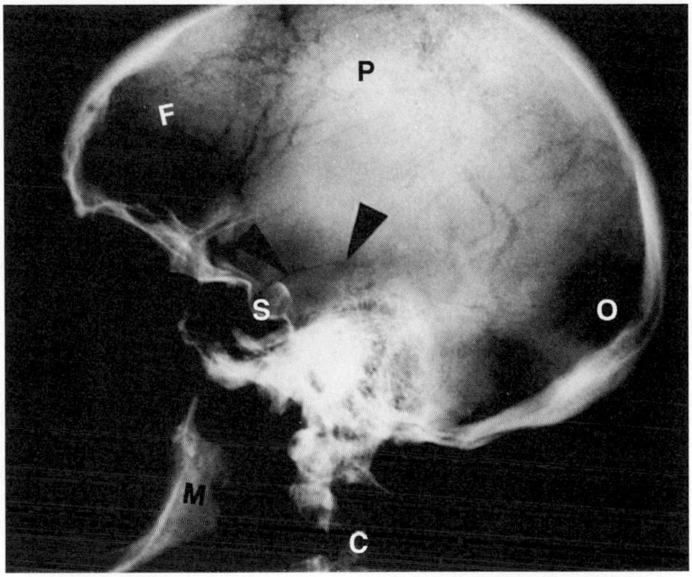

Figure 12-25 Skull x-ray. Lateral view. *Pointers* indicate fracture line in temporal bone. *F,* frontal bone; *P,* parietal bone; *O,* occipital bone; *S,* sella turcica; *M,* mandible; *C,* cervical vertebra.

The sella turcica is the bony structure surrounding and protecting the pituitary gland. Tumors of the pituitary gland may cause an increase in size or erosion of the sella turcica. These changes can be detected on skull x-ray films.

Procedure and Patient Care

Before

- Explain the procedure to the patient.
- Instruct the patient to remove all objects above the neck, because metal objects and dentures will prevent x-ray visualization of the structures they cover.
- Avoid hyperextension and manipulation of the head if surgical injuries are suspected.
- Tell the patient that no sedation or fasting is required.

During

- The patient is taken to the radiology department and placed on an x-ray table. Axial (submentovertical), half-axial (Towne), posteroanterior, and lateral views of the skull are usually obtained (Figure 12-26).
- A radiologic technologist obtains the skull films in a few minutes.
- Tell the patient that the test is painless.

After

- If a glass eye is present, note this on the x-ray examination request, because it can present a confusing shadow on the x-ray film.

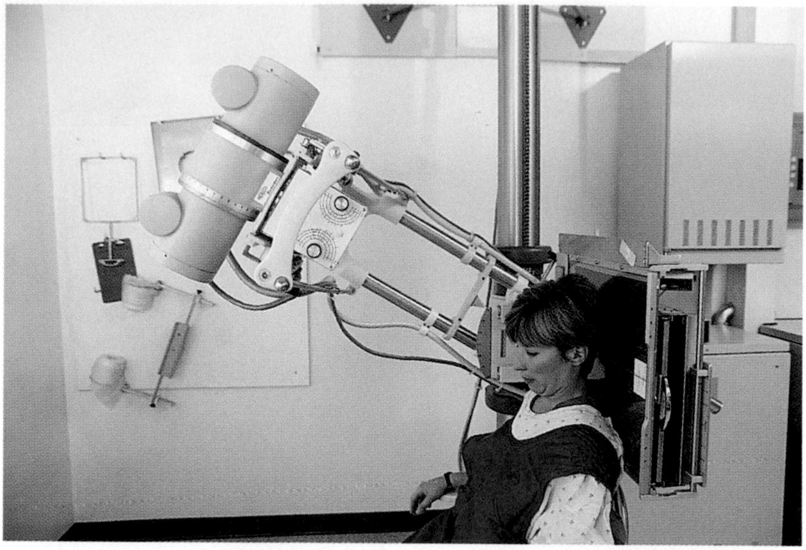

Figure 12-26 Patient positioned for a skull x-ray study (Towne view—anteroposterior projection with posterior view). A lead apron is placed on the patient to prevent unnecessary exposure to radiation.

Test Results and Clinical Significance

Skull fracture *This is seen as a radiolucent line in the skull. The normal bone sutures (where the bones have grown together during normal growth and development) can look like fractures to the untrained eye.*

Metastatic tumor *Breast cancer, Paget's disease, myeloma, and many other tumors can metastasize to the skull. Metastatic tumor can be osteolytic (radiolucent) or osteoblastic (radiopaque).*

Sinusitis *Swelling and mucus in the sinuses are evident as increased density on the x-ray film. Air-fluid levels may be evident also.*

Hemorrhage
Tumor
Hematoma
When unilateral, these abnormalities cause shift of midline structures (calcified pineal gland) to the opposite side.

Congenital anomaly *Many anomalies in the normal growth and development of the skull are obvious.*

Related Tests

- CT scan of the brain (p. 939): This test can be used to evaluate the skull. Its main purpose is to evaluate the brain.

Small Bowel Follow-Through
(SBF, Small Bowel Enema)

Normal Findings

Normal positioning, motility, and patency of the small intestine

Indications

This x-ray contrast-enhanced study of the small intestines is most often used to identify and determine the cause of small bowel obstruction. It is also used to identify tumors, strictures, inflammation, and other congenital or acquired diseases of the small intestine.

Test Explanation

The SBF study is performed to identify abnormalities in the small bowel. Usually, the patient is asked to drink barium; in patients who cannot drink, barium can be injected through a nasogastric tube. X-ray films are then obtained at timed intervals (usually 30 minutes to 1 hour) to follow the progression of barium through the small bowel. Significant delays in barium transit time may occur as a result of both benign and malignant forms of partial obstruction or diminished intestinal motility (ileus). On the other hand, the flow of barium is faster in patients who have hypermotility of the small bowel (e.g., malabsorption syndromes). Failure of the progression through the small bowel can be seen in patients with complete mechanical small bowel obstruction. Furthermore, SBF series are helpful in identifying and defining the anatomy of small bowel fistulas (abnormal connections between the small bowel and other abdominal organs or skin). Strictures due to Crohn's disease or radiation are also evident with SBF.

A more accurate radiographic evaluation of the small intestine is enabled by the *small bowel enema*. Barium is injected into a tube previously placed in the small bowel. This small bowel enema provides better visualization of the entire small bowel, because the barium is not diluted by gastric and duodenal juices, as when the patient drinks barium. This test is especially useful in the evaluation of partial small bowel obstruction of unknown cause. Tumors, ulcers, and small bowel fistulas are more easily identified and defined with the enema. Table 12-7 below lists x-ray studies used to visualize the GI tract. Note that this procedure is performed by a radiologist in the radiology department in approximately 30 minutes. Tell the patient that this test is not uncomfortable.

Table 12-7 ***X-ray visualization of gastrointestinal tract***

Study	Portion of GI tract evaluated
Barium swallow	Esophagus
Upper GI	Lower esophagus, stomach, and upper duodenum
Small bowel series	Duodenum, jejunum, and ileum
Barium enema	Rectum, colon, and distal ileum

Contraindications

- Complete small bowel obstruction
  The introduction of barium into an obstructed bowel may create a stonelike impaction; however, this is extremely rare.
- Suspected perforated viscus
  Barium should not be used in this situation because it may cause persistent and recurrent infections if it leaks out of the bowel. Meglumine diatrizoate (Gastrografin), a water-soluble contrast medium, can be used if perforation is suspected. However, it becomes diluted rapidly, minimizing the accuracy of the SBE.
- Unstable vital signs
  These should be monitored during the time required for this study.

Potential Complications

- Barium-induced small bowel obstruction

Interfering Factors

- Barium in the intestinal tract from a previous barium x-ray study may obstruct adequate visualization of the area of small bowel to be evaluated.
- Food or fluid within the GI tract may give the false sense of a filling defect due to a tumor or other mass.
- Morphine can significantly delay small bowel motility.

✓ CLINICAL PRIORITIES

- More accurate evaluation of the small intestines is provided by the *small bowel enema,* in which barium is injected through a tube placed in the small bowel.
- Barium should not be used in patients with suspected perforated viscus. In these patients, meglumine diatrizoate (Gastrografin), a water-soluble medium, is used.
- Cathartics are recommended after this test to aid in removal of the barium. Stools will return to normal color after evacuation of all the barium.

Procedure and Patient Care

Before

- Explain the procedure to the patient.
- Instruct the patient not to eat anything for at least 8 hours before the test. Usually, keep the patient NPO after midnight on the day of the test.
- Inform the patient that the SBF series may take several hours. Suggest that the patient bring reading material or some paperwork to occupy the time.
- Accompany the patient to the radiology department if vital signs are not stable.
- Arrange for transportation of the hospitalized patient back to the nursing unit between serial films.

During

- Note the following procedural steps:
  1. A specially prepared drink containing barium sulfate is mixed as a milkshake, which the patient drinks through a straw.
  2. Usually, an upper GI series is performed concomitantly (see p. 999).
  3. Barium flow is followed through the upper GI tract by means of fluoroscopy.
  4. At frequent intervals (15 to 60 minutes), repeated x-ray films are obtained to follow the flow of barium through the small intestine until barium is seen flowing into the right colon. This usually takes 60 to 120 minutes, but in patients with delayed progression of the barium, the test may take as long as 24 hours to complete.

Small Bowel Enema

1. Usually performed by placing a long, weighted tube transorally; however, a tube also can be placed into the upper small bowel endoscopically.
2. After the tube is in place, a thickened barium mixture is injected through the tube, and x-ray films are serially obtained as described for SBF.

After

- Inform the patient of the need to evacuate all the barium. Cathartics (e.g., magnesium citrate) are recommended. Initially, stools will be white, but should return to normal color with complete evacuation.

Test Results and Clinical Significance

Small bowel tumor *This may be evident as partial or complete small bowel obstruction. Usually, however, tumors are seen as filling defects in the column of barium in the small bowel.*

Small bowel obstruction *Adhesions are the most common cause of small bowel obstruction, followed by extrinsic tumor, hernia, and stricture from inflammatory bowel disease in adults. Hernias, intussusception, malrotation, bowel atresia, and volvulus are most common in children. Small bowel obstruction can be partial or complete. With complete obstruction, the barium column does not progress past the area of obstruction. With partial obstruction, the barium passes the area of obstruction, but abnormally slowly.*

Inflammatory small bowel disease (e.g., Crohn's disease) *Inflammatory bowel disease usually is apparent as a stricture causing partial small bowel obstruction.*

Malabsorption syndromes (e.g., Whipple's disease, sprue) *These are usually evident as rapid transit through the small bowel.*

Congenital or acquired anatomic anomaly (e.g., malrotation) *Malrotation usually causes the ligament of Treitz (junction of the duodenum and jejunum) to be in the right lower quadrant instead of its normal location in the left upper quadrant. Short bowel syndrome due to surgical small bowel bypass or resection is evident as rapid transit of barium through the small bowel.*

Congenital abnormalities (e.g., small bowel atresia, duplication, Meckel's diverticulum) *Bowel atresia or duplication can be noted as bowel obstruction in children. Meckel's diverticulum is evident as an outpouching of the ileum. It may not be apparent until adulthood, and may never cause symptoms.*

Small bowel intussusception *An upper segment of bowel becomes invaginated (swallowed up) into a lower segment. This usually causes bowel obstruction, and is most common in children.*

Small bowel perforation *When contrast leaks out of the intestine, perforation is present.*

Radiation enteritis *This becomes evident years after radiation therapy. It is demonstrated as a stricture of one or more segments of the small bowel.*

Related Tests

- Barium enema (p. 900): This test is contrast material–enhanced x-ray study of the colon. Often the distal small bowel is visualized.

Spinal Radiography (Cervical, Thoracic, Lumbar, Sacral, or Coccygeal X-Ray Studies)

Normal Findings

Normal spinal vertebrae

Indications

Spinal radiography is used to evaluate back or neck pain.

Test Explanation

Spinal x-ray studies may be performed to evaluate any area of the spine. They usually include anteroposterior, lateral, and oblique views of these structures. These x-ray films are often obtained to assess back or neck pain, degenerative arthritic changes, traumatic fractures, tumor metastasis, spondylosis (degenerative disease of the spinal structures), and spondylolisthesis (slipping of one vertebral disk over another). Cervical spine x-ray studies are routinely performed in cases of multiple trauma to ensure no fracture before the patient is moved or the neck is manipulated. Spinal x-rays are helpful in evaluating for spinal alignment abnormalities (e.g., kyphosis, scoliosis).

Contraindications

- Pregnancy

Procedure and Patient Care

Before

- Explain the procedure to the patient.
- Instruct the patient to remove any metal objects covering the area to be visualized.
- Immobilize the patient if a spinal fracture is suspected. Apply a neck brace if a cervical spine fracture is suspected.
- Tell the patient that no fasting or sedation is required; however, if a fracture is suspected, the patient may be kept NPO.

During

- Note that the patient is placed on an x-ray table. Anterior, posterior, lateral, and oblique x-ray films are obtained of the desired area of the spinal cord.
- A radiologic technologist obtains spinal x-ray films in a few minutes.
- Tell the patient that no discomfort is associated with this study.

After

- Patient positioning and activity depend on test results.

Test Results and Clinical Significance

Degenerative arthritis changes *Bone destruction or spurring is seen in patients with degenerative arthritic changes of the spinal joints.*

Traumatic or pathologic fracture *The cervical and lumbar portions of the spine are most frequently injured. Any portion, however can be affected by metastatic neoplasm (e.g., myeloma, Paget's disease, breast or lung cancer). Bone metastasis can lead to fracture without a traumatic event.*

Spondylosis
Spondylolisthesis
These are anatomic alterations of spinal alignment

Related Tests

- CT (p. 933) or MRI (p. 1009) of the spine: These studies demonstrate spinal anatomy and pathologic conditions better than spinal x-ray studies do. Alignment, however, is best evaluated with plain x-ray studies.

Swallowing Examination (Videofluoroscopy Swallowing Examination)

Normal Findings

Normal swallowing function and complete clearing of radiographic material through the upper digestive tract

Indications This test is performed to identify the cause of inability to swallow.

Test Explanation

Problems in swallowing may result from local structural diseases (e.g., tumors, upper esophageal diverticula, inflammation, extrinsic compression of the upper GI tract) or surgery to the oropharyngeal tract. Motility disorders of the upper GI tract (e.g., Zenker's diverticulum) and neurologic disorders (e.g., stroke syndrome, Parkinson's disease, neuropathies) also may cause difficulty in swallowing. Videofluoroscopy of the swallowing function allows the speech pathologist to delineate more clearly the exact pathologic condition in the swallowing mechanism, and to determine the most appropriate treatment and to teach the patient proper swallowing technique.

This test is performed by asking the patient to swallow barium or a barium-containing meal. With videofluoroscopy, the act of swallowing is visualized and documented. Structural abnormalities and functional impairment can be identified easily with the slow-framed progression and reversal possible with videofluoroscopy. This test is similar to barium swallow (p. 906), but finer details of swallowing can be evaluated with videofluoroscopy.

Contraindications

- Patients who aspirate saliva are not candidates for videofluoroscopy swallowing. Non-swallowing methods of alimentation will be required.

Procedure and Patient Care

Before

- Explain the procedure to the patient.
- Explain to the patient that no preparation is required.

During

- In the radiology department, the patient is asked to swallow a barium-containing meal. The consistency of the meal (e.g., liquid, semisoft [e.g., applesauce], or solid [e.g., a tea biscuit]) will be determined by the speech therapist and radiologist, to simulate foods to which the patient is to be initially reintroduced. While the patient swallows, videofluoroscopy is recorded in both the lateral and the anterior positions.
- The video is repeatedly examined by the radiologist forward and backward and by the speech pathologist.

After

- No catharsis is required.

Test Results and Clinical Significance

Upper GI tract disease
Neuromuscular disorder
Achalasia
Upper GI motility disorder (e.g., stroke syndrome, Parkinson's disease, peripheral neuropathy)
Diffuse esophageal spasms
Zenker's diverticulum
These disorders can be associated with swallowing dysfunction at various levels in the swallowing mechanism.

Related Tests

- Barium swallow (p. 906): This test is similar to videofluoroscopy except that multiple still x-ray films are obtained and the entire swallowing mechanism cannot be fully evaluated.

T-tube and Operative Cholangiography

Normal Findings

Normal common bile duct with no dilatation or filling defects
Good runoff of dye through the ampulla of Vater into the duodenum

Indications

Choangiography provides visualization of the bile ducts during and after surgery. It is most commonly used to identify common bile duct stones.

Test Explanation

In *operative cholangiography,* the common bile duct is directly injected with radiopaque material through the cystic duct. This is usually performed during cholecystectomy. Stones appear as radiolucent shadows. Gallstones, tumors, or strictures cause partial or total obstruction of the flow of dye into the duodenum. Visualization of the biliary duct structures enables the surgeon to see the surgical anatomy of the biliary tree. This reduces the possibility of inadvertent common bile duct injury during cholecystectomy. If common duct stones are demonstrated during operative cholangiography, a common duct exploration is performed. Some surgeons perform operative cholangiography in all patients who undergo cholecystectomy. Other surgeons use specific indications for operative cholangiography, including the following:

1. Jaundice
2. Abnormal liver enzyme levels
3. Dilated common bile duct
4. Evidence of pancreatitis
5. Evidence of small stones in the cystic duct during cholecystectomy

T-*tube cholangiography* is performed postoperatively following T-tube placement during a common duct exploration. Its main purpose is to detect retained common bile duct stones and demonstrate good flow of contrast dye into the duodenum. This test is performed, usually 5 to 10 days after surgery, with use of a T-shaped rubber tube placed in the common bile duct at surgery. If no stones are evident and there is good runoff of bile into the duodenum, the T-tube can be removed. If there are residual stones, the tube tract can be used to extract the stones.

Potential Complications

- Sepsis caused by increased ductal pressure with dye infusion

Interfering Factors

- Barium in the abdomen from a previous upper GI series or barium enema x-ray study precludes visualization of the bile duct.

Procedure and Patient Care

Before

- Explain the procedure to the patient when obtaining consent for the main biliary procedure.
- Tell the patient that no fasting or sedation is required for T-tube cholangiography. However, routine preoperative NPO status is necessary for operative cholangiography.

During

- Note the following procedural steps:

Operative Cholangiogram

1. Performed through catheterization of the cystic duct during cholecystectomy.
2. Alternatively, a needle or catheter is placed in the common bile duct.
3. The dye is injected directly into the common bile duct.
4. X-ray films are obtained while the patient is on the operating table, and are immediately reviewed by the surgeon.

T-tube Cholangiogram

1. The patient is taken to the radiology department.
2. A sterile dye solution is injected into the T-tube, previously placed by the surgeon.
3. X-ray films are obtained of the right upper quadrant of the abdomen with the patient placed in various positions.

- A radiologist or surgeon performs these procedures in approximately 10 minutes.
- Tell the patient that no discomfort is associated with these studies.

After

- Observe for signs of sepsis.
- If a T-tube has been surgically placed, establish a sterile, closed drainage system.

Test Results and Clinical Significance

Common bile duct stones *These appear as radiolucent rounded filling defects in the column of dye within the common bile duct.*

Anatomic variations *Many types of bile duct congenital anatomic variations can exist, and are demonstrated at cholangiography.*

Bile duct cysts *Though rare, these cysts appear as small to large outpouchings of the bile ducts.*

Stricture or tumor obstructing the common bile duct *Tumors of the bile duct (cholangiocarcinoma) or extrinsic tumors (e.g., pancreas, colon) can partially or completely obstruct the bile duct. Benign inflammatory or posttraumatic strictures also can cause varying degrees of obstruction.*

Bile duct surgical trauma *Ligation or laceration of the bile duct is obvious at the time of surgery with the use of cholangiography.*

Related Tests

- ERCP (p. 532): This is an endoscopic procedure performed to radiographically visualize the bile and pancreatic ducts.
- Percutaneous transhepatic cholangiography (PTC) (p. 976): This procedure provides visualization of the bile ducts by percutaneous access to the biliary tree through the liver.

Upper Gastrointestinal Tract Radiology
(Upper GI Series, UGI)

Normal Findings

Normal size, contour, patency, filling, positioning, and transit of barium through the lower esophagus, stomach, and upper duodenum

Indications

This x-ray contrast-enhanced study provides visualization of the mucosa of the esophageal, gastric, and duodenum lumens. It is indicated in patients with upper abdominal pain, dyspepsia, dysphagia, early satiety, or suspected gastroduodenal obstruction.

Test Explanation

The upper GI study consists of a series of x-ray films of the lower esophagus, stomach, and duodenum, usually using barium sulfate as the contrast medium. When there is concern for leakage of x-ray contrast through a perforation of the GI tract, however, meglumine diatrizoate (Gastrografin), a water-soluble contrast medium, is used. This test can be performed in conjunction with a barium swallow (p. 906) or small bowel (p. 991) series, which can precede or succeed the upper GI study, respectively.

The purpose of this examination is to detect ulcerations, tumors, inflammation, or anatomic malposition (e.g., hiatal hernia) of upper GI organs, as well as obstruction in the upper GI tract. The patient is asked to drink barium. As the contrast agent descends, the lower esophagus is examined for position, patency, and filling defects (e.g., tumors, scarring, varices). As the barium enters the stomach, the gastric wall is examined for benign or malignant ulcerations, filling defects (most often in cancer), and anatomic abnormalities (e.g., hiatal hernia). The patient is placed in a flat or head-down position, and the gastroesophageal area is examined for evidence of gastroesophageal reflux of barium.

As the contrast agent leaves the stomach, patency of the pyloric channel and the duodenum is evaluated. Benign peptic ulceration is the most common pathologic condition affecting these areas. Extrinsic compression caused by tumors, cysts, or enlarged pathologic organs (e.g., liver) near the stomach also can be identified by anatomic distortion of the outline of the upper GI tract.

A radiologist performs this procedure in approximately 30 minutes. The patient may be uncomfortable lying on the hard x-ray table, and occasionally may experience a sensation of bloating or nausea during the test.

Contraindications

- Complete bowel obstruction
- Suspected upper GI perforation
  Water-soluble meglumine diatrizoate should be used instead of barium.
- Unstable vital signs
  These patients should be monitored during the time required for this test.
- Patients who are uncooperative, because of the necessity of frequent position changes

Potential Complications

- Aspiration of barium
- Constipation or partial bowel obstruction caused by inspissated barium in the small bowel or colon

Interfering Factors

- Previously administered barium
  This may block visualization of the upper GI tract.
- Poor patient performance
- Incapacitated patients
  They cannot assume the multiple positions required for the study.
- Food and fluid in the stomach
  They give the false impression of filling defects in the stomach, precluding adequate evaluation of the gastric mucosa.
- Obtundation
  These patient cannot safely drink the barium.

✓ CLINICAL PRIORITIES

- When there is a concern for perforation in the GI tract, meglumine diatrizoate (Gastrografin) is used instead of barium. This may cause diarrhea after the procedure.
- For an *air contrast upper GI study,* the patient swallows a carbonated powder that creates CO_2 in the stomach and aids in visualization of the gastric mucosa.
- After the procedure, a cathartic is necessary to prevent impaction from the barium.

Procedure and Patient Care

Before

- Explain the procedure to the patient. Allow the patient to verbalize concerns.
- Instruct the patient to abstain from eating for at least 8 hours before the test. Usually, keep the patient NPO after midnight on the day of the test.
- Assure the patient that the test will not cause any discomfort.

During

- Note the following procedural steps:
  1. The patient is asked to drink approximately 16 oz of barium sulfate. This is a chalky substance usually suspended in milkshake form and drunk through a straw. Usually, the drink is flavored to increase palatability.
  2. After drinking the barium, the patient is moved through several position changes (e.g., prone, supine, lateral) to promote filling of the entire upper GI tract.
  3. Films are taken at the discretion of the radiologist as the flow of barium is observed fluoroscopically.
  4. The flow of barium is followed through the lower esophagus, stomach, and duodenum.
  5. Several films are obtained throughout the course of the test.
  6. For an *air-contrast upper GI study,* the patient is asked to rapidly swallow carbonated powder. This creates CO_2 in the stomach, providing air contrast to the barium within the stomach and increased visualization of the gastric mucosa.

After

- Inform the patient that if meglumine diatrizoate (gastrografin) was used, significant diarrhea may develop. This contrast agent is an osmotic cathartic.
- Instruct the patient to use a cathartic (e.g., milk of magnesia) if barium sulfate was used as the contrast medium. Water absorption may cause the barium to harden and create a fecal impaction if catharsis is not carried out.
- Instruct the patient to note the stools to ensure that all of the barium has been removed. The stools should return to normal color after the barium is completely expelled, which may take as long as a day and a half.

Test Results and Clinical Significance

Esophageal cancer *Most esophageal cancers occur in the lower esophagus. They are seen as a stricture or complete obstruction of the barium column.*

Esophageal varices *Serpiginous filling defects indicate esophageal varices.*

Hiatal hernia *There are two types of hiatal hernias. With a sliding hiatal hernia, the esophagogastric (EG) junction and upper stomach are in the chest. With the rolling type, the EG junction is normal but the fundus of the stomach rolls up into the chest. This latter type can become incarcerated and perforate. Surgical repair is required when identified.*

Diverticula *These can be in the upper esophagus (Zenker's) and due to spasm of the cricopharyngeus muscle (upper esophageal sphincter), or in the lower esophagus (epiphrenic) and due to paraesophageal infection.*

Gastric cancer *Cancers can be evident as large polypoid filling defects within the stomach or as ulcerative masses in the wall of the stomach.*

Gastric inflammatory disease (e.g., Menetrier's disease) *Thickened rugae or gastric folds are classic for chronic inflammatory changes of the stomach.*

Benign gastric tumor (e.g., leiomyoma) *Tumors can be small polypoid masses in the stomach or giant tumors that distort the entire upper abdomen.*

Extrinsic compression by pancreatic pseudocyst, cysts, pancreatic tumors, or hepatomegaly *Masses in the upper abdomen can distort the stomach. Because the stomach is a large sack, it is unusual for that structure to be obstructed by extrinsic compression.*

Perforation of the esophagus, stomach, or duodenum *Perforation is obvious when contrast material is evident outside the esophagus, stomach, or duodenum.*
Congenital abnormalities (e.g., duodenal web, pancreatic rest, malrotation syndrome) *These are congenital abnormalities that commonly cause duodenal obstruction in infants.*
Gastric ulcer (benign and malignant) *Malignancy can be ulcerative. Benign ulcers (stress or peptic) can also develop.*
Duodenal ulcer *Most duodenal ulcers are peptic ulcers. They are most commonly seen in the first portion of the duodenum, called the bulb.*
Duodenal cancer *This is very rare, and usually seen as a filling defect in the column of barium within the duodenum.*
Duodenal diverticulum *Not uncommon, these outpouchings rarely cause symptoms.*

Related Tests

- Esophagogastroduodenoscopy (EGD) (p. 536): This endoscopic procedure that provides better visualization of the upper GI organs. Further, biopsy can be performed with this procedure.

Venography, Lower Extremities
(Phlebography, Venogram)

Normal Findings

No evidence of venous thrombosis or obstruction

Indications

This x-ray contrast-enhanced study of the venous system of the lower or upper extremity is used to identify obstruction or thrombosis of the venous system in patients with a swollen arm or leg.

Test Explanation

Venography is an x-ray study designed to identify and locate thrombi in the venous system of the lower extremities. Dye is injected into the venous system of the affected extremity. X-ray films are then obtained at timed intervals to visualize the venous system. Obstruction to the flow of dye or a filling defect within the dye-filled vein indicates thrombosis. Positive study results accurately confirm the diagnosis of venous thrombosis; however, negative results although not so accurate, make the diagnosis of venous thrombosis unlikely. Often both extremities are studied, even when only one leg is suspected to contain deep-vein thrombosis. The normal extremity is used for comparison with the involved extremity. Unlike venous plethysmography (see p. 626), venography is accurate for thrombi in veins below the knee. Venography is also performed in the upper extremities to evaluate the more proximal axillary, subclavian, and innominate veins.

A radiologist performs this study in approximately 30 to 90 minutes. Venous catheterization is only as uncomfortable as a needle stick or a small incision in the foot. The dye may cause the patient to feel a warm flush (though not so severe as with arteriography).

Inform the patient that occasionally mild degrees of nausea, vomiting, or skin itching also may occur.

Contraindications

- Severe edema of the legs, making venous access for dye injection impossible
- Uncooperative patients
- Allergy to iodinated dye or shellfish
- Renal failure, because iodinated dye is nephrotoxic

Age-related concerns

- Elderly persons are particularly vulnerable to renal failure, especially if they are chronically dehydrated (e.g., chronic diarrhea).
- Dehydration after the test can be exacerbated by the diuretic action of the dye.

Potential Complications

- Allergic reaction to iodinated dyes
  Allergic reactions vary from flushing, itching, and urticaria to severe, life-threatening anaphylaxis (evidenced by respiratory distress, decrease in blood pressure, or shock). In the event of anaphylaxis, the patient may be given diphenhydramine (Benadryl), steroids, and epinephrine. Oxygen and endotracheal equipment should be available for immediate use.
- Renal failure, especially in elderly persons with chronic dehydration or mild renal failure
- Subcutaneous infiltration of the dye, causing cellulitis and pain
- Venous thrombophlebitis caused by the dye
- Bacteremia caused by a break in sterile technique
- Venous embolism caused by dislodgement of a deep-vein clot, induced by the dye injection

CLINICAL PRIORITIES

- Check the patient for allergy to iodinated dyes.
- During the dye injection, the patient may feel a warm flush.
- Fluids need to be encouraged after the test to prevent dehydration caused by the diuretic action of the dye.

Procedure and Patient Care

Before

- Explain the procedure to the patient.
- Obtained informed consent if required for this procedure.

- Assess the patient for allergy to iodinated dyes and shellfish. If a suspected allergy exists and venography is absolutely necessary, a steroid-antihistamine preparation should be used. Notify the radiologist of the potential for allergic reaction so that hypoallergenic, nonionic contrast material may be used.
- If needed, provide appropriate pain medication so the patient is able to lie still during the procedure.
- Ensure that the patient is appropriately hydrated before testing. Injection of the iodinated contrast may cause renal failure, especially in the elderly.

During

- Note the following procedural steps:
  1. The patient is taken to the radiology department and placed supine on the x-ray table.
  2. Catheterization of a superficial vein on the foot is performed. This may require a surgical cutdown.
  3. An iodinated, radiopaque dye is injected into the vein.
  4. X-ray films are obtained to follow the course of the dye up the leg.
  5. Frequently, a tourniquet is placed on the leg to prevent filling of the superficial saphenous vein. All of the dye therefore goes to the deep venous system, which contains the most clinically significant thrombosis that can embolize.

After

- Continue appropriate fluid administration to prevent dehydration caused by the diuretic action of the dye.
- Observe the puncture site for infection, cellulitis, or bleeding.
- Assess the patient's vital signs for signs of bacteremia (e.g., fever, tachycardia, chills).
- Evaluate the patient for signs of allergic reaction (e.g., rash, chills, fever, irritability). Treat with antihistamines or steroids.

Test Results and Clinical Significance

Obstructed venous system from thrombosis, tumor, or inflammation *This is evident as complete obstruction of dye flow in the main vein (usually femoral or iliac).*

Acute deep-vein thrombosis *This is evident as serpiginous filling defects in the column of dye on the wall of the vein.*

Related Tests

- Venous Doppler flow studies (p. 807): With the use of ultrasound, blood flow within the vein can be evaluated. Obstruction to flow is easily noted. This test is less invasive, equally accurate (above the knee), and associated with less risk than venography.
- Venous plethysmography (see p. 626): This is a manometric study of the venous system of the extremity. It enables identification of venous occlusion.

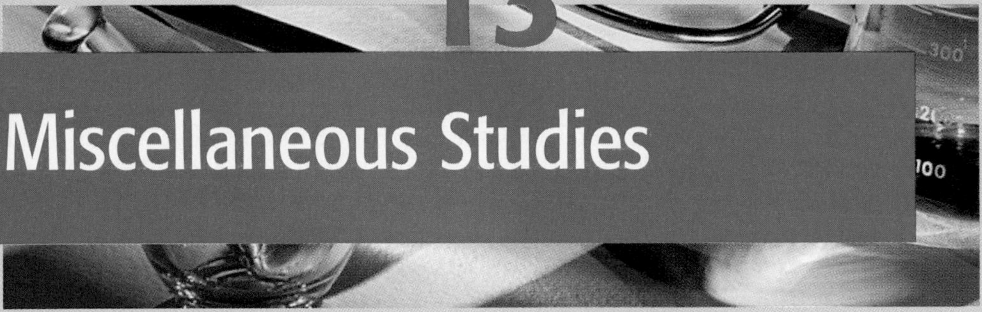

13 Miscellaneous Studies

TESTS

Overview

We have tried to organize a multitude of diverse diagnostic tests into groups based on the specimen on which the test was performed and the method of testing. This led to the development of chapters as presented in this text. However, a few tests could not readily be appropriated to any chapter. Therefore this chapter was created to include these important tests. There are no commonalities associated with these tests. All are described separately and in detail.

Chorionic Villus Sampling
(CVS, Chorionic Villus Biopsy [CVB])

Normal Findings

No genetic or biochemical disorders

Indications

CVS is performed in women whose unborn child may be at risk for a life-threatening or life-altering genetic defect. This includes women who (1) are older than 35-40 years at the time of pregnancy, (2) have had frequent spontaneous abortions, (3) have had previous pregnancies with fetuses or infants with chromosomal or genetic defects (e.g., Down's syndrome), or (4) have a genetic defect themselves (e.g., hemoglobinopathy).

Test Explanation

CVS can be performed at 8-12 weeks of gestation for early detection of genetic and biochemical disorders. Because CVS detects congenital defects early, first-trimester therapeutic abortions can be performed if indicated and desired.

A sample of chorionic villi from the chorion frondosum, which is the trophoblastic origin of the placenta, is obtained for analysis. These villi in the chorion frondosum are present from 8-12 weeks on and are believed to reflect fetal chromosome, enzyme, and DNA content. This permits much earlier diagnosis of prenatal problems than with amniocentesis, which cannot be done before 14-16 weeks. Further, the cells derived by CVS are more easily cultured for karyotyping (determination of chromosomal and genetic abnormalities). Although amniocentesis is the safer procedure, the cells obtained take longer to grow in culture, which further adds to the delay in obtaining results. At this point, therapeutic abortion for severe genetic defects is more difficult.

CVS requires significant experience to be performed safely. If the physician does not feel competent to safely perform the procedure, amniocentesis should be performed a few weeks later.

Potential Complications

- Accidental abortion
- Infection
- Bleeding

- Amniotic fluid leakage
- Fetal limb deformities

Procedure and Patient Care

Before

- Explain the procedure to the patient.
- Ensure that signed consent for the procedure has been obtained.
- Tell the patient that no food or fluid restrictions are necessary.
- Encourage the patient to drink at least 1-2 glasses of fluid before the test.
- Instruct the patient not to urinate for several hours before the test. A full bladder is an excellent reference point for pelvic ultrasound.
- Assess the vital signs of the mother and fetal heart rate before the test, and again during and on completion of the test.

During

- Note the following procedural steps:
  1. The patient is placed in the lithotomy position, and a sterile speculum is placed into the previously cleansed vagina to visualize the cervix.
  2. A cannula is inserted into the cervix and uterine cavity (Figure 13-1).
  3. Under ultrasound guidance, the cannula is rotated to the site of the developing placenta.
  4. A syringe is attached, and suction is applied to obtain three or more villous samples to ensure sufficient tissue for accurate sampling.
  5. If ultrasound indicates that the trophoblastic tissue is remote from the cervix, a transabdominal approach similar to that described for amniocentesis (p. 560) may be used.

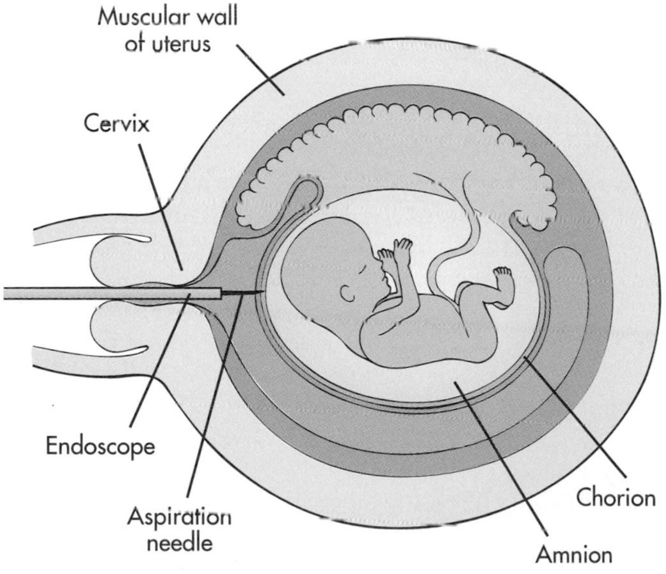

Figure 13-1 Chorionic villus sampling (CVS). Diagram of an 8-week pregnancy showing endoscopic aspiration of extraplacental villi.

- This procedure is performed by an obstetrician in approximately 30 minutes.
- Inform the patient that discomfort associated with this test is similar to that of a Papanicolaou test (Pap smear).

After

- Some mothers with Rh-negative blood may receive Rh_o(D) immune globulin (RhoGAM) because of the risk for development of maternal antibodies to the fetal blood cells, which could threaten fetal well-being.
- Monitor vital signs, and check the mother for signs of bleeding.
- Schedule an ultrasound in 2-4 days to affirm continued viability of the fetus.
- Assess the vaginal area for discharge and drainage; note the color and amount.
- Assess and educate the patient concerning signs of spontaneous abortion (e.g., cramps, bleeding) and endometrial infection (e.g., vaginal discharge, fever, crampy abdominal pain).
- Inform the patient how to obtain the results from the physician. Be sure she understands that the results are usually not available for several weeks (although they may be available much sooner if the test is performed at a major medical center).
- Inform the patient as to genetic counseling services if needed.

Home Care Responsibilities

- Instruct the mother to immediately report signs of spontaneous abortion (e.g., cramps, bleeding).
- Educate the mother to identify and report signs of endometrial infection (e.g., vaginal discharge, fever, crampy abdominal pain).
- The pregnant mother should be scheduled for an ultrasound 2-4 days after CVS to assure continued viability of the fetus.

Test Results and Clinical Significance

Chromosomal, genetic, and biochemical disorders *Many chromosomal and genetic defects are identified by karyotyping and genetic mapping. Genetic counseling is a vital part of this sort of testing. More research needs to be performed to develop accurate guidelines for therapeutic abortion. Further, religious, moral, and ethical aspects of these decisions need to be considered.*

Related Tests

- Obstetric ultrasonography (p. 796): This test is used to localize trophoblastic tissue.
- Amniocentesis (p. 560): Used to indicate fetal well-being and allows tissue sampling for karyotyping and genetic mapping.
- Fetoscopy (p. 540): During this test tissue can be obtained for karyotyping and genetic mapping.
- Non–stress, fetal (p. 304): This test is used to evaluate the viability of the fetus before, during, and after CVS.

Magnetic Resonance Imaging
(MRI, Nuclear Magnetic Resonance [NMRI])

Normal Findings

No evidence of disease

Indications

The indications for MRI change constantly as new uses for this technique are discovered. Its most important indications include evaluation of (1) headache or other neurologic signs of CNS lesions, (2) neck and back pain for disk herniation, and bones and joints (especially the knee) after traumatic injury or because of chronic pain.

Test Explanation

MRI is a noninvasive diagnostic technique that provides valuable information about the body's anatomy. MRI is based on how hydrogen atoms behave in a magnetic field when disturbed by radiofrequency signals. The unique feature about MRI is that it does not require exposure to ionizing radiation. MRI has several advantages over CT, including the following:

1. MRI provides better contrast between normal and pathologic tissue.
2. Obscuring bone artifacts that occur with CT do not occur with MRI.
3. Because rapidly flowing blood appears dark, many blood vessels appear as dark lumens. In MRI, this provides a natural contrast to the blood vessels.
4. Because spatial information depends only on how the magnetic fields are varied in space, it is possible to image the transverse, sagittal, and coronal planes directly with MRI.

Although the full usefulness of MRI is yet to be determined, it shows promise in evaluation of the following:

1. Head and surrounding structures
2. Spinal cord and surrounding structures
3. Face and surrounding structures
4. Neck
5. Mediastinum
6. Heart and great vessels
7. Liver
8. Kidney
9. Prostate gland
10. Bone and joints
11. Breasts
12. Extremities and soft tissues

The most common uses today, however, are visualization of the CNS,

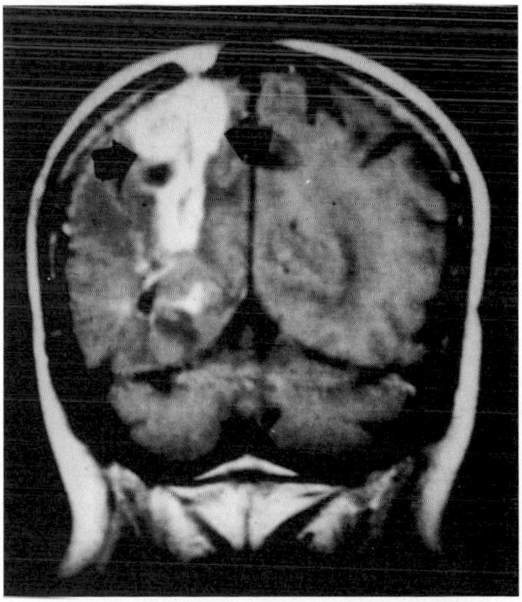

Figure 13-2 MRI with *arrows* indicating a brain tumor accentuated by Magnavist dye.

bony spine, joints, extremities, and liver (Figure 13-2). MRI is not useful for evaluation of the abdomen, because contrast agent is needed for good visualization of abdominal organs.

An important advantage of MRI is that serial studies can be performed without risk. This is useful in assessing the response of cancer to radiotherapy and chemotherapy. A major disadvantage is that fewer patients are eligible, compared with CT scanning. For example, examination of patients requiring cardiac monitoring or who have metal implants, pacemakers, or cerebral aneurysm clips will result in image degradation and possible danger to the patient.

This procedure is performed by a qualified radiologic technologist in approximately 30 to 90 minutes. The only discomfort associated with MRI may be from lying still on a hard surface and possible tingling in teeth containing metal fillings. In addition, claustrophobia is associated with being placed in the tube-like MRI unit. This problem is decreased if the newer, open MR imagers are used. Also, an injection is needed for administration of gadopentetate dimeglumine (Magnevist), used as contrast agent in MRI of intracranial and spinal lesions.

Contraindications

- Extreme obesity (>300 lb), because the table will not hold the weight
- Pregnancy, because the long-term effects of MRI are not known. Also there is risk of heating of the amniotic fluid and injury to the fetus
- Confused or agitated patients, because they cannot remain still
- Claustrophobia
- Unstable vital signs or requirement for continuous life-support equipment, because monitoring equipment cannot be used in the MRI room because it will be affected by the magnet
- Implanted metal objects such as pacemakers, infusion pumps, aneurysm clips, inner ear implants, and metal fragments in one or both eyes, because the magnet may move the object in the body, with possible injury to the patient

Interfering Factors

- Movement of the patient during MRI causes significant distortion of MR images.

✓ CLINICAL PRIORITIES

- The patient must remain motionless for long intervals during MRI, because movement can distort the images.
- Many patients experience a sense of claustrophobia during this test. Sedation may be necessary.
- This test cannot be performed in patients with any implanted metal objects (e.g., pacemakers). The magnet may move the object within the body and cause injury to the patient.

Procedure and Patient Care

Before

- Explain the procedure to the patient. Inform the patient that there is no exposure to radiation.
- Obtain informed consent if required by the institution.
- Tell the patient that he or she can drive without assistance after the procedure.
- Tell patients they may read or talk to a child in the imaging room during the procedure, because no radiation is used.
- Assess the patient for any contraindications to testing (e.g., aneurysm clips).
- If possible, show the patient a picture of the imaging machine (Figure 13-3), and encourage verbalization of anxieties. Some patients may experience claustrophobia. Antianxiety medications may be helpful for those with mild claustrophobia.
- Instruct the patient to remove all metal objects (e.g., dental bridges, jewelry, hair clips, belts, credit cards), because they will create artifacts on the scan. The magnetic field can damage watches and credit cards. Also, movement of metal objects within the magnetic field can be detrimental to anyone within the field.
- Inform the patient that he or she will be required to remain motionless during this study. Any movement can distort the scan. Young children often are sedated for this procedure. For head and neck MRI, the patient's head may be placed in a cradle that prohibits significant motion.
- Tell the patient that during the procedure he or she may hear a thumping sound. Earplugs are available if the patient wishes to use them.
- Remind the patient that a microphone inside the MRI tube allows the patient to communicate with personnel (Figure 13-4).
- Inform the patient that no fluid or food restrictions are necessary before MRI.
- For comfort, instruct the patient to empty his or her bladder before the test.

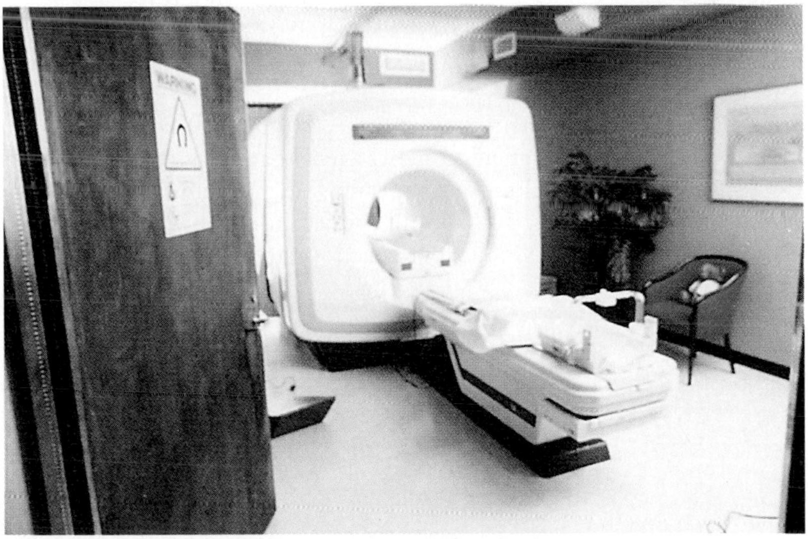

Figure 13-3 MRI equipment.

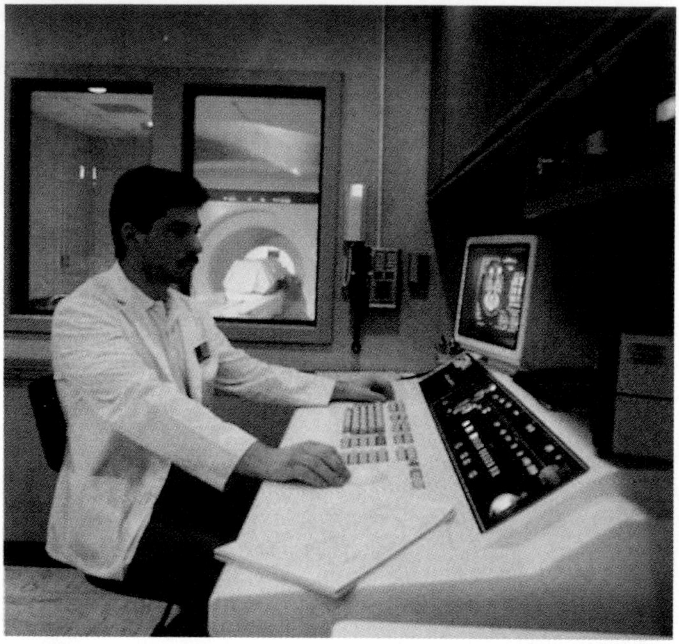

Figure 13-4 X-ray technician performs magnetic resonance imaging.

During

- Note the following procedural steps:
  1. The patient lies on a platform that slides into a tube containing the doughnut-shaped magnet.
  2. The patient is instructed to lie very still during the procedure.
  3. During the procedure, the patient can talk to and hear the staff via microphone or earphones in the imaging machine. Prism glasses can be worn so the patient can see outside the scanner.
  4. Gadolinium meglamine (Magnevist), approved by the U.S. Food and Drug Administration, is a paramagnetic contrast agent that can cross the blood-brain barrier. It is especially useful for distinguishing edema from tumors. If this is to be administered, approximately 10 to 15 ml is injected in the vein. Imaging can begin shortly after the injection. No dietary restrictions are necessary before using this agent.

After

- No special postprocedural care is needed.

Test Results and Clinical Significance

Brain

Cerebral tumor *Natural conrast can be accentuated by varying the MRI coil. Brain tumors can be specifically diagnosed. On T1-weighted images, tumors are radiolucent (dark), whereas on*

T2-weighted images they are radiopaque (white). MRI is particularly useful in evaluating the pituitary gland.

Aneurysm *This condition is evident as compression of normal brain tissue by a small, radiopaque, enlarged vascular abnormality. Bleeding or edema may be present with aneurysmal leak.*

Arteriovenous malformation *MRI angiography is a recent use of MRI, and its place in diagnostics is yet to be determined. However, large AV malformations can be seen with regular MRI as large radiolucent masses in the brain tissue.*

Hemorrhage

Subdural hematoma

Abscess

MRI can demonstrate intracranial hemorrhage or abscess.

Degenerating diseases (e.g., multiple sclerosis, hypoxic encephalopathy, encephalomyelitis) *Specific characteristics of these diseases can be detected with MRI.*

Hydrocephalus *This condition is evident as tremendous enlargement of the ventricular system of the brain.*

Other

Herniated lumbar and cervical disks *MRI is very sensitive for detection of these abnormalities.*

Tumor (primary or metastatic) *MRI is especially useful for detection of liver, lung, and soft tissue lesions.*

Joint disorders *MRI is especially useful for evaluation of knee injuries.*

Destructive lesion of bone *With multiple weighted images, tumors, osteomyelitis, and other destructive diseases of bone, and especially the spine, can be well demonstrated.*

Related Tests

- CT of the brain (p. 939): This is especially good for detection of bony abnormalities. MRI, however, provides better visualization of the CNS.

Oximetry (Pulse Oximetry, Ear Oximetry, Oxygen Saturation)

Normal Findings ≥95%

Critical Values ≤75%

Indications

Oximetry is used to monitor arterial O_2 saturation levels (SaO_2) in patients at risk for hypoxemia. This includes patients who are undergoing surgery, cardiac stress testing, mechanical ventilation, heavy sedation, or lung function testing, or who have multiple trauma. It is also used as an indicator of partial pressure of oxygen (PO_2) in patients who may experience hypoventilation, sleep apnea, or dyspnea. This test is commonly used to titrate O_2 levels in hospitalized patients.

Test Explanation

Oximetry is a noninvasive method of monitoring SaO_2 (i.e., ratio of oxygenated hemoglobin to total hemoglobin). SaO_2 is expressed as a percentage; for example, SaO_2 of 95% indicates that 95% of the total hemoglobin attachments for O_2 have O_2 attached to them. SaO_2 is an accurate approximation of O_2 saturation obtained from arterial blood gas study (see p. 97). By correlating SaO_2 with the patient's physiologic status, a close estimate of PO_2 can be obtained.

Oximetry is typically used to monitor oxygenation status during the perioperative period and in patients receiving heavy sedation or mechanical ventilation. This test is also frequently used in clinical situations such as pulmonary rehabilitation programs, stress testing, and sleep laboratories. Oximetry can be used to monitor response to drug therapy (e.g., theophylline). Pulse oximetry is constantly monitored during the perioperative period, and the results are one of the discharge criteria used in the post-anesthesia unit.

Interfering Factors

- Extreme vasoconstriction diminishes blood flow to the peripheral vessels, which decreases the accuracy of oximetry.
- Extreme alteration in temperature may diminish the accuracy of oximetry.
- Oximetry cannot differentiate carboxyhemoglobin saturation from O_2 saturation. Therefore, in cases of suspected smoke or carbon monoxide inhalation, oximetry should not be used to monitor oxygenation. The levels will be falsely elevated.
- Digital motion can alter accurate readings.
- Severe anemia affects the accuracy of comparison of oximetry and PO_2 levels.
- Fingernail polish will interrupt digital readings. The earlobe is used under these circumstances.

✓ CLINICAL PRIORITIES

- Oximetry is typically used to monitor O_2 status during the perioperative period, and in patients receiving conscious sedation. It is invaluable for titrating O_2 levels.
- Oximetry cannot differentiate carboxyhemoglobin from O_2 saturation. The level could be falsely elevated in patients with smoke or carbon monoxide inhalation.
- The oximetry probe cannot be used on fingertips with nail polish. In such cases, the earlobe is used.

Procedure and Patient Care

Before

- Explain, the procedure to the patient.
- Tell the patient that no fasting is required.

During

- Rub the patient's earlobe, pinna (upper portion of the ear), or fingertip to increase blood flow.

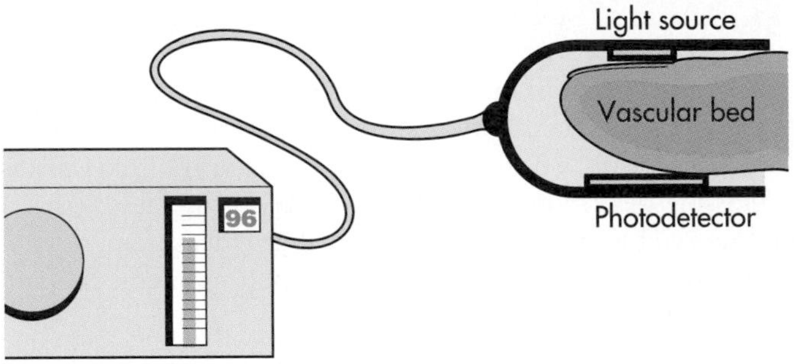

Figure 13-5 Oximetry. The pulse oximeter passes a beam of light through the tissue. The amount of light absorbed by the oxygen-saturated hemoglobin is measured by the sensor.

- Clip the monitoring probe or sensor to the ear or finger. The sensor warms and increases blood flow to the tissue. A beam of light passes through the tissue, and the sensor measures the amount of light the tissue absorbs (Figure 13-5).
- This study is usually performed by a respiratory therapist or nurse at the patient's bedside in a few minutes.
- Tell the patient that no discomfort is associated with this study.

After

- No special aftercare is needed.

Test Results and Clinical Significance

Increased levels

Increased fraction of inspired oxygen (FiO_2),
Hyperventilation
With increased alveolar O_2 caused by breathing more rapidly or increasing the O_2 in inspired air, PO_2 and O_2 can be expected to increase.

Decreased levels

Hypoventilation
Inadequate O_2 in inspired air (suffocation)
When ventilation is reduced enough to affect PO_2, oximetry values diminish.

Atelectasis, mucus plug, bronchospasm, pneumothorax, pulmonary edema, adult respiratory distress syndrome, restrictive lung disease *Nonaerated portions of the lung are still perfused with unoxygenated blood. This blood returns to the heart with little or no oxygen. The O_2 content is diluted, and oximetry values diminish.*
Atrial or ventricular cardiac septal defects *Unoxygenated blood gains access to oxygenated blood by direct shunting. By dilution, the O_2 content of the mixed blood returning to the heart is lowered, as is that of arterial blood.*
Severe hypoventilation states (e.g., oversedation, neurologic somnolence) *Without air exchange, PO_2 levels decrease.*
Pulmonary emboli

Related Tests

- O_2 saturation (p. 99): This is an indication of the percentage of hemoglobin saturated with O_2. This is part of arterial blood gas measurements.
- Po_2 (p. 99): This is a measure of the tension (pressure [P]) of oxygen dissolved in the plasma. This pressure determines the force of O_2 to diffuse across the alveolocapillary membrane. This is part of arterial blood gas measurements.
- O_2 content (p. 100): This is a calculated number that represents the amount of O_2 in the blood. The formula for calculation is:

$$O_2 \text{ content} = O_2 \text{ saturation} \times \text{Hemoglobin level} \times 1.34 + Po_2 \times 0.003.$$

Pulmonary Function Tests (PFTs)

Normal Findings Vary with patient age, sex, height, and weight

Indications

The primary reasons for performing pulmonary function studies include the following:

1. *Preoperative evaluation of the lungs and pulmonary reserve.* When planned thoracic surgery will result in loss of functional pulmonary tissue, as in lobectomy (removal of part of a lung) or pneumonectomy (removal of an entire lung), a significant risk of pulmonary failure exists if the preoperative pulmonary function is already severely compromised by other diseases, such as chronic obstructive pulmonary disease (COPD).
2. *Evaluation of response to bronchodilator therapy.* In some patients with a spastic component to COPD, long-term use of bronchodilators may be useful. Pulmonary function studies performed before and after the use of bronchodilators will identify this group of patients.
3. *Differentiation between restrictive and obstructive forms of chronic pulmonary disease.* Restrictive defects (e.g., pulmonary fibrosis, tumors, chest wall trauma) occur when ventilation is disturbed by limitation of chest expansion. Inspiration is primarily affected. Obstructive defects (e.g., emphysema, bronchitis, asthma) occur when ventilation is disturbed by increased airway resistance. Expiration is primarily affected.
4. *Determination of the diffusing capacity of the lungs (D_L).* Rates are based on the difference in concentration of gases in inspired and expired air.
5. *Performance of inhalation tests* in patients with inhalation allergies.

Test Explanation

Pulmonary function tests are performed to detect abnormalities in respiratory function and to determine the extent of pulmonary abnormality. Pulmonary function tests routinely include spirometry, measurement of air flow rates, and calculation of lung volumes and capacities. Gas diffusion and inhalation tests (bronchial provocation) are also performed when requested, but not routinely. Exercise pulmonary stress testing can also be performed to provide data concerning pulmonary reserve. During this staged test, the patient performs an aerobic function such as stationary biking or walking on a treadmill.

Spirometry is performed first. A spirometer is a machine that can measure air volumes. When a time element is added to the tracing, air flow rates can be determined. In the past, most spirometers worked on the bellows principle of water displacement. Now electronic spirometers are available that electronically measure these volumes and rates. Based on age, height, weight, race, and sex, normal values for volumes and flow rates can be predicted. Values greater than 80% of predicted values are considered normal. Spirometry provides information about obstruction or restriction of air flow. Spirometry supports the diagnosis of chronic obstructive pulmonary disease (COPD) and chronic restrictive pulmonary disease (CRPD).

Measurement of air flow rates provides information about airway obstruction. This portion of the study adds a time element to spirometry. When flow is plotted on the Y axis and volume is plotted on the X axis, flow/volume curves (isoflow loops) can be drawn when the patient is asked to maximally inhale, then forcefully exhale while being timed. The shape of the curve can be interpreted to identify and quantify airway obstruction. If air flow rates are significantly diminished (<60% of normal) or if requested by the physician, the test can be repeated after bronchodilators are administered by nebulizer. If the air flow rates improve by 20%, prolonged use of bronchodilators may be recommended for the patient. Emphysema or restrictive lung disease usually does not improve with bronchodilator therapy. Patients with an asthmatic component to COPD will benefit from bronchodilators. Changes in flow rate can be more accurately determined when isoflow loops are calculated with the use of a helium-air mixture.

Measurement of lung capacity (combination of two or more measurements of lung volume) can be performed by nitrogen or helium washout techniques. This provides further information about air trapping within the lung.

Gas exchange studies measure the diffusing capacity of the lung (D_L), that is, the amount of gas exchanged across the alveolar-capillary membrane per minute. Most laboratories use carbon monoxide (CO) to measure D_L, because CO has a great affinity for hemoglobin and only a small concentration is needed. Because of this affinity of hemoglobin for CO, the only limiting factor to the transfer of the gas is its rate of diffusion across the alveolar-capillary membrane (which is what is measured). Gas exchange is abnormal in congestive heart failure, pneumonia, and other diseases that fill the alveoli with fluid or exudate. Any disease that causes deposition of material in the interstitium of the lung (e.g., adult respiratory distress syndrome, collagen vascular disease, Goodpasture's syndrome, pulmonary fibrosis) will decrease gas exchange.

Measurement of arterial blood gas levels (see p. 97) is included in pulmonary function studies because the information obtained is used in calculations of lung function data. Pulmonary function tests routinely include the following:

Forced vital capacity (FVC): amount of air that can be forcefully expelled from a maximally inflated lung position. Less than expected values occur in obstructive and restrictive pulmonary diseases.

Forced expiratory volume in 1 second (FEV_1): volume of air expelled during first second of FVC. In obstructive pulmonary disease, airways are narrowed and resistance to flow is high. Therefore not so much air can be expelled in 1 second, and FEV_1 is less than the predicted value. In restrictive lung disease, FEV_1 is decreased because

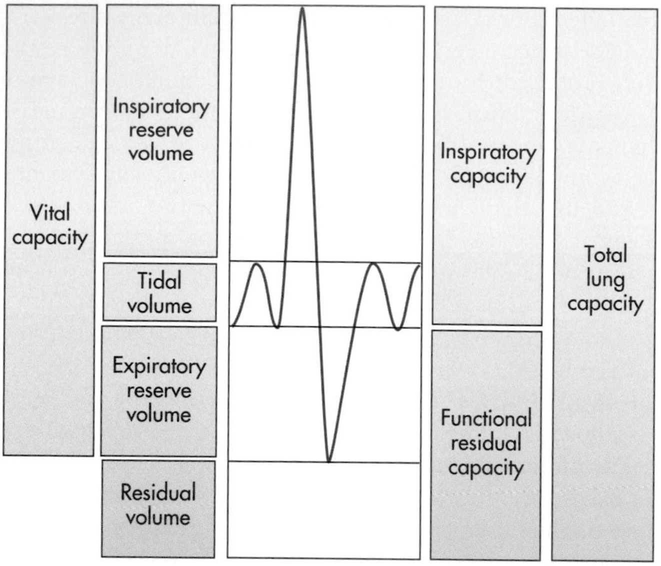

Figure 13-6 Relationship of lung volumes and capacities.

the amount of air originally inhaled is low, not because of airway resistance. Therefore the FEV_1/FVC ratio should be measured. In restrictive lung disease a normal value is 80%, and in obstructive lung disease this ratio is considerably less. The FEV_1 value will reliably improve with bronchodilator therapy if a spastic component to obstructive pulmonary disease exists.

Maximal midexpiratory flow (MMEF), or *forced midexpiratory flow:* maximal rate of air flow through the pulmonary tree during forced expiration. This test is independent of the patient's effort or cooperation. MMEF is less than expected values in obstructive pulmonary diseases and normal in restrictive pulmonary diseases.

Maximal volume ventilation (MVV) (formerly, *maximal breathing capacity*): maximal volume of air that a patient can breathe in and out during 1 minute. It is less than the expected value in both restrictive and obstructive pulmonary disease.

A comprehensive pulmonary function study also may include evaluation of the following lung volumes and lung capacities (Figure 13-6):

Tidal volume (TV or V_T): volume of air inspired and expired with each normal respiration.

Inspiratory reserve volume (IRV): maximal volume of air that can be inspired from end of normal inspiration. It represents forced inspiration over and beyond V_T.

Expiratory reserve volume (ERV): maximal volume of air that can be exhaled after normal expiration.

Residual volume (RV): volume of air remaining in the lungs following forced expiration.

Inspiratory capacity (IC): maximal amount of air that can be inspired after normal expiration. IC = TV + IRV.

Functional residual volume (FRV): amount of air left in the lungs after normal expiration. FRV = ERV + RV.

Vital capacity (VC): maximal amount of air that can be expired after maximal inspiration. VC = TV + IRV + ERV.

Total lung capacity (TLC): volume to which the lungs can be expanded with greatest inspiratory effort. TLC = TV + IRV + ERV + RV.

Minute volume (MV), or *minute ventilation:* volume of air inhaled and exhaled per minute.

Dead space: part of V_T that does not participate in alveolar gas exchange. Includes air within the trachea.

Forced expiratory flow (FEF): portion of air flow curve most affected by airway obstruction.

$FEF_{200-1200}$: rate of expired air between 200 ml and 1200 ml during FVC.

FEF_{25-75}: rate of expired air between 25% and 75% of flow during FVC.

Peak inspiratory flow rate (PIFR): flow rate of inspired air during maximum inspiration. It indicates large (trachea and bronchi) airway disease.

Contraindications

- Pain, because of patient inability to cooperate by deep inspiration and expiration
- Inability to cooperate because of age or mental incapability

Potential Complications

- Light-headedness during the test, due to relative hyperventilation
- Fainting during FVC maneuver, due to Valsalva effect
- Asthmatic episode, precipitated by inhalation studies; bronchodilators may be necessary for immediate treatment

✓ CLINICAL PRIORITIES

- Patient cooperation is essential for PFTs. These tests cannot be performed in patients with pain (e.g., from surgery, fractured ribs) or any problem (e.g., mental instability) that precludes cooperation.
- Because inhalation studies can precipitate an asthmatic episode, bronchodilators may be needed for immediate treatment.

Procedure and Patient Care

Before

- Explain the test to the patient.
- Inform the patient that cooperation is necessary for accurate results.
- Instruct the patient not to use any bronchodilators or to smoke for 6 hours before this test (if requested by physician).
- Withhold the use of small-dose meter inhalers and aerosol therapy before this study.
- Measure and record the patient's height and weight before this study to determine predicted values.
- List on the laboratory slip any medications the patient is taking.

During

- Note the following procedural steps:

Spirometry and Air Flow Rates

1. The unsedated patient is taken to the pulmonary function laboratory.
2. The patient breathes through a sterile mouthpiece into a spirometer, which measures and records the desired values.
3. The patient is asked to inhale as deeply as possible and then forcibly exhale as much air as possible. This is repeated several (usually two to three) times. The two best values are used for calculations. This test may be repeated with bronchodilators if values are deficient.
4. The machine computes FVC, FEV_1, FEV_1/FVC, PIFR, PEFR, and MMEF.
5. The patient is asked to breathe in and out as deeply and frequently as possible for 15 seconds. The total volume breathed is recorded and multiplied by 4 to obtain MVV.
6. The patient is asked to breathe in and out normally into the spirometer and then exhale forcibly from the end-tidal volume expiration point, to measure ERV.
7. The patient is asked to breathe in and out normally into the spirometer and then inhale forcibly from the end-tidal volume expiration point, to measure IC.
8. The patient is asked to breathe in and out maximally (but not forced), to measure VC and calculated TLC.

Gas Exchange: Diffusing Capacity of Lung (D_L)

1. The D_L for any gas can be measured as part of pulmonary function studies.
2. The D_L of CO is usually measured by having the patient inhale a CO mixture.
3. D_LCO is calculated by analysis of the amount of CO exhaled compared with the amount inhaled. Some methods require arterial blood gas tests to be performed at the same time as gas exchange tests.

Inhalation Tests (Bronchial Provocation Studies)

1. These tests may be performed during pulmonary function studies to establish a cause-and-effect relationship in some patients with inhalant allergies.
2. The *methacholine* or *histamine challenge* test is typically used to detect the presence of hyperactive airway disease. This test is not indicated in patients with known asthma. A positive result of methacholine challenge is >20% reduction in FEV_1.
3. Care is taken during this challenge test to reverse any severe bronchospasm with prompt administration of an inhalant bronchodilator (e.g., isoproterenol).

After

- Patients with severe respiratory problems occasionally are exhausted after PFTs, and will need rest.

Test Results and Clinical Significance

Pulmonary fibrosis
Interstitial lung diseases
Interstitial lung diseases are highlighted by perialveolar inflammation followed by fibrosis. Asbesto-

sis, ARDS, radiation fibrosis, collagen vascular diseases, Goodpasture's disease, amyloidosis, sarcoidosis, and end-stage hypersensitivity pneumonitis are some of the more common etiologic factors. Usually the FEV_1/FVC ratio is normal. Lung volumes and capacities are reduced. Hypoxemia is common. Diffusing capacity is markedly reduced.

Tumor *Cancers of the peripheral small bronchi may not cause any changes in pulmonary function studies. Tumors of the trachea (rare) and large bronchi (common) cause a reduction in PIFR.*

Chest wall trauma *Fractured ribs or recent surgery inhibits a patient's ability to fully cooperate with pulmonary requirements. As a result, most lung volumes and capacities will be reduced.*

Emphysema

Chronic bronchitis

Asthma

Patients with COPD can be expected to have reduced air flow rates (FEV_1, $FEF_{25\text{-}75}$, $FEF_{200\text{-}1200}$) and abnormal air flow curves (loops). RV and ERV are increased. VC is reduced. In patients with asthma, this is reversible to a large degree with the use of bronchodilators.

Inhalant pneumonitis (e.g., farmer's lung, miner's lung) *These patients have reduced lung volumes, impaired diffusing capacity, and exercise-induced hypoxemia. There is little air flow rate abnormality.*

Post-pneumonectomy *As expected, lung volumes and capacities are reduced. With no preexisting obstructive disease, no changes in air flow rates would be expected.*

Bronchiectasis *These patients, with chronic and recurrent bronchiole infection pockets, have reduced air flow rates (FEV_1, $FEF_{25\text{-}75}$, $FEF_{200\text{-}1200}$) and abnormal air flow curves (loops), which may be reversible. They also may have some reaction to methacholine challenge.*

Airway infection *Patients with acute bronchitis may experience transient air flow obstruction, as determined by reduced air flow rates (FEV_1, $FEF_{25\text{-}75}$, $FEF_{200\text{-}1200}$) and abnormal air flow curves (loops), which return to normal when the infection has resolved.*

Pneumonia *These patients may have reduced lung volumes and capacities. Without other concurrent lung disease, there is no air flow obstruction. Diffusing capacity is impaired.*

Neuromuscular disease *Patients with impaired muscle strength due to neuromuscular diseases (e.g., multiple sclerosis, myasthenia gravis) have reduced lung volumes and capacities.*

Hypersensitivity bronchospasm *These patients have reversible airway obstruction (FEV_1, $FEF_{25\text{-}75}$, $FEF_{200\text{-}1200}$) and abnormal air flow curves (loops) when induced by methacholine challenge. Air flow rates are reduced. Lung volumes may also be affected.*

Related Tests

- Arterial blood gases (p. 97): Measurements of arterial blood O_2 and CO_2 pressure and content are useful in determining pulmonary function and calculating lung volumes and capacities.
- Chest radiography (p. 924): Pulmonary function can, to a small degree, be assessed with x-ray films of the chest. Hyperexpanded lungs are evidence of chronic obstructive airway disease. Pulmonary fibrosis, pneumonia, and bronchiectasis may also be evident.

Sleep Studies (Polysomnography [PSG])

Normal Findings Respiratory disturbance index (RDI) <5-10 episodes per study

Indications

Sleep studies are indicated in any person who snores excessively, experiences narcolepsy, excessive daytime sleeping, or insomnia, or has motor spasms while sleeping, and in patients with documented cardiac rhythm disturbances limited to sleep time.

Test Explanation

Sleep apnea is a disease that is now becoming increasingly recognized because of its sleep time signs and daytime sequelae. Its economic impact on the workplace has demanded improved methods of diagnosis and treatment. Obstructive sleep apnea results from complete upper airway obstruction associated with no ventilation for at least 10 seconds. These apneic spells may be associated with significant oxygen desaturation, cardiac rhythm disturbances, muscle spasms or seizures (restless leg syndrome), sleep interruption, and insomnia. As a result of these symptoms, sleep is frequently interrupted. The preceding partial or near complete upper airway obstruction causes excessive snoring, which can be so severe that the home life of these patients may be severely affected. The daytime sequela of sleep apnea is excessive daytime sleeping or narcolepsy.

Sleep apnea can result from disorders other than airway obstruction. Central sleep apnea is highlighted by simple cessation of breathing not due to obstructed airway. Primary cardiac events that lead to significant and transient reduction in cardiac output can also cause apnea.

Testing for obstructive sleep apnea is performed in a specially constructed sleep laboratory. This is a well-insulated room in which external sounds are blocked and room temperature is easily controlled. During the observation period (usually during normal sleep hours), the patient is monitored by means of EKG (p. 478), pulse oximetry (p. 1013), EEG (p. 482), and electromyography (p. 486). Air flow in the mouth and nose is monitored. Chest and abdominal wall impedance as a measure of respiratory effort is also monitored.

Interfering Factors

- Psychologic insomnia associated with the laboratory environment compared with home
- Environmental noises, temperature changes, or other sensations

Procedure and Patient Care

Before

- Explain the procedure to the patient.
- Caffeine should be avoided for several days before testing.
- Reassure the patient that monitoring equipment will not interrupt the sleeping pattern.

- Allow the patient to express concerns about videotaping and other forms of monitoring.

During

- Electrodes for EKG, EEG, and electromyography are applied. Excessive hair may need to be shaved in male patients.
- Air flow, oximetry, and impedance monitors are applied.
- Once the patient is comfortable, he or she is allowed to sleep.
- The lights are turned off and monitoring begins before the patient is asleep.

After

- On completion of the sleep cycle, the monitors and electrodes are removed.
- Test results take several days to collate and interpret.

Test Results and Clinical Significance

Obstructive sleep apnea *Patients experience apneic episodes for >10 seconds, and hypoxemia; require significant effort to breathe; and may have muscle spasms or seizures.*

Central sleep apnea *Patients do not have the effort to breath during the apneic episode. Otherwise, the findings are nearly the same as for obstructive sleep apnea.*

Cardiac sleep apnea *Cardiac arrhythmia occurs before apnea, muscle spasm, and hypoxemia.*

Tuberculin (PPD Skin Test, Mantoux Test)

Normal Findings

Negative, reaction <5 mm

Indications

Tuberculin testing is performed in patients with suspected recent tuberculosis (TB) exposure or active TB infection. This includes patients with suspicious chest x-ray findings, productive cough with negative routine cultures, hemoptysis, or undetermined weight loss. PPD is also performed in patients who are at increased risk for development of TB (Box 13-1).

Test Explanation

Purified protein derivative (PPD) of the tubercle bacillus is injected intradermally. If the patient is infected with or has been exposed to TB (whether active or dormant), lymphocytes will recognize the PPD antigen and cause a local inflammatory reaction (see Box 13-1; Box 13-2). Although this test is used to detect TB infection, results do not indicate whether the infection is active or dormant. If test results are negative but the physician strongly suspects TB, testing with "second-strength" PPD can be performed. If these test results are negative, the patient has not been exposed to TB. (See p. 687 for tuberculosis culture.) Results of PPD skin testing usually become positive 6 weeks after infection.

Box 13-1 **Criteria for positive PPD test results in patients with no previous PPD results**

DIAMETER OF INDURATION 48-72 HOURS AFTER PPD INJECTION

≥5 mm (high risk)
- HIV infection
- Close recent contact with a person with active TB
- Patients with chest x-ray findings consistent with old, healed TB granulomatous infection

≥10 mm (moderate risk)
- Foreigners from continents with high TB rate (e.g., Asia, Africa, South America)
- IV drug abusers
- Economically poor in U.S.
- Nursing home residents
- Medical conditions associated with high risk for TB (e.g., malnutrition, post-gastrectomy, steroid use, cancer, diabetes)
- Long-term care facility worker

≥15 mm
- Persons who do not fulfill above criteria

Box 13-2 **Criteria for positive PPD conversion in patients with previously documented negative PPD**

<35 years old: Increase in PPD-induced induration of ≥10 mm within 2 years of last PPD test
>35 years old: Increase in PPD induration of ≥15 mm within 2 years of last PPD test

Box 13-3 **Conditions in which PPD test results may demonstrate no reaction despite patient exposure or will revert to negative**

Fully cured TB
Malnutrition
Immunocompromised (e.g., from AIDS, cancer therapy, advanced cancers [e.g., leukemia, lymphoma])
Overwhelming infection (e.g., bacterial, viral, or miliary TB)
Steroid therapy
Sarcoidosis

Box 13-4 **Skin tests for other diseases**

Schick test: shows previous exposure to diphtheria
Dick test: demonstrates antibody development to group A streptococci (scarlet fever)
Allergy skin testing: evaluates molds, dust, pollen, other allergens

Once positive, the reaction usually persists for life. Box 13-3 lists patients in whom test results may revert to negative or fail to become positive.

The PPD test also can be used as part of a series of skin tests performed to assess the immune system. If the immune system is nonfunctioning because of poor nutrition or chronic illness (e.g., neoplasia, infection, AIDS), PPD test results will be negative despite the patient having had active or dormant TB infection. Other pathogens used in skin tests to test immune function include *Candida,* mumps virus, and *Trichophyton,* organisms most people in the United States have been exposed to. It has been well established that any surgery is associated with greater mortality in patients with negative skin tests than in patients who react to these common pathogen skin tests. Box 13-4 lists skin tests for other diseases.

Laboratory testing for TB is usually performed as part of routine prenatal evaluation in pregnant women. Often this may be the mother's first contact with the health care system in several years.

PPD testing is associated with no complications, except in patients known to have active TB or who have been vaccinated against TB. In these patients, local reaction may be so severe as to cause complete skin slough, requiring surgical care. PPD testing will not cause active TB, because the test solution contains no live organisms.

Contraindications

- Active TB
- Immunization against PPD with *bacille Calmette-Guérin* (BCG)
  Patients will demonstrate a positive reaction to PPD vaccine even if they have never had TB infection.

Interfering Factors

- Subcutaneous injection of PPD may cause a negative reaction. The injection must be intradermal for induration to occur.
- Immunocompromised patients will not react to PPD despite exposure to TB.
- Improper storage of PPD can cause false-negative results.
- Improper dosage of PPD can cause false-negative results.

✓ CLINICAL PRIORITIES

- Positive PPD test results indicate previous exposure, not necessarily active infection. Active infection should be ruled out with appropriate cultures and other diagnostic tests.
- PPD testing should not be performed in patients with active TB or patients who have received BCG vaccine, because local skin reaction may cause complete skin slough requiring surgery.
- If the immune system is nonfunctioning because of poor nutrition or chronic illness, PPD test results may be negative even if the patient has active or dormant TB infection.

Procedure and Patient Care

Before

- Explain the procedure to the patient.
- Assure the patient that TB will not develop from this test.
- Assess the patient for previous history of TB. Report a positive history to the physician.
- Evaluate the patient's history for previous PPD results and BCG immunization.

During

- Prepare the volar (inner) forearm with alcohol, and allow it to dry.
- Intradermally inject PPD (Figure 13-7). A skin wheal (nearly 1 cm) should develop.
- Circle the area with indelible ink.
- Record the time when the PPD was injected.

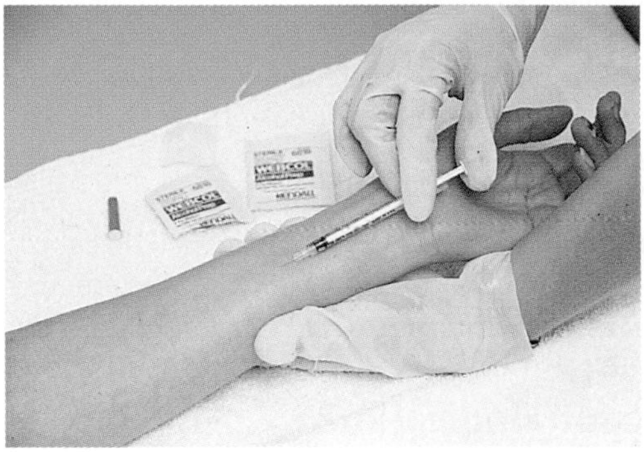

Figure 13-7 Intradermal injection in forearm for skin testing.

After

- Read the results in 48-72 hours.
- Examine the test site for induration (hardening), and encircle the area of induration. Measure the area of induration (not redness) in millimeters.
- If the test results are positive, ensure that the physician is notified and the patient is given appropriate treatment.
- If the test results are positive, check the patient's arm 4-5 days after the test to be certain that a severe skin reaction has not occurred.

Test Results and Clinical Significance

Positive results

TB infection

Nontuberculous *Mycobacteria* infection

Positive results indicate previous exposure, not necessarily active infection. Active infection should be ruled out with appropriate cultures and other diagnostic tests.

Negative results

Possible immunoincompetence in chronically ill patients *Immunocompromised patients and patients who have not been exposed to TB will not react to PPD. In other patients, positive results can revert to negative (see Box 13-3). Immunocompromised patients will not respond to other common pathogens.*

Related Tests

- Acid-fast bacilli (p. 636): This smear (usually sputum) is used to support the diagnosis of TB. By itself it cannot confirm a diagnosis of TB. This smear test is also used to monitor treatment for TB.
- TB culture (p. 687): This is the only way to confirm a diagnosis of TB. When TB is grown from culture of a specimen, the diagnosis of TB can be made and treatment based on drug sensitivities can be started.
- Chest radiography (p. 924): Because TB is most usually infective to the lungs, as a result of inhalation of airborne infectious material, the chest x-ray film often demonstrates the results (Ghon complex) of acute granulomatous infection.

Bibliography

Aspelin P: Ultrasound examination of soft tissue injury of the lower limb in athletes, *Am J Sports Med* 20(5):601-603, 1992.

Ball EM, et al: Diagnosis and treatment of sleep apnea within the community: the Walla Walla project, *Arch Intern Med* 157(4):419-424, 1997.

Barrick B, Vogel S: Application of laboratory diagnostics in HIV testing, *Nurs Clin North Am* 31(1):41-45, 1996.

Bates SE: Clinical applications of serum tumor markers, *Ann Intern Med* 115(8):623-634, 1991.

Behrman RE, et al, eds: *Nelson's textbook of pediatrics,* ed 15, Philadelphia, 1996, WB Saunders.

Bordow RA, Moser KM: *Manual of clinical problems in pulmonary medicine,* ed 3, Boston, 1991, Little, Brown.

Braunwald E, ed: *Heart disease: a textbook of cardiovascular medicine,* ed 5, Philadelphia, 1997, WB Saunders.

Brooks MI, et al: The infectious etiology of peptic ulcer disease: diagnosis and implications for therapy, *Primary Care* 23(3):443-454, 1996.

Brunzel NA: *Fundamentals of urine and body fluid analysis,* Philadelphia, 1994, WB Saunders.

Bubien RS, et al: What you need to know about radiofrequency ablation, *Am J Nurs* 93(7):30-36, 1993.

Carnaille B, et al: Scintiscans and carcinoid tumors, *Surgery* 116(6):1118-1122, 1994.

Casperson DS: Focus on oncology: prostatic specific antigen testing, *Urol Nurs* 11(1):31-34, 1992.

Cheney AM, Maquindang ML: Patient teaching for x-ray and other diagnostics, *RN* 56(4):54-56, 1993.

Coulter JS: Red blood cell distribution width and mean corpuscular volume: clinical applications, *Adv Clin Care* 6(6):13, 1991.

Creasy RK, Resnik R: *Maternal-fetal medicine: principles and practice,* ed 3, Philadelphia, 1994, WB Saunders.

Cupp MR, Oesterling JE: Prostate-specific antigen, digital rectal examination, and transrectal ultrasonography: their role in diagnosing early prostate cancer, *Mayo Clin Proc* 68:297-306, 1993.

Dalence CR, et al: Amniotic fluid lamellar body count: a rapid and reliable fetal lung maturity test, *Obstet Gynecol* 86(2):235-239, 1995.

Dearborn JT, Jergesen HE: The evaluation and initial management of arthritis, *Primary Care* 23(2):215-240, 1996.

De Veciana M, et al: Postprandial versus preprandial blood glucose monitoring in women with gestational diabetes mellitus requiring insulin therapy, *N Engl J Med* 333(19):1239-1241, 1995.

Frank AP, et al: Anonymous IV testing using home collection and telemedicine counseling, *Arch Intern Med* 157(3):309-313, 1997.

Gawlikowski J: White cells at war, *Am J Nurs* 92(3):44-51, 1992.

Greenberg LR, Moore TR, Murphy H: Gestational diabetes mellitus: antenatal variables as predictors of postpartum glucose intolerance, *Gest Diabetes* 86(1):97-101, 1995.

Gregor CL: Antepartum fetal assessment techniques: an update for today's perinatal nurse, *J Perinatal Neonatal Nurs* 5(4):1-15, 1992.

Halfman-Francy M: Recognition and management of bleeding following cardiac surgery, *Crit Care Nurs Clin North Am* 3(4):675-689, 1991.

Hancock RD: Venipuncture vs. arterial catheter activated partial thromboplastin times in heparinized patients, *DCCN* 12(5):238-245, 1993.

Henry JB: *Clinical diagnosis and laboratory management by laboratory methods,* ed 18, Philadelphia, 1991, WB Saunders.

Isselbacher KJ, et al, eds: *Harrison's principles of internal medicine,* ed 13, New York, 1994, McGraw-Hill.

Kee JL, Hayes ER: Assessment of patient laboratory data in the acutely ill, *Nurs Clin North Am* 25(4):751-759, 1990.

Kikuchi S, et al: Serum anti–*Helicobacter pylori* antibody and gastric carcinoma among young adults, *Cancer* 75(12):2789-2792, 1995.

Koepke JA, ed: *Practical laboratory hematology,* New York, 1991, Churchill Livingstone.

Kuhlman JE: Oral and IV contrast-enhanced abdominal CT, *Appl Radiol* 21(10):20-21, 1992.

Kvols LK, et al: Evaluation of a radiolabeled somatostatin analog (1-123 octreotide) in the detection and localization of carcinoid and islet cell tumors, *Radiology* 187(1):129-133, 1993.

Lancaster LE: Immunogenetic basis of tissue and organ transplantation and rejection, *Crit Care Nurs Clin North Am* 4(1):1-24, 1992.

Lavin J: Anergy testing: a vital weapon, *RN* 56(9):31-33, 1993.

Lee GR, et al, eds: *Wintrobe's clinical hematology,* ed 9, Philadelphia, 1993, Lea & Febiger.

Lensing AW, et al: A comparison of compression ultrasound with color Doppler ultrasound for diagnosis of symptomless postoperative deep vein thrombosis, *Arch Intern Med* 157(7):758-762, 1997.

Littrup PJ, Goodman AC, Mettlin CJ: The benefit and cost of prostate cancer early detection, *CA* 43(3):134-149, 1993.

Lowry WS: Tumor suppressor genes and risk of metastasis in ovarian cancer, *Br Med J* 307(6903):542, 1993.

McClatchey KD, ed: *Clinical laboratory medicine,* Baltimore, 1994, Williams & Wilkins.

Melillo KD: Interpretation of laboratory values in older adults, *Nurse Pract* 18(7):59-67, 1993.

Merva J: A closer look at the heart SAECG, *RN* 56(5):50-53, 1993.

Miller KE: Sexually transmitted diseases, *Primary Care* 24(1):179-193, 1997.

Miller PD, et al: Clinical utility of bone mass measurements in adults: consensus of an international panel, *Semin Arthritis Rheumatism* 25(6):361-372, 1996.

Mitlak BH, Nussbaum SR: Diagnosis and treatment of osteoporosis, *Annu Rev Med* 44:265-277, 1993.

Moore S: Screening for prostate cancer: PSA blood test, rectal examination, and ultrasound, *Urol Nurs* 12(3):106-107, 1992.

Morell V: Basic infertility assessment, *Primary Care* 24(1):195-204, 1997.

Mussolino ME, et al: Phalangeal bone density and hip fracture risk, *Arch Intern Med,* 157(4):433-438, 1997.

Norris MKG: Assessing fibrin-split products, *Nursing* 22(6):29, 1992.

Olaison L, et al: Fever, C-reactive protein, and other acute-phase reactants during treatment of infective endocarditis, *Arch Intern Med* 157(8):885-892, 1997.

Pagana KD, Pagana TJ: *Diagnostic testing and nursing implications: a case study approach,* ed 4, St Louis, 1991, Mosby

Pagana KD, Pagana TJ: *Mosby's Diagnostic and laboratory test reference,* ed 3, St Louis, 1997, Mosby.

Perkins A: An approach to diagnosing the acute sore throat, *Am Fam Phys* 55(1):131-138, 1997.

Rainwater LM, et al: Prostate-specific antigen testing in untreated and treated prostatic adenocarcinoma, *Mayo Clin Proc* 65(8):1118-1126, 1990.

Rao JK, et al: The role of antineutrophil cytoplasmic antibody (c-ANCA) testing in the diagnosis of Wegener granulomatosis, *Ann Intern Med* 123(2):925-932, 1995.

Resnick ML, Rifkin MD, eds: *Ultrasonography of the urinary tract,* ed 3, Baltimore, 1991, Williams & Wilkins.

Robie BH: Cardiovascular technology: noninvasive diagnosis of cardiovascular disease using ultrasound imaging, *J Cardiovasc Nurs* 6(2):36-42, 1992.

Rudolphi DM: Duplex scanning, *Am J Nurs* 90(4):123-124, 1990.

Ryan KJ, Berkowitz R, Barbieri R, eds: *Kistner's gynecology: principles and practice,* ed 5, St Louis, 1990, Mosby.

Sandowski DC, Rabeneck L: Gastric ulcers at endoscopy: brush, biopsy, or both? *Am J Gastroenterol* 92(4):608-613, 1997.

Schwartz SL, et al, eds: *Principles of surgery,* ed 6, New York, 1994, McGraw-Hill.

Sistrom C: Liver CT for cancer staging, *Appl Radiol* 21(6):19-24, 1992.

Spiro HM: *Clinical gastroenterology,* ed 4, New York, 1993, McGraw-Hill.

Stark JR: Tuberculosis in children, *Primary Care* 23(4):861-881, 1996.

Swezey RL, et al: Bone densitometry: comparison of dual energy x-ray absorptiometry to radiographic absorptiometry, *J Rheumatol* 23(10):1734-1738, 1996.

Tanagho EA, McAninch JW, eds: *Smith's general urology,* ed 13, Norwalk, Conn, 1992, Appleton & Lange.

Taylor A, Datz FL, eds: *Clinical application of nuclear medicine,* New York, 1991, Churchill Livingstone.

Thompson EJ: Transesophageal echocardiography: a new window on the heart and great vessels, *Crit Care Nurse* 13(10):55-56, 1993.

Thompson S: Ultrasonography: intraoperative diagnosis of choledocholithiasis, *AORN J* 51(4):983-985, 1990.

Tilton RC, et al, eds: *Clinical laboratory medicine,* St Louis, 1992, Mosby.

Tracker HL: Menopause, *Primary Care* 24(1):205-221, 1997.

Trate D, et al: Dysphagia: diagnosis and treatment, *Primary Care* 23(3):417-432, 1996.

Velos JC: A review of cardiac imaging modalities, *Nurse Pract Forum* 2(4):231-238, 1991.

Wozniak-Petrofsky J: Prostate specific antigen in prostate cancer, *J Urol Nurs* 12(3): 104-105, 1992.

Wozniak-Petrofsky J: Basics of urodynamics, *J Urol Nurs* 12(2):434-463, 1993.

Young DS: *Effects of drugs on clinical laboratory tests,* ed 3, Washington, DC, 1990, AACS Press.

Zoloth SR: Anergy compromise screening for tuberculosis in high-risk populations, *Am J Public Health* 83(5):749-751, 1993.

APPENDIX

A

Alphabetical Listing of Tests

A

B

C

K

L

M

S

T

U

V

W

X

APPENDIX

B

List of Tests by Body System

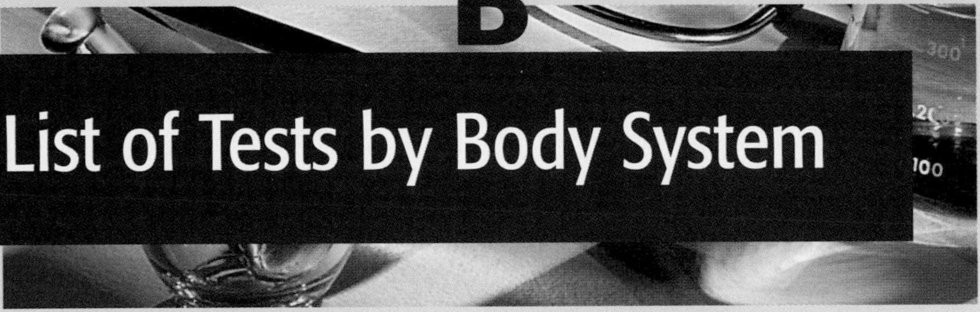

Tests in this list are grouped by the following body systems: cancer, cardiovascular, endocrine, gastrointestinal, hematologic, hepatobiliary, immunologic, miscellaneous, nervous system, pulmonary, reproductive system, skeletal system, and urologic.

Cancer Studies

Cardiovascular Studies

Endocrine Studies

Gastrointestinal Studies

Hematologic System

Hepatobiliary Studies

Immunologic Studies

Miscellaneous Studies

Nervous System Studies

APPENDIX B

Magnetic resonance imaging (MRI), p. 1009
Myelography, p. 908
Oculoplethysmography, p. 622
Positron-emission tomography (PET), p. 737
Skull radiography, p. 988
Spinal radiography, p. 994

Pulmonary Studies

Acid-fast bacilli smear, p. 636
Angiotensin-converting enzyme, p. 55
$Alpha_1$-Antitrypsin, p. 45
Arterial blood gases, p. 97
Blood gases, p. 97
Bronchography, p. 915
Bronchoscopy, p. 518
Carbon dioxide content, p. 133
Carboxyhemoglobin, p. 135
Chest radiography, p. 924
Chest tomography, p. 928
Computed tomography, chest, p. 942
Legionnaires' disease antibody, p. 284
Lung biopsy, p. 662
Lung scan, p. 726
Mantoux test, p. 1023
Mediastinoscopy, p. 548
Oximetry, p. 1013
Pleural biopsy, p. 670
Pulmonary angiography, p. 979
Pulmonary function tests (PFT), p. 1016
Sputum culture and sensitivity, p. 681
Sputum cytology, p. 683
Strep screen, p. 685
Thoracentesis and pleural fluid analysis, p. 606
Thoracoscopy, p. 555
Throat culture and sensitivity, p. 685
Tuberculin test (PPD), p. 1023
Tuberculosis culture, p. 687

Reproductive System Studies

Amniocentesis, p. 560
Antispermatozoal antibody, p. 82
Barr body analysis, p. 638
Biophysical profile, p. 792
Breast cyst and nipple discharge fluid analysis, p. 571
Breast ultrasonography, p. 783
Cervical mucus test, p. 573
Cervical, urethral, and anal cultures for sexually transmitted diseases, p. 677
Chlamydia, p. 649
Chorionic villus sampling (CVS), p. 1006
Colposcopy, p. 526
Contraceptive localization, p. 786
Contraction stress test (fetal), p. 474
Cytomegalovirus, p. 104
Endometrial biopsy, p. 653
Estrogen fraction, p. 202
Fetal biophysical profile, p. 792
α-Fetoprotein, p. 47
Fetoscopy, p. 540
Follicle-stimulating hormone (FSH), p. 296
Gonorrhea culture, p. 677
Herpes genitalis, p. 657
Herpes simplex, p. 657
Hysterosalpingography, p. 950
Hysteroscopy, p. 543
Infertility screen, p. 82
Karyotype, p. 149
Lamellar body count, p. 561
Laparoscopy, p. 545
Luteinizing hormone asay, p. 296
Mammography, p. 963
Nonstress test (fetal), p. 504
Papanicolaou test (smear test), p. 666
Pelvic ultrasonography, p. 796
Pelvimetry, p. 974
pH, fetal scalp, p. 324
Phenylketonuria (PKU), p. 326
Pregnancy tests, p. 348
Pregnanediol, p. 849
Progesterone assay, p. 351
Rubella antibody, p. 392
Semen analysis, p. 599
Sims-Huhner, p. 602
Syphilis detection, p. 403
Toxoplasmosis antibody titer, p. 430

Skeletal System Studies

Aldolase, p. 35

Alkaline phosphatase, p. 42
Arthrocentesis with synovial fluid analysis, p. 568
Arthrography, p. 398
Arthroscopy, p. 514
Bone densitometry, p. 908
Bones (long), radiography, p. 913
Lactic dehydrogenase (LDH), p. 278
Myelography, p. 968
Rheumatoid factor, p. 389
Spinal radiography, p. 994
Uric acid, blood, p. 446
Uric acid, urine, p. 857

Urologic Studies

ADH suppression, p. 65
Antegrade pyelography, p. 890
Antistreptolysin O titer, p. 85
Captopril renal scan, p. 745
Catecholamines, p. 877
Chloride, blood, p. 141
Chloride, urine, p. 827
Creatinine, blood, p. 178
Creatinine clearance, p. 180
Cystography, p. 948
Cystometry, p. 615
Cystoscopy, p. 528
Epithelial casts, p. 871
Granular casts, p. 871
Hyaline casts, p. 864
Intravenous pyelography, p. 953
Kidney, ureter, and bladder (KUB) radiography, p. 958
Leukocyte esterase, p. 863
Nitrites, p. 863
Osmolality, blood, p. 313
Osmolality, urine, p. 842
Pelvic floor sphincter electromyography, p. 506
Potassium, blood, p. 342
Potassium, urine, p. 847
Prostate/rectal ultrasonography, p. 799
Prostate-specific antigen (PSA), p. 356
Protein, blood, p. 357
Red blood cell casts and cells, p. 865
Renal biopsy, p. 674
Renal scanning, p. 745
Renin assay, plasma, p. 380
Renin assay, renal vein, p. 384
Retrograde pyelography, p. 982
Scrotal nuclear imaging, p. 753
Scrotal ultrasonography, p. 801
Urea nitrogen blood test, p. 443
Urethral pressure profile, p. 630
Uric acid, blood, p. 446
Uric acid, urine, p. 857
Urinalysis, p. 859
Urine culture and sensitivity, p. 873
Urine electrophoresis, p. 631
Urine flow studies, p. 631
Vanillylmandelic acid (VMA) and catecholamines, p. 877

APPENDIX

C

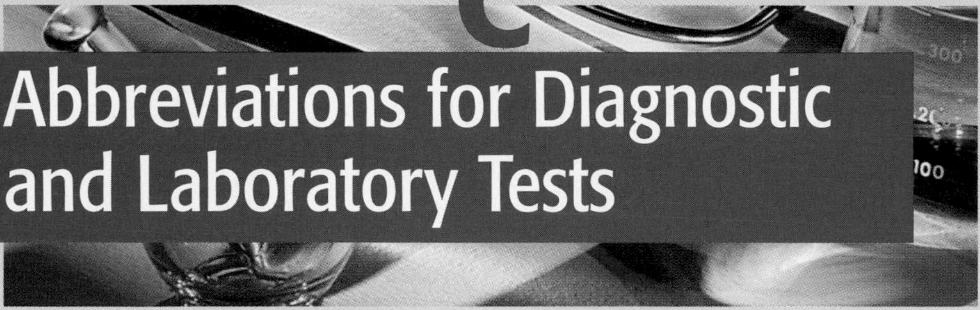

Abbreviations for Diagnostic and Laboratory Tests

A	ABEP	Auditory brainstem evoked potential
	ABGs	Arterial blood gases
	ACE	Angiotensin-converting enzyme
	ACTH	Adrenocorticotropic hormone
	ADH	Antidiuretic hormone
	AFB	Acid-fast bacilli
	AFP	α-Fetoprotein
	A/G ratio	Albumin/globulin ratio
	ALA	Aminolevulinic acid
	ALP	Alkaline phosphatase
	ALT	Alanine aminotransferase
	AMA	Antimitochondrial antibody
	ANA	Antinuclear antibody
	ANC	Absolute neutrophil count
	ANCA	Antineutrophil cytoplasmic antibody
	APTT	Activated partial thromboplastin time
	ASMA	Anti–smooth muscle antibody
	ASO	Antistreptolysin O titer
	AST	Aspartate aminotransferase
B	BE	Barium enema
	BMC	Bone mineral count
	BMD	Bone mineral density
	BPP	Biophysical profile
	BT	Bleeding time
	BUN	Blood urea nitrogen
C	C&S	Culture and sensitivity
	CAT	Computerized axial tomography
	CBC	Complete blood count
	CEA	Carcinoembryonic antigen
	CK	Creatine kinase
	Cl	Chloride
	CLO	*Campylobacter*-like organism
	CMG	Cystometrogram
	CMV	Cytomegalovirus
	CO	Carbon monoxide
	CO_2	Carbon dioxide
	COHb	Carboxyhemoglobin test
	CP, CPK	Creatine phosphokinase
	CRP	C-reactive protein
	CSF	Cerebrospinal fluid
	CST	Contraction stress test
	CT	Computed tomography
	CVB	Chorionic villi biopsy
	CVS	Chorionic villi sampling
	CXR	Chest x-ray

D	D&C	Dilation and curettage
	DIC	Disseminated intravascular coagulation
	DSA	Digital subtraction angiography
	DST	Dexamethasone suppression test
E	EBV	Epstein-Barr virus
	ECG, EKG	Electrocardiogram
	ECHO	Echocardiography
	EEG	Electroencephalogram
	EFS	Esophageal function studies
	EGD	Esophagogastroduodenoscopy
	ELISA	Enzyme-linked immunosorbent assay
	EMG	Electromyography
	ENG	Electroneurography
	EP	Evoked potential
	EPS	Electrophysiologic study
	ER	Estrogen receptor
	ERCP	Endoscopic retrograde cholangiopancreatography
	ESR	Erythrocyte sedimentation rate
	EUG	Excretory urography
F	FBS	Fasting blood sugar
	FDPs	Fibrin degradation products
	Fe	Iron
	FSH	Follicle-stimulating hormone
	FSPs	Fibrin split products
	FTA-ABS	Fluorescent treponemal antibody absorption test
	FTI	Free thyroxine index
	FUT	Fibrinogen uptake test
G	GB series	Gallbladder series
	GER scan	Gastroesophageal reflux scan
	GGT	γ-Glutamyl transferase
	GGTP	γ-Glutamyl transpeptidase
	GH	Growth hormone
	GHb, GHB	Glycosylated hemoglobin
	GI series	Gastrointestinal series
	G-6-PD	Glucose-6-phosphate dehydrogenase
	GTT	Glucose tolerance test
H	HAA	Hepatitis-associated antigen
	HAV	Hepatitis A virus
	Hb, Hgb	Hemoglobin
	HB_cAb	Hepatitis B core antibody
	HB_cAg	Hepatitis B core antigen
	HBV	Hepatitis B virus
	HCG	Human chorionic gonadotropin

	HCO_3^-	Bicarbonate
	HCS	Human chorionic somatomammotropin
	Hct	Hematocrit
	HDL	High-density lipoprotein
	5-HIAA	5-Hydroxyindoleacetic acid
	HIV	Human immunodeficiency virus
	HLA	Human lymphocyte antigen
	HSV-2	Herpes simplex virus, type 2
I	Ig	Immunoglobulin
	IGF	Insulin-like growth factor
	INR	International normalization ratio
	ITT	Insulin tolerance test
	IVC	Intravenous cholangiography
	IV-GTT	Intravenous glucose tolerance test
	IVP	Intravenous pyelography
	IVU, IUG	Intravenous urography
K	K	Potassium
	KS	Ketosteroid
	KUB	Kidney, ureter, and bladder x-ray study
L	LAP	Leucine aminopeptidase
	LATS	Long-acting thyroid-stimulator
	LDH	Lactic dehydrogenase
	LDL	Low-density lipoprotein
	LE	Lupus erythematosus
	LES	Lower esophageal sphincter
	LFTs	Liver function tests
	LH	Luteinizing hormone
	LP	Lumbar puncture
	Lp(a)	Lp(a) lipoprotein
	L/S ratio	Lecithin/sphingomyelin ratio
	LS spine	Lumbosacral spine
M	MCH	Mean corpuscular hemoglobin
	MCHC	Mean corpuscular hemoglobin concentration
	MCV	Mean corpuscular volume
	Mg	Magnesium
	MPV	Mean platelet volume
	MRI	Magnetic resonance imaging
N	Na	Sodium
	NMR	Nuclear magnetic resonance
	NST	Nonstress test

O	OB	Occult blood
	OCT	Oxytocin challenge test
	17-OHCS	17-Hydroxycorticosteroids
	O&P	Ova and parasites
	OPG	Oculoplethysmography
P	P	Phosphorus
	PAB	Prealbumin
	PAP	Prostatic acid phosphatase
	Pb	Lead
	PCO_2	Partial pressure of carbon dioxide
	PET	Positron-emission tomography
	PFTs	Pulmonary function tests
	pH	Hydrogen ion concentration
	PKU	Phenylketonuria
	PMN	Polymorphonuclear (type of WBC)
	PO_2	Partial pressure of oxygen
	PPBS	Postprandial blood sugar
	PPD	Purified protein derivative
	PPG	Postprandial glucose
	PR	Progesterone receptor
	PRA	Plasma renin assay
	PSA	Prostate-specific antigen
	PSG	Polysomnography
	PT	Prothrombin time
	PTH	Parathormone, parathyroid hormone
	PTC, PTCH	Percutaneous transhepatic cholangiography
	PTT	Partial thromboplastin time
R	RAIU	Radioactive iodine uptake
	RBC	Red blood cell
	RDW	Red cell distribution width
	RF	Rheumatoid factor
	RIA	Radioimmunoassay
	RPR	Rapid plasma reagin test
	RRA	Radioreceptor assay
S	S&A	Sugar and acetone
	SACE	Serum angiotensin-converting enzyme
	SBF	Small bowel follow-through
	SER	Somatosensory evoked responses
	SGOT	Serum glutamic oxaloacetic transaminase
	SGPT	Serum glutamic pyruvic transaminase
	SLE	Systemic lupus erythematosus
	SPECT	Single-photon emission computed tomography
	STS	Serologic test for syphilis

T	T_3	Triiodothyronine
	T_4	Thyroxine
	TBG	Thyroxine-binding globulin
	TBPA	Thyroxine-binding prealbumin
	T&CM	Type and crossmatch
	TDM	Therapeutic drug monitoring
	TEE	Transesophageal echocardiography
	TIBC	Total iron-binding capacity
	TPI	*Treponema pallidum* immobilization
	TPR	Tubular phosphate reabsorption
	TRAP	Tartrate-resistant acid phosphatase
	TRF	Thyrotropin releasing factor
	TRH	Thyrotropin releasing hormone
	TRP	Tubular reabsorption of phosphate
	T&S	Type and screen
	TSH	Thyroid-stimulating hormone
	TSIG	Thyroid-stimulating immunoglobulin
	TTE	Transthoracic echocardiography
U	UA	Urinalysis
	UGI series	Upper gastrointestinal series
	UPP	Urethral pressure profile
	US	Ultrasound
V	VDRL	Venereal Disease Research Laboratory
	VER	Visual evoked response
	VLDL	Very-low-density lipoprotein
	VMA	Vanillylmandelic acid
	VPS	Ventilation/perfusion scanning
W	WBC	White blood cell

Credits

Chapter 2
Figures: 2-1, 2-2, 2-3, Grimes DE: *Infectious Diseases*, 1991, Mosby; 2-4, 2-6, Wilson SF, Thompson JM: *Respiratory Disorders*, 1990, Mosby; 2-7, 2-10, 2-12, 2-13, 2-15, Pagana KD, Pagana TJ: *Mosby's Diagnostic and Laboratory Test Reference*, ed 3, 1997, Mosby; 2-8, 2-9, 2-11, 2-14, 2-19, Belcher AE: *Blood Disorders*, 1993, Mosby. Tables: 2-5, 2-13, 2-15, Pagana KD, Pagana TJ: *Mosby's Diagnostic and Laboratory Test Reference*, ed 3, 1997, Mosby.
Chapter 3
Figures: 3-1, 3-2, 3-10, 3-11, Canobbio MM: *Cardiovascular Disorders*, 1990, Mosby; 3-3a, 3-3b, Pagana KD, Pagana TJ: *Mosby's Diagnostic and Laboratory Test Reference*, ed 3, 1997, Mosby; 3-4, 3-5, 3-8, Chipps E, Clanin N, Campbell V: *Neurologic Disorders*, 1992, Mosby; 3-6, Mourad LA: *Orthopedic Disorders*, 1991, Mosby; 3-7, 3-9, Sigler BA, Schuring LT: *Ear, Nose, and Throat Disorders*, 1994, Mosby.
Chapter 4
Figures: 4-1, Doughty D: *Gastrointestinal Disorders*, 1993, Mosby; 4-2 courtesy Olympus Corporation; 4-3, 4-5, 4-6, 4-7, 4-8, 4-9, 4-10, Pagana KD, Pagana TJ: *Mosby's Diagnostic and Laboratory Test Reference*, ed 3, 1997, Mosby.
Chapter 5
Figures: 5-1, 5-2, 5-3, 5-4, 5-6, Pagana KD, Pagana TJ: *Mosby's Diagnostic and Laboratory Test Reference*, ed 3, 1997, Mosby; 5-7, Wilson SF, Thompson JM: *Respiratory Disorders*, 1990, Mosby; 5-5, 5-8 Beare PG, Myers JL: *Principles and Practice of Adult Health Nursing*, ed 2, 1994, Mosby.
Chapter 6
Figures: 6-1, Pagana KD, Pagana TJ: *Mosby's Diagnostic and Laboratory Test Reference*, ed 3, 1997, Mosby.
Chapter 7
Figures: 7-3, Pagana KD, Pagana TJ: *Mosby's Diagnostic and Laboratory Test Reference*, ed 3, 1997, Mosby; 7-6, 7-7, 7-8, Grimes DE: *Infectious Diseases*, 1991, Mosby.
Chapter 8
Figures: 8-2, 8-7, Mourad LA: *Orthopedic Disorders*, 1991, Mosby; 8-3, 8-4, 8-10, Chipps E, Clanin N, Campbell V: *Neurologic Disorders*, 1992, Mosby; 8-5, 8-6, Canobbio MM: *Cardiovascular Disorders*, 1990, Mosby; 8-9, Wilson SF, Thompson JM: *Respiratory Disorders*, 1990, Mosby.
Chapter 10
Figures: 10-1, 10-2, 10-9, 10-10, Canobbio MM: *Cardiovascular Disorders*, 1990, Mosby; 10-3, 10-4, Brundage DJ: *Renal Disorders*, 1992, Mosby; 10-6, Doughty D: *Gastrointestinal Disorders*, 1993, Mosby; 10-7, Belcher AE: *Cancer Nursing*, 1992, Mosby; 10-11, Pagana KD, Pagana TJ: *Mosby's Diagnostic and Laboratory Test Reference*, ed 3, 1997, Mosby.
Chapter 11
Tables: 11-1, 11-2, 11-3, Pagana KD, Pagana TJ: *Mosby's Diagnostic and Laboratory Test Reference*, ed 3, 1997, Mosby.

Chapter 12

Figures: 12-1, 12-13, 12-18, 12-24, Brundage DJ: *Renal Disorders*, 1992, Mosby; 12-2, 12-3, 12-26, Chipps E, Clanin N, Campbell V: *Neurologic Disorders*, 1992, Mosby; 12-4, 12-23, Pagana KD, Pagana TJ: *Mosby's Diagnostic and Laboratory Test Reference,* ed 3, 1997, Mosby; 12-5, 12-11, 12-17, Doughty D: *Gastrointestinal Disorders*, 1993, Mosby; 12-6, 12-20, 12-21, Edge V, Miller M, *Women's Health Care*, 1994, Mosby; 12-25, Pagana KD, Pagana TJ: *Diagnostic Testing and Nursing Implications: A Case Study Approach,* ed 4, 1994, Mosby; 12-8, Canobbio MM: *Cardiovascular Disorders*, 1990, Mosby; 12-10, Wilson SF, Thompson JM: *Respiratory Disorders*, 1990, Mosby; 12-14, Sigler BA, Schuring LT: *Ear, Nose, and Throat Disorders*, 1994, Mosby; 12-15, Gray M: *Genitourinary Disorders*, 1992, Mosby; 12-22, Belcher AE: *Cancer Nursing*, 1992, Mosby. Table: 12-2, Pagana KD, Pagana TJ: *Mosby's Diagnostic and Laboratory Test Reference,* ed 3, 1997, Mosby.

Chapter 13

Figures: 13-1, 13-5, 13-6, Pagana KD, Pagana TJ: *Mosby's Diagnostic and Laboratory Test Reference,* ed 3, 1997, Mosby; 13-2, Pagana KD, Pagana TJ: *Diagnostic Testing and Nursing Implications: A Case Study Approach,* ed 4, 1994, Mosby, courtesy Central Pennsylvania Magnetic Imaging, Williamsport, PA; 13-3, Brundage DJ: *Renal Disorders*, 1992, Mosby; 13-4, Sigler BA, Schuring LT: *Ear, Nose, and Throat Disorders*, 1994, Mosby; 13-7, Wilson SF, Thompson JM: *Respiratory Disorders*, 1990, Mosby.

Index

INDEX

F

G

INDEX

J

K

L

M

INDEX

T